VINTAGE
PAPERS FROM THE
LANCET

Front cover
The lancet blade shown on the front cover is photographed from an original instrument
kindly provided by The Royal College of Physicians. Photography by Nick Powell.

Endpapers
**From Kuroda *et al.:* Whole genome sequencing of meticillin-resistant *Staphylococcus
aureus. Lancet* 21.4.2001: 1225–1240.**
Genomic analysis of the pathogen MRSA: genetic elements presented in linear fashion
(colour adapted for this book).

VINTAGE
PAPERS FROM THE
LANCET

Ruth Richardson MA DPhil FRHistS

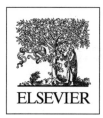

Edinburgh London New York Oxford Philadelphia St Louis Sydney Toronto 2006

ELSEVIER

First published 2006

ISBN 0-08-044683-3

British Library Cataloguing in Publication Data
A catalogue record for this book is available from the British Library.

Library of Congress Cataloging in Publication Data
A catalog record for this book is available from the Library of Congress.

Notice
Knowledge and best practice in this field are constantly changing. As new research and
experience broaden our knowledge, changes in practice, treatment and drug therapy may
become necessary or appropriate. Readers are advised to check the most current information
provided (i) on procedures featured or (ii) by the manufacturer of each product to be
administered, to verify the recommended dose or formula, the method and duration of
administration, and contraindications. It is the responsibility of the practitioner, relying on
their own experience and knowledge of the patient, to make diagnoses, to determine dosages and
the best treatment for each individual patient, and to take all appropriate safety precautions. To
the fullest extent of the law, neither the Publisher nor the Author assumes any liability for any
injury and/or damage to persons or property arising out or related to any use of the material
contained in this book.
The Publisher

While every effort has been made to contact authors of the more recent articles, due to the
passage of time and resulting movement of individuals this has not always proved possible.
The publishers would like to apologise to anyone who was unaware that their paper had been
included in this volume but would be happy to contact the relevant author(s) if provided with
the necessary details.

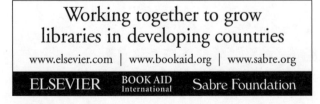

The
Publisher's
policy is to use
**paper manufactured
from sustainable forests**

The quality of the reproduction varies with the print/typeset quality of the original *Lancet* pages.

Printed in China.

DEDICATION

*This book
is dedicated to the memory of
Betty Bostetter
and
Roy Porter
two fine historians of medicine,
both greatly missed.*

For Elsevier

Commissioning Editor: Alison Taylor
Development Editor: Kim Benson
Project Manager: Elisabeth Lawrence
Production Manager: Yolanta Motylinska
Design: Merriton Sharp
Index: Jan Ross

FOREWORD

The Lancet owes a huge debt to Thomas Wakley, the journal's radical and occasionally reckless founding Editor. The style of medical journalism that he created in the 19th century continues to remind us why *The Lancet* is an idea that still matters in the 21st. He set a dauntingly high standard. Yet the ideals he stood for – science and enlightenment, criticism and influence, liberty and internationalism, clarity and engagement – remain very much alive now. This volume of papers, so ably compiled by Ruth Richardson, points to some of the milestones along this path of discovery and endeavour.

But I should also single out a man who was not only a governing influence on Wakley but also a figure of even wider importance in the history of ideas beyond medicine. William Cobbett (1763–1835) was, by all accounts, neither a perfect nor an easy man to know. He was quarrelsome. He took part in a multitude of libellous campaigns against individuals (such as Joseph Priestley) and nations (he wrote extensively about America). Cobbett was an acute observer and a garrulous critic of the industrial revolution. In 1802, he launched a weekly paper, the *Political Register*, to defend the rights of working people against the rise of an oppressive merchant class. He fought against all forms of authority. His writings caused so much trouble that he had to flee England. On his return he was tried for sedition. He spent much of his life poor and ignored. But somehow Cobbett's toil struck a nerve. After losing four elections, he was eventually elected to Parliament at the age of 69, where he continued to attack corruption and tyrany.

Wakley's life mirrored Cobbett's to a very large extent: a rural, non-aristocratic start; early radicalism; an astonishing ability to channel anarchic energies into the creation of a successful journal; repeated brushes with the law; and a strange final embrace with the establishment he had railed against for so long. As you turn the pages of this splendid collection, recall the spirit of these men. As Cobbett wrote in 1822, one year before Wakley published the first issue of *The Lancet*:

> "The man who can talk about the honour of his country, at a time when its millions are in a state little short of famine; and when that is, too, apparently their permanent state, must be an oppressor in his heart; must be destitute of all the feelings of shame and remorse; must be fashioned for a despot, and can only want the power to act the character in its most tragical scenes".

Such men still bear the burden for much of the preventable horror of disease and disability in the world today. Against them, we still stand.

Richard Horton
Editor, *The Lancet*

ABOUT THIS BOOK

The Lancet holds a singularly distinguished position in the world of medicine. Its pages are a rich resource for anyone with an interest in medicine, healthcare, the vicissitudes of infirmity, medical politics and medical education.

The journal has been edited by a series of remarkable men, and contributed to by a multitude of medical clinicians and researchers, and by the lives of myriad patients. Its pages stand witness to the history of its own times, from the cholera epidemics of the early 19th century to SARS.

Perhaps above all, *The Lancet* is a chronicle of the unfolding of knowledge in its most important human application.

This volume is a taster from this rich brew. It is a choice selection of historic clinical and scientific articles appearing in *The Lancet*'s pages over its publishing lifetime. It looks at the whole of modern medicine refracted through the pages of one of the finest medical journals in the world.

The book has four major sections:

▶ Wakley to Nightingale   (1820s to 1860s)
▶ Bacteria to blood groups   (1870s to 1910s)
▶ Iron lungs to ultrasound   (1920s to 1950s)
▶ Thalidomide to SARS   (1960s to 2005)

Each section, after a brief introduction, is internally arranged in chronological sequence. An index completes the volume.

Of course, as for any anthology of this kind, during the process of selection a vast amount of material has had to be excluded.

If there is a specific article you might like to see included were a second volume to be contemplated, do please let the author know.

A note about volumes, issues and pagination

The Lancet's first number appeared on the 5th October 1823. It took some time for *The Lancet* itself to establish what constituted an entire volume and to settle upon the intervals at which the journal should be indexed. The first few volumes spanned two calendar years, October to September, to suit the medical school year, listing themselves as 1823–4, or 1824–5, for example. With increasing success came expansion, more words per page, more pages per volume, and eventually two immense volumes every calendar year. The volume numbering is therefore confusing, especially in the early days, and although individual issue numbers are accurate, they are not particularly helpful in locating specific articles.

To avoid confusion, therefore, in this volume, *Lancet* articles are referred to simply by day, month, year and page.

The Lancet back-files on-line

Any reader who wishes to look up back issues of *The Lancet* may do so for themselves, as all its volumes since 1823 are now available on-line, at: www.sciencedirect.com.

Many public and academic libraries subscribe to *The Lancet* back-files. Local libraries should be able to advise those without access to on-line facilities. ●

THE AUTHOR

Dr Ruth Richardson is author of the introduction to this book, and has carefully selected the articles included here from the original volumes of *The Lancet*. She is an interdisciplinary historian and broadcaster who has published widely on the history of medicine, architecture, public health and periodical publication.

Dr Richardson has given lectures for academic and medical audiences across Europe and North America. Her history of the corpses in UK dissection rooms, *Death, Dissection and the Destitute* (Chicago University Press, 2000) is now a standard work and teaching text in medical history courses in the UK and USA. Her massive *Builder Illustrations Index* (co-authored with Robert Thorne) was awarded the Wheatley Gold Medal.

She has co-edited two volumes on medical humanities for the Royal College of Physicians of London, and is also the author of a new historical introduction to the latest edition of *Gray's Anatomy* (Elsevier, 2005).

Dr Richardson is a Scholar in the History of Science at the University of Cambridge, and Senior Research Fellow in History at the University of Hertfordshire at Hatfield. She is a Fellow of the Royal Historical Society and Examiner in the history of medicine at the Worshipful Society of Apothecaries, London. Dr Richardson has been a regular reader of *The Lancet* since 1975 and a contributor to the journal since 1995.

Most recently she has co-authored a paper with Professor Brian Hurwitz, for a recent *Lancet* Christmas issue, on *The Penny Lancet*. ●

ACKNOWLEDGEMENTS

Above all, I thank Professor Brian Hurwitz, who has lived with this project at home for a long time, and has been (as always) wise, helpful, encouraging and supportive. Our son, Josh, has been a sweet distraction.

I am deeply grateful for the hospitable welcome I was given by the editorial and other staff at *The Lancet*'s London office in Camden Town, especially from Richard Horton and Astrid James, Pia Pini, Bill Summerskill, David McNamee, Janna Palmer, Richard Lane, Andrew Bell, Hopelyn Goodwin, Rose Bryan and the incomparable John Bignall, who has been wonderfully generous with his time and good counsel. David Sharp advised and guided me, and has saved me from some howlers, for which I am extremely grateful. Of course, all remaining errors are my own.

I would also like to thank many people for help of various kinds during the creation of this book. The work of many historians has been of great assistance to me, as have my darling parents Hilda and William Richardson, and my four sisters.

Thanks also to Susan Armstrong, Paquita de Zulueta, Robert Bud, Rachel Calder, Dee Cook, Clive Coward, Dr Kiheung Kim, James Lefanu, Bridget Macdonald, Hilary Morris, Peter Razzell, Steven J Scheinman and Jane Wildgoose; and at Elsevier, Alison Taylor, Kim Benson, Yolanta Motylinska, Elisabeth Lawrence and Jan Ross. It has been a real pleasure to work with Dorothy Sharp on the book's design.

Staff at The British Library, St Pancras, at the Wellcome Library, at the Westminster Archive Centre, London, at the Royal College of Surgeons, London and at the Institute of Historical Research, University of London, have been unfailingly helpful. The book would have taken a great deal longer to assemble without the extraordinary efforts of *ScienceDirect* to create the on-line database of *The Lancet* back issues. ●

CONTENTS

Detailed listings appear at the start of each section.

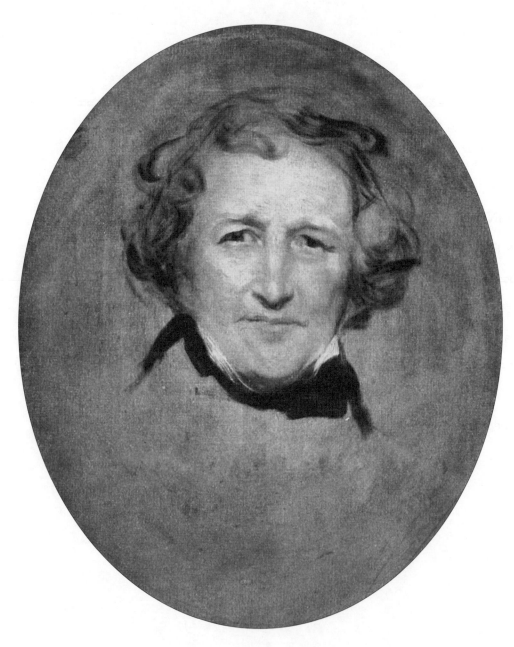

Thomas Wakley (1795–1862). Founder Editor of *The Lancet*.
From an oil sketch by Edwin Landseer.

THE LANCET: AN INTRODUCTION

Today there are thousands of biomedical journals. *The Lancet* is the only British weekly medical journal among them to have been continuously in print since 1823 – every week of every year for more than 180 years – an extraordinary achievement.

The international stature of *The Lancet* as a medical journal derives in part from its great age, which is in itself attributable to the journal's highly distinctive character.

The Lancet is deeply rooted in all things medical. It was founded – and by tradition is edited – by a medical doctor. It was created and designed for a broad medical readership, and it has always been committed to medical excellence.

Yet *The Lancet* has never regarded itself *only* as a medical journal. Medicine and science were not generally regarded as being synonymous at the time of its foundation, yet *The Lancet* has always been a vehicle for scientific and social ideas, innovation, and at one and the same time, for something greater: more imaginative, generous and inclusive.

The journal's editorial line is boldly independent: unconstrained by external influence, whether from professional medical organisations, pharmaceutical companies, politicians or from governments. It is also profoundly informed by its values. *The Lancet*'s honesty is uncompromising, and its compassion broad and active.

The Lancet's columns are a place where medicine addresses both itself and the human condition; where the conscience – indeed the consciousness – of the ameliorative impulse at the heart of medicine finds its bearings.

The Lancet's foundation

The early 19th century was a period of active entrepreneurial activity in newspaper and magazine publishing. A great many periodicals were being floated at that time. There was a hunger for reading matter of all kinds, and the application of steam to printing and papermaking made printed media cheaper, promoting a rising circulation of news, poetry, fiction and scientific thought.

However, government repression during the Regency period – provoked by an autocratic reaction against the French Revolution, and the ensuing Napoleonic Wars – rendered it a dangerous time to become a plain-speaking journalist and publisher.

Few periodicals of that era survived more than a short time, usually only months, rarely years. Many were forced out of business by government prosecution. Most were commercial failures which sank without leaving much trace.* Only those which somehow hit a winning formula lasted any time at all.

The Lancet was founded in October 1823 by Thomas Wakley, a London surgeon and general practitioner, then 28 years of age. It was the first successful medical weekly in the UK, and remains the only survivor from that time.

The Lancet is seen by historians – sometimes rather testily – as a publishing exception in every respect.* The only parallel to its success in the Anglophone world is its older sibling the *New England Journal of Medicine*, founded in Boston, Massachusetts in 1812, and like *The Lancet* still in weekly publication.*

The determining constituent in *The Lancet*'s early success was the spirited personality of Thomas Wakley himself. We shall look at him in a moment, but first, can his winning formula be analysed?

The title

The journal's chosen title was a curiosity, carrying layers of possible meaning. Most obviously, a lancet was the small but sharp instrument of choice for surgical practitioners in blood-letting, and used moreover to lance boils, to clean wounds, demarcate, isolate and relieve infection. The lancet was a hands-on practical instrument, one which symbolised decision-making and active intervention in the healing art.

As an old and esteemed correspondent later observed: "The action of the lancet was never punitive, but conservative of life and energy, and an agent used to purify the body from those deleterious products upon which its mortal ills depended. It occurred to Mr Wakley that, by using the quill for purposes similar to those for which surgeons used the lancet, he might, in the body medical, get rid of much that was harmful".*

There was also an architectural analogy. Tall pointed windows were admired by the neo-gothic modernist architects of that time who championed indigenous 'pointed' as against 'classic' in devotional architecture. To Wakley, the image of a lancet window throwing light in dark places is said to have been a favourite.*

Perhaps most significantly, though, a lancet is also a diminutive lance; a jousting weapon from the days of knights on horseback, used to unseat opponents, or of course, to thrust down the gorges (or between the ribs) of marauding dragons. The numerous playful appearances of incisive imagery in the early issues of *The Lancet* – in editorials, and in correspondence ("EZ may rest assured that Sir Billy Fretful shall shortly receive a pretty sharp cut from '*The Lancet*', as a chastisement for his unrelenting conduct ..."; "The Letter of MZ is much too sharp even for *The Lancet*") – make clear that Wakley and his readers very much enjoyed the cut and thrust his title implied.*

Immediate success

The Lancet's original 'bold and defiant' preface (republished in this volume) abjured medical obfuscation – especially in language – and renounced all pretension to medicine being a 'mystery'. Nor would the journal focus on medical esoterica: the intention was to look broadly at medical and surgical practice and research, the prevention of illness, appropriate diet and the promotion of human health.

* Notes on page 14; bold dates indicate papers in this volume.

The few medical journals then in existence were monthly, decidedly dull, costly, and with a narrow conventional 'establishment' focus, intended for a restricted and established medical audience. By contrast *The Lancet* appeared every week, had a genuinely radical anti-medical-establishment flavour and was exciting, challenging and unconventional. *The Lancet* repudiated limits to its readership, addressing itself to a constituency embracing everyone with an interest in medicine: past and current medical students, the entire profession, urban and country general practitioners, practitioners overseas and inquiring members of the wider public.

It rapidly became a paper weapon to expose and reform the abuses which existed in the hospitals and medical schools of the metropolis. At that time the granting of English medical qualifications was dominated by a London-based clique, whose appointments were obtainable only by family or money influence. Reform was no insignificant aim: it had sweeping national and, because of the colonial empire of the time, also international implications. The journal was soon available worldwide: in Edinburgh, Dublin, Paris, Strasbourg, Berlin, New York and Calcutta.

The new journal cost only sixpence an issue, which to those in employment was not exorbitant. The price included the stamp, at that time an important consideration. The government's imposition of a stamp tax on newspapers was intended to constrict adverse political comment in these years of political ferment. Payment of the tax protected a newspaper from prosecution for evasion (many publishers and vendors of unstamped papers were forced out of business), but imposed a bright red stamp, which was perceived by those who despised these 'taxes on knowledge' as a slavemark. Wakley always observed the law, even when he knew it to be an ass. *The Lancet* bore the red crest as a sign of its legitimacy as a weekly news publication, its freedom to be sold publicly and sent nationwide, and its freedom to speak without fear or favour.

Style and content

There are a good many other reasons for *The Lancet*'s immediate success, not least (as we shall see) that it offered excellent value.

The style and content of the new journal were crucial. Stylistically, *The Lancet* was accessible, honest, authoritative and bold. It looked professional. Its design emphasised accessibility: pocket-sized, with a clear typeface and good layout, its contents proved easy to read. Good engravers had been engaged for illustrations, and it had efficient distribution.

In tone *The Lancet* was optimistic, progressive, internationalist in outlook and character, hospitable to interdisciplinarity, and, in its interest in scientific experimentation it leaned towards Paris for its openness and scientific attainments. A decade or two earlier, this inclination might have been deemed semi-treasonous, but in 1823 the peace treaty had been signed 8 years and the long-banished Napoleon was in his tomb.

Ever since Waterloo in 1815, Paris had become the destination of choice for every medical student who could afford to get there. Experience of Parisian medical teaching gave a gloss of social sophistication to any young doctor, and an independence of thought, untrammelled by the dead weight of the almost feudal arrangements still so evident in England. On the English side of the Channel, many felt with good reason that French medicine

was both more dynamic and more scientific than the home variety. To some this opinion was grounds for trepidation, but not for *The Lancet*, which embraced scientific medicine with enthusiasm. "A new era has arisen in the history of medicine", it asserted, "mainly brought about by the zeal and industry of the French."*

The Lancet initially stated its aim, somewhat modestly, as "adding to the stock of useful knowledge... in these realms". Later it was more bold: "The object we have most at heart, is the advancement of our Profession". It would cover "... every subject connected with the progress of medical and surgical science, both in this country and on the continent", seeking to promote a genuine "republic of letters and of science".*

Early issues of *The Lancet* carried reports of animal trials of a new stomach pump (which it recommended for overdoses of laudanum), reports translated from French journals from the French physiologist Magendie, as well as good coverage of papers presented and discussions at a number of English medical societies. As the journal became more established, it carried articles and news from other eminent continental exponents of scientific medicine such as Liebig, Henle and Orfila, and from doctors around the world, from the United States to India.

The news *The Lancet* carried was fresh, every week. It could comment immediately on goings-on at teaching hospitals, report surgical operations, medical meetings or parliamentary findings within days. In addition to medical news it featured case histories, new remedies, physiological discoveries, and developed a lively correspondence section, carried reviews of new books, news of the contemporary arts scene, and is said to have been the first periodical in the world to carry chess problems and their solutions. This sort of breadth was what cemented *The Lancet*'s appeal, both initially, and in the longer term.

Reading through the early issues, one is struck by how swiftly the journal got off the ground. Interesting and important case histories were freshly reported as they developed from week to week. A sense of pressure of space becomes evident in the manner in which articles had to be cut short and held over for completion in later issues. Communications were soon arriving from all over the country, and abroad. Lack of space swiftly became a recurrent theme. One gains a strong sense of the journal as a conduit, trying to hold a flood of material, bursting to get into print. *The Lancet* clearly answered a need which had been entirely unmet before it went into production, and served to grant ideas that had been repressed (probably for years) legitimacy and momentum.

The Lancet opened the door to a new world for forward-looking medical men, who, the historian Betty Bostetter has observed, had been "trying to do nineteenth century scientific work in a medical world still controlled by... medieval guilds".*

Because *The Lancet* was intent on medical reform, it certainly acquired enemies as well as friends. The journal saw itself as fulfilling the role of a public prosecutor: working for the public good, on behalf of the offended laws of physic.* Its arrival was greeted with alarm in some quarters, which is understandable perhaps, when we consider its refusal to reverence rank without merit. The modern analogy might be closer to the present-day *Private Eye* – a UK weekly magazine devoted to lampooning the political establishment – than with the current *Lancet*.* The journal was... "dreaded and hated by one section of the Profession [hospital consultants and the medical College elites] whilst it was encouraged and supported by the other [students, alumni, general practitioners]". An old employee later said that for several years it was carried on "at the point of the bayonet".

The journal has been criticised for going at its reforming agenda like a bull at a gate, but we must not forget several important and related points. *First*, there genuinely was much that needed reforming. *Second*, there have always been those who believed doctors ought to stick together in a sort of professional conspiracy against patients. *The Lancet* was unusual in being emphatically not of this party. *Third*, the idiom of the times: in the 1820s political and other caricature could be very robust, often crude and even cruel. *The Lancet* was often blunt, but always fair. *Finally*, criticism of *The Lancet* derives largely from those who opposed it, or those whose generation – or whose memoirs – date from a later era, when Victorian gentility had toned down the vigour of language and imagery available to reformers of any kind.

Other Victorians continued to celebrate *The Lancet*'s temerity, notably a correspondent who observed in 1892, that although the journal started as a "tiny instrument", its effect was "startling in the extreme"; "so sharp and penetrating were the articles... and withal so bold, that many were astonished... The comfortable hospital doctors beheld [*The Lancet*'s] appearance with trepidation. Quacks held their breath, malpractitioners were in alarm, and the medical public were quiet and expectant. Its statements and criticisms were courageous and full of manly vigour, and it sounded in medical literature a stirring note altogether different from the tone of its tame predecessors".

Some contemporaries may well have had their reservations as to *The Lancet*'s style, but numbers welcomed and supported *The Lancet*'s reforming ardour. Certainly enough bought it, and contributed to it, to keep it economically and intellectually buoyant. An early correspondent expresses a little of the excitement: "there has been quite a revolution in the professional discipline of the hospitals"... "all the physicians, surgeons, midwifers, and apothecaries within the scope of my acquaintance, read [*The Lancet*] with avidity".*

And because *The Lancet* possessed such vitality, no-one in the field could afford to miss reading it. Friends and enemies alike purchased it, and of course the discussion it generated in other journals and newspapers prompted wider curiosity, further promoting its success. Before long, competitors were advertising in its pages.

The Lancet prospered so well, so swiftly, that within months even its young proprietor was able to express pleasurable surprise: "Our success has exceeded our most sanguine expectations".* Subscribers were soon clamouring for the reprinting of the journal's earliest numbers, so they could complete their own sets for library binding. There was an awareness that *The Lancet* was a phenomenon, and a presentiment that it would last.

Wakley himself

Thomas Wakley was tall, well built, energetic and pugnacious – a sporting pugilist in his youth (boxing was more reputable in the Regency era than now) and a man with both a resolute sense of justice and a genial sense of humour. He emerges from surviving documents as a presence to be reckoned with. A contemporary friend described him as "brave, determined and manly".

His life experience was considerably greater than most of his contemporaries, since, at the age of 10, he had already worked his way to India and back under sail.

The attraction to the 10-year-old was perhaps not simply that of the sea, but its contemporary aura of heroism. Wakley was 10 in 1805, the year in which Napoleon's planned invasion of Britain was triumphantly thwarted when the combined French and Spanish fleet was utterly vanquished by Nelson at Trafalgar. This was the era of the fearless English Tar, whose courage Horatio Nelson exemplified: famous for his intrepidity, for losing an eye and an arm in miscellaneous skirmishes, for ignoring orders and for brilliant tactical manoeuvres. Nelson was loved by the British people because he was known to have risen to the pinnacle of the British Navy from the ranks, not by influence, but by native born merit. His death, from a sniper's bullet at Trafalgar, was a national calamity.

Wakley had been born in 1795 to a comfortable Dorset farming family, the youngest son of 11 children. He was well educated, attending good junior and (after the cabin-boy escapade) senior schools. His teenage years were years of war abroad and political repression at home. His apprenticeship as a surgeon-apothecary complete, Wakley enrolled as a pupil at the United Hospitals of Guy's and old St Thomas's (then occupying land now beneath London Bridge Station) in Southwark. He had just turned 20. It was 1815: the year of Waterloo, the final downfall of military dictatorship in France and the toppling of Napoleon's numerous relatives from assorted thrones across Europe. The peace brought crowds of demobbed servicemen seeking work, extensive poverty and pressure for change.

Wakley had probably been warned about inadequacies in the institutional medical tuition at the United Hospitals, because he signed up for a private course, too, at a well-known anatomy school nearby. The school was run by Edward and Richard Grainger, brothers known for their teaching, and for their medical reforming sympathies.

Unfortunately, Wakley did not live long enough to leave any memoirs, so very little is known directly about his personal experience during this formative part of his life. The derivation of his radicalism is uncertain – it may have been a family inclination, or personal, from being a put-upon youngest boy in a large family (he had six older brothers), he may have acquired it at school, or at sea, at medical school, or perhaps simply absorbed it from 'the air' as he was growing up. Wakley's natural inclination was to side with the powerless, to champion justice, to square up to what he perceived as the bully.

From *The Lancet*'s later campaigns we can deduce that by the time he qualified, Wakley had developed a strong notion of scientific rigour, of the standards good medicine should attain, and of the gulf between these standards and the realities of medical school. His profound disgust with the corruption he witnessed, the bungled surgery and the negligent attitudes towards students, and towards patients' suffering (indeed, towards their very survival), fuelled him for much of the rest of his life.

Wakley's dedication to human rights and to practical reform in medical governance are clear from the earliest issues of *The Lancet*. Feature articles and letters focused upon public health and humanitarian issues of wide geographical scope, including the appalling sanitary conditions inside English prisons, and the poor treatment of hospital and mental patients, expressed in headlines such as "Barbarous Mode of Punishing Criminals in Russia"; "Nottingham Lunatic Asylum. Abolition of Bodily Restraint in all Ordinary Cases. Example to Bethlem".

Although he toned down his youthful rhetoric as he matured, Wakley held to his convictions all his life. Whatever their source, it looks to have run deep.

High standards

The Lancet's reputation for setting high standards in medicine began at the outset with its first issue, which opened with a full transcript of the opening lecture of the doyen of British surgery, Sir Astley Cooper.

The publication of entire lectures in this way was highly innovative. Cooper, like many of his contemporaries, had hitherto regarded his lectures as his stock in trade, to be transmitted to suitable witnesses only after the payment of appropriate fees. Wakley argued in print (and later in court when another lecturer objected) that *The Lancet's* coverage of lectures delivered in a public institution were akin to court or parliamentary reports.

In reality, few enough of those who actually attended Cooper's famous lectures possessed shorthand swift enough to take down every word. Surviving student notebooks suggest the interest of the lectures was often too great to be recorded at the time. *The Lancet's* transcripts rendered Cooper's lectures as contemporaries might have heard them, and are a good read even today: informative and engaging. Students at other medical schools read them to see what they were missing, rival lecturers to see what made Cooper so famous, and many more potential readers, of course – who might never attend a lecture at any medical school – were probably intrigued to find *The Lancet* could satisfy their curiosity with what it described as probably the finest surgical lectures in Europe.

Not unexpectedly, standards which fell short of *The Lancet's* hopes for the profession also emerged in the journal's pages. When, for example, students complained to the journal of the foolish behaviour by part of the audience at Charles Bell's lectures, the disruption was censured in no uncertain terms.

Poor standards of care in public hospitals met with criticism, too. An early issue of *The Lancet* addressed what we would now call the 'quality of care' meted out to patients. The case report of a drayman whose leg had to be amputated in a London teaching hospital, after being crushed under a carriage wheel, offers an instance. His post-operative care provoked a remark which reveals the practical nature of *The Lancet's* reforming compassion. *The Lancet* noticed that the lack of bed-pan equipment for the patient's comfort had resulted in haemorrhage: simply for the "lack of a simple contrivance" which would allow the patient's stump to remain horizontal for a period after the operation.

> "We have seen so many instances of this kind in the Borough hospitals, that we shall take every opportunity of giving publicity to them when they occur, in the expectation that a cause of so much mischief will soon be remedied. It is however, melancholy to state that this is but one out of many evils in the metropolitan hospitals, which are a disgrace to those who allow them to exist. In due time we shall expose them all."*

This is hospital reform with a nursing eye and a significant agenda, 30 years before Florence Nightingale. Wakley understood the institutions he was criticising, and knew that no reform in small matters would occur without a greater change: it was in details

like this – the lack of decent bed-pans – that more fundamental shortcomings were apparent. That the best medical care must also be humane was a deeply held conviction, and it was nourished by another: the remedial authority of an independent and free medical press, acting via what Wakley termed "the potent influence of public indignation".

Exposing imposture

Alongside Astley Cooper's famous lectures, the journal's early issues also carried the first of many startling news exclusives. This one unfolded gradually over several weeks, exposing the story of a churchman known as "Dr Collyer", who had posed as a medical doctor to lure away and effect sexual abuse upon young working class boys at a public bathing pool.

Child abuse did not then have a name, nor was it something which could easily be spoken about. *The Lancet's* ire was directed at the fact that Collyer had used the guise of a medical doctor, and the pretence of a medical examination, to effect the abuse.

Wakley was greatly affronted that the offer of medical help might be traduced by predation, and he worked for years against sham doctors and their deceptions. The journal's "avowed object", according to an 1824 editorial, was "to expose all unfounded pretensions to medical skill, whether originating in fraud, hypocrisy or fouler motives."* The General Medical Council and the UK Medical Register were to be the eventual result, the fruit of 35 years effort and agitation.

The Collyer case is not typical of later exposés by *The Lancet*, in that it had a sexual component, something the journal abjured thereafter. Yet the manner in which the story was dealt with exemplifies *The Lancet's* later campaigns against other abuses: righting wrongs by naming and shaming offenders. Verifiable identification of culpable individuals and their locus and style of activity appeared in the journal, with plenty of convincing first-hand evidence to substantiate and justify *The Lancet's* position. This strategy served either to goad guilty parties to sue for libel; apologise and reform; or leave the field, the journal having thoroughly blown their cover.

A parallel aspect of *The Lancet's* endeavour to expose imposture was its insistence on ethical pharmacy, initially by publishing, in plain English, the recipes of what it called 'quack' – patent and other proprietary – medicines, so all readers could see that their main ingredients were invariably flour, salt, sugar, sulphur, mercury, alcohol and/or opium.

Medical impostures extended upwards to the governing bodies which oversaw medical qualifications. To *The Lancet*, the Royal Colleges of Surgery and Physic were run by self-perpetuating cliques, oligarchies "bloated with wealth and blustering with power... musty receptacles of ignorance and imbecility [where] every abuse is to be found". They were referred to as "turnpikes on the way to improvement" which blighted the careers of talented men.*

The Worshipful Company of Apothecaries also came in for ridicule, as the "Old Hags at Rhubarb Hall". Reformers believed the apothecaries sustained their monopoly over dispensing, and their control over the qualification of dispensing doctors, by cultivating an atmosphere of almost cabalistic mystery about the constituents of medicines that were – to the new generation of scientific doctors – straightforward compounds. In fact, the apothecaries were running a complex battle (which they ultimately lost) for the control of the drugs business, at least partly out of genuine concern for the purity of drugs. Their activities, at the time, looked more like empire-building than public spirit, which was why Wakley did not support them.

Audit

What we would now call audit was another key area in which *The Lancet* was actively interested. Leading articles tackled the misuse of charitable donations to 'voluntary' (charitable) hospitals, by the careful examination of bed numbers and expenditure between comparable institutions, revealing institutional mismanagement and poor value for money. To Wakley, the disparity looked very much like peculation, and it was this which most concerned him:

> "There is more of downright hypocrisy, humbug and intrigue practised in [charity hospitals] than can possibly be imagined. At least half the money which is now subscribed for the benefit of the afflicted in our hospitals never reaches, in any form, the persons of the poor."*

This sort of scrutiny of management probity was unheard of in a medical journal at the time, and called forth reams of defensive reports from enquiries headed by worthy bigwigs, whom *The Lancet* respected no more than incompetent managers. Hospital governors and their supporters suffered considerable discomfiture at this sort of public oversight.

In *The Lancet*'s eyes, a great many second-rate doctors were operating in public hospitals, so surgical audit also became a topic for which the journal became well known, and greatly feared.

The Lancet brought the issue of differential death rates to public attention in 1824, publishing a comparison of the fatality rates among patients undergoing the same operation in the same institution (Guy's) but under different surgeons.

There is good reason to suppose that *The Lancet* received its information from insiders. Wakley had trained at the United Hospitals, and was well aware of the snobbery against poorer students, who – whatever their talents or inclinations – were forced to become general practitioners because surgical jobs were awarded only by money or favour, not by merit. One observer described the situation at the Borough hospitals as "a snug family party".

Wakley clearly felt it his public duty to publish the results he had been given. Many contemporary medical men considered it bad form to reveal a colleague's incompetence and *The Lancet*'s conduct was deprecated in some circles. Soon afterwards, Magendie, the great French physiologist, personally visited *The Lancet* office, and Wakley published the following defiant declaration:

> "We take this opportunity of publicly returning our acknowledgements for the polite and flattering manner in which M. Magendie, during his short stay in this metropolis, presented us with his most valuable journal. *The Lancet* can afford to have Messrs Travers, Green and Tyrrell [surgeons at the United Hospitals] for enemies, when it can rank the first physiologist in Europe, among its friends."*

Long after Wakley's death, Sir John Erichsen observed that medical professionals are "for the most part ignorant how much they owe to him for exposing and fearlessly attacking the manifold abuses that existed in every department of the profession" at that time. Wakley's labours: "cleared the road to fame and fortune" for many other doctors, by establishing the principle of genuine merit-based professionalism in medicine. Erichsen may have had his own glittering career in mind.

Fearless of prosecution

The Lancet's propensity to uncloak surgical ineptitude and institutional corruption rendered it the friend of reforming doctors nationwide. It also resulted in a celebrated court case in 1828. The stimulus for the case was a report, written by a medical eye-witness, of a bungled operation at Guy's Hospital. *The Lancet* concluded that the patient had died because the surgeon, Bransby Cooper, had been elevated beyond his competence only because he was a nephew of Sir Astley Cooper.

The subsequent court case for malicious libel was widely reported, exposing to public view exactly what *The Lancet* had been campaigning against: the nepotism of the metropolitan surgical elite. Wakley acted as his own advocate to defend *The Lancet*'s coverage.

The opposing barrister, an ex-Attorney General, was an implacable opponent of press freedom, who demanded £2000 exemplary damages. This enormous sum of money – probably equivalent to over £1m today – was set with the clear intention of bankrupting Wakley, and silencing *The Lancet* for ever. By the end of the case, even the judge demurred as to the justification for such a sum in damages, and the jury awarded only £100 instead.

Wakley's courage in reporting on this and other cases will perhaps be better appreciated in the context of government prosecutions of contemporary journalists like the poet Leigh Hunt and Wakley's own friend William Cobbett, both imprisoned in 1812, or of William Hone – prosecuted three times and acquitted by stalwart London juries on each occasion – in 1817; or, if we recollect the sufferings of the Dickens family when Charles Dickens's father was incarcerated in the Marshalsea Debtors Prison between 1822 and 1824. *The Lancet*'s costs in this case were amply covered by a public subscription, the surplus of which was sent to the patient's widow. The case was a landmark in investigative medical reporting, the freedom of the press, and in medical accountability.*

The Lancet was subsequently involved in other court cases, and many more were threatened, Collyer's being among them. In the journal's first decade there were 10 cases, in which a total of £8,000 was claimed against *The Lancet*, only £155 and a farthing in fact being awarded. Wakley remained cool and fearless, and continued to publish when he knew it right to do so. He did become more cautious: choosing his subjects with considerable care, and using defensive devices such as ostensibly denying allegations so as to be able to air them, utilising satire and nicknames more extensively so those he exposed would appear absurd if they took up a case, or avoiding direct allegation while publishing extensive data from which readers might draw their own conclusions.

There can be little doubt that fear of *The Lancet*'s scrutiny, and of medical whistleblowers, caused a great many institutions and individuals to adjust behaviour, not always in the public-spirited manner Wakley might have hoped.

At St Thomas's Hospital, for example, great notices threatened with immediate expulsion any medical student who reported on lectures to *The Lancet*. Of course this was greeted at the journal with hilarity and derision: some of its anonymous columnists were members of the hospital's staff.

Opinion former

Wakley perceived at quite an early stage in *The Lancet*'s development that any piecemeal reform resulting from skirmishes like the Cooper case would be too slow for his liking. The era was one of reforming pressure in politics, and Wakley turned his prodigious energies towards parliamentary legislation.

At first he worked behind the scenes with sympathetic politicians, such as Henry Warburton during the 1834 Select Committee on Medical Education. Having witnessed how the system worked, Wakley saw he could do it himself. Doubtless, too, he appreciated Members' traditional immunity from prosecution for allegations made inside the House.

Ultimately Wakley stood for election as an independent radical, and in 1835 was elected Member of Parliament for Finsbury, a large north London constituency newly created under the 'Great' 1832 Reform Act. Wakley used his maiden speech to attack the vindictive punishment of the Tolpuddle Martyrs, six Dorset labourers who, in trying to prevent a further cut in their starvation wages, fell foul of government anti-trade union legislation, and were sentenced to transportation.

Wakley spoke well on a wide variety of matters – lifting taxes on knowledge, property qualifications, the state of factories, legal representation for prisoners, military flogging, the cruelties of the workhouse system, cutting the cost of bread by repealing the hated Corn Laws and opening museums on Sundays. A contemporary portrait described him as "an open, candid and honest denouncer of invidious distinctions between rich and poor, especially in legislation" mentioning that he exercised his parliamentary right of "keeping on his hat in the presence of the King". Wakley was a great believer in the Christian notion of the equality of men's souls, and was not seeking a title.

Much parliamentary work took place in the evenings and at night, and after 1839, Wakley's daylight hours were divided between *The Lancet* and another important post to which he devoted similar energy: as elected Coroner for West Middlesex. This, too, was the result of a campaign. Wakley believed coroners should be medically qualified, that many accidents attributable to hardship, negligence or cruelty, or to secret homicide, had been overlooked by the lawyers who had previously held such posts, because they were essentially unqualified to discover cause of death.

As coroner, Wakley was as compassionate and courageous as he was Editor and MP. We know this because on one occasion he was closely observed by one of the best witnesses alive at the time. Many years later, Charles Dickens described how, in 1840, he had been summoned to serve as a juryman at Marylebone workhouse at an inquest concerning a newly dead baby. The jury was called to decide whether the mother – a young orphan maid-of-all-work – had concealed the birth, or had committed infanticide. Concealment was punishable with imprisonment, whereas infanticide was a hanging offence.

The post-mortem findings seemed inconclusive, and the harder-hearted members of the jury held sway, until Dickens himself:

> "... took heart to ask a question or two which hopefully admitted of an answer that might give a favourable turn to the case. ... it did some good, and the Coroner, who was nobly patient and humane, cast a look of strong encouragement in my direction. I tried again, and the Coroner backed me again, for which I ever

afterwards felt grateful to him, as I do now to his memory. At last we found for the minor offence. The poor desolate creature, who had been taken out during our deliberation, being brought in again to be told of the verdict, then dropped upon her knees before us, with protestations that we were right – protestations among the most affecting that I have ever heard in my life – and was carried away insensible."

Afterwards, Wakley personally confirmed to Dickens the correctness of the jury's verdict of 'found dead'. As a surgeon himself, Wakley had perceived the existence of "some foreign matter in the windpipe, quite irreconcilable with many moments of life". Dickens, who was already a well-established author, was haunted by the woman's face in his dreams that night, and could afford to arrange for:

> "... extra care to be taken of her in the prison, and counsel to be retained for her when she was tried at the Old Bailey. Her sentence was lenient, and her [later] history and conduct proved it was right".

Dickens makes it clear that, without the fortuitous conjunction of a discerning coroner and a benign intelligence among the jurymen, an irrevocable miscarriage of justice might have transpired. Dickens admired Wakley ever afterwards.*

Among Wakley's best known cases was that of Private Frederick White, an army recruit flogged to death at Hounslow Barracks in 1846.* Acting on information, Wakley ordered the soldier's exhumation from the grave in which those responsible had hurriedly buried him, and a fresh post mortem: which revealed that Private White had died not of heart failure as recorded on his death certificate, but from complications deriving from a prolonged and vicious flogging. With the jury's support, a more accurate verdict was arrived at. The case was widely reported, and Wakley's efforts helped bring about the control, and ultimately the withdrawal, of flogging in the services.

Like Charles Dickens, Wakley was also an effective critic of the heartlessness of the New Poor Law, exposing its many shortcomings: most memorably perhaps, in the scandal at the Andover workhouse, where the pauper inmates were so starved that they fought each other for fragments of rancid meat on bones they were crushing to manufacture fertiliser.* Wakley also ran a *Lancet* campaign for fair play – specifically decent pay and conditions – for Poor Law medical officers, and for naval surgeons, both often shabbily treated by their employers.

Wakley's policy of raising matters in *The Lancet* and in Parliament resulted in several investigative Select Committees and, Dr Bostetter estimates, "at least ten recommendations for measures that... later became the law of the land".*

For a number of years, Wakley worked tirelessly at these three interrelated roles – journalist, politician and coroner – routinely cutting sleeping hours to accommodate late nights at Westminster, and the long journeys he often had to undertake to attend inquests, and perform constituency work. His work, said a close observer, "was incessant and gigantic". But his punishing schedule eventually told on his health, and Wakley retired from Parliament in 1852 after a collapse.

The next decade was an important one for *The Lancet*, as Wakley's sons James and Thomas Henry (both young doctors) came to work in the office, the latter on a part-time basis. This move served to provide for the long term future continuity and stability of the journal, both by taking weight from Wakley's shoulders, and by training up the next generation in the business of editing and management. After his recovery, Wakley himself returned with renewed vigour, and the appointment of a celebrated *Lancet* Analytical Sanitary Commission to investigate the adulteration of food.

The work was undertaken by a careful investigative scientist, Dr Arthur Hassall, of the Royal Free Hospital, assisted by Dr Henry Lethaby (later Medical Officer of Health for the City of London). Thousands of rigorous chemical and microscopic analyses were undertaken on food samples purchased at random, and the results published in *The Lancet* by food type – tea, bread, beer and so on. Between 1851 and 1854, reports on 30 or so common foodstuffs appeared in the journal, ultimately being collected in a substantial volume in 1855.

Once again *The Lancet* decided to name and shame. Hassall's shocking findings obtained enormous public exposure, being picked up by newspapers nationwide, provoking national disgust. Shamed manufacturers and tradesmen were forced to think again about the profitability of adding alum to bread, water and salt to beer, and poisonous colourings (such as white lead) to children's sweets. None of the hundreds of guilty tradespeople revealed by *The Lancet* to have polluted foodstuffs for profit took the journal to court. According to a historian of British diet, *The Lancet*'s efforts had a significant cultural impact, both on the provision of pure foodstuffs and purchasing habits, as well as the advertising of food, even before parliamentary intervention.* *The Lancet*'s influence is hardly to be wondered at when we consider that the journal was telling advertisers in the mid-1850s that its circulation was double that of any other medical journal in the Universe.

In the same decade, Wakley's long campaign for a General Medical Council, and for a national Medical Register of all qualified doctors, at last came to fruition in 1858.

For much of his adult life, Wakley suffered from periodic bouts of ill health, but always seemed able to throw them off. In his last years, however, he seems to have become seriously consumptive, and in the winter of 1861 he travelled to Madeira for its climate. He died there in May 1862, aged only 66. His body was returned to London for burial beside his wife and daughter at Kensal Green.

The Lancet's voice

The prodigious energy and principled commitment with which Wakley infused the journal from its inception renders it difficult to distinguish *The Lancet*'s voice from Wakley's own, even after his death. But workaholic though he was, Wakley could not possibly have written everything in the journal without a by-line. The convention of anonymous editorials – to which *The Lancet* (like the London *Times*) long adhered – conceals the fact that the journal's voice was a team effort even in Wakley's time.

Some of the more caustic of the journal's early editorials were written by surgeon William Lawrence, and many had an added sparkle of wit inspired by William Cobbett.

One of the most memorable columns in the early journal, the hilarious series of 'Intercepted Letters', purported to be genuine correspondence between members of the medical elite. The letters were well-informed and clever spoofs, signed only by the hapless victims of their jests, but their real author was a friend of Lawrence's, the surgeon James Wardrop. Both these medical men served the royal family as well as *The Lancet*, which indicates the breadth of the desire for medical reform, even among 'insiders', at the time.

Wakley commissioned much of the copy originating from other hands, and chose what to publish of what might arrive unsolicited at *The Lancet*'s office. His sub-editorial staff – like his assistant and deputy coroner – were highly efficient. Besides Lawrence and Wardrop, a number of medical men who wrote anonymously for *The Lancet* have been identified, among them JF Clarke, William Coulson, John Elliotson, William Farr and Erasmus Wilson. There were certainly many others who advised the journal's Editor, and shared expertise and inside knowledge with *The Lancet*'s readership, without identifying themselves.

Wakley kept an editor's eye on everything appearing under *The Lancet*'s name, tweaking the prose himself where necessary. He liaised every evening with his printer, who worked on the premises. On printing nights a lawyer was on hand with others, for a merry editorial session before the journal went to press. Charles Dickens and George Godwin – both well known editors of successful weeklies contemporary to Wakley's *Lancet* (*Household Words* and *The Builder*) – ran their offices in a similar way. All three were workaholic reformers with more than one job. Only Godwin lived beyond 70.

Because he had written and addressed so much, and had campaigned so actively and successfully for so long, Wakley left behind him a richly creative journalistic legacy. *The Lancet* had published lecture texts, news exclusives, Royal Charters, the texts of entire legislative or draft enactments, had appointed special commissions (sanitary and otherwise), featured regular and irregular columns of various kinds, statistical and chemical analyses, scientific papers, verbatim coverage of debates, hypotheses, whistleblown secrets, arts and leisure articles, descriptions of new treatments and technologies, detailed case histories, research letters and other correspondence, transcripts of court proceedings, satires, pseudonymous and anonymous texts, reports of experiments, special supplements, architectural plans, fictional documents, translations, rhymes and snatches of dramatic dialogue, announcements, formulae, news of medical dinners and ceremonial events, book reviews, witness statements from inquests and Select Committees, obituaries, fundraising testimonials, quips, spoofs and petitions.

The Lancet had intervened in many imaginative ways to educate, inform or cajole the profession, the public and parliament in reforming directions. Wakley's practical, tactical agility and creative investment in the journal had led him to devise and adapt a remarkable variety of instruments and techniques between the journal's wrappers during his lifetime, such that his successors had any number of templates to take up again if and when it suited them to do so. Having once been used in *The Lancet*'s columns, there was in a sense a permissive sanctioning by precedent of adaptive, pro-active, investigative medical journalism, its impelling force consistently ameliorative.

Staff at *The Lancet* during the founder's lifetime, and since, may often have asked themselves what Wakley might have thought or said in particular circumstances, composing and editing their own prose accordingly, perpetuating its tone – or at least an echo of it – for many years.

Publication in *The Lancet* remains a genuine accolade for any medical author, and standards are maintained by the questioning process. In *The Lancet* office today the most frequently heard question (often out loud) concerns manuscripts: "Is this a *Lancet* piece?" meaning, is it *Lancet* calibre?

The variety of genres *The Lancet* has historically published allows for considerable elasticity in the kind of articles that will be given consideration, but the real test is the standard of the work.

The journal's international prestige both demonstrates and depends upon the high quality of submissions by authors world wide, the good advice the journal receives from its peer reviewers and the decisions taken at weekly editorial meetings.

After Wakley

After Wakley, his sons continued to maintain the standards *The Lancet* had set, publishing many first rate medical and scientific articles, good commentary on medical and medico-political matters, and intervening when necessary to support reform. In the 1860s, a laboratory was established on the premises, for the independent analysis of drug and bacterial samples.

One of *The Lancet*'s most effective interventions came shortly after Wakley's death, in fact. In 1865, with the active support of staff member Dr Ernest Hart (later a distinguished Editor of the *British Medical Journal*), Wakley's sons James (the new Editor) and Thomas Henry (*Lancet* part-timer) together established a new *Lancet* Commission to investigate the treatment of the sick in London's workhouses.

James Wakley saw the Commission as an editorial legacy from his father, who had referred to workhouse wards as "ANTE-CHAMBERS OF THE GRAVE". Although he probably had an inkling as to what might emerge, perhaps no-one else had an adequate overview of quite how bad things were until *The Lancet* began publishing its Commissioners' reports, at intervals during 1865–1866.*

They found overcrowding so bad in some places that cubic space per patient was half the legal limit allowed for convicted prisoners: patients had to share beds, or could gain access to them only from the foot end. They found doorless latrines on the wards lacking toilet paper or handwashing facilities, infestations, epidemics, high death rates and no professional nursing whatsoever. These historic reports were so shocking that the government swiftly established its own enquiry in 1866 which verified *The Lancet*'s findings and passed the Metropolitan Poor Act the following year. The next decade saw the creation of 10,000 beds in the London region, in 20 newly constructed hospitals, and a nationwide campaign which established similar schemes across the country. Many of these great new hospital buildings were later adopted by the National Health Service: some, indeed, remain in use.

In this, as in many other things, *The Lancet* was active in the right direction, but of course the journal did not possess a monopoly on good sense, and has occasionally blundered: "We have no sympathy for the notion of making lady physicians" commented an editorial on the London Female Medical College in 1866, revealing the limits to James Wakley's reforming tendencies. Only later, when women doctors' scientific and clinical value became obvious, did *The Lancet* rectify that silly statement, by publishing their work.

Editorial control of *The Lancet* remained in the hands of the Wakley family until the 20th century, for after James's death in 1886, his older brother, Thomas Henry (a recent President of the Royal College of Surgeons), took the reigns jointly with his own son, 'Young Tom'.

Another key intervention came in the 1890s, when *The Lancet* established a special Analytical Commission to investigate the standards of purity and potency of the new antitoxins against the killer disease diphtheria. At the time, this enquiry was seen by some as contentious, and it was feared that *The Lancet* was playing into the hands of anti-vaccinationists. But the variability in antigenicity and the high levels of contaminants exposed by *The Lancet*'s enquiry served to improve safety in the long term by establishing sound manufacturing standards.

The 20th century

The editorship of *The Lancet* was eventually delivered into the safe hands of Squire Sprigge, a literary-minded doctor well groomed for the post. When he had first joined the staff in 1892, Sprigge's first project had been to write a history of the journal and its founder. The work on his substantial volume, which took 5 years to research and write, had given him a clear idea of what he was taking on when, after the death of 'Young Tom' in 1909, Sprigge accepted the editorial chair. Sprigge remained in harness until his own death in 1937, seeing the journal through the First World War, and almost up to the outbreak of the Second.

Continuity has been maintained since Sprigge's day by the same policy. All but one of the subsequent editors (and the exception was the briefest in *The Lancet*'s history) have been selected from experienced existing staff. The table given here shows that there have been only six editorial generations at *The Lancet* since Wakley's time: the current Editor, Richard Horton, was recruited by Robin Fox, who was recruited by Ian Douglas-Wilson. From him the chain goes back to Theodore Fox, to Sprigge, to TH Wakley and to Wakley himself. So even today, over 180 years since the start of *The Lancet*'s success, Wakley is only six handshakes away.

Editorial generations at *The Lancet*

1823	☛	Thomas Wakley	Founding Editor
1852		James Wakley joins staff	
1852		TH Wakley joins staff, part-time	
1862		James Wakley	Editor
1880		'Young Tom' joins staff	
1886	☛	TH Wakley and 'Young Tom'	joint Editors
1892		Squire Sprigge joins staff	
1905		Egbert Morland joins staff	
1908	☛	Squire Sprigge	Editor
1925		Theodore Fox joins staff	
1937		Egbert Morland	Editor
1944	☛	Theodore Fox	Editor
1944		Ian Douglas-Wilson joins staff	
1951		Ian Munro joins staff	
1964	☛	Ian Douglas-Wilson	Editor
1968		Robin Fox joins staff	
1976		Ian Munro	Editor
1988		Gordon Reeves	Editor
1990	☛	Robin Fox	Editor
1990		Richard Horton joins staff	
1995		Richard Horton	Editor

☛ Chain of direct training relationships.

Each of the 20th century editors has remained true to the spirit of the journal in individual ways. Sprigge, for example, was a great supporter of free school meals to nourish the 'half-starved' schoolchildren of the slums, and he also activated the idea of a new *Lancet* Sanitary Commission in the early 1930s to examine (with Bradford Hill) the state of British nursing.

In 1938, the journal spoke out in support of the idea of family allowances to lift families out of dire poverty. So concerned was Egbert Morland, then Editor, at the effects of the poverty of the Great Depression in widespread child and maternal malnutrition, that the journal issued a pamphlet on this issue. Under Morland, too, the journal took the courageous step, in 1938, of publishing a letter expressing solidarity with European doctors victimised under the Nazis. Morland steered the journal through the Second World War (four of them from outside London, because of the Blitz), publishing some splendid scientific articles, including the momentous work by Chain and Florey on penicillin.

The next Editor, Theodore Fox, presided over an exciting era of *The Lancet*'s history, 1944–1964, publishing thoughtful editorials on the trials of Nazi doctors at Nuremberg, and the arrival of both the National Health Service in the UK and the international World Health Organisation. Alongside much intelligent commentary, the journal accommodated some superb clinical work, such as the Charnley hip, and the development of ultrasound scanning. Fox, like his predecessor, was a Quaker, and was known for his wit, word-play and tight editing.

He was followed by Ian Douglas-Wilson, who made a determined effort to reduce delays in the process of peer reviewing articles, resulting in a significant speeding up of the process. Having served in the Royal Army Medical Corps during the Second World War, Wilson was accustomed to efficiency and swift reactions to events. In his era (1964–1976) the journal published some key papers on pharmacological advances (propranolol, salicylates, diphosphonates, L-dopa) as well as the much-cited paper on the 'Inverse Care Law', by Julian Tudor Hart.

Another RAMC man followed Wilson into the editorial chair: Ian Munro, in whose era (1976–1988) the journal became known for its coverage of international human rights issues. There followed the shortest editorship in the journal's history, under an editor chosen by the publishers Hodder & Stoughton, which was not a conspicuous success as it lasted less than 2 years. When Robin Fox took the helm in 1990, he and his deputy David Sharp garnered a lively editorial team.

Fox held the journal steady during its acquisition in 1992 by its current publisher, Elsevier, and in 1995 relinquished the post to the current Editor, Richard Horton. Almost as youthful as Wakley had been when he founded the journal, Horton has now been in post a decade, and has shown himself a worthy successor, sustaining the journal's world class reputation with important scientific articles and fine commentary, particularly in the field of global health.

The Lancet has moved home, from its founding premises at 201 Strand, to other addresses in the purlieus of Fleet Street, in the Strand and its vicinity [for the next 150 years], and more recently, from Bloomsbury to Camden Town. Richard Horton has overseen the last two of these moves, and other significant changes including the founding of offshoot journals, *Lancet Neurology*, *Lancet Oncology* and *Lancet Infectious Diseases*, and the

computerisation of the entire editorial and production process. He too has added to the editorial team, while appreciating the mature voices of longer serving staff.

Alongside all the long term changes of personnel, the public visage of *The Lancet* has also been influenced by changes in printing technology, and by contemporary aesthetic perceptions of good design, as the changing page layouts which appear in this volume bear witness.

In Wakley's day the entire journal was written and typeset by hand. Now the editorial process is done largely on computer, as also is its typesetting and design. We have seen that in Wakley's day a printer was on hand to typeset and correct galleys in the editorial office. Today, the editorial and production staff are again housed under one roof – on a single large open plan floor. The office at Jamestown Road, Camden Town, has an atmosphere of vitality and busy camaraderie, underpinned by a keen sense of collective effort and responsibility for a noble enterprise.

The Lancet's breadth

The prime challenge involved in selecting highlights of *The Lancet*'s achievement has been addressing the extraordinary extent and breadth of the journal's output. Indeed, Squire Sprigge – despite being Wakley's biographer and a long-standing Editor of *The Lancet* himself – declined to make any attempt to outline the journal's content at the time of the first centenary in 1923, on the grounds that he regarded such a project as impossible. We are in the fortunate position of having a further 80 years' output to consider, so the challenge is proportionately greater.

So, what is presented here is an indication, no more, of the journal's richness and breadth: a sort of wine-tasting for readers' relish and enjoyment.

For simplicity, the material has been divided into four great tranches:

► 1820s–1860s: the era of the development of anaesthetics
► 1870s–1910s: the era of the development of antisepsis
► 1920s–1950s: the era of the development of antibiotics
► 1960s–2005:   the era of the development of clinical trials

More space has been allocated to the most recent of these periods, since medical and scientific output has increased in the last 50 years or so. Papers and their titles have become longer, along with the number of collaborators listed as having created them, and the number of acronyms appearing in them. Fortunately, in recent times, *The Lancet* has substituted for the old concluding summary at the end of scientific papers, a good abstract at the top. This sensible change has allowed the essence of many more papers to be included here than would otherwise have been the case, as we have chosen to reproduce only the front pages in many instances.

The Lancet's international stature, and its success as an independent voice in the world of medical publishing, rests not only on the publication of important clinical and scientific papers, but in major part on its commentaries on unfolding events. Our selection therefore includes several choice examples of these, either because they comment on key events, or because they reveal something of the journal's evolving character.

Certainly many good things are missing, but those selected to represent their time in this volume are all remarkable, and in very different ways.

1823–1860s

This first great era of *The Lancet*'s work embraces the interval from the foundation of the journal in 1823 to the end of the 1860s. This is Thomas Wakley's time, during which the character of the journal was established. Here are included typical Wakley pieces, his opening manifesto and other materials by which the personality of the journal in his day is made evident (*1823, 1826, 1835, 1858*).

Wakley's reforming stance encompassed all of medicine, promoting debate, and particularly, promoting innovation, scepticism towards pretension and scientific openness.

The manner in which clinical and scientific reports were then presented differs quite markedly from what we would expect today, indeed, part of the interest in looking at the early *Lancet* is in appreciating the contrast.

In this section we find some remarkable papers, including the major historic discovery of the entire era – anaesthesia by sulphuric ether – a full report of which was published in *The Lancet* within weeks of its public demonstration in Boston, and within days of its first demonstration in London (*1847*). *The Lancet* also received James Young Simpson's report on his discovery in the same year (*1847*) of chloroform, which was later administered to Queen Victoria during one of her many confinements (*1853*).

Other important early materials include blood transfusion (*1829*), the use of saline infusion in cholera (1831, *1832*) and a fine article on fracture repair using plaster of Paris (*1834*).

Marshall Hall was not the first to try to resuscitate victims of drowning, but his work on artificial respiration (*1856*) was based on physiology, and in this respect influenced later attempts even into our own time.

Extensive *Lancet* coverage of continental medical developments attracted medical attention to the use of the stethoscope in diagnosis (*1826*), new work in physiology (*1828*) and toxicology (*1829*) and the groundbreaking work of Louis on the medical value of statistics (*1834*).

Serious public health and dietary concerns came to the fore in O'Shaughnessy's work on adulteration of foods, particularly the use of dangerous substances such as white lead in the manufacture of children's sweets (*1831*), and in *The Lancet*'s own investigation of the adulteration of staple foods (*1862*).

Wakley's enthusiasm for preventive medicine is shown in his efforts to gain parliamentary passage for his Smallpox Prevention Bill (*1840*). Advocacy of public baths (*1835*) and attention to slum housing conditions (*1849*) testify to *The Lancet*'s active involvement in the great 'Health of Towns' movement, while the journal was also mindful of the care of the unfortunate – the underclass of the poor (*1837, 1865*) and the mentally ill (*1846*).

Transmissible disease coverage includes cholera (*1832, 1854*), puerperal fever (*1848*), yellow fever (*1861*) and the unexpected (and long unexplained) death of Prince Albert at Windsor (*1862*), later believed to have been caused by typhoid. *The Lancet* later published a sanitary survey of Windsor, revealing its grossly insanitary infrastructure and polluted water supply (*1885*).

Reports of remarkable public events associated with medical education and the history of surgery from *The Lancet*'s pages include the first ever public dissection before a lay audience of working people (*1827*), the Burke and Hare murders (*1829*) and the UK visit of the famous American doctor Mary Walker (*1866*).

All these – and the establishment of the General Medical Council (*1858*) – were key events in public perceptions of professional conduct.

Military medicine is represented by the Private White flogging case (*1846*) and by disparagement of Florence Nightingale's work in the Crimea by a *Lancet* correspondent (*1854*) who represents hostile medical attitudes at the time, and provides us a notion of what she and Mary Walker were up against.

1870s–1910s

This second section of *The Lancet*'s history covers the remarkable era in which antisepsis and then asepsis rose to importance, in which bacteriology came of age. It represents the editorship of Wakley's sons and their handover to Sprigge, up to the time of the influenza pandemic of 1918–1919.

Inaugurated with the publication of Lister's work on antisepsis (*1870*), this section includes material from some distinguished figures, such as Florence Nightingale on the need for sanitary reform in India (*1870*), Pasteur himself on germ theory (*1881*), Ross on the mosquito (*1898*) and Koch discussing tuberculin and tuberculosis (*1890, 1906*).

The laboratory techniques which took on great importance at this time, are exemplified here by an article by Patrick Manson (*1884*). New biological products emerging from laboratory-based exploration meant that science could at last grapple with ancient foes such as leprosy (*1884*), tuberculosis (*1890*), cholera (*1893*), puerperal fever (*1895*), diphtheria (*1896*), malaria (*1898*), typhoid (*1901*) and plague (*1903*). Other work deriving from the logic of public health intervention had a significant impact on yellow fever (*1902*).

Integral to many of these discoveries was a burgeoning understanding of disease transmission, represented in this part of the volume by papers on mosquitoes (*1898*), flies (*1907*) and doctors' hands (*1906*).

Careful clinical studies also generated some remarkable new findings, such as Paget's description of osteitis deformans (Paget's disease) (*1876*), Beatson on hormonal influence on breast cancer (*1896*) and Garrod on inherited metabolic diseases (*1908*). Interest in inheritance (what we would now call genetics) is also evident in a study of the international distribution of blood groups (*1919*).

A growing understanding of the physical impacts of dietary deficiency is noticeable, too, with important work on iodine deficiency and cretinism (*1893*), beri-beri (*1906, 1909*) and rickets (*1919*). Concern with nutrition, however, was not the main consideration of those who inflicted forcible feeding upon women suffragette prisoners in English prisons. *The Lancet* published the views of three concerned doctors who criticised the use of this procedure as tantamount to torture (*1912*).

Medical technology and imaging developed apace in this era. Nitze's report of his electro-endoscopic cystoscope (*1888*) conveys the thrill of exploration that the development of scopes allowed, as does the initial excitement – and then the anxiety – about X-rays (*1896, 1910*).

Two interesting short papers giving real time recordings of human physiological phenomena must both have felt very new when they were published in *1918*. The first, a galvanometric study of a normal (English) person's reaction to an air raid; the other, an electrocardiogram recording made during an attack of angina pectoris.

In an earlier paper (*1879*), Murrell had described his work on nitro-glycerine for angina pectoris, using sphygmographic heart tracings showing the influence of this powerful drug. Other significant drug developments make an appearance in *Lancet* reports in this era. Clinical logic and observation led to the discovery of antimony as a new treatment for bilharzia (*1918*), and the antipyretic effects of salicylates (*1876*), while laboratory-based investigation yielded the German discoveries of heroin (*1898*) and aspirin (*1899*). We have a clinical case history on the life-saving attributes of adrenaline (*1906*), reasoned advocacy for the prevention of shock in surgical operations by the use of pre-medication relaxants (*1913*) and the attempt to battle with puerperal fever using a new streptococcal antitoxin (*1895*). Ehrlich's 'Salvarsan', or '606', was described in *The Lancet* by Ehrlich himself, by courtesy of a British naval surgeon who went to Germany to see for himself (*1910*).

This sort of cooperation between German and British scientific doctors came to an abrupt end in 1914. Thereafter, the extent to which war dominated the profession's attention for the duration of the First World War is evident in the number of papers appearing in *The Lancet* on war-related issues, including trench fever (1915), trench foot (*1915*), war heart (*1917*) and shell shock (*1915*) – although this last had also been discussed in the journal during the Boer War (*1900*).

The mental image of staff trying out a new stretcher in a corridor in *The Lancet*'s old premises in the Strand emerges in *1915*, and there is also a report of some good work on the value of salicylic acid in the treatment of war wounds (*1916*). One of the most memorable of these war-related contributions is the text of an address on the repression of war experience by WHR Rivers, of Craiglockhart War Hospital, a model of humane medical understanding (*1918*).

A number of the great names of medical history appear here, from Manson, Ross and Haffkine to Almroth Wright, Gorgas and Takaki. But an obscure name which deserves to be better known is that of JAB Hammond, who described an epidemic of a rapidly fatal 'purulent bronchitis' among British soldiers in France (*1917*). It was shown subsequently (also in *The Lancet*) that the virus involved in Hammond's epidemic was the same as that which caused the 1918–1919 influenza pandemic which followed the Great War, and is thought to have caused 50 million deaths worldwide. Hammond's work is now believed to have described a 'herald wave' outbreak in the pandemic's course, perhaps offering a clue to its derivation.* A parallel, and possibly related epidemic, was that of 'epidemic stupor' in children: a meningitis-like illness, followed by statue-like freezing, now known as encephalitis lethargica (*1918*).

1920s–1950s

The third great era of *The Lancet*'s work presented here stretches from 1920 to the close of the 1950s. This period spans the latter half of Squire Sprigge's long editorship, Egbert Morland's entire era and most of the 20 year period during which Theodore Fox was at the helm.

This was an eventful 40 years in historical terms: the inter-war years (including the Great Depression), the Second World War, followed by the inauguration of the UK National Health Service, and the establishment of the World Health Organisation. These two last events occurred so closely together that both were greeted on the same editorial page in *1948*.

In the pre-penicillin era, infection and measures to counter it were major preoccupations, represented by Ethel Cassie's excellent work on the prevention of puerperal sepsis (*1925*); and Collier's face mask for accoucheurs (*1931*) which shows that by the 1930s an understanding that normal throat organisms might kill women after childbirth was at last being taken on board. A memorable paper by Bourdillon (*1941*) demonstrated (with accompanying pictures made using the newly available flash-light photography) how a sneeze spreads germs.

This period also saw the successful use of curare in the treatment of the rigors of tetanus, from which patients at that time generally died (*1934*), hastening its modern use in anaesthesia. There was also solid work in fracture care using plaster of Paris (*1935*), practical improvements in hospital equipment (*1939*) and the innovative use of electro-encephalography to locate otherwise completely inaccessible brain tumours (*1936*).

Some major work on disease aetiology/diagnosis was accomplished in this period: for example, on asbestosis/mesothelioma by Wood and Gloyne (*1930*), on the causative organisms of psittacosis by Coles (*1930*), and Cicely Williams described the nutritional deficit disease Kwashiorkor in Ghana, where affected children had a 90% mortality (*1935*). Closer to home, Wilson argued forcefully for a safer milk supply – one which would not transmit tuberculosis, diphtheria or typhoid. He was addressing the UK situation, but similar concerns were active in the United States in the same period (*1933*).

In the 1930s, difficulties were encountered in trying to eradicate a somewhat larger organism: the scabies mite. The medical officer to a large public mental hospital contributed a clinical report (*1935*) describing his experience. The inadequacy of existing sulphur treatment obviously came as a surprise to him, and dealing with an infestation among institutionalised mental patients made his task no easier. His admirably controlled exasperation makes this paper a classic of its type.

Even doctors felt the pinch during the deep trade depression of the 1930s. A *Lancet* letter described the "gentle art of bilking the doctor" – avoiding payment for treatment given – revealing the realities of life for British doctors before the National Health Service ensured steady incomes (*1930*). During that difficult decade, *The Lancet* urged the government to assist poorer families, so as to help prevent deficiency diseases among mothers and their offspring (*1938*) in the UK, where rickets was not uncommon.

Also in *1938*, *The Lancet* published a courageous letter signed by 18 well known British doctors, in support of colleagues suffering victimisation by the Nazi regime in Austria.

Maternal death rates remained a serious concern despite the arrival of sulphonamide drugs (see *1936*, *1937*) which did not always counteract coccal infections. Alexander Fleming co-authored a *Lancet* paper in *1939* expressing alarm about the problem of toxicity and bacterial resistance to sulphonamide drugs, farsightedly recommending the idea of a combination of drugs to counteract the problem. *Staphylococcus aureus* was a dangerous organism then, as it is today. An excellent paper (*1939*) shows how it was dealt with in hospitals before the arrival of penicillin and its derivatives.

That same year, Murray visited London to describe his pioneering work on heparin (*1939*), which was picked up and developed after the war by Bauer (*1946*). Gibson's modest letter suggesting salicylic acid might be of value in coronary thrombosis appeared in *The Lancet* in *1948*.

Probably the most renowned medical milestone in this entire period was proof of the chemotherapeutic value of penicillin, accomplished by a team working in Oxford during the Battle of Britain, and published in *The Lancet* in August that year, *1940*. Ernst Chain and Howard Florey had revived Fleming's decade-old finding of the efficacy of penicillin as a bactericide, and proved its therapeutic value in laboratory experiments and tests on animal models (mice, rats and cats). Subsequent work on human patients (*Lancet* 16.8.1941: 177–189) was assisted by Peter Medawar, working close by with JZ Young during that crucial summer, on the regeneration of severed nerves using concentrated blood plasma as a matrix (*1940*).

At this time there are reports of the psychiatric effects of air raids on civilians (*1941*), of neurological work on mis-perceptions of the body and phantom limbs (*1942*), and an excellent summation of first aid burn treatment, by McIndoe (a plastic surgeon in an RAF burns unit) when incendiary bombs were a major preoccupation (*1941*). Bourdillon's work on sneezing (*1941*) mentions inhibiting germ spread in air raid shelters. But in general, the Second World War seems to have been less preoccupying to *The Lancet* than the First World War had been.

The war did, however, bring to the surface a matter which had been simmering for a long time, and which burst forth in 1946, with the Nuremberg trials of doctors implicated in Nazi atrocities. Typically, *The Lancet* faced the issue head-on in an editorial (*1946*) which provoked a considerable correspondence. There had nevertheless been moments when even *The Lancet* had published questionable research findings, as for example, when a team researching rheumatoid arthritis decided to try the therapeutic value of deliberately infecting a series of 'volunteers' with hepatitis (*1944*).

The Nuremberg debate may have been partially responsible for a sporadic series of introspective essays by different hands, represented here by Lord Platt and Richard Asher (*1947, 1951*).

An effective non-toxic medication for the tuberculosis bacillus, another formidable organism, emerged with the discovery by Lehman (*1946*) of 'PAS' (*para*-amino-salicylic acid). Administered in combination with streptomycin, PAS was subsequently proven effective in a therapeutic trial in *1949*, and it still remains of therapeutic value in tuberculosis. Of course, vaccination was preferable. Ascertaining a patient's immune status was a lengthy business until Heaf developed his multi-puncture test (*1951*) which significantly accelerated the process.

Polio and other inoculations assumed great importance in this era, too, particularly after a serious polio epidemic in Copenhagen (*1953*) and an MRC investigation confirming a curious associa-tion of polio paralysis with other inoculations (*1956*).

A turning point for general practice in the UK occurred in 1950, with the publication in *The Lancet* of *The Collings Report* – an unflattering analysis of the state of the general practice

standards of care and premises inherited by the National Health Service from the pre-existing private sector (*1950*).

Within the next decade, reforming general practitioners had begun to assert their worth, establishing their own College, and mounting research efforts such as that demonstrating the efficacy of pre-emptive screening in general practice for cervical cancer (*1958*).

An outspoken 'point of view' piece by Learoyd, entitled 'The Carnage on the Roads' put road traffic accidents firmly on the public health agenda (*1950*); while two fine articles appeared side-by-side in *1953*, confronting the health effects of the dire environmental pollution of London smogs.

Bradford Hill had tried before the war to enthuse colleagues with the value of the statistical approach (*1937*). Later, he endeavoured to confirm an Australian finding correlating birth defects and maternal rubella in pregnancy by undertaking a retrospective analysis of UK National Health Insurance records to trace affected women (*1949*), with qualified success. Statistics were becoming increasingly important in medical papers, and were also being more carefully scrutinised: witness, for example, Cochrane's analysis of observer error (*1951*), which led to the recognition of the need for controlling for bias in this respect.

An urgent preliminary publication in *1956*, from a team led by Alice Stewart, warned of an association between exposure to X-rays in utero and childhood cancer, based on a statistical analysis of exposure among children who had died of leukaemia or other malignancies. Fortunately, a landmark paper reporting the successful use of ultrasound scanning appeared shortly afterwards (*1958*).

This era also saw *Lancet* reports concerning the development of mechanical means to support failing human organs. The 'iron lung' was the earliest (*1931*) followed after the war by kidney dialysis (*1948*) and heart bypass (*1958*). The development of lens implants after cataract removal was described in *1952*.

The Lancet commented wisely in *1954* on the recently reported structure of DNA (the findings of Watson and Crick were originally published in *Nature*) and a series of key *Lancet* papers appeared later the same decade concerning chromosomal sex (*1955*), blood groups (*1956*), foetal blood groups (*1956*) and Down syndrome (*1959*).

1960s–2005

This is the final tranche of papers representing *The Lancet's* publishing history. This section has proved the most difficult to select, as it remains perhaps too soon to discern the full significance of many articles published in recent times. Admiration for editors' perspicuity rises accordingly!

The era since 1960 has seen six editors: Ian Douglas-Wilson took over from Theodore Fox in 1964, remaining in post for 12 years. Subsequently Ian Munro served as Editor for a similar period. His retirement in 1988 was followed by the briefest editorship in *The Lancet's* history (less than 2 years duration): that of Gordon Reeves. Robin Fox took over in 1990. His successor, Richard Horton, has been Editor of *The Lancet* since 1995.

Newly discovered disease aetiologies in this period are many, among which may be mentioned Farmers' Lung (*1963*), viral African lymphoma by Epstein and Barr (*1964*), the relationship of kuru and cannibalism (*1968*), isolation of the Ebola virus (*1977*), Hepatitis 'C' (*1978*), Kaposi's sarcoma and HIV (*1981, 1994*), the extraordinary discovery of Helicobacter (*1983*), New Variant CJD (*1996*), the coronavirus in severe acute respiratory syndrome (SARS) (*2003*) and the re-emergence of a fatal influenza virus (*2004*), the last two by the same remarkable team.

The Lancet has been host to a number of important papers on methicillin-resistant *Staphylococcus aureus* (MRSA) (*1968*), including its entire genetic profile (*2001*). Other important papers concern sickling in malaria (*1970*), chemotherapy for tuberculosis in East Africa (*1978*), the carriage of Creutzfeldt-Jakob disease in cadaver-derived growth hormone (*1985*), the effect of unemployment on mortality (*1984*), the relationship of sleeping position in infants and risk of Sudden Infant Death Syndrome (SIDS) (*1989*), the importance of listening to parents in the diagnosis of childhood cancers (*2001*) and analysis of risk factors for heart attack (*2004*). The effect of salicylates on human blood platelets was reported in *1968*, 20 years after Gibson raised its therapeutic possibilities in a letter to *The Lancet*.

Therapeutic drugs described in the pages of *The Lancet* include the first beta-blocker propranolol (*1964*), L-Dopa (*1969*), cyclosporin (*1978*) and the first successful anti-herpes drug, acyclovir (*1979*). *The Lancet* was the journal of choice for those urgently reporting iatrogenic associations, such as those of the contraceptive pill and near-fatal emboli (*1961*) and the mutagenic deformities caused by thalidomide (*1961*).

Antenatal screening developed apace in this era, through the analysis of human amniotic fluid cells extracted via amniocentesis (*1966*) and subsequently by maternal serum analysis (*1973, 1984*), allowing the development of genetic counselling in some hereditary conditions (*1979*).

A long awaited explanation for spina bifida was published in *1965*, although the association with folic acid took a generation to be accepted by some in the profession. Other key nutritional relationships elucidated in *The Lancet* include dietary roughage (*1969*), dietary fat (*1973*) and the life-saving importance of Vitamin A (*1986*). A startling finding – from a study of 26 years duration – of a dose-related negative health impact of television watching (*2004*) awaits confirmation.

The development of understanding concerning the complexities of human fertility resulted in the modest letter (*1978*) from Steptoe and Edwards which announced the momentous news of the first live birth of a child conceived by *in vitro* fertilisation. More recently, the development of techniques for the cryo-preservation and re-transplantation of human ovarian tissue has resulted in the birth of a live child, after its mother had undergone treatment for stage 4 Hodgkin's lymphoma (*2004*).

Persistent vegetative state (PVS) after brain damage was first defined and named in *1972*. Jennett, one of the authors of this paper, went on to co-create what became known as the 'Glasgow Coma Scale', designed to assess depth of coma and impaired consciousness, and which has had considerable practical long term impact on intensive care for the comatose patient since it was published in *The Lancet* in *1974*.

Significant improvements in imaging in this period are represented by reports of the development of fibre optics (*1961*) and nuclear magnetic resonance (*1981*).

Research in human biochemistry in this era revealed the existence of natural endorphins in spinal marrow and blood plasma (*1978*), and pioneering work on the natural mechanisms of the immune system (*1968*) paved the way for immune suppression (*1978*) crucial to the development of transplant surgery, such as the hand transplant reported in *2000*. Less complicated surgery for hip replacement devised by Charnley (*1961*), and for angina by balloon angioplasty developed by Grüntzig (*1978*), have remained beneficial ever since publication.

In the honourable tradition of Lister, Charnley also drew attention to the role of permeable surgical gowns in infection spread (*1969*). A more recent editorial in *The Lancet* on hand-washing (*1994*) made the controversial suggestion that patients might more effectively police hospital hygiene.

One of the most notable developments in this era has been the evolution of research trials and the increasingly sophisticated use of statistics to analyse and review results. Research tends increasingly to be conducted co-operatively by workers in different locations, and increasingly by teams of researchers with collective – rather than individual – names: so more multi-authored, multi-centred trials. Papers are on average longer, too. In some large trials and meta-analyses, lists of authors and of references alone stretch to several pages.

In useful counterbalance to this process has been the innovation of simple first page summaries, which (happily) has allowed the appearance here of the essence of more papers than would otherwise have been possible, including, among others, reports of trials concerning radical versus simple mastectomy (*1973*); the effects of a modified fat diet (*1973*); short course treatment for tuberculosis (*1978*); the GISSI trial of thrombolysis in heart attack (*1986*); the effect of vitamin A supplementation on child mortality (*1986*); breast cancer screening (*1990*); the SALT trial of aspirin and stroke (*1991*); the drug zidovudine in HIV (*1994*); the cholesterol-lowering drug simvastatin (*1994*); the UKPDS trial of diabetes control (*1998*); the effects of antioxidants (*2002*); the Magpie trial concerning the prevention of pre-eclampsia (*2002*); the Million Women study looking at the relationship of hormone replacement therapy (HRT) and breast cancer (*2003*); and recent trials of a much-awaited vaccine effective against malaria (*2004*).

In the midst of these trials, the Editors of both *The Lancet* and the *British Medical Journal* jointly wrote an editorial (*1999*) arguing that the time had come to register randomized controlled trials, both to obviate duplication and to prevent the misuse of trial results.

We are in the era of 'evidence-based medicine' and it is widely understood to be important that publication does not simply 'cherry-pick' positive results. The development of systematic reviews/meta-analyses of trial results can – by the amalgamation of results – reveal more than individual trials alone. One of the most powerful of such studies (*2004*) compared published and unpublished data concerning selective serotonin reuptake inhibitors (SSRIs) in childhood depression, and found that while the results showed that risks mostly outweighed benefits, materials so far published gave the opposite impression, indicating apparent benefit. In such a field as the medication of children, such findings give serious pause for thought.

The Lancet's ongoing interest in medical education is represented by a report concerning a medical school experiment in *1972*, in which medical students were led to expect sedative or stimulant effects from placebo capsules. Thirty percent experienced drug-associated changes. Despite its educational value, whether such an experiment would nowadays be considered ethical leads to consideration of the growing importance of medical ethics, represented here by several papers: one describing the human relations in obstetric care (*1960*); a key essay on the 'Inverse Care Law' which looks at the contrasting distributions of healthcare need and healthcare services (*1971*); a justifiably indignant editorial in the Wakley spirit concerns the routinised use of electro-convulsive treatment (ECT) on institutionalised mental patients (*1981*); and an analysis of a survey concerning what sort of people donate their bodies for dissection in medical schools, and their motivations for doing so (*1995*).

Historically, *The Lancet* has always been internationalist in character, and issues of global health well represented in its pages. This aspect of its coverage is shown here by three recent papers: the report of a field trial in a poor rural part of India, in which a simple intervention – the training of local birth attendants in neonatal care and hygiene – cut the number of neonatal deaths by 50% in the study region at a cost of only $5.3 per child (*1999*); an essay arguing for cheap insulin for the world's poorest countries, whose poorest inhabitants have none (*2000*); and an influential article asking 'Where and why are 10 million children dying every year?', and provides an answer by showing that of all worldwide deaths of children under 5, half occur in a handful of countries, blighted by disease overload and under-nutrition (*2003*). When I asked the current Editor, Richard Horton, which paper he was most proud of having published so far, this was the article he chose.

Envoi

Editorial meetings in *The Lancet*'s office at Jamestown Road, London, are lively affairs around an enormous table piled with manuscript folders. The room is lined with bookcases, heavy with old volumes of *The Lancet*. Wakley's portrait makes him a silent, somewhat quizzical presence among those who come to consider the latest manuscripts, along with editors' and external reviewers' comments, and to make decisions together. Discussions are sometimes straightforward, often intense, never dull, and invariably good humoured. Just as in Wakley's day, there can be gales of laughter.

Wakley would be surprised and pleased to see the journal today, for *The Lancet* remains true to the instincts of its founder, a uniquely free spirit in medical publishing. It draws its vitality from the continuity of spirit embodied in the current staff, and from the great medical endeavour beyond its walls.

The Lancet's historic voice, and the solid and historic accomplishment embodied in its many great volumes, nourishes the journal's work, and maintains its fundamental principles in more modern circumstances: the highest standards in medicine, science and public service; justice, honesty, liberty, independent thought, compassion and human dignity. ●

Notes

The Lancet's foundation: For the journals which sank without trace, see: Loudon J, Loudon I (1992) Medicine, politics and the medical periodical. In: Bynum WF, Lock S, Porter R (eds) *Medical Journals and Medical Knowledge*. London: Routledge, pp. 49–69; Hurwitz BS, Richardson R (2004) The Penny Lancet. *Lancet* 18/25.12.2004: 2224–2228. The testy comments of modern historians can be sampled in: Bynum WF, Lock S, Porter, R (eds) (1992) *Medical Journals and Medical Knowledge*. London: Routledge, pp. 2, 9, 33, 44, 45, 58–61. For *The Lancet*'s sibling status with the *New England Journal*, see Bostetter M (1985) The journalism of Thomas Wakley. In: Weiner, J (ed) *Innovators and Preachers: The role of the Editor in Victorian England*. Westport, Connecticut: Greenwood Press, pp. 275–292.

The Lancet's title: For the old correspondent, see *Lancet* 2.1.1892: 58–59; and for the favourite image, see Bostetter, mentioned above. For Billy Fretful and MZ see *Lancet* 5.10.1823: 36; 12.10.1823: 72.

Style and content: For *The Lancet* on the industry of the French see *Lancet* 1.5.1824: 138–152; and for its own aims, see *Lancet* 5.10.1823: 1–2; 4.1.1824: 1, 5; 22.1.1825: 82. The mediaeval guilds quote comes from Betty Bostetter, see above. The 'offended laws of physic' is a *Lancet* quote, see: 19.8.1826: 663–667. The analogy with *Private Eye* has also been made by the Loudons, see above. 'Dreaded and hated/encouraged, supported' derive from Clarke JF (1874) *Autobiographical Recollections of the Medical Profession*. London: Churchill. For the early correspondent with avid friends, see *Lancet* 26.2.1825: 249–250, and *The Lancet*'s pleasurable surprise at its own success, see *Lancet* 4.1.1824: 1.

High standards: For the passage about the Borough hospitals, see *Lancet* 30.11.1823: 311.

Exposing imposture: The journal's avowed object is described in *Lancet* 4.1.1824:1. The passage about the Colleges being bloated with wealth is from *Lancet* 22.1.1825: 82.

Audit: The humbug quote is from *Lancet* 1.5.1830: 179, as also is the passage concerning Magendie: 28.12.1823: 441–446; 3.7.1824: 1.

Fearless of prosecution: The views concerning the landmark Bransby Cooper case, see Richardson R (2000) *Death, Dissection and the Destitute*. Chicago: Chicago University Press, pp. 44–48; and Betty Bostetter mentioned above.

Opinion former: For Dickens at the inquest, see Richardson R (2001) Coroner Wakley: two remarkable eyewitness accounts. *Lancet* 22.12.2001: 2150–2154. For the Private White case, see Hopkins H (1977) *The Strange Death of Private White*. London: Weidenfield. For Andover, see Anstruther I (1973) *The Scandal of the Andover Workhouse*. London: Bles. The historian of British diet is John Burnett (1979) *Plenty and Want*. London: Scolar, pp. 240–255.

After Wakley: For *The Lancet*'s workhouse investigation, see Richardson R, Hurwitz BS (1997) Dr Joseph Rogers and the reform of workhouse medicine. *History Workshop Journal* 43: 218–225.

The Lancet's breadth: The investigators who realised that the same virus had been at work were: Abrahams, Hallows and French, *Lancet* 4.1.1919: 1–11. For the recent views concerning Hammond and the 1918–1919 influenza epidemic, see Oxford JS *et al.* (2005) A hypothesis: the conjunction of soldiers, gas, pigs, ducks, geese and horses in Northern France during the Great War provided the conditions for the emergence of the "Spanish" influenza pandemic of 1918–1919. *Vaccine* 23(7): 940–945.

1820s–1860s
From **WAKLEY** to
NIGHTINGALE

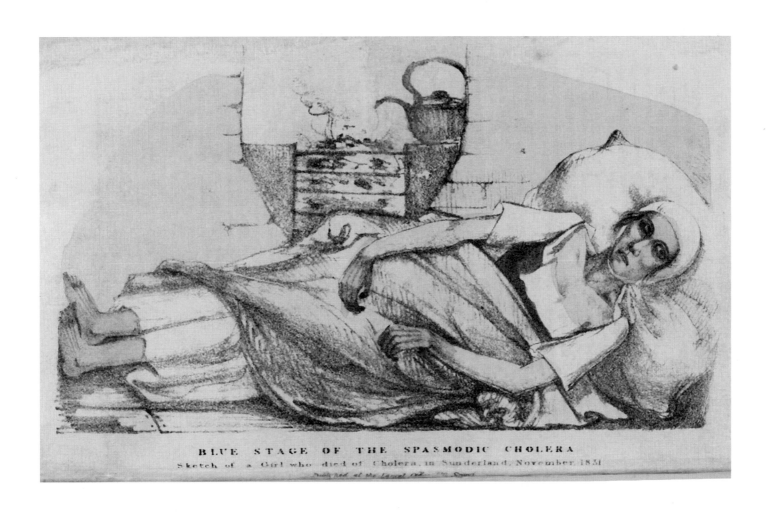

BLUE STAGE OF THE SPASMODIC CHOLERA
Sketch of a Girl who died of Cholera, in Sunderland, November 1831

1820s–1860s

1841   **West: On a peculiar form of infantile convulsions.**   65
13.2.1841: 724–725
Dr WJ West wrote to *The Lancet* to seek the assistance of his fellow doctors in the case of his own child's infantile spasms, a previously undescribed form of epilepsy, now known as West Syndrome. West records that in consultation concerning this case, Dr Charles Clarke had called the child's bobbing spasms 'salaam' convulsions. A poignant letter.

1844   **Liebig: Lectures on organic chemistry.**   67
6.7.1844: 463–465   (Extract: first two pages only)
Liebig was probably the biggest name in European scientific medicine at this time. *The Lancet* was delighted to have his lectures, translated swiftly and corrected by the man himself, for its new redesigned and more capacious format, launched in 1844. The lectures had already been trailed, with running headlines: "Liebig a contributor to *The Lancet*". The opening pages of this lecture provide a flavour of Liebig's teaching technique.

1846   **Conolly: Lectures on the construction and government of lunatic asylums.**   69
4.7.1846: 1–2   (Extract: first two pages only)
Conolly was a leading figure in the humane care of the mentally ill.

1846   **Military flogging, and its effects.**   71
15.8.1846: 172–179   (Extract: pages 176–179 only)
Private Frederick White's case was one of Wakley's flagship coroner cases. His death certificate said he had died of congestion of the heart. Exhumed, a new post mortem revealed that he had died from complications following a flogging. This was an influential case in the eventual cessation of flogging in the services. This extract covers the evidence of Erasmus Wilson and the jury's verdict.

1847   **Boott, Bigelow, Liston: Surgical operations performed during insensibility, produced by the inhalation of sulphuric ether.**   75
2.1.1847: 5–8
Hot news. First reports from America of the use of ether as an anaesthetic and a description of its first successful use in Britain, by Robert Liston himself. (Later communications gave credit for the discovery to Horace Wells of Connecticut; see *Lancet* 13.3.1847: 265–267.)

1847   **Bence Jones: Papers on chemical pathology.**   79
24.7.1847: 88–92   (Extract: pages 91–92 only)
Bence Jones was a life-long enthusiast for chemical understanding of the body. As a mature student he studied under a hospital apothecary, qualified as a doctor and then studied in Europe under Liebig. Florence Nightingale later called him "the best chemical doctor in London". A colleague had sent him a curious sample of a patient's urine, containing a material which behaved strangely on heating, with the question "what is it?". Bence Jones tested it and found it to be a protein. The urine was from a patient with the fatal disease multiple myeloma. The substance – 'Bence Jones protein' – remained a medical curiosity for over a century, when it was found to derive from a malignant change in the part of the bone marrow involved in the production of antibodies, now known as 'light-chains'. This is the text of a lecture in which Bence Jones first publicly described the phenomenon.

1847   **Simpson: On a new anaesthetic agent, more efficient than sulphuric ether.**   81
20.11.1847: 549–550
Chloroform announced by the doctor whose discovery it was.

1848   **Beecroft: Illustrations of the contagious nature of puerperal fever.**   83
24.6.1848: 684–685
Beecroft argued that there was no practical difference between contagion and infection, and that puerperal sepsis was a communicable disease. The work of Oliver Wendell Holmes and of Semmelweis were not yet known in Britain at this time. Maternal mortality was high. Beecroft's paper was a laudable attempt to alert doctors to treat the condition as contagious, and to their own possible carrier status.

1862   *The Lancet* **Analytical Sanitary Commission: Bread and its adulterations.**   102
15.2.1862: 182–183
A simple and devastating analysis of the adulteration of bread at this time.

1865   *The Lancet* **Sanitary Commission for investigating the state of the infirmaries of workhouses: Bermondsey.**   104
4.11.1865: 513–515
Exemplary behind-closed-doors investigative journalism. This was the eighth of a highly influential series of investigations which changed healthcare for the poor in Britain for the long term. Bermondsey was among the best of the establishments examined. This enquiry, which followed Florence Nightingale's work in the Crimea, effected the creation of thousands of new hospital beds and better nursing for the poor.

1865   **Brunton: A new otoscope or speculum auris.**   107
2.12.1865: 617–618
New technology. Scopes develop apace in the 19th century. This one, by John Brunton, was a good attempt to get light down the ear canal.

1866   **Dr Mary Walker.**   109
24.11.1866: 593–594
The famous American woman army doctor lectured in London, and according to this report, was greeted with boorish behaviour by male medical students. "We cannot say much for her lecture", reports *The Lancet* correspondent.

THE LANCET.

Vol. I.—No. 1.]   LONDON, SUNDAY, October 5, 1823.   [Price 6d.

PREFACE.

It has long been a subject of surprise and regret, that in this extensive and intelligent community there has not hitherto existed a work that would convey to the Public, and to distant Practitioners as well as to Students in Medicine and Surgery, reports of the Metropolitan Hospital Lectures.

Having for a considerable time past observed the great and increasing inquiries for such information, in a department of science so pre-eminently useful, we have been induced to offer to public notice a work calculated, as we conceive, to supply in the most ample manner, whatever is valuable in these important branches of knowledge ;—and as the Lectures of Sir Astley Cooper, on the theory and practice of Surgery, are probably the best of the kind delivered in Europe, we have commenced our undertaking with the introductory Address of that distinguished professor, given in the theatre of St. Thomas's Hospital on Wednesday evening last. The Course will be rendered complete in subsequent Numbers.

In addition to Lectures, we purpose giving under the head, Medical and Surgical Intelligence, a correct description of all the important Cases that may occur, whether in England or on any part of the civilized Continent.

Although it is not intended to give graphic representations with each Number, yet, we have made such arrangements with the most experienced surgical draughtsmen, as will enable us occasionally to do so, and in a manner, we trust, calculated to give universal satisfaction.

The great advantages derivable from information of this description, will, we hope, be sufficiently obvious to every one in the least degree conversant with medical knowledge ; any arguments, therefore, to prove

Printed and Published by A. Mead, 201, Strand, opposite St. Clement's Church.

2   THE LANCET.

these are unnecessary, and we content ourselves by merely showing in what directions their utility will be most active : To the Medical and Surgical Practitioners of this city, whose avocations prevent their personal attendance at the hospitals—To Country Practitioners, whose remoteness from the head quarters, as it were, of scientific knowledge, leaves them almost without the means of ascertaining its progress— To the numerous classes of Students, whether here or in distant universities—To Colonial Practitioners—And, finally, to every individual in these realms. Consequently, we shall exclude from our pages the semibarbarous phraseology of the Schools, and adopt as its substitute, plain English diction. In this attempt, we are well aware that we shall be assailed by much *interested* opposition. But, notwithstanding this, we will fearlessly discharge our duty. We hope the age of " *Mental Delusion* " has passed, and that mystery and concealment will no longer be encouraged. Indeed, we trust that mystery and ignorance will shortly be considered synonymous. Ceremonies, and signs, have now lost their charms; hieroglyphics, and gilded serpents, their power to deceive. But for these, it would have been impossible to imagine how it has happened that medical and dietetical knowledge, of all others the most calculated to benefit Man, should have been by him the most neglected. He studies with the greatest attention and assiduity the constitutions of his horses and his dogs, and learns all their peculiarities; whilst of the nature of his own he is wholly uninformed, and equally unskilled as regards his infant offspring. Yet, a little reflection and application would enable him to avert from himself and family half the constitutional disorders that afflict society ; and in addition to these advantages, his acquirements in Medical learning would furnish him with a test by which he could detect and expose the impositions of ignorant practitioners.

In conclusion—we respectfully observe, that our Columns will not be restricted to Medical intelligence, but on the contrary we shall be indefatigable in our exertions to render " THE LANCET " a complete Chronicle of current Literature.

THE COLLEGE CHARTER.   663

THE LANCET.

London, Saturday, August 19, 1826.

———

It will be recollected, that at a most numerous Meeting of the Members of the College of Surgeons, held at the Freemasons' Tavern in February last, a Committee was appointed to attain the objects expressed in the following resolution: "That THE CHARTER of the College, by conferring on the Council and Court of Examiners the unqualified and unconstitutional privilege of electing those who are to be their colleagues in office, has been the sole cause of the injuries and grievances detailed in the foregoing resolutions. *With a view of effectually preventing* a RECURRENCE of those numerous evils, and of rendering the Royal College of Surgeons in London a benefit to the public, and an honourable distinction to ALL its members, we further resolve, *That a Petition founded on the adopted Resolutions be immediately prepared and presented to the House of Commons,* praying for the appointment of a Committee to inquire into the abuses of the said College, with a view of ultimately obtaining from His Majesty a NEW CHARTER, which shall provide that the officers of the College be annually chosen by the Members, so that EACH MEMBER may have a voice in the election of those persons who are to regulate the proceedings of that College, in the prosperity of which he must feel a personal, as well as a national interest."

Six months have now elapsed since this Committee was appointed to prepare the above Petition, yet it has not been accomplished. A feeling of very general dissatisfaction pervades the profession, in consequence of the Petition not having been presented to the House of Commons during the last Session of Parliament. In this feeling we do not participate; on the contrary, we rejoice that this delay has occurred, although the circumstances which produced it are not calculated to give satisfaction. Had the Petition been presented to the Legislature in the last Session, there would not have been time for it to have undergone that investigation and discussion, which its nature so justly merits; and had a dissolution of Parliament occurred whilst the proceedings were pending, we must, before a new House of Commons, have commenced *de novo;* and we should therefore have gained nothing by our previous labours but expense.

We thought also that a reasonable delay might prove beneficial to our cause, by affording the Committee and the Members of the profession ample time to investigate the nature of the abuses which exist in the College, and the source whence they spring; we expected that the Committee would take every opportunity of communicating with the influential members of the college in our principal cities and towns, and that they would pursue those measures which were best calculated to insure a long list of signatures to the Petition. We shall not, however, state on the present occasion whether we are satisfied or dissatisfied with the general conduct of the Committee, as it will be matter for discussion at a future period. And indeed, we should not have noticed the subject in this day's Journal, had it not been for the report of the Meeting of the Trustees of the Hunterian Museum, which we insert in another page, and had we not been given to understand that another Meeting of the Committee is shortly to be held at the Freemason's Tavern. We are almost afraid that the Committee for some time past have been on the wrong scent; in fact, that they have altogether lost sight of the substance, and are in full chase after the shadow. Instead of sending a Petition to the Legislature, they forward their resolutions to the Trustees of the Hunterian Museum, in which they reproach the Curators, whilst in strict justice the reproach belongs to the Trustees themselves; they are the Governors of the Museum, and it is *their* duty to see that the public should derive from it that benefit which they have a right to expect from so valuable a collection. The Curators act merely under the directions of the Trustees, and neither the Counsel of the College nor the Court of Examiners, have, *ex-officio*, any control over the management of the Museum. As far then as the Museum is implicated, the Council of the College stands in a great measure exculpated, whilst the Trustees deserve a vast deal of censure for their extreme negligence, in not having rendered this unique Museum available to the purposes of surgical science.

Had the great body of the profession participated in the government of the College, the Trustees would not have been permitted for so long a time to have slumbered at their posts; they would have been made acquainted with their peculiar duties, and the manner in which these could be rendered beneficial to the country, would have been pointed out to them. They are men of high character; many of them are men of talent, and their minds only require to receive a proper direction to accomplish all that the science can deserve.

We will ask one question here, and which we should very much like to see answered; *who advised Government to purchase the Hunterian Collection,* WHILST THERE WAS NO CATALOGUE? There was a something in this transaction, either very *corrupt* or exceedingly *stupid*, and we will endeavour to become acquainted with its history.

We hope the gentle hints given above will be sufficient to convince our Committee, that they have not kept their eye steadily fixed upon the great engine of our injuries, and of our insults, and of the profession's degradation; (viz.) the CHARTER! and let them bear in mind, that every improvement they effect in the government of the College, will in an exact ratio weaken their cause when before the Legislature; let the College be taken into the House of Commons, surrounded by all its hideousness; let its unjust, tyrannous, and imbecile regulations remain in full force; let the whole of its corruption and its incapacity to do any thing for science, as at present constituted, be clearly illustrated in our Houses of Parliament; and then let the imbecility of its Governors, and their infamous measures, be traced to their detestable and detested CHARTER.

––––––––––

There are great changes contemplated amongst the Metropolitan Medical Teachers; "a Holy Alliance" is formed in *Windmill-street*, composed of the shattered and decaying materials of some of the Western Lecturers, and some of those reptiles, the "Hole and Corner gentry." Sir Astley is likely to increase his troops, and quite overwhelm poor Joe Green, notwithstanding his ill-gotten Museum; but our readers will be astonished when we tell them that JOHN ABERNETHY, notwithstanding all his former protestations of the incapacity, inability, and stupidity of men at his time of life, still clings to the loaves and fishes, and has expressed his determination to go on lecturing as long as he is able, i. e. as long as pupils will attend him, which we suspect will not be of very great duration, if the report be true that Mr. LAWRENCE is now determined to give a course of lectures on surgery, upon a scale much more extended than the *pure Surgeons* of this metropolis have hitherto been pleased to present to their pupils. But more of this hereafter.

DIRECTIONS FOR USING THE STETHOSCOPE.   667

sufficient to originate the rumour in question, setting aside the studied accuracy of the style in which the cases are written. But he did not write them, it seems; and however humble his pretensions may be, is desirous of letting the world know it, not wishing to " appropriate to himself the blunders of others,"—having enough of his own. He says he has no connexion with Dr. Macleod's Journal, that he has never read a page of it, that he has never reported cases, &c., and we suspect if he had told us what else he has *not* read, and what else he has *not* done, he would have used several quires of paper; at all events he may be assured that we *know* him, and that if we hear any more of his vagaries the public shall know him too.

AUTHOR GUTHRIE feels sorry that he should have been represented as saying any thing with a " modest air," and was so cut at the imputation of " *not writing English*," that he had determined to send to us forthwith for an explanation. He was restrained, by the interference of a cool good-natured friend. Perhaps Sir Anthony !

JEMMY COPLAND we understand relinquishes the office of Undertaker to the Mausoleum, and is to be succeeded by little BRODIE—a hopeful substitute.

We insert the letter of a Yorkshire Farrier precisely as it has been sent to us, because we happen to have enough of York in us to know who the writer is; we shall probably turn his production to account on some future day.

DIRECTIONS FOR THE USE OF THE STETHOSCOPE.

———

Almost seven years have now elapsed since LAENNEC proposed mediate auscultation as a mode of exploring the diseases of the thoracic viscera : a period sufficient in this busy age of investigation to try the merits of any hypothesis; and to outlive such a probation is almost enough to ensure permanent popularity. After various trials with materials of different density, a perforated cylinder of moderately light wood has been found the most convenient; and what may appear at first in opposition to an axiom in physics, in the present case the most accurate conductor of sound. To this cylinder the name *stethoscope* has been given; a name which very well expresses its principal use. The stethoscope merited, and has now obtained the patronage of the majority of scientific practitioners, and up to the present time has had the rare fortune of being without one decided public opponent. It is employed almost universally in France, and extensively in Germany, but as yet not so frequently in this country as it deserves; we are therefore glad to find that Sir JAMES MACGREGOR has recently ordered the army surgeons to use it generally, and to report the results of their investigations.

The appointment of LAENNEC to La Charité gave to him and to the numerous students who attend his clinic from all parts of Europe, more frequent opportunities of studying auscultation, than they could ever have hoped for at the Necker Hospital; and it is to this circumstance we are principally indebted for the improved shape in which the present edition of his work has appeared*. We regret to say that his health is in a very precarious state; he is obliged to leave the clinic to the superintendence of others, and is gone into Brittany, where he will pass the summer.

The first edition of Laennec's work has been translated into German, under the superintendence of Dr. FRORIEP, at Weimar, and into English by Dr. FORBES ; it has also found its way into the Italian and Russian languages. The last edition

———

* Traité de l'Auscultation Mediate et des Maladies des Poumons et du Cœur. 8vo. Paris, 1826.

of the valuable work of BERTIN*, edited by his friend Bouillaud, on the diseases of the heart and large vessels, and the clinical reports published by LERMINIER and ANDRAL,† contain many facts illustrative of the use of the stethoscope. Dr. FORBES,‡ also, in 1824, published a considerable number of cases observed at the Chichester Dispensary; but the greatest number of interesting facts has been collected by Dr. LOUIS of Paris, who during the past year has published a very respectable work on pulmonary consumption§. It is true that Andral has given a negative testimony against some of the signs said to be afforded by the stethoscope, but this is of no great weight, since Laennec had before admitted the existence of the same objections, under certain circumstances.

Many persons have inquired why Laennec has called it *mediate* auscultation; it is to distinguish it from *immediate* auscultation, or the direct application of the ear to the chest; a mode of examination with which the father of physic was so well acquainted, that he thought he could distinguish a serous from a purulent effusion in the thorax. " You will know by that," says he, " that the chest contains water and not pus, if by applying the ear for some time to the parietes, you hear a sound like to that of boiling vinegar."‖ It is singular enough that the passage never arrested the attention of physicians, so as to induce them to make any use of it; the commentators of Hippocrates passed over it as a matter of little consequence, and Laennec confesses that many years before the idea of mediate auscultation suggested itself, he had read the same passage without exciting any particular attention.

In the summer of 1816, Laennec was called to a young lady who presented the general symptoms of disease of the heart; the application of the hand to the chest, and percussion, afforded very little assistance, and immediate auscultation was interdicted by the sex and *embonpoint* of the patient. The recollection of the well known fact, that the tap of a pin at one end of a beam could be heard distinctly at the opposite end, induced him at the moment to avail himself of this acoustic phenomenon. He took a quire of paper, rolled it tightly together, applied one extremity over the region of the heart, and putting the ear to the other, was surprised to find that he could distinguish the pulsation of the heart in a more distinct manner than he could before do with the naked ear. Having hit upon the principle, he extended its application to the investigation of the various sounds produced in the chest by the respiration, the voice, and the accidental presence of fluids in the lungs, pleural sacs, and pericardium. He immediately commenced a series of observations at the Necker Hospital, which have afforded a large number of new and safe signs, easy to be understood for the most part, and calculated to make the diagnosis of almost all the diseases of the lungs, pleura, and heart, more circumstantial and certain than the surgical diagnostics established by the aid of the probe or the finger.

Many persons who are not able to avail themselves of Laennec's works, feel anxious to learn his late opinions on the subject of mediate auscultation; to such, the following abstract on the use of the stethoscope will prove an acceptable boon.

Shape of the Stethoscope.—Some alterations have been made in the shape of the stethoscope, of which the following are the principal: The diameter of the cylinder is sixteen lines, or one inch and a third English; of the tube which passes longitudinally through its centre, one quarter of an inch. The usual length of the cylinder is one foot, divided generally in the middle, but sometimes at different distances, by the contrivance known to mechanics, as the tenon, or tenet, and mortoise; the tenet is about one inch and a half long, rounded at its extremity, and made to fit tightly by passing a waxed thread around it. The two pieces are hollowed at one of their extremities to the depth of one inch and a half, the one to receive exactly the tenet just described,

---

* Traité des Maladies du Cœur et des gros vaisseaux redigé par Bouillaud. Paris, 1824. For an analysis of which, see THE LANCET, Vol. V. No. 7.

† Clinique Medicale, tome III. Paris, 1826.

‡ Treatise on Percussion; an extended analysis of this work, which contains also a translation of Avenbrugger's, will be found in THE LANCET, Vol. V. Nos. 4 and 5.

§ Recherches Anatomico-Pathologiques sur la Phthisie Pulmonaire, Paris, 1825.

‖ The passage is as follows:—Τούτω ἤν γνοίης, ὅτι οὐ πυον, ἀλλὰ ὕδωρ ἐςι. καὶ ἤν πόλλον χρόνον προσεχων τὸ οὐς ἀκουαζη προς τὰ πλευρα ξέει ἔσωθεν οἶον ψόφος. Hipp. de Morbis, II. Sect. 59, according to the text of Froben and Mercurialis; but Vanderlinden has ὄζει for ξέει; we know not upon what authority.

DIRECTIONS FOR USING THE STETHOSCOPE.   669

and the other to receive the *obturateur* or stopper of the same size and shape as the tenet, furnished with a brass tube passing through its centre, which extends about an inch into the tube of the adjoining piece. The extremity of the cylinder formed by the stopper, or obturateur, should be slightly concave, as it is less liable to slip when applied on the chest, and the skin, with a very slight degree of pressure, entirely fills up the space. The upper part of the tube, or that to be applied to the ear, is also slightly concave, and Laennec has lately used a plate of horn slightly concaved, of a larger diameter than the cylinder fitted on this end, for the purpose of adapting the ear more accurately, and thus shutting out external sounds. In the Charité, however, a rim of horn, fitted on the edge of the cylinder, of about a quarter of an inch in width, is more generally employed than the plate. The wood most frequently used is the walnut; some stethoscopes are made of cedar; in this country the ash or maple would be fit woods. Thus made, the cylinder is used without the stopper, for the exploration of the respiration and the rattles; and with it, when it is intended to examine the voice and the pulsations of the heart.

General remarks.—The cylinder should be held like a writing pen, and the hand should be placed near the chest of the patient, in order to be certain that the extremity is in direct apposition with it. When excessive emaciation has caused furrows between the ribs by the absorption of the pectoral muscles, the spaces may be filled up with lint or charpie, covered with a bit of linen. The interposition of the charpie between the instrument and the skin by no means impedes the transmission of sound.

The diagnostic signs afforded by mediate auscultation in diseases of the lungs and pleura, are derived from certain variations afforded by the respiratory murmur, the resounding of the voice and of the cough within the chest, as well as the rattle or *rhoncus*, a term which Laennec has lately substituted for *râle*, and some other accidental sounds which may be heard in that cavity. The stethoscopic signs of the diseases of the heart and large vessels, form altogether a particular class, and will therefore be mentioned separately.

The *general precautions* necessary to be observed in practising mediate oscultation are, 1st, to apply the stethoscope accurately and perpendicularly on the part to be examined, so that there may be no hiatus between the surfaces of the instrument and the chest. 2dly, Too great pressure must be avoided, particularly when the stopper is not employed, and when the chest of the patient is thinly covered. 3dly, It is not necessary that the chest should be entirely naked, all the positive stethoscopic signs, and often the negative, may be observed through thick garments, provided that they are accurately applied to the chest. It is, however, better if the chest be slightly covered, as for example with a flannel waistcoat, or a shirt. Silks and woollen stuffs are objectionable, on account of the crackling noise which is produced by their friction on the instrument. The person examining the patient ought to place himself in an easy and unrestrained position, without bending or extending the head; since the rush of blood to the head in such positions would impede the delicacy of hearing. The best position, if the patient be in bed, is to have one knee on the ground. To examine the anterior parts of the chest, the patient ought to be lying on the back, or seated, inclined slightly forwards; to examine the back the patient must stoop forward, the arms at the same time being firmly crossed; for the side it is sufficient to incline the body a little to the opposite side, and to allow the head to rest upon the hand.

Auscultation of the Respiration.—To examine the respiration, the cylinder must be used without the stopper, and the patient must make some inspirations of a moderate force and frequency, followed by equal expirations.

It happens sometimes that some persons whose lungs are very sound only afford a very weak, and sometimes almost no respiratory sound. Ordinarily the weakness of the respiratory noise is with them in direct ratio to the effort which they have made to respire. At other times, patients imagining that some extraordinary thing is required of them, try to dilate the chest with all their power, or they make several inspirations more and more strong, without expiring in the interval, and in these cases one scarcely ever hears any thing. In these and in all other cases where the respiratory noise is feeble, the patients must cough, the cough is succeeded by a full and deep inspiration, the air rushes into the lungs, and one is often surprised to find the air pass readily through lungs deemed from the first experiment almost impermeable. Or the same object may be accomplished by making the patient speak, read, or repeat several phrases in succession.

The noise caused by the respiration presents different characters in the pulmonary tissue and in the larynx, the trachea. and in the large bronchial trunks.

The Pulmonary Respiratory Sound.—If the stethoscope without the stopper be applied to the chest of a healthy man, a slight but extremely distinct murmur is heard, which denotes the entrance of the air into the pulmonary tissue, and its expulsion. This murmur may be most accurately compared to the noise made by a man in health, when during a sound but tranquil sleep, he from time to time takes a full and deep respiration. This pulmonary respiratory murmur is best distinguished on all those points of the chest where the lungs are nearest in contact with the parietes, namely, on the anterior superior, lateral and inferior posterior parietes. The armpits, the space between the clavicle and the superior edge of the trapezius muscle, are the points where it is heard with the most force. The sort of restraint and fear which the patient feels on the first examination, should deter any one from giving a decided opinion as to its results ; the examination should be repeated after the patient has been somewhat accustomed to the method, and then a judgment may be fairly given. No noise must be allowed in the chamber, in the ward, or among the bystanders, since it confuses a beginner; but after a time, when the ear has become habituated to the different sounds, this is not so important. Laennec has asserted over and over in his clinic, that he has tuned his ear so nicely to the study of minute sounds, that he can distinguish at the same moment the pulsations of the heart, the noise of the respiration, of the various rattles, of the borborygmi in the intestines, and a muscular noise made either by himself or the patient; and that although the students move about him and sometimes talk in a half voice, he is seldom obliged to demand silence.

The respiratory murmur is distinct in proportion to its rapidity ; a deep inspiration slowly made, is scarcely audible, whilst an incomplete inspiration scarcely sensible to the eye, made briskly, produces much more noise. Many causes may vary the intensity of the respiratory noise ; *age*, particularly. In infants the respiration is very sonorous and noisy, it can easily be heard through several thick garments. It is not only in intensity that the respiration of infants differs from that of adults : the nature of the sound itself is different; this, like all simple sensations, is difficult to describe, but is easily recognized by comparison. It appears as if in infants all the air cells dilated

themselves to their full extent, whilst in the adult they appear only to do so partially, or that their structure in the adult age does not allow of any equal proportionate extension. This difference is more marked in inspiration than in expiration. This characteristic respiratory sound continues from infancy, more or less, to puberty, and some adults retain this peculiarity to an extreme age. These are principally women or men of a nervous constitution, who present something of the mobility and especially of the irascibility of infancy. To this sound of the respiration in adults, the name of *puerile* is given. Some such persons have not, properly speaking, any real disease, but they pant after taking exercise, although thin ; and they take cold easily. Some others who present the puerile respiration, are affected with chronic catarrhs, with dyspnœa, and such a case constitutes one of the diseases to which the name asthma has been given. Whether this puerile respiration be the result of asthma, or of a certain hardening of the pulmonary tissue, is not yet decided, but on this point the following remark is made. It appears to me, says Laennec, quite certain that the constitution of the pulmonary organ, the most favourable for the preservation of health and long life, is that in which only a moderate expansion of the lungs is necessary, and the respiratory murmur less loud than in infants. That state ought therefore to be considered the natural and healthy state: *Id est maximè naturale, quod natura fieri optimè patitur.*

HOSPITAL REPORTS.

HOSPITAL OF SURGERY,

Panton Squar , St. James's.

STAPHYLOMA OF THE CORNEA.

A countryman, 50 years of age, had a violent attack of inflammation in his right eye, occasioned by the beard of a barley-corn getting within the eyelids, which terminated in a staphyloma of the cornea. The whole cornea is white and opaque, and projects so considerably, as to prevent the eyelids closing over it. As he suffered much inconvenience from this eye, Mr. Wardrop deemed it ex-

PUBLIC ANATOMICAL DEMONSTRATIONS.   349

LONDON MECHANICS' INSTITUTION.

——

We announced in a former Number, that Dr. Birkbeck had commenced a course of Lectures on Anatomy to the members of this Institution. Six lectures have been already given; in the first four the bones were considered, in the last two the muscles. The descriptions of the particular bones were very concise, but the different articulations were minutely pointed out, and their motions illustrated by reference to subjects with which all present were familiar, and which could not fail to make an impression on those who heard them. For instance, the Lecturer compared the lower jaw to a sledge striking upwards against a suspended anvil (the upper jaw,) and the action to that of a lever of the third kind, the prop being at one end, the weight at the other, and the power applied between them. Again, the nature of the articulation between the occiput and atlas, and atlas and dentata, was ingeniously explained; the Lecturer also availed himself of the illustration employed by Paley in his Natural Theology, to show the two distinct motions permitted in these parts. The first, that of nodding between the head and first vertebra. The next that of rotation between the first and second vertebræ. This author says, ",We see the same contrivance, and the same principle employed, in the frame or mounting of a telescope. It is occasionally requisite that the object end of the instrument be moved up and down, as well as horizontally or equatorially. For the vertical motion, there is a hinge upon which the telescope plays; for the horizontal or equatorial motion, an axis upon which the telescope and the hinge turn round together. And this is exactly the mechanism which is applied to the motion of the head." Dr. Birkbeck, however, showed the impropriety of Paley's comparison of the adaptation of the tooth-like process of the dentata into the atlas, with a tenon and mortice, observing, that had Paley worked at the bench, he would never have made so unmechanical a comparison. The Lecturer, in his description of the hip-joint, alluded to the very great difficulty with which the head of the thigh bone is removed from the acetabulum, after the ligaments have been divided; this, Dr. Birkbeck stated, was owing to the attraction of cohesion, which in this part of the body is very great; a circumstance that has been overlooked by most anatomists. The simple fact may be easily shown, by putting the flat surfaces of two bodies well lubricated in contact with each other, when it will be found that their separation cannot be easily effected. In speaking of the origin of the ligamentum teres, the lecturer gave it different from the mode in which it is usually said to arise; even Sir A. Cooper, in his work on Fractures and Dislocations, describes this ligament as arising from the upper and inner part of the acetabulum. Dr. Birkbeck, however, described it as being triangular, the base of which is bifurcated, and attached on each side of the notch at the lower and inner part of the acetabulum to the cotyloid ligament. In short, the bones, and particularly those parts relating to the mechanism of the joints, were well described, and the audience, which has been always crowded, appeared to take great interest in the whole of the lectures.

In the two last the muscles were described from the human subject. This was to us one of the most gratifying scenes we ever witnessed; the introduction of the human subject before so numerous and mixed an audience without the slightest mark of disapprobation, nay, with every appearance of satisfaction, is a striking proof of the good sense of the members of this institution. The benefit resulting from an exhibition of this nature, does not consist so much in the information communicated, as the feeling and taste which it engenders. Human dissection, which is so indispensably necessary to the successful cultivation of medical science, has received in this country such determined opposition, that until the public feel the importance of anatomy, and see with what little violation of feeling it may be cultivated, very few of the difficulties which now retard its prosecution will be removed. The profession, which from its superior knowledge of the value of anatomy, should have spared no exertions in attempting to remove the difficulties which impeded its cultivation, has remained, if not an indifferent, yet a silent observer of all, and takes no means to effect a change. The legislature has shown but little disposition to advance the study of anatomy, its great object having always been to pass enactments, only characterised by the severity of the punishment destined for those concerned in the exhumation of the dead. In this state of things, the only chance of amelioration which we possess, is by the diffusion of information among the public; by teaching them the value of dissections, and preparing their minds for the introduction of those measures, by which the difficulties attending the cultivation of anatomy in this country would soon be removed. To the mechanics of London much credit is due for the example they have set, an example which ought to be followed by similar bodies throughout the country.

The muscles were well shown, and could be seen at a remote part of the theatre; the arrangement of the tendon of the hand and foot was very much admired, and the audience on both nights, appeared much entertained by the exhibition.

DR. BADHAM.

To the Editor of THE LANCET,

SIR,—In reply to your inquiries about Dr. Badham, and his competency to fill the chair in the University of Glasgow, to which he is, I believe, appointed, I have no hesitation in assuring you, that he is *highly* qualified for it; and I am much surprised that you should have been unable to procure any information respecting him.

Dr. Badham has published a most excellent Treatise on Bronchitis; is the author of a beautiful and correct translation of Juvenal, which may be classed with Pope's Homer, and Dryden's Virgil. He has lately also written a most classical little poem on Warwick Castle, and has evinced himself a scientific physician, an elegant scholar, and a man of very extensive literary attainments.

The University of Glasgow will in short have reason to be proud of its Professor.

I am, Sir,
Your most obedient,
J. C. B.

June 9, 1827.

We have the best authority for stating, that the information contained in this letter is correct.—*Ed. L.*

HOSPITAL REPORTS.

HOSPITAL OF SURGERY,

Panton Square, St. James's.

CONGENITAL DIVISION OF THE PALATE.

E. M., æt. 21. Her soft palate is divided vertically into two symmetrical portions, the cleft extends completely through the soft parts, but the bones are entire. The uvula is likewise split into two parts, which are situated on each side of the fauces.

The edges of the palate are separated from one another to a considerable distance, particularly in their posterior aspect.

The power of articulating the guttural sounds is almost entirely lost: she has however, command over those formed by the lips. During deglutition, fluids occasionally pass into the nares. The disease was congenital. It is remarkable that this girl, who is passionately fond of music, is able to sing with considerable execution.

Operation.

Mr. Wardrop, availing himself of Mr. Alcock's experience in this operation, requested his assistance. Three broad ligatures were first introduced through the soft palate, about a quarter of an inch from its edges, and at regular distances; this part of the operation was readily accomplished by means of Mott's needle. Mr. Alcock cut off the callous edges, with a pair of common curved eye scissors. The edges were then brought into contact, except at the upper portion of the cleft, where they could not be made to meet. A considerable degree of inflammation supervened, followed by bleeding from the edges of the wound, but no adhesion took place.

ABSCESS OF THE LIVER.

J. S., ætat. 57, residing at Harrow Weal, presented himself at the Hospital about six weeks ago, with a globular tumour, the size of the fœtal head, extending in the course of the linea alba, from the ensiform cartilage, nearly to the umbilicus. The swelling was soft and elastic, and afforded a distinct, though deeply seated sense of fluctuation. There was little pain on pressure, and the integuments were not discoloured. He experienced a constant uneasiness in the loins and right shoulder, with occasional rigors. His stools were white, and his skin and conjunctiva of a yellow tinge.

Six weeks after an attack of jaundice, followed by symptoms of acute inflammation of the liver, he noticed the swelling, which had rapidly increased. Mr. Wardrop stated, that he had no doubt the tumour was an abscess formed in, or connected with, the liver. In these affections, he observed, it is much better to avoid making any opening with the view of discharging the purulent matter, for he was sure he had seen many bad consequences arise from puncturing swellings of a similar nature. He accordingly directed the following treatment:—

℞ *Hydrarg. submur.* gr. i., to be taken every night; and,

℞ *Pil. rhei comp.* ii., every morning.

OPTIC NERVES.—AMAUROSIS.   103

FOREIGN DEPARTMENT.

MAY VISION BE PRESERVED, NOTWITH-
STANDING THE DESTRUCTION OF THE
OPTIC NERVES?

BY M. MAGENDIE.[*]

WE have given an account in this Journal
of an experiment which clearly shows, that
the fifth pair of nerves is the principal organ of the general sensibility of the head,
that it is positively the agent of smell, and
that the senses of vision and hearing are dependent on it for a peculiar kind of influence,
their special sensibility. Hence, when the
fifth pair is divided on both sides, the animal loses its sight, notwithstanding that the
iris is still acted on by the sudden admission of light. But, although analogy might
lead us to suppose, that the fifth pair could
even temporarily supply the action of the
optic nerve, some facts have recently come
under our own observation, which set the
matter beyond doubt.

AMAUROSIS; DEVELOPMENT OF A CYST BE-
HIND THE COMMISSURE OF THE OPTIC
NERVE.

On the admission of the patient into the
Hôtel Dieu, the pupils were very much
dilated; the right possessed slight motion,
the left none. The power of the left eye
was completely destroyed, but the right retained the power of vision in a slight degree.
It was about eighteen months that the patient, whose business was that of writing,
had been obliged to give up his occupation,
on account of violent pains in the head and
gradual loss of sight. The usual means were
resorted to, but without any relief, and the
patient one day expired suddenly; a few
days, however, before his death, he could
see objects distinctly.

Inspectio cadaveris.—Between the decussation of the optic nerve, and the pons varolii,
in fact within the circle of Willis, there was
a cyst of the size of a hen's egg, partly
fibrous, and partly osseous in its structure,
which corresponded to the tractus opticus.
The cyst was filled with a yellowish matter,
mixed with blood. Laterally and superiorly
the cyst corresponded to the optic nerves,
which it had flattened and nearly destroyed.
The remains of the nerves adhered internally to the cyst, by the cerebral matter,
and anteriorly were lost in a white spot on
the osseous part, which corresponded to the
commissure. Still nearer to the optic foramina, the nerves were found in a state of

[*] Journal de Physiologie, Jan. 1828.

atrophy. There was no trace of the pituitary gland. The retina was thin, red, and
nearly transparent.

There are some points worthy of attention in this case; the patient could see
objects distinctly a few days before death,
and there was nearly complete interruption
of the optic nerve from the brain to the
eye. The optic nerves were also in a state
of atrophy anterior to the cyst, and the retina
was thin and transparent, appearances which
are only observed in individuals who have
been blind for many years, and in whom
the optic nerves have not suffered any diminution of size, or any apparent alteration in
their central medullary part. The same
phenomena may be observed in mammalia
who have become blind, and in whom there
is no apparent alteration of the optic nerve.
In birds, on the contrary, loss of sight is
followed in fifteen days by atrophy of the
optic nerve. If we admit, therefore, as
true, the preceding account, it is scarcely
possible to attach in that the exercise of
vision to the retina, since, on neither side,
was it in a fit state to act. We must,
therefore, have recourse to the fifth pair, to
understand how the impression of light was
transmitted to the brain. I am aware that
this conjecture may appear strange to most
of my readers, who have been accustomed
to regard the optic nerve as essential to
vision as the heart is to the circulation.
I must, however, state, that my experiments
(Journal de Phys., vol. iv.) on the optic
nerves were not favourable to this opinion,
for if a nerve be divided in the cranium,
anterior to its decussation, the eye of the
same side does not act. And, lastly, if the
point of decussation itself be divided on the
median line, the animal becomes completely
blind. From these experiments, then, it is
evident that the optic nerve is indispensable to vision, but then here the lesion of
the nerve is sudden, whilst in the case related, its alteration was slow.

CASE.—A woman, seventy years of age,
who had died of some complaint unconnect-
ed with the nervous system, was brought
into the theatre at Salpetriere to be examined. For a long time she had been
blind on the right eye, and the lens of this
side had been opaque; she had been able
to see on the left side. The right optic
nerve was of the usual size; that on the
other side was much smaller, thin, and in
a state of atrophy. This alteration was so
distinct, that those who were present imagined that the person must have been blind
on the right eye.

We do not see how either of the above
cases goes to prove that the power of vision
is not dependent on the optic nerves; in the

first case, the optic nerves were not completely destroyed; and, in the second, although vision was more perfect on the side where the optic nerve was affected than on the other where it was not, still there was a very apparent cause in the right eye, perfectly independent of the nerve, viz., opacity of the lens. M. Magendie regrets that he was not present himself at the examination of the last case.

A CASE OF SUFFOCATION PRODUCED BY THE PRESENCE OF A LEECH IN THE LARYNX.

BY DR. LACRETELLE.*

A soldier suddenly felt a sense of suffocation, and the surgeon of the regiment was sent for in great haste. The fact was, that passing through a country during great heat, the men drank, without the least precaution, in most of the streams, or even pools, which they met with. We found our patient with a red and swollen face; his mouth frothy, his eyes turned up, and his breathing almost entirely suspended. After this paroxysm, he came to his senses; he soon fell, however, into the same state. No symptom of apoplexy was present; his breathing only appeared embarrassed, and the obstacle which opposed the entrance and exit of air, appeared to us the sole cause of all these symptoms. On attemping to answer any questions, a fresh paroxysm came on, and he was compelled to desist. The introduction of a foreign body into the trachea, appeared to us as the probable cause of his sufferings, hence we decided on performing laryngotomy. Whilst we were making preparations for this operation, our patient breathed his last.

On opening the body, we discovered a leech in the right ventricle of the larynx; it was only with great trouble, that we detached it from its situation. Its body, rather large, obstructed the glottis, and rendered the entrance of air, by this opening, almost impossible.

OPENING OF THE FORAMEN OVALE, WITH GENERAL CONTRACTION OF THE AORTA AND ARTERIES, WITHOUT CYANOSIS.

BY M. MIGUEL.†

This case tends to prove, that the blue disease does not depend on the communication of the right with the left cavities of the heart, and confirms what MM. Fougier, Breschet, Marc, &c., have published on this subject. This is a case of a man thirty-six years of age, who entered the Hospital of Charité in 1826, under the care of M. Cayol, for difficulty of breathing, and continual sense of suffocation. His countenance was of a bluish colour; great pain in the heart and head, accompanied with strong beatings of the heart and arteries, which lasted for about a minute; he then became pale, and fainted. He experienced much less pain after blood-letting; and he asserted that, in six years, more than six thousand leeches had been applied, and that he had been bled about seventy-one, or two times. This disease terminated in dropsy. There was a dull sound in the region of the heart; the pulse small, unequal, intermittent, which was a contrast with the great violence of the heart's pulsation; the extremities were cold; breathing was short, laborious, but there was no violet or blue colour in the lips, cheeks, or any other part of the body.

From these symptoms, Mr. Cayol thought that there was *considerable hypertrophy of the left ventricle, with contraction of the orifice of the aorta, by a commencement of ossification of the sygmoid valves.* After remaining in the hospital fifteen days, the man died in a state of suffocation. On opening the body, the heart was found to be of twice its natural size; the parietes of the left ventricle and the auricles, were doubled in thickness and capacity; the two auricles communicated together by an opening of the size of half a crown, thin, and rounded; this was evidently the foramen ovale, not obliterated. The pulmonary veins were dilated; the aorta, and all the arteries of the body were, on the contrary, of smaller size than usual.

CASE OF HEMATEMESIS OCCASIONED BY A LEECH IN THE STOMACH.*

BY M. VANDERBACH.

A soldier, after having experienced for fifteen days pain in the stomach, accompanied with vomiting of blood, *felt something* which ascended along the œsophagus, and which attached itself to the left side of the pharynx, producing a tumour which impeded deglutition and respiration. The vomiting ceased a little; but the patient continually expectorated, and his expectorations were mixed, both with black and red blood: two days after, when the patient was lying down, he was awakened by a sense of pain in the pharynx, as well as in the back of the fauces; he introduced his hands to this spot and drew out a leech, which was alive. The patient stated, that he had drank several times from streams, but he had never observed any foreign body in the water. From this time the symptoms all disappeared.

---

* Gazette de Santé, 25 Fevrier, 1823.
† Revue Medicale

* Journ. Univ.

THE EDINBURGH MURDERS.   433

THE LANCET.

London, Saturday, January 3, 1829.

———

WE approach with horror the subject which has lately occupied the High Court of Justiciary at Edinburgh. It was most truly said, by Lord MEADOWBANK, that in the history of civilised society there was nothing parallel in atrocity to the crime of which one of the wretches, who has trafficked in the bodies of his murdered victims, has just been found guilty. The crime, or rather series of crimes, which the late trial has brought to light, indicates, no doubt, the existence of a state of deep-rooted moral disease among the lower orders of the population in Edinburgh; but we shall not occupy the time of our readers by speculating on the dreadful traffic, which has been carried on in the Scottish capital, as a symptom of moral disease. What we shall mainly insist upon is the necessity of putting an end, at once, to this horrid trade between the murderer and the anatomist. The perpetration of such crimes is a stain upon human nature, but the repetition of them may be effectually prevented. It is fearful and humiliating to reflect on the enormities of which wretches wearing the human form are capable; but the murder of men for the sake of obtaining the price of their dead bodies, is a crime which the Government may at once prevent. The remedy is in the hands of the Government, and that remedy it is the bounden duty of the Government to apply. The crime may not be confined to Scotland. Murderers, like Burke, may be, and probably are, at our own doors. While the temptation to commit the crime is suffered to remain, no man can say, with certainty, that it may not be his own fate, or the fate of his children, or kindred, to be marked out as victims for the dissecting table, and to perish beneath the poignard, or the gripe of an assassin,

No. 279.

eager to receive the price of his victim's corpse from the hands of the anatomist. Our first proposition, therefore, is, that it is the bounden duty of the Executive Government to see that all THE DISSECTING ROOMS IN THE KINGDOM BE FORTHWITH CLOSED.

The immediate closure of all dissecting-rooms is the only measure which will effectually prevent the repetition of the crime, by removing all temptation to the perpetration of it. The injury to medical science, the inconvenience to medical teachers, the interruption of anatomical studies, are all utterly insignificant considerations, compared with the overwhelming necessity of protecting the public against assassins, who traffic in the dead bodies of their victims. It is evident that some measure must be adopted by the Legislature, without delay, for the supply of our anatomical schools with subjects; but, until such a measure shall be adopted, it is of paramount importance that the traffic between the murderer and the anatomist shall, at all events, be put an end to. Let it not be hastily supposed that we are raising an alarm not justified by the circumstances under which bodies are furnished to the anatomical schools in this country, or that we are suggesting a remedy against a contingency which is not likely to happen. No man, who reads attentively the evidence given before the Parliamentary Committee on anatomy, can say, that murders similar to those brought to light at Edinburgh are not likely to be committed in this country. No man, who weighs that evidence attentively, can feel assured that such murders have not already been committed in this metropolis. It was proved before that Committee, both by the testimony of surgeons, and by that of individuals who had themselves supplied the schools of anatomy with subjects for dissection, that the resurrection-men belonged to the lowest dregs of society, that they were, for the most part, thieves, house-breakers, men of the most abandoned

2 F

434   THE EDINBURGH MURDERS.

character, and capable of committing the most atrocious crimes. Sir ASTLEY COOPER, upon being questioned as to the character of the resurrection-men, stated, that he considered them " the lowest dregs of degradation. I do not know," says the worthy Baronet, " that I can describe them better; there is no crime they would not commit; and, as to myself, if they would imagine that I should make a good subject, they really would not have the smallest scruple, if they could do the thing undiscovered, to make a subject of me!" (*Minutes of Evidence taken before the Committee of Anatomy*, p. 18.)—The flippancy and bad taste of this answer may have deprived it of the weight which is really due to it; but the recent dreadful disclosures have demonstrated that the worthy Baronet's opinion of the resurrection-men is too well-founded. In another part of his evidence, Sir ASTLEY COOPER states that there is no person, however exalted his rank, whose body, if he (Sir ASTLEY) were disposed to dissect it, he could not obtain. The worthy Baronet is probably ignorant of the state of the law on this subject; but the appalling transactions at Edinburgh prove that he was too well founded in his fact, and that he made no miscalculation as to the desperate resolution of the class of men engaged in supplying the anatomical schools with subjects for dissection. The following is the part of Sir ASTLEY COOPER's evidence to which we allude :—

" Does the state of the law actually prevent the teachers of anatomy from obtaining the body of any person which, in consequence of some peculiarity of structure, they may be particularly desirous of procuring ?—The law does not prevent our obtaining the body of an individual, if we think proper; FOR THERE IS NO PERSON, LET HIS SITUATION IN LIFE BE WHAT IT MAY, WHOM, IF I WERE DISPOSED TO DISSECT, I COULD NOT OBTAIN."—*Minutes of Evidence before the Committee on Anatomy,* p. 18.

We observed, in commenting on this part of Sir ASTLEY COOPER's testimony, (THE LANCET, No. 262, p. 727,) that this extraordinary declaration was well calculated to produce an effect on the fears of persons to whose understanding reason could find no access; and that the worthy Baronet had, with his wonted felicity of diction, made his threat of dissection apply rather to the LIVING than to the dead; little anticipating,—as indeed the worthy Baronet could have little anticipated,—the possibility of such a declaration admitting of a literal interpretation. It is our firm conviction, that, unless the executive government take immediate steps for putting a stop to all dissection, until the legislature shall have placed the supply of the schools of anatomy under due regulations, no man in the country is completely secure from the knives of the assassin and the anatomist. The present price of a corpse offers a stronger temptation to desperate and reckless villains than that for which they are in the constant habit of risking their lives; and the ready mart for their victims renders the chance of impunity after the commission of murder with a view to the sale of the corpse, greater than after the commission of any other crime. The burglar is never sure of obtaining as much as the value of ten or twelve pounds in the house into which he breaks; he encounters the risk of losing his life in the commission, or on conviction of the offence; and he commonly goes prepared to destroy life in case of resistance. Is it likely that such a man would be much moved by the consideration of the greater or less enormity of a crime, or that he would hesitate to commit a murder at once, if he could not only secure a profit upon his crime, but be nearly certain of escaping with impunity? It is from the calculation of the chances of escape in the event of conviction that robbery is now seldom combined with acts of violence to the person; but if thieves and burglars perceive that there is a mode of committing murders

SUBJECTS FOR DISSECTION. 435

with a sure profit and small chance of detection, what security does the conscientiousness of these abandoned characters afford to the public against the frequency of such murders? And who shall say that such murders have not been already committed? In the present state of the law, surgeons have no means of ascertaining,—they cannot even inquire, without risk, into the mode whereby the persons whose bodies are brought to the dissecting-rooms have come by their death. It is the state of the law, and not the medical profession, that is to be blamed for all the evils which have been produced by the existing system. The traffic between the teacher of anatomy and the vendor of dead bodies is an illegal and, therefore, a secret traffic, excluding from its nature the means of investigating the circumstances under which the subjects sold for dissection have been obtained. We have ourselves, within a recent period, seen bodies brought into dissecting-rooms in this metropolis, exhibiting none of the appearances usually found in the bodies of persons who had died from disease, but with all the indications presented by the bodies of men who had died within a few hours, and in a state of PERFECT HEALTH. One *head* in particular—subjects are now frequently sold piecemeal—attracted our attention, and that of other gentlemen present. It was the head of a perfectly *fresh* subject; not the slightest indication of disease could be traced; it was, apparently, the head of a man who had lived in health and vigour within a few hours. We could not learn whence it was brought, nor how the man (from whose trunk it had been severed) had come by his death. He might possibly have expired suddenly from natural causes; he might have destroyed his own life; but the late horrible disclosures prove that he might also have been slaughtered for the price of his corpse. Again we say that, until the legislature shall provide the means of supplying our anatomical schools with subjects from an unexceptionable source, there is but

one way to prevent the possibility of a repetition of such atrocities as those which have been detected at Edinburgh, and that is, by causing every dissecting-room in the kingdom to be closed. Such a measure cannot fail, under the circumstances, to be cheerfully acquiesced in by teachers and students themselves; and there will be the less difficulty in carrying it into effect, since, as the law stands at present, all dissection, except that of criminals executed for murder, and except such partial dissections or *post-mortem* examinations as may be assented to by the friends of deceased persons, is, in effect, illegal. According to the decision of Baron HULLOCK, a surgeon, or other person, having a body in his possession for the purpose of dissection, except under the circumstances above excepted, is liable to be tried and punished for a misdemeanour. The executive government, therefore, in order to suppress a nefarious traffic during the interval between the detection of the crimes to which it has led, and the period at which the legislature can interpose, has only to take measures for effectually preventing a practice which, though hitherto connived at from the supposed necessity of the case, has been declared to be illegal.

The readers of this Journal must be too sensible of the zeal which we have ever shown for the advancement of anatomical science to suppose, that the foregoing observations have been dictated by a diminished sense, on our part, of the necessity of affording due facilities to the study of anatomy. We were among the first to point out the impolicy of the existing laws regarding dissection, and to suggest the means of affording an ample supply of subjects to our schools of anatomy from an unexceptionable source. Week after week, while the Select Committee of the House of Commons was sitting, we discussed this subject in all its bearings, and we had the satisfaction of seeing most of our arguments and suggestions repeated by the witnesses, and

2 F 2

embodied in the recommendations of the Committee, as published in the Parliamentary Report. The first measure which we suggested, as an indispensable preliminary to any effectual legislative provision for the supply of our anatomical schools, was the repeal of the enactment (25 Geo. II,) which subjects the bodies of persons executed for the crime of murder to dissection—an enactment which, by associating the idea of dissection with that of punishment for crime, has created, in this country, an artificial prejudice against dissection, perfectly distinct from that natural aversion with which we all regard it, as applied to the bodies of those whom, when living, we have esteemed and loved. In this recommendation, nearly all the witnesses examined before the Parliamentary Committee concurred, and it has been adopted by the Committee in their Report. We recommended the application of the bodies of *unclaimed* persons to the purposes of dissection, as an unexceptionable source for the supply of our anatomical schools, since it would meet the demand of science without violating the feelings of surviving relatives and friends, against which feelings it would be as unavailing as it would be impolitic to attempt to legislate, and since it would effectually put an end to the disgusting offence of body-snatching. We also suggested, that all the bodies of unclaimed persons should, after they had undergone dissection, be interred at the expense of the parties, for whose benefit they had been dissected; and that the offence of body-stealing should be made a felony, punishable with not less than fourteen years' transportation. We would now further suggest the expediency of appointing an officer, or officers, whose functions might be similar to those of the *chef des travaux anatomiques* at Paris, and under whose authority alone the bodies of unclaimed persons might be distributed to the anatomical schools. Neither should a body, otherwise obtained, be dissected, unless a Coroner's Inquest had been previously held upon it, and the probable cause of death duly certified. And, as a further precautionary measure, we would recommend that the *possession* of a body for the purpose of dissection, not obtained through the regular officer, should be made a misdemeanour, punishable with not less than FOURTEEN YEARS TRANSPORTATION. This would effectually rid society of resurrectionists and trading assassins; for let it be recollected, that if there were no receivers, there would be no thieves, and, in this case, no murderers.

The view taken of this question by the Select Committee on Anatomy, of which the Home Secretary was a member, is so sound and enlightened, that we look forward with confidence to the result of a parliamentary discussion. In the meantime, we cannot help regretting that some writers, who appear to have given less of their attention to this subject than to most of the topics to which they apply their powerful minds, should have given currency to propositions wholly at variance with the views of the Committee, and incompatible with the measures recommended by that body to the adoption of the Legislature. Among some recent suggestions, the proposal to make dissection a punishment for the offence of suicide, is one of the most objectionable, because it is neither more nor less than a proposal to sanction and perpetuate an absurdity, which, in the opinion of nearly all the witnesses examined before the Committee, is the very cause of the evil to be provided against, namely, the absurdity of identifying dissection with punishment, and associating it with crime. The following passage appeared this week, in a leading article of *The Times*:—

" But the thing which is of most consequence, is to devise some legal method of supplying the medical profession with subjects for *examination* (as *The Scotsman* newspaper properly terms it) by legal means. We have before recommended, that all persons who destroy themselves should, by the Coroner's warrant, be consigned to the sur-

THE LANCET.

Vol. II.]   LONDON, SATURDAY, JUNE 13.   [1828-9.

OBSERVATIONS

ON

TRANSFUSION OF BLOOD.

By Dr. Blundell.

With a Description of his Gravitator.*

States of the body really requiring the infusion of blood into the veins are probably rare; yet we sometimes meet with cases in which the patient must die unless such operation can be performed; and still more frequently with cases which seem to require a supply of blood, in order to prevent the ill health which usually arises from large losses of the vital fluid, even when they do not prove fatal.

---

* The instrument is manufactured by Messrs. Maw, 55, Aldermanbury.

In the present state of our knowledge respecting the operation, although it has not been clearly shown to have proved fatal in any one instance, yet not to mention possible, though unknown risks, inflammation of the arm has certainly been produced by it on one or two occasions; and therefore it seems right, as the operation now stands, to confine transfusion to the first class of cases only, namely, those in which there seems to be no hope for the patient, unless blood can be thrown into the veins.

The object of the Gravitator is, to give help in this last extremity, by transmitting the blood in a regulated stream from one individual to another, with as little exposure as may be to air, cold, and inanimate surface; ordinary venesection being the only operation performed on the person who emits the blood; and the insertion of a small tube into the vein usually laid open in bleeding, being all the operation which it is necessary to execute on the person who receives it.

The following plate represents the whole apparatus connected for use and in action :—

Tab. 1.

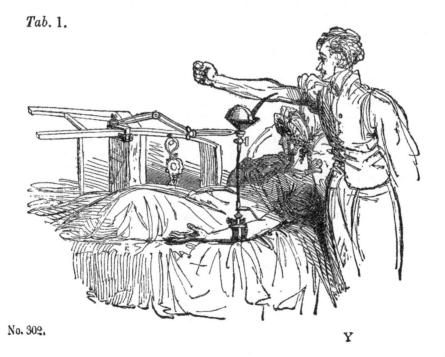

No. 302.   Y

When the apparatus has been put together for use, the following points of management require the attention of the operator :—

First, an ounce or more of clean water (better if milk-warm) is to be poured into the coniform blood receiver, the stop-cock being at the same time shut. Secondly, the vein of the patient who is to receive blood is to be distinctly exposed to the extent of half an inch, or more, the integuments and cellular web being laid open by the scalpel; an operation which may be performed by those who are dexterous at a single stroke of the knife. Thirdly, the venous tubule, see Table 2, Fig. *a*, being plugged into the angular tube which terminates the flexible canula, the operator ought to arrange the apparatus so as to place the tube immediately over the vein of the patient, and then laying hold of the tubes moveably suspended above the vein, he ought to bear down and adjust the flexible arm support, Table 2, Fig. *e*, until the venous tubule is brought into *light* contact with the vein, so that the horizontal extremity of the tube may lie externally along the course of the vessel to the extent of half an inch. This tubule, it should be observed, is of very pure silver, and flexible, and may, therefore, if necessary, be altered a little in its curves, so as to adapt it with nicety to any accidental variation in the direction of the vessel which receives it; but the less tampering with the silver the better. Of course the point of the tubule ought to be directed towards the heart, and its whole length ought to be adjusted to the direction of the vein with great exactness, so that the extremity of the tube may lie within the cavity of the vessel, without straining or otherwise injuring it; indeed, throughout the whole of the operation, the vein must be spared as much as possible.

These preliminary measures taken, the operator, moving the arm a little aside, ought next to lay open the vein with a lancet, to such an extent (say the tenth of an inch) as may ensure the easy entrance of the pipe; and if any blood issues, a small probe may be slid transversely underneath the vein, between the venous orifice and the inferior extremity of the cutaneous wound, so as to enable the operator to close the vein at pleasure, by gently pressing it down upon the probe.

The arm being prepared in this manner, the bracelet, or spring clasp, Table 2, Fig. *i*, (its cup resting rather behind the middle of the screw which supports it, say at point *x*, Table 2,) ought now to be put upon the arm of the patient, to which it will cling, and then the ball and cap, Table 2, Fig. *h*, being adjusted to the cup, but rather lightly, that they may be easily separated again, the

operator, taking a firm hold, right and left, of the two springs which form the clasp of the bracelet, he opens them a little, when he may easily advance or retract the clasp along the arm, so as to bring the silver tubule (disarranged by these previous operations) to its just bearings and light contact with the vein externally as before. At this time the nuts of the flexible arm-support, Table 2, Fig. *d*, ought, if necessary, to be screwed tight, so as to give stability to the whole apparatus, and preserve the adjustment.

This accomplished, the operator ought now to open the ball and socket-joint by separating the cap and cup, and laying hold of the apparatus at this part, he should, *with all gentleness*, pass and repass the silver tubule (moveable because suspended by the flexible canula) into the cavity of the vein, so as to satisfy himself that it really does enter the vessel, and that it is not unawares inserted between the vein and its sheath of cellular web, an accident which may easily occur, not without a risk of frustrating the whole operation. After this, again withdrawing the tubule from the cavity of the vein, he may open the stop-cock, when the water in the coniform receiver above will gravitate through the tubes, and being suffered to run for two or three seconds, will completely expel the whole of the air; after which the stop-cock being again closed, the tubes will remain full, (if this part of the operation has been well performed,) a small quantity only of water lodging in the point of the receiver, part of which may be removed, if necessary, by means of a piece of *clean* sponge, a convenience which should always be at hand.

The operation being brought to this point, the venous tubule may now be easily deposited in the cavity of the vessel; when, by turning the screw, Table 2, Fig. *e*, the small cup may be made to pass backward and forward, in the direction of the venous orifice, until it is brought exactly under the cap and ball, to which it is to be afterwards screwed down, care being taken not to derange the vein or venous tubule, neither of which are, on any account, to be disturbed.

The tubule being now retained in the vein at the proper degree of obliquity, the cap may be screwed home upon the cup; and if it be thought necessary to advance or withdraw the tubule a little, as it lies within the cavity of the vessel, this of course may be easily effected by the action of the screw support, Table 2, Fig. *e*, as before.

The hood, Table 2, Fig. *k*, being now mounted upon the receiver, Tab. 2, Fig. *f*, a vein should be opened in the arm of the person who emits the blood, and this arm ought then to be held over the receiver in the usual manner, so that the blood may

DR. BLUNDELL'S GRAVITATOR.   323

flow into it, when the cock may be turned, and the transfusion will immediately begin; the blood flowing along the tube directly from the arm of the person who emits the blood, to the arm of the person who receives it. In this mode of operating, the small quantity of water which fills the tubes will, as a matter of course, enter the veins along with the blood; but though this is certainly undesirable, it does not appear to cause any obvious hurt.

As the operation proceeds, if the blood flow freely, it ought to be collected in the receiver; if it dribble down the arm, it is better not to make use of it. If the pipes become clogged in consequence of the inspissation of the blood, the operation will be arrested: the stoppage of the operation, when this accident occurs, is an excellence of the instrument, not a defect. To clear the apparatus, a syringe is provided, fitting the opening of the stop-cock, by means of which warm water may be forced through the tubes before the blood hardens in them.

In the progress of the operation watch the countenance; if the features are slightly convulsed, the flow of blood should be checked: and if the attack is severe, the operation must be suspended altogether. On the other hand, so long as no spasmodic twitchings of the features, or other alarming symptoms are observed, we may then proceed without fear.

If there be occasion to suspend the operation, all the blood which lies in the apparatus, during the interruption, ought to be cleared away, and warm water being passed through the tubes, the transfusion ought to be commenced afresh.

Throughout the whole process, only a small quantity of blood should be allowed to collect in the receiver at once, nor should its level ever rise above the line drawn around its interior. This line indicates the measure of two fluid ounces.

If the blood collect in the receiver too fast, this may be easily remedied, either by placing a finger below the orifice in the arm of the person who supplies it, so as to check the stream; or else, by requesting him to withdraw his arm, so that the blood may no longer reach the receiver.

In cases requiring transfusion, the heart and vascular system being feeble, there is reason to believe that their action might be arrested by too rapid an influx, and that sudden death might, in that manner, be produced. It is necessary to guard against this accident with care; and it is to be recollected, that by means of the flexible arm-support, the receiver may be placed at any level above the arm of the patient, and that the rapidity of the influx may thereby be increased or retarded accordingly. It should too be observed, the force of the stream may be diminished at pleasure, by means of a partial closure of the stop-cock: and although this tends to produce a slight suction, yet it may, notwithstanding, be the best mode of regulating the impetus of the stream. The force of the stream may also be ascertained, by pouring water into the receiver before the operation is begun, and the elevation of the receiver, or the turn of the cock, may be adjusted accordingly before the operation begins.

The following plate represents the several parts of the apparatus referred to as Table 2 :—

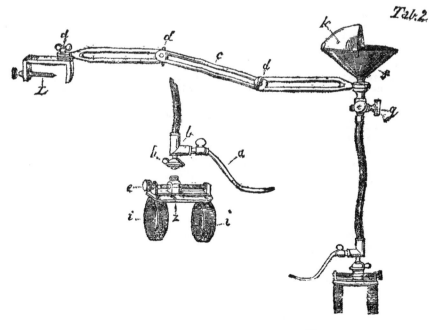

THE LANCET.

Vol. II.]   LONDON, SATURDAY, SEPTEMBER 12.   [1828-9.

ON PRUSSIC ACID.

By M. Orfila.

M. Orfila's memoir, of which the following is an abridgment, gives a very clear exposition of the best methods of discovering, by means of chemical reagents, the presence of hydrocyanic acid in various liquids; of determining the proportion in which it is contained in them, and its effects on the animal economy; and, lastly, of the most efficacious treatment in cases of poisoning by it.

If the acid be mixed with a liquid, the best reagent is the nitrate of silver, which indicates even a very small quantity of it, by a curdly white precipitate, consisting of the cyanuret of silver. This substance has the following properties: it is insoluble in water and nitric acid, at a low temperature, but very soluble in the latter at a boiling heat, and in ammonia; it has a very slight tendency to become of a violet colour, is decomposed by the action of heat, and the free contact of air, so as to give cyanogen and metallic silver, the former of which being easily recognised by the smell, the cyanuret of silver can hardly be confounded with any other substance. The deuto sulphate of copper, with a little potash, which was proposed by M. Lassaigne as a test for prussic acid, is much more sensible than the sulphate of iron, but less so than the nitrate of silver; moreover it gives a precipitate, which may be confounded with a great many other substances. The persulphate of iron, with a small addition of potash, gives a precipitate of blue colour, (or which becomes so by adding a few drops of sulphuric acid,) but it is by far too little sensible to serve as a test for prussic acid.

In those cases where the acid is mixed with coloured fluids, so as to produce, on the addition of nitrate of silver or persulphate of iron, brown precipitates, a piece of writing paper, impregnated with a solution of caustic potash, is dipped into the fluid for about two or three minutes, and after having become dry in the air, a saturated solution of the persulphate of iron is sprinkled over it, by which the paper immediately turns of a blue colour, with a slight greenish hue. Sometimes it will be sufficient to destroy the colour of the fluid, by the addition of purified animal charcoal. If either of the two methods prove ineffectual, the fluid must be distilled, and then submitted to the action of nitrate of silver.

The best method of ascertaining the relative quantity of prussic acid in a fluid is the following:—a certain portion of the fluid having been mixed with water, an excess of the solution of nitrate of silver is added guttatim, by which the whole of the prussic acid is precipitated as cyanuret of silver. Numerous experiments have shown that syrup, and the mucilages of gum arabic, and althæa, with which the hydrocyanic syrup is generally prepared, form no precipitate with the nitrate of silver; the cyanuret of silver, in the above experiment, is consequently to be considered as perfectly free from the admixture of any other substance. This method is greatly preferable to distilling the fluid, and collecting the vapour over, or letting it pass through, a solution of the nitrate of silver. In an experiment of that kind, which was made last year in consequence of an order from the "Procureur du Roi," by MM. Barruel, Gay-Lussac, Magendie, and the author, not more than 3.73 grains of the cyanuret were obtained, from a syrup which, by dropping the solution of nitrate of silver in the manner above recommended, was found to furnish 4.558 grains of the cyanuret. From the latter substance, the absolute quantity of hydrocyanic acid is easily obtained by calculation. The cyanuret of silver consists of 32.900 cyanogen, and 135.160 silver, and hydrocyanic acid of 96.34 cyanogen, and 3.66 hydrogen. The quantity of cyanogen in the cyanuret of silver, serves, accordingly, to determine the relative quantity of the prussic acid.

In order to appreciate the quantity of hydrocyanic acid mixed with muriates, carbonates, phosphates, &c., the solution of the nitrate of silver is added, which gives a precipitate, consisting of the cyanuret, muriate, phosphate, carbonate, &c., of silver. The phosphate and carbonate of silver are dissolved by the admixture of diluted

738   M. ORFILA ON PRUSSIC ACID.

nitric acid, the remainder, consisting of the cyanuret and muriate of silver, is boiled for half an hour with nitric acid, by which the cyanuret of silver is completely taken up, the muriate remaining undissolved. The cyanuret of silver, during its dissolution in the nitric acid, undergoes the following change : the water being, by the action of the acid, decomposed, its oxygen combines with the metal, which thus becomes a nitrate, while the hydrogen unites to the cyanogen, and forms hydrocyanic acid, which is disengaged by the action of heat. In order, therefore, to appreciate the quantity of the cyanuret of silver, a sufficient quantity of hydrocyanic acid is added to the nitrate obtained, to convert the whole of the metal into a cyanuret, the weight of which, together with that of the muriate, will serve to determine the relative quantity of acid in the fluid.

To the above method, it might be objected that the cyanuret of silver obtained, affords no sufficient reason to suppose the existence of *free* hydrocyanic acid in the fluid, and that the same result would have taken place if it had existed in the form of a hydrocyanate or cyanuret; the distillation of a portion of the fluid in a closed vessel, is sufficient to settle this question, by the condensation of hydrocyanic acid in the receiver, in case it existed free in the fluid, while the cyanurets and hydrocyanates (except the hydrocyanate of ammonia) are not volatilised or decomposed at the temperature of boiling water.

With respect to the morbid alterations produced in the animal economy by the ingestion of large doses of prussic acid, it appears, from numerous experiments upon dogs, that there is no inflammation of the stomach or intestinal canal; while, in the human subject, several *post-mortem* examinations have shown the contrary: this difference may, perhaps, be accounted for, by the circumstance of the dogs having been killed almost suddenly in the greater number of the experiments. MM. Adelon, Marc, and Marjolin, give the following results of the *post-mortem* examinations of seven patients of the Salpêtrière, who, some years ago, died between twenty-five and thirty minutes after having each of them swallowed about nine drachms of the hydrocyanic syrup. The mucous membrane of the stomach and smaller intestines was evidently inflamed, and its folliculæ mucosæ were more than usually developed; the external surface of the stomach and intestinal canal was injected, the spleen softened, and, in some of the bodies, almost diffluent ; the veins of the liver were gorged with black fluid blood, the kidneys of a violet colour, softened, and filled with blood; the substance of the heart was rather firm ; its cavities, as well as the larger arteries, empty, the larger veins, on the contrary, being gorged with very black liquid blood, without exhibiting any trace of coagulum. The mucous membrane of the larynx, trachea, and bronchia, was injected, and of a deep red colour; and the bronchia filled and surrounded by spurious liquid blood ; the mucous membrane of the bladder, as well as that of the œsophagus and pharynx, was of a white colour, but appeared healthy ; the cerebral membranes were injected, the sinûs of the dura mater was filled with black fluid blood; the substance of the brain was somewhat softer than usual, but, in other respects, as well as the spinal chord, healthy ; no smell of bitter almonds was perceptible in any of the tissues ; all the bodies were extremely rigid.

Although we know as yet of no direct antidote for prussic acid, there are many cases where the poisonous effect of a small dose of it has been obviated by means of proper treatment ; and some which M. Orfila observed in his own practice, place it beyond all doubt, that the ingestion of a dose which otherwise would have caused death within fifteen to eighteen minutes, in consequence of the treatment employed, did not prove fatal. M. Orfila having convinced himself, by numerous experiments, that neither the infusion nor decoction of coffee, nor the essential oil of turpentine, nor any of the other remedies recommended, had any effect, came, at last, to the following result :—

1. The inhalation of the vapour from a weak solution of ammonia in water, is to be considered as one of the most efficacious means of checking the poisonous effects of prussic acid. The solution must not be stronger than about one part of the caustic liquor of ammonia to twelve of water, or it will cause a spasmodic contraction of the glottis, and inflammation of the trachea ; the internal use of ammonia appears to have no effect whatever.

2. The inhalation of the vapour from a weak solution of chlorine, (four parts of water to one of chlorine,) which was first proposed by M. Simeon, of the Hopital St. Louis, is not less efficacious than ammonia. M. Orfila asserts that dogs, after having swallowed prussic acid in a quantity sufficient to kill them within fifteen minutes, had been saved from perishing by the inhalation of chlorine, even if it had been employed four or five minutes after the ingestion of the poison.

3. Lastly, the affusion of cold water over the head and along the back, according to the experiments of M. Herbst: of eight dogs, to which this method was applied, three survived the administration of a sufficient quantity of prussic acid to kill them within a short time ; the other five died, but the destructive effect of the poison had evidently been retarded by the cold affu-

sions. One of the dogs, after a dose of acid sufficient to kill him within twelve minutes, continued to live for two hours and a half; of two others, who, without the use of cold affusions, would, most probably, have died within two or three minutes, the one remained alive for twenty, the other during fourteen, minutes after the ingestion of the poison.

Besides the above remedies, M. Orfila recommends the use of ice to the head, leeches to the temples, and bleeding; the latter of which, however, he remarks, has, in no case, been sufficient to destroy the effect of the poison, if unassisted by the other remedies above recommended.

HYDATIDS AND DROPSY OF THE UTERUS.

To the Editor of THE LANCET.

SIR,—I beg to forward to you the following interesting cases: one of hydatids in the uterus, the other of dropsy in the uterus, treated by my friend Mr. W. WILDSMITH, *of Leeds.* I am, Sir, your wellwisher,

JOHN EPPS.

2, Seymour Place, Bryanstone Square.

CASE OF HYDATIDS OF THE UTERUS.

June 2, 1828. Mrs. A. applied to me respecting a disease which had long resisted the use of domestic remedies. She had diarrhœa, as if from impaired biliary secretion, a paucity of urine, and enlargement of the abdomen. She had not menstruated for four months, but had suffered some pain at the usual periods, attended by a slight serous discharge, and three or four times had experienced a sudden gush of water, as if from the escape of liquor amnii. It was her opinion, and that of her friends, that she was pregnant. She had two children living, and during the latter pregnancy had menstruated till the fourth month. Being of a lax habit, and debilitated by occasional sickness—in addition to the paucity of urine, swelling of the legs, general distress over the whole body, with the absence of quickening and enlargement of the breasts, I thought it most probable that she was dropsical. I endeavoured to regulate the bowels, and to establish a freer flow of urine. On the 7th the diarrhœa was checked, but the urine continued scanty. The legs were swelled to a great degree, and tenderness of the abdomen was now felt, for which latter the sp. tereb. was applied. On the 14th, I commenced giving small doses of calomel, which, in four days, occasioned slight salivation. On the 20th I was sent for in haste, and was informed that she had flooded for two hours, and uterine pains were frequent and tolerably strong. On examination, I encountered what I conceived to be the placenta, and, at every pain, large coagula seemed to be expelled. The external parts were quite lax, and my hand readily passed within the vagina. It was my desire to seize the fœtus and placenta, and so terminate the labour and hæmorrhage together; but the further I pushed my hand, the more interminable appeared the mass which filled the uterus; and my fears relative to what appeared the continued hæmorrhage in so delicate a woman, increased as I proceeded. It now occurred to me to examine the matter which was expelled, and I was greatly surprised to find it to consist of that peculiar fabric called hydatids. The hæmorrhage which had preceded their discharge had ceased. I therefore withdrew my hand, and awaited their final expulsion, to assist which I gave a Əj. dose of the secale cornutum. This somewhat increased the pains, but failed in expelling more hydatids. Having given a little brandy and water, I again introduced my hand, and cautiously broke the mass into fragments, which gradually escaped by my hand, until I could feel the sides of the uterus, which had become a little tender. I now desisted, and gave her a dose of tinct. opii. No bad symptoms followed, and, in a fortnight, she was quite recovered. About a month afterwards she menstruated, and became pregnant about October, and was delivered of a healthy child in July of the present year.

Remarks.—Many cases of hydatids are recorded in obstetrical treatises; but occurring so seldom, they scarcely attract the notice of the practitioner; to me it was perfectly novel. The symptoms which attended were of a most ambiguous character, and the difficulty of obviating them by the usual methods, determined me to employ mercury: to this I attribute the disorganisation of the hydatids, and their consequent disgorgement. If, from the accompanying symptoms, a correct diagnosis could be formed, I have no doubt that mercury would prove a certain remedy, and which, if used early, would save the patient much distress and anxiety. But the most curious circumstance attending this case is, that the uterus should so far regain its full and healthy powers, and in so short a time as to give birth to a child within thirteen months after this most formidable disease, and that no trace of hydatids has since appeared in the patient.

My friend Mr. Batty, of this town, witnessed the case during the final discharge of the hydatids. In quantity, there were between three and four quarts, varying in size from the smallest seed to a moderate sized grape, and when detached from the large mass, being, together, not unlike bunches of the latter.

3 B 2

THE LANCET.

VOL. II.]   LONDON, SATURDAY, MAY 14.   [1830-31.

POISONED CONFECTIONARY.

DETECTION OF GAMBOGE, LEAD, COPPER, MER-
CURY, AND CHROMATE OF LEAD,

In various articles of Sugar Confectionary.

By W. B. O'SHAUGHNESSY, M.D.

IN the following observations, it is my principal aim to lay before the public and the medical profession, a calm, dispassionate statement of the existence of the various poisons enumerated above, in several articles of confectionary, the preparation of which, from their peculiar attractions to the younger branches of the community, has grown into a separate and most extensive branch of manufacture. I am fully aware of the hazardous task that individual undertakes, who ventures in this country to signalise such abuses. The wrath of the particular trade is, of course, especially excited. The sneers and ridicule of the ignorant are also abundantly provoked, principally through the recollection of the indiscreet and mischievous efforts, which overzealous or designing alarmists have occasionally made to terrify the public mind by topics of this description. I hope, however, by a plain narrative of facts, and by reference to justly-accredited authorities, to avoid at the same time these unpleasant imputations, and to show the real extent of the danger in question.

I had, as far back as a year since, been requested, by the Editor of this Journal, to undertake a series of analytic investigations into the truth or inaccuracy of various alleged adulterations, with the view that the authenticated information thus obtained might either dissipate needless apprehension, by pointing out the falsity of many alarming statements, or might lead to the efficient protection of the public health, by showing, as far as analysis could teach, what were the admixtures really prejudicial and essential to be prohibited. Different circumstances, unnecessary to particularise here, combined to delay the commencement of these inquiries until a fortnight since,

No. 402.

when I received from Mr. Wakley the numbers of the *Journal de Chimie Medicale* for the preceding three months, to an article in which (*Janvier*, No. 2) he requested me to direct my attention.

The article alluded to is from the pen of the distinguished *Chevallier*, whose labours in this department of medical police have acquired for him the highest reputation as a philanthropist and physician ; it is entitled, " Note sur la vente des sucreries, coloriées, bonbons, &c.," and as it places the importance of the subject in the most striking light, and shows, at the same time, the enlightened measures adopted by the French government on the occasion, I subjoin a sufficient abstract of its contents.

M. Chevallier commences by observing,[*] that at several times he had related in the *Journal de Chimie*, various serious accidents produced by the consumption of sugar confectionary coloured by mineral poisons. Of these he particularises the *schweinfurt green*, a compound of arsenious acid (arsenic) and copper ; the *chromate of lead*, and the *sulphuret of mercury*. Lastly ; he enumerates *gamboge*, a drastic purgative, and consequently an active irritant poison. Despite of the notification of this dangerous practice, made in nearly all the journals, literary, political, and medical, this mode of colouring was persevered in, till at length the Council of Health was consulted on the subject. This body lost no time in investigating it as it deserved, and the result was, an ordonnance of police for the suppression of the nuisance. The following document, which led to the ordonnance, is well worth attention :—

Report, addressed by M. Andral to the Prefect of Police, on the dangers which may result from the use of coloured sugar confectionary.

" M. le Prefet,—You have instructed the Council of Health to report to you, on the danger which may result from the consumption of coloured confectionary, and on the measures necessary to be adopted to prevent the manufacture and sale of any such per-

[*] Journal de Chimie, tome vi, p. 608.

O

nicious articles. The delegates of the Council have the honour to submit to you the following propositions :—

" 1. It will be important to specify in the ordonnance, what are the colouring substances which should be prohibited. These are, in the first place, all those derived from the mineral kingdom, except the oxides of iron, ferruginous lakes, or Prussian blue, all of which may be safely employed. Of vegetable substances, *gamboge* should be severely proscribed, as being a drastic cathartic, which even in minute doses necessarily occasions violent intestinal irritation. *Litmus* should be equally prohibited, as well on account of its being occasionally incorporated with putrified urine, as that some manufacturers mix it with common *arsenic* and the peroxide of *mercury*.

" The most diversified colours may be obtained by the confectioners from totally harmless compounds. Thus from the lakes of cochineal and carmine, they can prepare all the reds; the lakes of logwood will afford them the violet; the lakes of dyer's broom (*genista tinctoria*), &c. will give the yellow; the lake of Persian grain (*polygonum Persicaria*), with Prussian blue, form a more beautiful green than any mineral can produce; finally, by the mixture of these harmless colours all the intermediate tints and shades will be obtained.

" 2. The papers used for wrapping up sugar confectionary should also be strictly attended to, since they are coloured with the same poisonous materials, and *children invariably will suck or eat these papers*, from which it is evident the most fatal accidents may occur. *A member of the Council of Health, a short time since, snatched a coloured paper of this description from an infant's mouth, and by analysis obtained from it both* ARSENIC AND COPPER.

" 3. The delegates of the Council are of opinion, that to ensure the observance of the ordonnance, you should determine, M. le Prefet, that a committee be appointed to visit the workshops of the manufacturers of this species of confectionary : all the poisoned articles should be seized and their venders fined. Lastly; the delegates of the Council recommend, as a measure of great utility, that on the day following the seizure, the names of the confectioners should be published in all the journals and placarded over the walls of the city.

" In conclusion, the delegates of the Council believe, that an ordonnance, founded on the principles thus pointed out, will prove of essential service, by suppressing a practice so pernicious to the public health."

The immediate result of this pointed and satisfactory report, was the issuing of an ordonnance from the prefecture of police, dated the 10th of December, 1830, and signed by the Comte Treilhard, in which the practice is denounced in the most energetic terms, the poisonous ingredients specified, the harmless enumerated, and in addition to the proposals of M. Andral, orders are given that no confectionary shall be sold, unless wrapped up in paper, stamped with the name and address of the confectioner. Further, by this edict, the venders are held personally responsible for all accidents occasioned by the confectionary or liqueurs sold in their establishments.

Pursuant to these resolutions, the visits were made, and several poisoned specimens destroyed. Generally speaking, the confectioners gladly banished from their laboratories the pernicious materials, and availed themselves of the harmless substitutes recommended in the report. Lastly, M. Chevallier describes the mode in which the sulphuret of mercury (vermilion), the chromate of lead, and the arsenite of copper (Schweinfurt green), may be detected by chemical analysis.

The preceding abstract, sanctioned by the name of M. Chevallier, and of that illustrious pathologist M. Andral, is amply sufficient to entitle me to the attention of the public, while I describe the extent to which the practice of using poisonous colours is carried on in London, and thence disseminated over the united kingdom, and its foreign colonies and possessions.

On the subsequent day to that on which I perused the article just alluded to, I purchased, in company with my friend Dr. Green, at several shops, different specimens of coloured confectionary, and of colourless articles, wrapped in stained paper. Of the coloured articles, the greater number (class 1) were sold expressly for eating, some (class 2) cast into small figures of cards, &c., were *apparently* rather intended for ornament, but were sold without restriction; and, lastly, some (class 3) were expressly designed for ornament alone. Of the first class I examined about thirty different kinds, and found the *reds* tinted as follows:

Ten Specimens of Red Comfits, &c.

1 Minium, or red oxide of lead.
2 Red sulphuret of mercury (vermilion).
1 Mixture of both the former.
1 *Of a yellowish or orange tint,* chromate of lead, and a vegetable lake of lime.
2 Cochineal alone.
1 Cochineal, with a trace of *vermilion*.
2 Vegetable lakes of alumina and lime.
—
10

It is seen here, that of the ten specimens of comfits sold for eating expressly, six contained mineral poison; all these specimens, with one exception, were only coloured externally.

DR. O'SHAUGHNESSY ON POISONED CONFECTIONARY. 195

Of the *yellows*, class 1, seven specimens of different forms and tints. 4. *Gamboge*, coloured externally ; 1. Coloured throughout a vegetable lake of lime ; 1. *Coloured throughout*, oxide of lead, and traces of antimony, or Naples yellow. Six of the seven consequently contained deleterious substances.

Of the *greens*, class 1, several specimens, all were coloured by Prussian blue, and a vegetable yellow lake of alumina mixed with the sulphate of lime, except one specimen, of which I had only two comfits, and which gave me a mixture of copper and lime.

The *blues*, class 1, were chiefly Prussian blue, and contained no hurtful compound.

In the second class, or those *apparently* intended for ornament, but sold without restriction, and formed in all sorts of fantastic shapes, of eight forms of yellow, three contained chromate of lead ; one Naples yellow ; one massicot or yellow lead, and three vegetable lakes of alumina and lime. All these were coloured throughout, and contained moreover sugar, and the sulphate of lime or plaster of Paris.

The *reds* in this class were, of six specimens, three vegetable lakes of alumina or lime, one chromate of lead, with a red vegetable lake, two red lead.

The *greens* and *blues* were composed as I described in class 1.

In the *third* class the composition was precisely the same, and the proportion little different from class 2.

The papers were next examined, especially those used for enveloping the sugar drops called " kisses." Without exception the reds were coloured by the RED SULPHURET of MERCURY, the yellows by the CHROMATE of LEAD, and many of the greens by VERDEGRIS, or the carbonate of copper.*

With respect to the quantities of the poisonous substances, I had not leisure to submit the various products to the tedious process of delicate weighing. Moreover, it appears to me to be altogether unnecessary to take the trouble, as the mere presence of the minutest possible quantity of any such substance should not be allowed. In this opinion I entirely coincide with MM. Chevallier and Andral. It is perfectly unnecessary for me to occupy the pages of this Journal with any observations on the *nature* of the danger which thus threatens the junior branches of the community, and which indisputably exercises the most pernicious effects on their constitutions ; I will merely

remark that one concern in the city, from which I have obtained the greatest number of poisonous specimens, employs eleven men daily in the preparation of these articles, furnishes immense quantities of them to country confectioners, supplies many of the minor shops in the metropolis, and, if I am rightly informed, exports to our foreign possessions to a considerable amount. Extent of manufacture always implies extent of sale, and in this case the ratio of the consumption of course equals both. I cannot, therefore, be accused of exaggeration, when I assert that millions of children are thus daily dosed with metallic and vegetable poisons, in minute quantities it is true, but in quantities dependent on their amount on the caprice of a workman or a machine, and sufficient in the minutest degree to exercise their peculiar insidious effects, if taken as a practice from day to day. Neither are these effects chronic alone, for not long since an *acute* case of poisoning arising from the use of confectionary of this description occurred in the children of a highly respectable family in Southwark, and on analysis the comfits were found to contain minium, or the red oxide of lead.

The next topic remaining for me to notice is the

MODE OF ANALYSIS OF SUSPECTED SPECIMENS.*

This varies, in its first step, according to the extent to which the colouring matter pervades the specimen. *If entirely external*, it should be agitated in water in a wine glass till the colour is washed off, which takes place usually in a few seconds. The solid part, or body of the article, should then be removed by decantation into another vessel, and the liquid if transparent and coloured filtered through paper and preserved. If the colour be throughout as seen on the fracture, the specimen should be reduced to powder, and boiled in a small flask in distilled water, which dissolves the sugar, and leaves the mineral substance, vegetable lake, &c., which should next be transferred to a watch-glass, and dried in the water-bath.

If the supernatant liquid in either case remain transparent and colourless, it is an indication that the colouring matter is either a mineral substance, or a vegetable lake ; in this case the fluid may be rejected, and attention confined to the deposit alone. If again we obtain a coloured fluid and a considerable residuum, it indicates a vege-

---

* Sealed phials, containing specimens of the poisoned comfits, are left at THE LANCET Office for public inspection in order to supersede the necessity of a description of their forms, which could at best communicate a very faint idea of the pernicious kinds.

* M. CHEVALLIER merely describes the mode of detecting vermilion, the arsenical greens, and chromate of lead. I have ventured to recommend different processes in this paper, under the conviction that those employed by M. Chevallier were not detailed with sufficient minuteness to be of practical utility.

O 2

274 DR. LATTA ON THE TREATMENT OF MALIGNANT CHOLERA

following symptoms : pulse 125, almost imperceptible ; surface dry and cold ; hands shrivelled ; the lips, chin, hands, and feet, blue ; eyes sunk and surrounded with a dark areola ; countenance expressive of great anxiety ; cramps of the lower extremities ; voice feeble ; thirst excessive ; tongue slightly furred and warm ; sickness and purging of a fluid resembling rice-water ; urine suppressed. Two grains of calomel, with three drops of tincture of opium, to be taken every five minutes for one hour, and then every ten minutes ; hot bricks to be applied to the feet.

Five p.m. The symptoms still continue, but are less severe. One drop and a half of the tincture of opium with the calomel, to be taken every ten minutes for one hour ; and afterwards every fifteen minutes.

Eight p.m. Was joined by Dr. Ayre ; pulse 100, and stronger ; surface warm ; blueness disappeared ; countenance regained its natural appearance ; cramps less severe ; purging entirely abated ; sickness continues ; has not yet passed any urine. Repeat the calomel, with one drop of the tincture every half hour.

Saturday, half past twelve a.m. Sickness nearly abated ; thirst not so troublesome ; has passed no urine. The pills to be taken every hour.

Seven a. m. Pulse 90 and strong ; sickness entirely ceased ; no urine yet ; has had some sleep during the night. The pills to be continued and taken every two hours.

Two p.m. Has had two liquid stools void of bile ; urine still suppressed. Continue the pills as before.

Half past nine p.m. Improved in all her symptoms. Has passed a little urine, after 36 hours suppression. A powder of jalap and rhubarb to be taken immediately, and repeated in three hours.

Sunday, ten a.m. Appears much improved ; has just passed another stool, but not altered in appearance. Urine passes freely. The powders of rhubarb and jalap to be repeated.

Nine p.m. Has been rather affected with sickness ; in other respects much better ; has passed some bilious stools ; the mouth slightly affected. An effervescing draught to be taken occasionally. She may be considered as quite convalescent.

R. SHARPE.
Monday, May 21st.

In the cases above given, and in those to which I have referred, as at once illustrating my views of the nature of the disease, and of the treatment demanded for it, I desire not to push my conclusions beyond what the facts will legitimately warrant. The four cases are the only ones in which I knew the practice has been pursued in strict accordance with my views, and without any admixture of other means. They were all severe cases, and they all recovered, and without being followed by any consecutive fever, which happens in so many cases of recovery, but which did not happen here, and could not happen if my views be correct concerning the mode by which the calomel acts upon the disease. The treatment and results of every case I may hereafter have shall be reported, and I hope, in the mean while, that others may be induced to make the same trials, and duly report the issue of them.

JOSEPH AYRE.
Hull, May 23d, 1832.

MALIGNANT CHOLERA.

DOCUMENTS

COMMUNICATED BY THE

CENTRAL BOARD OF HEALTH, LONDON,

RELATIVE TO THE TREATMENT OF CHOLERA BY THE COPIOUS INJECTION OF AQUEOUS AND SALINE FLUIDS INTO THE VEINS.

No. 1.

Letter from DR. LATTA* *to the Secretary of the Central Board of Health, London, affording a View of the Rationale and Results of his Practice in the Treatment of Cholera by Aqueous and Saline Injections.*

Leith, May 23, 1832.

SIR,—My friend Dr. Lewins has communicated to me your wish for a detailed account of my method of treating cholera by saline injection into the veins, with which I now most willingly comply. My scope for observation, since I commenced this treatment, has been too limited to allow me to be very copious on the subject, but I think I can adduce sufficient proof to the unprejudiced, not only of its safety, but of its unquestionable utility. I have never yet seen one bad symptom attributable to it, and I have no doubt that it will be found, when judiciously applied, to be one of the most powerful, and one of the safest remedies yet used in the second stage of cholera, or that hopeless state of collapse to which the system is reduced.

---

* Dr. Latta having signified his wish that this communication should be published in THE LANCET, the Central Board of Health have accordingly forwarded it to this Journal.—ED. L.

BY AQUEOUS INJECTIONS INTO THE VEINS.   275.

Before entering into particulars, I beg leave to premise that the plan which I have put in practice was suggested to me on reading in THE LANCET, the review of Dr. O'Shaughnessy's report on the chemical pathology of malignant cholera, by which it appears that in that disease there is a very great deficiency both of the water and saline matter of the blood. On which deficiency, the thick, black, cold state of the vital fluid depends, which evidently produces most of the distressing symptoms of that very fearful complaint, and is, doubtless, often the cause of death. In this opinion I am abundantly borne out by the phenomena produced on repletion by venous injection.

So soon as I learnt the result of Dr. O'Shaughnessy's analysis, I attempted to restore the blood to its natural state, by injecting copiously into the larger intestines warm water, holding in solution the requisite salts, and also administered quantities from time to time by the mouth, trusting that the power of absorption might not be altogether lost, but by these means I produced, in no case, any permanent benefit, but, on the contrary, I thought the tormina, vomiting, and purging, were much aggravated thereby, to the further reduction of the little remaining strength of the patient; finding thus, that such, in common with all the ordinary means in use, was either useless or hurtful, I at length resolved to throw the fluid immediately into the circulation. In this, having no precedent to direct me, I proceeded with much caution. The first subject of experiment was an aged female, on whom all the usual remedies had been fully tried, without producing one good symptom; the disease, uninterrupted, holding steadily on its course. She had apparently reached the last moments of her earthly existence, and now nothing could injure her—indeed, so entirely was she reduced, that I feared I should be unable to get my apparatus ready ere she expired. Having inserted a tube into the basilic vein, cautiously — anxiously, I watched the effects; ounce after ounce was injected, but no visible change was produced. Still persevering, I thought she began to breathe less laboriously, soon the sharpened features, and sunken eye, and fallen jaw, pale and cold, bearing the manifest impress of death's signet, began to glow with returning animation; the pulse, which had long ceased, returned to the wrist; at first small and quick, by degrees it became more and more distinct, fuller, slower, and firmer, and in the short space of half an hour, when six pints had been injected, she expressed in a firm voice that she was free from all uneasiness, actually became jocular, and fancied all she needed was a little sleep; her extremities were warm, and every feature bore the aspect of comfort and health. This being my first case, I fancied my patient secure, and from my great need of a little repose, left her in charge of the hospital surgeon; but I had not been long gone, ere the vomiting and purging recurring, soon reduced her to her former state of debility. I was not apprised of the event, and she sunk in five and a half hours after I left her. As she had previously been of a sound constitution, I have no doubt the case would have issued in complete reaction, had the remedy, which already had produced such effect, been repeated.

Not having by me the Number of THE LANCET containing Dr. O'Shaughnessy's analyses, I adopted that of Dr. Marcet, only allowing a smaller proportion of saline ingredients. This I now find to be considerably less than natural, according to the more recent analyses. I dissolved from two to three drachms of muriate of soda and two scruples of the subcarbonate of soda in six pints of water, and injected it at temperature 112° Fah. If the temperature is so low as a hundred, it produces an extreme sense of cold, with rigors; and if it reaches 115°, it suddenly excites the heart, the countenance becomes flushed, and the patient complains of great weakness. At first there is but little felt by the patient, and symptoms continue unaltered, until the blood, mingled with the injected liquid, becomes warm and fluid; the improvement in the pulse and countenance is almost simultaneous, the cadaverous expression gradually gives place to appearances of returning animation, the horrid oppression at the præcordia goes off, the sunken turned-up eye, half covered by the palpebræ, becomes gradually fuller, till it sparkles with the brilliancy of health, the livid hue disappears, the warmth of the body returns, and it regains its natural colour,—words are no more uttered in whispers, the voice first acquires its true cholera tone, and ultimately its wonted energy, and the poor patient, who but a few minutes before was oppressed with sickness, vomiting, and burning thirst, is suddenly relieved from every distressing symptom; blood now drawn exhibits on exposure to air its natural florid hue.

Such symptoms, so gratifying both to the sick and the physician, must never allow the latter to relax in his care—the utmost vigilance is still necessary. At first the change is so great that he may fancy all is accomplished, and leave his post for a while. The diarrhœa recurring, he may find his patient, after the lapse of two or three hours, as low as ever. As soon as reaction by the first injection is produced, mild

276   DR. LATTA ON AQUEOUS INJECTIONS IN CHOLERA.

warm stimulants, such as weak gin-toddy, mixed with some astringent, should be freely and assiduously administered. An attempt should be made to fill the colon with some astringent fluid. That such is requisite, is evident from the watery diarrhœa returning with violence, and if not restrained, death will ultimately make sure of his victim, therefore so soon as the pulse fails, and the features again shrink, the venous injection must be repeated, taking care that the fluid in use retains its proper temperature. The injection should be carried on very slowly, unless the patient is much exhausted, when it may be used more rapidly at first, until a little excitement is produced, after which it should not exceed two or three ounces per minute, and now is the time for the exhibition of astringents by the mouth, which will be retained, for in general the sickness entirely leaves during the operation.

Such remedies must be persisted in, and repeated as symptoms demand, or until reaction is permanently established. I have witnessed no violent symptoms accompanying the rapid injection of the fluid, but I have thought that the hasty repletion of the system was followed by great increase of the evacuations, and consequently a more sudden depression of the powers of life. The quantity to be injected depends on the effect produced, and the repetition on the demands of the system, which generally vary according to the violence of the diarrhœa; the greater the degree of collapse, the greater will be the quantity needed, though not uniformly, for a very slight loss produces much depression in some systems; hence there is often great collapse, without much vomiting, purging, or cutaneous discharge.

Although in every case, even the most desperate, the cholera symptoms were removed, some of my cases failed, which I attributed to one or other of the following causes; either the quantity injected was too small, or its effects were rendered abortive by extensive organic disease, or its application was too late.

I have already given an instance where deficiency in quantity was the cause of failure, which I will now contrast with one in which it was used freely. A female, aged 50, very destitute, but previously in good health, was on the 13th instant, at four a.m., seized with cholera in its most violent form, and by half-past nine was reduced to a most hopeless state. The pulse was quite gone, even in the axilla, and strength so much exhausted, that I had resolved not to try the effects of the injection, conceiving the poor woman's case to be hopeless, and that the failure of the experiment might afford the prejudiced and the illiberal an opportunity to stigmatise the practice; however, I at length thought I would give her a chance, and in the presence of Drs. Lewins and Craigie, and Messrs. Sibson and Paterson, I injected one hundred and twenty ounces, when like the effects of magic, instead of the pallid aspect of one whom death had sealed as his own, the vital tide was restored, and life and vivacity returned; but diarrhœa recurred, and in three hours she again sunk. One hundred and twenty ounces more were injected with the same good effect. In this case 330 ounces were so used in twelve hours, when reaction was completely reestablished; and in forty-eight hours she smoked her pipe free from distemper. She was then, for better accommodation, carried to the hospital, where probably, from contagion, slight typhoid symptoms were produced. She is now, however, convalescent.

The second cause of want of success is the presence of organic disease; this, probably, renders the possessor very liable to attacks of cholera; and the latent evil, which previously gave but little uneasiness, suffers aggravation in all its symptoms, more especially after reaction has been produced, and has evidently, in many cases, been the cause of death. A delicate young female, of strumous habit, who had been for some years subject to pectoral complaints, was rescued from a state of collapse by the injection of sixty ounces of the saline fluid, administered in separate portions, within the space of twelve hours. After lingering for ten days she died; the heart was found in a state of atrophy, covered with strong evidence of the existence of ancient disease, and floating in eight ounces of pus. In another case every internal organ was diseased; some of them so much so, that it was astonishing the individual lived so long.

The third cause of the occasional want of success, is the late application of the remedy. Hitherto I have had opportunity of injecting only in extreme cases, after every other means had entirely failed, cases which apparently would have soon proved fatal. Here the obstacles to be overcome have been of no ordinary kind, notwithstanding the result of the practice is of the most encouraging nature, and the number of cases now convalescent or doing well highly gratifying. In every fatal case we have had an opportunity of examining, independent of organic disease, I have found a large quantity of fibrin in the cavities of the heart, especially on the right side, where it had extended from the auricle through the ventricle into the pulmonary artery. Such deposition must have formed a certain obstacle to recovery, and is, no doubt, from the interruption it gives to the

DR. LEWINS ON AQUEOUS INJECTIONS IN CHOLERA,   277

pulmonary circulation, the cause of the heavings of the chest, and the inordinate action perceptible in the centre of circulation many hours before death. Now surely it is reasonable to suppose, that if this, the most simple of all remedies, were applied early, before the blood drained of its water has collected in the larger vessels, in fact before such fibrinous depositions have taken place in the cavities of the heart, is it not reasonable to suppose that such would be entirely prevented?

But not only is early injection advisable on this account, not only is stagnation of the blood prevented by it, and the laborious breathing, and the præcordial oppression, the intense sickness, the burning thirst, the extreme depression of the vital powers, and the chances of aggravating chronic disease, or of producing new organic lesion, in a great measure avoided; but it is rational to suppose that the consecutive fever will be rendered much milder, and that this is the case, is supported by my own experience, even though the remedy has not been applied earlier, indeed the fact is very evident. In an ordinary attack of cholera, much fluid is lost; and if the individual is so fortunate as to get out of the stage of collapse, if consecutive fever of typhoid type comes on, the system, left to its own resources to replace the lost serum, must be but ill fitted for the task, for the debility is extreme, absorption goes on slowly, the fever will be much aggravated by the irritation of internal congestion; local inflammation will thereby be produced, and the chance of recovery will be but small. Much of this evil is to be mitigated or entirely avoided by injection into the veins, of which circumstance I can adduce living instances; and where the patient, who had been injected, has sunk under organic disease, the usual marks of congestion are not perceptible.

The apparatus I have used, is Read's patent syringe, having a small silver tube attached to the extremity of the flexible injecting tube. The syringe must be quite perfect, so as to avoid the risk of injecting air; the saline fluid should never be injected oftener than *once* into the same orifice, and the vein should be treated with much delicacy to avoid phlebitis. The wound should be poulticed and carefully watched, if it does not heal by the first intention.

I am, Sir,
Your most obedient servant,
THOMAS LATTA, M.D.

――――

No. 2.

Letter from DR. LEWINS *to the Secretary of the Central Board of Health.*

Results of the Injection Practice in the Drummond-street Cholera Hospital, Edinburgh.

SIR,—You will receive from Dr. Latta the details of two or three cases treated by saline injections. We have both been so much occupied to-day, that we have not had leisure to get our communications ready to be sent in the same envelope. We steal an hour from the time usually allotted for rest to write to you. In case Dr. Latta should omit to mention the circumstance, I beg to mention that his patient, Cousins, the woman who was injected to the amount of 376 ounces, and who promised to do well, for a considerable time, was a person of very dissipated habits.

In the Drummond-street Hospital six patients have been injected, and three recovered, or are recovering. In the three that died, extensive organic disease was found on dissection; disease that had existed previously to the attack of cholera.

I send herewith the report of two cases, treated by Dr. Craigie of this place, which, at my request, he furnished me to-day for the perusal of the Board.

I intended to have sent an account of an interesting fatal case, the only one in which the venous injection may be said to have fairly failed where it was fairly used; that I shall do to-morrow. I have the honour to be, Sir, your most obedient servant,
ROBERT LEWINS, M.D.
Leith, May 27th.

――――

No. 3.

Details of Two Cases of Malignant Cholera treated by Venous injection, by DR. CRAIGIE, *of Leith.*

No. 1. *Case successful.* 15 *lbs. injected at intervals in nine hours.*—Martha Smith, aged 38, a noted drunkard, thin and debilitated, in sixth month of pregnancy, admitted into the hospital at 8 p.m., May 16th, 1832.

It appears she had had vomiting and purging since Sunday morning, 12th inst. Cramps came on about four hours ago in both legs; great evacuations both upwards and downwards like dirty water. The countenance is now collapsed; eyes sunk; tongue cold; pulse imperceptible at wrists; very small in brachial artery; 124.

℞ *Muriat. sodæ* ʒij;
Carbon. sodæ ʒi;
Aq. calid. ℔vj. *solve.* Ft. *Enema statim injiciend.*

Sinapisms to spine and epigastrium; let her be placed on heated tin mattress.

its race without being endowed with this common property of feeling,—without being capable of receiving some sensible impressions from the contact of surrounding objects. The effect of those impressions in exciting perceptions of touch, must greatly depend upon the delicate structure and sensibility of the parts with which the external objects come into contact; so that in the naked and soft forms of invertebrated animals we must naturally expect, ceteris paribus, the sense of touch to be most general and most acute, and those which have the surface of their bodies covered with dense substances will necessarily possess a much less acute sense of touch, though their other organs of sense may enable them, by the delicate sensibility which they retain, to provide for all their necessary wants. Indeed we observe, even from the polygastric animalcules, that organs are developed at the anterior part of the body which appear to be adapted to communicate sensations corresponding with those of touch in the higher animals. They have long *cilia* almost already developed into tentacula, and those *tentacula* so common in the class of zoophytes appear to be endowed with great delicacy of feeling. These fleshy and sensitive tentacula and tubular feet of the radiated animals continue up through many of the succeeding classes of animals, becoming jointed in the articulated classes, where they form *palpi* and *antennæ*; and in the soft molluscous classes they again assume the form and name of *tentacula*,—soft, sensitive, and fleshy, without any jointed appearance. We observe remnants of those sensitive organs even in the class of fishes in the form of processes or filaments still disposed as organs of touch around the mouth.

In the vertebrated classes of animals we observe a great difference in the sensibility and exposure of the exterior surface of the body to impressions of touch. Many fishes and higher animals are covered with dense scales, which must deaden the general sense of touch over the surface of their bodies. Other fishes have the lower part of the head, the lower part of the abdomen, the circumference of the mouth, and other exposed parts, covered with a naked, delicate, and soft integument, which will compensate for the want of development of the arms and hands as organs of touch. But in the land amphibious animals, and in all the higher vertebrata, we observe the anterior extremities to become more delicately organized, and fit for communicating delicate impressions of the forms, densities, temperature, and other physical qualities of external bodies; and in proportion to the high nervous sensibility, the

vascularity, the flexibility, and the softness of the hands and other external cutaneous parts, will that common sense of of touch become increased as we pass up through the vertebrated classes to man, who surpasses all inferior animals in the exquisite and equal development of all his organs of sense, and in the perfection of all those higher organs of relation by which animals are more immediately connected with outward nature.

USE OF

PLASTER OF PARIS

IN THE

TREATMENT OF FRACTURES.

To the Editor of THE LANCET.

SIR,—The extensive circulation which your Journal so deservedly enjoys, affords us the best means of communicating to the medical profession a mode of treating simple oblique fractures (particularly those of the thigh), which, although not unknown, has never hitherto been brought into practice. The mode of treatment alluded to is, that of confining the limb by means of plaster of Paris. A recent successful case induces us to submit the subject to the consideration of the profession, at the same time anticipating a difference of opinion as to the expediency of the plan. We recollect, indeed, reading an article, some time since, in one of the medical periodicals, in which a method, proposed for treating fractures with plaster of Paris, was strongly condemned by the editor as *impracticable* and *injudicious*; but as we have heard Baron Larrey say, that during the Egyptian campaigns of Napoleon, he had with benefit employed it in small quantities round fractured limbs, with the idea of preventing irritation during travel, we considered it might be tried without incurring a charge of rashness.

—— *Tinney*, of Walton, near this place, æt. 19, of muscular habit, in the month of December last, broke the right femur, in the upper part of the lower third, by a fall from a cart. The patient was put in Mr. Amesbury's splints. On the following day, the limb being much shortened, gradual extension was made; the pulleys were used a second and third time during the five following days, notwithstanding which the ends of the bones could not be kept in apposition, from the extreme obliqueness of the fracture. Finding, on the sixth day after the accident, that it would be impossible to prevent a shortening of

WITH PLASTER OF PARIS.   517

the limb, we determined on the application of the plaster of Paris. A deal box or trough was prepared, six inches in depth, and of sufficient length to take the whole of the limb from the pelvis, and in this box the leg was placed. A hole being made through the end of the box to admit of the pulleys, and the limb being strapped with soap-plaster from the heel to the nates, and well smeared with oil, extension was made from the foot, and the fractured bones were brought in apposition. The plaster of Paris, in a liquid state, was then poured into the box, until it covered the limb to the depth of an inch.

To guard against possibility of inconvenience from tension, as soon as the plaster on the surface had assumed such a consistence as to admit of its being divided by a spatula, a groove, an inch and a half in width, was made in it on the anterior part, extending the whole length of the limb, so that any change which took place might be distinctly observed. The plaster, of course, within five minutes from its first application, assumed a perfect consistence and hardness, and thus the limb remained during five weeks, at the end of which period the apparatus was removed, and the leg found to be perfectly straight and not shortened. The box and plaster mould we have sent to the College of Surgeons, where it may be seen. On inspection of the mould it will be obvious, that, if necessary, the plaster could have been at any moment removed from the limb without the slightest inconvenience to the patient, and in much less time than a bandage.

It has been suggested, that the heat given out by the plaster during the process would be so great as to prove inconvenient; this, however, is not the case. The only inconvenience which arose from the last time of reduction till the union of the fracture, was a little tenderness of the skin, just over the tendo achillis, produced by the web of the pulleys being moulded with the limb, which in future might be avoided by slackening or removing it after securing the thigh.

In consequence of the success which attended this experiment, we have since made several moulds, and are so thoroughly convinced of the superiority of the plan of treatment, that we should not hesitate to apply it to compound fractures. As these observations may, we hope, induce other surgeons to adopt this practice, a few hints will not, perhaps, be wholly undeserving of attention. By mixing *chalk* or *whiting* with plaster of Paris, the composition remains from four to ten minutes, according to the quantity of chalk used, as manageable with the trowel as common

mortar. The limb being placed on a board, and extension kept up gradually, till the fracture be reduced, a tolerable quantity of the plaster of Paris and whiting is to be placed far enough round the thigh to include the trochanter major, and to pass between the pubes and scrotum, the latter being protected by means of oiled lint. These two resisting points being secured, the condyles of the femur are to be managed in like manner; the operator may then cover the thigh as much as he pleases in a *simple* case, but in *compound* fracture the plaster should merely be applied so as to unite the points of resistance at the groin with those at the knee. As by possibility inflammation or erysipelas might supervene, the two bodies of plaster of Paris above and below, covering the limb, should be united with a greater or less quantity of the plaster, according to the injury done to the soft parts, so as to admit conveniently of the application of poultices or lotion in case of need.

In fractures of the upper third of the femur, if the bent position should be thought necessary, a single inclined plane will be found most easy to manage, by making extension from the *foot*, the pulleys being fastened to the ceiling; but should the comfort of the patient require relaxation of the flexors of the leg, the condyles might be secured first, and the knee bent afterwards. We have alluded more particularly to fractured *thighs*, as they are the most unmanageable, and most often the cause of shortened limbs.

Although the detail of this mode of treatment has necessarily encroached somewhat on your valuable columns, we hope it will not be thereby inferred, that in its application it is attended with more than ordinary trouble to the operator; on the contrary whilst the benefit to the patient is so great the surgeon will not find it consume more of his time than the ordinary and more familiar method. This remark arises from the desire we feel to obviate every objection which might be urged against the remedy; but we are confident that the members of our profession are far too alive to the calls of suffering humanity, to allow personal inconvenience to influence them in their selection of a remedy.

Before concluding, we may express our opinion that, in fractures of the neck of the thigh bone, motion of the limb would be more readily prevented by confining both trochanters by means of the plaster of Paris than by any other plan hitherto adopted.

We are, Sir, your obedient servants,
BOND AND GALE, Surgeons.
Glastonbury, Somersetshire.

and are carried out of the intestinal tube along with the fecal matter.

It must be admitted, that a certain degree of difficulty is experienced in performing the second part of the operation, namely, in sheathing the end of the elder tube provided with threads, in the end of the intestine held open by the assistant. The membranes double upon themselves, forming a constant obstacle to the introduction (*invagination*) of the tube. This operation upon the dead subject offers flattering results, inasmuch as the intestines, under such circumstances, do not contract. To obviate this difficulty, Dr. Alexander Thomson has devised the following method, proposed by him at a late sitting of the "Anatomical School of the Hospitals of Paris," but which has as yet only been applied upon the dead subject.

M. Amussat's instrument, consisting of one piece, is, according to Dr. Thomson's suggestions, divided into two portions. The two cones are moveable one upon the other, and are united by means of an ebony tube three or four lines in length. The base of each tube is separated by a groove two lines in depth, and a line and a half wide. Besides, each base is hollowed. When united, they present a ridge of two or three lines.

The moveable cone is pierced with two holes at its border, for allowing the introduction of two ligatures. Two other waxed threads pass through the substance of the tube, upon which the other cone is fixed. The end of the groove formed by the union of the two cones is made somewhat rough, for the purpose of keeping a more firm hold upon the intestine. The moveable cone is fixed upon a handle, which extends about three quarters of an inch beyond its truncated extremity. At the middle of the handle is a small permanent stud, for the purpose of holding the ligatures which are coiled around it. The extremity of the handle serves to open a free passage into the intestine, until it has reached two-thirds of an inch beyond the base of the cone fixed upon the said handle. Close to the stud are two steel arms, furnished with hooks and springs for securing the intestine. A ligature is then placed over the groove in the base of the cone, and it is tightened so as to produce strangulation of the intestine, the operator cutting off a portion of the extremity beyond the constricted part. The two ligatures are then loosened, by which the cone is set at liberty, a needle is put on each, and they are passed through the strangulated portion of intestine. The same method having been adopted with respect to the other end of the intestine, the two cones are then united in such a way that the ligatures applied for fixing them may be in immediate contact. They are tied, and cut off near the knots, and the intestine is returned into the abdomen.

In the thesis presented to the Faculty of Paris this year by M. Choisy, previously to taking out his diploma, he describes a method of suture which does not differ from that of his instructor M. Amussat.

The substitution of a tube of elder wood is not a new invention, it is mentioned in the writings of Fabricius de Aquapendente. * Guy de Chaulac says, "Some surgeons place a tube of elder in the intestine, to prevent the feces from rotting the suture." He was quite unconcerned with regard to the expulsion of the tube, since he adds at the conclusion of the same page,† "For nature, awake to the necessity of removing those foreign bodies, expels them from the suture, and carries them out of the intestinal canal."

However, the mode of using the elder tube adopted by M. Amussat, resembles in no respect that of the ancients, and must be considered as a very ingenious application of the material, originating with that skilful surgeon.

Paris, Oct. 1834.

ON THE

NUMERICAL METHOD

OF ARRANGING THE

PHENOMENA OF DISEASES.

By E. Ch. A. Louis, *M.D., Phys. to the Hosp. of La Pitie, Paris.*‡

To know with precision the value of each symptom of a disease, we ought in the first place to seek for the proportion of cases in which it is observed, and this is to be done by *counting*. For the words "more or less," so often employed, and now consecrated by custom, signify, it will be agreed, either nothing, or very little. When it is said, for instance, that a symptom is frequently observed in a disease, does that mean that it is observed twenty, thirty, forty, sixty, or eighty times in a hundred? Evidently it is uncertain; an expression is used, the meaning of which is not known, and which it is not possible to replace by one more exact, except by the method of counting. Thus, it was

---

* Opera Chirurgica, p. 224, lib. ii.
† La Grande Chirurgie composée en 1363, edit. 1632, p. 306.
‡ See page 221.

THE PHENOMENA OF DISEASES.   205

known that diarrhœa is common during the course, or at the commencement, of typhoid fevers, but to ascertain the real meaning of this word " common," it was necessary to *count;* and it is only after having done so, after having ascertained that diarrhœa occurs in two thirds of the cases, at their commencement, that this symptom has become of great importance in the history, and especially in the diagnosis, of fevers. The same may be said of the rose-coloured lenticular spots observed in the same disease; little notice was taken of them in its history, until after it was ascertained that they appeared almost constantly, so as to be wanting 'scarcely twice in a hundred cases.' So that if one of these two symptoms, the diarrhœa or the typhoid maculæ, were wanting at the commencement, or in the course of an affection which should otherwise in some points resemble typhus fever without having the characteristic symptoms of any other disease, we should almost entirely lay aside the idea of typhus.

If there exists an exception to a general law, the most general possible, under the point of view which we are now considering, I mean the just appreciation of the symptoms, how are we to know it except by means of the numerical method? Rusty, viscous, semitransparent sputa form one of the most remarkable and constant symptoms of pneumonia, and are very rarely absent, at least when the disease attacks a person previously in good health, and of mature years. Still this symptom has been absent, and in the circumstances just indicated; but in what proportion of cases? What is the value of this exception? It is not known; the numerical method has not extended so far.

Those who are inclined to oppose the numerical method, for this method has its adversaries, and among them men of real merit, will perhaps object that the proportion of cases in which the same symptom is observed, is not the same in sporadic and in epidemic cases of disease; that, thus, to count, is a thing at least useless. It may happen, indeed, that the proportion is not the same in epidemic diseases and in those which are not so; but that can only be rigorously proved by the numerical method: and the objection supposed, would be one of the most conclusive arguments in its favour. It is on purpose that we may know the difference which may exist between epidemic cases, and the same disease developed sporadically, that the numerical method is necessary. For, to speak only of the symptoms, the difference can only be in their degree of violence, or in the proportion of cases in which they show themselves; in fact, in their *more or less* frequent appearance: and wherever we have to do with the words *more or less*, to count is indispensable.

Suppose that this task had been completed for all diseases; that we had for each of them the proportion of cases in which a symptom presents itself, with the modifications produced by age, sex, strength or weakness; that we knew also in what proportion of cases this symptom is slight or severe under the circumstances mentioned, (the disease being sporadic or epidemic,) to what a height would pathology be raised, as regards our knowledge of symptoms!

And it is not merely to the study of symptoms that the numerical method is applicable; the other points in the history of diseases are equally capable of being enlightened by it; I mean their progress, their termination, and the causes which preside over their development.

It is known beyond a doubt, that peripneumony is more frequent than nephritis, but in what proportion is the difference? We are ignorant. Peripneumony and typhoid fever are frequent; but is one more frequent than the other, and if so, in what proportion? Inflammation of the various serous membranes is not rare, but what difference is there between them in this respect? We know not: for to obtain this knowledge it would be necessary to enumerate all the facts of the same sort which are well authenticated; and this has not been done. Nevertheless, this knowledge would not be superfluous, since it would indicate what difference there is between issues which appear in all respects similar; it would probably put an end to much prejudice, and would show the degree of connexion which exists between diseases of the viscera, of whatever nature they may be, and those of the serous membranes which cover them.

The numerical method is not less useful in the research of the causes of diseases, whether in giving us the means of recognising serious errors, or in enabling us to avoid them. Thus, it is an opinion still very generally prevailing, that tubercles in the lungs are the result of inflammation of the bronchi, or of the parenchyma of the organ in which they are disseminated. But ought not that physician to feel himself much shaken in his opinion, who learns that bronchitis, at least in the severe form, is more frequent in the male than in the female, in the proportion of three to one; that it is the same with peripneumony; whilst phthisis, on the contrary, is less frequent in the male than in the female? Similar remarks may be naturally applied to cancer.

This disease can scarcely be considered as a termination or consequence of inflammation, by him who knows, from the inspection of a great number of bodies, that whilst pulmonary and intestinal inflammations are the most frequent, cancer appears most commonly in the uterus and stomach; that the liver is next in frequency, and then at a considerable distance, the lungs and kidneys;* that of eight hundred subjects whose viscera have been examined with care, only two examples of cancer of the rectum have been found, and not a single case of that affection in the small intestine.

Whether then we wish to appreciate the value of symptoms, to know the progress and duration of diseases, to assign their degree of gravity, their relative frequency, the influence of medical constitutions upon their development, to enlighten ourselves as to the value of therapeutical agents, or the causes of disease, it is indispensable to count. The only reproach which can be made to the *numerical method*, if we may give that name to the assistance which addition lends to medicine, is, that it offers real difficulties in its execution. For, on the one hand, it neither can nor ought to be applied to any other than exact observations, and these are not common; and, on the other hand, this method requires much more labour and time than the most distinguished men of our profession can dedicate to it. But what signifies this reproach, except that the research of truth requires much labour, and is beset with difficulty?

Some practitioners, however, and among them men recommendable by the solidity of their understanding, think that medicine, and especially practical medicine, is not susceptible of that degree of certainty to which, it appears to me, a profound study of facts would tend to elevate it; and, perhaps, these practitioners, if they cast their eyes on this little essay, will say, " This science, which you are rendering so sure and so firm with your figures, will abandon you at the bedside of the patient." Without doubt, the science will abandon the practitioner at the bedside, if he make a bad application of it; but how can the science desert him if he employ it with discernment, I mean the *true* science, which is only a summary of particular facts ? Thus, for example, a case of pneumonia presents itself; a physician is called in, who prescribes that treatment which the numerical method has shown him to be most efficacious in the affection at present under his observation. Nevertheless this patient dies, contrary to the first prognosis. Can it be said that the science has abandoned the physician? By no means. The science has demonstrated, that in cases of this disease, and under circumstances nearly similar, the method employed is the best, that it succeeds ten times out of eleven; whilst the most efficacious of the other methods succeeds only nine times out of eleven; so that it was right to prefer the first. But the science has not yet taught us, and probably never will teach us, to designate beforehand, almost at the commencement of the disease, the subject who is to sink under it. The science then has not abandoned the physician : it is only a little in advance of his art; and that is all which the supposed fact proves. But, supported upon science thus constructed, the art will, assuredly, advance with security; the physician, after having carefully studied the circumstances in which a patient is placed, will act with confidence, and will not change his method of treatment, unless he finds that that which hitherto he was bound to consider the best, is really inferior to another, not less conscientiously studied than the first.

MERCURIAL INUNCTION IN ERYSIPELAS.—Lately I have tried the plan of mercurial inunction, as recommended in THE LANCET of July 14th, 1832, p. 480, and of Sept. 1834, p. 739, and upon the whole am led to consider that it is a most valuable application in this disease. To ascertain as much as was possible the value of this mode of treatment, it has been employed nearly to the exclusion of other remedies, the bowels being merely regulated, and the diet attended to. In two cases where there was much sinking, tonics and stimulants were combined; in most of the cases, mercury applied in this manner affected the mouth. Understanding that this plan had been used in Mercer's Hospital, I applied to Mr. Reid for information, and was favoured with the following communication :—" It certainly would appear to me from a number of instances to have considerable power in limiting the extent, and generally checking the progress, of the disorder; two, three, or four applications have usually sufficed."—*Dr. M'Dowel in Dublin Med. Journ.* Nov. 1834.

---

* We live in a day in which " exact observation " is, indeed, wanting, when, for instance, the subjoined passage from the journal of a contemporary, dated eighteen months since, may be placed in juxta-position with the above statement :—" It is a question if real scirrhous disease has ever been found in the liver ; and if we abide by the definition of scirrhus, as it occurs in the breast and uterus, we shall probably be forced to acknowledge that this morbid change of structure is seldom or never seen in parenchymatous viscera."—REV.

456   CATALEPSY.—KINNERTON-STREET SCHOOL.

not confer the power of granting licenses to practise medicine.

One wing of the North London Hospital is to be erected immediately, the late subscriptions being large enough to cover the expense. Although we do not regard great hospitals as essential to the perfection of medical education, yet the attendance of medical students is likely to be so abundant at this Institution, that we are glad at the increased means of judiciously distributing the attention of pupils in the wards.

THE case of catalepsy recorded (to such extent as it has as yet advanced) at page 413 of this week's LANCET, is one of a most singular character, from its complications with pregnancy, jactitation, and a heaving of the chest and abdomen, the protraction of the fits, and the long sustentation of nutrition through the agency of the stomach pump. We should have been glad if Dr. HANNAY had stated at the close of his remarks, his impressions as to the period of conception. The patient was married in October 1833, was attended by a medical practitioner under the expectation of a speedy delivery in the middle of June 1834, and bore a healthy child on the 23rd day of the month of October following. At the date of the last report of the progress of the case, the catalepsy still persisted, though it was "less frequent; the jactitation, however, being almost constant."

INTERCEPTED LETTERS.

"DEAR SIR BENJAMIN,—It grieves me most exceedingly that an express from Kensington Palace will unavoidably prevent me from enjoying the high gratification I had anticipated in being present at the stripping of the mummy. Your talents have contrived a most admirable occasion for opening your new School of Medicine. It would afford me excessive pleasure if you could order any one of the best writers on our Journal to draw up an account of the interesting phenomena, whether vital or physical, which the dissection of the mummy may bring to light, that I may have it read at the next College meeting, for we run very short of papers. Excuse this hasty note, though I must find time and room to beg that you will accept of my warm and hearty congratulations and good wishes for the success of your new building. I am the more earnest in the expression of these wishes, because I am fully aware of the high feelings which have caused you to embark in so expensive, thankless, and I fear profitless a speculation, and of the difficulties which men, who are eager in the diffusion of knowledge, like yourself, have in realizing anything like a moderate pecuniary recompense for all their outlay and their numerous cares. Whatever gratification the establishment of this new company may afford you as a scientific man, I much fear that you will not realize one per cent for your money.

"Ever Yours,   H. H.

"May Fair, Wednesday morning.

"P.S. I shall take occasion to congratulate the public and the profession generally on the happy prospect of your being induced to resume your valuable lectures, which you had, unfortunately for medical science, resigned for some years past; lectures which for the perspicuity and elegance of their composition, their profound research, the originality of their views, their acumen, the eloquence of their delivery, their everything else in short, which is desirable in lectures,—have never been surpassed, seldom equalled."

"DEAR DR. TURNER,—Although it is probable that Sir Benjamin has sent you an invitation to attend the opening of a mummy at his new building, it is my wish that none of the Fellows of our College should attend, as I have just learned, for certain, what indeed I had suspected was true, namely, that it is one of the little baronet's jobs, and that nobody will be present but the members of his own clique at *St. George's,* a herd of subordinates, his immediate dependants, along, no doubt, with some of the tag-rag of the licentiates.

You know my dislike of every species of quackery, and how deeply its indulgence affects the respectability of our profession; and had Sir BENJAMIN only come openly forward to revenge the wrongs done to him by his opponent at the hospital, and manfully declared himself the projector, proprietor, and upholder of a new school, how much more respectable would it have been than working like a mole under ground! He might then have got some of the respectable portion of his brethren to have joined him, in place of the lame and decrepid coadjutors on whom he must now rely. Indeed, it always has appeared to me to be a mad scheme altogether, as there is no opening for anything like a new establishment. The number of pupils they were able to congregate when they were all pulling in the same boat, was too small to enable them to make, as Mr. GUTHRIE said, a commonly decent appearance in society. What will it be when split in two?

"Ever yours,   H."
"May-fair, June 30th."

———

"DEAR SIR HENRY,—I regret that I did not receive your letter in time to prevent me from attending the opening of the mummy in Kinnerton-street. Except myself there was scarcely a respectable and independent member of the profession present; but I do not regret going, as it turned out to be a fine intellectual comedy. You would notice in your card of invitation, that the mummy was presented to the school by no less a man than Sir FREDERICK FITZCLARENCE, but on inquiring I found that, like BRODIE's other trickeries, it had not been presented to the school at all, but that Lord FITZ had given it to BOBBY KEATE ages ago. This chicanery is, therefore, a bad start.   T."

———

REMUNERATION OF MEDICAL MEN AT INQUESTS.

———

To the Editor of THE LANCET.

SIR,—The following is a copy of a petition which is to be presented to the House of Commons against a clause in the Coroner's Bill, which it is believed would tend to the injury of medical practitioners.

I am, Sir, your obedient servant,
J. M. PENMAN.

Sunderland, 29 June, 1835.

———

To the Honourable the Commons of the United Kingdom of Great Britain and Ireland in Parliament assembled.

The Humble Petition of the undersigned Members of the Medical Profession resident in the borough of Sunderland,

Sheweth,—That your petitioners have read with regret the twelfth clause of the Coroner's Bill now before your Honourable House, which clause limits the remuneration of medical men to one pound, for performing a post-mortem examination, and denies them any remuneration for their professional evidence.

That the performance of post-mortem examinations is in many cases attended with great danger to health and life (and several of your petitioners have suffered severely from making such examinations), and after exhumation the service is peculiarly unpleasant and disgusting.

That with regard to professional evidence, not connected with post-mortem examinations, your petitioners beg to remind your Honourable House, that it is the peculiar lot of medical men to be immediately summoned on the occurrence of accidents and sudden illness (a refusal to accede to which summons would be stigmatized as the grossest inhumanity), for which, if the cases terminate fatally, they seldom receive any reward; whilst by this very compliance with the demands of humanity, they become liable to be called upon for further sacrifices of their time in giving unremunerated professional evidence at a coroner's inquest; that these duties press much more heavily on medical men than the simple office of witness does on other classes of the community. Your petitioners further submit, that there is a wide distinction between the evidence and opinions of professional men on the one hand, and the mere casual evidence of bystanding citizens on the other; that although the latter are not rewarded for their casual evidence, it is but right that medical men, whose education and skill (like those of lawyers) are intended for their maintenance, should be remunerated when professionally employed and consulted.

That, lastly, it appears from the above-mentioned clause, that any medical man is liable, at the summons of a coroner, to be dragged from his home, however inconvenient it may be, compelled to perform an examination, however unpleasant or dangerous, and then to give his professional opinion on the case; and that independently of the inadequate remuneration, the compulsion to qualify himself as a witness in the first instance, in order to give evidence, is an unparalleled breach of the liberty of the subject.

Your petitioners, therefore, humbly submit the propriety of fixing one pound as the minimum instead of the maximum fee for post-mortem examinations; to admit of increase at the discretion of the coroner, according to the circumstances of the case; and that in all cases where medical men are summoned to give professional evidence at a coroner's inquest, whether or not they may have made a post-mortem examination, their professional services shall be recompensed.

And your petitioners will ever pray, &c.
(Signed by twenty-nine physicians and surgeons.)

———

602   MR. HYTCH ON PUBLIC BATHS.

phers whose wisdom would have been much better employed in the observation of facts and natural analogies.

In considering the whole animal kingdom, from the aquatic animalcules up to intellectual men, we are convinced that the various yet regular degrees of perfection and capability of enjoyment with which they are endowed, result from a corresponding degree of development of one great system—the nervous. Wherever we find a marked accession of strength, of complicated mechanical arrangement, of sensibility to external impressions, and an incipient power of judgment (or instinct), in any family, or individual animal,—there do we as certainly discover an increase of nervous matter, and a more complex and artificial arrangement of its parts.

In the higher vertebrata we have at last a docility, and an absence of *vegetative* existence—nay, in some instances a fondness for the society of man himself—all indicative of an intellect, and marked by a corresponding *cerebral* development, which is gradually rising to its perfection in the mind of man. I would particularly lay stress upon the development of cerebrum as the only true criterion of perfect existence; as upon this depends the validity (or otherwise) of the opinion to which I have come, viz., that the distinction of sex in the human family is originally made by the greater or less deposition of *cerebral* matter in the embryo.

Phrenologists have proved that the difference in character of man and woman is caused entirely by the development of the intellectual and emotional faculties— the latter being more considerable in women, and vice versâ—and that the more a man's *cerebellic* faculties are enlarged, the more does he partake of the warm feelings and passionate temperament of the female sex; who, on the other hand, when their *cerebral* organs happen to be most developed, gradually approach in intellectual power to man's standard; but at the same time lose the peculiarly feminine softness and grace of their less intellectual (cerebral) sisterhood.

From these and other considerations, it appears to me that we may conclude the difference in sex, so remarkable in the adult, to be owing to the original cerebral development, and consequently that every male is, during one period of foetal existence, in a state of cerebral development, which, if retarded, or only perfected, by the end of the period of gestation, would constitute a female—in other words that a female is an imperfect but a near approach to a male—and a necessary gradation between man and the higher classes of intellectual animals. We know that the foetus in utero proceeds, from a mere point of animal matter, through all the various degrees of existence enjoyed by lower animals, until it reaches at last that perfection of vitality which cannot exist but in a rarer medium than the liquor amnii, and that therefore it is thrust forth by the action of the uterus, induced probably by some change in the placental blood, acting as the proper stimulus to the nerves which supply the contracting muscular fibres of the uterus.

Also we know that until an advanced stage of foetal existence there is no apparent difference of sex; in fact, that this difference is not settled until a certain point of cerebral development is attained.

These two facts of the gradual perfection of existence in the foetus, and its late distinction into a settled sex, would seem to favour the opinion I have formed; and I doubt not that there may be many other circumstances which would bear upon the subject, which either I am ignorant of, or do not just now remember, but which may be familiar to some of your readers who are better able to form a correct decision on the matter than I am. I remain, Sir, your very obedient servant,

PHILONEURON.

Leeds, July 26, 1835.

PUBLIC BATHS.
——

To the Editor of THE LANCET.

SIR,—If there be any position in physical science which cannot be doubted, it is that which says that cleanliness is essential to the preservation of health. However other doctrines may be disputed, this cannot be; and whoever may have visited the habitations of the poor, must have seen that a large proportion of those diseases which are *supposed* to be incident to their station, have been caused by the neglect of personal cleanliness. I do not say that they do not wash their hands, faces, and feet, at stated times; but the doing of these things, and they are neglected by too many, does not constitute cleanliness; for a man may wash his face and hands, and keep them perfectly clean, whilst the other parts of his body are neglected altogether. This arises in a great degree from a dread of water, which many persons possess; but in most cases it arises from the want of public baths,—a want which has engaged the thoughts of many; but their advocacy has not produced the desired effect.

It may be said that there are several places open to the public, such as "the

Serpentine," &c., and that there are, I cannot deny. But it must be recollected that they are only open to the public at certain hours which are most inconvenient to the labouring population,—that the distance is too great for a working man to compass within his "spare hours," and that there are many disadvantages connected with them. The Serpentine, for instance, is above two miles from the most central part of London, and no one is allowed to enter the water before nine in the evening, or after eight in the morning. And besides this it is one of the most dangerous pieces of water with which I am acquainted; deep hollows are constantly entrapping him who stays near the shore; cold springs are so frequent, that the swimmer invariably becomes acquainted with the cramp, if he was never introduced to it before; and, in short, the constant attendance of the Humane Society's boats, shows that it is an unfit place for bathing. Such is the Serpentine, and the picture will be found to embody correctly the characteristics of all similar places.

There are, it is true, subscription baths where these evils do not exist; but to all who are acquainted with the wages of a working man, it must be evident that the charge for admittance is far beyond the limits of his purse. Were he to bathe each day, he would have to deduct seven shillings per week from his scanty earnings, and thus the benefit derived would be purchased at the expense of the necessaries of life.

I have thus shown the evils which are connected with the present bathing places, —evils which I think might be obviated by the establishment of Public Baths, through the aid afforded by a Parliamentary grant. The necessaries for bathing are all around us; even the most insulated manufacturing town is not without them, whilst in agricultural districts they abound. In London the expense would not be great. Much less than has been wasted on crude empirical schemes would serve to perpetuate them. Springs abound: the cost would consist in digging them and in building places to screen the bathers from public view. But if there be no probability of our obtaining a Parliamentary grant for this object,—and this question must be agitated before there will be,—a society might be established for this purpose. Of course a small charge might be made for bathing,—such as would meet the pockets of the people, and pay a small interest on the capital invested. That such a plan, if carried into effect, would pay, I have no doubt; all subscription baths have prospered,—why should not one established on a more popular scale succeed?

Much more might be said on this subject, but let what I have written suffice. The advantages of bathing are evident to all in a moral and physical view. The people are not a pigmy race. As fine forms and noble proportions are to be found amongst Englishmen, as ever Phidias modelled or Raphael drew; but how much more would this beauty be increased by personal cleanliness! True beauty of form may be preserved without, but it would be increased and rendered durable by bathing. I trust that these remarks will meet with your approval and support, and I remain, yours truly,

E. J. HYTCH.

New-court, Carey-street,
August, 1835.

REPLY OF

DR. FOSBROKE TO DR. COX

RESPECTING

COMA SOMNOLENTUM AND THE CAUSES OF LETHARGY.

SIR,—I find in THE LANCET, of June 27, some strictures on my case of lethargy (LANCET, June 13), by Dr. Cox, of Great Yarmouth.

Instead of controverting my opinions, he has misunderstood and misrepresented them; and, unless he had done so, there could not have been so much as an attempt at controversy. So plainly do the misunderstanding and misrepresentation speak for themselves, that I cannot help thinking he has not read what he is writing about, or read as

" —— swift Camilla scours the plain,
Flies o'er th' unbending corn, and skims along
    the main,"

with a rather dim and shadowy view of objects in his flight.

"England and France," says Voltaire, "went to war about a window." *Componere magna cum parvis*, I suppose two doctors must go to war about a word; for Dr. Cox seems to dwell much on the term "Coma Somnolentum," which I placed after the word Trance, with an [" or "] between, in the title only of the case, and nowhere else, as if I attached great importance to it; a point completely assumed by him, apparently to give full effect to a definition which he has quoted from Boerhaave, and of which he is enamoured. I will give,—-

I. *Boerhaave's definition.*—Coma Somnolentum, a disease in which *the eyes are*

264 TREATMENT OF THE STARVED CHILDREN IN THE

lithotrity, which succeeds when proper attention is paid to the evil disposition of the organs. It will then be well to make one or two trials, not injurious to cystotomy, if at last that be necessary.

In a fourth series we must place the cases for which lithotrity is generally contra-indicated; a single stone, but voluminous and hard, quantity of gravel of middling size, encysted stone, horny bladder, bloody, and very painful; prostate hypertrophied, painful, strong deviation of the urethra, persisting coarctation of long standing; urine purulent, ammoniacal; kidneys diseased, patient irritable, weak, and worn out.

Originally, paralysis and chronic catarrh of the bladder were looked on as contra-indications of lithotrity. Experience has proved that these are not of great consequence in lithotrity. Most calculous patients are affected with catarrh of the bladder, more or less intense. Instead of this complication being increased by lithotrity, it improves during the treatment, and generally disappears with the principal disease.

THE EVIDENCE

RELATING TO THE

MEDICAL RELIEF OF THE SICK POOR IN THE PAROCHIAL UNIONS,

GIVEN BEFORE THE

SELECT COMMITTEE OF THE HOUSE OF COMMONS, IN 1837.

TENTH DAY.

Wednesday, April 14.

Mr. FAZAKERLEY in the Chair.

MR. THOMAS BOURNE.

4324. *Examined by the* CHAIRMAN.] You are master of the Fareham workhouse?—Yes.

4328. In what state were the boys Cooke, Warren, and Withers, when they were sent to you?—They appeared healthy.

4330. Who is the medical man of that house?—Mr. John Blatherwick.

4332. Had those children dirty habits?—They commenced their dirty habits the first or second night after their admission.

4334. What observation did the medical man make upon hearing of that?—None in particular.

4336. What did you do to correct those habits?—Withheld part of the food.

4342. Were the visiting guardians made acquainted with the food being diminished?—Yes, they did not object to it. Half of the food for the day was stopped.

4348. Was any punishment also had recourse to?—The children were placed in the stocks frequently, both standing and sitting, and were kept in them from meal to meal, at the same time that their food was diminished, I believe. When the schoolmistress intimated to me that it did not appear to have any effect upon their filthy habits, I desired her to discontinue withholding their food, or any other punishment.

4359. How soon after they were in the house did the schoolmistress observe to you that their health appeared to decline?—I suppose a month.

4362. Did you communicate it to the medical officer?—Yes, he saw them; he did not direct anything; they were obliged to be put to bed in consequence of their dirty habits.

4365. Do you mean to say, that those circumstances being made known to the medical man he gave no directions as to their diet or general treatment?—None at all; he said he could give no sort of medicine for it. About ten days before they were removed to Droxford again they were, by the order of the medical man, removed to an out-building, in consequence of their filth, that it should not affect the health of other children.

4392. Are you aware of a resolution passed by the Board of Guardians on the subject, of this nature: "Fareham Union, 3rd of March, 1837. Resolved, that the master of the workhouse has not used a sound discretion in so extensively and repeatedly reducing the food of the three children in question, without specially reporting to the Board"?—Yes.

4400. *By* Mr. GORDON.] Were there many other children whose food was diminished?—Yes; it was very frequent for beds to be dirted and wet amongst so many children, and it was the custom to diminish the quantity of their food.

4402. Have you ever known illness produced from the food being diminished?—No; the visiting committee, or such part of it as did visit, were acquainted with the diminution, and they did not object to that mode of punishment.

4419. *By* Mr. WALTER.] Were those children beaten also?—I have done it once or twice with a small birch rod.

4420. Have any of the paupers beaten them?—I do not know.

4421. Recollect?—One of the girls, Susan Axford, had beaten one of them.

4428. Did any of the guardians ever see the children in the stocks?—Yes.

4429. Did the chaplain?—Yes. The chaplain is Sir Henry Thompson, Bart.

4437. Did the porter ever punish any children?—I complained of him to the Board for severity which I had heard it was general for him to use. He superintended, with his wife, in the school.

4442. Did he punish them severely?—Yes; he hurt their hands a good deal with his ferule.

4445. Two of those dirty boys slept together?—Yes, in a large bed; the other slept with his sister generally, who was 12 years of age, and she became very ill indeed in consequence of the filthy habits of her brother. She continued to sleep with him the whole time.

4466. Does the same medical gentleman now attend the workhouse as before?—Yes.

4639. Will you read the dietary of the workhouse for young children?—On the Sunday, children under nine years of age have three ounces of bread for breakfast, and one pint of gruel with milk; the dinner is one pint of meat soup, half a pound of potatoes, and three ounces of bread; supper, four ounces of bread, one ounce of cheese, or half an ounce of butter; Monday, for breakfast, five ounces of bread, one pint of gruel with milk; dinner, eight ounces of suet pudding; supper, five ounces of bread, one ounce of cheese, or half an ounce of butter.

4641. On Monday were these children almost always deprived of half that sustenance?—The Monday was the same as any other day; they were not punished more than twice or three times a week. (The dietary of the other days in the week was detailed by the witness.)

4643. By Mr. MILES.] Are the Committee to understand that, with this dietary those dirty children were punished frequently three times a week by half that allowance being stopped?—Yes.

4645. Give the number of ounces of food for the whole week?—286; nine ounces of which is meat; potatoes, 32 ounces; cheese, 7 ounces; pudding, 8 ounces; three pints of soup; and a pint of gruel every morning.

4689. By Mr. HARVEY.] You received back one-half of the allotted food of the diminished meals of children?—Yes.

4694. What is done with it?—It is put up for the next meal.

4696. Is it at the discretion of the mistress to withhold food as a punishment?—Yes, and also to put children in the stocks.

4717. You have stated that the children were taken to an outhouse; is it a room, or a stable, or a washhouse?—It is a plastered room on the other side of the yard, originally intended for a workshop, with a stone floor.

4720. Is there any fire-place in it?—No.

4722. At what period of the year were the children confined in that room?—In January.

4738. So you had three dirty boys in the same bed in a room where there were many other boys in beds who were of cleanly habits?—Yes.

4778. By Mr. HODGES.] After they were removed to that out-building, did they ever come out of it into the school?—No; they were confined in that place 10 days prior to their removal to Bishop Waltham.

4790. By Mr. WAKLEY.] What were the dirty habits of the children?—Wetting, as well as dirtying themselves, night and day; they would stand in the school and do it; they would not ask to go out.

4802. Did you ever know a young infant that was not dirty?—No.

4803. Do you consider that those children, with regard to information, were in a state of infancy?—No, I should hardly state so; they were big boys, breeched all three, and capable of knowing the calls of nature.

4805. When you found their habits so exceedingly dirty, were breeches still continued to them?—Yes.

4810. Had they but one suit of clothes?—Only one suit.

8411. So that, when they were not dirtying their clothes, they were kept in bed to dirty the bed?—When their clothes were dirty they had to be cleaned.

4813. How soon can a woman wash and dry a pair of trowsers?—In not less than four or five hours, at that time, and they were obliged to be dried in doors.

4814. Did the medical man, while they were in the out-building, prescribe no medicine for them, or attempt to explain the cause of the malady?—No.

4819. Did it not occur to you that there was something extraordinary in the constitution of their minds?—I considered that they were not so sharp as the generality of children.

4821. Were any means, therefore, used to give them information?—Not that I am aware of.

4831. Did it not appear to you that as you were weakening the body by continuing the short allowance, you were increasing the cause of the evil?—As soon as I found that it had no avail I ordered it to be discontinued.

4834. You say that the porter punished boys with much severity; has that porter been dismissed?—No.

4947. By Mr. WALTER.] Have you had much illness among the children?—Latterly we have had the typhus fever. Three died of the typhus.

4949. Has the itch been prevalent in the workhouse?—Since the removal of those children we discovered that there was a complaint; but the medical officer said it was not the itch, and it was allowed to go on for some time, and at last it was treated as the itch.

4950. By the CHAIRMAN.] Was it cured when treated as the itch?—It has been cured.

4951. By Mr. WALTER.] Does it exist now?—There are some cases now in the house.

4981. By Mr. CHICHESTER.] What salary has the medical officer?—I am not aware.

SMALL-POX PREVENTION BILL.   235

elementary form, would admit of any classification, combination, or tabular arrangement that might afterwards be deemed advisable. When the abstracts were made by the overseers, they could only be arranged in the form originally prescribed. When the errors of the last census, in the omission of the ages, and the failure of the return of occupations, were discovered, they could not be rectified, as all the original facts were destroyed, if they ever existed in a correct form.

We shall take an early opportunity of discussing, in detail, some of the more important points in the census; and in the machinery by which it is carried into effect. The division of the country into districts by the Registrar-General, and the existence of a class of officers who are habitually accustomed to record similar facts, as well as to communicate with a central office, present facilities which did not before exist.

SMALL-POX PREVENTION BILL,
FRAMED BY MR. WAKLEY.

THE following is a draught of a Bill which it is probable would have been proposed to the House of Commons on Monday evening last, May 4, if the discussion on the Bill which has been passed by the House of Lords had taken place at that time.

The motion for going into Committee on the Lords' Bill was postponed by Sir JAMES GRAHAM from Monday last to the 11th of May. Additional time, therefore, is afforded for the consideration of this highly-important national question. In inserting the communication of Mr. DODD, of Chichester, Mr. WAKLEY hopes that other practitioners who may have suggestions to offer on the same subject, will make them at a sufficiently early period to render the facts which they may contain available in the House of Commons at the proper period. The members of the profession will observe that the "Order for Vaccination" attached to this Bill has been constructed so as to render it ffectual, perhaps, for all the purposes for

which an Act of this kind could be framed. It is, for instance,

1st, An order for the vaccination of the person requiring that operation.

2nd, It shows the name, age, and residence of the person to be vaccinated, and the occupation of the parents.

3rd, Who was the vaccinator.

4th, When the operation was performed.

5th, Whether successfully or not.

6th, It contains the testimony of two witnesses to the correctness of the foregoing statements.

7th, It becomes, first of all, a voucher that the charge for the vaccination is due to the operator.

8th, And, afterwards, when in the possession of the parochial officer, it is a receipt (or voucher) for the payment of that charge.

9th, Placed on a file, these orders render unnecessary the trouble of keeping a book of account, or register, of the vaccinations.

10th, The order affords the opportunity of recording practical remarks on the case, for future collation and use.

The free distribution of these Orders among the medical men of every district of the kingdom, on the application of the medical practitioners themselves, and the prevention, by legal ordinance, of all inoculation for small-pox, will seem to secure, by the simplest means that can be devised, an effectual machinery for ensuring the general practice of vaccination throughout this country. Such a Bill will not be the less acceptable to the profession in consequence of its admitting of no interference whatever with the proposed arrangements, on the part of the Poor-Law Commissioners.

Respecting the reduction of the vast mass of important practical matter which the occasional contributions of even a few lines, only, from each vaccinator, in the last column of the "Order," must supply a form available for the purposes of science, we shall offer a few suggestions on another occasion. At present, the proper means do not exist. The entire medical institutions of the three kingdoms do not offer to notice one competent, efficient, trustworthy body in whose hands to confide materials of scientific value, the property of the nation, requiring industrious collation and analysis. A NATIONAL FACULTY OF MEDICINE would at once present a safe depository for such documents. Until possessing such an institution, the Vaccine Board may be made to serve the purpose.

A BILL
INTITULED
AN ACT TO EXTEND THE PRACTICE OF VACCINATION, AND TO PROHIBIT INOCULATION FOR THE SMALL-POX.

WHEREAS it is expedient to extend the Practice of Vaccination, and to prevent Inoculation for the Small-pox; Be it therefore enacted by the Queen's most excellent Majesty, by and with the consent of the Lords Spiritual and Temporal, and Commons in this present Parliament assembled, and by the authority of the same, that from and after the passing of this Act, every relieving officer, or clerk of any board of guardians, of any union in Great Britain and Ireland, and every overseer of any parish in England and Wales, wherein relief to the poor is not administered by guardians, shall, on application being made to him, deliver to the applicant an Order, framed according to the form contained in the Schedule hereunto annexed, for the vaccination of any person on whose account it may be required.

And be it further enacted, That from and after the passing of this Act, any person who shall inoculate with variolous matter for the purpose of causing the disease called small-pox, or shall use in any other manner any variolous matter for such purpose, in any part of Great Britain or Ireland, shall be liable to be summarily proceeded against and convicted before a justice of the peace, or a magistrate, on proof of such offence having been committed in England or Wales, or in case such offence shall have been committed in Ireland, then, before the magistrates assembled in petty sessions; and for every such offence such person shall be sentenced by such justice of the peace, or magistrate, or magistrates in petty sessions, as aforesaid, to be imprisoned in the common gaol, or House of Correction, for a term of not less than seven days, or for a longer term than three months, with or without hard labour.

And be it further enacted, That any legally qualified medical practitioner who may, by the authority of such Order, as aforesaid, vaccinate any person in any parish or union, he shall, on presenting the said order, within two calendar months from the date thereof, to the guardians or overseers of the unions or parishes, as aforesaid, be paid by the said guardians or overseers the sum stated in the Schedule, marked B, hereunto annexed. Provided always, That if the said Order be not presented within the period of two calendar months, as aforesaid, the payment of the sum stated shall not be made.

And be it further enacted, That the guardians of every union, and the overseers of every parish, as aforesaid, are hereby empowered and directed to pay such sums as are specified in any such Order, as aforesaid, out of the monies which are in their possession, from time to time, collected as rates for the relief of the poor. Provided always, That no such payment shall be made to any vaccinator who is not a legally-qualified medical practitioner, or to any person who holds the office of vaccinator under the National Vaccine Board.

And be it further enacted, That such guardians of any union, or overseers of any parish, as aforesaid, shall, in the month of January in every year, prepare from the Orders returned to him by vaccinators, a summary of the numbers of persons vaccinated, and of the ages of such persons, and of the instances in which the operation was unsuccessful, and shall forward the said summary to * * *

B.—The sum to be named in the Vaccination Order, shall not be less in amount than two shillings, or more than three shillings.

———————————

AT the Septenniary Festival of the LONDON HOSPITAL, in the Mile-end-road, held the other day at the London Tavern, the Duke of CAMBRIDGE in the chair, the subscriptions announced in the room, at the conclusion of the dinner, amounted, incredible as it may appear, to the noble and generous contribution of TEN THOUSAND AND NINE POUNDS, and, in addition to this enormous sum, as a general subscription to the hospital, it was announced that a sum of One Thousand Eight Hundred Pounds had just been subscribed, by gentlemen of the Jewish persuasion, towards the erection of an additional wing to the building, for the reception of destitute and afflicted Jews.

Facts of this description are calculated to raise the character of this nation above that of all others on the face of the globe. Where, beyond our own shores, could be found a company,—simply, almost, a private meeting,—at which a sum of ELEVEN THOUSAND EIGHT HUNDRED POUNDS would be subscribed in charity over the dinner table? Who shall say that England is poor, when such tales as these can be truly related?

724   PECULIAR INFANTILE CONVULSIONS.

laudanum and ammonia, were again administered, with the most beneficial effect; after
which he rested tolerably well. The dressings were this morning removed, and the
wound looks healthy; water-dressings and
bandage as before were applied. From this
period the sickness did not return. He took
porter, which was gradually increased to one
pint daily; had a nutritious diet; took aperient medicine when required, with ℥iss,
decoction of bark, and 20 drops of dilute
sulphuric acid, three times a-day; the wound
dressed as often as it was needful. He continued to get well gradually; and after ten
weeks the wound was quite healed, and his
general health much improved. It is now
more than nineteen months since the operation; the leg has continued quite well; and
he can walk eight miles without much inconvenience, which he frequently does. I
have seen him to-day; he still wears a bandage, which, he says, supports the leg. On
measuring it round the portion of fibula remaining, above, it is eleven inches; the sound
leg, at this point, measures also eleven inches; below, just above the ankle, each leg
measures the same, viz., seven inches; the
foot turns inwards a little, with a slight inclination upwards.

The dry diseased bone removed, in length
measures eight and a half inches, and round
its widest circumference four inches and
three-quarters. Its weight Troy is four
ounces two drachms; a healthy fibula weighs
about one ounce six drachms. The length of
the surface of attachment to the tibia is one
inch and three-quarters; its breadth at its
widest part three-quarters of an inch.
Above this surface is a cavity large enough
to hold a small nutmeg, rough at the bottom,
which contained a very small portion (not
more than ten grains in weight) of detached
carious bone; this cavity communicated
with a canal, extending three inches down
the centre of the bone, somewhat larger than
a goose-quill.

After the wound was healed, he wore, for
twelve months, a spring, which was fixed in
a strong boot, having a joint opposite the
outer ankle. This spring passed up close
to the leg; and was fastened above, just below the knee, with a strap. This supported
the leg, and, with the boot, obviated the
turning in of the foot, and enabled him to
work and walk much more comfortably.
He has left off this for some months.

This case is interesting, from the increased
size of the bone, the great density of its
structure, and firm attachment to the tibia;
the necessity of an operation, by affording
more permanent relief than had hitherto
been done, as well as the comparatively
trifling inconvenience experienced in walking
and using his leg, after the loss of so large
a portion of the fibula; also the distressing
sickness and extreme nervous exhaustion
following the operation, so effectually relieved, three successive nights, by the stimulating and opiate glysters, in conjunction
with the creosote draughts.
Dec. 5, 1840.

ON A PECULIAR FORM OF INFAN-
TILE CONVULSIONS.

To the Editor of THE LANCET.

SIR:—I beg, through your valuable and
extensively circulating Journal, to call the attention of the medical profession to a very
rare and singular species of convulsion peculiar to young children.

As the only case I have witnessed is in
my own child, I shall be very grateful to any
member of the profession who can give me
any information on the subject, either privately or through your excellent Publication.

The child is now near a year old; was a
remarkably fine, healthy child when born,
and continued to thrive till he was four
months old. It was at this time that I first
observed slight *bobbings* of the head forward,
which I then regarded as a trick, but were,
in fact, the first indications of disease; for
these *bobbings* increased in frequency, and
at length became so frequent and powerful,
as to cause a complete heaving of the head
forward towards his knees, and then immediately relaxing into the upright position,
something similar to the attacks of empros-
thotonos: these bowings and relaxings would
be repeated alternately at intervals of a few
seconds, and repeated from ten to twenty or
more times at each attack, which attack
would not continue more than two or three
minutes; he sometimes has two, three, or
more attacks in the day; they come on whether sitting or lying; just before they come
on he is all alive and in motion, making a
strange noise, and then all of a sudden down
goes his head and upwards his knees; he
then appears frightened and screams out: at
one time he lost flesh, looked pale and exhausted, but latterly he has regained his
good looks, and, independent of this affection, is a fine grown child, but he neither
possesses the intellectual vivacity or the
power of moving his limbs, of a child of
his age; he never cries at the time of the attacks, or smiles or takes any notice, but looks
placid and pitiful, yet his hearing and vision
are good; he has no power of holding himself upright or using his limbs, and his head
falls without support.

Although I have had an extensive practice
among women and children, and a large circle of medical friends, I have never heard or
witnessed a similar complaint before. The
view I took of it was that, most probably, it
depended on some irritation of the nervous
system from teething; and, as the child was
strong and vigorous, I commenced an active

treatment of leeches and cold applications to the head, repeated calomel purgatives, and the usual antiphlogistic treatment; the gums were lanced, and the child frequently put into warm baths. Notwithstanding a steady perseverance in this plan for three or four weeks, he got worse, the attacks being more numerous, to the amount of fifty or sixty in the course of a day. I then had recourse to sedatives, syrup of poppies, conium, and opium, without any relief: at seven months old he cut four teeth nearly altogether without any abatement of the symptoms, and, up to this period, he was supported solely at the breast; but now, at the eighth month, I had him weaned, as he had lost flesh and appeared worse; I then only gave him alteratives, and occasionally castor-oil. Finding no benefit from all that had been done, I took the child to London, and had a consultation with Sir Charles Clarke and Dr. Locock, both of whom recognised the complaint; the former, in all his extensive practice, had only seen four cases, and, from the peculiar bowing of the head, called it the "salaam convulsion;" the latter gentleman had only seen two cases; one was the child of a widow lady, it came on while she was in Italy, and, in her anxiety, she consulted the most eminent professional gentlemen of Naples, Rome, Florence, Genoa, and Paris, one of whom alone seemed to recognise the complaint. In another case, mercury, corrosive sublimate, opium, zinc, and the preparations of iron, were tried without the slightest advantage; and, about six months from the commencement of the symptoms, a new one was added; there began a loss of motion in the whole of the right side, and the child could scarcely use either arm, hand, or leg. Sir Astley Cooper saw the child in this state; he had never seen or heard of such a case, and gave it as his opinion, that "it either arose from disease of the brain and the child will not recover, or it proceeds merely from teething, and, when the child cuts all its teeth, may probably get well;" some time after, this child was suddenly seized with acute fever; the head became hot, and there were two remaining teeth pressing on the gums; the child was treated accordingly; leeches to the head, purged, and lowered; the gums were freely lanced; in a few days the teeth came through, and the child recovered, and from that time the convulsive movements never returned. Sir C. Clarke knows the result of only two of his cases: one perfectly recovered; the other became paralytic and idiotic; lived several years in that state, and died at the age of 17 years. I have heard of two other cases, which lived one to the age of 17, the other 19 years, idiotic, and then died. I wrote to Drs. Evanson and Maunsell, of Dublin; the former gentleman being in Italy, the latter very kindly replied, he had seen convulsive motions in one finger, arm, or leg, but had never witnessed it to the extent of my poor child. As there has been no opportunity of a post-mortem examination, the pathology of this singular disease is totally unknown.

Although this may be a very rare and singular affection, and only noticed by two of our most eminent physicians, I am, from all I have learnt, convinced that it is a disease (*sui generis*) which, from its infrequency, has escaped the attention of the profession. I therefore hope you will give it the fullest publicity, as this paper might rather be extended than curtailed. I am, Sir, one of your subscribers from the commencement, your faithful and obedient servant,

W. J. WEST.

Tunbridge, Jan. 26, 1841.

P.S.—In my own child's case, the bowing convulsions continued every day, without intermission, for seven months; he had then an interval of three days free; but, on the fourth day, the convulsions returned, with this difference, instead of bowing, he stretched out his arms, looked wild, seem to lose all animation, and appeared quite exhausted.

EPISTAXIS.

PLUGGING THE NARES WITH PUTTY.

To the Editor of THE LANCET.

SIR:—William Wells, a painter, 8, Little Exeter-street, Lisson-grove, aged 44, was seized about three, A.M., on Friday, the 8th, with epistaxis. The blood flowed four or five hours. Next day, about ten, A.M., it burst out again, and flowed freely for about twenty minutes. During Sunday it recurred and ceased several times. On Monday it burst out anew; and then Mr. Cunningham, surgeon, Salisbury-street, was called in, who plugged the nostrils with lint; and that not sufficing, bled him to about eight or ten ounces. On Tuesday, two, P.M., bursting out afresh, a surgeon from the Marylebone Infirmary attended him, and plugged the nostrils through the mouth. The bleeding was not arrested; the pressure and material used, no doubt, being insufficient. At eight, P.M., on Tuesday, I saw him. The blood had been flowing since two; he was faint, his lips pallid; he said he could scarcely see. An order had arrived to take him to the infirmary. He prayed not to be removed. He begged the plugs to be withdrawn; I did so; and the nostrils being freed from blood, as much as possible, the left one, from which it chiefly flowed, was plugged with glazier's putty, inclosed in linen, by forcing, twisting, and pressing it up. The same was done to the right nostril. The mouth and throat were then several times gargled with water. No trace of blood.

At eight, A.M., next morning, I was sent for. The putty had shrunk; the bleeding

LECTURES

ON

ORGANIC CHEMISTRY;

DELIVERED DURING THE WINTER SESSION, 1844, IN THE
UNIVERSITY OF GIESSEN.

BY

JUSTUS LIEBIG, M.D., PH.D., F.R.S., M.R.I.A.,

Professor of Chemistry in the University of Giessen.

THEORY OF ORGANIC RADICALS.
THEORY OF TYPES.

GENTLEMEN,—Organic chemistry, upon which we are now about to enter in a course of lectures, has been defined, THE CHEMISTRY OF COMPOUND, OR, ORGANIC RADICALS. I deem it, therefore, necessary in the first place, to give you an explanation of the term *organic radical*.

In comparing the number of compound bodies which come within the domain of inorganic chemistry with those belonging to organic chemistry, we are at once struck with their great disproportion, the number of the latter compounds being apparently infinitely great; at least, so far as our knowledge extends, it is illimitable. At the same time we observe that nearly all organic compounds consist of the same elements, and yet how astonishing is the variety of their properties!

By far the greater number of organic substances contain only three elements, namely, *oxygen, hydrogen*, and *carbon*. A less numerous class contain four elements having *nitrogen* added to the former three; and a few consist of five, namely, *carbon, hydrogen, nitrogen*, and *sulphur*.

We have, as I have just observed, in these combinations of the same elements, the greatest variety of chemical properties, and the question naturally arises, what is the *rationale* of this? How is it that compounds, consisting of the same elements, nay, many of them of the same elements in exactly the same relative proportions, can manifest such different chemical properties? *Sugar*, for example, is composed of carbon, hydrogen, and oxygen. *Acetic acid* is a compound of the same elements. It might be here alleged that the difference in the relative proportions in which carbon, hydrogen, and oxygen enter into and form sugar and acetic acid, causes the differences in their chemical properties. But there are many compound substances, consisting of the same elements, combined in precisely the same relative proportions, the chemical properties of which, nevertheless, manifest a most extraordinary variety. A solution of this difficulty is possible only by assuming that the chemical properties of organic compounds depend upon a certain peculiar arrangement of their ultimate particles or *atoms*.

What, we may here inquire, is the manner in which such an arrangement can be represented most intelligibly? The hypothesis assumed,—and which, indeed, forms the very foundation of organic chemistry,—is, that organic substances are combinations of simple bodies with compounds, in which the latter act the part of simple bodies, and that thus there exists no ternary or quarternary compound, but that those combinations, which are usually designated *ternary* or *quarternary*, are in reality *binary* compounds.

Thus we assume that all organic substances are either combinations of a simple body with a compound, the latter performing the part of a simple body, or combinations of two compound bodies, both functioning like simple bodies, or, finally, combinations of those double compounds with each other. To all such compound bodies as are found to act the part of a simple body the term *radical* is applied. In the course of these lectures I shall have frequent occasion to advert to examples illustrative of the existence and properties of such radicals. In this term we include substances which perform the part either of metalloids or of metals. CYANOGEN is an example of a radical acting as a metalloid. CACODYL is one of the most remarkable of those organic radicals

which function as metals. It was discovered and isolated a few years ago by Professor Bunsen, and is a compound of arsenic, carbon, and hydrogen. Cyanogen and cacodyl, therefore, may be taken as the representatives of the two classes of organic radicals; the former representing those acting as metalloids, the latter those acting as metals.

Now a great number of organic bodies consist of combinations of these radicals with oxygen, sulphur, &c. Thus, for instance, cyanogen combines with oxygen, what is the result of this combination? An acid is formed. Now, what is the characteristic property of metalloids in their combination with oxygen? We know that it is never to form bases with that element, not even in the lowest degree of oxidation, but invariably *acids*. The characteristic property of a metal, on the contrary, is (of course we disregard here the physical properties of metals altogether), that its lowest degree of oxidation does not form an acid, but a substance, the properties of which are quite opposite to acids, that is, are *basyle*.

CYANOGEN, therefore, with regard to its chemical character as a radical, belongs to the class of the metalloids.

CACODYL ETHYL, &c., according to these chemical properties, *i. e.* their properties they manifest in relation to other bodies, and inasmuch as in their lowest degree of oxidation they form *bases*, belong to the class of *metals*. In this manner we obtain a division of compound radicals into two great groups or classes, namely, 1st. Those which form with oxygen compounds acting as *acids*, and, 2nd, those forming with oxygen substances which perform the function of *bases*.

Again, compound radicals are capable of combining with each other; thus, for instance, cyanogen and cacodyl combine and form a body in which two compounds enact the part of simple substances.

If I were to present to you merely the relative proportions of the elements forming this double compound,

$$\begin{array}{lll} C_4 & H_6 & As_2 = \text{Cacodyl,} \\ C_2 & N & = \text{Cyanogen,} \end{array}$$

$$C_6 \quad H_6 \quad As_2 \quad N, \quad \text{Empirical formula of cyanide of cacodyl,}$$

you would not be able to deduce any conclusion as to its chemical constitution. But if you consider this compound as a combination of two radicals, you will at once clearly understand its character and relations. For when this substance is brought into contact with hydrochloric acid, it will form with it hydrocyanic acid and chloride of cacodyl, whilst, when brought into contact with potass, it will form cyanide of potassium and oxide of cacodyl,—

1. Cyanide of cacodyl : $Cy + Kd$

   Hydrochloric acid : $Cl + H$

2. Cyanide of cacodyl : $Cy + Kd$

   Potash : $O + K$

These illustrations will demonstrate to you the great advantages we derive from our theory of organic radicals. It enables us to form accurate notions respecting the properties and relations of organic compounds, to understand their true constitution, and to divide them into groups corresponding to the divisions of the substances met with in inorganic chemistry.

We assume, therefore, that organic substances are neither ternary nor quaternary compounds, but that they owe their origin to combinations either of simple with compound bodies, or of two compound bodies with each other (the compound bodies in all these cases acting as simple bodies), and, finally, to a union of these double compounds.

The aim of chemistry in investigating organic substances is to ascertain to which class of radicals, or of compound radicals, the substance, the nature and properties of which we are desirous to examine, belongs.

When comparing the composition of butyric acid, of acetic ether, of aldehyde, elaldehyde, and metaldehyde,

$$\begin{array}{llll} C_8 & H_8 & O_4 & \text{Butyric acid,} \\ C_8 & H_8 & O_4 & \text{Acetic ether,} \\ C_4 & H_4 & O_2 & \text{Aldehyde,} \\ C_4 & H_4 & O_2 & \text{Elaldehyde,} \\ C_4 & H_4 & O_2 & \text{Metaldehyde,} \end{array}$$

R 2

we find the relative proportion of atoms the same in all these five compounds, whilst the absolute number of atoms in butyric acid and acetic ether is double the number contained in the other three.

Now, in order to arrive at any intelligible idea respecting the manner in which the three elements carbon, hydrogen, and oxygen, are arranged in these bodies, possessed, as they are, of such different properties, or, to form a notion of their true constitution, it is not sufficient arbitrarily to assume any given arrangement of atoms; but we must study their reactions and examine carefully the phenomena which are manifested when they are brought into contact with other chemical compounds.

For example, butyric acid with hydrate of potass yields a crystalisable salt, and water is separated.

Acetic ether with the same substance decomposes into alcohol and acetate of potass.

Aldehyde is converted into a brown resin by hydrate of potass.

Metaldehyde and elaldehyde undergo no change when brought into contact with the same substance and under precisely the same circumstances which decompose aldehyde.

From these relations we conclude that we ought to describe butyric acid by the formula

$$C_8 \, H_6 \, O_3 + H \, O,$$

and acetic ether, as

$$C_4 \, H_3 \, O_3 + C_4 \, H_5 \, O;$$

and finding that aldehyde, when exposed to the air, absorbs two equivalents of oxygen, and becomes converted into acetic acid, we represent it by the formula

$$C_4 \, H_3 \, O + H \, O,$$

which expresses the lowest degree of oxidation of the radical of acetic acid.

Elaldehyde and metaldehyde have not hitherto been very minutely examined; we consider them isomeric bodies, and we express their composition by an empirical formula, which implies no theoretical notion as to their true chemical relations.

Further: if we compare the composition of oxalic acid with that of mellitic acid, we shall find that both contain the same quantity of oxygen, but different amounts of carbon. Assuming carbon to be the radical of the oxalic and mellitic acids, the following are the relative proportions of their elements.

$$C_2 \, O_3 = \text{anhydrous oxalic acid,}$$
$$C_4 \, O_3 = \text{anhydrous mellitic acid;}$$

thus, there is double the amount of the radical in the latter that there is in the former.

In like manner we may suppose that succinic acid contains the same radical (carbon and hydrogen) as formic acid, but double the quantity, whilst both contain the same proportion of oxygen; and, further, that succinic acid, malic acid, and racemic acid are compounds of the same radical in the same relative proportions, but with different proportions of oxygen.

$$(C_2 \, H) \, O_3 = \text{formic acid}$$
$$2 \, (C_2 \, H) \, O_3 = \text{succinic acid}$$
$$2 \, (C_2 \, H) \, O_4 = \text{malic acid}$$
$$2 \, (C_2 \, H) \, O_5 = \text{racemic acid.}$$

Moreover, many acids, in the form of hydrates, contain equal relative proportions of carbon and hydrogen, combined with the same proportion of oxygen.

$$C_4 \, H_4 \, O_4 = \text{acetic acid}$$
$$C_8 \, H_8 \, O_4 = \text{butyric acid}$$
$$C_{10} \, H_{10} \, O_4 = \text{valerianic acid}$$
$$C_{14} \, H_{14} \, O_4 = \text{œnanthic acid}$$
$$C_{24} \, H_{24} \, O_4 = \text{lauric acid}$$
$$C_{26} \, H_{26} \, O_4 = \text{cocinic acid}$$
$$C_{32} \, H_{32} \, O_4 = \text{ethalic acid}$$
$$C_{34} \, H_{34} \, O_4 = \text{margaric acid}$$

These acids unquestionably exhibit a certain analogy of composition; they differ from each other, inasmuch as some of them contain one, two, three, four, &c., more or less, equivalents of carbon and hydrogen than others, combined with exactly the same amount of oxygen.

We may readily apprehend how one acid may, by the loss of oxygen, be converted into another acid; and, as the combination of the same elements gives origin to atoms of a higher order, so the division of such complex atoms may be the means of forming more simple radicals.

When we have once admitted the existence of organic radicals it must follow as a necessary consequence that the decomposition of an organic substance, its resolution into other compound bodies, must tend to form new and, for the most part, less complex radicals than existed in the primary compound. Thus, as the decomposition of nitrate of ammonia at a high temperature gives rise to the formation of water and nitrous oxide,—two oxides of simple radicals,—so the decomposition of sugar by fermentation,—that is, the division of its constituent atoms, —gives rise to the formation of carbonic acid, on the one hand, and a hydrate of an organic oxide, the oxide that is, of a compound radical, on the other (namely, alcohol, which is hydrate of oxide of ethyle).

When the theory of organic radicals was first promulgated the question of their existence or non-existence in organic compounds gave rise to much discussion. The opponents of that theory exclaimed, " Exhibit to us your compound radicals and we will believe you." The isolation of every one of these radicals may, perhaps, be for ever impossible, but happily for the progress of science, it is quite unnecessary to isolate them in order to be sure of their existence. For theoretical purposes, if the existence of some of them is absolutely certain, and their chemical character and relations are known, we have abundant reason to conclude, when we find the same chemical character and relations manifested by other compounds, to conclude that they also possess an analogous chemical constitution, that they contain similar radicals, although we may not be able to isolate them. Those who have, upon this ground, denied their existence are chargeable with much inconsistency. Long before the *isolation* of aluminum, of magnesium, of yttrium, the existence of those metals was admitted as an undeniable fact.

No one entertains the slightest doubt of the existence of hyposulphurous acid, although no one can pretend to have seen that substance.

The multitude of organic acids in the state they are presumed to exist in their anhydrous salts, are at present mere conceptions, or, if the phraseology please you better, " compounds only created by the imagination."

By a close and satisfactory train of reasoning the existence of innumerable organic radicals, which have not hitherto been isolated, is rendered indisputable, whilst that of the anhydrous organic acids is really very problematical, as we must recollect that the so-called anhydrous acids want entirely the chemical characters attributed to them, and that most of them obtain their characteristic mode of action only after their combination with water or with its elements.

But that cyanogen possesses chemical characters precisely analogous to chlorine, that cacodyl must, according to its relations and properties, be considered a metal (if we were not able to decompose it into several elements), are facts which admit of no controversy. And when we meet with compounds which manifest properties and relations exactly analogous to those of the compounds of cyanogen and cacodyl, the inference is logically irresistible that they involve similar radicals, *i. e.* substances analogous to the known radicals in their chemical character, although no one has yet succeeded in isolating those theoretical radicals.

THEORY OF CHEMICAL TYPES.

In the oxidation of many organic compounds, or in their decomposition by chlorine, it frequently happens that one of their constituent elements, their *hydrogen*, is withdrawn from its combination, and is replaced by its equivalent amount of oxygen, of chlorine, or of hyponitric acid, so as to leave the substance possessed of the same number of equivalents which it had originally.

When this takes place, and the new product to which the decomposition has given birth, has a constitution analogous to the original compound, the latter is said to be the TYPE, since it represents, in the number and mode of arrangement of its elements, all the ensuing combinations.

In this manner certain classes of compound bodies may

THE LANCET, July 4, 1846.

LECTURES
ON THE
CONSTRUCTION AND GOVERNMENT
OF
LUNATIC ASYLUMS,
SUPPLEMENTARY TO CLINICAL LECTURES DELIVERED IN THE MIDDLESEX LUNATIC ASYLUM AT HANWELL.

BY JOHN CONOLLY, M.D.,
PHYSICIAN TO THE ASYLUM.

LECTURE I.

Site and general plan best suited to an asylum.—Errors of existing plans.—Arrangement of galleries and sleeping-rooms, and for the classification of the patients.—Inconveniences of large dormitories.

THE construction, arrangement, and government of asylums for the insane are subjects at this time so important, in consequence of the many new asylums about to be built in England and in Ireland, as well 'to deserve very careful consideration. They are also, like everything connected with asylums, of great consequence in relation to the treatment of the patients, and to their bodily as well as mental health. In offering some observations on these subjects, I would first remark, that a lunatic asylum is intended to be, not merely a place of security, but a place of cure, and that every case is curable or improvable up to a certain point. The cure of the curable, the improvement of the incurable, the comfort and happiness of all the patients, should steadily be kept in view by the architect, from the moment in which he commences his plan, and should be the constant guide of the governing bodies of asylums in every law and regulation which they make, and every resolution to which they come. At present this is very far from being the case.

As it is scarcely possible to construct a building intended for the residence of several hundreds of human beings, in a state of unsound mind, without finding that some inconveniences are inherent in its design, a new plan is at present generally adopted whenever a new asylum is built, and, generally, some new inconveniences are incurred. In building and in governing asylums, it is just the same, and partly from the same cause. Nothing appears to be viewed with so much dislike as an appeal to the authority of medical men who have lived in asylums, and among the insane, and who alone know what the insane require. So no two plans are alike, and almost all asylums are under regulations, several of which are injudicious, often interfering with the comfort of the officers, and sometimes directly impeding the improvement of the patients.

There are scarcely any works written expressly on this subject with which the English reader is familiar, or to which he can safely be referred. Several sound observations concerning the plan of asylums are, however, scattered through the writings of M. Esquirol, and many valuable remarks are published in Sir William Ellis's work on Insanity. A work, by the celebrated Dr. Jacobi, of Siegburg, entirely devoted to the construction and management of asylums, has also been translated into English by Mr. Kitching, under the superintendence of Mr. Tuke, of York, who, although not a medical man, is known all over the world as one of the most enlightened friends of the insane. Mr. Tuke has contributed to the translation a valuable preface, and notes. The work itself contains a great number of useful suggestions; but the reader should be cautioned that they were written thirteen years ago, and are all conformable to the old system of restraint and force, although tempered by the author's evident kindness of heart and sound understanding.

In most of the old asylums the architects appear to have had regard solely to the safe keeping of the inmates, and the buildings resemble prisons rather than hospitals for the cure of insanity. Even now, high and gloomy walls, narrow or inaccessible windows, heavy and immoveable tables and benches, and prison-regulations applied to the officers and attendants, attest the prevalence of mistaken and limited views. It appears to me, that not only should no general plan of a lunatic asylum be determined upon without being submitted to the consideration of a physician acquainted with the character, habits, and wants of the insane, but that no alteration should be made in an asylum without a reference to its resident medical officers. They alone at once see, or at least appear much to regard, the effects of rash and unadvised modifications. The building of a wall, the raising of a roof, the alteration of

a door or window, may materially affect the daily comfort of numerous patients. What an anxiety for mere safety has suggested, may at once be seen by them to be inconsistent with light and cheerfulness, and apparent conveniences will to them always appear objectionable if purchased by a diminution of proper ventilation and warmth.

The only way to avoid the defects apparent in so many existing asylums, without incurring new ones, would be, to take a careful preparatory survey of the character and requirements of the insane, so that a just estimate might be formed of what is generally desirable, and what is wanted in particular portions of the building only. To render this survey effective, the aid of medical men who have lived in asylums should be required at every step.

To escape an error against which all the world would cry out more than against any other, it must, however, be remembered, that the first thing demanded by society, when we undertake to relieve it of the presence of those who cannot be at large consistently with the safety of themselves or others, is their perfect security. But security does not require gloom, or a frightful apparatus. We require that the building should be on a healthy site, freely admitting light and air, and drainage. Space should be allowed for summer and winter exercise, for various employments, and for all the purposes of domestic economy. Warmth must be provided for during the winter, light for the winter evenings, coolness and shade in the summer. Separate wards and bed-rooms for the tranquil, for the sick, for the helpless, for the noisy, the unruly, or violent, and the dirty; a supply of water so copious, and a drainage so complete, that the baths, water-closets, and building in general, may always be kept perfectly clean and free from bad odours. There should be work-shops, and work-rooms, and school-rooms, separate from the wards, and cheerfully situated; a chapel, conveniently accessible from both sides of the asylum; as also a kitchen, a laundry, a bakehouse, a brewhouse, and rooms for stores, and all the requisites for gardening and farming; and also a surgery and all that is necessary for the medical staff. All these are indispensable in every large public asylum.

There can be no doubt that the best site for an asylum is a gentle eminence, of which the soil is naturally dry, and in a fertile and agreeable country, near enough to high roads, a railway, or a canal, and a town, to facilitate the supply of stores, and the occasional visits of the friends of the patients, and to diversify the scene without occasioning disturbance. A very elevated situation is often attended with the disadvantage of a deficient supply of water, and a difficulty in adding to the extent of the building. Mr. Tuke justly points out the ineligibility, in this climate, of a site level with a running stream; and observes, that a moderate elevation does not necessarily induce the evils of exposure and publicity, as supposed by Jacobi. Patients of all classes derive advantage from the circumstances of situation just mentioned; and if it is intended to receive patients of the educated classes into the house, it should unquestionably be situated amidst scenery calculated to give pleasure to such persons when of sane mind. Those whose faculties have never been educated derive little satisfaction from the loveliest aspects of Nature, and experience little emotion amidst the grandest. The sun rises and sets, the stars shine and fall, the hills reflect all the variety of brightness and shadow, of wildness and of verdure, and yet are scarcely noticed with more than mere passing attention. But when education has called the higher faculties into life, impressions upon them, even from external Nature, become powerful for good or ill, and in the case of a mind diseased, may act as remedies, or aggravate the malady. The celebrated Robert Hall attributed much of his unhappy state of mind, and even his temporary insanity, to a change of residence from a picturesque and interesting part of the country to a cheerless plain, of which the dulness, flatness, and invariable monotony, saddened his heart. Cowper, all of whose writings indicate exquisite sympathy with the sights and sounds of common rural retirement, and who, like Robert Hall, was occasionally afflicted with insanity, felt awe-struck and overwhelmed when visiting a friend whose house was situated among lofty hills covered with trees. There are few persons of any degree of education, much of whose daily and habitual pleasure does not arise from the view of the objects around them; and the first desire of all who can quit the crowd and toil of business, is to be where they can enjoy "a prospect," or to surround their houses with shrubs and flowers. Even in the populous city, the pent-up artizan has a bird, to sing to him whilst he works, and a few flowers, which he cultivates with care. We must not neglect such instincts and capacities if we profess to cure the

B

diseased mind. Our practice can only securely rest on the consideration of everything, great or little, capable of affecting the mind beneficially or hurtfully.

The more experience I have of the duties to be performed in a lunatic asylum, the more strongly I become impressed with the inconveniences attending any part of the building consisting of more than two stories. The third story is difficult of access and egress for the patients; it is unavoidably dull, and it becomes almost unavoidably neglected. It is equally opposed to good classification and to proper superintendence; and it causes too many insane persons to be included on the same measure of ground, rendering ventilation more difficult, and decreasing the healthiness of the establishment. There should be no inhabited attics; no bedrooms or dormitories in the basement of the building. All the rooms should be above ground, so as easily to be visited, and to make it easy for the patients to go out of doors. Wide and easy stone staircases, with good square landing-places, and without acute-angled steps, should connect the upper and the lower story. Light and air should pervade every part of the building; water and warmth should be everywhere equally supplied.

It is particularly necessary to observe that almost every desirable quality, both in the construction and government of an asylum, becomes more difficult to be obtained or preserved in an asylum, of which the size is greater than is required for 360 or 400 patients. This preliminary observation will apply to all the suggestions I shall have to make. In an asylum of a larger size, the architect must sacrifice much to expediency, and the government of the asylum can scarcely preserve any uniformity of character.

A great fault is generally committed in the original construction of county asylums, which subsequently entails many other faults. The asylum is usually erected merely for the supposed actual number of lunatics within a county; and, in consequence of the incurable patients not being discharged, the building becomes, in the course of ten years, crowded with nearly double the number first provided for; first, by means of the erection or extension of wings, to which, if the original plan has been well devised, there exists no objection, but afterward, by piling a third story wherever it can be raised, or by excavating rooms and wards under ground. These arrangements have all the disadvantages which I have mentioned. They make proper classification, either within doors or without, almost impossible, and by the accumulation of so many persons, day and night, in a lofty building, many of whom can seldom leave the wards, and none of whom is in perfect health, the asylum becomes subject to every atmospheric and terrestrial influence unfavourable to life. If no epidemic outbreak alarms the governors into an investigation and reform of buildings so arranged, or ill-placed, or otherwise unhealthy, the inmates are merely all brought to a low standard of health, to uneasiness, suffering, and a disposition to illness. There is always a risk of more active disease; and this may not only depopulate the institution to a great extent, but spread pestilence around it. Lessons of this kind are learnt with unwillingness, because they are opposed to the strong avarice which governs mankind; and they are also soon forgotten. The terrible examples afforded in 1832, when the malignant cholera last visited us, are so unheeded, that when the malady comes again, it will find almost every asylum, public and private, equally unprepared with reasonable preservatives against it.

Among the various forms of asylums adopted by architects, I believe there is none so convenient as one in which the main part of the building is in one line, the residence of the chief physician or other officers being in the centre, and also the chapel, and a large square room in which the patients may be occasionally assembled from either side of the asylum on the occasion of an evening entertainment, and which may also be capable of division for schools: the kitchen, laundry, workshops, and various offices, being arranged behind these central buildings. To this main line, wings of moderate extent being added at right angles in each direction, the building assumes what is called the H form; but it is desirable that the length of front should be more extended than that of the wings; and it is better still if the wings only extend in one direction, and away from the front, or northward, supposing the front of the asylum to be to the south. At Hanwell, the wings advance from the main front at right angles in one direction only, and new wings have been added at right angles with the first, in the same direction as the main front. It is evident that a building of this shape, long and narrow, consisting of a succession of galleries or corridors, with bedrooms on one side only, may be moderately perflated by every wind that blows—an advantage extremely salutary to those who pass their whole time in it. The want of proper ventilation is chiefly incidental to the angles of the building, and to the centre, and should be carefully provided against. In hot climates, exposure to the sun is a frequent cause of cerebral excitement, and many of our patients persist in exposing their bare heads to the sun in the hottest weather, until it is scarcely possible to touch their heads with one's hand. But in this country the hot season is of short duration, and it is especially necessary to consider that no gallery within the house, and no airing-ground exterior to it, should be deprived of some share of sunshine in the winter, as well as of free access of air, and some shade in summer. Quadrangular buildings, (unless the quadrangle is very large, and the buildings are very low,) and circular buildings, and central towers or crescents with radiating wings in three or more directions, are open to the greatest objections on every account. A north and south aspect is perhaps as convenient as any other, and the galleries and day-rooms should certainly face the south, or south-east. If the houses of the officers are also to the south, and the kitchen and other offices behind the centre, the principal approach to the asylum must be on the south likewise, and, being exposed to the windows of all the galleries and day-rooms, should be screened by an avenue or a semicircular plantation of trees or shrubs. If the central house projects a little from the main front, and has the kitchen, &c. behind it, the projection and the approach will form a complete division between the east and west galleries, and the male and female patients will be effectually separated, both in the front and at the back of the asylum; those of one sex being out of sight of those of the other, both in the galleries and airing-courts.

Much ornament or decoration, external or internal, is useless, and rather offends irritable patients than gives any satisfaction to the more contented. In some of the Italian asylums, busts, pictures, and ornaments abound, and the walls are painted with figures representing various allegories or histories. These would appear more likely to rouse morbid associations than to do any good. I also disapprove of painting numbers and titles on the walls of airing-courts, by which the walls are disfigured, and the patients are reminded of their confinement as insane persons when walking out for relaxation, or led to consider themselves prisoners. The wards and bedrooms also should only be designated by simple numbers.

When it is remembered that many patients are sent to an asylum whose senses are as perfect, and whose feelings are as acute, as those of sane people, and that from the moment they enter the outer gate everything becomes remedial with them, or the reverse, the reason will at once be seen why the outer aspect of an asylum should be more cheerful than imposing, more resembling a well-built hospital than a place of seclusion or imprisonment. It should be surrounded by gardens, or a farm. Even the part of the building to which the patient is first admitted is important. In the new asylum about to be built, I feel sure that the magistrates will anxiously avoid an inconvenience which is very much felt in the present building, where the reception rooms open directly into large towers, in which a circular staircase is so guarded with iron palisades as to give the patients looking through them, in the three different stories, the appearance of persons shut up in tiers of iron cages. A most painful impression is often made by this prospect being suddenly presented to the new comer; and it is strongest in those in whom the hope of recovery renders the avoidance of all counteracting agencies of the most consequence. The reception-room should be a cheerful and neatly-furnished sitting-room, and so situated that the newly-admitted patients can proceed from it to whatever part of the asylum it is thought best they should be sent. Thus, violent and noisy patients would not be led shouting and struggling through tranquil wards; and timid and quiet patients would not have to pass along corridors containing patients whose unfamiliar looks agitate or affright them.

In all building arrangements for the insane, a very liberal space should be allowed. The galleries should be spacious, and the doors wide, particularly those through which a crowd of patients must often pass. The same rule should be observed in the kitchens, laundry, storerooms, &c., of which, in many respects, the Hanwell asylum presents an excellent example. The galleries at Hanwell are, however, only ten feet wide; those of Bethlem are much wider. The galleries in the Kent asylum are fourteen feet wide, and those at Siegburg twenty feet. A width of twelve feet, with a height of eleven, seems to be suitable for the galleries of a county asylum. A public asylum is ordinarily a series of galleries, out of which almost all the bed-rooms open on one side, whilst on the other large windows

176   MILITARY FLOGGING, AND ITS EFFECTS.

lowing as proofs that what Dr. Hall called endocarditis in the deceased was really so:—The lining membrane of the heart was of a deep-red colour, not from blood contained in the cavity of the heart; it was a true inflammation; it was not from decomposition, because the heart was not decomposed, but really from inflammation, because the membrane was thickened by effused fibrin, soft, and slightly adherent. The membrane was readily separated from the heart, showing a diminution in the strength of the cohesion. There were polypi-formed concretions, of uncoloured fibrin, interlacing and attached to the cordæ tendineæ and the carneæ columnæ, which was a proof that the inflammation was recent. There was also the first stage of pneumonia in the left lung. The marks of pleurisy on the right side were old. The pericardium was not inflamed. The pleuræ costalis and pulmonalis of the left side were agglutinated in front, and laterally, by recently effused fibrin. It is very difficult to say what was the cause of the inflammation of the heart, or the endocarditis; but witness can say what was not the cause. The punishment he thinks was not; because it would be the first case on record that witness knows of in which such a connexion is proved. Witness cut off a portion of the skin from the back; it was loaded with blood, and shrank away greatly directly that he put the knife into it. Witness saw a beautiful bright red muscle beneath it, with no inflammation at all in it.

Horatio Grosvenor Day, Member of the Royal College of Surgeons of England, and a Licentiate of the Society of Apothecaries, being sworn, saith that he lives at Church-street, Isleworth, in the parish of Isleworth, Middlesex, and that, by the direction of the coroner, he made an examination of the body of deceased on the first Thursday after his death, (July 16th,) at the barracks at Hounslow Heath. The body had already been opened by some surgeon. The contents of the chest and abdomen were very much decomposed, and were out of their usual position. The heart appeared to be rather smaller than usual, and the muscular fibres softer. The lining membrane was rather redder than usual; but he saw in it no trace of inflammation; this might have been in consequence of the previous examination of that organ, as it had been divided in several places. The lungs were gorged with blood on both sides, particularly the left. There were traces of inflammation in the left pleura. Witness cannot speak of any adhesions there, but he understood that some had been divided there at the first examination. The portion of the pleura covering the ribs, the pleura costalis, was much inflamed. The liver was larger than usual, and rather paler; otherwise it was quite healthy. Witness did not then examine the spine. Witness thinks that the death was produced by pleurisy and pneumonia. How they were caused witness cannot tell, but supposes they were owing to the exposure of deceased to a change of the weather from heat to cold. The piece of skin corresponded with the space on the back, with the exception of a small portion on the left side.

Erasmus Wilson, being sworn, saith that he resides at No. 55, Charlotte-street, Fitzroy-square, St. Pancras, London, and is a Fellow of the Royal College of Surgeons of England, Consulting Surgeon to the St. Pancras Infirmary, London, and Lecturer on Anatomy and Physiology in the Middlesex Hospital School, and has written two works on the Anatomy, Physiology, and Diseases of the Skin. By order of the coroner, witness made, on Wednesday, July the 22nd, an examination of the back of the deceased. The body had already been twice examined by other surgeons, and was in too bad a state for an examination of the contents of the chest and abdomen. Mr. Day accompanied witness at the inspection. Witness's attention was especially directed to deceased's back and spine. On the skin over each shoulder there were marks of lashes, and on the right of the middle line, between the shoulders, there was a large gap occasioned by the removal of a portion of the skin. A small bottle, containing a piece of skin, was handed to witness by the sergeant of police. Witness took the skin from the bottle, and found, that although much shrunk by immersion in spirits of wine, while the gap from which it had been removed was stretched to its utmost, yet that it corresponded with the gap, with the exception of the side nearest the middle line, where a part had been cut away and lost. Witness was informed that the lost piece had been cut away in order to make the remainder sufficiently small to enter the bottle. From the position which the lost piece occupied, witness believes that it was more protected from the lashes than the preserved portion, and therefore, being less interesting in a medical point of view, had been cut off. On the preserved portion of skin there were several marks made by the lashes; the marks were red, and upon cut-

ting into one of them, witness found that the redness, which was indicative of inflammation, extended through the entire substance of the skin. On raising the muscles or flesh from off the ribs and spine, witness found a part of the deepest layer of muscles—namely, that which lay in contact with the bones, in a state of disorganization, and converted into a soft pulp. In medical language, witness should call this a pulpy softening of the muscles. The seat of this pulpy softening was upon and between the sixth and seventh ribs, near their attachment to the spine, together with their intervening space, and the hollow between the sixth and seventh pieces of the dorsal portion of the spine. The extent of the disorganization was about three inches in length, by about one inch and a half in greatest breadth, and between a quarter and half an inch in thickness. In the space between the ribs, the muscle had undergone this pulpy alteration even so deep as the lining membrane of the chest, the softened muscle being in absolute contact with the lining membrane. That portion of the flesh which occupied the groove of the spine, and had undergone a similar disorganization, was one of the little muscles known to medical men under the name of multifidus spinæ. In addition to softening, this little muscle was partly surrounded with blood; it was in the state medically called ecchymosed. The interior of the spine was in a state of extreme decomposition. The tissue between the spinal canal and spinal sheath was filled with a dark-coloured fluid, resulting from decomposition. The sheath itself was smooth and polished on its internal surface—a state indicative of health. It was perfectly devoid of nervous substance, which had been converted into fluid by decomposition, and had flowed away. The nerves remained, and presented a healthy appearance. So that, as far as the spine is concerned, witness says that he discovered no indications of disease. Witness considers that two questions naturally arise out of the examination, which he has now described—namely, first, What was the cause of the pulpy softening of the muscles? Secondly, Could the state of disorganization preceding the pulpy softening influence the disease existing in the chest? The cause of the pulpy softening witness believes to have been the excessive contraction of the muscles taking place during the agony of punishment. This excessive contraction would produce laceration and subsequent inflammation of the muscles; and the inflammation, instead of being reparative, would, in consequence of the depressed state of the powers of the nervous system of the deceased, and the injury of the muscles, be of the disorganizing kind which results in pulpy softening. Had the man lived, the disorganization of the muscles would in time have been repaired. As regards the second question, witness says, that there can be no doubt that although the common cause of inflammation of the contents of the chest is cold, acting in conjunction with physical and moral depression, and might have been the cause in the case of the deceased, yet the presence of a portion of muscle in a state of disorganization and inflammation, in close contact with the lining membrane of the chest, might be adequate to the production of the same effect. Witness says, that certainly no surgeon would feel comfortable with regard to the state of his patient if he were aware of such dangerous proximity. Witness says, that the morbid appearances of the muscles of the back, which he described, are a new observation in the science of pathology, and, so far as he knows, has not been alluded to in any printed work extant. It was one which he was wholly unprepared to find, and he is not surprised that the medical witnesses whose depositions he has heard given in this court were not conversant with the occurrence of such a change under the influence of the injuries of the skin such as deceased is said to have received on the 15th of June. The morbid change in the muscles found by witness corresponded with the side upon which the inflammation of the pleura was found; and since hearing the evidence given before this Court, witness is still more convinced, than he was, that a relation subsisted between that disorganization and the disease which was found within the chest, and that the morbid change in the muscles lying in contact with the pleura had a prominent share in exciting the inflammation of that membrane. The pulpy softening of the muscles was not near the surface of the back, nor on the side from which the skin had been removed; it was situated deeply, and, witness believes, resulted from involuntary contraction of the muscles: witness repeats, that he considers that the immediate cause of the death of deceased was the inflammation of his heart, pleura, and lung; that that inflammation was caused by the injuries produced by the flogging of the deceased; and that deceased would have been alive now but for the punishment which he received on the 15th of June, 1846; witness has no doubt of that whatever. Witness having heard it said by Mr. Clarke, an attorney now in this court, on the part of Colonel Whyte, that the depositions of the medical witnesses who preceded him in their evidence were diametrically opposed to that of witness on the subject last mentioned, witness therefore says, that until his evidence was concluded the other medical witnesses did not know the whole of the post-mortem changes which existed in the body of deceased. Those witnesses had not examined the deep muscles of the back adverted to by witness; those changes were of a most serious nature, and place the punishment of flogging in an entirely new position in a medical point of view. The change in the muscles was of a more intense kind than the softening of the heart, which latter, according to the medical witnesses, amounted only to friability. Witness has been a lecturer on anatomy for twelve years, and during that time has examined between five hundred and one thousand bodies, and never saw a similar change to that which he has now described existing in the muscles of the back of deceased. Witness considers that the contraction which caused the rupture of the muscles must have been involuntary : no voluntary action on the part of deceased could have occasioned it ; neither could a blow directly upon them, because the injured muscles were in a position of the spine by which they were peculiarly and sufficiently protected from such an injury, and the superficial or superincumbent muscles were not similarly affected. Nor, in the opinion of witness, could a fall forward, such as witness has heard described in this court, have done it. Witness says that death generally results from a suspension of the function of the lungs ; that the disease of the heart and lung caused that suspension in the deceased man; and that the punishment of deceased on the 15th of June, and the moral prostration caused by that punishment, rendered him susceptible of atmospheric changes which would not otherwise have affected him. Whether any such atmospheric changes did affect deceased or not, witness cannot tell, as he did not see the man during life.

On the 3rd of August, the same witnesses made the following additional statements :—

Dr. Warren—Witness says, that having heard the depositions of all the medical witnesses examined at this inquest, up to Monday, August 3rd, 1846, he still says, that he believes that the death of deceased was not caused by, and was in no way connected with, the punishment that he received on the 15th of June, 1846.

Dr. Reid—Witness has now heard the whole of the depositions of the medical witnesses and all the other evidence given in this court up to August 3rd, 1846, and he now states that the inflammation of the lungs, the heart, and the pleura, which was found in deceased at the post-mortem examination, was the cause of his death, and that he cannot, with satisfaction to his own mind, connect the disease with the punishment that the deceased man received on the 15th of June, 1846, because and for these reasons:—Witness thinks that this inflammation was more likely to have been produced by sudden atmospheric changes affecting deceased than by anything that he had heard described in the depositions of the witnesses at this inquest. It is very difficult to state the cause of the inflammation which was found in the thorax of the deceased man. Witness considers that the disease was in nowise connected with the punishment which deceased received on the 15th of June, 1846.

Mr. Day—Witness was present at an examination of the back of the deceased man, made by Mr. Erasmus Wilson, on Thursday, July 16th, 1846, and he has heard the evidence of Mr. Wilson given in this court, and now, witness, on his re-examination by the court, says that he verifies the statements of Mr. Wilson as to the character of certain parts of the muscles of the back; but he is not prepared to go the length that Mr. Wilson has done, in connecting the disorganized state of the muscles with the cause of death. Witness thinks that the cause of the change of the muscles is a mere matter of conjecture. Witness does not ascribe it to the blows from the flogging, but he thinks that it may have been caused by the struggles of the deceased man, from the agony caused by his punishment. The disease in the chest was sufficient to cause the death. The flogging may have indirectly caused the disease. The confinement of deceased to the hospital during his treatment for wounds in the back, and the depression of spirits produced by the punishment, may have rendered the deceased man less able to bear the disease which he already had, independently of the injurious effect produced upon him by the flogging itself. When the examination was completed, witness signed a paper, conjointly with Mr. Wilson, as follows:—

"The muscles of the deep layer of the back covering the sixth and seventh ribs, and corresponding intercostal spaces, were softened and converted into a puriform pulp, (pulpy degeneration;) the same change extended to the intercostal muscles, and to one of the fasciculi of the multifidus spinæ. The latter was also ecchymosed. The extent of the morbid change was about three inches in length, by about one inch and a half at the broadest part ; in thickness it occupied about quarter of an inch.

The cellular tissue of the theca vertebralis was loaded with a dark brown fluid of the consistence of cream, which most probably resulted from softening of the tissue and cadaveric transudation. There was no trace of disease within the theca.   (Signed)   HORATIO G. DAY,
July 22, 1845.   ERASMUS WILSON."

Mr. Day further made this additional statement :—

Wednesday, July 22nd, 1846.

I accompanied Mr. Erasmus Wilson to Heston Church-yard to examine the state of the spine of the late Frederick John White, the body having been exhumed by order of the coroner for that purpose.

On the body being removed from the coffin, the piece of integument which had been dissected from the back was again compared with the exposed space, and found to correspond in shape, with the exception of a small portion ; but from the circumstance of the removed part having shrunk, and the opening expanded, there appeared considerable difference in size.

The external layers of muscles were perfectly healthy, but on dissecting downwards, nearer the spine, we found near the sixth and seventh dorsal vertebræ, or bones of the spine, and the corresponding ribs on the left side, a portion of muscle in a softened or pulpy state, the fibres being infiltrated with a fluid resembling matter in its early stage. This appearance extended about three inches in length, by one and a half in breadth, and barely a quarter of an inch in depth.

The external covering of the sheath of the spinal cord was loaded with a thick brown fluid, the result of decomposition or infiltration.

The contents of the spinal canal were much decomposed, but there was no trace of disease or inflammation perceptible on the most minute investigation.

The softening of the muscular fibre had extended into the intercostal muscles immediately subjacent, but had not penetrated the internal intercostals,* and therefore could not produce the slightest effect upon the pleura, or any of the contents of the thorax.

The portion of lungs brought into view by removing part of the sixth and seventh ribs, presented the gorged and blackened appearance noticed at the previous examination.
    (Signed)   HORATIO GROSVENOR DAY.

Mr. E. Wilson—Witness having heard the whole of the depositions of the witnesses made in this court on the 27th of July and the 3rd of August, 1846, says, that he considers that the death of deceased was produced by the flogging which he had received, and its consequences upon his system. Witness has formed that opinion, because he believes that death from flogging is not an uncommon occurrence. The diseases which attend flogging in general are identical with those which existed in the deceased. Painful and extensive injuries of the skin are liable to produce inflammation of the internal organs. A burn, though not extensive, will give rise to fatal disease of the internal organs of the body, the stomach and bowels, the heart and lungs, the liver and the kidneys. External injuries are not unfrequently followed by secondary diseases. A consequence of flogging is newly brought to light in the examination of the muscles of the back of deceased. Often, in hospitals, when there appears to be no danger to patients from the primary disease, there exists some internal inflammation, which suddenly becomes violent, and rapidly ends in death. Witness has no doubt whatever that the death of deceased was caused by the flogging which he received.

The Coroner having summed up the evidence, the Jury returned the following

VERDICT:—

"That on the 11th day of July, 1846, the deceased soldier, Frederick John White, died from the mortal effects of a severe and cruel flogging of one hundred and fifty lashes,

---

* At a subsequent stage of the inquiry, Mr. Wilson explained that there was no internal intercostal muscle in the situation referred to by Mr. Day, and, therefore, that a penetration of one layer of muscle necessarily reached the pleura.

178   MILITARY FLOGGING, AND ITS EFFECTS.

which he received with certain whips on the 15th day of June, 1846, at the cavalry barracks on Hounslow Heath, at Heston; and that the said flogging was inflicted upon him under a sentence passed by a district court martial, composed of officers of the 7th regiment of hussars, duly constituted for his trial. That the said court martial was authorized by law to pass the said severe and cruel sentence; and that the said flogging was inflicted upon the back and neck of the said Frederick John White by two farriers, in the presence of John James Whyte, the lieutenant-colonel, and James Low Warren, the surgeon, of the said regiment; and that so and by means of the said flogging the death of the said Frederick John White was caused."

In returning this verdict, the jury stated that they "could not refrain from expressing their horror and disgust at the existence of any law amongst the statutes or regulations of this realm which permits the revolting punishment of flogging to be inflicted upon British soldiers; and, at the same time, the jury implore every man in the kingdom to join, hand and heart, in forwarding petitions to the legislature, praying, in the most urgent terms, for the abolition of every law, order, and regulation, which permits the disgraceful practice of flogging to remain one moment longer a slur upon the humanity and fair name of the people of this country."

The subject of the inquest having been incidentally noticed in the House of Commons on Friday night last, August 7th, and an insinuation having been directed against the manner in which the Coroner conducted the inquiry, Mr. Wakley, in self-vindication, read the two following letters—the first having been received from Mr. Clark, the solicitor, who so ably appeared at the inquest on behalf of the officers of the regiment, and the second from the Rev. H. S. Trimmer, a magistrate of the county, who so honourably deferred the application for the burial of the body to the Coroner's court. Until the inquest, both of those gentlemen were entire strangers to Mr. Wakley. The third letter was not read in the House of Commons, but was mentioned by Mr. Wakley. It is from Mr. Twining, magistrate of Twickenham, a member of the bar, and who for many years was a judge in India. With this gentleman Mr. Wakley had not the honour of being acquainted, never having had the pleasure of seeing him but once before, and then on a public occasion. With the testimony of gentlemen of such authority and undoubted respectability, in favour of the manner in which he discharged his duty during the most protracted investigation, and under circumstances of most peculiar and extraordinary excitement, he cannot condescend to notice the animadversions of persons who were not present at the inquiry.

"Sion-place, Isleworth, Aug. 6, 1846.

"SIR,—You request me to state to you what was my impression as to the manner in which the inquest on late Private White, of the 7th Hussars, was conducted by you; and as I conclude your inquiry to have reference only to your own conduct on that occasion, I have no hesitation in saying, that you allowed us to have any witnesses examined we pleased, and to make any statements we thought either necessary or desirable, and the ends of justice demanded: and you certainly conducted the investigation with extraordinary patience and attention.

"And it seems that it does not remain with me to answer the latter inquiry in your letter—namely, whether I consider your charge to the jury to have been fairly made; as I find that, on reference to the *Sun* newspaper of Tuesday last, your charge is there set out most correctly; and of its merits the public can therefore judge, and whom my opinion, consequently, will not in the smallest degree influence.

"I am, Sir, your most obedient servant,
"Thomas Wakley, Esq., M.P."   "G. CLARK.

"Heston Vicarage, August 6, 1846.

"MY DEAR SIR,—I am favoured with your letter, in which you request me to state to you my impression as to the manner in which the inquest on Frederick John White, of the 7th Hussars, was conducted, and whether I consider your charge to have been fairly made?

"In reply to these questions, I have great pleasure in stating, that having been present (with the exception of about one hour) during the whole of the proceedings, and having heard your charge, from its commencement to its close, I cannot but express my decided opinion, that throughout the inquiry there appeared the greatest readiness and anxiety on your part to receive and fairly examine all legal evidence, without respect

to the parties bringing it forward, which might tend to ensure an impartial verdict; and that nothing could be fairer towards all parties, or better calculated to assist the jury in coming to a correct conclusion on the whole evidence, than your charge; of which, on my return to my family after the inquest, I expressed my admiration, considering it, as I really did, as at once judicious, luminous, and impartial.—I beg to remain, my dear Sir, very faithfully yours,
"Thos. Wakley, Esq."   "H. S. TRIMMER.

"Perryn House, August 6, 1846.

"MY DEAR SIR,—I feel considerable difficulty in answering your inquiry, it being quite impossible for me to express my admiration—my sincere and unqualified admiration—of the fair, able, and dignified manner in which the important proceedings at Hounslow, on Monday, were conducted. Having, almost from my first, to this my second childhood, had a predilection for judicial business, I have been rather a great frequenter of courts of justice; and I certainly have never, in any court in any country, been more gratified than on the late occasion;—I allude more particularly to your charge, where your calm and dignified repression of all bias and excitement, amidst circumstances so calculated to bias and excite; your own example of this equanimity—your discriminating and fair and clear exposition of the law, and of the facts of the case—nothing extenuating, nor setting down aught in malice; the application of your remarks rather to the system than to the involuntary and degraded agents of its cruelties;—the whole of this I thought at the time, and still think, above all praise.

Speaking of these proceedings yesterday to some gentlemen here, I said that I doubted whether any man but Mr. Wakley could have so ably conducted this affair.—My dear Sir, yours very truly,
"Thomas Wakley, Esq."   ———   "THOMAS TWINING.

The remarks made at this inquest on the mischief liable to accrue to internal organs at an uncertain period, after injury to the skin, are quite in accordance with evidence given on cases of almost weekly occurrence in the coroner's court. Death from disease of the viscera (and particularly those of the thorax) is continually found to result from slight injuries in even remote parts of the body, and especially after those involving any portion of the surface, as burns, bruises, &c. An instance, eminently in point, happened during the interval between two of the sittings at the above inquest, the leading facts of which were the following:—

J. C——, aged twenty-eight, footman to a family residing at 36, Russell-square, and of sober habits, was alarmed, about half past ten on the night of the 12th of July last, by a violent screaming and cries of "fire" from several persons in the house, and on hastening up stairs he found that the clothes of a lady in the house were on fire. He instantly ran to her, and succeeded in extinguishing the flames. The event greatly agitated and excited him; and the fingers of both his hands were severely burned, the whole of one hand being considerably scorched. About an hour after he had been in bed, whither he retired as soon as he could, he felt severe pain in his right side, which persisted throughout most part of the night. In the morning he was visited by a surgeon of the neighbourhood, who ordered a liniment of oil and lime-water, under the use of which, to the parts immediately affected, in the course of a week, he became "marked off the list as well," and he had then fully returned to his duties. He had complained of nothing further during his treatment up to this time, beyond a sharp pain in his stomach, which had occurred when his fingers were dressed; but this was not regarded by his attendant as of any moment, and he took no medicine of any description. On the 20th of July, he complained of some relaxation of the bowels to the surgeon, who sent him "something to quiet the bowels," which he continued to use during the remainder of that and the following day. On the evening of the 21st, however, he complained of a great deal of pain at the pit of the stomach, and was seized with vomiting, which being encouraged by draughts of warm water, in the course of the night he brought up "a large quantity of green bile." On the morning of the ensuing day, (22nd,) he was better; but in the evening his wife called on the surgeon, and stated that he appeared to be "out of his head," and not to know what he was saying. His attendant now found him suffering under fully marked delirium tremens, for which a large dose of opium was given, perfect quietude enjoined, beef tea, arrow-root, &c., ordered. Next day, (23rd,) the sickness and purging were aggravated, and the patient complained of pain extending from the region of the liver to the pit of the stomach; delirium and hurried breathing were also present. For these symptoms a blister was placed on the scrobiculus cordis, and five grains of calomel with a grain and a half of opium were administered. On the ensuing day he was removed, at his own request, to his wife's lodging in Milton-street, Euston-square; and on the following, (25th,) to University College Hospital. At this period he was found to be labouring under severe pleuro-pneumonia of the right, and probably also of the left, side of the chest. For this, cupping, and tartar emetic, were the chief remedies employed; but during the next day he was occasionally delirious, countenance livid, pulse full, skin very hot, &c. These symptoms were somewhat abated by a bleeding to sixteen or eighteen ounces, but he died suddenly about eight o'clock P.M.

At the post-mortem examination, made seventeen hours afterwards, the following notes were taken:—

Body moderately fat. The right pleura contains about half a pint of turbid serum, and the whole of that membrane, both costal and visceral, is covered by an irregular layer of thick lymph, beneath which the membrane is vascular. The left pleura contains the same quantity of serum, and the appearance in it is nearly the same.

In the right lung, where resonance was distinctly heard during life, a portion of the substance is found permeable to air, but almost the entire of the remaining portion of the lung is solidified, of a greyish-red colour and granular, and sinks in water.

The left lung is coated with lymph, like the right. On the posterior surface there are many superficial hæmorrhagic spots, not extending into the lymph. The texture is permeable to air, and contains a quantity of frothy mucus and water, showing that the lung was not inflamed. The pericardium contains a large quantity of turbid fluid, and both of its surfaces were coated with rough, shaggy lymph. The stomach is distended with a brown turbid fluid. The mucous membrane towards the cardiac orifice is very dark-coloured, the colour depending on punctiform redness. The mucous membrane is soft; the peritonæum healthy. The liver projects a good deal below the ribs, and into the left hypochondrium; it weighs five pounds, nine ounces. Nothing very unusual in its appearance is observable, excepting its size. The spleen weighs nine ounces and a half, and is softer than usual. The right kidney weighs eight ounces; the capsule separates easily; the substance is large and flabby. The cortical part is paler than natural, and yellow, and evidently contains deposit. The left weighs eight ounces; the capsule is easily separable, large, flabby, coarse in texture, smooth on the surface, and mottled. (Bright's disease.) The bladder contains ten ounces of urine, of the specific gravity of 1017, and containing albumen.

This man, previously to the injury of the skin of his hands, was regarded by every person who knew him to be in perfectly good health, and up to that time, he had never been hindered from performing his daily duties. He himself attributed his illness solely to the accident he had met with, and the state of excitement he had been put into at the time of its occurrence. The surgeon who had first attended him (but who had lost sight of him for at least two days before his entrance into the hospital,) was present during the post-mortem examination by Dr. Quain. According to his evidence, delivered by him at the inquest, he " disbelieved in any connexion between the burn and the disease which caused the man's death." He considered " that the patient had no disease in the chest during the first week, nor a complication of any sort until the bowel complaint occurred." He thought, however, that " nothing he saw in the chest in the form of disease had existed in the chest, in any stage, before the 12th of July. The pain in the stomach (he considered) was probably caused by the burn. But he does not in any way connect the burn with the death, he (the patient) having appeared perfectly recovered during a week from any affection of the body consequent on that he had received on the night of the burn."

LIABILITIES OF THE MUSCLE IN DISEASE.

(CLINICAL REMARKS IN ST. GEORGE'S HOSPITAL.)

HERE, in Crayle ward, on the water-bed, is a young unmarried woman, (E. B——, admitted Dec. 17th, 1845;) her intellect, memory, and sense of feeling, in no degree impaired, yet motionless as an unstrung puppet, more helpless than an infant,—paraplegia, the result of a summer-day's pleasuring, four years ago, in Epping Forest. She cannot raise, cannot turn, herself in bed; is unable, by any effort of her will, to bend either toe or finger; has lost all command of the rectum and bladder; articulates with extreme slowness and difficulty, and is in fear of choking by every morsel she swallows; there is divergence of both eyes from their central axis of vision, and she suffers much at times from painful flexion of the legs, both above and below the knee.

Damp and fatigue have, in this case, determined, by slow degrees, the effects of palsy to the fibre, which, by the young Scotch baker in York ward, were obtained at once from his mess of arsenic and verdigris. Sixty grains of sugar of lead failed, you will remember, on the other hand, to paralyze a single muscle of the young girl, self-poisoned, in the Burton ward. The case of E. B., now before us, is too chronic to be promising; but let us not condemn it without a thought.

Paraplegia, in spite of bad treatment, not unfrequently surprises us by recovery. We are too apt to renounce these cases of double palsy as hopeless, under the belief that they of necessity imply organic change of structure in corresponding portions of the brain and spinal marrow. Many of them, be assured, are merely functional in the muscle, and are consistent with entire soundness of the appended nervous structure, from its origin, in triple union with the blood and fibre, to its final organization, in the central nervous column. The proprietor and director of a large fashionable hotel at the west-end of the town, who had been long paraplegic, first came under my care on Oct. 26th, 1843. At that time, he could not raise himself from the chair without assistance, was confused to the last degree in his intellect, and was unable to prevent a continual dribbling of water from his bladder. By the accounts given to me by his family, he had become continually worse, under various plans of treatment addressed to supposed organic disease of the brain and spinal marrow. In the course of the winter, 1843-44, he gradually recovered, by the use of mild, alterative, and tonic remedies, that were general in their operation through the system. For more than two years past, he has now been able to walk a considerable distance in the street, and to assist in the management of his large domestic affairs.

How strange and inconsistent in modern pathology is this exclusive reference to the nerve, in all questions relating to the nature and treatment of muscular disorders! In the operations of disease, every organ, excepting the muscle, is supposed to originate its own symptoms, and to maintain its own process of damage or cure. Heart, liver, lungs, kidney, are thus made responsible, by name and in their complete structure, for the disorders affecting their several functions. The muscle alone—of all organs, in truth, the most independent—is never suffered in the lists of nosology, under its proper designation, but finds a place, by right of spasm and palsy, in the loose catalogue of the " neuroses," as a mere part and offset of the so-called " nervous system." By most practitioners, when in consultation on disorders of the contractile function, " muscular" and " nervous" are used as convertible terms, for the expression of their views in the treatment of the case. In the physic of 1846, there is no greater, no more mischievous, error, than this substitution, in the complete organ, of a part for the whole,—this degradation, in the nosology of spasm and palsy, of the blood and the fibre, by distinction, undue and exclusive, of the nerve. In the instance of paraplegia now before us, by routine, and as a matter of course, the treatment has had reference almost exclusively to the brain and spinal marrow, and here, it may be, is the true principle of the case; but I see no warrant, by alleviation of the symptoms, or from the early history of the illness, for a further use of blisters, setons, and other counter-irritants. There has been no pain in the head or back, no fit, no direct evidence of disease in the central nervous structures. The patient is as much alive as ever to the stimulus of pinching, pricking, or tickling, on any part of the cuticular surface. Her illness began with a " severe cold," after exposure to wet, with fatigue, on a long holiday, enjoyed " al fresco," four years ago, before which time she had been " perfectly well." She is now without fever, has appetite sufficient for her life of motionless repose, and is regular in all her functions. She has never lost her senses, or failed in her memory. If the case be insisted on as one essentially " nervous,"—as a result, that is, of palsy in the limbs, from effects of congestion, inflammation, or thickening of the brain and spinal marrow, or of their investing membranes,—then, on this same exclusively " nervous" theory, it would be assumed that the disturbing agencies of damp, chill, and fatigue, were first brought into operation on the outer surface of the body,—on the skin, that is, by its expanded nerves, and so on from them to the spinal marrow, and back by reflex action, in the phrase of the day

ON SURGICAL OPERATIONS PERFORMED DURING INSENSIBILITY.   5

pleura over the pericardium. The whole internal surface of the left pleura was drawn and puckered like old strumous scars, and deeply and profusely inlaid, and elevated with flattened white malignant tubercles. The floor of the cavity was contracted and drawn up. The pericardium contained about two ounces of clear serum; its reflected surface was marked with small flattened nodulated elevations, and the subjacent structure was much thickened and indurated; the attached surface, except a large point of attrition anteriorly, was healthy. The substance, cavities, and valves of the heart, were generally healthy, except perhaps a little thickening of the mitral valve. Right side distended with fibrinous coagula; aorta natural; around and in the muscular substance of the œsophagus were found points of hard malignant matter; the mucous membrane was healthy; no trace of any rib having been broken.

Abdomen.—Peritonæum healthy; mesenteric glands enlarged, one consisting of a hardened cretaceous mass. The stomach was distended; vessels on the inner aspect somewhat injected and arborescent; mucous membrane softened here and there, of a dull greyish-white colour, and easily scraped off; in several parts irregularly dotted, of a dusky colour. Liver rather large, dark, firm. Spleen healthy. Kidneys rather large and congested; structure healthy.

Remarks.—The symptoms for the relief of which this patient first applied were clearly to be attributed to the stomach, and the result of the necropsy showed the justice of this opinion. No history of any acute attack was given, nor any symptom, other than to be accounted for by a state of chronic inflammation of the mucous membrane of the stomach, and which, from his occupation, I was induced to think likely, with probably some chronic disease of the liver. His cough was but cursorily mentioned, as he considered it of secondary importance to the suffering caused by the stomach derangement. Though very excitable, he was, withal, most unwilling to give way, and avoided rather than willingly imparted any extended account of himself or his feelings. The relief was but slight, and on his cough beginning to assume a more prominent position, I examined his chest carefully, and was at once convinced of the presence of advanced disease on the left side. Leading questions and the statement of his wife furnished the additional history, which was, however, with difficulty obtained, even in its incomplete form. The succession of symptoms seem to be, a blow some months ago on the left side, followed by pain there for a day or two, exposure to wet, and after an interval, dry cough of a very severe character, occurring in paroxysms, dyspnœa, inability to lie on the sound side, scanty and clear expectoration, without febrile symptoms, or anything to indicate active mischief. In the course of the attack, gastric symptoms arose, which for a time were very prominent. Lastly, universal dulness, and fixed condition of the left chest, and altered position of the heart, the very faint sounds of which induced me to suspect a preternatural quantity of fluid in the pericardium.

The symptoms, so far, were those commonly met with in pleurisy of a sub-acute or chronic form, succeeded by persistent effusion; they were, however, equally compatible with a solid growth in the chest, of malignant character, and to this opinion I was inclined throughout, and for the following reasons: the veins of the chest were enlarged; a scirrhous tubercle followed the blow; it is not general to have much pain on lying on the affected side in mere effusion; the dulness on percussion was perfectly wooden; and the peculiar sounds elicited by the stethoscope appeared to require more than mere effusion to account for them. The existence of enlargement in the axillary glands would have been an additional reason for suspecting malignant disease, but I did not notice this fact during life. The voice also was peculiar, and showed great obstruction to respiration, and the inability to sit up in bed is not a usual sign in effusion. The heart may be displaced in either case, and malignant disease may exist without characteristic expectoration.

With this uncertainty in my own mind I was desirous of another opinion, and Dr. Addison was kind enough to examine this patient's chest, and investigate his case, the result being that the presence of fluid alone did not satisfy him, and he was inclined to suspect malignant disease to be the cause of the peculiar symptoms.

Increased severity of the weather, and perhaps debility from insufficient nourishment, owing to his gastric mischief, tended to accelerate and rapidly bring on the more urgent symptoms.

On the 30th, Dr. Birkett (to whom I am also greatly indebted for valuable assistance in recording the appearances found after death) saw him with me, and examined his chest as far as could be without distressing the patient—indeed, only anteriorly,—and was rather inclined to the belief that there was fluid present. In the evening of that day, I again visited the patient, in company with my father and Dr. Birkett, and took with me the tapping instruments, intending, should our examination of his chest seem to justify it, to explore at least, and if fluid were present, to remove it, as affording the only hope of relieving the extreme oppression. The reasons which deterred me from this were—1st. The inability to find by auscultation any one spot where the sounds conveyed to the ear might seem, as far as could be, to ensure the safety of exploring. 2nd. The heart was more audible in the left infra-mammary region, and its sounds clearer than heretofore. (Could this have been at all occasioned or influenced by the accession of a tympanitic condition of the stomach?) And 3rd. On applying the ear briefly to the posterior parietes of the left chest, the sounds were too close to the ear. Careful examination was out of the question, as in the semi-recumbent position alone did he seem able to breathe, I may almost say, at all. The exploration was reluctantly abandoned, and death soon terminated the patient's sufferings.

In concluding, it may be well briefly to consider the connexion between the symptoms during life and the morbid condition displayed by the post-mortem examination.

1st. The presence of the extensive collection of fluid, the result of that form of disease denominated by Laennec hæmorrhagic pleurisy, fully explained all the symptoms supposed during life to indicate effusion; and the commencement of this, I think, may justly be assigned to a period shortly after the blow. The effusion on the right side was evidently very recent.

2ndly. The condition of the contents of the posterior mediastinum will explain the sounds heard in the left infra-clavicular region, and account for the transmission of the sounds of the opposite lung, or apparent laryngeal respiration.

3rdly. The density of the fluid rendered it a better conducting medium for sound; and the position of the lung against the posterior parietes, and its not being quite impermeable to air, will explain the sounds posteriorly. And

4thly. The gastric symptoms are fully and sufficiently accounted for. What, then, would have been the effect of tapping? Unquestionably, relief, but only temporary, for the malignant disease would have very probably been excited to increased action by the withdrawal of the fluid, and speedily terminated life, even supposing his powers had rallied, and his cough had been subdued. I am, however, quite convinced, that though the position of the lung was against the ribs, yet had exploration been performed, (where it was intended, if possible, to have done so—viz., in the posterior lateral region, five or six inches from the spine, and not low down,) that the whole of the fluid might have been removed also, with perfect safety, as regards any injury likely to have been inflicted by the trocar.

Original Papers.

SURGICAL OPERATIONS PERFORMED DURING INSENSIBILITY,

PRODUCED BY THE INHALATION OF SULPHURIC ETHER.

(Communicated by FRANCIS BOOTT, M.D.*)*

To the Editor of THE LANCET.

SIR,—I beg to call your attention to the report of an anodyne process, by means of which surgical operations have been performed without pain. I think it would be interesting to the profession if published in THE LANCET. I also send a letter from Dr. Bigelow, bearing date more than three weeks after the report drawn up by his son. I wish to add, that Dr. Bigelow is one of the first physicians of Boston, a Professor of the Medical School of Harvard College, and a man of great accomplishment.—Yours sincerely,

Gower-street, Bedford-square, Dec. 1846.   F. BOOTT.

Extract from a private letter from Dr. BIGELOW *to* Dr. FRANCIS BOOTT.

"Boston, Nov. 28, 1846.

"MY DEAR BOOTT,—I send you an account of a new anodyne process lately introduced here, which promises to be one of the important discoveries of the present age. It has rendered many patients insensible to pain during surgical operations, and other causes of suffering. Limbs and breasts have been amputated, arteries tied, tumours extirpated, and many hun-

6   ON SURGICAL OPERATIONS PERFORMED DURING INSENSIBILITY.

dreds of teeth extracted, without any consciousness of the least pain on the part of the patient.

"The inventor is Dr. Morton, a dentist of this city, and the process consists of the inhalation of the vapour of ether to the point of intoxication. I send you the *Boston Daily Advertiser*, which contains an article written by my son Henry, and which is extracted from a medical journal, relating to the discovery.

Let me give you an example. I took my daughter Mary, last week, to Dr. Morton's rooms, to have a tooth extracted. She inhaled the ether about one minute, and fell asleep instantly in the chair. A molar tooth was then extracted, without the slightest movement of a muscle or fibre. In another minute she awoke, smiled, said the tooth was not out, had felt no pain, nor had the slightest knowledge of the extraction. It was an entire illusion.

"The newspaper will give you the details up to its date, since which other operations have been performed with uniform success.

"*Dr. F. Boott.*"

The following paper, by HENRY JACOB BIGELOW, M.D., one of the Surgeons of the Massachusetts General Hospital, was read before the Boston Society of Medical Improvement, Nov. 9th, 1846, an abstract having been previously read before the American Academy of Arts and Sciences, Nov. 3rd, 1846.*

IT has long been an important problem in medical science, to devise some method of mitigating the pain of surgical operations. An efficient agent for this purpose has at length been discovered. A patient has been rendered completely insensible during an amputation of the thigh, regaining consciousness after a short interval. Other severe operations have been performed without the knowledge of the patients. So remarkable an occurrence will, it is believed, render the following details relating to the history and character of the process, not uninteresting.

On the 16th of October, 1846, an operation was performed at the hospital, upon a patient who had inhaled a preparation administered by Dr. Morton, a dentist of this city, with the alleged intention of producing insensibility to pain. Dr. Morton was understood to have extracted teeth under similar circumstances, without the knowledge of the patient. The present operation was performed by Dr. Warren, and though comparatively slight, involved an incision near the lower jaw, of some inches in extent. During the operation, the patient muttered, as in a semi-conscious state, and afterwards stated that the pain was considerable, though mitigated; in his own words, as though the skin had been scratched with a hoe. There was probably, in this instance, some defect in the process of inhalation, for, on the following day, the vapour was administered to another patient with complete success. A fatty tumour, of considerable size, was removed by Dr. Hayward from the arm of a woman, near the deltoid muscle. The operation lasted four or five minutes, during which time the patient betrayed occasional marks of uneasiness; but upon subsequently regaining her consciousness, professed not only to have felt no pain, but to have been insensible to surrounding objects—to have known nothing of the operation, being only uneasy about a child left at home. No doubt, I think, existed in the minds of those who saw this operation, that the unconsciousness was real; nor could the imagination be accused of any share in the production of these remarkable phenomena.

I subsequently undertook a number of experiments, with the view of ascertaining the nature of this new agent, and shall briefly state them, and also give some notice of the previous knowledge which existed of the use of the substances I employed.

The first experiment was with sulphuric ether, the odour of which was readily recognised in the preparation employed by Dr. Morton. Ether inhaled in vapour is well known to produce symptoms similar to those produced by the nitrous oxide. In my own former experience, the exhilaration has been quite as great, though perhaps less pleasurable, than that of this gas, or of the Egyptian *haschish*.† It seemed probable that the ether might be so long inhaled as to produce excessive inebriation and insensibility; but in several experiments the exhilaration was so considerable that the subject became uncontrollable, and refused to inspire through the apparatus. Experiments were next made with the oil of wine, (ethereal oil.) This is well known to be an ingredient in the preparation known as Hoffman's anodyne, which also contains alcohol, and this was accordingly employed. Its

* From the Boston Medical and Surgical Journal.
† Extract of Indian hemp.

effects upon the three or four subjects who tried it were singularly opposite to those of the ether alone. The patient was tranquillized, and generally lost all inclination to speak or move. Sensation was partially paralyzed, though it was remarkable that consciousness was always clear, the patient desiring to be pricked or pinched, with a view to ascertain how far sensibility was lost. A much larger proportion of oi of wine, and also chloric ether, with and without alcohol were tried, with no better effect.

It remains briefly to describe the process of inhalation by the new method, and to state some of its effects. A small, two-necked glass globe contains the prepared vapour, together with sponges, to enlarge the evaporating surface. One aperture admits the air to the interior of the globe, whence, charged with vapour, it is drawn through the second into the lungs. The inspired air thus passes through the bottle, but the expiration is diverted by a valve in the mouth-piece, and escaping into the apartment is thus prevented from vitiating the medicated vapour. A few of the operations in dentistry, in which the preparation has as yet been chiefly applied, have come under my observation. The remarks of the patients will convey an idea of their sensations.

A boy of sixteen, of medium stature and strength, was seated in the chair. The first few inhalations occasioned a quick cough, which afterwards subsided; at the end of eight minutes the head fell back, and the arms dropped, but owing to some resistance in opening the mouth, the tooth could not be reached before he awoke. He again inhaled for two minutes, and slept three minutes, during which time the tooth, an inferior molar, was extracted. At the moment of extraction the features assumed an expression of pain, and the hand was raised. Upon coming to himself he said he had had a "first-rate dream—very quiet," he said, "and had dreamed of Napoleon—had not the slightest consciousness of pain—the time had seemed long;" and he left the chair, feeling no uneasiness of any kind, and evidently in a high state of admiration. The pupils were dilated during the state of unconsciousness, and the pulse rose from 130 to 142.

A girl of sixteen immediately occupied the chair. After coughing a little, she inhaled during three minutes, and fell asleep, when a molar tooth was extracted, after which she continued to slumber tranquilly during three minutes more. At the moment when force was applied, she flinched and frowned, raising her hand to her mouth, but said she had been dreaming a pleasant dream, and knew nothing of the operation.

A stout boy of twelve, at the first inspiration coughed considerably, and required a good deal of encouragement to induce him to go on. At the end of three minutes from the first fair inhalation, the muscles were relaxed and the pupil dilated. During the attempt to force open the mouth he recovered his consciousness, and again inhaled during two minutes, and in the ensuing one minute two teeth were extracted, the patient seeming somewhat conscious, but upon actually awaking, he declared "it was the best fun he ever saw," avowed his intention to come there again, and insisted upon having another tooth extracted upon the spot. A splinter which had been left afforded an opportunity of complying with his wish, but the pain proved to be considerable. Pulse at first 110, during sleep 96, afterwards 144; pupils dilated.

The next patient was a healthy-looking, middle-aged woman, who inhaled the vapour for four minutes; in the course of the next two minutes a back tooth was extracted, and the patient continued smiling in her sleep for three minutes more. Pulse 120, not affected at the moment of the operation, but smaller during sleep. Upon coming to herself, she exclaimed that "it was beautiful—she dreamed of being at home—it seemed as if she had been gone a month." These cases, which occurred successively in about an hour, at the room of Dr. Morton, are fair examples of the average results produced by the inhalation of the vapour, and will convey an idea of the feelings and expressions of many of the patients subjected to the process. Dr. Morton states, that in upwards of two hundred patients, similar effects have been produced. The inhalation, after the first irritation has subsided, is easy, and produces a complete unconsciousness at the expiration of a period varying from two to five or six, sometimes eight minutes; its duration varying from two to five minutes; during which the patient is completely insensible to the ordinary tests of pain. The pupils in the cases I have observed have been generally dilated; but with allowance for excitement and other disturbing influences, the pulse is not affected, at least in frequency; the patient remains in a calm and tranquil slumber, and wakes with a pleasurable feeling. The mani-

ON SURGICAL OPERATIONS PERFORMED DURING INSENSIBILITY. 7

festation of consciousness or resistance I at first attributed to the reflex function, but I have since had cause to modify this view.

It is natural to inquire whether no accidents have attended the employment of a method so wide in its application, and so striking in its results. I have been unable to learn that any serious consequences have ensued. One or two robust patients have failed to be affected. I may mention as an early and unsuccessful case, its administration in an operation performed by Dr. Hayward, where an elderly woman was made to inhale the vapour for at least half an hour without effect. Though I was unable at the time to detect any imperfection in the process, I am inclined to believe that such existed. One woman became much excited, and required to be confined to the chair. As this occurred to the same patient twice, and in no other case as far as I have been able to learn, it was evidently owing to a peculiar susceptibility. Very young subjects are affected with nausea and vomiting, and for this reason Dr. Morton has refused to administer it to children. Finally, in a few cases, the patient has continued to sleep tranquilly for eight or ten minutes, and once, after a protracted inhalation, for the period of an hour.

The following case, which occurred a few days since, will illustrate the probable character of future accidents. A young man was made to inhale the vapour, while an operation of limited extent, but somewhat protracted duration, was performed by Dr. Dix upon the tissues near the eye. After a good deal of coughing, the patient succeeded in inhaling the vapour, and fell asleep at the end of about ten minutes. During the succeeding two minutes, the first incision was made, and the patient awoke, but unconscious of pain. Desiring to be again inebriated, the tube was placed in his mouth and retained there about twenty-five minutes, the patient being apparently half affected, but, as he subsequently stated, unconscious. Respiration was performed partly through the tube, and partly with the mouth open. Thirty-five minutes had now elapsed, when I found the pulse suddenly diminishing in force, so much so, that I suggested the propriety of desisting. The pulse continued decreasing in force, and from 120 had fallen to 96. The respiration was very slow, the hands cold, and the patient insensible. Attention was now, of course, directed to the return of respiration and circulation. Cold affusions, as directed for poisoning with alcohol, were applied to the head, the ears were syringed, and ammonia presented to the nostrils and administered internally. For fifteen minutes the symptoms remained stationary, when it was proposed to use active exercise, as in a case of narcotism from opium. Being lifted to his feet, the patient soon made an effort to move his limbs, and the pulse became more full, but again decreased in the sitting posture, and it was only after being compelled to walk during half an hour that the patient was able to lift his head. Complete consciousness returned only at the expiration of an hour. In this case the blood was flowing from the head, and rendered additional loss of blood unnecessary; indeed, the probable hæmorrhage was previously relied on as salutary in its tendency.

Two recent cases serve to confirm, and one, I think, to decide, the great utility of this process. On Saturday, November the 7th, at the Massachusetts General Hospital, the right leg of a young girl was amputated above the knee, by Dr. Hayward, for disease of this joint. Being made to inhale the preparation, after protesting her inability to do so, from the pungency of the vapour, she became insensible in about five minutes. The last circumstance she was able to recall was the adjustment of the mouth-piece of the apparatus, after which she was unconscious until she heard some remark at the time of securing the vessels—one of the last steps of the operation. Of the incision she knew nothing, and was unable to say, upon my asking her, whether or not the limb had been removed. She refused to answer several questions during the operation, and was evidently completely insensible to pain or other external influences. This operation was followed by another, consisting of the removal of a part of the lower jaw, by Dr. Warren. The patient was insensible to the pain of the first incision, though she recovered her consciousness in the course of a few minutes.

The character of the lethargic state which follows this inhalation is peculiar. The patient loses his individuality, and awakes after a certain period, either entirely unconscious of what has taken place, or retaining only a faint recollection of it. Severe pain is sometimes remembered as being of a dull character; sometimes the operation is supposed to be performed by somebody else. Certain patients whose teeth have been extracted, remember the application of the ex-

tracting instruments; yet none have been conscious of any real pain.

As before remarked, the phenomena of the lethargic state are not such as to lead the observer to infer this insensibility. Almost all patients under the dentist's hands scowl or frown; some raise the hand. The patient whose leg was amputated, uttered a cry when the sciatic nerve was divided. Many patients open the mouth, or raise themselves in the chair, upon being directed to do so. Others manifest the activity of certain intellectual faculties. An Irishman objected to the pain that he had been promised an exemption from it. A young man taking his seat in the chair and inhaling a short time, rejected the globe, and taking from his pockets a pencil and card, wrote and added figures. Dr. Morton supposing him to be affected, asked if he would now submit to the operation, to which the young man willingly assented. A tooth was accordingly extracted, and the patient soon after recovered his senses. In none of these cases had the patients any knowledge of what had been done during their sleep.

I am, as yet, unable to generalize certain other symptoms to which I have directed attention.* The pulse has been, as far as my observation extends, unaltered in frequency, though somewhat diminished in volume, but the excitement preceding an operation has, in almost every instance, so accelerated the pulse that it has continued rapid for a length of time. The pupils are, in a majority of cases, dilated; yet they are in certain cases unaltered, as in the above case of amputation.

The duration of the insensibility is another important element in the process. When the apparatus is withdrawn, at the moment of unconsciousness, it continues, upon the average, two or three minutes, and the patient then recovers completely or incompletely, without subsequent ill effects. In this sudden cessation of the symptoms, this vapour in the air tubes differs in its effects from the narcotics or stimulants in the stomach, and as far as the evidence of a few experiments of Dr. Morton goes, from the ethereal solution of opium when breathed. Lassitude, headach, and other symptoms, lasted for several hours when this agent was employed.

But if the respiration of the vapour be prolonged much beyond the first period, the symptoms are more permanent in their character. In one of the first cases, that of a young boy, the inhalation was continued during the greater part of ten minutes, and the subsequent narcotism and drowsiness lasted more than an hour. In a case alluded to before, the narcotism was complete during more than twenty minutes; the insensibility approached to coma.

The process is obviously adapted to operations which are brief in their duration, whatever be their severity. Of these, the two most striking are, perhaps, amputations and the extraction of teeth. In protracted dissections, the pain of the first incision alone is of sufficient importance to induce its use; and it may hereafter prove safe to administer it for a length of time, and to produce a narcotism of an hour's duration. It is not unlikely to be applicable in cases requiring a suspension of muscular action, such as the reduction of dislocations or of strangulated hernia; and finally, it may be employed in the alleviation of functional pain, of muscular spasm, as in cramp and colic, and as a sedative or narcotic.

The application of the process to the performance of surgical operations, is, it will be conceded, new. If it can be shown to have been occasionally resorted to before, it was only an ignorance of its universal application, and immense practical utility, that prevented such isolated facts from being generalized.

It is natural to inquire with whom this invention originated. Without entering into details, I learn that the patent bears the name of Dr. Charles T. Jackson, a distinguished chemist, and of Dr. Morton, a skilful dentist, of this city, as inventors,—and has been issued to the latter gentleman as proprietor.

It has been considered desirable by the interested parties that the character of the agent employed by them should not be at this time announced; but it may be stated that it has been made known to those gentlemen who have had occasion to avail themselves of it.

I will add, in conclusion, a few remarks upon the actual position of this invention as regards the public.

No one will deny that he who benefits the world should receive from it an equivalent. The only question is, of what nature shall the equivalent be? Shall it be voluntarily ceded

---

* Since the above was written, I find this irregularity of symptoms mentioned in the case of poisoning by alcohol. Dr. Ogston, according to Christison, has in vain attempted to group together and to classify the states of perspiration, pulse, and pupil.

by the world, or levied upon it? For various reasons, discoveries in high science have been usually rewarded indirectly by fame, honour, position, and occasionally, in other countries, by funds appropriated for the purpose. Discoveries in medical science, whose domain approaches so nearly that of philanthropy, have been generally ranked with them; and many will assent with reluctance to the propriety of restricting by letters patent the use of an agent capable of mitigating human suffering. There are various reasons, however, which apologize for the arrangement, which I understand to have been made with regard to the application of the new agent.

1st. It is capable of abuse, and can readily be applied to nefarious ends.

2nd. Its action is not yet thoroughly understood, and its use should be restricted to responsible persons.

3rd. One of its greatest fields is the mechanical art of dentistry, many of whose processes are by convention, secret, or protected by patent rights. It is especially with reference to this art, that the patent has been secured. We understand, already, that the proprietor has ceded its use to the Massachusetts General Hospital, and that his intentions are extremely liberal with regard to the medical profession generally; and that so soon as necessary arrangements can be made for publicity of the process, great facilities will be offered to those who are disposed to avail themselves of what now promises to be one of the important discoveries of the age.

To the Editor of THE LANCET.

SIR,—I forwarded a few days ago, for publication in THE LANCET, Dr. H. J. Bigelow's report on the anodyne effects of the inhalation of the vapour of strong, pure sulphuric ether; and since that time I have received an Address, delivered by the Hon. Edward Everett, (late Minister from the United States to the Court of St. James's,) at the opening of the new Medical College in Boston, an extract from which will be interesting, as affording his high testimony to the safety and efficacy of the process. In a note, Mr. Everett, the President of Harvard College, says—"I am not sure that, since these remarks were delivered, a discovery has not been announced which fully realizes the predictions of the text. I allude to the discovery of a method of producing a state of temporary insensibility to pain, by the inhalation of a prepared vapour. I witnessed a very successful instance of its application, on the 18th of November, and was informed at that time by Dr. Morton, that he had employed it in several hundred cases of dentistry. It has also been made use of with entire success at the Massachusetts General Hospital, and elsewhere in Boston, in capital operations of surgery. The few cases of failure may, perhaps, be ascribed to irregularities in the process of inhalation, or to peculiarities of temperament or constitution on the part of the patient. I understand that great confidence is placed in the discovery by the most distinguished members of the medical profession of this vicinity, and that they are disposed to regard it as an effectual method of inducing complete insensibility under the most cruel operations, by means easily applied, entirely controllable, and productive of no subsequent bad consequences. It seems not easy to overrate the importance of such a discovery."

I beg to add, that on Saturday, the 19th, a firmly fixed molar tooth was extracted in my study from Miss Lonsdale, by Mr. Robinson, in the presence of my wife, two of my daughters, and myself, without the least sense of pain, or the movement of a muscle. The whole process of inhalation, extracting, and waking, was over in three minutes; yet the same apparatus was used in three or four cases afterwards, and failed in each case to produce insensibility. I attribute the failure to the defect in the valve of the mouthpiece, by which the expired air was returned to the bottle, instead of passing into the room. The valve was a ball-and-socket one, and required a very strong expiration to make it act freely. I would add, that the efficacy of any apparatus must depend upon the facility of breathing the vapour, and the perfect action of the valve, admitting the expired air to pass easily into the room. In Miss Lonsdale's case, we all observed she breathed strongly, and thus, no doubt, opened the valve. In all the other cases, we had great difficulty in making the patients breathe through the mouthpiece.

Yours sincerely, F. BOOTT.

ower-street, Dec. 21, 1846.

To the Editor of THE LANCET.

Gower-street, Dec. 22, 1846.

SIR,—If you have not heard of Mr. Liston's success in the se of the inhaled ether, the following note I have received

from him will interest you, as confirming the American report:—

"Clifford-street, Dec. 21, 1846.

"MY DEAR SIR,—I tried the ether inhalation to-day in a case of amputation of the thigh, and in another requiring evulsion of both sides of the great toe-nail, one of the most painful operations in surgery, and with the most perfect and satisfactory results.

"It is a very great matter to be able thus to destroy sensibility to such an extent, and without, apparently, any bad result. It is a fine thing for operating surgeons, and I thank you most sincerely for the early information you were so kind as to give me of it. "Yours faithfully,
"To Dr. Boott." "ROBERT LISTON.

I hope Mr. Liston will report of these cases more fully.
Yours sincerely, F. BOOTT.

To the Editor of THE LANCET.

SIR,—Having noticed, in several periodicals and newspapers, reports of two operations recently performed by Mr. Liston, at the University College Hospital, upon patients under the anodyne influence of inhaled vapour of ether, in which amputation of the thigh in one case, and evulsion of the nail of the great toe in the other case, were effected without pain to the patients, I take this earliest opportunity of giving notice, through the medium of your columns, to the medical profession, and to the public in general, that the process for procuring insensibility to pain by the administration of the vapour of ether to the lungs, employed by Mr. Liston, is patented for England and the Colonies, and that no person can use that process, or any similar one, without infringing upon rights legally secured to others.

I am aware that doubts exist in the minds of some as to the liberality of rendering inventions or improvements, which tend to alleviate suffering, subjects of patents; but I cannot see why the individual who, by skill and industry, invents or discovers the means of diminishing, or, as in this instance, annihilating human suffering, is not full as much entitled to compensation as he who makes an improvement in the manufacture of woollen or other fabrics. Indeed, he is entitled to greater compensation, and for a stronger reason,— he has conferred upon mankind a greater benefit.

With this view, I have accepted from the American inventors, or their representatives, the agency of affairs connected with the English patent; and it is my intention, while I hold the trust, to adhere to such a course, that the charge of illiberality shall rest upon any persons rather than upon the proprietors of the patent, or upon their agent,

Duke-street, St. James's, Dec. 28, 1846. JAMES A. DORR.

ON

CRITICISMS UPON PHRENOLOGY.
A REVIEW REVIEWED.
By GEORGE COMBE, ESQ., Edinburgh.

(Remarks on an article in the British Quarterly Review, for November, 1846.)

(Concluded from last volume, p. 663.)

DR. SKAE does not quote Mr. Noble's work, or allow him fairly to speak for himself on these topics; but as if, in the fifty years before mentioned, no step had been made in the investigation, either by friend or foe, he comes forward with new principles, new measurements, and new results, all of his own devising; and he does so under the pretence that his method is one of strict scientific accuracy, fairly entitled to supersede all the others. Let us, then, briefly consider its merits.

First, he asks, " What, then, is the size of an organ in the estimate of a phrenologist's eye?" The true answer has already been given— *Its length* AND *its breadth.* But Dr. Skae's answer is different. He informs us, that " It can be *only* its degree of prominence, as compared with the neighbouring surface of the cranium, *or* its distance from some central point. Of the breadth of the organ, it is impossible that he can form any estimate, except such as depends upon the breadth or size of the entire head; for if the organs do not always occupy the same relative part of the surface of the entire cranium, it is impossible for any phrenologist to define the precise surface of their cranial limits. Will any phrenologist undertake to say that the organ of Benevolence occupies a greater relative portion of the surface of the cranium in one

DR. BENCE JONES ON CHEMICAL PATHOLOGY.   91

there were small chalky deposits at the apices of both lungs; some pleurisy of right side.

In the worst cases of delirium tremens, I observed the most marked contrast to cases of inflammatory disease. The following case, also under Dr. Nairne, is the best example I can adduce:—

David D——, aged thirty-five, hair-dresser, was admitted at five P.M., 18th of June, 1845. Said to have had some dropsy for the last six weeks, and for three days to have been in a very excited state, without sleep. Two hours after admission he had a fit, which lasted ten minutes; snoring and convulsion; did not fall asleep after it. At night had half a grain of morphia, and was quiet.

19th, (fourth day.)—Quiet; face injected; answers sensibly; much tremor; only four ounces of water passed during twelve hours of the night; specific gravity, 1019.1, and contained total phosphates, 2.41. In the evening he began to be very restless, up, and running about the ward.

20th, (fifth day.)—No food; pulse 110, not weak, soft; tongue furred, moist; skin warm and perspiring; obliged to be confined; seven ounces of water, specific gravity, 1019.3, contained only .15 total phosphates. A second experiment with the same water gave only .12.

21st, (sixth day.)—Continued in the same state; very violent; six ounces of water in the morning had, specific gravity, 1017.9, and contained total phosphates, only .06. Six ounces obtained in the evening had, specific gravity, 1019.7, and contained total phosphates, .24.

22nd.—In the evening he had two fits, and died. Examined fifteen hours after death.

The dura mater was more than usual adherent to the calvaria; the subarachnoid cellular tissue and the pia mater were filled with large quantities of clear fluid; the cineritious substance was pale, and the white substance presented slight venous congestion; the ventricles were not enlarged; the structure of the brain appeared to be pretty healthy; liver was rounded and granular; blood was fluid and very thin. There were several tubercular deposits in the apices; there was red hepatization of the back of the right lung.

In another case of delirium tremens, I found at one time the urine of specific gravity, 1018.0, contained no alkaline phosphates whatever, and only .10, earthy phosphates.

The power of alcohol to stop the production of phosphoric acid—that is, to hinder the oxidation which usually takes place in the nervous substance—is not less interesting than the production of an excess of phosphoric acid in inflammation of the brain.

The experiments I have made can be considered only as the first steps in the investigation of this action of oxygen. Should they be confirmed, they will furnish the strongest evidence of the action of ordinary chemical forces within the human body. An action similar to the oxidation of the vegetable salts in the blood, and depending on the same causes as the production of carbonic acid in respiration—namely, the absorption of oxygen by the lungs, and the power which that gas possesses of combining with other elements, as carbon, hydrogen, phosphorus, sulphur, or the iron, which, in my first lecture, I brought before you.

I am unable, from want of time, to mention other supposed instances of oxidation, as in the iron of the red globules, as conjectured by Liebig, or of the fibrin, as stated by Mulder. I can only refer you to the last experiments of Magnus on the absorption of atmospheric air by the blood, in opposition to the theories of respiration which these physiologists have published. I would at the same time refer, also, to Professor Scharling's experiments on the production of carbonic acid in disease. Of these, the most interesting are those on six patients with phthisis. Five of these expired less carbonic acid than healthy persons of the same sex and age would have done. The sixth patient showed no marked diminution. Four patients with chlorosis showed no increase or diminution whatever in the amount of carbonic acid excreted. Such experiments deserve the most careful repetition, and promise the most valuable results.

I must pass on now to other chemical processes in the body; and here I must allude to those most interesting relations in composition between the albuminoid substances which analysis has made known to us. I use the term albuminoid, not because they have reactions like albumen, but because they have an elementary composition closely agreeing with that of albumen. These substances contain carbon, hydrogen, oxygen, nitrogen, sulphur, and phosphorus. Mulder states that he separated the sulphur and phosphorus, and found then that white of eggs, serum, fibrin, and casein, all agreed in composition exactly. They all, then contained the same quantity of carbon, hydrogen, oxygen, and nitrogen. This common quantity of carbon, hydrogen, oxygen, and nitrogen, Mulder named protein; and he considered the albumen, the serum, the fibrin, and the casein, all consisted of protein, combined with different quantities of phosphorus and sulphur:—

Crystalline	$= 15$ eq. protein $+$ sulphur S
Casein	$= 10$ „ „ $+$ „ S
Gluten	$= 10$ „ „ $+$ „ S_2
Fibrin	$= 10$ „ „ $+$ „ S $+$ phosp. ph.
Egg albumen	$= 10$ „ „ $+$ „ S $+$ „ ph.
Blood albumen	$= 10$ „ „ $+$ „ $S_2 +$ „ ph.

So that for the conversion of albumen of blood into casein, sulphur and phosphorus must be separated; and for the conversion of the fibrin of the blood into casein, phosphorus alone need be separated. If the formulæ are true, such a separation, in fact, must take place in the lacteal glands, in order to produce milk; and to the casein of the milk, the sulphur and phosphorus must again be added, to produce the albumen in the infant's blood; or phosphorus alone requires to be added to produce the fibrin. The object attained is probably the regulation of the escape of nutriment from the mother, and its absorption by the child. The quantity of casein present in the milk formed may depend on the activity of this separation of phosphorus and sulphur from albumen.

In addition to these combinations of protein with sulphur and phosphorus, Mulder, in a later paper, has stated the existence of two oxides of protein—a binoxide and tritoxide; the first insoluble in water, the last very soluble. These exist in inflammatory blood, and may be formed, in various ways, from albumen and fibrin; by treating albumen with chlorine, the tritoxide may be formed; or fibrin, if treated with hydrochloric acid, will give binoxide.

Protein consists of carbon, hydrogen, oxygen, and nitrogen; the binoxide and tritoxide must therefore contain only two or three equivalents more oxygen than protein does: there must be no other difference—no sulphur and no phosphorus. Liebig has digested fibrin in hydrochloric acid to obtain the binoxide of Mulder; but he says he always finds sulphur in the compound, and that therefore, in this way, no binoxide of protein is formed, but some substance containing sulphur. It may be an oxide of albumen. Moreover, Liebig says, when trying to make protein itself, some sulphur always remains combined with the carbon, hydrogen, oxygen, and nitrogen. In the new edition of his "Animal Physiology," the accuracy of Mulder's first experiments regarding the formation of the common principle of protein, as well as the latter ones regarding the oxides of protein, will, it is said, be doubted. I have not been able to make the experiments I wished to make on the subject; but when it is remembered that Mulder was the first to determine the existence of sulphur and phosphorus in these substances—the first to analyze them, to determine the quantities of the elements present—and, moreover, that these first analyses were all made by Mulder himself, and bear internal marks of the greatest accuracy,—it will appear most probable that he obtained the substance which he calls protein free from sulphur and phosphorus, as he, the discoverer of the sulphur and phosphorus in the albuminous substances, states that he did.[*]

Whether the albumen, casein, and fibrin, are formed by the addition of sulphur and phosphorus to protein, as Mulder thinks, protein itself being first formed, is a totally different question; and as the sulphur and phosphorus are found in the albuminoid constituents of plants, and are merely absorbed into the human body, according to Liebig, this is a question which vegetable chemistry may possibly be able to determine; but it is a question altogether different from the one which Mulder has, I consider, solved—that all these albuminoid bodies can have the sulphur and phosphorus separated from them, and then give the same results on analysis. Thus much regarding the analyses made by Mulder himself. The analyses relating to the formation of the oxides of protein were made by others in his laboratory; and though I believe it to be probable that there may be oxides of protein such as Mulder gives the formulæ for,—substances containing no sulphur and phosphorus,—still, I think the substances analyzed in his laboratory, in some cases, (certainly in the one stated by Liebig—the solution of fibrin in hydrochloric acid,) were oxides of albumen, rather than oxides of protein, for this reason—that I have found another oxide of albumen in the

* Professor Liebig, in his late work on the "Chemistry of Food," pp. 18 to 28, states the principal facts on which his own views are founded. I would also refer to a letter of Professor Mulder, in *Jameson's Journal*, April, 1847, p. 355; and to a paper read at the meeting of the British Association, at Oxford, June 25th, 1847; or *Jameson's Journal*, July, 1847, p. 162.

urine, in a case of mollities ossium. The patient was a wealthy tradesman, aged forty-five. I saw him on the 15th of November, 1845, with Dr. Watson and Dr. Macintyre. Rather more than a year previously, he was first taken ill. Dr. Watson first saw him in the spring of 1845, after he had been actively treated for pleurisy. In June he had œdema of the legs. He improved in Scotland during the summer, the legs continuing to swell, and the appetite being ravenous—he expressed it as being so much so, that he dreamed of eating dogs and cats. On the last day of October, a peculiar state of urine was discovered, through the carefulness of Dr. Macintyre. When I saw the patient, there was excessive emaciation; yellowish skin; clear conjunctivæ; lips dry; tongue fissured, moist, furred at the back; pulse 85, small; skin moist; bowels, tendency to diarrhœa; motions reported not unhealthy; urine not passed in large quantities; no urgency—no frequency; pinkish urates deposited; much mucous râles in the chest; over-strong pulsation of the heart; complained of pains in the left shoulder and side; was obliged to be moved most gently in bed on account of the pain.

He died about six weeks afterwards, and the only marked disease was mollities ossium. The kidneys were healthy to the eye, with and without the microscope. But to return to the water. This note of Dr. Watson shortly describes its state.

Saturday, Nov. 1st, 1845.

"DEAR DR. JONES,—The tube contains urine of very high specific gravity. When boiled it becomes slightly opaque. On the addition of nitric acid, it effervesces, assumes a reddish hue, and becomes quite clear; but as it cools, assumes the consistence and appearance which you see. Heat reliquifies it. What is it?" . . . .

This test-tube shows what I first saw. The specific gravity never was below 1031, and twice I found it above 1042. It was generally acid, sometimes much so, and remaining so for many weeks. Usually thick from urate of ammonia and crystalline phosphate of lime. Boiling gave no immediate precipitate, though the slightest boiling produced some change; for after it, nitric acid gave a precipitate, which, in the un-boiled urine, it would not do for many hours. Long boiling produced a further change, and coagulation ultimately took place, (immediately with carbonated alkali.)

This urine then contained an enormous quantity of this substance, something like albumen, but differing in very many things from albumen, more especially in the solubility of the nitric acid precipitate by heat. The peculiar substance I separated by means of its insolubility in alcohol. I obtained it in this quantity and form. The substance so obtained had all the reactions which the urine had after it had been heated. Soluble in cold, very soluble in boiling water, not coagulating by heat, but coagulating on long boiling, and coagulum again ultimately soluble by continued boiling; giving a precipitate with acids soluble by heat, and becoming again thick on cooling. I purified this substance with alcohol and ether, and have analyzed it at 212° and 300° over and over again. It differs entirely from the oxides of protein. It contains phosphate of lime, sulphur, and phosphorus. The quantity of carbon, hydrogen, oxygen, nitrogen, differ also remarkably from fibrin and albumen, but agree very nearly with tritoxide of protein. I consider the substance, therefore, as an oxide of albumen, and the enormous quantities which the urine contained is best seen by considering the serum of the blood as the nutritious part of it; then each ounce of this urine contained as much nutritive matter as an ounce of the blood. No supply of food could compensate for such a loss.—(See "Proceedings of the Royal Society," April 22nd, 1847.)

The well-marked solubility of the nitric acid precipitate, and the silence of Mulder on this point, made me immediately try what was the reaction of nitric acid on his so-called tritoxide. I obtained some inflammatory fibrin, and treated it with boiling water; nitric acid gave a precipitate soluble by heat, and refalling on cooling. Moreover, sulphur was present in this substance.

I also passed chlorine into serum and into albumen from eggs, and so obtained the so-called tritoxide; and here also is the precipitate with nitric acid soluble by heat; and the whole of the albumen of the blood, by the action of chlorine and ammonia, can be changed into this substance.

It will immediately be asked, what is the connexion between mollities ossium and this state of urine? and to such a question I am as yet unable to give a positive answer. But I may here mention a conjecture which I have formed, that chlorine may have been the cause of the formation of this

substance, and also the cause of the solution of the earthy matter of the bone.

If this be the case, then, the cells in the bone and the kidney must take on the same decomposition of chloride of sodium as the cells in the stomach in the state of health do. I believe that the production of this substance must take place in the cells of the kidney and bone, because I found albuminous fluid in the pericardium, after death, reacted in the ordinary way, and the blood itself was coagulable by heat and acids. (The pericardium fluid was feebly alkaline, specific gravity, 1015.3, and coagulated immediately.) I need hardly remark on the importance of seeking for this oxide of albumen in other cases of mollities ossium. The white, solid, fibrin-like coagula in some urine, looking like blancmange, will probably also be found to be another oxide of albumen.

But why do the cells take on this peculiar action? On this question, the whole of secretion and nutrition are involved. The formation, by cells, of nervous matter, that highest of all the animal functions, seems little likely to be understood at present as a merely chemical process. The decomposition of phosphoric acid appears, at first sight, to be requisite. Still less can we conceive how the power of sensation, and all the intellectual and moral powers, are united to this peculiar compound, and this no chemical and no microscopical research will help us to explain.

Such, then, is the outline of the separate forces in action in organized beings. But the separate action of forces is not found in Nature to take place. Although it has been necessary to separate and distinguish actions, for the purpose of obtaining clearer ideas of each force, yet such a course of necessity involves the loss of that union, of that association of forces, which throughout inorganic as well as organic nature is so apparent.

If the forces of heat, electricity, and magnetism, are called into action, not only by chemical forces, but most decidedly also by the most opposite class of mechanical forces, as by friction; if even in quantity these forces are related to each other, a certain quantity of chemical action, producing, probably, a definite quantity of heat, a definite quantity of electricity, and this a fixed quantity of magnetic force; or, if the expression may be so applied, supposing that an equivalent of mechanical force produces an equivalent of heat, an equivalent of electricity, and this its equivalent of magnetism again;—if there be such union and relation in inorganic forces, how probable must the existence be of an analogous association in organic forces; and not only are sensation, contraction, and chemical forces most closely related to each other, and dependent on each other in animal life, but the cell-forming force, the cell-modifying force, and chemical forces, are in no less intimate relation throughout all life; and even in the highest of all created beings how often can we trace the inordinate action of the higher mental functions exaggerating the contractility and sensibility of the body, and deranging the action of those lower forces which it has been my attempt in these lectures more especially to bring before you.*

The phenomena which result from the joint action of all the forces we sum up in the word life, and the cessation of the most chemical of these phenomena in animals—namely, respiration, is the ordinary meaning of the word death, as the word to expire shows; and as the expiring taper is rekindled when placed in oxygen gas, so life may be restored by artificial respiration renewing those chemical changes on which the circulation through the lungs chiefly depends.

Lastly. It is, then, in the addition of the forces of sensation and contraction to the cell-modifying and cell-forming forces that animal life differs chiefly from vegetable life; whilst the highest of all life—that is, human life, is characterized by the further addition of the higher moral and intellectual powers. And as, on the one hand, in proportion as these powers, with sensation and motion, may be lost by accident or disease, does man approximate to a state of vegetation, to the state of those fungi which, not being peculiarly acted on by light, absorb oxygen, and respire carbonic acid. So, on the other hand, when the higher faculties are developed, may man attain not only to the doing good to others, as is the object of our own profession, but he may increase his affinity, or attraction, or love, for the never-ceasing and unlimited good, which is the highest of those forces whose united action I might perhaps venture to designate as Eternal Life.

---

* The endeavour to establish by experiment the convertibility of the forces will doubtless lead to important discoveries. So the alchymists, in searching after the transmutation of matter, became acquainted with those truths which, now that the equivalent relations of substances are made known to us, appear as the necessary results of a universal law.

PROFESSOR SIMPSON ON A NEW ANÆSTHETIC AGENT.   549

placenta in their natural state, under water, and when the uterine vessels were filled with injection, having led to no conclusive and satisfactory results respecting the connexion of the placenta and uterus, it occurred to me, soon after the publication of my paper in the *Philosophical Transactions*, in 1832, that the most likely means of discovering the real connexion of these parts would be to examine the placenta when the vessels of the uterus were filled with their own blood, and coagulated. On the 24th of May, 1833, such an opportunity presented itself, through the kindness of Mr. Girdwood, of Paddington; and that no doubt might exist in the minds of anatomists, as to the accuracy of the description, I requested Mr. Lawrence carefully to examine the parts with me, and to draw up an account of the appearances which we observed. It was my wish immediately to have published the memorandum containing an account of these results, but I was dissuaded from doing so by Mr. Lawrence, who thought it better to wait until another opportunity should occur of verifying the observation, and still further elucidating the subject. The facts were, however, immediately made known to Sir Astley Cooper, Professor Owen, Mr. Mayo, and many other members of the profession, who felt interested in the subject, and they were thus stated, about a month after, in the review of 'Velpeau's Embryology,' in the *Medical Gazette:*—'About a month ago, before the preparation at the College of Surgeons was examined by Messrs. Stanley and Mayo, we understand that Dr. Robert Lee, in order as far as possible to obviate every fallacy, examined a gravid uterus, in the eighth month, in which he had previously coagulated the maternal blood. He was able to satisfy himself and Mr. Lawrence, who was present at the examination, that coagula of the maternal blood extended from some of the openings in the lining membrane of the uterus, into canals formed by the deciduous membrane, on the margin of the placenta. These vessels or channels in the decidua could be traced only a short distance along the margin of the placenta, and between the lobes.'"

Paul Portal's cases were omitted in Old Mortality Table; Dr. Simpson has assigned the following reason for this omission, which, independently of the other flagrant errors, vitiated the whole—"In the Table, as originally published," he says, "I erroneously relied on Dr. Lee's accuracy, when, in his 'Clinical Midwifery,' he stated that Portal's work contained an account of eight cases *only* of unavoidable hæmorrhage." In spite of all the errors which are stated by Dr. Simpson to have been committed by Dr. Lee, Dr. Simpson placed such unbounded reliance on "Dr. Lee's accuracy," while constructing "Old Mortality Table," in 1845, that he did not consider it necessary to consult Portal's original work. Being ignorant of the number of cases of placental presentation in Portal's work, or, more probably, knowing that the mortality was one in eighteen, and not one in three, Portal's cases were excluded altogether, and this culpable act, committed for the purpose of exaggerating the mortality in placental presentation, is thrice falsely imputed to an erroneous "reliance on Dr. Lee's accuracy," when in his 'Clinical Midwifery' he stated that Portal's work contained an account of eight cases only of unavoidable hæmorrhage." My "Clinical Midwifery" contains no statement bordering upon such an assertion as this, which is utterly false and unfounded, and obviously made for the purpose of convicting me of an error which I never committed, and which I have proved, by the most conclusive evidence, it was impossible for me to commit. The words in my "Clinical Midwifery," are "Portal's Treatise (1686) contains an account of eight cases of uterine hæmorrhage, in which he found the placenta not merely 'at the mouth of the womb,' but adhering to the whole neck of the uterus."

My object throughout this discussion has not been to bandy abuse with Professor Simpson, nor to correct charges of misrepresentation which are either without foundation, or which have been refuted again and again, but my aim has been, to prove, before the face of the profession, that the practice of tearing away the adherent placenta from the neck of the uterus, either by the hand, or by an iron or other instrument, is a murderous practice· and, furthermore, that the physiological assumption of the escape of the maternal blood from the vessels of the placenta in unavoidable hæmorrhage is a gross, unparalleled, and unretracted blunder! I am content to leave it to the profession to decide whether these things are or are not so? We shall see whether scientific accoucheurs abide by the old established rules of practice, and whether Dr. Simpson himself does not flee off to some new marvel, some fresher novelty, to attract public notoriety, and to cover his defeat in this BATTLE OF PLACENTA PRÆVIA!

Savile-row, Nov. 1847.

ON
A NEW ANÆSTHETIC AGENT, MORE EFFICIENT THAN SULPHURIC ETHER.

By J. Y. SIMPSON, M.D.,

PROFESSOR OF MIDWIFERY IN THE UNIVERSITY OF EDINBURGH, PHYSICIAN-ACCOUCHEUR TO HER MAJESTY IN SCOTLAND, ETC.

AT the first winter meeting of the Medico-Chirurgical Society of Edinburgh, held on the 10th of November last, I had an opportunity of directing the attention of the members to a new agent which I had been using for some time previously, for the purpose of producing insensibility to pain in surgical and obstetric practice.

This new anæsthetic agent is chloroform, chloroformyle, or perchloride of formyle.* Its composition is expressed by the chemical formula $C_2 H Cl_3$. It can be procured by various processes, as by making milk of lime, or an aqueous solution of caustic alkali, act upon chloral; by distilling alcohol, pyroxylic spirit, or acetone, with chloride of lime; by leading a stream of chlorine gas into a solution of caustic potass, in spirit of wine, &c. The resulting chloroform obtained by these processes is a heavy, clear, transparent liquid, with a specific gravity as high as 1.480. It is not inflammable. It evaporates readily, and boils at 141°. It possesses an agreeable, fragrant, fruit-like odour, and a saccharine, pleasant taste.

As an inhaled anæsthetic agent, it possesses, I believe, all the advantages of sulphuric ether, without its principal disadvantages.

1. A greatly less quantity of chloroform than of ether is requisite to produce the anæsthetic effect—usually from a hundred to a hundred and twenty drops of chloroform being sufficient, and with some patients much less. I have seen a strong person rendered completely insensible by seven inspirations of thirty drops only of the liquid.

2. Its action is much more rapid and complete, and generally more persistent. I have almost always seen from ten to twenty inspirations suffice—sometimes fewer. Hence the time of the surgeon is saved, and that preliminary stage of excitement which pertains to all narcotizing agents, being curtailed, or indeed practically abolished, the patient has not the same degree of tendency to exhilaration and talking.

3. Most of those who know, from previous experience, the sensations produced by ether inhalation, and who have subsequently breathed the chloroform, have strongly declared the inhalation and influence of chloroform to be far more agreeable and pleasant than those of ether.

4. I believe that, considering the small quantity requisite, as compared with ether, the use of chloroform will be less expensive than that of ether—more especially as there is every prospect that the means of forming it may be simplified and cheapened.

5. Its perfume is not unpleasant, but the reverse, and the odour of it does not remain, for any length of time, attached to the clothes of the attendant, or exhaling, in a disagreeable form, from the lungs of the patient, as so generally happens with sulphuric ether.

6. Being required in much less quantity, it is much more portable and transmissible than sulphuric ether.

7. No special kind of inhaler or instrument is necessary for its exhibition. A little of the liquid, diffused upon the interior of a hollow-shaped sponge, or a pocket-handkerchief, or a piece of linen or paper, and held over the mouth and nostrils, so as to be fully inhaled, generally suffices, in about a minute or two, to produce the desired effect.

I have had an opportunity of using chloroform with perfect success in several surgical operations, (removal of tumours, of necrosed bone, partial amputation of the great toe,) and in tooth-drawing,† opening abscesses, for annulling the pain of

---

* In making a variety of experiments upon the inhalation of different volatile chemical liquids, I have, in addition to perchloride of formyle, breathed chloride of hydrocarbon, acetone, nitrate of oxide of ethyle, benzin, the vapour of iodoform, &c. I may probably take another opportunity of describing the result. It is perhaps worthy of remark, that in performing his experiments upon inhalation, Sir Humphry Davy confined his attention to the inspiration of gases, and does not seem to have breathed any volatile liquid.

† A young dentist, who has himself had two teeth extracted lately,—one under the influence of ether, and the other under the influence of chloroform,—writes me the following statement of the result:—"About six months ago, I had an upper molar tooth extracted, whilst under the influence of ether, by Mr. Imlach. The inhalation was continued for several minutes before I presented the usual appearance of complete etherization; the tooth was extracted; and although I did not feel the least pain, yet I was conscious of the operation being performed, and was quite aware when the crash took place. Some days ago, I required another molar extracted, on account of toothach, and this operation was again performed by the

dysmennorrhœa and of neuralgia, in two or three cases where I was using deep and otherwise very painful galvano-puncture for the treatment of ovarian dropsy, and in removing a very large fibrous tumour from the posterior wall of the uterus by enucleation, &c.

I have employed it also in obstetric practice, with entire success. The lady to whom it was first exhibited during parturition had been previously delivered in the country by perforation of the head of the infant, after a labour of three days' duration. In this, her second confinement, pains supervened a fortnight before the full time. Three hours and a half after they commenced, ere the dilatation of the os uteri was completed, I placed her under the influence of the chloroform, by moistening, with half a teaspoonful of the liquid, a pocket-handkerchief, rolled up in a funnel shape, and with the broad or open end of the funnel placed over her mouth and nostrils. In consequence of the evaporation of the fluid, it was once more renewed in about ten or twelve minutes. The child was expelled in about twenty-five minutes after the inhalation was begun. The mother subsequently remained longer soporose than commonly happens after ether. The squalling of the child did not, as usual, rouse her; and some minutes elapsed after the placenta was expelled, and after the child was removed by the nurse into another room, before the patient awoke. She then turned round, and observed to me that she had " enjoyed a very comfortable sleep, and, indeed, required it, as she was so tired,* but would now be more able for the work before her." I evaded entering into conversation with her, believing, as I have already stated, that the most complete possible quietude forms one of the principal secrets for the successful employment of either ether or chloroform. In a little time, she again remarked, that she was afraid her " sleep had stopped the pains." Shortly afterwards, her infant was brought in by the nurse from the adjoining room, and it was a matter of no small difficulty to convince the astonished mother that the labour was entirely over, and that the child presented to her was really her " own living baby."

Perhaps I may be excused from adding, that since publishing on the subject of ether inhalation in midwifery, seven or eight months ago,† and then for the first time directing the attention of the profession to its great use and importance in natural and morbid parturition, I have employed it, with few and rare exceptions, in every case of labour that I have attended, and with the most delightful results. And I have no doubt whatever, that some years hence the practice will be general. Obstetricians may oppose it, but I believe our patients themselves will force the use of it upon the profession.‡ I have never had the pleasure of watching over a series of better and more rapid recoveries, nor once witnessed any disagreeable result follow to either mother or child, whilst I have now seen an immense amount of maternal pain and agony saved by its employment. And I most conscientiously believe, that the proud mission of the physician is distinctly twofold—namely, to alleviate human suffering, as well as preserve human life.

In some remarks which I published in the *Monthly Journal of Medical Science* for September, 1847, p. 154, relative to the conditions for insuring successful etherization in surgery, I took occasion to insist upon the three following leading points: —"First, the patient ought to be left, as far as possible, in a state of absolute quietude and freedom from mental excitement, both during the induction of etherization, and during his recovery from it. All talking, and all questioning, should be strictly prohibited. In this way any tendency to excitement is eschewed, and the proper effect of the ether-inhalation more speedily and certainly induced. And, secondly, with the same view, the primary stage of exhilaration should be entirely avoided, or at least reduced to the shortest possible

limit, by impregnating the respired air as fully with the ether-vapour as the patient can bear, and by allowing it to pass into the lungs both by the mouth and nostrils, so as rapidly and at once to induce its complete anæsthetic effect on the patient, a very common, but certainly a very unpardonable error, being to exhibit an imperfect and exciting, instead of a perfect and narcotizing, dose of the vapour. Many of the alleged failures and misadventures are doubtless entirely attributable to the neglect of this simple rule; not the principle of etherization, but the mode of putting it in practice, being altogether to blame. But, thirdly, whatever means or mode of etherization is adopted, the most important of the conditions required for procuring a satisfactory and successful result from its employment in surgery, consists in obstinately determining to avoid the commencement of the operation itself, and never venturing to apply the knife until the patient is under the full influence of the ether-vapour, *and thoroughly and indubitably soporized by it.*"

In fulfilling all these indications, the employment of chloroform evidently offers great and decided advantages in rapidity, facility, and efficiency over the employment of ether. When used for surgical purposes, I would advise it to be given upon a handkerchief, gathered up into a cuplike form in the hand of the exhibitor, and the open end of the cup placed over the nose and mouth of the patient. For the first inspiration or two it should be held at the distance of an inch or so from the face, and then more and more closely applied to it. To insure a full and perfect anæsthetic effect—more especially when the operation is to be severe—a tea-spoonful of the chloroform should at once be placed upon the hollow of the handkerchief, and immediately held to the face of the patient. Generally, a snoring sleep very speedily supervenes; and when it does, it is a perfect test of the superinduction of complete insensibility. But many patients are quite anæsthetic without this symptom.

As an illustration of the influence of this new anæsthetic agent, I will select and append notes of two operations performed with it, on Friday last, by Professor Miller—the first in the Royal Infirmary,* the other in private practice. The notes and remarks are in Mr Miller's own words.

CASE 1.—" A boy, four or five years old, with necrosis of one of the bones of the fore-arm. Could speak nothing but Gaelic. No means, consequently, of explaining to him what he was required to do. On holding a handkerchief, on which some chloroform had been sprinkled, to his face, he became frightened, and wrestled to be away. He was held gently, however, by Dr. Simpson, and obliged to inhale. After a few inspirations he ceased to cry or move, and fell into a sound, snoring sleep. A deep incision was now made down to the diseased bone; and, by the use of the forceps, nearly the whole of the radius, in the state of sequestrum, was extracted. During this operation, and the subsequent examination of the wound by the finger, not the slightest evidence of the suffering of pain was given. He still slept on soundly, and was carried back to his ward in that state. Half an hour afterwards, he was found in bed, like a child newly awakened from a refreshing sleep, with a clear merry eye, and placid expression of countenance, wholly unlike what is found to obtain after ordinary etherization. On being questioned by a Gaelic interpreter who was found among the students, he stated that he had never felt any pain, and that he felt none now. On being shown his wounded arm, he looked much surprised, but neither cried nor otherwise expressed the slightest alarm."

CASE 2.—" A young lady wished to have a tumour (encysted) dissected out from beneath the angle of the jaw. The chloroform was used in small quantity, sprinkled upon a common operation sponge. In considerably less than a minute she was sound asleep, sitting easily in a chair, with her eyes shut, and with her ordinary expression of countenance. The tumour was extirpated, and a stitch inserted, without any pain having been either shown or felt. Her sensations throughout, as she subsequently stated, had been of the most pleasing nature; and her manageableness during the operation was as perfect as if she had been a wax doll or a lay figure.

" No sickness, vomiting, headach, salivation, uneasiness of chest, in any of the cases. Once or twice a tickling cough took place in the first breathings."

Edinburgh, November, 1847.

---

same gentleman. I inhaled the vapour of chloroform, half a drachm being poured upon a handkerchief for that purpose, and held to my nose and mouth. Insensibility took place in a few seconds, but I was so completely *dead* this time, that I was not in the very slightest degree aware of anything that took place. The subsequent stupifying effects of chloroform went off more rapidly than those of ether, and I was perfectly well, and able again for my work, in a few minutes.

* In consequence of extreme anxiety at the unfortunate result of her previous confinement, she had slept little or none for one or two nights preceding the commencement of her present accouchement.

† See Monthly Journal of Medical Science for February, p. 639; and for March, pp. 718 and 721, &c.

‡ I am told that the London physicians, with two or three exceptions only, have never yet employed ether-inhalation in their midwifery practice. Three weeks ago, I was informed, in a letter from Professor Montgomery, of Dublin, that he believed that in that city, up to that date, it had not been used in a single case of labour.

* Professor Dumas, of Paris, Mr. Milne Edwards, Dr. Christison, Sir George Ballingall, and a large collection of professional gentlemen and students, witnessed this operation, and two others, performed, with similar success, by Professor Miller and Dr. Duncan.

684   MR. BEECROFT ON THE CONTAGIOUS NATURE OF PUERPERAL FEVER.

reference to his hair, nearly the same opaque white condition as in the last case. His habits are most dissolute, particularly in spirit drinking; and the district in which he resides is famous for its calcareous productions. Original colour of the hair, black.

Remarks.—In Cases 2 and 6 we perceive that albinism of the hair set in about the same period, and that both subjects were drinkers of ardent spirits to an immoderate extent. I have nothing to do with the question of temperance, and never interdict the moderate use of spirit, unless upon some professional grounds.

Now, alcohol, added to a solution of the sulphate, or of the acid phosphate of lime, precipitates it in an insoluble form; and if the same decompositions transpire in, as out of the system,—and we have no evidence to support a contrary hypothesis,—the imbibition of alcoholic drinks may be rightly regarded as one cause of osthexial formations generally.

That the abnormal excess of lime in the system, irrespective of its causes, is the essentially proximate excitant of such formations, must be looked upon as capable of being supported by more efficient evidence than any other; and until absolute demonstration shall usurp the place of hypothetical, or probable reasoning, is it not an indication of the soundest reason, to stand on that foundation, supported by strong evidence of truth?

Braunston, Northamptonshire. May 1847.

ILLUSTRATIONS OF
THE CONTAGIOUS NATURE OF PUERPERAL FEVER.
WITH REMARKS ON ITS TREATMENT, AND ON CONTAGION AND INFECTION.

By SAMUEL BEECROFT, Esq., M.R.C.S.E., Hyde.

I LAY the following cases and remarks before the profession, from a desire to render my mite towards elucidating the true nature of contagious diseases. I think that of late there has been manifested a disposition to decry the influence of contagion; this probably arises from all epidemic diseases having been considered, by our earlier predecessors, to have been propagated thereby. I am afraid we are acting equally rashly with them, by rushing into the opposite extreme, and proportionally denying its agency. I do not apply such remarks to the class of cases I am about to relate, for I believe that most of us agree in the contagious character of puerperal fever, but I wish to show how careful we ought to be in refusing to acknowledge the influence of contagion. For some time it was denied to this class of diseases, and even now is by the French school. Not long since, there was the same disposition to deny that typhus was capable of being communicated by contagion, but I think, from the number of medical men who have lately fallen its victims, that question is finally set at rest.

I would state my opinion that all diseases originating from a pestiferous virus entering into the body, and poisoning the blood, should be set down as capable of transmitting the same virus to others, and thus communicating the disease. I cannot see why the animal body cannot expel from it that which enters it, and thus become the medium of infection. And here I would observe that the distinction made by some of our medical authors, between contagion and infection, is unnecessary, for we know that the skin (though in a minor degree than the lungs) has the property of absorption, and therefore we must come to the opinion that infection may enter the body by contact. There can be no doubt that depraved food, bad air, want of cleanliness, &c., are powerful means of propagating epidemic disease; but I question if it is generally generated by these agents. It may be owing to our ignorance, that we lay such stress on these perceptible causes, and trust not the unknown, merely from not being able to detect them in our present imperfect knowledge of chemistry. The preceding remarks arose from reading that the Sanitary Commission had come to the opinion that cholera is not contagious, which opinion appears to me to be rash and not trustworthy, until we better know what the true principle of contagion is. Having already encroached much on the valuable space of THE LANCET, I shall condense the following cases, and therefore shall not enter minutely into the symptoms of each case:—

CASE 1.—Mrs. H——, aged thirty-four years, of a gross, lax habit, troubled with erysipelas nasi, was delivered, after an easy labour of her fifth child, on Saturday, Nov. 28, 1846, (the

night of a violent snow-storm, and when extreme cold set in.) She was seized with vomiting and purging, and died on morning of the eighth day after delivery. I attributed her death to exhaustion caused by the vomiting and purging, which I thought was brought on by carelessness in living—taking fermented liquor, and eating goose, beef, &c., on the second and third days after delivery.

I had permission to make a post-mortem examination, which was instituted fifty-five hours after death, but it was not so minute as it otherwise would have been, from my assistance being urgently requested at the case of convulsions which I will shortly describe. The body was in good condition; redness about the nose, of a slight dingy hue; the right side was contracted; the lungs and heart were healthy; blood very dark and fluid; the stomach large, with considerable redness of its mucous coat, near the pylorus; liver enlarged, very dark, easily stripped of its peritonæal coat, and breaking up like a soft coagulum; gall bladder contained some dark fluid similar to what had been ejected; peritonæum perfectly healthy; not the least effusion in the abdomen, nor any signs of inflammation of the peritonæum covering the viscera; bowels healthy, in some parts congested; kidneys healthy; uterus contracted, containing nothing, but its internal surface coated with a dark viscid substance; its walls were perfectly healthy, and I perceived no condition of any of the organs to account for death, unless it was the diseased state of the liver.

CASE 2.—Mrs. G——, aged twenty-six years, troubled with erysipelas nasi; delivered of her third child, labour easy, twelve P.M., Dec. 6th. She slept well during the night; in the morning, about eight o'clock, complained of headach, and soon after vomited some bilious, dark-looking fluid. At ten o'clock, after vomiting, convulsions set in, and my attendance was required, whilst making the previous post-mortem examination. Although active treatment was resorted to, the convulsions continued, and she died at ten P.M. the same day, twenty-two hours after delivery.

CASE 3.—Mrs. B——, aged twenty years, healthy; delivered of her first child, at two A.M., Dec. 9th. Rigors came on during the following day, with well-marked symptoms of puerperal fever, and she died on the 15th, six days from delivery, pus being deposited in the shoulder and elbow the day prior to death.

CASE 4.—Mrs. N——, aged thirty-one years; not well for some weeks; suffering from cough and occasional abdominal pains, which resembled those of labour; but for some days before labour came on she went about her usual household duties. I went with the husband from the previous case, and she was delivered, after an easy labour, of her fourth child, about three o'clock the same morning. Puerperal fever came on, and she died on the 11th of December, the day but one after delivery.*

I now thought the cases to be contagious, and did not attend another labour until the 20th. After using every precaution, I on that day attended Mrs. E——, who did well, and Mrs. H——, the subject of the following case:—

CASE 5.—Mrs. H——, aged thirty, suffering from varicose ulcer of the leg, surrounded with considerable redness, of an erysipelatous nature, was delivered of her third child, after an easy labour, on the morning of Dec. 20th. On the fourth day after confinement, fever set in, and she died the following Sunday, (Dec. 27th.)†

CASE 6.—I was called to attend Mrs. M——, aged twenty-seven years, of her third child. The child was born, and the cord divided, when I arrived at the house; and on placing my hand on the abdomen, the uterus contracted, and the placenta was expelled. Her sister, who lived in the house, was suffering from typhus; but this patient ailed nothing prior to delivery. Puerperal fever set in the day after delivery, and she died on the same day as the preceding case.

I now gave up attending midwifery, went from home for a time, and again attended a labour on Jan. 16th, 1847, from which time to Jan. 31st I attended seven cases. Two of them difficult, and required turning, and the other the use of the forceps, which I employed for a medical friend. All of these cases did well. The weather had been warmer; but at the

---

* Mrs. F——, nearly sixty years of age, who nursed Mrs. N——, had at the time old-standing ulcers of the left leg. Erysipelas of the leg came on, rapidly spreading to the groin, and attended with low fever and sloughing of the diseased leg; and she died on December 22nd, thirteen days after Mrs. N——'s death.

† Mrs. H——'s child died on Jan. 11th, from erysipelas of the head and face, being three weeks old, and fifteen days after the death of its mother.

latter part of the month it became very cold. On the morning of Jan. 31st I attended

CASE 7.—Mrs. W——, aged twenty-five years; disfigured with erysipelas nasi spreading to the cheeks; had seven rigors during labour, and chills the day previous; labour easy. Adynamic puerperal fever set in, and she died on the morning of Feb. 5th, the face looking horrible from the extreme blackness of the erysipelatous parts.

I saw no more of the disease, though occasionally alarmed by rigors following delivery, excepting an anomalous case which occurred to a Mrs. F——, who was delivered on the 1st of April, she having just recovered from fever. The woman did well for the first fortnight, but was forced to exert herself in her household duties, being unable to pay for a nurse. She sent for me on April 23rd, and stated that she had been out for a distance of two miles the week before, and had not been well since. The lochia had not ceased, and for some days she said that the discharge was very copious and disagreeable. She was then suffering from phlebitis, a phlegmon existing over the right elbow and hip, and she died on the 29th, having every symptom of puerperal fever.

In considering over the preceding cases, I think there cannot be any doubt that a contagious principle was generated by Mrs. H——, (the first case,) which was conveyed to my third case, and thus the puerperal fever was originated; and I cannot help thinking that the second case (convulsion) had some connexion with that of Mrs. H——. The third, fourth, fifth, and sixth cases show the contagious nature of the disease, and the seventh and last cases, also, that puerperal fever may be propagated either by direct contagion, or by atmospheric influence acting on those who may be predisposed to the disease. The prevalence of erysipelas at the same time, and the tendency manifested to it in the cases related, strengthen the opinion, that puerperal fever and erysipelas are the same disease, one being capable of producing the other. The symptoms presented by these puerperal cases evidenced that the disease was dependent on a poisoned state of the blood, and not in any particular organ. There were a small, feeble, and very rapid pulse, anxiety, and a sense of uneasiness about the heart, hurried breathing, cough; in some of the cases, purulent expectoration, and profuse sweating. Some were troubled with vomiting and purging; no tenderness of the abdomen, but on pressing the uterus, which was rather larger than usual, pain was produced. There was no swelling or tympanitis when death took place within the fourth day; but in those who lived longer, the abdomen began to enlarge a short time before death. The lochia was deranged, and occasionally scanty, and in one case retention of urine existed. The cases were distinctly of the adynamic kind, presenting signs of a violent shock to the whole system. With respect to the treatment of such a form, (not puerperal peritonitis,) I should be inclined to follow the advice of those who do not recommend bleeding. I tried it in two cases, but it did no good. I would assist nature by acting on the principle of elimination. A mild emetic might be serviceable at the commencement by unloading the biliary ducts, followed by frequent doses of calomel; for I believe the liver is the most important organ to call to our aid in expelling the poison, and it is probable, from its office as a depurative of the blood, that it presents a morbid appearance after death, and thus in various diseases, (cholera, for instance,) this has been said to be the cause, when it ought only to rank as the effect of the disease. Diaphoretics also might assist; Dover's powder I found useful in calming the patient, and relieving pain; indeed, every means of eliminating the poison from the blood might be employed, whilst at the same time the system must be supported by ammonia, wine, beef-tea, &c.

Hyde, 1848.

ON A CASE OF
MECHANICAL INJURY OF THE KIDNEYS,

FOLLOWED BY COMA, SUPPRESSION OF THE SECRETION OF UREA BY THE KIDNEYS, AND ITS ABSORPTION INTO THE BLOOD.

BY E. J. SHEARMAN, M.D., Rotherham.

IN consequence of death in general so speedily following the suspension of the excretion of urea by the kidneys, owing to its consequent quick absorption into the blood and poisonous influence on the brain and nervous system, it rarely happens that time is given for a practitioner to determine decidedly, both chemically and pathologically, that the comatose symptoms depend altogether on the non-elimination of urea by the kidneys. The following case, from the attending circum-

stances, elucidates this point so simply and fully, that I cannot refrain from putting it on record:—

On the 23rd of last September, Edward C——, aged eight years, in perfect health, while at play, was run over across the loins by a heavy truck. In two hours after the accident I saw him. He was then in a state of collapse, and my impression was, that some internal hæmorrhage was then going on, for he was blanched, cold, and pulseless. He complained of acute pain in the left lumbar region, which was very tender to the touch, spreading to both the inguinal and the pubic region. I gave him stimulants, and kept him warm, by which means, in the course of thirty-six hours he gradually improved; and he then passed a large quantity of blood with his urine, not having previously voided any urine since the accident. This was repeated several times during the next twenty-four hours.

I examined this urine and blood most carefully, but failed to detect the least particle of urea or urates in it.

My little patient became more restless; fever set in, with a pulse at 130; and the pain in the region of the kidneys increased, notwithstanding the application of leeches &c. But these symptoms, in the course of two days, were succeeded by coma; he could not be kept awake.

I now bled him in the arm, and reapplied leeches to the tender part. On examining this blood, urea was most distinctly detected in it, and in considerable quantity. The urine, at the same time, contained not a particle of urea, urates, uric acid, or albumen, and its specific gravity was only 1,005.

I got him under the influence of mercury as quickly as possible; as soon as its specific effect was apparent, urea gradually reappeared in the urine, and its specific gravity increased. By degrees the comatose symptoms subsided, and in the course of five weeks usual health was re-established. He continues quite well.

The mode of detecting urea in the blood which I adopted was the one recommended by Dr. G. O. Rees, (" On the Analysis of Blood and Urine, in Health and Disease," second edition, page 40,) and which I will describe shortly, as some readers may not have that useful work in their possession.

The first quantity of serum analyzed was 400 grains by weight, which were evaporated to dryness over an open steam bath. I broke up the dry extract, added two ounces of distilled water, and digested it over a steam bath for an hour, occasionally supplying the loss of water; then filtered the digested fluid, washing the residue on the filter with distilled water, which I added to the mother liquor. I then evaporated the whole over an open steam bath, and digested the residue with eight times its bulk of absolute alcohol, at a gentle heat, for half an hour, taking care not to diminish materially the bulk of the fluid. It was then filtered a second time, evaporated to dryness, and dissolved in a little lukewarm distilled water, and again evaporated to the consistence of a thin syrup. I now added a few drops of nitric acid, and set it aside to crystallize.

Previously to adding the nitric acid, a very strong odour of urea was perceptible. On examining the fluid under the microscope, to which the nitric acid had been added, tabular crystals of nitrate of urea were easily perceived, commencing in appearance as transverse lines across the watch-glass.

On examining afterwards a larger quantity of serum, (600 grains,) a more considerable quantity of the nitrate of urea was observed.

Although the quantities of serum analyzed were, in both cases, small, undeniable proof of the existence in them of urea, in considerable quantity, presented themselves; there must, then, have been a large quantity of urea in the blood.

It was my intention to have ascertained the amount of urea in a certain portion of serum, but I was obliged, from existing circumstances, to suspend my examinations at this point.

It is well known that, in youth, the quantity of urea in the urine is much larger than in the adult, owing to the more rapid disintegration of the tissues. In this case, a considerable portion of that excretion must have been circulating through the system.

In the absence of an actual examination of the organs affected, it appears to me that the ramifications of the renal arteries, which form the external vascular portion of the kidneys, were ruptured by the accident, which would be followed by congestion and inflammation of the Malpighian bodies and tubuli uriniferi, thus preventing all real secretion, and merely allowing the watery part of the blood to percolate through the tubular portion of the organs.

Rotherham, February, 1848.

204   OSSIFICATION OF THE PLACENTA.—UNHEALTHY CONDITION OF PADDINGTON.

the centre, and, at times, the stricture is on one side. The middle of a long stricture is sometimes larger in diameter than at the ends, and frequently the urethra assumes a tortuous direction; or a membrane, denominated a bar, will extend across the canal. All these remarks on the variety of strictures,—which require different modes of treatment,—by bougies, catheters, natron exsiccatum, argenti nitras, kali purum, and unguentum hydrargyri fortis, are introduced, in order to show the enormous amount of irritation which would be produced in an already excited state of the urinary organs, where extraneous deposits are of too stimulating a nature to require any addition of inflammatory excitement to remove the cause. With a view of mitigating the existing symptoms by the removal of all unnatural secretions, and relaxing spasmodically contracted canals and passages, the soothing effects of heat and moisture are employed, as being well-known agents for the purpose. Nothing but an easy and perfectly controllable method of administering them is wanted, a desideratum which I have found attained by means of the instrument referred to, a diagram of which may in some measure serve to point out its construction and mode of application.

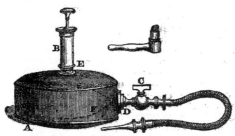

A, is a vessel made sufficiently strong, and of material impervious to air in a condensed state; B, a syringe for compressing atmospheric air into the said vessel; C, is a stopcock which screws into the opening at D, and, in conjunction with the valve, E, serves to secure the injection, after being poured into the vessel through the opening, and to regulate the stream by diminishing or increasing the power from one drachm to the weight of several pounds; G, is one of the vessels for containing compressed air, or any of the gases. When the injector is to be used, unscrew the stopcock, C, and fill the vessel quite full of the liquid to be injected, then return the stopcock into the opening tolerably tight. The air-syringe, B, must now be screwed into E, which, being worked to the extent of twenty or thirty strokes, renders it ready for use. On introducing the ivory pipe in the usual way, the injection can be administered with any required degree of force, and in any position of the body, without the aid of a second person, and without the introduction of the slightest particle of atmospheric air.

Carlisle-street, Soho, 1849.

A REPORT OF TWO CASES OF OSSIFICATION OF THE PLACENTA.

By JAMES ROBERTSON, M.D., F.R.C.S.,
SURGEON TO THE HITCHIN INFIRMARY.

OTTO says, that " even the dead child, with its membranes, if it have been retained for a long time in the mother's womb," is sometimes ossified; but I suppose this, or even the ossification of a part, as the placenta, is rare, for I am not able to find any case recorded of late. Even Rokitansky omits to mention ossification amongst his " Abnormities of the Ovum," and appears not to have seen ossification of the placenta; for he says, " Foreign observers have given instances of osseous deposits in, or ossification of, the placenta; they are gibbous, nodulated, or cordate formations, which are probably developed in the placental tissue after it has been obliterated by inflammation, or in the fibrinous coagula caused by hæmorrhage."

As the instances are few, I have noted the two following, which have occurred in my practice:—

Mrs. ——, the mother of several children, supposed herself pregnant; but when about six months gone, her abdomen diminished in size, and she knew no more about it till about nine months afterwards, when suddenly, early one morning, she thought herself in labour, and quickly gave birth to a withered, leather-like fœtus and placenta, of average size for a full-grown child, but which was entirely composed of an

aggregation of spiculæ of bone. There was scarcely any discharge. The fœtus was probably six months old, and had been retained in the womb nine months after its death.

Mrs. —— supposed herself about five months gone with child, when the abdomen began to lessen in size. She consulted me about two months after this, when a tumour, having all the appearance, on examination, of the pregnant womb, was evident. Three months after she suddenly aborted a withered, leather-like fœtus, and a placenta which was bloodless, gristly, and had numerous spiculæ and plates of bone scattered over both free and attached surfaces. There was considerable flooding. The fœtus was probably about five months old, and had been retained in the womb five months after its death.

Hitchin, Herts, August, 1849.

ON THE
NEGLECTED AND UNHEALTHY CONDITION OF A PART OF PADDINGTON.
INEFFICIENCY OF THE BOARD OF HEALTH, AND INGRATITUDE TOWARDS THE MEDICAL PROFESSION.

By JOHN GRAY, Esq., Surgeon, London.

OBSERVING that an inquest was lately held on the body of a man who died of cholera in the Wharf-road, Paddington, and as you invariably expose the neglect of sanitary measures by the accredited authorities, I trust you will afford a niche in your paper for this letter, whereby the public may be made aware of the neglected and disgraceful state in which that locality is left by the parish authorities, and the utter inefficiency of the so-called board of health. I have frequent occasion to visit the neighbourhood where the attacked person died, and never could it be believed, except by actual inspection, that such a mass of filth could be allowed to accumulate and rot amidst a densely crowded population. Why, Sir, there is a dust-heap of garbage, of the most disgusting description, that has been lying for years, consisting of many thousand tons, with herds of swine luxuriating on this decomposed offal; the smell is so abominable, that the highly respectable inhabitants of Eastbourne-terrace, several hundreds of yards distant from it, and opposite, are obliged to keep their windows shut when the wind blows from that quarter. Besides, a vast amount of dung is allowed to be brought there by the Grand Junction Canal Company; and when it is turned over to be rotted for conveyance, the stench is so abominable that every one in the neighbourhood is instantly forced to close every aperture to shut out the horrid effluvium. If the ancient Egyptians were visited with plagues, surely the inhabitants of Dudley-grove have as much reason to complain as they had, for of all the places that ever I saw, this certainly is the place for the plague of flies, and such flies as are nowhere to be seen but there—they are not the ordinary flies, but great long fellows, with snouts like elephants, and stings in their tails as long as stocking needles. If I said they swarmed in myriads I should be infinitely behind the mark; they are myriads and tens of myriads; and to preserve a piece of meat beyond a day is out of the question, for the bluebottle flies keep up a perpetual buzz, and hum around your ears as if a whole congregation of Welch ranters were catechising. Another and very serious matter for reflection is that of the Paddington churchyard, which is so filled with dead that it has actually risen upwards of four feet above the footpath with the remnants of mortality; but so long as the clergy, who have fees from the living and the dead, are allowed to bury there, so long will the danger to the living be permitted. Frequently as I pass through the churchyard when graves are being dug, the effluvium is disgustingly perceptible. What, I ask, is the value of the sanitary board, when they allow such abominations? What is the use of Mr. Edwin Chadwick's statistics to society, by detailing the number of deaths, if no stop is put to the cause of them? Where is the pretended philanthropy of Dr. Southwood Smith, if he merely prates, and does not act? In short, I believe Mr. Edwin Chadwick has sucked the brains of the credulous and easily led medical profession for his own advantage; and Dr. Southwood Smith, after trying many dodges—viz., sanatoriums, &c., has not been slack in bayoneting him in the rear. And then, in reference to that excellent and open-hearted good nobleman, Lord Carlisle, full of tenderness, and plastic in disposition, he would do much if greater firmness were characteristic of his mind.

No real rectification of malarious influences can or ever will be achieved, until persons are appointed by authority to remove all nuisances; and who, I ask, are so fitted as those of the medical profession?—and for why? because they are in the hourly and daily habits of visiting the lowest and densest haunts of the poor and needy. But it seems the design of the government invariably to humiliate the medical profession, and make them subservient; and for what reason? why, because the profession has forgotten and neglected its value and position in society—it has been the tool and adjutor of corrupt ministration—it has not shown its strength and influence in political affairs—it has no recognised status as a body, like the church and the law, who are eternally in the front rank of beseechers for their own advantage. If the medical profession were true to themselves, and endeavoured to place a few more like Mr. Wakley in parliament, they then would have that just and proper weight which becomes their value and importance in the political community. I need not to apprise your mind of the many obligations the public owe to the profession for advantages they already possess. To us alone any progress in cleansing is due—not one syllable has emanated from the clergy or law to advance sanitary measures; to us belong the honour, to us the merit is denied. We are the fools by which the cunning weave their webs to procure to themselves warm comforts and independence.

Howley-place, Harrow-road, August, 1849.

THE POISONED FLOUR AT STOURBRIDGE.

REMARKS ON CASES OF POISONING BY THE ACETATE OF LEAD; AND ON DR. AYRE'S TREATMENT OF ASIATIC CHOLERA.

By WILLIAM NORRIS, M.D.,

LATE PHYSICIAN TO THE STOURBRIDGE DISPENSARY.

ACUTE and chronic diseases of the abdominal viscera form a large class of the most violent and dangerous character that come under the treatment of the medical practitioner; and without early and decisive measures they too often terminate fatally; and any opportunity that may occur to throw the least additional light on their pathology or treatment should be zealously cultivated.

As an awful occurrence has taken place in the towns of Stourbridge and Kidderminster, and the neighbouring villages, from the mistake of a miller's servant, who mixed about thirty pounds of acetate of lead, in the place of alum, with seventy or eighty sacks of flour, nearly a thousand persons having suffered from its poisonous effects, I shall make a feeble attempt to place before the profession anything new or striking, with the hope that it may induce eminent toxicologists to investigate the alarming disease more minutely. The sufferings of the patients, in consequence of eating the poisoned bread, have been unusually severe, and protracted for some weeks after the violent symptoms first commenced; the strongest and most robust men (from long suffering, and from the frequent occurrence of violent paroxysms) have been reduced to the most emaciated and feeble state.

The persons who ate the bread, after a few weeks, complained of a peculiar taste; some compared it to soda, others to rusty needles, or copper. The tongue was covered with a darkish, cream-coloured mucus, and was soft and flabby; the gums were swollen, with a blue line on the margin, and in many cases the blue tinge extended nearly over the gums, and occasionally on the inner side of the lower lip, and in a faint degree over the mucous membrane of the mouth, and towards the fauces. The tonsils were in some cases enlarged, producing soreness of the throat; and in other cases there was salivation, a clear fluid flowing from the mouth many days after convalescence.

These symptoms were accompanied by loss of appetite, nausea, vomiting, flatulency, and obstinate constipation, with a sense of constriction in the throat and epigastrium, and a violent spasmodic pain and twisting around the umbilicus, which was retracted. The pain was sometimes increased by pressure, occasionally extending over the abdomen; and when the paroxysms were violent, the muscles of the abdomen were contracted spasmodically.

A most frequent symptom was pain in the loins, about the situation of the lumbar fascia; also in the deltoid muscles. The patients were chilly, with great languor and lassitude; the cutaneous secretion was diminished; the intellect was clear, but there was generally depression of the nervous, sanguiferous, and muscular systems; the pulse was low and feeble; the features were sallow and shrunk; and the muscles were soft and flabby. The fluid vomited was often mixed with bile, and occasionally coffee-ground secretion; the fæces were dark, and highly offensive, with scybala; the secretion from the kidneys was scanty, and of a dark-red colour, almost like porter.

Treatment.—The bowels were in general so obstinately costive, that large and frequently-repeated doses of the strongest cathartics were often necessary. Sometimes I began with a large dose of calomel, followed by sulphate of magnesia or castor oil. When these did not produce sufficient effect, croton oil and voluminous enemata were used with manifest advantage. Croton-oil frictions were useful when vomiting was excessive; to allay the sickness, hydrocyanic acid, or small doses of calomel-and-opium. By the omission of the daily purgative the symptoms would in many cases return. The patients were directed to take light, nutritious food, and milk, during convalescence. Some cases were so slight (although the gums were blue) that the patients would not take medicine.

In violent cases, when other remedies had failed, the warm bath relaxed the spasms very speedily. Opiate frictions and bran poultices were useful in milder cases. The soothing effects of the warm bath in some instances were quite astonishing, and in violent cases it should never be omitted, for it not only relieves the abdominal pain, but allays the spasms and irritation in other muscles of the body. When there was tenderness in the abdomen on pressure, leeches were beneficial, and in one case venesection was absolutely necessary.

A young woman, Phœbe W——, aged twenty-two, who had suffered severely from peritonitis three years before, had been ill from the effects of lead (with very blue gums) more than a week, when the pain in the abdomen much increased, with great tenderness on pressure, feverish excitement, and rapid pulse. Venesection and leeches were used, and the sufferings were mitigated; the symptoms returned with increased violence, and bleeding and other antiphlogistic remedies were repeated. The blood was buffed and cupped. As the inflammatory symptoms subsided she became almost maniacally hysterical on several successive nights, and yet she recovered many weeks sooner than any of the family, so that I am inclined to believe that in strong subjects venesection may be useful.

In very severe cases there was great exhaustion, and a slight leaden hue in the countenance; then stimulants became absolutely necessary.

It was melancholy to observe ten or twelve patients in poor families, all suffering at the same time, and scarcely able to assist each other, without funds, and without necessaries.

In one of the last numbers of the *Provincial Journal* I found iodide of potass, recommended in small doses, as a remedy for the poisonous effects of lead and mercury, by forming a soluble salt, which is readily eliminated. The experiments were performed by M. Natalis Guillot, read before the Académie des Sciences, Paris. I have tried this remedy in some cases, and certainly, gums that had been blue for months in a few days changed to a more natural appearance, and no symptoms of severity have since occurred; in fact, the patients appear now quite convalescent.

The poison of lead appears to exert its deleterious effects mostly on the muscular system. One of the most frequent symptoms was an acute or chronic pain in the muscles of the loins, and perhaps in the fascia lumborum; and in many cases the larger muscles of the body were affected with pain. Probably the abdominal pain is occasioned by the spasmodic constriction of the muscular fibres of the larger bowels, thus diminishing their contractility of tissue; and this may, in part, be the cause of constipation, though in some cases the spasm may be confined to the abdominal muscles.

In a youth eighteen years of age, with blue gums, the pains were confined to the muscles of the arms and legs, and he suffered most severely from violent contraction in all the extremities, without pain of abdomen or loins.

In this neighbourhood we have numerous glass-houses, and many hundreds of men are constantly employed in the fumes of lead, whom we know by a sallow, thin, unhealthy aspect, with soft and flabby muscles. The relapses in some constitutions were very frequent and very severe, sometimes after several weeks had elapsed, and patients thought themselves well.

Mr. S——, aged forty-seven, an irritable man of nervous temperament, had suffered from several severe paroxysms; the pains begun gradually to return a month after the onset of the disease, and increased like the pains of labour, every ten minutes, or a quarter of an hour; there was great difficulty in relieving his bowels, (which, in many instances, were locked up for a week or nine days.) When the bowels were cleared, large and repeated doses of laudanum only mitigated his sufferings, till at length, at the end of thirty-six hours, the pains

ADMINISTRATION OF CHLOROFORM TO THE QUEEN. 453

office of the College into contempt. This must be the effect of the absurd plan proposed in the Charter. We might go on to compare the last fifty extra-licentiates with the fifty ancients, but we forbear, though their names are quite as well-known as the ancient WHITTERS and FITTONS and YONGES and DUNNES. If the fifty old men of the College under the present *régime* are most of them fit for superannuation, how will it be under a new Charter, when the " Catalogue" must contain as many thousands of names as it now contains hundreds ?

A VERY extraordinary report has obtained general circulation connected with the recent accouchement of her most gracious Majesty Queen VICTORIA. It has always been understood by the profession that the births of the Royal children in all instances have been unattended by any peculiar or untoward circumstances. Intense astonishment, therefore, has been excited throughout the profession by the rumour that her Majesty during her last labour was placed under the influence of chloroform, an agent which has unquestionably caused instantaneous death in a considerable number of cases. Doubts on this subject cannot exist. In several of the fatal examples persons in their usual health expired while the process of inhalation was proceeding, and the deplorable catastrophes were clearly and indisputably referrible to the poisonous action of chloroform, and to that cause alone.

These facts being perfectly well known to the medical world, we could not imagine that any one had incurred the awful responsibility of advising the administration of chloroform to her Majesty during a perfectly natural labour with a seventh child. On inquiry, therefore, we were not at all surprised to learn that in her late confinement the Queen was not rendered insensible by chloroform or by any other anæsthetic agent. We state this with feelings of the highest satisfaction. In no case could it be justifiable to administer chloroform in perfectly ordinary labour; but the responsibility of advocating such a proceeding in the case of the Sovereign of these realms would, indeed, be tremendous. Probably some officious meddlers about the Court so far overruled her Majesty's responsible professional advisers as to lead to the pretence of administering chloroform, but we believe the obstetric physicians to whose ability the safety of our illustrious Queen is confided do not sanction the use of chloroform in natural labour. Let it not be supposed that we would undervalue the immense importance of chloroform in surgical operations. We know that an incalculable amount of agony is averted by its employment. On thousands of occasions it has been given without injury, but inasmuch as it has destroyed life in a considerable number of instances, its *unnecessary* inhalation involves, in our opinion, an amount of responsibility which words cannot adequately describe.

We have felt irresistibly impelled to make the foregoing observations, fearing the consequences of allowing such a rumour respecting a dangerous practice in one of our national palaces to pass unrefuted. Royal examples are followed with extraordinary readiness by a certain class of society in this country.

WE observe that the authorities of the University of St. Andrews complain that the diplomas of graduation issued by them are charged with a stamp duty. They represent that this is an impost pressing unfairly upon their University, inasmuch as the University of London is exempt from it. It may, we think, be very justly contended that the imposition of a stamp duty on the granting of a diploma is objectionable on the general ground that it must operate as a tax upon education, than which no tax can well be worse in principle or more mischievous in operation. But we think the authorities of St. Andrews, in forsaking that fundamental objection, and seeking to strengthen their position by an endeavour to show a special grievance, have not acted with due consideration or full knowledge of facts. There is a wide difference between their relation to the State and that occupied by the University of London, which renders all comparison as to this question inapplicable. In the case of the University of St. Andrews, the professors, the examiners, and the University chest are directly interested in passing candidates for degrees; to each a share of the fees is awarded; and, regarding the matter in a strictly fiscal point of view, the Chancellor of the Exchequer may with some show of reason maintain that an institution conducted with a view to private or corporate profit should contribute to the public necessities. The relation of the University of London is totally different. No examiner, nor other person is directly or indirectly interested in the passing of candidates; nor does the University itself benefit in the slightest degree. The senate is amenable to Parliamentary responsibility. A Parliamentary grant provides the funds necessary for its government, and in the yearly estimate of what is required the income from fees is taken into account. It would be a simple absurdity to burthen degrees conferred by a body holding such a relation to the State with a stamp duty. It would be passing money from the left pocket into the right.

This is why the University of London is exempted from the stamp duty on its diplomas, and it will be seen at once that the case is altogether exceptional. At the same time we are far from entertaining the opinion that the other British Universities are in any degree placed at a disadvantage as regards competition with the metropolitan University. In addition to the necessarily heavy expences attending a professional education and examinations spread over a period of six, seven, or in some cases nine years, the fees for the M.D. degree amount to £22, and the severity of the examinations must still further limit the number of candidates. That the northern Universities have not suffered in consequence of the foundation of a University in London is, moreover, conclusively proved by the fact that the number of applicants for degrees has of late years been greater than in former times.

A MORNING paper lately gave a report of a meeting held at a house in Bloomsbury-square which is dignified with the title of ' hospital," and is appropriated to the globulistic humbug. Who do the respectable and legally-qualified medical practitioners of Middlesex think occupied the chair on the occasion ? We must tell them. It was no less a person than Lord ROBERT GROSVENOR, their county member. In the course of the proceedings the noble lord said that " he re-" gretted there was not a more numerous attendance at the " meeting. He could not account for it; but he believed " there was an apathy on the part of the public with regard " to the support of these hospitals. He hoped, however, that '' this institution had done nothing to cause the public to

snuff them occasionally, and lend instantaneous aid in the event of any inflammable matter being accidentally ignited, by sparks or otherwise.

Great care must indeed be taken that no loose tow be permitted to lay about, especially when the passages and doors of the magazine or light-room are open, because, from its inflammable texture, the most dreadful consequences might arise should the smallest portion take fire.

An intelligent boy, or woman, if on board, may be stationed to offer pins, shift bloody water, hand and wash sponges and hold lights, under the direction of the purser and chaplain.

Civilians after the Action.—To order cots to be got ready for wounded officers, and hammocks for the men who can be safely taken from the platforms, and aid in their gentle removal to whatever place may be appropriated for their reception, kindly cheering and encouraging them the while.

In moments of leisure to examine those on whom the tourniquet has been applied; if any one is found to bleed, to screw the tourniquet as tight as possible, and acquaint one of the medical officers.

General Surgical Suggestions.—The principal objects of the surgeon during a naval action, are to stop all hæmorrhages and to dress wounds not seeming to require any important operation. If possible, therefore, he should content himself with endeavouring to save life, and restraining the effusion of blood, until he be less hurried.

Immediate amputation may, however, become necessary, from a limb being shattered so high that a tourniquet cannot be well retained, or where a limb has been completely destroyed. But, even in this latter case, if the wounded are numerous and crowding fast upon him, I should judge it better to apply the tourniquet, and wait till after the action.

All gun-shot wounds should be dressed, at first, in the most simple manner. When every extraneous substance is removed, the parts are cleaned and the bloodvessels secured; pledgets of lint or tow spread with ointment should be applied, and a compress of linen, the whole being gently secured by two or three turns of a roller; or, if the wound or fracture be on the lower limb, with a tailed bandage.

If balls, splinters, portions of clothing, loose spiculi of bone, or other extraneous bodies can be easily removed, they should be extracted at once; but if from the seat or direction of the wound there arises much difficulty it will generally be better to defer their removal until a calmer interval succeeds.

Wounds penetrating the thorax or abdomen, when not immediately fatal, are to be treated as in the last suggestion;—foreign bodies must be removed, protruded parts returned, bleedings moderated, and the most simple dressings applied.

In cases of fractured cranium, with a depression of a portion of the bone, the elevator must be applied so as to relieve the brain from pressure if possible; but the more delicate use of the trephine must be deferred until after the action.

If fractured or dislocated limbs are hastily set or reduced during the engagement, they should be carefully examined as soon as possible afterward, and the bones properly re-placed.

Bloodvessels are best secured with the tenaculum and noose, care being taken to avoid the inclusion of nerves; but where there is difficulty from the depth of the parts, or the minuteness of the arteries, the needle may be employed.

It is a good general rule to apply the tourniquet as high as possible—*i. e.*, in the upper extremity, immediately below the shoulder; and in the lower near the groin; excepting when amputation is to be performed above the ankle, or below the knee, when the pad of the tourniquet may be placed in the ham.

The wounded, when dressed, should in general be removed from the cockpit to the platforms, previously prepared, but officers and those requiring capital operations, or frequent attention, may be put into the adjacent berths and cabins.

In engagements with fleets there are often intervals of firing, occasioned by necessary evolutions, and these intervals may afford time for urgent operations, especially if there be more than two medical officers on board, and the wounded are not overwhelming.

But as an action between single ships, in close combat, usually terminates within two hours, and seldom exceeds three, a great deal of confusion and mischief might arise from commencing to operate without requisite assistance, when no harm could happen from a short delay.

Amputation.—The surgeon must amputate generally.

When, together with extensive and contused wounds of the soft parts, the bones are much broken and splintered.

When the principal bloodvessels of a limb are destroyed.

When a joint is considerably injured.

When the whole or very great portion of the muscles and integuments have been totally carried away by ball or splinters.

When part of a limb has been carried away.

It is desirable to preserve as much of a limb as can be saved without hazard, with one exception, however—viz., that it is better to amputate immediately above than directly below the knee-joint, where the bones are large and the soft parts are deficient; but it should also be borne in mind that in gun-shot and severe sabre wounds, the integuments and muscles may be injured and the bones splintered far beyond the first apparent extent of the mischief.

N.B. A great part of these arrangements being applicable to line-of-battle ships, they must be modified according to locality, space, and other circumstances, for frigates and smaller vessels.

ON THE NATURE AND CAUSES OF THE DISEASES OF EMIGRANTS.

By C. COOPER, Esq., M.R.C.S.E., Dublin.

In these times of railroad enterprise and steamboat travelling, a voyage across the wide Atlantic, or still wider Pacific, is spoken as lightly of, and thought as little about, as a pleasure trip on one of our large rivers; but the time was, and it has not long gone by, when even a voyage across the channel, or a visit to the Continent, was thought almost an heroic accomplishment. In those days an accouchement at sea was counted a wonder; the babe and its mother were noticed as prodigies, and a birth at sea has even formed the subject of a novel; but at the present time few, if indeed any, of our emigrant packet-ships cross the ocean without at least one birth; and so common has this become, that no notice is now taken of it, except merely to mention the fact in the ship's manifest or the passengers' way-bill.

Of late the tide of emigration has progressed, and is still progressing, to an amazing extent, particularly from Great Britain and Ireland, and we find in every good seaport town in the United Kingdom packet-ships for the conveyance of emigrants to various foreign ports; and as this tide of emigration has gone on, has there been no improvement in the means and ways adopted for the transportation of so many of our fellow-countrymen to foreign countries? Most decidedly there has; but although much has been done, still much, very much, remains to be done, and there are many and vast improvements yet wanting even in our finest and best packet-ships.

In THE LANCET, published about last April, I saw an article by Mr. T. Westropp upon "Emigrants and their Diseases," in which he made several remarks on the accommodation for passengers in the ship he sailed in. His remarks are undeniable as far as respects most, if not all, the passenger-ships from Irish ports. I myself have visited many of them when ready to sail, and have always found the accommodation miserable. But the regular lines of packets from English ports are more neatly and permanently fitted up, and the difference is evident to any one who may go on board one in Dublin, and then visit one in Liverpool and London. Just to show a difference, I will allude to two points Mr. Westropp mentions concerning the ships he was in—viz., the water-closets, and the means of cooking for passengers. What are these on board a Liverpool liner, not to go to other ports in England? Here we have the water-closets for steerage passengers permanent fixtures, forming a portion of the ship, as it were built in with her bows, always kept clean, and from which you never get an unpleasant or an unhealthy effluvia; and then what are means of cooking on board these packet-ships? Regular passengers' gallies as good as the cabin galley, supplied with fine large stoves, ovens, and boilers, and, in addition to this, provided with passenger cooks and stewards. But this arrangement I never saw, nor do I believe that it is to be found, in any of the ships from Irish ports. From thence the only water-closets I ever saw were mere temporary places—boxes of wood made by nailing a few boards together, and that in so flimsy a manner, that they could not possibly exist even half a voyage; and from the way in which they were made, they could not but become dirty and offensive, and would be far from conducive to health or cleanliness. And what is the passengers' cooking apparatus on board one of our Irish emigration ships? A comfortable galley, a good stove supplied with oven and boiler?—nay, this would be too good for poor Irishmen. Their galley is a case of wood, lined with bricks and fronted with bars—a common kitchen-grate erected on deck. It may answer for cooking; but the smoke from these must, as it is wafted by

EMIGRANTS—THEIR FOOD, HABITS, AND DISEASES. 299

the wind along the deck, (and not carried as it should be by a chimney over the heads of the passengers,) be conducive to health, and fine food for ophthalmia.

Thrice have I crossed the Atlantic to New York, in charge of emigrants, and it was my good fortune to get into ships of the first class. They were American built, of upwards of 2000 tons burthen, and possessed the best, or at least I should say as good, accommodation as any going; yet with the best accommodation there is wide scope for improvement in every respect, and it is this has led me to write on the subject.

Let us for a few moments look at the diseases that I have met among the emigrants on my passages out to New York, and then examine the means for the relief or cure of the same which I had on board.

The first trip I made across the Atlantic was in the month of December, 1852. On board we had upwards of four hundred passengers, including second-cabin and steerage. I had some cases of ophthalmia on board, but they were all of a trivial nature, and arose from cold caught from exposure after embarkation, and just before starting. I found it very easily subdued by a collyrium of sulphate of zinc, or a little opium wine. In this trip we had no sickness to speak of. The seasickness was soon over, and we had only, in addition, a few cases of diarrhœa, which, however, soon gave way to the opium-with-chalk mixture, or a few powders composed of tannin and compound chalk powder. We had one death—a German child; it died of starvation. Such a death may appear strange to any who have not had German passengers, or do not know what the lower order of them are; but I am sorry to have to say it is no uncommon occurrence for a German child to be starved in the midst of plenty on board our emigrantships. I had one case of this in the first ship I was in, and though I watched closely, I had also one case in the last trip I made. How, you may inquire, is it that a mother will suffer her child to die of starvation? and how is it that such a thing is permitted to pass unnoticed in our ships? The answer to these queries I cannot well give from my own knowledge; but the captain told me it was a common occurrence, and could not be helped; and the reason he gave was, that these Germans were going to a strange country; that any of their children who were able to work they would take care of; but they felt that those who were not able to work would be an incumbrance; they could not leave them behind; they dare not make away with them on shore, because of the law; but they could at sea and on board ship, and excuse themselves by saying that the child could not or would not eat the ship's provisions. I know, in my last trip, notwithstanding threats from the captain, officers, and myself, and in spite of all our watching, a German child of five years of age, a fine child when she came on board, died of starvation. Her legs measured five inches and a half in circumference, her thighs nine, and her arms five. There was a state of emaciation for a girl of five! and the excuse was that given above. It is rather strange that a child wont eat rice, gruel, bread, or even arrow-root, with which last I myself supplied her. After making away with her, the mother tried her best to starve her infant, but was unable, as too good a watch was kept over her, and I would take food to the little one myself, and see it eaten. This is most unnatural in a mother—scarcely to be credited. " Can a woman forget her sucking child, that she should not have compassion on the son of her womb?" Yes, hard as it is to believe it, yet it is true that in some cases, as the above, she may—she can—she does; and yet she is permitted to land with impunity, and no notice taken of the circumstance—and why? I cannot tell, unless it be that a trial would cause too much delay and loss of time, and it is no easy matter to catch them after they leave the ship.

The second trip I made was in the month of May, 1853. We had 844 passengers with us, and except a little sea-sickness, and that was very shortly got rid of, we had not a single case of sickness the whole passage out. The passengers were healthy and happy, and their time was pleasantly spent in dancing, singing, or reading. We had no Germans on board, and I had the satisfaction of landing them all safe, without a single loss, but with an addition to their number; and here I may mention that I had one birth in each trip.

I would that I could say the same of the last trip I made out, but, alas! it was otherwise. I left this in the same ship I had made my second trip in, about the 11th of August, 1853. On board we had as steerage passengers a number of Poles and Germans, (these are never celebrated for their cleanliness;) we had also English, Welsh, and Irish passengers, both in the steerage and second-cabin, to the number of 800, and they were as clean and respectable a set of emigrants as I had ever seen cross the Atlantic. The ship was inspected, the emigrants passed, and we sailed. The second day we were out I was sent for to see a German woman, whom I was told was dying. I hastened to the lower deck, where she was, and I found her speechless, pulseless, livid, and icy cold; a cold, clammy sweat bedewed the surface of her skin, and she was gasping for breath. I saw little or nothing could be done for her. I could learn nothing about her. They told me she had not been ailing before, and that she was suddenly seized as I saw her. I confess I could not understand it; and knowing the messes Germans feed on, I thought she might have taken something poisonous; however, no time was to be lost. I gave at once a mustard emetic, used sinapisms, and hot-water applications to the body and extremities, but to no purpose. I then gave brandy and Cayenne pepper, but she died in about two hours after I first saw her. After this I was continually sent for by German after German, and never saw them till they were in the state last described. My opinion of poisoning was strengthened, not only by the state I found them in, but also by the suddenness of the attack, the statement that they did not feel sick at the stomach, and that their bowels were confined; they also seemed to suffer no pain; and also I had seen some of them not very long before sitting on the deck in apparent health and spirits. I tried almost everything that I could lay my hands on, and that I thought might benefit—even purgatives—till at last I told the captain I thought they were poisoned. My opinion was told to them by an interpreter on board, but it produced no change. At length a Frenchman, a steerage passenger, told us that they were " eating stinking flesh," and a search was instituted, the result of which was that some ten or twelve kegs of flesh, and some thirty or forty large loaves of bread, were brought up on deck for the captain's inspection. The bread was originally intended for brown bread; it, however, was so hard that you could stick neither knife or marling-spike into it; and when one of the men broke it across one of the stanchions, it flew off in smoke, and presented to your view, on the inside, all the colours of the rainbow in their richness, it was so stale and mouldy.

As to the meat, what shall I say? Evidently it was meant for beef—corned beef, or pickled beef; but I dare not say whether it was ox or horse flesh! It was shipped as corned meat for the German passengers. When the kegs were brought on deck for inspection, the flesh contained in them was as green as grass, and sufficient to poison a dog; nay, a dog would not eat it. Then they had pickles too, and they were also decomposed.

All this we hove overboard, greatly to the annoyance of the Germans, but certainly for their good; and we hoped that we had gotten rid of all, but it was not so. Finding what we were about to do, they managed to hide some of the bread and flesh, wrapped up in aprons or other cloths, under their pillows and berths, and when they could not get it cooked in the passengers' galley, (for I had given orders to the passengers' cook not to cook any of it for them,) they have been seen sitting on the decks and eating the flesh,—yes, eating that green flesh that a dog would not eat—eating it raw on the decks! and this, bad as it seems, would not have been so much to be wondered at, had they nothing else; but when we took their meat and bread, we supplied them with ship's provisions, and those of good quality.

Having at length got rid of all these wretched provisions—for the sale of which the maker and supplier richly deserves prosecution and punishment—and after losing a good number of the Germans, the disease seemed to abate, and we were earnestly hoping that we were done with any further sickness or death, when, in two or three days after, a Welshman in the upper deck of the steerage was attacked, and the disease spread among the English and Irish passengers, and then it was that I learned in reality that the disease was cholera. I now saw the cramps, the vomiting, and the purging in their full power, but still I never could see a case at its commencement. I have gone round from berth to berth four and five times a day, asking them how they were, and begging that the moment they felt diarrhœa coming on they would let me know; but it was of no use. As I would inquire singly how they were, the invariable answer I would receive was) " Oh, we are quite well, thank God!" and shortly after, perhaps before I could get to my state-room, I should be sent for to see some of them, seized with cramps, &c., and would find them that they had been suffering from diarrhœa for, some of them, twenty-four hours or more, but thought to battle it off, till at last the cramps would seize them, and they would have to give in. The cases we had may be thus described:—Diarrhœa set in; in the first instance it was slight and neglected. In this stage

I never saw a case. The diarrhœa increased, and vomiting and cramps succeeded; then it was that I would be sent for; no longer could the disease remain hidden; the agony of the patient betrayed him; his groans and cries he could not suppress. The body and extremities became cold and livid, and the pulse, if not gone, was rapidly sinking; the thirst was excessive, and the patient was always craving for water! water! water! but the more they drank the more they retched and vomited. While the cholera was in Dublin I had seen calomel and opium used with great benefit, and I determined to try it now, but found that it would not answer in every case, so that I had to try other measures also. I tried all that could be well tried in such cases, at least everything that lay within my reach,—and on board we had a good assortment of medicines, and were not restricted to a medicine chest. I tried the submuriate of mercury and powdered opium, and also the submuriate and tincture of opium, the acetate of lead, &c. &c. I generally commenced by giving a strong mustard emetic, which seemed to rouse the patients a little, and then followed it up by giving large doses of calomel—say one scruple or half a drachm, and either one grain of powdered opium or ten drops of tincture of opium every ten minutes, along with sinapisms, hot stupes, embrocations, and hot bricks or jars of hot water to the feet, thighs, arms, &c. The embrocations I used were chiefly composed of spirits of turpentine, and I was successful in saving some lives, even beyond my expectations.

But, as I said before, I did not confine myself to this treatment. I tried charcoal in drachm and half-drachm doses, but found it of little use after a time; (it is largely used in this and yellow fever in America.) I repeatedly gave brandy and Cayenne pepper made hot; and to the children, wine mulled and heated with various spice. Of wine and brandy there happened to be a good store on board, and it was not restricted when it was necessary. The fresh meat and other provisions, from the tables of the first cabin, were liberally distributed by the captain to any of the sick whom it was fit for, and that with an unsparing hand, till, on our arrival in quarantine at Staten Island, we had not for our own use in the cabin a bit of fresh meat till we could get it from shore. As it was, it was well that we got in as soon as we did. Had we been longer out, more lives must have been lost, for we had run out of medicine, wine, and brandy. As it was, we ran so short that I was glad to have recourse to a couple of bottles of an American cholera mixture, and even to the captain's private case of homœopathic medicines, from which, according to the directions in their book, I selected the medicines marked ipecacuanha and veratrium, and used them according to the rules laid down. I used these sooner than let the sick drop and die before my eyes without making at least an effort to save them. But the use of these was not attended with much benefit. After our arrival, I landed fifteen sick at quarantine. We lost thirty-six on board, and two died at Staten Island, making in all thirty-eight. One woman, who was not expected to live on her landing, was saved by injecting salt and water into the veins of her arm.

(*To be continued.*)

ON HEADACHE AND ITS VARIETIES.

By PATRICK J. MURPHY, M.D.

(*Continued from p. 210.*)

UNFORTUNATELY a great difficulty of diagnosis exists in our profession when co-existing symptoms arise from different diseases. The anæmic headache may exist for years, and then have the neuralgic superadded, but this is not of so much practical importance, as the remedies for the one form do not make the other worse; on the other hand a delicate female, long suffering from anæmia and its headache, is often attacked with fever, and the anæmic is thus replaced by the congestive headache. If stimulants be now given, serious mischief may be the consequence, while, on the contrary, a practitioner who sees her for the first time may deplete too largely and produce a tedious convalescence. These mistakes can occur only on the invasion of the fever, for in a few days, the thirst, heat of skin, and loaded tongue, point out clearly what is to be contended with. Cupping or leeching will relieve the head for a few hours, but if the fever be ataxic a degree of prostration may be induced from which the patient can never be roused. I have never seen the anæmic and rheumatic headache combined, the combination is rare, but there is no reason why such may not occur.

Treatment.—As debility not only attends, but is often the sole cause of this form of headache, the treatment must, of course be directed in accordance with this view. The diet is most important, and the proper kind at once suggests itself; it should be nutritious, and as the muscular coats of the stomach and intestinal tube have lost their tone, or, more correctly speaking, have their contractile power weakened, common sense points that it should be easy of digestion. Animal food is indispensable, it may be taken twice a day. Mutton is to be preferred. Beef, unless stewed, lies heavy on the stomach of weak people. The lean of roast pork may be permitted, it is a variety and digestible. The flesh of young animals is neither as nourishing nor digestible as those of mature age. Wild fowl, hare, or rabbit, seldom disagree. Roast meat contains more nutritious matter than boiled, but either may be taken according to the fancy of the patient. The richest soups and strongest jellies are in every way inferior to the meat from which they are produced, even in a healthy stomach they cause flatulence and distention, and, *a fortiori*, the weak stomach cannot escape. The more solid fish, such as sole, turbot, &c., may be permitted. Stewed eels are wholesome and agreeable. Oysters fresh, uncooked, and cut into three or four portions never disagree. Vegetables, unless potatoes, should be cautiously used. Bread should be stale, nothing is more indigestible than fresh bread or buttered toast. An excellent evening meal can be made with tea and rusks. Of fruits, strawberries, raspberries, gooseberries, pears, peaches, and plums are agreeable and aperient; uncooked apples usually disagree. Nuts, almonds, and raisins frequently give rise to painful feelings in the stomach. There is a craving for stimulants, which ought to be indulged in moderation. Ale or porter may be allowed at dinner and supper; perhaps porter is preferable, as it usually contains a chalybeate. Bitter ale is useless. A glass of wine between breakfast and luncheon, with a biscuit, is always found grateful and invigorating. To alcoholic drinks the objections are self-evident, especially when young females are the patients. Very delicate females are much benefited by breakfasting in bed. The meals should be light, and repeated whenever the faintness or sinking of the stomach is approaching. Many cases, however, will occur, more particularly in young men, where no directions for diet will be needed, almost all kinds of food being digestible.

All causes of exhaustion should be guarded against. There is nothing more injurious to a flaccid heart than smoking, many cases being traceable to this cause alone.

The medicine on which the greatest reliance may be placed is iron. Fortunately, this remedy can be exhibited in various forms and combinations. The formulas in the Pharmacopœia are as numerous, as those of mercury. Griffith's mixture is an excellent mode of prescribing iron, but as the myrrh is unpalatable and useless, it may be omitted; or a form for which we are indebted to Mr. Donovan may be more advantageously substituted; it is as follows: pure sulphate of iron, one drachm; magnesia, ten grains; purified sugar, one ounce, rose or cinnamon water, eight ounces; mix. This is a scientific prescription; and if the iron be free from red oxide, the green colour is preserved for eight or ten days. The magnesia neutralizes the sulphuric acid, and converts the sulphate into a protoxide. The sugar prevents decomposition, and it may be flavoured with mint or peppermint water. In hospital practice it would be found most economical, and treacle might be used instead of sugar. In the hysterical female, infusion of valerian adds to its value; and if there be great sense of exhaustion, ammonia in combination is most beneficial. Persons will take pills who object to fluid medicines. The compound iron pill might be improved by using treacle and potash, which keep the pill soft; and by omitting the myrrh, which only adds to the size. If the cause of the debility be from leucorrhœa, perspirations, or hæmorrhage, the tincture of sesquichloride of iron, in doses of fifteen drops, three times a day, will be the most certain form to employ at first. Young unmarried females, from about their 22nd year, are very subject to a chronic gastritis, or rather irritable stomach; for these the best preparation is the carbonate of iron, with sugar, of the Edinburgh Pharmacopœia. If the appetite be bad, sulphate of quinine may be combined with iron. The occasional constipation which is caused by the loss of tone the sulphate of zinc, with small doses of sulphate of strychnia, relieves. In severe chlorosis, the crystallized citric acid aids the iron; and in scrofula, iodide of potash may be joined with the iron mixture. If there be a periodical neuralgia, the most effective form is the precipitate of carbonate of iron. In a severe case of chorea and anæmic headache, Fowler's solution of arsenic

THE HEIGHAM HALL ASYLUM: THE CASE OF THE REV. E. HOLMES.   449

Mr. Cann, jun., *produced by the proprietors*, and which infer-ences Mr. Cann utterly disclaims and repudiates. That re-port you will observe perfectly exonerates the proprietors of the asylum from all blame, except for appointing Mr. Holmes as chaplain, which appointment the justices considered im-proper.

A copy of this report was forwarded by the justices to the Commissioners in Lunacy, who acknowledged its receipt, but paid no further attention to it.

The Rev. E. Holmes was at this time, and in consequence of the report, *suspended* from the performance of his duties in the house; but the proprietors could not, upon what they considered unfounded and insufficient evidence, allow the matter to rest here, and obtained the evidence *of all the parties* connected with the case, and laid it before the chairman (Sir Samuel Bignold) of the visiting justices, as well as before the Commissioners in Lunacy. Sir Samuel Bignold appointed a time for re-hearing the case, but subsequently considering the re-hearing unneces-sary, wrote the following letter to a friend of the proprietors.

"Surrey-street, Norwich, August 10th, 1854.

"DEAR SIR,—The affair of the Rev. E. Holmes having been alluded to in the House of Commons, I think you would do right to request some member to explain that the case was inves-tigated by the visiting justices, at whose meeting I acted as chairman, that the fullest evidence was tendered to them, and that they agreed to a report, which was signed by every justice, and forwarded to the Commissioners in Lunacy, who have acknowledged the receipt, but have not suggested any further steps as called for. Some additional evidence has been placed before me touching the sanity of Mr. Holmes, in June, 1852, when the transaction referred to occurred, and the impression produced upon my mind in reading such evidence is, that *he was rightly placed in Heigham Hall Lunatic Asylum*, at the period when he was lodged there. I am now urged by the family and friends of Mr. Holmes, to summons afresh the visiting magistrates to go again into the inquiry, but in my opinion, the case is so clear that any renewed inquiry would be superfluous. I do trust that the matter will now be suffered to drop. Mr. Holmes' family are an opulent family, and they deem it best that he should continue a boarder at the asylum, though in a state of convalescence, and this disposal of him is, I think, most wise and proper.

"SAMUEL BIGNOLD, Mayor of Norwich."

This letter speaks for itself, and I considered the affair terminated, having the sanction of the chairman of the visiting magistrates to Mr. Holmes' residence as chaplain. During this interval the Rev. Mr. Holmes was suspended, but continued to reside in the asylum, efforts being continually made to have the case re-opened.

On the 27th of September last the visiting magistrates made a report, to the effect that the Rev. E. Holmes was a boarder in the house, in variance with the Act of Parliament of 16 and 17 Vic., cap. 96, which, be it observed, came into operation on the 1st of November, 1853, more than a year after Mr. Holmes was appointed resident chaplain, upon which application was made to the Commissioners in Lunacy to legalize his residence as such; but they considered Mr. Holmes did not come under the clause of the Act, and therefore refused the permission. Mr. Holmes immediately left the house. If the breach of this law be the breach complained of, I can only say it occurred in perfect in-nocence on our part; and the Commissioners, in reference to it, state, in a letter dated the 5th of October, 1854, as follows:—

"The Commissioners are satisfied that, in retaining Mr. Holmes as a boarder since the cessation of his services as chaplain, consequent upon the inquiry by the visitors, you acted under a misapprehension of the provisions of the Act 16th and 17th Vic., cap. 96, and that you did so under the ex-pectation that Heigham Hall would be shortly visited by some of the Commissioners, and that they would sanction the arrangement.

(Signed) "R. W. S. LUTWIDGE, Secretary."

And on the 11th of October they further wrote as follows:—

"19, Whitehall-place, October 11th, 1854.

"GENTLEMEN,—With reference to the correspondence and discussion which has taken place with reference to the Rev. E. Holmes, the Commissioners in Lunacy deem it only fair towards you to say that they are satisfied that when sent to Heigham Hall he was insane, and a proper person to be placed, as such, under medical care in an asylum.

(Signed) "R. W. S. LUTWIDGE, Secretary.

"To Messrs. Nichols, Ranking, and Watson, Heigham Hall."

At the last sessions, application was made for the renewal of the license, and opposed by Mr. Palmer, one of the magistrates,

on the grounds of an infraction of the law, on which occasion Mr. Sultzer, another of the magistrates who had taken an active part in the inquiry, made the following remarks upon the *management* of the asylum :—

" I have great pleasure in taking this opportunity to state, that so far as the internal arrangements of this institution and the treatment of the patients are concerned, they reflect the highest credit upon the resident proprietor. I have never gone through the establishment without feeling great satisfac-tion that persons reduced to the deplorable condition of lunatics are so well cared for, and so well treated, with a view to their restoration to society. This circumstance would certainly induce me to give my vote in favour of the renewal of the licence."

These proceedings at Quarter Sessions were reported at length in the local papers, and upon such reports the *Daily News* and *Examiner* formed articles, not too severe were the facts such as would appear from the reports furnished to them. Permit me to add that the proprietors had no desire to conceal this appointment of chaplain, but the reverse, for they caused to be made a conspicuous chaplain's book, in which, on the 21st of September, 1852, the chaplain made his first entry, and to which he signed his name. And, moreover, on the follow-ing 16th of November, this chaplain's book was exhibited to the visiting magistrates, read by them, and signed by them.

That the visiting magistrates were not ignorant *who* the chaplain was is proved by an entry made in the visitors' book, on the 16th of September, 1852—viz., that "divine service is performed on Sunday by a clergyman of the Church of England, recently discharged as a *patient* from the establishment, but still residing there."

To show their perfect knowledge and appreciation of this fact, the word "patient" was underlined by *the visitors*.

The visiting magistrates should not plead ignorance of Mr. Holmes's case, since his case was minutely stated in the case-book, and which case-book was exhibited to, and signed by, them and the Commissioners in Lunacy no less than ten times during the period Mr. Holmes officiated as chaplain; in addi-tion, this chaplain's book continued to be exhibited to the visitors, and signed by them, and a similar number of entries with reference to the performance of Divine service were made in the visitors' book, in which disapprobation was not even hinted at. It must be admitted, if the appointment was im-proper, it was at least sanctioned by those whose authority should at once have pointed out its lately discovered flagrancy; but it is a singular fact that it was not until Dr. Ranking be-came a proprietor at Heigham Hall, that Dr. Hull's sense of public justice induced him to make known that he (a magistrate himself) had, two years before, become acquainted with what he calls a rescue from the gripe of the law, and that this should have been concealed by him while on friendly terms with Mr. Nichols, and only published when that gentleman united him-self with a too successful rival to Dr. Hull in public estimation. Was not this concealment as improper as the alleged offence itself ?

Permit me to say, in conclusion, that we alike court and challenge inquiry, and are sure that a full, public, and search-ing investigation into the admission and appointment of Mr. Holmes, and the alleged infraction of the law, will end in a complete exoneration of the proprietors, and disappointment to the originators of this malicious attack.

I am, Sir, your obedient servant,
JOHN FERRA WATSON,
Resident Medical Proprietor of Heigham Hall Asylum.
Heigham Hall, November, 1854.

NURSES FOR THE SICK AND WOUNDED AT SCUTARI.

To the Editor of THE LANCET.

SIR,—In reference to the subject of nurses for the East, to which your attention has lately been drawn by a correspondent signing himself " One Interested," I have been anxiously look-ing for your opinion on the plan adopted by the Government. In his celebrated letter to Miss Nightingale, our sentimental Secretary-at-War says—"There is but one person in England that I know of who would be capable of organizing and super-intending such a scheme;" and " I must not conceal from you that upon your decision will depend the ultimate success or failure of the plan." So then, according to this, had not Miss Nightingale been coaxed and flattered into compliance, our sick and wounded soldiers would have been left without nurses. Mr. Sidney Herbert speaks of the difficulty of finding nurses at all versed in their business, but I have yet to learn that such were properly sought for. Amongst the many plans and suggestions from the various parties who seem to have considered it their province to interfere in a matter which ought, in my humble opinion, to have been left altogether in the hands of the Director-General of the Army Medical Department, I have not heard of the simple one of applying to all the large hospitals in the United Kingdom. Had Dr. Smith, instead of listening to so much sentimental twaddle, despatched a circular something like the following— " Wanted, two matrons and forty nurses for the hospital at Scutari," I have very little doubt that two ladies, capable of "organizing and superintending, directing and ruling," and the requisite number of nurses thoroughly versed in their business, would speedily have been forthcoming; at least, this would have been the proper way to have " tested the willingness of trained nurses." It would seem, from most of the letters which have appeared in the daily papers on the nurse scheme, that devotion and self-sacrifice are to be found only in nunneries and sisterhoods, and that it is to such establishments as that of Miss Sellon, and not to our hospitals, that we are in future to look for nurses. Just fancy a number of these young ladies, *uniformed* in black, doing duty at Scutari! The whole scheme is bad, *un-English*, unbusiness-like; and yet it is said the authorities are determined to adhere to it. There are at present a number of young ladies anxiously expecting the word of command from the official with " plenary authority over all the nurses," and " of unlimited power in drawing upon the Government," to start for the East. Some of these would-be nurses are to walk the hospitals for two or three weeks for the purpose of becoming " *certificated*," and then there will be as little doubt of their qualification as of their " *call*" to go forth for the sake of their country and their church.

Do, Mr. Editor, let your voice be heard in support of a better system, ere another batch of incapables be sent out. If more nurses are wanted, let such as are physically and in every other way qualified be despatched—good, sturdy Englishwomen; and let us hear no more of the necessity of lady nurses in order to prevent the ribald jokes of the sick soldiers.

November, 1854.   ANOTHER INTERESTED.

DEATH OF MR. KNIGHT HUNT.—This gentleman, so well known on the London and provincial press, expired on the 18th instant at his residence, Forest-hill, near Sydenham. The career of this gentleman has been an instructive one, exhibiting how much may be done by honourable industry. At an early age the subject of this brief notice found himself entirely dependent on his own exertions, not only for the support of himself, but for a widowed mother, younger brothers and sister. He therefore entered himself a medical student at the Charing-cross Hospital. On the 13th of November, 1840, he was admitted a Member of the Royal College of Surgeons. Shortly after this the health of Mr. Hunt became considerably impaired. He retired into the country, where he commenced the practice of his profession, and in the active duties of surgeon to the Docking Union, Norfolk, and by the invigorating country breezes, his health was soon recruited. Finding, however, that his professional receipts were not equal to the increasing wants of his family, he again returned to town, and was appointed editor of the *Pictorial Times*, and became the "London Correspondent" to several provincial papers, in addition to which he established *Hunt's London Journal*. On the establishment of the *Daily News*, he was appointed sub-editor, and during the last two or three years had the entire management of that journal. But it soon became evident to his friends that the intense application he devoted to his literary occupations was preying seriously on a naturally delicate constitution; and a few weeks since, on his return home after an unusually busy night at the office, he complained of a slight cold, which soon became a severe attack of bronchitis. From this, however, he was recovering, when he attacked by typhus fever of so bad a character as to leave no hopes of recovery, notwithstanding the unremitting attention of his old and valued friend, Dr. Paul, of Camberwell house, assisted by Sir John Forbes and Mr. Wells. He died on Sunday evening, aged forty-one. at a small freehold estate he had only lately purchased, situated at Forest-hill. The deceased was well known as the author of " The History of the Fourth Estate," 2 vols.; " The Book of Art; or Cartoons, Frescoes, Sculptures, &c.," 4to; " History and Scenery of the Rhine;" and many other works; and several popular Guide Books. Indeed, Mr. Hunt could never remain idle at any place he visited for the restoration of his shattered health. He accordingly made himself thoroughly acquainted with the history and antiquities and other objects of interest to the tourist, and before returning to town a book was ready for the publisher.

Medical News.

ROYAL COLLEGE OF SURGEONS—The following gentlemen having undergone the necessary examinations for the diploma, were admitted Members of the College at the meeting of the Court of Examiners on the 17th inst.:—

BOND, JOHN SULLIVAN, William-street, Dublin.
DARBY, EDMUND, Bath.
HALE, THOMAS EGERTON, Macefen, Cheshire.
LANE, WILLIAM RALPH, Army.
MAYNE, ROBERT FURLONG, Newton-Abbot, Devon.
REYNOLDS, THOMAS, Necton, near Swaffham.
SEWARD, THOMAS, Petersfield, Hants.
SHUTER, HENRY, North-end, Fulham.
TAYLOR, CHARLES GIBSON, Australia.

At the same meeting of the Court, Mr. ROBERT SPROULE passed his examination as Naval Surgeon. This gentleman had previously been admitted a Member of the College, his diploma bearing date 20th of December, 1850.

APOTHECARIES' HALL.—Names of gentlemen who passed their examination in the science and practice of Medicine, and received certificates to practise, on—

Thursday, November 16th, 1854.
DYSON, EDWARD, Almondbury, Yorkshire.
NEWMAN, WILLIAM, Bradfield, Sheffield.

Names of the gentlemen who passed their examination in Classics and Mathematics, on Tuesday and Wednesday, the 21st and 22nd of November, 1854:—

ABBEY, WALTER, Queen's College, Birmingham.
BELL, JAMES VINCENT, Rochester.
BROWNE, HENRY ERNEST, 13, Berkeley-square.
DAVY, JOHN SWEET, Chulmleigh.
FACER, JOHN HENRY, Rugeley, Staffordshire.
FERGUSON, GEORGE, Giltspur-street.
GODDARD, LEONARD, 5, St. John's-street-road.
GRIFFIN, RICHARD WILLIAM W., Weymouth.
HAMMOND, SAMUEL, Lower Edmonton.
HORNIBLOW, WILLIAM R., Shipston on-Stour.
HOSKINS, EDMUND J., College, St. Bartholomew's Hospital.
HUNTSMAN, THOMAS, 6, Mount-street.
LEACHMAN, ALBERT WARREN, Compton-terrace.
MACY, ERNEST A., West-town, Somerset.
MILLIGAN, PERCY, Keighley.
MOXON, WALTER, Belitha-terrace, Islington.
PHILLIPS, DANIEL WELD, Queen's College, Birmingham.
POWELL, WILLIAM L., Macclesfield.
RAULSTON, WILLIAM HENRY, Helperby, Boro'bridge.
SANSOM, ARTHUR ERNEST, King's College.
SHEA, JOHN, Blackfriars-road.
SIMONDS, THOMAS, Abbots Barton, Winchester.
SPRAGUE, CHARLES GORDON, Ashford, Kent.
WILLIAMSON, HENRY, Sherborne.
WINTERBOTHAM, W. L., Strand.

HUNTERIAN SOCIETY.—At the next meeting, on Wednesday, the 29th inst., Dr. Hughes will read a paper " On some Cases of Paracentesis Thoracis."

HARVEIAN SOCIETY.—Dr. Sieveking will read a paper " On Epilepsy," on Thursday, December 7th.

The ST. MARY'S HOSPITAL SCHOOL has received the recognition of the Royal College of Surgeons.

SOCIETY FOR THE WIDOWS AND ORPHANS OF MEDICAL MEN.—The following gentlemen have been elected directors of this Society: Sir J. Eyre, M.D.; Dr. J. Clarke; R. L. Thorn, Esq.; G. Pilcher, Esq.; J. Propert, Esq.; H. Blenkarne, Esq.

APOTHECARIES TO THE FORCES.—We have been requested by the Director-General of the Army Medical Department to publish the following memorandum: " It is understood that apothecaries to the Forces will be selected from the dispensers of medicines who are already employed with the army in the East."

APPOINTMENT.—Mr. Eubulus Williams has been appointed resident surgeon to the Royal Berkshire Hospital.

ELECTION AT ST. BARTHOLOMEW'S.—Dr. Martin has been elected assistant-physician to St. Bartholomew's Hospital. The time has not yet come for the "average man," or perhaps it has gone by. We think it must at length be acknowledged, even by those to whom the truth is unwelcome, that THE LANCET has rendered the most signal service to this institution, and to those whose hope of advancement rests on their scientific merit.

THE LANCET,]   DR. MARSHALL HALL ON ASPHYXIA.   [APRIL 12, 1856.

ASPHYXIA,

ITS RATIONALE AND ITS REMEDY.

BY MARSHALL HALL, M.D., F.R.S.

THE term Asphyxia, which ought to be exchanged for Apnœa, designates that condition of the animal system which results from the suspension of respiration.

Respiration involves two processes—the inhalation of oxygen, and the exhalation of carbonic acid.

The remedy for the suspension of respiration is, on every principle of common sense, the restoration of respiration. This view might be considered, irrespective of physiological inquiry and proof, as self-evident; but that proof is amply supplied by physiology.

Of the two functions suspended, it is certain, from physiological inquiry, that the retention of the carbonic acid is by far the more fatal, and that, in a word, asphyxia is the result of carbonic acid retained in the blood, which becomes, in its excess, a blood-poison.

If this view be correct, it is evident that restored respiration is to the blood-poison in asphyxia what the stomach-pump is to poison in the stomach; and that it is *the* special remedy, the *sine quâ non*, in asphyxia.

But this blood-poison is formed with a rapidity proportionate to the circulation, which is, in its turn, proportionate to the temperature. To elevate the temperature, or to accelerate the circulation, *without* having *first* secured the return of respiration, is therefore *not to save*, but in reality *to destroy life!*

Now, let me draw my reader's attention to the *Rules* for treating asphyxia, proposed and practised by the Royal Humane Society. They are as follow:--

"1. Convey the body carefully, with the head and shoulders supported in a raised position, to the nearest house.

"2. Strip the body, and rub it dry; then wrap it in hot blankets, and then place it in a warm bed in a warm chamber free from smoke.

"3. Wipe and cleanse the mouth and nostrils.

"4. In order to restore the natural warmth of the body,—

    Move a heated covered warming-pan over the back and spine.

    Put bladders or bottles of hot water, or heated bricks, to the pit of the stomach, the arm-pits, between the thighs, and to the soles of the feet.

    Foment the body with hot flannels.

    Rub the body briskly with the hand; do not, however, suspend the use of the other means at the same time; but, if possible, immerse the body in a warm bath at blood heat, or 100 deg. of the thermometer, as this is preferable to the other means for restoring warmth.

"5. Volatile salts or hartshorn to be passed occasionally to and fro under the nostrils.

"6. No more persons to be admitted into the room than is absolutely necessary."

My first remark on these rules for treating asphyxia, is, that "to convey the body to the nearest house," is doubly wrong. In the first place, *the loss of time* necessary for this purpose is—*loss of life!* on the contrary, not a moment should be lost; the patient should be treated instantly, on the spot, therefore. In the second place, except in very inclement weather, the exposure of the face and thorax to the breeze is an important auxiliary to the special treatment of asphyxia.

But most of all, the various modes of restoring the temperature of the patient, the warm-bath especially, are objectionable, or more than objectionable; they are at once inappropriate, unphysiological, and deleterious.

If there be a fact well established in physiology, it is that an animal bears the suspension of respiration in proportion, not to the warmth, but, within physiological limits, to the lowness of the temperature, the lower limit being about 60° Fahr. A warm-bath of 100° Fahr. must be injurious.

All other modes of inducing warmth are also injurious, if they divert the attention from *the one remedy* in asphyxia—artificial respiration,—or otherwise interfere with the measures to be adopted with the object of restoring this lost function.

Such, then, are the views which the scientific physician *must* take in regard to the late rules for treating asphyxia promulgated by the Royal Humane Society.

I now proceed to state the measures by which those rules must be replaced.

I revert to a proposition already made: as asphyxia is the result of suspended respiration, the one remedy for the condition so induced is, self-evidently and experimentally, the restoration of respiration.

But there is an impediment to artificial respiration never before pointed out. It is the obstruction of the glottis or the entrance into the windpipe, in the supine position, by the tongue falling backwards, and carrying with it the epiglottis—an event which can only be effectually remedied by adopting *the prone position.* That position is displayed by the subjoined figure.

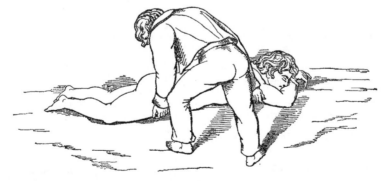

In this position the tongue falls forward, drawing with it the epiglottis, and leaving the ingress into the windpipe *free.*

But even when the *way* is patent, there remains the question, how is respiration to be effected? The syringe or the bellows may not be at hand, and if they were, the violence used by them is apt to *tear* the delicate tissue of the lungs. The mode proposed by Leroy, of compressing the thorax by means of a bandage, and allowing its expansion by the resilience of the costal cartilages, is proved by experiment to be futile, chiefly, no doubt, from its being attempted in the supine position, with the glottis obstructed.

The one effectual mode of proceeding is this: let the patient be placed in the prone position, the head and neck being preserved in their proper place. The tongue will fall forward, and leave the entrance into the windpipe free. But this is not all the thorax and abdomen will be *compressed* with a force equal to the weight of the body, and *expiration* will take place. Let the body be now *turned* gently on the side. (through rather more than the quarter of a circle,) and the pressure on the thorax and abdomen will be removed, and *inspiration*—effectual *inspiration*—will take place! The expiration and inspiration are augmented by timeously applying and removing alternately pressure on the spine and ribs.

Nothing can be more beautiful than this life-giving—(if life *can* be given)—this breathing process.

In one series of experiments, twenty cubic inches of air were expelled on placing a corpse in the prone position, and ten cubic inches more by making pressure on the thorax and ribs, the *same* quantities being *in*haled on removing that pressure, and on rotating the body on its side. But I must give the experiments in detail:—

A subject was laid on the table, and pressure made on the thorax and ribs, so as to imitate the procedure of Leroy. There was no result; a little gurgling was heard in the throat, but *no inspiration* followed. The tongue had fallen backwards, and closed the glottis or aperture into the windpipe! All inspiration was prevented.

Another subject was placed in the *prone* position. The tongue having fallen *forwards*, and the glottis being free, there was the *expiration* of twenty cubic inches of air, a quantity increased by ten cubic inches more on making pressure along the posterior part of the thorax and on the ribs. On removing this pressure, and turning the body through a quarter of a circle or rather more, on the side, the whole of the thirty cubic inches of air were *in*spired!

These manœuvres being repeated, ample respiration was performed!

Nay, there may be a question whether such considerable acts of respiration may not be too much.

It is to be observed, however, that, in this mode of artificial respiration, *no force* is used; the lung therefore is not injured; and that, as the air in the trachea and bronchial tubes undergoes little or no change in quantity, the whole inspired air passes into the air-cells, where the function of respiration is alone performed.

It deserves to be noticed, that in the beginning of this experiment in the prone position, the head had been allowed to hang over the edge of the table: all respiration was frustrated! *Such is the importance of position.*

Reserving the full exposition of this method of *postural respiration*, this theseopnœa, (from θεσις, position,) for another occasion, I will conclude by reducing these views into the simplest *Rules* for the treatment of asphyxia.

New Rules for the Treatment of Asphyxia.

I. Send with all speed for medical aid, for articles of clothing, blankets, &c.

II. Treat the patient on the spot, in the open air, exposing the face and chest freely to the breeze, except in too cold weather.

I. *To excite Respiration,*

III. Place the patient gently on the face, (to allow any fluids to flow from the mouth.)

IV. Then raise the patient into the sitting posture, and endeavour to *excite* respiration,

    1. By snuff, hartshorn, &c., applied to the nostrils;

    2. By irritating the throat by a feather or the finger;

    3. By dashing hot and cold water *alternately* on the face and chest.

If there be no success, lose no time, but

II. *To imitate Respiration,*

V. Replace the patient on his face, his arms under his head, that the tongue may fall *forward*, and leave the entrance into the windpipe free, and that any fluids may flow out of the mouth; then

    1. Turn the body gradually but completely on the *side, and a little more*, and then again on the face, alternately (to induce *inspiration* and *expiration*);

    2. When replaced, apply pressure along the back and ribs, and then remove it (to induce further *expiration* and *inspiration*,) and proceed as before;

    3. Let these measures be repeated gently, deliberately, but efficiently and perseveringly, *sixteen times* in the minute, *only;*

III. *To induce Circulation and Warmth,*

    1. *Continuing* these measures, rub all the limbs and the trunk *upwards* with the warm hands, making *firm pressure* energetically;

    2. Replace the wet clothes by such other covering, &c., as can be procured.

VI. *Omit the warm-bath until respiration be re-established.*

To recapitulate, I observe that—

1. If there be one fact more self-evident than another, it is that artificial respiration is the *sine quâ non* in the treatment of asphyxia, apnœa, or suspended respiration.

2. If there be one fact more established in physiology than another, it is that within just limits, a *low* temperature conduces to the protraction of life, in cases of suspended respi-

ration, and that a more elevated temperature destroys life. This is the result of the admirable, the incomparable, work of Edwards.

3. Now the *only* mode of inducing efficient *respiration* artificially, at all times and under all circumstances, by the hands alone, is that of the postural manœuvres described in this paper. This measure *must* be adopted.

4. The *next* measure is, I have stated, to restore the *circulation and warmth* by means of pressure firmly and simultaneously applied *in the course of the veins*, therefore *upwards*.

5. And the measure *not to be adopted*, because it tends to extinguish life, is *the warm bath, without* artificial respiration. This measure *must* be relinquished.

These conclusions are at once the conclusions of common sense and of physiological experiment. On these views human life may, nay, must, sometimes depend.

Practical Contributions
ON THE
DISEASES OF FEMALES.

BY HENRY BENNET, M.D.,
PHYSICIAN-ACCOUCHEUR TO THE ROYAL FREE HOSPITAL.

No. X.

A REVIEW OF THE PRESENT STATE OF UTERINE PATHOLOGY.

The Displacement Theory.—In my preceding communication I drew attention—to the smallness of size and lightness of weight of the uterus; to the great laxity of its means of support and fixity; to the extreme mobility which it consequently evinces; to the ease with which it obeys the many physiological causes of displacement to which it is subjected; and to the complete immunity from pain, or even inconvenience, with which these displacements are borne.

I explained the immunity from pain evinced by the uterus when displaced under the influence of physiological causes, by referring to the law through which all our viscera bear, without inconvenience, any amount of displacement compatible with their means of fixity, and any amount of pressure to which they can be exposed from the proximity and functional activity of surrounding organs. I pointed out that this capability of our organs to bear considerable pressure without inconvenience is not only observed in the temporary physiological conditions described, but is also found to exist under the permanent pathological pressure of *non-inflammatory* morbid growths, such as tumours, aneurisms, &c. I then laid stress on the very important fact, that when once inflammation supervenes, this immunity from pain and inconvenience on pressure ceases;—as evidenced by the inability of patients suffering from inflammation of the abdominal or thoracic viscera to lie otherwise than on their back: or as evidenced by the pain which is experienced on the pressure of an inflamed finger. Finally, I recalled the rapidity with which the uterus increases in size and weight under the influence of the physiological stimulus of pregnancy, and reverts to its natural size and weight when that stimulus is removed.—This brief recapitulation of my last communication is necessary, as in the above facts is found the key to the history of uterine displacements or deviations, as I have interpreted them.

The uterus may be displaced or deviated in various ways. Its position and form may be modified with reference to its own axis, or with reference to its conventional anatomical pelvic axis, which corresponds, as we have seen, to that of the upper pelvic outlet. When the axis of the uterus itself is modified, the uterus is said to be flexed, anteriorly, posteriorly, or laterally; and we have thus antero-flexion, retro-flexion, and latero-flexion. When the uterus is displaced *in toto*, without any abnormal bend or flexion taking place, so that its axis is

THE NEW MEDICAL COUNCIL.

AT London, on the 23rd day of November, and within the Hall of the Royal College of Physicians there, the members of the General Council of Medical Education and Registration of the United Kingdom having met, pursuant to a summons by the Secretary of State, there appeared for

The Royal College of Physicians of London...	Dr. Thomas Watson.
The Royal College of Surgeons of England	Mr. J. Henry Green.
The Apothecaries' Society of London...	Mr. John Nussey.
The University of Oxford	Dr. H. W. Acland.
The University of Cambridge	Dr. H. J. H. Bond.
The University of Durham	Dr. Dennis Embleton.
The University of London	Dr. John Storrar.
The Royal College of Physicians, Edinburgh	Dr. Alexander Wood.
The Royal College of Surgeons, Edinburgh	Dr. Andrew Wood.
The Faculty of Physicians and Surgeons, Glasgow	Dr. James Watson.
The Universities of Aberdeen and Edinburgh	Professor Syme.
The Universities of Glasgow and St. Andrews	Dr. J. A. Lawrie.
The King and Queen's College of Physicians in Ireland	Dr. Aquila Smith.
The Royal College of Surgeons of Ireland	Dr. Robert Carlisle Williams.
The Apothecaries' Society of Ireland ...	Dr. Charles H. Leet.
The University of Dublin	Dr. James Apjohn.
The Queen's University of Ireland ...	Dr. John D. Corrigan.

Sir James Clark, Bart.
Sir Charles Hastings.
William Lawrence, Esq.
Mr. Thomas Pridgin Teale.
Professor Robert Christison.
Professor William Stokes.
} Nominated by Her Majesty, with advice of her Privy Council.

Dr. Thomas Watson was elected Chairman *ad interim*; Dr. Alexander Wood was elected Secretary *ad interim*; and Sir Benjamin Brodie was elected President of the Council on the motion of Dr. ACLAND, seconded by Dr. APJOHN.

The Committee adjourned at a quarter past three till four o'clock.

At the adjourned meeting at four P.M. Sir BENJAMIN BRODIE took the chair, and returned thanks.

On the motion of Dr. ALEXANDER WOOD, seconded by Dr. JAMES WATSON, the following gentlemen were appointed a committee to examine and classify the letters addressed to the Council now on the table:—Dr. Alexander Wood, Mr. Teale, and Dr. James Watson.

On the motion of Dr. ANDREW WOOD, seconded by Dr. WILLIAMS, the following gentlemen were appointed a committee to estimate the amount of revenue likely to accrue under the Medical Act, and also the expenditure necessary to carry out its provisions, and to report to the Council at the next meeting:—

Dr. Andrew Wood, Chairman.	Dr. Storrar.
Dr. Williams.	Dr. Aquila Smith.
Dr. Christison.	Dr. Lawrie.
Dr. Alexander Wood.	Dr. Embleton.

On the motion of Dr. ALEXANDER WOOD, seconded by Dr. BOND, the committee last appointed were requested to prepare an outline of the order of business to come before the Council.

On the motion of Dr. CHRISTISON, seconded by Sir CHARLES HASTINGS, the following gentlemen were appointed a committee to report to next meeting as to the recommendation of a committee for preparing the *National Pharmacopœia*, and the powers to be conferred on that committee:—Dr. Christison, chairman, Sir James Clark, and Dr. Apjohn.

On the motion of Sir CHARLES HASTINGS, seconded by Sir JAMES CLARK, it was agreed.—

"That the minutes of each meeting of the Council, as well as all notices of motions, be printed and transmitted to each member of the Council."

Sir Benjamin Brodie having been obliged to vacate the chair, Dr. Thomas Watson, on the suggestion of Mr. GREEN, was requested to take it.

Dr. WATSON intimated that Dr. Mayo, President of the College of Physicians, had requested him to inform the Council

that the rooms of the College were fully placed at the disposal of the Council until they acquired more permanent accommodation.

Dr. STOKES, seconded by Dr. STORRAR, moved that the thanks of the Council be given to the College of Physicians for their courtesy.

The interim Chairman and interim Secretary were appointed to intimate to the Secretary of State for the Home Department the election of Sir Benjamin Brodie as President of the Council.

The committees nominated this day were appointed to meet at 11 A.M. on the 24th.

The Council then adjourned till 3 P.M. on the 24th of November.

JAMES CLARK, Bart.,
Interim Chairman.

Correspondence.

"*Audi alteram partem.*"

THE NEW CHARTER OF THE COLLEGE OF PHYSICIANS AND THE UNIVERSITY OF LONDON.

[LETTER FROM DR. HENRY SAVAGE.]

To the Editor of THE LANCET.

SIR,—"Hear both sides" has ever been a leading principle with THE LANCET. Your report of the proceedings of the recent meeting of the University of London medical graduates is incomplete. As one of the minority then present, I send you the following additional particulars, essential for a correct view of one side of the question. I must depend on your character for fair play to give immediate insertion to them.

Dr. Brinton having introduced his violent resolution by all sorts of vague personalities, we put the question to him direct, —What is the nature of the objections to Dr. Storrar? Dr. Brinton, in the name of his coadjutors, declared that he founded his resolution on the following objections:—

1st.—Dr. Storrar was not a member of the College of Physicians.

2nd.—He was unknown to scientific or professional fame.

3rd.—He did not possess adequate *social qualifications*.

4th.—His genius, as shown on our graduates' committee, was merely polemic.

We pressed for further explanation of the objection—social qualifications. His reply was, "He meant that Dr. Storrar was not in intimate and frequent acquaintance with the heads of the profession."

Dr. Brinton said he himself was in the habit of meeting and associating with the individuals he called heads of the profession, not one of whom failed, even in ordinary gossip, to shake their heads, with the most ominous astonishment, at Dr. Storrar's selection by the Senate of the University of London as its representative on the Medical Council !

I have ever contended that a College of Physicians and the University of London must necessarily be antagonistic. Here is a remarkable instance of it. Forty-six of our graduates having too little faith in the efforts of our graduates' committee, secede from time to time into the College of Physicians. They lost their money; they are, *quasi* College—nowhere at all, and their first step after the new Medical Act is to go dead against the Senate. More than this: Dr. Storrar was returned by a triumphant majority at Convocation as eligible for a seat in that body, so their next step was to form a deputation personally to request Mr. Walpole to pass him over !

In the name of the minority at the meeting above referred to, I protest in the strongest manner against this conduct of the forty-six, because—

1. They are influenced by party bias, or why wait till Dr. Storrar's appointment, to urge the objections now for the first time brought forward. The leaders in the movement against him were actually his colleagues on the graduates' committee.

2. The leaders of the forty-six are now engaged in contriving a new charter for the College of Physicians, which notoriously persevered to the last moment in a systematic opposition to the just privileges of the London University Graduates.

3. It is mainly to Dr. Storrar's skill and unwearied vigilance that the privileges now enjoyed by University medical graduates in the new Medical Act were secured to them, and the

an excellent auxiliary to our treatment; but, it must also be borne in mind, that in every case treated by camphor, except one, (Dr. Pidduck's, in which the dose of strychnia was comparatively small,) other remedies—and amongst them emetics—were given. It can, therefore, scarcely be said to answer all our requirements. Charcoal is said to act upon poisons by their adhering to its surface, and so being removed from contact with the stomach; and tannin by producing an insoluble compound with the strychnia. Neither of these, therefore, can exert any beneficial effect beyond what takes place with the unabsorbed poison. The experiments of Dr. Hammond, of Fort Riley, show that no reliance can be placed on *fat* as an antidote.

I now proceed to examine the claims of emetics to effect our object—or rather I would say vomiting; and to prove that this is the agent I will draw attention to its effects in some diseases manifesting phenomena not very dissimilar from those caused by the poison under consideration. I allude to those disorders having a paroxysmal or spasmodic character—namely, whooping-cough, hysteria, and infantile convulsions. In all these, in common with strychnia poisoning, we have, first, the periodical return of the paroxysm or spasm; secondly, the intermittent and irregular performance of the function of respiration; and, thirdly, a dark and highly carbonized condition of the blood. My attention was many years ago directed to a fact which is no doubt familiar to the profession, that the paroxysm of whooping-cough is almost invariably cut short by a good fit of vomiting, and that the countenance, which before was dusky from the circulation of highly carbonized blood, soon becomes florid and animated; the respiration, which before the fit was laboured and irregular, now becomes free and easy, and the child returns to its play or its meals. In the convulsions of children we have the same irregular, intermittent, and imperfect performance of the function of respiration, and the same irregular distribution, generally diminution of animal heat.

Reflecting on the results of vomiting on the paroxysm of whooping-cough, I was induced to try it in convulsions, and, where I could obtain it, have never found it fail in removing the convulsion.

In the allied disease of hysteria, where a very similar condition of the respiratory organs and functions exists, the breathing here being irregular, imperfect, and often at distant intervals, and where the external manifestations very much resemble those we have been considering, I have for many years looked upon vomiting as the remedy above all others to be relied on to remove the paroxysm or fit.

In the cases above mentioned it would be unfair to regard the mere emptying of the stomach as the *ratio medendi*. I have long since come to the conclusion that the return to healthy respiration has more to do with the relief of these diseases than is generally admitted. I believe the experiments of Dr. Harley have led him to the conclusion that strychnia produces death, not by its action on the nerve substance, but on the blood, by destroying its capability to absorb oxygen. This theory appears to derive considerable strength from the fact of the blue or dusky condition of the skin in the subjects of poisoning by strychnia, indicating a highly carbonized state of the blood. It has been suggested by Dr. Brown-Séquard, that in many cases of poisoning the loss of animal heat tends to a fatal result. Now, what is the meaning of this fact but that it is in consequence of the respiration being imperfectly and insufficiently performed, and, the circulation through the lungs having been thereby impeded, that the blood is not passing with its accustomed energy through the capillaries, and this tendency to death takes place? A similar condition to this must exist in the cold stage of fevers; and here we give emetics—and what for, if not to bring about, by the action of vomiting, a more complete and full respiratory action, and a more perfect series of that action, by which the blood is more quickly driven through the lungs, causing an increased absorption of oxygen, and a consequent greater development of animal heat, with its more general diffusion over the body? These results of vomiting, which are self-evident, cannot be the effect of the mere evacuation of the contents of the stomach; they must therefore be accomplished by the physiological action of vomiting. If this be true, then, *we have, in vomiting, a real and true antidote to poisoning by strychnia; and it is by the maintenance of the condition of system thereby induced that we must reasonably hope to combat the two morbid effects of the poison which are said to tend to death—I mean the diminished capacity of the blood for oxygen, and the consequent falling of the animal heat.*

But although I believe we have sufficient evidence to prove that this alone, when freely accomplished, is of itself sufficient to prevent death, yet I would not limit the treatment entirely to its production; for after the evidence we have had of the power of chloroform to subdue the spasms, I think we shall consult the comfort and ease of our patients by its careful exhibition, but I do not think it should be carried to the pitch of producing complete insensibility, nor, indeed, beyond the degree which causes the breathing to become regular. When the sickness has somewhat subsided, we may give camphor, suspended in almond emulsion, or any other fitting vehicle. With a view of assisting to maintain the animal warmth, I would place the patient near a good fire, or keep him well covered with blankets. It is of the utmost importance that the most perfect quiet should be observed by the patient and those about him, since it is obvious that any touch of the surface, or movement of any attendant in contact with the patient, may bring on a paroxysm of tetanic spasm, which might prove fatal. During the very severe fit, I believe we derived most timely aid from cold affusion, which appeared to bring on inspiration, and restore the then suspended animation. These remedies, though useful auxiliaries, are quite subordinate to the more important act of vomiting.

When once vomiting has been brought on, we should assist it by copious draughts of warm water, which will prolong the sickness, and also render it less painful. As regards the kind of emetic to be used, of course we give the preference to those of a non-depressing character; and were I to see another case, I should be disposed to use mustard, as being quicker in its operation than all others. Sulphate of zinc and ipecacuanha, however, afford a very appropriate form.

Camden-road Villas, March, 1861.

ON THE CONTAGION OF YELLOW FEVER.

BY W. BUDD, M.D., Clifton.

AFTER the vague platitudes to which we have so long been accustomed whenever the subject of epidemics is in question, it is a pleasure to read the remarks made by Dr. M'William in his manly and sensible speech on the interesting account, lately given to the Epidemiological Society by Dr. Bryson, of the introduction of yellow fever into Port Royal, Jamaica. The two precautions on which he so ably insisted, in their application to future outbreaks, do not, however, comprise all that may be done in the way of prevention. To run infected ships out of the tropics, and, whether on board ship or on shore, to maintain as strict a separation as possible between the sick and the healthy, are not the only precepts of first-rate importance suggested by the contagious nature of this fearful malady and the known thermometrical conditions required for its propagation. To destroy the contagious properties of the black vomit, and of the other excretions, immediately on their issue from the body, is, to say the least, as essential in many cases, if we wish to limit the sphere of the infection. Whenever a contagious disorder is attended by discharges that are characteristic of it, these discharges are always (as I have elsewhere endeavoured to show) the chief vehicle of the morbid poison. They originate, in fact, in, and are the outward mark of, the very act of elimination. It is from this intimate connexion with the specific poison, in each particular case, that such discharges derive their special character. I need scarcely add that yellow fever offers no exception to this law. It would occupy too much space to give in detail the decisive evidence by which it may be shown that the black vomit and the secretions of the same kind which issue from the bowel have a very large if not the principal part in the propagation of this pestilence. It may be sufficient to state, here, that this conclusion may be deduced with the utmost certainty from already existing data. By their nature as well as their amount, these discharges are eminently fitted to spread and carry out, over a wide sphere, the work of dissemination. In malignant attacks the quantity of fluid thrown off by the stomach, in the shape of the characteristic black vomit, is often absolutely enormous. In many subjects a similar fluid is discharged in floods by the bowels also. At sea, it saturates not only the bedding and the other furniture, but the timbers of the ship also, which it infects with a long-abiding taint. On shore, it poisons the latrine or privy, or, worse still, some drain, gutter, or open ditch that may happen to be at hand. In either case, the noxious matter, once cast forth, fills the air with contagious exhalations.

It is essential to a true view of the events to understand that the atmosphere thus generated is, in all probability, immeasurably more infectious than that which immediately surrounds the fever patient. In many instances, not only is the air poisoned, but the virus, percolating through the soil, finds its way into the drinking water also.

The circumstances here pointed out explain perfectly all that is most characteristic in the dissemination of this fatal malady. They explain—

1st. The well-ascertained relation of this dissemination to defective drainage.

2nd. The frequent occurrence of the disease in persons who have held no communication with the sick, and under circumstances that not only do not bear the common resemblance of contagion, but seem at first sight to preclude its operation.

3rd. The entire failure experienced in so many cases of the mere separation of the sick from the healthy, however strictly carried out, in preventing the spread of the disorder.

4th. The peculiar fatality of yellow fever in barracks and other establishments, a part of whose economy it is to have common privies for the use of large numbers of persons, and *which are at once the receptacles of discharges from the sick and the daily resort of the healthy.*

5th. The frequent decimation of the inmates of one wing of a barrack or other public building, while in an adjoining or nearly contiguous wing, identical with the other in every sanitary condition except in having a latrine of its own, all the inmates have remained perfectly healthy.

And, lastly, they explain perfectly the still more striking fact, (inexplicable on any other grounds,) of which there have, I believe, been many examples, in which, in large public establishments containing persons of both sexes, one sex has suffered from the fever in an extreme degree, while the other has entirely escaped.

To separate the healthy, however strictly, from the fever patients, but to allow them still to come into intimate contact with the most specific of all the fever exuviæ, is a proceeding that may be described as worse than futile. It is much as if, in the case of small-pox, we should take the utmost care to separate the uninfected from the small-pox patient, and still to allow them to come into contact with things and places tainted in the highest degree with the small-pox virus.

In the spring of 1859, when yellow fever committed such havoc amongst the troops at Trinidad, I drew up, for the use of a friend who was about to join his regiment there, a little code of precautionary measures, from which the following are extracted :—

a. All discharges from the sick (including especially the characteristic black vomit) to be received, on their issue from the body, if possible, into vessels containing a saturated solution of chloride of zinc. Such portions of these discharges as may be unavoidably spilt, or scattered about, to be covered at once with peat charcoal and chloride of lime.

b. The latrines, or other places which serve as the final receptacles of these discharges, *to be reserved exclusively for that use.*

c. All latrines or privies to be thickly strewed night and morning with a mixture of equal parts of peat charcoal and chloride of lime.

d. All tainted linen to be burnt immediately on its removal from the sick.

e. The hands of all attendants on the sick to be frequently and carefully washed, especially after being soiled by black vomit or other discharges.

f. The utmost care to be taken in providing pure drinking-water, and where any doubt may exist as to its quality, the water to be boiled and filtered through charcoal before use.

g. The interior of infected barracks and other places to be well fumigated with chlorine, and afterwards white-washed and painted. Existing privies, and all drains connected with them, if infected with yellow-fever discharges, to be built over or otherwise abolished, after a preliminary disinfection.

h. The attendants on the sick, and those engaged in disinfecting operations, to be chosen (in accordance with Sir W. Pym's suggestion) from persons who have had the fever before, when such persons are to be had.

i. Convalescents to be kept for some time in strict separation from the uninfected.

Do what we may, it will probably be impossible to prevent the spread of yellow fever in all cases. But by combining the measures here described with the precautions suggested by Sir W. Pym and other writers, and so ably enforced by Dr. M'William, there can be little doubt that its ravages may be very greatly limited.

March, 1861.

A Mirror

OF THE PRACTICE OF

MEDICINE AND SURGERY

IN THE

HOSPITALS OF LONDON.

Nulla est alia pro certo noscendi via, nisi quam plurimas et morborum et dissectionum historias, tam aliorum proprias, collectas habere et inter se comparare.—MORGAGNI. *De Sed. et Caus. Morb.*, lib. 14. Procemium.

WESTMINSTER HOSPITAL.

TWO CASES OF CYNANCHE TRACHEALIS ; TRACHEOTOMY IN THE SECOND, FOLLOWED BY DEATH TWENTY-FOUR HOURS AFTER.

(Under the care of Dr. RADCLIFFE.)

OF the seven cases of croup now recorded, three were submitted to tracheotomy, with the recovery of but one. In the other four no operation was resorted to, and only two recovered. They are not selected to illustrate any special point in the history of croup, but as examples of the disease ordinarily occurring in hospital practice. We may remark that tracheotomy in the young child seems a very uncertain operation, although it cannot be denied that cases here and there do recover in which it has been performed. Many physicians hesitate to recommend its adoption until too late. To be o service, it should be had recourse to at an early period, when the vital powers have not become too much depressed by the exhausting effects of the disease.

The notes of the two following cases were taken by Mr. Middleton, house-physician to the hospital :—

CASE 1.—Sarah B——, aged two years and four months, admitted at eleven A.M. on December 3rd, 1860. Two nights previous to admission she went to bed apparently well ; but on the following morning, after a somewhat restless night, she was observed to breathe with some difficulty, and to have a cough, which gradually became more troublesome during the day, and in the evening was noticed to have a harsh, ringing sound.

At the time of admission to the hospital, the countenance was anxious, flushed, and inclined to be dusky ; skin hot and dry ; extremities warm ; pulse quick ; respiration 60. The cough was frequent, and had a loud brassy tone ; the inspiration had the distinctive ringing sound of croup. Bowels open ; secretion of urine free ; thirst considerable ; appetite not entirely lost. Chest well formed ; resonant everywhere in front ; posteriorly, marked dulness on percussion over the whole lower third of each lung. Vocal fremitus strongly felt over the whole chest ; ordinary sounds of respiration for the most part masked by the tracheal sounds ; coarse crepitus occasionally distinguishable both in inspiration and in expiration. To have a hot bath containing mustard immediately, and a mixture of two grains of sulphate of copper in two ounces of water: two teaspoonfuls to be taken every ten minutes till vomiting is produced. Hot sponges, changed frequently, to be kept applied to the throat. Vomiting soon occurred, expelling a considerable quantity of flaky matter.—Three P.M.: Pulse 152 ; respiration 48 ; skin warm and perspiring freely ; countenance improved, and free from duskiness ; cough unaltered. To have five minims of dilute nitric acid in three drachms of water every half hour ; beef-tea (double strength) and milk to be given every hour, hot.

Dec. 4th.—Ten A.M.: Slept but little, but has not been very restless ; takes the medicine and nourishment regularly. Inspiration more prolonged, with much less of the ringing tracheal noise ; pulse 120 ; respiration 28 ; skin warm and moist ; countenance calm and of natural colour. In the course of the afternoon the respiratory sounds became more audible throughout

what is more, these calculations are marvellously correct. Life, so uncertain in the individual, is very remarkably subject to unseen and inflexible laws in the mass; so that the mathematicians easily deal with it in gross. This is singularly verified in the history of the rise and progress of insurance companies. Life is infinitely more certain than fire; and so great have been the advantages which this gives to the offices, that it appears from recent statistics that the profits of the companies on life insurance have been by far more steady and considerable than on fire insurance. Where the two have been combined, often all the profits of the company have been derived from the life department; and some ninety-three companies for insurance solely against fire have been broken up altogether.

AN EPIDEMIC CHECKED.

A REMARKABLE proof of what may be done in removing causes of disease by careful supervision and skilled medical direction has been afforded at the Central London District School. The children at that school were, as we stated lately, suffering most extensively from defective domestic arrangements. Putting aside some minor causes of complaint, they were the subjects of an epidemic affection of the eye. Upwards of a hundred of them were so affected. Mr. Haynes Walton was called into consultation as an ophthalmologist of scientific reputation, and decided that the affection was catarrhal ophthalmia; that the dust of the courtyards and other conditions brought under review were not the causes of it, but that it was due to an injudicious method of ventilation. Over the head of each bed was a great hole, through which the air was constantly renewed; and thus each child was continually exposed, when lying in bed, to a direct draught of cold air. The result was almost universal catarrhal ophthalmia. These holes he advised to be stopped up, and other methods of ventilation introduced as a substitution. The result has been, that ophthalmia has disappeared from the school, and so completely that a recent committee have intimated a doubt whether it had ever existed. This is just one of the instances of the useful preventive functions which medical men may be called to fill; great good would result if public institutions were more thoroughly and generally supervised in this way.

THE ILLNESS OF THE LATE PRINCE CONSORT.

As yet we have not obtained permission to furnish the medical profession with an authentic account of the illness of his late Royal Highness the Prince Consort, but we feel bound to repeat the appeal for such an authorized publication. The mass of our correspondence on this subject, and the unanimity with which the entire body of the press endorsed that appeal by copying it in their impressions, indicate sufficiently the extent to which the mind of the profession and the nation is unpleasantly affected by the injudicious reticence observed in this matter up to the present time. The only argument which has been addressed to us in favour of the abstinence from such publication is, that the nature and progress of an illness is a private matter—a confidence which the public cannot ask the physicians to surrender. If this were so here, it would certainly not be the voice of this journal which would be heard calling upon the physicians to supply such an account, however desirable it might be on public grounds: the duty would have rested with other departments of the press, and with them it should have remained. But since this illness affected a person so near to us all that we have clad ourselves in mourning for its fatal result, that we have suspended our business, and given all the outward tokens of the grief that has reigned in our hearts—so near to us that we were, so to say, summoned to the bedside of the illustrious patient by his physicians during its progress; since we were called daily and publicly to hear

their opinions, to accept their statement of the character of the malady and the prognosis as to its duration; and since they thus took the whole body of Englishmen, laymen and physicians, into their confidence--no doubt under the highest sanction and command,—it cannot surely be said that the profession are disentitled to ask that the account given of the malady shall be coherent and satisfactory. Let us look at the accounts already furnished to us officially on this head. Let us put together the bulletins:—

"*Sunday, Dec. 8th.*—His Royal Highness the Prince Consort has been confined to his apartments for the last week, suffering from a feverish cold, with pains in the limbs. Within the last two days the feverish symptoms have rather increased, and are likely to continue for some time longer; but there are no unfavourable symptoms."

"*Wednesday, Dec. 11th.*—His Royal Highness the Prince Consort is suffering from fever, unattended by unfavourable symptoms, but likely from its nature to continue for some time."

"*Thursday, Dec. 12th.*—His Royal Highness the Prince Consort has passed a quiet night. The symptoms have undergone little change.—James Clark, M.D.; Henry Holland, M.D.; Thomas Watson, M.D.; William Jenner, M.D."

"*Friday, Dec. 13th.*—His Royal Highness the Prince Consort passed a restless night, and the symptoms have assumed an unfavourable character during the day.—James Clark, M.D.; Henry Holland, M.D.; Thomas Watson, M.D.; William Jenner, M.D."

"*Saturday, Dec. 14th*, 9 A.M.—His Royal Highness the Prince Consort has had a quiet night, and there is mitigation of the severity of the symptoms.—James Clark, M.D.; Henry Holland, M.D.; Thomas Watson, M.D.; William Jenner, M.D."

"*Saturday, Dec. 14th*, 4.30 P.M.—His Royal Highness the Prince Consort is in a most critical state.—James Clark, M.D.; Henry Holland, M.D.; Thomas Watson, M.D.; William Jenner, M.D."

"*Saturday Night, Dec. 14th.*—His Royal Highness the Prince Consort became rapidly weaker during the evening, and expired without suffering at ten minutes before eleven o'clock.—James Clark, M.D.; Henry Holland, M.D.; Thomas Watson, M.D.; William Jenner, M.D."

Finally, the death was certified to be "Typhoid fever: duration 21 days."

Now we will not sum up coherently these scattered documents, because in doing so we might seem to accuse the physicians, which we certainly desire not to do. But we will ask those distinguished men just to consider what effect upon the mind of the profession such a series of documents are likely to produce if unexplained. Here is an account of a disease which begins on the 8th with "feverish cold;" which on the 11th is unattended by unfavourable symptoms; and on the 14th kills, the term "typhoid fever" then first officially appearing. It would be wrong to infer that this disease, being "typhoid fever (21 days)" from the first, was mistaken for a "feverish cold" until the 11th December, or eighteenth day of the disease: but so the medical attendants seem here to represent to the world. Indeed it is clearly impossible to give a fair clinical history of a disease in five bulletins addressed to the public, and therefore necessarily drawn up in very general, if not even vague, terms. The medical attendants of the Prince, therefore, cannot have fairly represented themselves to the world in the accounts thus published. It must be remembered that during the illness of so illustrious and beloved a personage, the greatest desire prevailed to modify the language describing his malady, so as to keep clear of raising anxieties and fears that might not be justified by final events. It is in the highest degree desirable to satisfy the reasonable demands of the profession and of the public, by permitting the physicians to place upon record an authentic medical history of the fatal illness, which, as affecting a personage of national and historical interest, ought without delay to be removed from all shadow of doubt or ambiguity.

THE LANCET, February 15, 1862.

A Lecture

ON THE

FOSSIL REMAINS OF MAN.

Delivered at the Royal Institution, Feb. 7th, 1862,

By PROFESSOR HUXLEY, F.R.S.

IT is the object of this lecture to explain why those persons who look at Man from a scientific point of view as the great final term of animal development, regard two skulls not very long since discovered as the most venerable and the most interesting specimens of humanity. Of those two skulls (of which casts were on the table), the one belongs to the oldest man of whom we have any knowledge, and the other seems to be the lowest and most degraded in rank of any which can claim humanity. In order to explain how these skulls possess that interest, why one of them may be regarded as the most ancient relic of man, and what are their relations to the existing races, many preliminary details must be reviewed.

And first, a few words as to the terms much used by the students of craniology—High Organization and Low Organization, Elevation and Degradation. The variations to which these terms are applied are best seen in running through the mammalian scale, and comparing the brain-receptacle of man with those of lower animals. Degradation is a relative term. In comparing the brain-case of man with those of the great anthropoid apes, the relative differences which indicate degradation are easily seen. First of all, they differ in absolute capacity: the human cranium has absolutely the greatest contents. In man, we observe that the brain-case is large, the facial element small. In a gorilla the cranium is small, and quite outweighed by the vast development of jaw, and of the massive bony prominences over the orbits and those to which the muscles, and especially those muscles which move the head and jaws, take attachment. In the chimpanzee we have, similarly, a small cranium, large jaw, and very prominent supra-orbital ridges, so that the eyes are deep set, and the face projects, outweighing the head. Thus we observe a gradually-diminishing brain-case, and an increase of facial development and of the bony ridges over the eye, which overhang the face and obscure the characters of the skull. These are the characters of degradation.

It is the more necessary to consider carefully the features of the skull of man in the present inquiry, because we have little else than the skulls left from which to decipher the nature of those early men of whom we speak.

Among the races of men, as they vary, we find a certain approximation to one of two types. If, on the one hand, we take such a skull as that of the negro, we find it long and narrow. The longitudinal diameter greatly predominates, so that the transverse is not more than from six-tenths to seven-tenths of the longitudinal measurement. This type of skull is known as the "dolicho-cephalic" or long-headed; and the negro is of a long-headed race, although long-headed only in this technical anatomical sense, and by no means fitted to compete in the contests of life with the "long-headed" and astute members of European society. Examine, on the other hand, the skull of a Turk or a Tartar, and we shall observe another type of conformation. The transverse measurement here more nearly approaches the longitudinal, of which it constitutes from eight-tenths to more than nine-tenths. This is the brachy-cephalic character. These characters have been systematically examined and explained by Retzius. The standard of brachy-cephalism is when the transverse is eight-tenths or more of the longitudinal diameter.

These differences are, however, quite apart from physiological distinctions of character. We may find, for example, two races, such as the Caffre and the Calmuc, with very opposite measurements, but yet very similar in morals and manners, or rather in the total want of both morals and manners.

Next, if we take the skull of a Turk, Greek, or European,

we may observe that the face hardly projects beyond the level of the forehead; but in an African skull the face projects, the nose projects, and so does the jaw. These are the characteristic differential qualities, of which the first is known as orthognathism—a character of elevation; and the second as prognathism—a character of degradation. On these the illustrious Camper, with the luminous and far reaching intelligence for which he was distinguished, founded his facial angle, and saw his way to a scientific craniology. The indications so furnished are valuable, but insufficient.

In inquiring into the shape and structure of the skull, ethnologists have at the same time connected these varieties with geographical distribution. It may be greatly doubted whether these varieties of form can be mapped out with the accuracy that has been assumed. But certain broad and sure results have been obtained which may be safely stated. If we take a map of the world, and draw a line from Russian Tartary to the Bight of Benin, at the northern and eastern end we shall find that the brachy-cephalic type prevails. Here are the Mongolian races, the Turks and Tartars, who are the most perfect specimens of brachy-cephalism. At the south-western extremity, the Bight of Benin, are found the dolicho-cephalic people, of the purest negro type. Furthermore, at the north-east extremity of the line, we find orthognathous people, and at the south-western extremity of the line we find the tribes who are most eminently and markedly prognathous. This is one of the broadest and most indisputable truths which ethnology has contributed to science.

This distinction accompanies a prodigious contrast in the conditions of life. At the northern extremity of the line we have a cold, dry, and barren clime; at the southern, a country heated, steaming and crowded with a rank and reeking vegetation. They are the two ethnological poles. In whichever direction you pass, you will find that as you go to the west and the south from the northern pole you get amongst a longer-headed people, with faces more or less projecting; and as you pass towards the north and the east from the southern pole, you become mixed up with tribes gradually approximating to the type of brachy-cephalism. Pass southward from the northern pole, through Cochin China, and we find a gradual tendency to prognathism. Take the other pole, and pass from West Africa northward or to the east, and an opposite tendency to orthognathism is perceived, until we come to a people, along a line from the British Islands to Hindostan, oval-headed, more or less prognathous or orthognathous, and standing half way in the scale.

This is a broad statement, open to many exceptions and variations, but affording a fair view of the cranial characters of the tribes of men as they are distributed over the earth. But has this distribution been always the same? Has the human frame been invariable? Does palæontology, in its application to ethnology, show here also incessant changes and successions? or does it exhibit a uniform state of things through all the ages in which we have traces of man? The answer differs in different regions. There are no materials for saying that Asia was ever inhabited by a different race; none as to the Polynesian Archipelago or the Australian continent; none as to North America or the extreme southern parts of America. But there is a certain amount of evidence that, in the valley of the Mississippi, there once existed a race differing from the recent Indian tribes; that the marvellous race of men who constructed those great mounds, replete with proofs of an older civilization, were of another type. These mounds do not afford much evidence on this matter; but when skulls are found there they are those of a round-headed people. But pass from America to the Old World, and the indications of older races than those now occupying the territory are well marked.

Passing beyond the middle ages, we find everywhere traces on the earth of the great Roman race. Leaving them behind, we come, in Western Europe, to the relics of a long-headed people, the parents of the Germanic race, and allied to the Scandinavian races. They were workers in iron, and their epoch of occupation lasted a long time. Before these we find the evidences of the pre-existence of a smaller race of long-headed men, like the Hindoos; not workers in iron, but in bronze, and who possessed a certain cultivation and domesticated for their use certain animals. Archæologists can go further than this. Behind these there is a third race—a ruder people, in whose tombs are found certain weapons, but no domesticated animals; they are characterized by fashioning for themselves weapons of stone, flint, serpentine, and the like materials. They buried their warriors in the tumuli, sitting, and, each provided with his heavy axe, ready to meet either friend or foe when he passed through the solemn portals of death into the blessed regions, of which they formed their own rude and savage notions. These weapons were always made of the same stony material, and always ground to a sharp edge. The Danish archæologists, who have examined very carefully the cranial character of the human relics here interred, have found that they belonged to a much rounder-headed people than those of the succeeding period. Mr. Busk, who has personally repeated, and added to, those investigations in Denmark, has confirmed these statements. These skulls are rather below the average bulk, they are somewhat rounded, the transverse amounting to eight-tenths of the longitudinal diameter, and some of them are remarkable for the flatness of the forehead and the prominence of the supra-orbital ridges; the jaws are large, but not prognathous. These characters belong to all the skulls of the men of the stone epoch.

How far is this stone epoch distant from us in time? This is a question always difficult to answer, and to which a cautious reply must needs be given. Distant it was indeed—far beyond any records of history. But some singular means exist of estimating the space of time which separates those races from us. Denmark possesses great peat-bogs in various parts of the country, in which are embedded forests of trees. In the more superficial layers of the soil are imbedded fallen trunks of beech-trees—great trunks of beech like those which now adorn the surface of the country, and are its chief and most graceful decoration. Beneath these beech-trees we come to a lower forest—a forest of oak-trees, fallen with their tops to the centre, of noble size—oaks which had taken centuries to grow, and which have been centuries in the ground. Dig deeper again, and you come to another forest of large and splendid pine-trees—noble trunks of three feet in diameter, of great age and magnificent proportions. Now, in the memory of man there has been nothing in Denmark but beech-trees. Past the memory of man grew and flourished those giant oaks; they had centuries of growth, and for centuries they have been buried. Past these centuries we must look down the vista of ages for the time when the pine-trees stood erect, and slowly gathered their bulk, and fell into the lowest part of this deep peat, to be again covered with the wrecks of succeeding epochs of vegetation.

Now, in the beech forests of the bog we find only traces of the men of iron; amongst the oaks, only of the men of bronze; and amongst the pines, only of the men who worked in stone, and nothing but stone. Beneath the pines we find only peat, and no remains of man of any kind whatever.

What is meant by this lapse, not so much of time, but of facts? We cannot number the ages that saw the rise and fall of these monarchs of the vegetable world, and the succession of these races of man. But great as the range of time thus traversed must have been, it is inappreciable when compared with the chronology of geology. Contrasted with the distance of the earlier geological epochs, it is as the diameter of our earth compared to our distance from one of the fixed stars.

In the time of the men of the stone epoch the physical geography of Europe was as it is now. What was dry land then is dry land now; the caves and fissures which are now high and dry were then high and dry: but beyond that epoch lies the age when the physical features of the land were very different. What is now sea and seashore was then dry land, covered with thick forests; what is now the channel of a river was then far distant from any watercourse. It is in caves such as these that, associated with the bones of mammalians now extinct, and of others that could only have existed under totally different climatal conditions—associated with the bones of the *Elephas primigenius*, the urus, and the great cave-bear, we find those wonderful stone axes which have been lately so carefully examined and discussed—stone axes not polished and ground, but hacked and chipped to a sharp edge. These are the work of human hands, yet they are found in European soil, together with the remains of the mammoth, the cave-bear, the hyena, and hairy rhinoceros. What manner of man was this?

An approximative answer may be given from the result of the examination of the two human skulls which form the subject of the present inquiry. The one of them was found by Schmerling in 1833, in the Cave of Engis, near Liege, in the Valley of the Meuse, high and dry, covered with a deposit of red earth and beneath stalagmite. In the same position, and at the same time, were found associated with these human skulls, bones of the cave-bear and its contemporaries. The skulls of the man and of these early animals were alike in condition, and equally deprived of their gelatine. Now the anatomist cannot, in virtue of his science, enter into any discussion as to the age of these skulls and the age of the strata in which they were found. This is the province of the geologist, and I take the evidence of Sir Charles Lyell on this point. Sir Charles has revisited this cave, and re-examined the ground in which the relics were discovered, and he has staked his reputation as a geologist on the coexistence of the skull of the man with the bones of the animals. I take the evidence of Sir Charles Lyell as conclusive, and assume that the man who made those stone axes was coeval with the brutes, and that here is the skull of one of that race. No axes were found in this precise cave, but the shaped flints which have been found belong to this epoch. In this cave stone flakes were found, but no shaped axes. It is certain, however, that the two belong to the same period. This is the skull of one of those primeval men who flourished when over England ranged the bison, the cave-bear, and the hairy rhinoceros.

What are the characters of this brain-case? What are the deviations from the highest human character of skull? What are its relations to the present race of men? It is a skull not badly shaped; it is long; the transverse diameter is considerably less than the longitudinal diameter; the forehead is fairly and well developed. But the supra-orbital ridges are rather prominent. This is, indeed, a character of degradation; but a vast number of European skulls have the same peculiarity. Schmerling thought the skull one of low race; but others have ranked it high. And Schmerling certainly condemned it on insufficient grounds. Every variety of peculiar dolicho-cephalic skulls may be found in a large collection, such as that of the College of Surgeons; and there may be seen a skull from Mozambique in one case, while opposite to it is an equally degraded cranium of very marked form, indeed one of the worst that I have seen, and which is that of a Celtic Highlander. In fact, extremely exceptional conditions may be observed amongst perfectly recent skulls. I should mention in connexion with the Engis skull, that with the adult skull were found others, some of quite young persons.

The second cranium, known as the Neander-thal skull, was found in a cave in the valley of that name, overlooking the Düssel, a tributary of the Rhine. There is no definite record of the age of this skull. It was buried in the mud, and with it were bones of the extremities. It is the lowest and most degraded of all human skulls. There is a marvellous low forehead; the supra orbital ridges are enormous, and the skull flat and low; the supra-occipital ridges are not overhung at all. This skull is degraded, and of so low a type that the inspection of a cast of it suggested to me the question whether it was not deformed or abnormally modified. I caused, therefore, a careful examination to be made of the interior of the skull, in order to ascertain whether the lateral sinuses were normally placed. I found that they were, and photographs of the interior of the skull show that the channels and markings of the interior of the cranium have the ordinary relations. The depressed vertex, shallow forehead, and sloping occiput,—the signs of degradation which it bears,—are the indications of the depressed and low character of the brain which it enclosed.

Taking these two skulls of the Engis and Neander-thal Caves as the oldest known vestiges of man, I asked, What are the relations which can be observed between them and the skulls of existing races? Did they belong to two different races? They present, indeed, very strongly-marked differences of shape; and looking at the two skulls of Engis and of the Neander-thal, it would be difficult to find any other two which differ from each other more strongly. But I am not willing to draw any definite conclusion as to their specific variety from that fact. I inquire rather, are not the variations amongst the skulls of a pure race to the full as extensive?

I take the pure Australian as an example for this inquiry; and here we may observe how great is the range of variation in that pure race. The Engis skull may be easily matched by an Australian skull. The following table shows how closely the measurements approximate :—

	Horizontal Circumference.	Vertical Arc.	Transverse Arc.	Length.
Engis	$20\frac{1}{2}$ ...	$13\frac{1}{2}$ ...	$13\frac{1}{2}$ ...	$7\frac{3}{4}$
Australian ...	$20\frac{1}{2}$ ...	13 ...	13 ...	$7\frac{1}{2}$
English... ...	$21\frac{3}{4}$ ...	$13\frac{1}{2}$ ...	14 ...	$7\frac{3}{4}$

With the Neander-thal skull, however, we shall not find much more difficulty, for in the College of Surgeons there are a number of skulls of Southern Australians, and one or two of these are wonderfully near the degraded type of the Neander-thal skull. The differences are inconsiderable; and, except that in the supra-orbital ridges and the occipital ridges the Neander-thal skull retains characters of degradation which go beyond those of the South Australian, or any others that I have met, the resemblance is perfect. Seeing that the variations of conformation in a pure race, such as the Australian, are so great, it cannot be safely inferred that these two skulls, which vary very little more, are even of different races.

It is remarkable that the habits of these men of the age of stone clearly resembled, in several respects, those of the Australian savage tribes. The evidence of the mode of life of the ancient men consists in the great collection of bones found with traces of their industry—bones of the urus, the bison, and other creatures, which they split, to extract the marrow from them, and which they worked up into implements. These bones &c. are found also amongst the piles at the bottom of some of the lakes in Switzerland. The Australian savages similarly utilize the bones of the kangaroo, and their universal weapon is the rudely-fashioned stone axe; while the nearly allied people of New Guinea build houses on piles like those of the ancient population of the Swiss lakes. So that in that most remote epoch, as at the present day, we may believe that savage man was a creature of similar habits and mode of life.

These conclusions have not been arrived at by an easy or uncontested path. Those who believed, from the evidence of their senses, that there were men the contemporaries of the *Elephas primigenius* and his co-mates, had to breast a tempest of stormy opposition. And now that men are generally agreed to accept these facts, we find that this has been after all only a battle of outposts, and that we must go far back beyond even these primeval times to meet with the oldest of men.

THE

Lettsomian Lectures on Surgery

FOR THE YEAR 1862.

◆

ON

PRACTICAL LITHOTOMY AND LITHOTRITY.

BY HENRY THOMPSON, ESQ., F.R.C.S.,

ASSISTANT-SURGEON TO UNIVERSITY COLLEGE
HOSPITAL.

No. I.

AFTER some preliminary observations relative to the occasion of the Lettsomian Lectures, and on the choice of the subject determined on, the lecturer enumerated various sources of information which had been specially placed at his disposition for the purpose of this course. Very valuable results of practice had been furnished from the hospitals of Norwich, Cambridge, Oxford, Leicester, and Leeds, for which he was deeply indebted to Mr. Cadge, Mr. Humphrey, Mr. Hussey, Mr. Smith, Mr. Paget, and Mr. Nunneley. The results of practice of University College Hospital had been afforded him, by the kindness of his colleagues. And from such sources 1500 cases had been available,—every one of complete authenticity,—forming the most perfect data obtainable in connexion with the subject. Next, the manuscript notes of the late Mr. Crichton, of Dundee, who had left records of the greater number of his cases, containing much matter hitherto unpublished, had been placed at his disposal by his son, Mr. J. R. Crichton—upwards of 200 cases more. Dr. Keith, of Aberdeen, who had already cut or crushed 300 cases of calculi, had afforded him much valuable information. The unrivalled experience of Civiale had been unreservedly communicated, and especially with a view to these lectures. Lastly, to the President himself, as well as to others too numerous to mention, he was under considerable obligations in various ways.

The subject of lithotomy is by no means so simple and so limited at the present day as it was considered to be a few years ago. If we take the writings of our best surgeons of the last fifty or sixty years who have devoted themselves to it, we cannot but be struck with the fact that no other mode of performing lithotomy is alluded to—except for occasional trial or as a matter for speculative remark—than the lateral operation. Most assert that it is the only method which should be employed, except in certain circumstances which are extremely

unusual; and it is right to add, that some great authorities appear still to hold the same opinion. The last ten or fifteen years, however, have witnessed some change in this respect in England, and several attempts have been made to remove the stone by other modes of incision; while the surgical practice of Paris has exhibited similar endeavours for a longer period of time. The introduction and progress of lithotrity have, in a great measure, been the cause of this. Lithotrity has achieved such indisputable success with small stones, that those whose habits and inclinations lead them to prefer the use of the knife, have endeavoured to find a method of employing it which should enable them to compete on equal terms with the crushing operation. But where no such feelings exist, the conviction has forced itself on the minds of most surgeons, that the difference between a large stone and a small one is so great, both as regards the prognosis of the case and the difficulty to the operator, that it is impossible to regard even all calculous patients who are to be submitted to the knife as belonging to one category, and as amenable but to one remedy. It is believed to be neither philosophical nor politic to apply to every stone—whether it be no bigger than a nut or as large as an apple—invariably one and the same proceeding. We have learned the importance, in the first place, of ascertaining, before deciding on any operation, the physical characters of the calculus—that is, as regards its size and hardness; and, secondly, the condition of the patient in relation to the state of his urinary organs and his general susceptibilities. Hence the student of our subject, in these modern times, has several modes of lithotomy to understand, and several questions presented to his consideration, in order that he may arrive at a practical solution of the question when a patient comes before him—viz., what is the best operation for this particular case? Hence also it is that, up to the present time, there has been little attempt to offer a comprehensive appreciation of the various methods now in vogue. The choice has hitherto been mainly limited to the alternatives of lateral lithotomy and lithotrity, with recently, in some quarters, the added resources of the median operation. An attempt to supply this desideratum will occupy a considerable portion of the concluding lecture.

The various procedures employed under the name of lithotomy must be ranged in two separate classes—namely:

1st. Operations by which the bladder is reached from the perineum; and among these I shall notice several principal methods, which will sufficiently include minor modifications.

2nd. An operation performed above the pubes, and known as the high or supra-pubic operation.

I. *Operations performed in the Perineum, or Perineal Lithotomy.*

These are of various kinds, but all may be classified either as lateral or as central operations.

Lateral operations are those which are confined within one of the lateral divisions of the perineum. The incisions are directed between the central and lateral muscles of the perineum. They necessarily approach the pubic ramus, the pubic artery and its branches, and are directed transversely to these latter near to their origin from the arterial trunk. They involve one side of the prostate gland—it may be nearly to its full extent; while in children, and in exceptional adult cases, they go beyond it.

Central operations are those in which the incisions are limited to the central part of the perineum, are made in the line of the raphé itself or transverse to it, and lie mainly between the anus and the symphysis pubis. They do not approach the rami or the great vessels, nor do they run transversely near to the origin of the branches from the pudic artery. In no case do the incisions reach the external limits of the prostate gland. The distinction is important, and has an intimate relation to all that follows. It indicates a principle by which to distinguish and classify all the proposals made for the performance of lithotomy in the perineum.

Lateral operations.—There is one proceeding only which will be regarded as the type of this class—namely, the operation at present most generally practised in this country, and universally known as the lateral operation. Although in different hands some of its details vary, the general outline and character are the same in all.

Central Operations.—The "median" operation: The stone was removed by a median incision in the perineum, made close to and parallel with the raphé in the old Marian operation during the sixteenth century and long afterwards. But the far greater success which the lateral method realized led ultimately to the total extinction of the Marian. The disastrous results of this procedure were due, however, to the vio-

was carrying out a work of public utility and benevolence. The tragedy of "Hamlet" is not commonly considered to be otherwise than an honour to our national literature; and if the Bishop of Exeter entertains other than the usual views on this subject, it was yet a particularly unfortunate and ill-chosen occasion for punishing the public reading of that masterpiece, when the effort was made on behalf of a cause of the most unadulterated good, and the most unsectarian charity.

SECONDARY EFFECTS OF ACCIDENTS.

A case was tried in the Court of Common Pleas on Wednesday, in which a lady's-maid of the Duchess of Montrose, who received a severe blow upon the right side in a collision on the London and North-Western Railway, Nov. 15th, 1860, claimed damages for the secondary effects of the injury sustained. She was able to attend to her duties until the following January. Dr. Tyler Smith said that a swelling formed on the right side; that consumptive disease of the lung had set in, and would, in his opinion, ultimately cause her death. The patient was the subject of recent phthisis, which had apparently set in since the accident. There was now spitting of blood, and, in his opinion, she would never again be fit to fill her former situation. Damages were awarded to the extent of £700.

Another case tried this week in the Court of Queen's Bench, before Mr. Justice Blackburn, illustrates the important bearing of the remarks recently made in The Lancet Report on the subject of Secondary Effects of Accidents. In this case (English v. the North London Railway Company) it was shown that while the immediate effects of the fracture of ribs, bruising and wounding of the knee and back, were relieved by proper care within a short time, the results of the serious concussion were the really important source of disablement. Loss of memory, giddiness, and defective sight, still existed, and the general health appeared to be affected. Damages of £200 were given.

It is clear that the attention of surgeons must in these cases be directed carefully to the examination of the nervous system; and concussion enters so largely into the ultimate and permanent injuries sustained, that the companies will find their pecuniary account in padding their seats and carriages of all classes, so as to limit to the utmost the violence of the shock occurring at the moment of accidents. Meantime the health of the travelling public would be favourably influenced by this reform.

MORTALITY IN THE LONDON AND PARIS HOSPITALS.
To the Editor of The Lancet.

Sir,—In your able leading article in last week's journal, on the comparative rates of mortality in the London and Parisian hospitals, one important item is omitted in the estimate,—namely, the comparative strength of constitution or vital endowment of the class of patients admitted. The superiority of the English over the French, arising from the more nutritious diet in health, is alone sufficient to account for the difference in the rate of mortality; just as the death-rate in the population of London is lower than that of Paris.

Upon the subject of warming and ventilating the wards of an hospital, the combination of two modes will be found effectual. The one is by means of large inverted basins inserted on a level with the ceiling, with an aperture in the apex connected with an horizontal tube extending between the joists to the chimney or the open air, for the middle wards; and through the roof, for the attics. The other mode is by the adoption of Cundy's open firegrate stove, which warms and ventilates, by the admission of a volume of fresh air, through an air-channel, equal to that which passes off by the combustion of the fuel. Both are perfectly automatic. The advantages of this combined plan are: warmth without closeness; ventilation without draughts; economy of fuel with a cheerful open fire.

I am, Sir, yours &c.,

February, 1862.   M.D.

THE
ANALYTICAL SANITARY COMMISSION.

RECORDS OF THE RESULTS OF
MICROSCOPICAL AND CHEMICAL ANALYSES
OF THE
SOLIDS AND FLUIDS
CONSUMED BY ALL CLASSES OF THE PUBLIC.

BREAD,
AND ITS ADULTERATIONS.

THE following analyses were undertaken for the purpose of determining whether alum is still commonly added to Bread, and also the proportions in which it is used:—

Results of the Analysis of Thirty-two Samples of Bread for Alum.

At the time of analysis the breads had become dry and stale. This should be borne in mind, as, in consequence, the amount of alum in 1000 grains of the bread, which was the quantity subjected to analysis, was proportionately increased.

1st Sample.
Purchased at the establishment of—Mr. Stevens, Cambridge-road, Hackney.
No Alum.

2nd Sample.
Purchased at the establishment of—Mr. Hill, Red House, Bishopsgate-street Within.
No Alum.

3rd Sample.
Purchased at the establishment of—Mr. G. Elphinstone, 21, Throgmorton-street, City.
No Alum.

4th Sample.
Purchased at the establishment of—Mr. Nevill, Central Depôt, 16, Holborn-hill.
Contains *alum* in the proportion of 82·91 grains to the 4 lb. loaf.
A second loaf purchased some days subsequently, contained a still larger amount of alum.

5th Sample.
Purchased at the establishment of—Mr. Robb, 79, St. Martin's-lane.
No Alum.

6th Sample.
Purchased at the establishment of—Mr. W. Cook, 199, Piccadilly.
No Alum.

7th Sample.
Purchased at the establishment of—Mr. Stewart, 46, Bond-st.
No Alum.

8th Sample.
Purchased at the establishment of—Mr. Bonthron, 106, Regent-street.
Contains a small quantity of *alum*—namely, 25·91 grains to the 4 lb. loaf.
A second loaf purchased a few days afterwards furnished a nearly similar result.

9th Sample.
Purchased at the establishment of—Mr. J. Elphinstone, 227, Regent-street.
No Alum.

10th Sample.
Purchased at the establishment of—Mr. Bragg, 2, Wigmore-street, Cavendish-square.
No Alum.

THE LANCET,]   BREAD, AND ITS ADULTERATIONS.   [FEBRUARY 15, 1862. 183

11th Sample.

Purchased at the establishment of—Mr. Sapsford, 20, Queen Anne-street, Cavendish-square.
No ALUM.

12th Sample.

Purchased at the establishment of—Mr. J. Cook, 48, Edgware-road.
No ALUM.

13th Sample.

Purchased at the establishment of—Mr. Weston, 128, Edgware-road.
No ALUM.

14th Sample.

Purchased at the establishment of—Mr. Withers, 86, Black-man-street, Borough.
Contains *alum* in the proportion of 82·91 grains per 4 lb. quartern loaf.

15th Sample.

Purchased at the establishment of—Mr. Cowan, 76, Blackman-street, Borough.
Contains 152·88 grains of *alum* to the 4 lb. loaf.

16th Sample.

Purchased at the establishment of—Mr. Bailey, 207, High-st., Borough.
Contains 62·18 grains of *alum* to the 4 lb. loaf.

17th Sample.

Purchased at the establishment of—Mr. Bishop, 172, High-st., Borough.
No ALUM.

18th Sample.

Purchased at the establishment of—Mr. Hills, 78, St. George's-road, Southwark.
Contains 85·50 grains of *alum* to the 4 lb. loaf.

19th Sample.

Purchased at the establishment of—Mr. H. Blake, 26, West-minster-road.
Contains 103·65 grains of *alum* to the 4 lb. loaf.

20th Sample.

Purchased at the establishment of—Mr. Goedecker, 27, Bridge-road, Lambeth.
Contains 106·24 grains of *alum* to the 4 lb. loaf.

21st Sample.

Purchased at the establishment of—Mr. Blatchley, 10, Chel-tenham-place, Westminster-road.
Contains 85·50 grains of *alum* to the 4 lb. loaf.

22nd Sample.

Purchased at the establishment of—Mr. Harnor, 6, Lower Marsh, Lambeth.
Contains 82·91 grains of *alum* to the 4 lb. loaf.

23rd Sample.

Purchased at the establishment of—Mr. Wertzell, 8, Crawford-street, W.
No ALUM.

24th Sample.

Purchased at the establishment of—Mr. Schwenk, 75, Craw-ford-street, W.
Contains 98·46 grains of *alum* to the 4 lb. loaf.

25th Sample.

Purchased at the establishment of—Mrs. Wyman, 105, Craw-ford-street, W.
No ALUM.

26th Sample.

Purchased at the establishment of—Mr. Zoller, 14, Homer's-row, Crawford-street, W.
Contains 69·96 grains of *alum* to the 4 lb. loaf.

27th Sample.

Purchased at the establishment of—Mr. Fuchs, 37, Crawford-street, W.
No ALUM.

28th Sample.

Purchased at the establishment of—Mr. Kirkby, 45, Crawford-street, W.
Contains 38·86 grains of *alum* to the 4 lb. loaf.

29th Sample.

Purchased at the establishment of—Mr. Kirkby, 45, Crawford-street, W.
Contains 158·06 grains of *alum* to the 4 lb. loaf.

30th Sample.

Purchased at the establishment of—Mr. Robinson, 30, Skinner-street, Somers-town.
Contains 98·46 grains of *alum* to the 4 lb. loaf.

31st Sample.

Purchased at the establishment of—Mr. Burrows, 21, Skinner-street, Somers-town.
Contains 44·05 grains of *alum* to the 4 lb. loaf.

32nd Sample.

Purchased at the establishment of—Mr. Bate, 80, Brewer-street, Somers-town.
Contains 90·69 grains of *alum* to the 4 lb. loaf.

These results will be more readily appreciated by an examination of the subjoined table :—

Table showing the quantities of alum detected in the 4 lb. loaf, and calculated to the sack of ninety-two 4 lb. loaves.

Name.	Per 4 lb. loaf. Grains.	Per sack of ninety-two 4 lb. loaves. Oz.	Drs.
Nevill	82·91	17	4
Bonthron	25·91	5	4
Withers	82·91	17	4
Cowan	152·88	32	2
Bailey	62·18	13	1
Hills	85·50	18	0
Blake	103·65	21	8
Goedecker	106·24	22	4
Blatchley	85·50	18	0
Harnor	82·91	17	4
Schwenk	98·46	20	7
Zoller	69·96	14	7
Kirkby	38·86	8	1
Kirkby	158·06	33	2
Robinson	98·46	20	7
Burrows	44·05	9	2
Bate	90·69	19	1

It thus appears, that of the thirty-two samples subjected to analysis, *seventeen, or more than one half,* contained *sulphate of alumina and potash,* commonly known as ALUM.

The quantities ranged per quartern loaf between 25·91 grains and 158·06 grains, and per sack of ninety-two 4 lb. loaves between 5 oz. 4 dr. and 33 oz. 2 dr.

It appears further, that as the rule, to which there are some exceptions, the more respectable high-priced bakers, who buy the best flour and sell superior bread, do not make use of alum, for the employment of which no necessity whatever exists.

The principal reason why alum is so generally used by the bakers who sell cheap bread, is, that they are thereby enabled to impart to much less costly flour, when made into bread, the colour and appearances which, without the alum, can only be obtained by means of a flour of superior quality and higher price.

That the addition of a powerful substance like alum, and in the large quantities detected in the above analyses, is prejudicial to health, and is productive of dyspepsia and other derangements of the digestive organs, is well ascertained.

The adulteration of bread with alum is contrary to law, and bakers using that substance are liable to punishment. This offence is punishable not only under the Bread Act, but under the recent Act for the prevention of adulteration. The former Act is sometimes—that is, rarely and at long intervals—enforced, but the latter is, as respects the adulteration of bread, as of other articles, inoperative. It is, therefore, obvious that the law is at present wholly ineffectual in putting a stop to a very scandalous and injurious adulteration of a prime article of daily consumption.

struck, fracture of the distal table only, without injury to the proximal one, can be produced in either case, and that such fracture occurs in obedience to a well-known physical law—that fracture commences in the line of extension, which is the distal side, and not in that of compression.

Mr. BAKER BROWN exhibited a large Ovarian Tumour. The actual cautery had been successfully applied to the pedicle. He stated that he had had thirteen successes out of fifteen cases.

Dr. MURCHISON read a paper

ON HYDATIDS OF THE LIVER, THEIR DANGERS, THEIR DIAGNOSIS, AND THEIR TREATMENT.

The paper was elaborate and exhaustive. It commenced with a report of twenty cases, including all that had been the subject of post-mortem examination at the Middlesex Hospital during the last eleven years, and others that had occurred in the author's own practice. In the course of the paper also, reference was made to all the cases recorded in the Pathological Transactions and others in the medical journals. Dr. Murchison pointed out that, owing to the sudden termination of fatal cases of hydatid disease, hospital records hardly gave a fair view of the ratio of deaths from this cause. Although there could be no doubt that an hydatid cyst might become arrested in its growth, shrivel up, and undergo what is called a spontaneous cure, this result rarely happened when the tumour was large enough to be diagnosed during life. In the large majority of cases it went on increasing, and ultimately burst, and when this happened death was the usual result. Attention was directed to the remarkably latent character of hydatid tumours of the liver: in most cases they gave rise to no uneasiness until they had attained such a size as to compress adjoining organs, or until they were on the point of bursting, and peritoneal inflammation was excited on their surface. The directions in which an hydatid tumour of the liver might burst were various. 1. Into the cavity of the chest. 2. Into the peritoneum. 3. Through the abdominal parietes or lower intercostal spaces. 4. Into the stomach or intestine. 5. Into the bile-duct. 6. Into the vena cava inferior. Independently of rupture, hydatids might destroy life—1st. By compressing important organs and interfering with their functions. 2nd. By suppuration of the cyst, or external to the cyst, and pyæmia. 3rd. By the formation of secondary hydatid tumours in different parts of the body. It followed that the risks to which a person with a large hydatid tumour of the liver was liable were many, and the chances of his escaping them were few. Although the tumour might remain stationary for years, an accident might at any moment cause death. Turning to treatment, little benefit could be expected from medicines. Chloride of sodium and iodide of potassium, the two most vaunted remedies, were of no use. It was difficult to conceive how chloride of sodium could destroy an hydatid, seeing that hydatid fluid always contained such a large amount of this salt, which, indeed, appeared to be essential to the life of the parasite. With regard to iodide of potassium, there was not only no proof that it could cause absorption of an hydatid, but there was positive evidence that the drug never reached the hydatid. Not a trace of iodine could be discovered in the hydatid fluid of a patient of Dr. Murchison's, who had taken fifteen grains of iodide of potassium daily for several weeks before. Puncture of the cyst was of much greater promise, and had been attended with great success. The dangers were peritonitis and suppuration of the cyst, but by the employment of a fine trocar these dangers might in a great measure be avoided. The error of using a large trocar, or of making an incision with a scalpel, lay at the root of most of the accidents that had occurred. The evacuation of the fluid through a fine canula sufficed to destroy the life of the hydatid. Of twenty cases of hydatid tumour of the liver tapped as described, and collected by the author, all but three had recovered; and of the three fatal cases, death in one was due to secondary tumours, in a second to a miscarriage, and in the third case the cyst had suppurated and the patient was moribund at the time of the operation. In all cases, therefore, where an hydatid tumour of the liver was large enough to be diagnosed during life, and was increasing in size, the operation of puncture and evacuation of the cyst in the manner described was advisable. But before resorting to puncture, it was of course necessary to be certain of the nature of the tumour. The diseases most liable to be mistaken for hydatid tumours of the liver were, abscess of the liver, a distended gallbladder, extensive effusion into the right pleura, an aneurism of the aorta or of the hepatic artery, and cancer of the liver. The points of diagnosis from these lesions were carefully considered, but the author believed that what was called

"hydatid vibration" was a sign of little importance in diagnosis. In a doubtful case there could be no objection to making an exploratory puncture of the tumour. If the tumour was hydatid the fluid drawn off would at once reveal its nature, even if it contained no echinococci. Hydatid fluid was clear and colourless as water; it had a specific gravity of 1009 or 1010; and it contained not a trace of albumen, but a large quantity of chloride of sodium : these characters applied to no other fluid in the human body, whether healthy or morbid. If the tumour turned out to be cancer, or even aneurism, there was ample evidence that no harm would result from a minute puncture. The paper concluded with the details of a case under the author's care, where paracentesis had been performed with complete success. The patient at the end of a year was in perfect health.

In the discussion which followed, Dr. GIBB mentioned examples of hydatid disease in the young, and a case in which hydatids between the rectum and bladder had been diagnosed and cured.

Dr. ALTHAUS referred to the saline treatment with favour, and as deserving of trial first.

Dr. COBBOLD declared that treatment useless; and referred at length to the great importance of the subject, bearing testimony to the accuracy of Dr. Murchison's results and observations.

Mr. BROWN suggested that, after puncture of hydatids of the liver, a firm, many-tailed bandage should be applied to secure rest and apposition, and prevent effusion into the peritoneal cavity.

The Lancet Sanitary Commission
FOR
INVESTIGATING THE STATE
OF THE
INFIRMARIES OF WORKHOUSES.

REPORTS OF THE COMMISSIONERS.
No. VIII.
METROPOLITAN INFIRMARIES.

BERMONDSEY INFIRMARY.

THE large parish of Bermondsey, containing 100,000 inhabitants, adjoins the borough of Southwark, and is the seat of many of the principal manufactories of the metropolis. Many of the trades carried on here are of the class which cause nuisances; as, for instance, tanneries, skin and hide dressing establishments, and offensive chemical works, besides a great skin market. There are also many most noxious tidal ditches within the district, which are calculated to favour epidemic diseases, although in this respect there has been some improvement of late years, which may be chiefly attributed to the fears excited by the cholera epidemics of 1832 and 1848, the mortality in the latter year having been altogether unprecedented according to the experience of other districts.

The workhouse, a four-storied brick building with a basement, forms an almost square block, intersected by several airing yards, the south side being partially open, and the east and north sides somewhat irregular. The building dates from 1791, but additions were made in 1844; it is surrounded by various erections, except on the south side. The western portion is devoted to the infirmary proper; the infirm wards are in the east. The soil is clay, with peat beneath. The whole site is below high-water mark, and formerly was part of the bed of the Thames. The consequence of this is that the house is often flooded, the water standing two feet deep in the basement! This accident can only be prevented by closing the mouth of the house-drain or sewer, in which case there is of course no escape for rain-fall or sewage at such times. It is unnecessary to say a word more to condemn the site as utterly unfitted for a residence for the sick. The water-supply is derived from Thames Ditton, and seems to be pure and abundant; it is stored in brick tanks, which are periodically cleansed.

The house was built for 900 inmates, and at the time of our visit contained only 470. The classification is by no means complete; amongst other particulars we noted that there is no ward for the separation of "foul" cases. The children are all sent, when they reach the age of five years, to the Sutton Schools.

As regards the sick wards (seven in number, three for males, and four for females), we are able to speak generally in terms of commendation. There is a decided deficiency in the allowance of cubic space, as is the case in nearly all workhouse infirmaries; but a great deal of attention is paid to subsidiary ventilation, and a tolerably free circulation of air seems to be secured. Moreover, the wards are well lighted, and the arrangements for warming are good. The bedsteads and bedding, with the single exception of the employment of flockbeds, to which we have objected on several previous occasions, are thoroughly good, and in particular there is excellent provision made for "wet" cases; the bed-linen is good and clean, and the personal cleanliness of the patients is thoroughly well cared for; in fact, it is evident that the master, Mr. Hodgkins, carries out good discipline among his subordinates. The water-closets, lavatories, and water-supply to each ward also appeared well ordered and well kept.

The lying-in ward, in which from thirty to forty births take place annually, is strikingly free from odour, and the beds are clean; moreover, the labour-bed is well contrived for the purpose of preventing stains on the floor, as it stands on lead sheeting, with an elevated rim around its margin. There is some danger, however, that without close watching the boards beneath might rot and become offensive. We were assured by the medical officer, Dr. Cuolahan, who obligingly accompanied us, and gave us free access to his records and books, that he has not lost one case from puerperal fever or any other cause connected with parturition.

The wards for the infirm present a marked contrast with those for the sick; in fact, they are excessively bad. Two of them especially, which are called "Lazarus" and "Aaron" respectively, are very dirty, and deficient in both light and air. The occupants were the most thoroughly "pauperized" set we have seen in any of our visitations, herding together in a miserable manner in the midst of conditions which must render any medical treatment of their chronic diseases of little avail. Their watercloset and urinal (abutting on the deadhouse) stink so offensively as to poison the whole atmosphere of their airing-court, and must, doubtless, have had a share in aggravating the epidemics from which the establishment has formerly suffered.

The arrangements which are made for the accommodation of the wayfaring class, or "tramps," in Bermondsey, have already attracted the indignant notice of the Poor-law Board and the public press, and may be shortly and justly described as altogether brutal. The peculiar conditions of the parish render it inevitable that this class of paupers should exist in great numbers, the fluctuations of commercial and manufacturing operations frequently throwing many working people at once out of employment; and as these poor folk are not distinguished by provident habits, their application for casual relief follows as a necessary consequence. Of this the guardians must be well aware. Yet the fact is that, although as many as forty or fifty persons have been known to apply for shelter in a single night, the authorities have only provided accommodation for twenty-four persons, and even such shelter as they give is *not fit for a dog*. We use these words advisedly, and we are sure our readers will endorse them when they learn that the beds provided consist simply of bunks, or long orange-boxes, with a wooden log for a pillow, a blanket and rug to cover the sleeper, *and not even a bit of straw for him to lie on!* We believe that the guardians of Bermondsey are entitled to

the distinction of being entirely singular in their mode of lodging the houseless poor.

The peep which these facts give us into the psychology of the Bermondsey authorities quite prepares us for the discovery that the nursing department, including night-nursing, in defiance of common sense and the recommendation of the Poor-law Board, is committed exclusively to twenty-two pauper inmates, who are remunerated merely by improved diet, and, in some cases, a special dress. But we were not a little astonished and pained to find both the master and the surgeon arguing in favour of this state of things, which the general voice of the medical profession, equally with the Poor-law Board, has loudly condemned; and we know of no better argument to convince all reasonable persons that the central board should, without delay, be armed with powers sufficient to enable it to compel this disgraceful state of things to cease.

With regard to the quality of food supplied and the cooking, we are able to speak on the whole with satisfaction. But when we examine the *amounts* of nourishment allowed (except to the sick, with respect to whom the medical officer is allowed all proper freedom of action), our satisfaction ceases. 15 oz. of meat, 24 oz. of potatoes, three pints of soup, 84 oz. of bread (besides gruel for the able-bodied, and tea, sugar, and butter for the aged and infirm) per week, is an altogether insufficient allowance, and, to the infirm class especially, must be considered as hard treatment.

The medical officer of Bermondsey Workhouse has arduous duties; for, in addition to 100 sick and infirm in the house, he has medical charge of a parish district. For all the labour involved in these two offices, and for all drugs and extras, he receives £150 per annum! He attends the house daily, recording his visits, and also the whole of his orders and directions, in a book, which is well and regularly kept.

The diseases admitted into the infirmary are chiefly chronic affections of the heart and lungs, diseases of the brain and nervous system, scrofulous affections, and ulcers of the leg—disorders attributable, to a large extent, to privation and distress. The cholera outbreaks of 1832 and 1848 told severely on the Bermondsey poor, and in all probability a new epidemic would have similar effects; meantime the workhouse, in its present condition, could not with safety receive cases of this terrible malady, and indeed is in a state to foster epidemic diseases generally. In 1863, a wardsman contracted "typhus" (or more probably typhoid) fever, in consequence, it was believed, of sleeping near the deadhouse and the offensive closet already denounced; and subsequently a nurse was attacked, and died in the Fever Hospital. There can be no doubt that the infirm department constitutes a potential "fever-nest" of a very dangerous kind. An analysis of the mortality for seven years has been kindly made for us by the officials, and shows the following causes of death. The total mortality was 855; of these, 95 came under the zymotic class (including 34 cases of Asiatic cholera* in the last epidemic), 167 under tubercular diseases, 139 under diseases of the brain and nervous system, 174 under diseases of the respiratory organs, 156 under "decay of nature," 35 under heart diseases, 23 under diseases of the digestive organs, 10 under kidney diseases, 9 under uterine disorders, 8 under cancer, 6 under dropsy, 5 under abscess, 6 under premature birth, 6 from deficient supply of breast-milk, 4 from diseases of the joints &c., besides 10 sudden deaths, of which the causes are not specified. There is nothing on the face of this table of deaths which seems to challenge particular observation; yet we cannot but think that an exact analysis, if such were possible, of the causes of the various deaths from "diarrhœa," "tabes," "convulsions," &c., might reveal serious mischief resulting from an improper dietary. We are strongly tempted to entertain this idea by one feature of the diet-tables as yet unmentioned—viz., the reckless disregard

---

* During the months of July, August, and September, 1849, there were 61 deaths in the infirmary, 29 being inmates.

which they evidence of the necessity of supplying *milk* in good quantity to young children; in this point of view the dietary of Bermondsey is extremely reprehensible, *only half a pint of milk-and-water per diem* (with an additional allowance, twice a week, of half a pint of rice-milk) being allowed to children between two and five years. This is a very grave defect, and one which can scarcely fail to be very mischievous.

To conclude:—

1. The infirmary of Bermondsey occupies an entirely improper site, and ought to be rebuilt in an elevated situation.

2. In view of the needs of the parish, a separate fever-house should be built adjoining such new infirmary.

3. Properly trained and paid nurses are required.

4. The medical officer ought to receive the amount of his present salary for the workhouse duty alone, the guardians also finding all drugs, &c.

5. The sanitary arrangements of the infirm department are scandalously bad, and require immediate and thorough revisal.

6. Altogether new arrangements are needed for the casual poor, who are at present treated with great cruelty and neglect.

New Inventions
IN AID OF THE
PRACTICE OF MEDICINE AND SURGERY.

NEW DENTAL FORCEPS.

THE accompanying woodcut represents a new extracting forceps, the invention of Mr. A. E. Harris, Dentist, Mile-end-road. The object was, to obtain an instrument by which to faci-

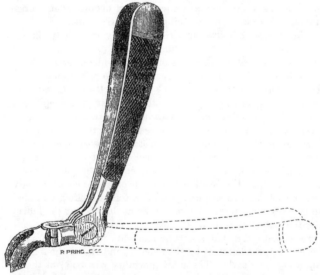

litate the extraction of the lower molar teeth. The instrument is so designed as to render easy insertion of the claws of the forceps between the tooth and alveolar process. The forceps is composed of the hawk's-bill claws, with the usual circular joint, behind which is a vertical hinge-joint allowing the handles of the instrument to be raised to a position perpendicular, and almost at right angles, with the patient's mouth; so that the claws of the instrument, as it were, "drop" into the required position, slight direct downward pressure being all that is required on the part of the operator. The direction of the extracting or raising force is directly above, and in a perpendicular line with the tooth, so that the least movement of the hand will immediately remove the tooth without any chance of an imperfect operation. This second hinge consists of a centre circular part placed vertically, like a wheel, between the blades of the handles of the forceps, and the latter being compressed by the hand during extraction, renders this joint fixed and immovable, and the tooth is literally "lifted" out of its socket.

COLLINS'S BINOCULAR DISSECTING MICROSCOPE.
(DR. LAWSON'S PLAN.)

THIS is a cheap, handy, and convenient instrument. We would particularly allude to the great advantage of binocular vision for low powers in dissecting; and to the superiority of this little instrument over others at present employed, on account of its portability and great efficiency when in use. The case, when closed, measures 6 in. by 3¾ in. The top and front let down by hinges, and on them can be fitted the instruments requisite for dissecting, as shown in the diagram. The sides draw out 5 in., and serve the purpose of rests for the hands. A circle of glass is in the centre of the gutta-percha trough, so that light can be transmitted from the mirror.

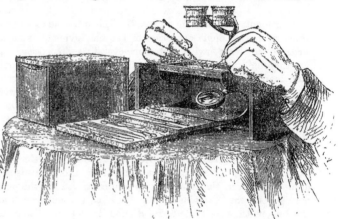

Altogether it is the best and most useful instrument we have seen. It is made by Mr. Charles Collins, 77, Great Titchfield-street, Oxford-street, from the plan of Dr. Lawson, Professor of Histology at St. Mary's Hospital.

POOR-LAW MEDICAL REFORM.
To the Editor of THE LANCET.

SIR,—I am sure it will be the almost unanimous desire of the Poor-law medical officers that Mr. Griffin remain at the post he has filled so long and so ably. I for one will be most happy again to subscribe any sum that may be necessary to advocate our claims. I would therefore impress on all my brother medical officers the necessity of putting aside all past lukewarmness, and of showing that we are in earnest by sending the subscription asked (five shillings). I am sure we have only to unite and act together to ensure success. In previous appeals for pecuniary help, Mr. Griffin has not met with that response which his disinterested endeavours on our behalf merited. A majority of our number never contributed anything towards his expenses, which must of necessity have been considerable. This no doubt cramped his efforts and did the cause much injury.

For the better collecting of subscriptions, I would suggest that one medical officer in every district of union should be appointed to canvass his brethren for the money needful to defray the necessary expenses that will be incurred in printing &c. By so doing, a larger amount than Mr. Griffin has ever yet received could be raised.

I hope therefore that this time we shall all work together heartily and with a will, and if we do so I have no doubt of our success.

I am, Sir, your obedient servant,

Oct. 28th, 1865.   J. H.

ROYAL COLLEGE OF SURGEONS.—The first examination this session in Anatomy and Physiology at the above institution commences this day (Saturday); and it is stated that the numbers are in excess of the corresponding period of last year. The gross number of pupils registered at this institution as pursuing their studies at our eleven metropolitan hospitals now amount to 1036, being an increase of 47 over the number of last session. This includes also those gentlemen pursuing their studies for the diploma in Dental Surgery of the College.

THE LANCET,]   DR. BRUNTON ON A NEW OTOSCOPE OR SPECULUM AURIS.   [DEC. 2, 1865. 617

spheric changes which acclimatization in an uniform medium gradually begets; to such an extent that settlers of old standing positively shiver and catch cold at a variation of two degrees and a half in Fahrenheit's scale, of which the recent immigrant is only agreeably, if at all, conscious. It is usual to meet these slight alterations by moving to a higher or lower point on the steep incline of rock which forms the hemispherical valley of Funchal. Without rising beyond the limits of the town, a barometer shows upwards of an inch in depression; and in an evening's ride you may easily cause the aneroid in your pocket to fall twice that amount. All local varieties, however, are subordinate to the dominant character of the climate, which is warm, equable, and moist almost to saturation. There is one great exception to this rule: at variable intervals the climate is suddenly and abruptly changed for a short time while the "leste" wind blows. The physical causes of this phenomenon seem variously and imperfectly explained; but it essentially consists of a hot dry sirocco, coming in the direction of the African coast, and at once separating the readings of the wet and dry bulb thermometers, previously nearly on a level, by a space of from ten to twenty degrees. Fortunately, this unpleasant visitor arrives rarely, and seldom lasts more than a few days at a time.

The above description embraces the simpler elements of heat and moisture; but it is far from improbable that further researches into questions of radiation and electricity may develop some important peculiarities as yet unsuspected, except from the subjective indications of that most sensitive of all meteorological instruments, the human body.

Now a few corollaries from the preceding statements may prove of interest, the more so as they have hitherto hardly been published with sufficient breadth and simplicity.

Madeira is *au pied de la lettre*—a gigantic greenhouse, facing the south, sheltered on the north by a natural wall of enormous height; and the climatic conditions which foster the fig, the banana, the yam, and the sugar-cane, may be of incalculable benefit to delicate and half-exotic organizations in our own species. But they do not suit all and every one; they may do harm as well as good. There will be some constitutions which, like the deciduous trees of our country, when transplanted into that region of perennial verdure, still cling to their old habits, still droop at their wonted season, and seem by a strange instinct or memory to protest against the excess and surfeit of good things.

Moreover, the climate, by the very fact of its sedative and tranquillizing power, is devoid of any stimulant or tonic activity. It stands at the very opposite pole from the dry pungent heat of Algiers or Upper Egypt, and is of service to invalids who would be utterly unable to live in those localities. Yet the first remark one usually hears in ordinary conversation on this subject maintains the importance of going early, and in the first stage of pulmonary disorder. With rare exceptions, this is the very reverse of the truth; and a trip to Switzerland, to the Isle of Man, or to either of the places before named, would be a far more judicious recommendation. Perhaps a long sea-voyage destined to last for several months, such as that to Australia, is a more satisfactory prescription than any.

There is another error on this subject, which can be exposed without entering into details of a medical nature; and that is the unkindness of sending a declining, fading invalid far from home and friends without some *à priori* indication that the malady is curable even by change of climate. Everyone knows that some sufferers drop slowly but steadily into their graves in spite of treatment, and seemingly unaffected by external influences; the poison is too strong—the morbid cause has sunk too deep into the system to be touched by our remedies. Let such stay at home, and let us in pity save them from dying in the solitude of unfamiliar scenes and strange faces. This is the mistake which has given Madeira the name in some mouths of "the grave of English consumption"—a designation which in its essential attributes no place deserves less. It will be easily understood that the presence of digestive disturbance or great nervous depression are strong arguments against so relaxing a residence; and a recent gallant writer in a fortnightly contemporary has contributed a pathetic lamentation on this topic from personal experience, which, though one-sided, is to a certain extent true, and forms a valuable addition to the literature of hypochondriasis.

What then, it may be asked, is the favourable side of the question? Who are the fit subjects for Madeira? The answer may be given best under two heads. Firstly, invalids who, although undoubtedly suffering from phthisis, have, by careful management and favourable circumstances, been enabled to produce a temporary check in the advance of the morbid pro-

cess. Instances are not rare where this arrest of disease is for a while established, and where, if nature be given time, with the removal of all accidental causes of irritation, the necessarily slow process of repair will be accomplished. In our trying climate such favourable conditions can hardly be obtained, and each winter bears away with it the small accumulated capital of health which has been realized during the summer. But a journey south offers a succession of three consecutive summers, and in this period there is abundant evidence to prove that material and permanent amendment can be brought about. Secondly, even in the presence of advanced and perhaps incurable disease, so much palliation may be secured as to come very nearly up to the curative standard. Plenty of authentic cases are on record where, even under these unfavourable conditions, lives have been prolonged for periods so considerable as twenty-five years and under. It will be matter of comparative indifference to the sufferer whether such a renewed lease of life be considered as an absolute pardon or merely as a temporary reprieve.

It is to be hoped that additional facts may ere long be obtained on this important subject. There is no reason why the therapeutic power of climate should not be ascertained and recorded as accurately as that of any medicinal substance; up to the present time, however, efforts in this direction have been scanty and unsystematic. Careful observation of the cases sent this winter to Madeira from our hospital will help to supply the deficiency; and, pending their publication, I have purposely thrown my own impressions into a tentative and untechnical form.

Vigo-street, Nov. 1865.

A NEW OTOSCOPE OR SPECULUM AURIS.

BY JOHN BRUNTON, M.A., M.D.

IN the spring of 1861, while examining a patient's ears with the ordinary aural instruments, two serious difficulties arose to me in forming a correct diagnosis with such instruments—viz.: 1. That the observer's head very greatly obstructed the light; 2. That the eye could not get near enough the object to permit of minute examination, and more so if *sunlight* instead of *artificial* light was used. The instrument of which a description and drawing are here given then suggested itself to me.

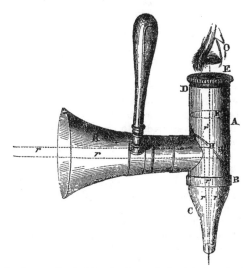

The instrument consists of a brass tube (A), two inches long and three quarters of an inch in diameter, to one end of which (B) is made to fit on, by sliding, an ear-piece similar to Toynbee's aural speculum. At the other end (D) is an eye-piece (E), with a lens (F) of moderately magnifying power; the eye-piece slides so as to admit of focal arrangement to suit the eye of the observer. In the body of the instrument, near the ear-piece end, and set at an angle of 45°, is a concave mirror (G) with a hole in the centre (H); this aperture in the mirror is in the line of the axis of the tube and ear-piece. At a right angle to the body of the instrument, and opposite to the mirror, is adapted a sliding funnel-shaped polished silver reflector (K) for collecting and concentrating the rays of light, so that the rays (r r) are let in at the side, and, falling on the mirror (H), are reflected and concentrated into the ear, and carried back (r' r') to the eye of the observer (o) through (H), the hole in the mirror, and are magnified by the lens of the eye-piece (E, F). There is also a handle attached to the light-reflector, which works on a sliding band, and can be turned about to suit either hand of the observer as he may wish, when looking at the right or left ear.

With this instrument the observer's eye is brought in close contact with the patient's ear, and the light coming in at the side is in no way obstructed. The otoscope is easily used, and with best advantage by sunlight. It is applied thus: With the left or right hand, as the case may be, the surgeon pulls directly outwards the auricle, inserting the ear-piece into the external meatus. He then desires the patient to turn his head round till the light falls directly upon the mirror, when the meatus, membrane of the tympanum, &c., will be observed very clearly, the smallest change of structure may be noted, and the movement of the membrane readily seen. If the membrane and ossicles are gone, the tympanic cavity can be observed and noted. With this instrument the bloodvessels that traverse the membrane of tympanum can be seen in the healthy ear.

The advantages of the instrument are—

1. Simplicity of construction.
2. Ease of application, a few trials sufficing to make the observer expert.
3. Precision and minuteness with which the ear can be examined.
4. That it can be used with artificial or sun light (the latter preferred).
5. That it can be used with the magnifying power or not at pleasure.

The instrument was made for me by Mr. White, of Renfield-street, Glasgow, optical and mathematical instrument maker to the University. It was shown some time ago to the Medical Society of London. It is used in Glasgow.

The principle of the instrument can be adapted in many ways. I have used the otoscope with advantage in examining the nasal passages.

Caledonian-road, November, 1865.

NOTES

ON A CERTAIN FORM OF HÆMOPTYSIS, UNASSOCIATED WITH PULMONARY TUBERCULOSIS.

BY RICHARD PAYNE COTTON, M.D., F.R.C.P. LOND.,
PHYSICIAN TO THE HOSPITAL FOR CONSUMPTION AND
DISEASES OF THE CHEST, BROMPTON.

HÆMORRHAGE from the lungs, to a greater or less degree, is so frequently found in connexion with a tubercular condition of the chest, that its diagnostic value, as a separate symptom, is very apt to be overrated. In the early period of my attendance at the Brompton Hospital for Consumption, I saw so much hæmoptysis amongst the unmistakably phthisical out-patients, that I was sometimes tempted to the general conclusion that hæmoptysis was, practically, but another name for phthisis. Subsequent and more extensive observation has, however, very much changed my views in this particular; and I am now fully convinced that hæmoptysis is met with in a very considerable number of non-tubercular cases. Simple pulmonary congestion, whether the result of inflammatory action, or arising from mechanical obstruction consequent upon heart-disease; pneumonia, whether acute or chronic; bronchitis; general plethora,—may at any time give rise to hæmorrhage from the lungs. I have seen, indeed, most active bleeding where some of these conditions have been combined — as in congestive bronchitis in persons of plethoric habit. To this list, congested states of the pharynx, tonsils, and gums might fairly be added; but I wish my present observations to apply to hæmoptysis, not in its literal sense, but as it is now usually employed—as hæmorrhage *from the lungs*. In a future communication I propose to enter upon the various forms which hæmoptysis, under these several conditions, is disposed to assume. In the present instance I am anxious only to draw attention to a not unfrequent, but, so far as I know, little re-cognised form of non-tubercular hæmoptysis, met with chiefly in the female sex, but sometimes also amongst males, generally in the early period of life.

It may simplify my description of this variety of hæmoptysis if I give a brief account of two or three cases in point.

A young lady, aged eighteen, recently arrived from a residence in one of the West India islands, was supposed to be phthisical. I was requested to see her, and report upon the nature of her disease, about which several very conflicting opinions had already been given. She was anæmic, nervous, and out of health; had a dry cough, but had not become thinner; her catamenia were regular, but scanty; her appetite was capricious; and she had had frequent hæmoptysis, which there was every reason to believe did not proceed from either the mouth or fauces. The blood, upon examination, was found to be thin and watery, of a dark colour, free from coagulum, unassociated with either bronchial or salivary secretion, and in general appearance much resembling a mixture of *red-currant jelly and water.* I was informed that this was its general character. Sometimes it had been considerable—as much as half a pint in twenty-four hours; at others, it would not exceed a teaspoonful or two during the same period; sometimes it would be scarcely enough to tinge a pocket-handkerchief, and often it would disappear for days together. This state of things had existed for nearly two years, causing great anxiety to the patient and her friends, from a belief that it was indicative of pulmonary disease. Careful examination of the chest, however, failed to elicit any evidence that such was the case. Rest, change of air, and the tincture of sesquichloride of iron, entirely restored this patient to health. It is now more than three years since I was consulted, and I heard a short time back that the young lady was in perfect health.

A case very similar to this came under my notice two years ago in consultation with Mr. Humpage, of Upper Seymour-street. A young lady, aged twenty-four, had long been delicate, and was supposed by her family to be consumptive. She had become thinner; had had a dry cough for some length of time; and had spat blood. Upon examination, this was found to present an appearance very similar to that described in the preceding case; it looked, in fact, more like watery red-currant jelly than anything else. As in the other patient, there were no decided physical signs of tubercular disease; and we came to the conclusion that the patient was not phthisical. Time has justified our diagnosis; Mr. Humpage having lately informed me that the young lady had, for many months, lost the symptom which had caused so much alarm, and was in good health.

Another case, which I shall even more briefly relate, came under my notice about eighteen months back. It was that of a young lady, twelve years of age, of slender and somewhat delicate appearance, but free from every symptom of tubercular affection. Mr. J. N. Winter, of Montpelier-road, Brighton, frequently saw this patient, and quite agreed with me as to the nature of her disease. She first alarmed her parents by spitting up, just after going to bed one night, a considerable quantity of blood. This was found upon examination to be watery and dark-coloured—in fact, of the *thin red-currant jelly character* already described. This symptom has recurred at various intervals with more or less intensity, and the child still remains delicate, but without any indications of tubercular disease. At the time of her attacks her tonsils and pharynx are somewhat congested, her gums spongy, and her fingers even have sometimes exuded a little watery blood, just as one sometimes sees in extreme cases of purpura. It is evident that, in this instance, the blood escapes not only from the mucous membrane of the respiratory passages, but also from that of the throat, tonsils, and gums.

Other cases of this form of hæmoptysis have fallen under my observation; but I shall not specially refer to them in consequence of not knowing their sequel. At least twelve or thirteen have happened in my own wards at the Hospital for Consumption. Two only of these were males; the rest were females, generally of delicate and nervous appearance, and under the age of thirty. Several had very suspicious symptoms of phthisis; but the physical signs failed to exhibit any evidence of pulmonary tuberculosis, and most of them improved in health under appropriate treatment. In every case the expectoration was of the same general character; sometimes it was mixed more or less with bronchial mucus, slightly tinged perhaps with blood, and sometimes with salivary secretion; but more frequently it was simply watery blood, resembling, as I have described, a mixture of red-currant jelly with water.

The following are the conclusions at which I have arrived from a consideration of the preceding notes:—

is in the highest degree inimical to the best interests, not of the medical service only, but of the entire army.

We print the two following circulars by way of an appendix to our Report: the direct contradiction implied therein tells its own tale, and needs not a word of comment from us.

Circular Memorandum, addressed to General and other officers commanding at Stations at Home and Abroad.

Horse-Guards, Aug. 28th, 1865.

His Royal Highness the Field-Marshal Commanding-in-Chief desires to draw the attention of general officers in command of districts, and commanding officers of corps in general, to the necessity of examining into the sanitary state of all barracks and cantonments occupied by troops.

A permanent Sanitary Committee should be appointed at all camps and garrisons, consisting of a field officer, or captain when no field officer is present, an officer of the Royal Engineer Department, if available, or an officer of the Barrack Department, and a medical officer, whose duty it should be to visit, periodically, all barracks or cantonments at the station, and satisfy themselves that the barracks are not occupied to a greater extent than authorised, that the barracks are clean, and that all the orders on the subject of ventilation are carried out, that the drains, cesspools, &c., are in good order, that no accumulation of filth is allowed in the barracks or cantonment.

The Boards will also visit the neighbourhood of all barracks or cantonments, and place themselves in communication with the civil authorities and local boards of health, in order that any nuisance that may exist, tending in any manner to prejudice the health of the troops, may be removed.

His Royal Highness trusts that the cordial co-operation of the civil and military authorities in this important matter, may benefit the population of the towns where troops are quartered.

The Sanitary Committees will make reports to the general officers commanding the districts in which they may be serving upon any subject that may require their immediate attention.

A journal of the proceedings of each Committee will also be kept, which is to be forwarded monthly for the perusal of the general officers in command, who will in like manner report to the quarter-master general, for the information of the Field Marshal Commanding-in-Chief, any circumstances requiring his Royal Highness's immediate attention, and make a monthly report of the general proceedings of the various Committees under their orders.

By command,
RICHARD AIREY, *Quarter-master General.*

Circular Memorandum, addressed to General and other Officers Commanding at Stations at Home.

Horse Guards, 12th May, 1866.

With reference to the Circular Memorandum from this Office, No. 164, dated 28th August, 1865, respecting the appointment of permanent sanitary committees at all camps and garrisons, his Royal Highness the Field Marshal Commanding-in-Chief, with the concurrence of the Secretary of State for War, directs it to be notified that in future *no communications are to be made by the sanitary committees to the civil authorities or local boards of health which might result in the War Department being called upon to expend money.*—By command,

J. HOPE GRANT, *Quarter-master General.*

DR. MARY WALKER.

THE large room at St. James's Hall was crowded on Tuesday evening to hear a lecture from Dr. Mary E. Walker upon "The Experiences of a Female Physician in College, Private Practice, and in the Federal Army." The audience was of a very mixed description, the greater portion being evidently actuated by curiosity to see and hear the lecturess; whilst a certain section, which mainly occupied the upper gallery, was as evidently bent upon getting the greatest possible amount of fun out of the proceedings. To beguile the tedium incident upon a little delay which took place ere the lady appeared, this compact body chanted with stentorian voices the Federal army chorus—

"Glory, glory, alleluia !
As we go marching on."

Any slight monotony which the constant repetition of this war-song might have created was avoided by interspersing it

with "Rule Britannia," and the more familiar but less refined "Slap bang !" So noisy and demonstrative was this part of the assembly, that it seemed likely every now and then that the lady-doctor would not be able to get through her discourse; but by the aid of a couple of stalwart policemen a moderate amount of attention was preserved.

We are so little in the habit of describing the costume of our professional brothers—or sisters—that we shall be pardoned for any little errors in our description of Miss Walker's dress. So far as we could judge, she wore a long dark cloth tunic, reaching nearly to the knees, fitting closely to the figure above and expanding below, open to a certain extent in front, so as to disclose an inner garment, which we dare not attempt to name, but which served the purpose of a waistcoat, and carried a watch and chain disposed as is usual among men. Dark trousers ("pantalettes" she called them) and boots like those ordinarily worn by the male sex completed the essentials of her costume. She had, besides, a light wreath of dark-green leaves upon her hair, a turn-down collar and neckerchief; whilst shirt wristbands peeped from her sleeves and partially concealed the white kid gloves upon her hands. She wore an order given her by the United States Government. She described her own costume as "a physiological dress with moral bearings" (taken, we presume, from the shoulder).

Considering that she is *petite* and feminine in appearance, her delivery sustained the trying ordeal of the large hall very fairly. Nor was she wanting in self-possession, a quality which was tested in no ordinary manner in the course of the evening. Her action was somewhat awkward and constrained, the frequent uplifting of her hands towards the ceiling in the sentimental parts of her lecture having anything but a graceful effect.

We cannot say much for her lecture. The early part was as prosy as anything we had the ill fortune to hear in our student-days. The description of the obstacles she met with in her course of study chiefly harped upon one string—dress. Indeed this essentially feminine trait disclosed itself throughout her discourse. One could discern the tone of a woman in whom an otherwise laudable desire for a convenient and reasonable costume was swallowed up by the little feminine vanity which accompanies singularity. And so there was enough talk of short petticoats, pantalettes, and ankles to cause considerable surprise amongst the female portion of the auditory as yet unaccustomed to the "go-a-headedness" of our Yankee cousins.

After graduating in 1855, Dr. Mary Walker was seized, it appeared, with a burning desire to go out to the Crimea, and obtain the post of assistant-surgeon in our army. Happily, perhaps, for the hearts of our gallant army surgeons, she did not achieve this object of her ambition, and subsided into the less romantic but more profitable position of a female physician in New York. And here, she said, she desired it to be understood that she practised exclusively among women and children. Nevertheless, if she chanced to be the nearest doctor, she was often sent for to attend men. Wives to whom she had been of service would entreat her to see their husbands; and she was very liable to be called up at night because she "got her clothes on quicker than the 'men-doctors.'" She also frequently extracted teeth for old men. Like the rest of us, she had to encounter difficulties about fees. On one occasion a gentleman came to pay his bill, and supposed that because she was a woman her account would be less than that of a "man-doctor." But she soon disposed of this troublesome gentleman, and convinced him that as she had gone through all the usual studies and expenses of a medical education, and more than the usual difficulties, owing to her sex, if she made any difference at all, it would be to charge at a higher rate than the men. Whereupon there was great applause from her hearers, who doubtless one and all, thus reminded of their obligations, wrote long-looked-for cheques for their doctors before going to bed. Perhaps, also, they were amused at finding that the fascinations of a bloomer costume and the romantic adventures of camp life had not entirely sufficed to quench the attractions of the "almighty dollar."

From private practice, Dr. Mary Walker passed to her war experiences. Not directly, however; for she thought fit to improve the occasion by a tolerably long digression into American politics. Whether the audience included some slaveholders who objected to hearing a national institution stigmatised, or whether they thought politics a more improper subject for a lady than the diseases of men and women, they showed considerable impatience at this point, which called forth a very characteristic remark from the lecturess. "In a very few moments," she said, "I am going to say something about wounded soldiers." It was her pleasure to pronounce the diphthong in "wounded" as we do in "rounded," and the constant repetition of this word was somewhat singular to English ears. Her career in camp and hospital seems to have been more feminine than one might have expected from so strong-minded a lady. She appeared not a little proud of the influence which her sex commanded amongst the "wounded" soldiers. Many would not submit to operation, she said, without her opinion respecting its advisability, or her presence during its performance. She described, with much woman's tact, her tender care of the wounded,—how she would convey a warrior with his head resting in her lap; and asked her hearers whether, if they had a father, brother, or son wounded or sick, away from home, they would not like to know that he was being looked after so carefully. Some of her most pathetic stories, however, convulsed the audience with laughter. She told how a poor yellow-faced soldier said to her, "Let me kiss you twice!" and when she hesitated, a fine young soldier who stood by his side said, gallantly perhaps, but somewhat illogically, "Let him kiss you; he is a nice young man; and the reason is that he has not slept for twenty-four hours!" whereupon, we believe (and hope), the request was granted.

Now all this was very kind and tender on the part of Miss Walker, but we can scarcely think that it proves either the necessity or advisability of the presence of young-lady doctors in an army. It is the sort of thing which appeals with great force to the feelings of hearers who have derived their ideas of war-suffering from pictures of a snug hospital-ward, with a fair lady smoothing the pillows of the wounded soldiers. It hardly represents the stern requirements of actual service, the physical labour and mental exertion of tending wounds, and deciding when a wrong decision may mean death. And we could not help feeling, as we listened to the fair lecturess, that however good and meritorious her performance of the part of doctor had been, she was after all but an *amateur*, with all the weak points which must ever separate such a position from the hard realities of active professional work.

We cannot pass over without an expression of regret and censure the riotous conduct of some of the young gentlemen in the gallery said to be students of medicine; and we notice with pain that some of them made a subsequent and most discreditable appearance in the police-court.

THE VISITATION OF EXAMINATIONS.
To the Editor of THE LANCET.

SIR,—In your journal of the 3rd instant you make some important remarks on the "Visitation of Examinations" by members of the General Medical Council. You very reasonably wish to know why a member of that body should object to co-operate in these visitations; and you ask my distinguished colleague, Dr. Acland, to state his reasons for declining, if he has declined, to perform the duty.

The difficulties felt by more than one member of the Council in undertaking this duty were well described by Dr. Allen Thomson in our last session (see THE LANCET, June 9th, 1866, p. 625), when he also protested against "the assumption that all the members of the Council were qualified to fill the judicial position of inspectors."

Possibly Dr. Acland may think, with the great Duke, that it is safer simply to act upon one's own judgment than to give one's reasons for so acting. With less prudence, perhaps, I did explain my reasons for requesting the English Branch Council to excuse my taking any part in their arrangements for visitation. Those reasons found their way indirectly into print; and, after your notice of the subject, I think it better, with your permission, that they should now appear in THE LANCET. The greater portion of what I wrote was as follows:

"I have uniformly objected to the measure, both in principle and in detail; and the results of the recent visitation have in no degree removed my objections.

"Although a majority of the General Council has so interpreted the last sentence of section 18 of the Medical Act, as to found on it a resolution (April 6th, 1865) that the Branch Councils, or such of their members as may be deputed by them, *shall* visit the examinations, preliminary and professional, conducted by the qualifying bodies, and report thereon to the General Council,—there still exists a minority who do not so understand that provision of the Act, which, in their

opinion, is merely permissive, and not intended to supersede any more correct or efficient method of attaining the object in view.

"I believe that had it been left to each Branch Council to decide *for itself* whether it should depute its members to visit the examinations of the licensing bodies within its jurisdiction, the English Branch would not have agreed to undertake such visitation, and the Irish Branch would have peremptorily negatived the proposal. I believe that, in fact, we owe the adoption of this very questionable measure, by the General Council, to the unanimity and energy of our Scottish colleagues.

"The manifest diversity of opinion on this point among the three nationalities in the Council may, I think, justify any individual member in declining to accept his share of responsibility in this proceeding.

"But, if I am mistaken, and if it were to be decided by legal authority, not only that the minority are in error, but further that they are bound to aid the majority in the performance of these visitations, undertaken voluntarily, and on a disputed interpretation of the Act, I for one should feel it my duty—though with much regret—to resign my seat in the Council.

"I will now state, as briefly as I can, my principal objections to the present system of visitations.

"If it be granted that the examinations of candidates by any of the qualifying bodies, represented in the Medical Council, are so defective in their nature and so fallacious in their results as to require the employment of some external agency to inspect them and report to a controlling and reforming authority (which I by no means assert), it would, I think, be obvious to every intelligent and impartial observer that the *representative* members of Council ought not themselves to constitute that agency.

"Even were the theoretical objection set aside, it does not yet appear how *any* members of Council can do the work at all satisfactorily or effectively: (1) because, with their utmost diligence and their largest possible expenditure of time and labour, they can be present at only a very small proportion of the many examinations held annually by the medical licensing bodies; (2) because the same gentlemen, however able and accomplished, can hardly be expected to superintend with equal thoroughness and efficiency those examinations in all branches of knowledge—general, scientific, and professional—which, at various stages of his education, each medical student has to pass through; and (3) because the representatives of the licensing bodies, though themselves free from corporate bias or interested motive, are not likely to satisfy the requirements of the profession, the public, and the Government, by undertaking a duty *which makes them, as a body, judges in their own case.*

"Here, however, I beg not to be understood as supporting an objection which has been lately (and forcibly) made to 'reciprocal visitation by the representatives of rival bodies,' as though such attendances must necessarily degenerate into a mere exchange of empty courtesies, if not of invidious remarks. For this objection seems to assume what is not the fact—viz., that the licensing bodies are really 'rivals,' similarly constituted for similar purposes, conferring similar qualifications, and alike open to the same kind of criticism. It also implies a suspicion—not to be entertained for a moment—of the honour and justice of the visitors.

"Assuming, for the sake of argument, that the regular attendance of appointed visitors or assessors is a sound and true method of securing the thorough efficiency and trustworthiness of examinations, it follows that such visitors ought to be constantly (or at least frequently) present; each devoting his attention to those subjects with which he is most conversant, and on which his authority is unquestionable. Such a system, as I have said, cannot be carried into effect by members of the Council. Yet there is no reason why the Council should not be empowered to appoint and to regulate the duties of visitors not belonging to their body."

So far, then, I agree with you that it would be better to appoint "one or two visitors, not officials of any corporation, properly paid, properly instructed, and working on a given system."

But it cannot be denied that the grievously defective character of some of the qualifying examinations has already been proved, and the nature and extent of their defects pretty accurately ascertained, by the additional examinations which the Army and Navy Medical Boards enforce, with infinite advantage to their respective services and to medical education in general. I cannot doubt that if some such practical test of the efficiency of the recognised examinations were applied to appointments

1870s–1910s
From **BACTERIA** to
BLOOD GROUPS

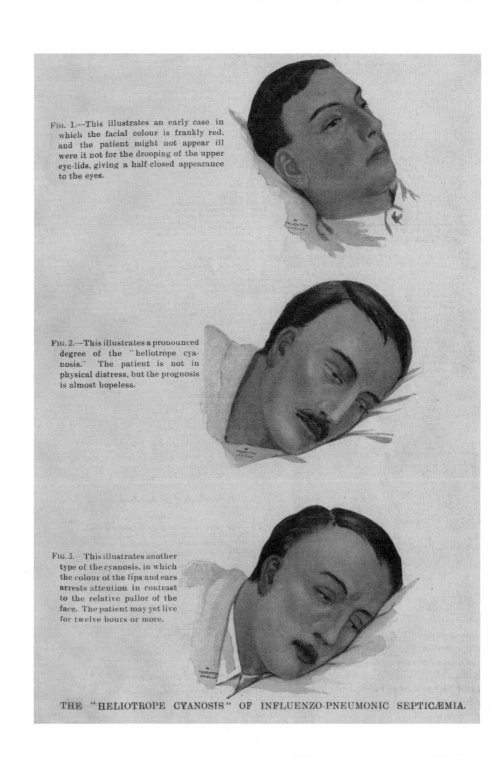

FIG. 1.—This illustrates an early case in which the facial colour is frankly red, and the patient might not appear ill were it not for the drooping of the upper eye-lids, giving a half-closed appearance to the eyes.

FIG. 2.—This illustrates a pronounced degree of the "heliotrope cyanosis." The patient is not in physical distress, but the prognosis is almost hopeless.

FIG. 3.—This illustrates another type of the cyanosis, in which the colour of the lips and ears arrests attention in contrast to the relative pallor of the face. The patient may yet live for twelve hours or more.

THE "HELIOTROPE CYANOSIS" OF INFLUENZO-PNEUMONIC SEPTICÆMIA.

1870s–1910s

1870 **Lister: On the effects of the antiseptic system of treatment upon the salubrity of a surgical hospital.** 120
1.1.1870: 4–6
Joseph Lister contributed a number of major articles to *The Lancet*. This example is the first part of a great broadside on the issue of antisepsis, and justly famous. The entire debate on antisepsis is well chronicled in the pages of *The Lancet*, with Lister himself contributing articles on (among many other things) antiseptic ligatures, the use of antiseptic methods to save limbs with compound fractures and compound dislocations, and letters and articles confirming his system's value from supporters, as well as opponents' attacks. Constant striving to improve patient care meant that Lister had often moved on before most people had caught up with him. His relationship with Pasteur is mentioned with self-gratification by Pasteur himself (see *1881*).

1870 **Nightingale: Sanitation in India.** 123
19.11.1870: 725
The views of this remarkable woman herself. Florence Nightingale spent much of her energy (after the Crimea and the establishment of her school of nursing) on improving sanitary conditions in India. This letter was written in the context of continued argument about the mechanism of cholera transmission, and shows her intense attachment to practical matters, and her insistence that men in power keep their minds focused above all on the practical matter of saving life.

1876 **Cavafy: On the antipyretic action of salicylate of soda.** 124
4.11.1876: 633
The salicylates (now thought of as aspirin compounds) were the subject of interest at this time. This paper notes the value of salicylate of soda in lowering temperature in fever, an important observation which would have long term effects. Aspirin (see *1899*) capitalised on this attribute, as much as on the effect on pain. The value of salicylates in antisepsis (see *1916*) and blood thinning took longer to be appreciated (see *1948*, *1968*, *1991*).

1876 **Paget: On a form of chronic inflammation of bones.** 125
18.11.1876: 714–716
Sir James Paget's description of osteitis deformans (Paget's disease) was delivered at a meeting of the Royal Medical and Chirurgical Society in London on the 14th November 1876. This report appeared in *The Lancet* only 4 days later and well conveys the buzzing atmosphere of active engagement and debate during this important Victorian medical meeting.

1879 **Murrell: Nitro-glycerine as a remedy for angina pectoris.** 128
25.1.1879: 113–115
Murrell undertook self-experiments using nitro-glycerine, making careful notes of its action, and a colleague recorded his pulse on a sphygmograph. Murrell then administered it to 12 male and 23 female patients. The variety of their reactions, too, was carefully noted, including temperature and pulse tracings, headaches, nausea, vomiting, drowsiness, weakness and loss of consciousness. Murrell's desire to push others as far as himself in such experiments was not questioned in *The Lancet* at the time. In some cases here, doses were doubled and redoubled on out-patients, to see whatever effects they might report the following week, over several weeks. Murrell regarded nitro-glycerine as preferable to nitrite of amyl (also announced in *The Lancet* 27.7.1867: 97–98) for angina because of its longer-lasting effects on the heart. He also noted the chemical's diuretic effect, carefully measuring output. Nitro-glycerine is still prescribed for angina.

1881   **Pasteur: An address on the germ theory.**   131

13.8.1881: 271–272

Pasteur gave this keynote address at the 1881 International Medical Congress, which took place in London. He discussed the varying virulence of cultures of chicken cholera, the value of vaccines, the nature of attenuation, the investigations of himself and his 'savants' (Chamberland and Roux) concerning splenic fever (anthrax), the failure of burial to inactivate it and mentioned the vast demand in France for his anti-anthrax sheep vaccine. Pasteur concluded with a genuflexion to Jenner.

1884   **Manson: The demonstration of the bacillus leprae.**   133

23.8.1884: 342–343

The leprosy bacillus had been discovered by Hansen in 1872. This paper described a method by which other researchers could isolate and demonstrate it: a good paper on lab technique from the man who helped resolve the puzzle of malaria (see *1898*). Laboratory and microscope science were fundamental to the development of bacteriology, and underpinned many of the developments in medicine in the second half of the 19th century. This paper encapsulates the spirit of painstaking striving evident in many *Lancet* articles at the time.

1885   **Report of *The Lancet* Special Commission on the sanitary condition of Windsor.**   135

15.8.1885: 306–308   (Extract: first page only)

A *Lancet* special investigation showing intolerably low standards of public health in this place, including permeation of Windsor's water courses and soil with sewage. These findings served to help explain Prince Albert's demise at Windsor Castle, 20 years after the event.

1888   **Nitze: Fifteen cases of tumours of the bladder, diagnosed by means of the electro-endoscopic cystoscope.**   136

21.4.1888: 763–766

"One look into the bladder, illuminated as if by daylight, is generally sufficient to afford means for forming an opinion". Excellent, well illustrated article by the inventor of this exciting new scope.

1889   **Paget: The distribution of secondary growths in cancer of the breast.**   140

23.3.1889: 571–573

In attempting to account for the particular distribution of metastases from breast cancer, Stephen Paget was continuing his father James's interest in mortality from this disease (see *Lancet* 19.1.1856: 62–63). The puzzle is still unanswered: but chemical markers have very recently been analysed, suggesting an answer may not be far off (see Eccles SA and Paon L. Breast cancer metastasis: when, where, how? *Lancet* 19.3.2005: 1006–1007).

1890   **Koch: A Remedy for tuberculosis.**   143

22.11.1890: 1085–1086

Koch was not at all happy about publishing the information in this address, wanting more time to investigate, but the "currency of inaccurate and distorted reports" pushed him into premature publication. At this stage, Koch believed his 'tuberculin' a cure. It turned out to be a useful test of immune status. A great many people tried it as a cure, however, only to be bitterly disappointed. Koch was a grand figure and this was a key discovery – wrong application here, but important nevertheless. The original paper appeared in two German periodicals on 15th November 1890 and was translated into English in *The Lancet* only a week later. *The Lancet* later featured Ehrlich on tuberculin (*Lancet* 24.10.1891: 917–920) and Koch's later, more realistic, views (see *1906*).

1893   **Haffkine: Injections against cholera.**   145

11.2.1893: 316–318

Haffkine was a world leader in creating vaccines for epidemic killer diseases (see also plague *1903* below). This paper was given on 8th February 1893, at a laboratory meeting during a visit to England, and appeared in *The Lancet* within days. It is followed by the opening column of a fine report on seamen's diet from a special *Lancet* Commission.

1893   **Carmichael: Cretinism treated by the hypodermic injection of thyroid extract and by feeding.**   148

18.3.1893: 580–581

This report conveys the excitement of a new treatment, and the illustrations emphasise its success.

1895 **Kennedy: Puerperal septicaemia: use of streptococcus antitoxin.**   150
2.11.1895: 1106
Antitoxins were undergoing a vogue at this time: a great many doctors had acquired laboratory experience and developed the ability to isolate strains and use them as vaccines. Not all worked, however. In this case, the antitoxin was supplied by Dr Armand Ruffer. The patient, from Plaistow, is said to have been the first recipient in England of the antitoxin.

1896 **Jones and Lodge: The discovery of a bullet lost in the wrist by means of the Roentgen rays.**   151
22.2.1896: 476–477
First published use in Britain of X-rays to locate a foreign body. The sense of excitement in the use of the rays is apparent. The bullet was a lead pellet and could not be located by surgical exploration, partly because of swelling. The boy's hand was exposed to the rays for over 2 hours, no-one at this early stage having any notion what ill effects might ensue (see *1910*).

1896 **Beatson: On the treatment of inoperable cases of carcinoma of the mamma: suggestions for a new method of treatment, with illustrative cases.**   153
11.7.1896: 104–107
Having studied lactation in sheep for his MD thesis, Beatson had discerned a relationship between lactation and cancer formation in the female breast. He had noted the association of ovaries and breast tissue after hearing of the farming practice of ovariotomy to prolong lactation in cows. The doctor's logical process of reasoning, his discussion of the ethical issues, and the patient's courage in agreeing to the untried operation, are all evident. Hormones were not then understood, but this was a step on the way.

1896 **A report of *The Lancet* Special Commission on the relative strengths of diphtheria antitoxic serums.**   157
18.7.1896: 182–195   (Extract: first page only)
The Lancet intervenes to insist on vaccine safety, setting standards of purity and potency by demonstrating the opposite in the various vaccines available at that time.

1898 **Ross: The role of the mosquito in the evolution of the malarial parasite. The recent researches of Surgeon-Major Ronald Ross.**   158
20.8.1898: 488–489
Part of this report was read by Patrick Manson, on Ross's behalf, to a medical meeting in Edinburgh; and part was sent direct by telegraph to *The Lancet* by Ross himself. The article features his momentous discoveries concerning the life-cycle of the malarial parasite, most particularly its passage from mosquito to host via the salivary glands of the mosquito. Ross explained his reasons for believing mosquito bite was the sole route of transmission in a later letter to *The Lancet* (7.7.1900: 48–50).

1898 **A new hypnotic: 'heroin'.**   160
3.12.1898: 1511
The Lancet report of early clinical trials of Dreser's discovery of an important new substance, 'heroin'.

1899 **Analytical records from *The Lancet* laboratory: 'aspirin'.**   161
22.7.1899: 219
The Lancet reports on its own analysis of this new salicylate drug, 'aspirin', just launched by Bayer.

1900 **Finucane: General nervous shock, immediate and remote, after gunshot and shell injuries in the South African Campaign.**   162
15.9.1900: 807–809
Early description from the Boer War of the phenomenon of shell-shock, now more generally associated with the First World War. The doctor's fellow-feeling for the men under his care is unmistakable. See also *1915* and *1918* below.

1909 **Fraser and Stanton: An inquiry concerning the etiology of beri-beri.**   183
13.2.1909: 451–455   (Extract: first three pages only)
The study of deficiency diseases contributed to Casimir Funk's discovery of 'vitamines'. This was a definitive paper confirming that the key to the aetiology of beri-beri was dehusked white rice. The crossover study was undertaken in a Malaysian setting, with groups of Japanese indentured labourers working on road construction projects in remote districts, each group fed different types of rice [dehusked white and pre-cured parboiled (brown/red) rice]. Those fed on white rice developed beri-beri, but the others did not, and when brown rice was later given to those with beri-beri, they rapidly got well, whereas beri-beri developed among the previously healthy group when fed white rice.
A later *Lancet* article by Gowland Hopkins summarised the field just before the First World War (Diseases due to deficiencies in diet, 8.11.1913: 1309–1310).

1910 **Alexander: "A victim to science": X ray martyr.**   186
22.1.1910: 267
Medicine comes down to earth. The dire effects of X-ray exposure were then becoming evident.
The purpose of this letter was to solicit donations to a fund for a Mr Cox, who had worked "... day and night testing the appliances to ensure the utmost value of the X-ray apparatus for the use of the English surgeons at the front in the South African War". With a colleague, Cox had invented means to indicate depth as well as the surface coordinates of bullets in the body. Both men had developed X-ray carcinoma; the colleague's hands had been amputated and Cox was "pitiable", having lost his right arm and with his face badly affected.
The development of X-ray carcinoma was discussed by Cecil Rowntree in *The Lancet* (20.3.1909: 821–824).

1910 **Home and Ehrlich: Ehrlich-Hata "606".**   187
8.10.1910: 1096–1099
Not the first report from *The Lancet* concerning the "astonishingly effective" new drug Salvarsan, but the most interesting. Home was a naval surgeon, with a strong interest in the treatment of syphilis, who had pitched up in Germany to see things for himself. His article contains the translation of a talk given by Ehrlich himself describing how the discovery was made, followed by an essay by Home describing all he had witnessed on his visit, imparting the sense of a miracle drug phenomenon in progress.

1912 **Savill, Moullin and Horsley: The forcible feeding of suffrage prisoners.**   191
24.8.1912: 549–551
History and human rights in *The Lancet*'s pages: great concern expressed for prisoners under a 'treatment' described here as a torture.

1913 **Crile: The kinetic theory of shock and its prevention through anoci-association (shockless operation).**   194
5.7.1913: 7–16   (Extract: first three pages only)
Crile argued that deaths from operative shock could be prevented by therapeutic drug-induced relaxation of patients before anaesthesia. Origin of 'pre-med' idea. Good mix of theory and effective practice.

1915 **Myers: A contribution to the study of shell shock.**   197
13.2.1915: 316–320   (Extract: first page only)
Myers is now recognised as a key figure in the history of shell-shock, or battle neurosis, which was still disputed as a diagnosis at this stage. Mott's Croonian lectures, looking at the effect of high explosives on the central nervous system, appeared in *The Lancet* in 1916. For WHR Rivers's work on the repression of war experience, see *1918* below.
The army's refusal to accept shell-shock/battle neurosis as a genuine phenomenon in the First World War has since been described by retired judge and former soldier Anthony Babington in *The Lancet* as "a stain on army medicine" (20.11.1993: 1253–1254).

1915 **A new folding stretcher.**   198
23.10.1915: 928
Interesting and potentially useful invention: a folding stretcher, portable as a backpack, for use in the trenches. *The Lancet* staff endorsed it after trying it out in "a tortuous communicating passage" in the Strand premises.

1915   **Osler: Cold-bite + muscle-inertia = trench-foot.**   199
18.12.1915: 1368
A short letter on an important matter from a distinguished physician. Its message is in the title.

1916   **Garrett Anderson, Chambers and Lacey: Treatment of septic wounds, with special reference**
to the use of salicylic acid.   200
3.6.1916: 1119–1120
A splendid paper by three women doctors caring for war-wounded soldiers away from the front in a
London hospital, showing the value of salicylates in antisepsis. The work was based on the cases of men
transported to the military hospital, Endell St, London, within days of being injured in France.

1917   **Garrod: A variety of war heart which calls for treatment by complete rest.**   202
30.6.1917: 985–986
This was an important article in the development of understanding concerning the "irritable heart of
soldiers": a major problem in the First World War and other conflicts. Rest and graded exercise were
developed as therapy.

1917   **Hammond, Rolland and Shore: Purulent bronchitis. A study of cases occurring amongst the**
British troops at a base in France.   204
14.7.1917: 41–45
Hammond's work, on a rapidly fatal 'purulent bronchitis' among British soldiers in France, is now
thought to describe a 'herald wave' outbreak of the subsequent influenza pandemic of 1918–1919 which
killed more people than the First World War. The virus involved was later found to be the same
(Abrahams, Hallows and French: *Lancet* 4.1.1919: 1–11).

1918   **Rivers: An address on the repression of war experience.**   209
2.2.1918: 173–177
WHR Rivers is well known as having worked at Craiglockhart War Hospital and as an exceptionally gifted
anthropologist. Rivers conveys his thoughtful concern for the mental life of those affected by the carnage
of war, and does not shirk from relating to a medical audience the genuine horror of his patients' war
experiences, and the torment of their dreams. He argues that repression had (sometimes serious) dangers,
and that the best way to deal with traumatic war experience was to confront it while not dwelling upon it,
to deliberately endeavour to regard it in a new way and to move on. This process is now known as
'reframing'. Rivers died unexpectedly in 1922. Obituary notices in *The Lancet* make clear that many felt
his loss was a catastrophe both for anthropology and for psychotherapy.
In her '*Regeneration*' trilogy of novels, Pat Barker has created a literary portrait of Rivers caring for
(among others) both Wilfred Owen and Siegfried Sassoon. For a good recent article on Rivers, see *Lancet*
19.7.1997: 205–209.

1918   **Batten and Still: Epidemic stupor in children.**   214
4.5.1918: 636
Report of an illness which seems to have been a manifestation of the 1916–1926 encephalitis pandemic.
Symptoms "at first sight suggested the diagnosis tuberculous meningitis", but the anomalous course of
the illness prompted this article, describing it as a new disease. Affected children became frozen, statue-
like, but even when apparently comatose, were often acutely aware of their surroundings. The condition
became known as encephalitis lethargica (see *1969*).

1918   **Waller: Galvanometric observation of the emotivity of a normal subject (English) during the**
German air-raid of Whit-Sunday, May 19th, 1918.   215
29.6.1918: 916
Extraordinary little paper. Palmar measurement of emotivity contributed to the development of lie
detectors. The nationality of the subject was clearly considered to be important.

1918   **Christopherson: The successful use of antimony in bilharziosis administered as intravenous**
injections of antimonium tartaratum (tartar emetic).   216
7.9.1918: 325–327   (Extract: first page only)
Important discovery for the treatment of this cruel tropical parasitic disease.

1918 **Bousfield: Angina pectoris: changes in electrocardiogram during paroxysm.**   217
5.10.1918: 457–458   (Extract: first page only)
Another interesting paper. The patient just happened to be in the right place at the right time, with doctor present and the equipment attached! Possibly an early instance of 'white-coat hypertension', the phenomenon of patient anxiety generated by the presence of a doctor.

1919 **Mellanby: An experimental investigation on rickets.**   218
15.3.1919: 407–412   (Extract: first page only)
Investigation on dogs revealing the dietary cause of this deprivation condition and the value of cod liver oil in reversing it. Mellanby's wife May did some impeccable work on malnutrition and dentition, published in an earlier issue of *The Lancet* (7.12.1918: 767–770).

1919 **Hirschfeld and Hirschfeld: Serological differences between the blood of different races.**   219
18.10.1919: 675–679   (Extract: first two pages only)
Paper on international variations of blood groups, showing, for example, that "Russians in Siberia have the same proportion of (blood group) B as the natives of Madagascar". The authors suggest cooperation between anthropologists and serologists to attempt systematic mapping of blood groups. Such a study (they suggested) should include the great apes.

leave a trace of their existence than those local affections of organs which appear at the time much more formidable. Thus I am now seeing a gentleman who had a bad attack of gout a short time ago, and a distinct mark is visible on his nails, corresponding to the time of the illness. In another gentleman there exists a mark on his nails at about one-eighth part distant from the root; he had an attack of acute rheumatism about six weeks ago. I have also lately seen another patient with these markings well formed after a severe attack of diphtheria.

Amongst the many interesting communications which have come to hand, I may mention one from Sir Thomas Watson, in which he informs me that he had several years ago an interesting conversation with Dr. Maclean, of the Colchester Hospital, on this subject; the latter gentleman having observed transverse depressions on men's nails in consequence, as he thought, of temporary starvation or arrest of nutrition of the tissues during a bygone acute disease, and these he called "hunger traces." Dr. Maclean had also noticed similar furrows on the hoofs of horses, and indentations or traces on the wings and tail feathers of domestic fowls and of wild birds living in captivity under similar conditions. Mr. Salter also informs me that some illnesses leave indelible traces on the teeth; and, if I have not misunderstood him, he has known a severe attack of whooping cough in childhood leave its traces on the teeth for ever. Dr. Mackaye, of Ardgay, informs me that he was much interested in the subject many years ago, not only in reference to the nails, but as to the changes which the hair undergoes; and he was led more especially to the investigation by the allusions made to the subject by Professor Alison in his lectures at the Edinburgh University. Dr. Washbourn, of Gloucester, also sent me a very interesting account of his own case, which was one of a most severe choleraic attack, accompanied by an alarming prostration and a sensation of icy coldness at the epigastrium; this was succeeded on his recovery by markings on all his nails, which he watched creeping on to the edge, when they finally disappeared.

There seems, then, to be sufficient facts to prove that during a severe illness a partial cessation of the nutritive processes takes place, as shown by the markings on the nails, by the falling off of the hair, or by the furrows on the teeth. Further observation may show in what affections these changes are more likely to occur, and thus may afford some indication of the amount of prostration which the system has undergone. It is remarkable that the first case in which I observed the nail-marks was one identical with that of Dr. Washbourn, one where a sudden and almost fatal prostration succeeded to a choleraic attack. The whole subject is suggestive of a wide field of physiological and pathological inquiry; at present it remains rather within the range of clinical study.

Grosvenor-street, W., Dec. 1869.

ON THE

EFFECTS OF THE ANTISEPTIC SYSTEM OF TREATMENT UPON THE SALUBRITY OF A SURGICAL HOSPITAL.

BY JOSEPH LISTER, F.R.S.,

PROFESSOR OF CLINICAL SURGERY IN THE UNIVERSITY OF EDINBURGH.

THE antiseptic system of treatment has now been in operation sufficiently long to enable us to form a fair estimate of its influence upon the salubrity of an hospital.

Its effects upon the wards lately under my care in the Glasgow Royal Infirmary were in the highest degree beneficial, converting them from some of the most unhealthy in the kingdom into models of healthiness. The interests of the public demand that this striking change should be made generally known; and in order to do justice to the subject, it is necessary, in the first place, to allude shortly to the position and circumstances of the wards.

Each of the four surgeons of the infirmary had charge of three large wards, two male and one female, besides several small ones for special cases. Of these, the most important were the male accident ward and that for female patients, the former containing the chief operation cases as well as those of injury. The third main ward of each surgeon was devoted to chronic male cases, and was in the old infirmary building; but the other two were in the "New Surgical Hospital," erected nine years ago. This consists of four stories above a basement, each floor containing two large wards communicating with a central staircase, besides several smaller apartments. The wards are spacious and lofty, and in the centre of each are two open fireplaces, in a column which runs straight up to the roof, conveying the chimneys of all the floors, and also collateral ventilating shafts, which are warmed by the chimneys that accompany them, and, communicating with various apertures in the ceilings, form excellent means of carrying off the vitiated atmosphere, while fresh air is amply supplied by numerous windows at both sides, the beds being placed in the intervals between them, at a considerable distance from each other. Except the serious defect that the waterclosets in many cases open directly into the wards, the system of construction seemed all that could be desired.

But, to the great disappointment of all concerned, this noble structure proved extremely unhealthy. Pyæmia, erysipelas, and hospital gangrene soon showed themselves, affecting, on the average, most severely those parts of the building nearest to the ground,[*] including my male accident ward, which was one of those on the ground-floor; while my female ward was on the floor immediately above. For several years I had the opportunity of making an observation of considerable, though melancholy, interest—viz., that in my accident ward, when all or nearly all the beds contained patients with open sores, the diseases which result from hospital atmosphere were sure to be present in an aggravated form; whereas, when a large proportion of the cases had no external wound, the evils in question were greatly mitigated or entirely absent. This appeared striking evidence that the emanations from foul discharges, as distinguished from the mere congregation of several human beings in the same apartment, constitute the great source of mischief in a surgical hospital. Hence I came to regard simple fractures, though almost destitute of professional interest to myself and of little value for clinical instruction, as the greatest blessings; because, having no external wound, they diminished the proportion of contaminating cases. At this period I was engaged in a perpetual contest with the managing body, who, anxious to provide hospital accommodation for the increasing population of Glasgow, for which the infirmary was by no means adequate, were disposed to introduce additional beds beyond those contemplated in the original construction. It is, I believe, fairly attributable to the firmness of my resistance in this matter that, though my patients suffered from the evils alluded to in a way that was sickening and often heartrending, so as to make me sometimes feel it a questionable privilege to be connected with the institution, yet none of my wards ever assumed the frightful condition which sometimes showed itself in other parts of the building, making it necessary to shut them up entirely for a time. A crisis of this kind occurred rather more than two years ago in the other male accident ward on the ground-floor, separated from mine merely by a passage 12 ft. broad; where the mortality became so excessive as to lead, not only to closing the ward, but to an investigation into the cause of the evil, which was presumed to be some foul drain. An excavation made with this view disclosed a state of things which seemed to explain sufficiently the unhealthiness that had so long remained a mystery. A few inches below the surface of the ground, on a level with the floors of the two lowest male accident wards, with only the basement area, 4 ft. wide, intervening, was found the uppermost tier of a multitude of coffins, which had been placed there at the time of the cholera epidemic of 1849, the corpses having undergone so little change in the interval that the clothes they had on at the time of their hurried burial were plainly distinguishable. The wonder now was, not that these wards upon the ground-floor had been unhealthy, but that they had not been absolutely pestilential. Yet at the very time when this shocking disclosure was being made, I was able to state, in an address which I delivered to the meeting of the British Medical

---

* Statistics collected by desire of the managers established the fact that the ground-floor wards were, on the average, most liable to pyæmia, whoever might be the surgeon in charge; and that those on the floor immediately above came next in this respect.

Association in Dublin, that during the previous nine months, in which the antiseptic system had been fairly in operation in my wards, not a single case of pyæmia, erysipelas, or hospital gangrene had occurred in them; and this, be it remembered, not only in the presence of conditions likely to be pernicious, but at a time when the unhealthiness of other parts of the same building was attracting the serious and anxious attention of the managers. Supposing it justifiable to institute an experiment on such a subject, it would be hardly possible to devise one more conclusive.

Having discovered this monstrous evil, the managers at once did all in their power to correct it. The extent of the corrupting mass was so great that it seemed out of the question to attempt its removal; but it was freely treated with carbolic acid and with quick lime, and an additional thickness of earth was laid over it; and, further, a high wall at right angles with the end of the building, and reaching up to the level of the first floor, so as necessarily to confine the bad air most prejudicially, was pulled down, and an open iron railing was substituted for it.

There can be no doubt that these measures must have proved salutary. But even if it were admitted that they cured completely the particular evil against which they were directed, it would still have to be confessed that the situation of the surgical hospital has been far from satisfactory. Besides having along one of its sides the place of sepulture above alluded to, one end of the building is conterminous with the old Cathedral churchyard, which is of large size and much used, and in which the system of "pit burial" of paupers has hitherto prevailed. I saw one of the pits some time since, having been requested to report upon it by one of the civic authorities, who is also a manager of the infirmary, and who, having accidentally discovered what was going on, at once took steps to prevent for the future the occurrence of anything so disgraceful. The pit, which was standing open for the reception of the next corpse, emitted a horrid stench on the removal of some loose boards from its mouth. Its walls were formed, on three sides, of coffins piled one upon another in four tiers, with the lateral interstices between them filled with human bones, the coffins reaching up to within a few inches of the surface of the ground. This was in a place immediately adjoining the patients' airing ground, and a few yards only from the windows of the surgical wards. And the pit which I inspected seems to have been only one of many similar receptacles, for THE LANCET of Sept. 25th contains a statement, copied from one of the Glasgow newspapers, that "the Dean of Guild is said to have computed that five thousand bodies were lying in pits, holding eighty each, in a state of decomposition, around the infirmary."* Just beyond the churchyard rises an eminence covered by an extensive necropolis, which, however, from its greater distance, must have comparatively little deleterious influence. When I add that what is called the fever hospital,† also a long four-storied building, extends at right angles to the new surgical hospital, separated from it by only eight feet, and that the entire infirmary, containing 584 beds, stands upon an area of two acres, and that the institution is almost always full to overflowing,‡ I have said enough to show that the wards at my disposal have been sufficiently trying for any system of surgical treatment. Yet, during the two years and a quarter that elapsed between the Dublin meeting and the time of my leaving Glasgow for Edinburgh, those wards continued in the main as healthy as they had been during the previous nine months. Adding these two periods together, we have three years of immunity from the ordinary evils of surgical hospitals, under circumstances which, but for the antiseptic system, were especially calculated to produce them.§

* I doubt if even my sense of the importance of the subject I am dealing with would have induced me to enter into these disagreeable details, were I not able at the same time to bear my testimony to the zealous manner in which the managers of the Infirmary and the Town Council are exerting themselves to correct the evils referred to. I understand that it is in contemplation to abolish entirely intra-mural interment in Glasgow.

† About half the wards of the fever hospital are used for surgical cases.

‡ The rapid increase of Glasgow has rendered the Infirmary, in spite of considerable additions of late years, quite inadequate to the wants of the population; but this evil will shortly be remedied by the construction of a general hospital in connexion with the new College.

§ The antiseptic system was commenced nearly five years ago, but was for the first two years employed almost exclusively in compound fractures and abscesses, which form but a small proportion of surgical cases, so that the system cannot be said to have been in operation for more than three years with reference to the subject of the present paper.

It may be well to mention in detail some facts regarding the comparative frequency, before and after the period referred to, of the three diseases to which surgical wards have hitherto been peculiarly liable—namely, pyæmia, erysipelas, and hospital gangrene.

And first of pyæmia. This fearful disease used to occur principally in two classes of cases—namely, compound fractures and the major amputations. In compound fracture, it was so rife just before the introduction of the antiseptic system that I had one of the sulphites administered internally as a prophylactic, in accordance with Polli's views, to every patient admitted with this kind of injury; though I cannot say that we observed any distinct evidence of advantage from the practice. But since I began to treat compound fractures on the antiseptic system, while no internal treatment has been used, I have not had pyæmia in a single instance, although I have had in all thirty-two cases—six in the forearm, five in the arm, eighteen in the leg, and three in the thigh. These cases do not include those in which the injury was so great as to demand immediate amputation. But it must be remarked that many of the limbs saved were so severely injured that I should formerly have removed them without hesitation. I almost forget the kind of considerations which used to determine me to amputate under the old treatment; though I know that experience taught us that it was only in comparatively mild cases that it was justifiable to attempt to save the limb. Now, however, there is scarcely any amount or kind of injury of bones, joints, or soft parts which I regard as inconsistent with conservative treatment, except such destruction of tissue as makes gangrene of the limb inevitable as an immediate consequence.

But I may take this opportunity of observing that the attempt to save a limb which, under ordinary treatment, would be subjected to immediate amputation, ought not to be made lightly, or without a thorough acquaintance with some trustworthy method of carrying out the antiseptic system; by which I mean, not the mere use of an antiseptic, however potent, *but such management of the case as shall effectually prevent the occurrence of putrefaction in the part concerned.* Without this such endeavours are far worse than useless; for by the time that local disturbance and constitutional disorder have made it apparent that the antiseptic means have failed, the patient is so much prostrated by irritation and blood-poisoning, that the operation, if performed, is probably too late; and thus a loose and trifling style of "giving the treatment a trial" swells the death-rate at once of compound fracture and of amputation.

On the other hand, the surgeon will not on this account be justified in contentedly pursuing the old practice of primary amputation; for the antiseptic means which it has been the main labour of the last five years of my life to improve are now so satisfactory* that anyone duly impressed with the importance of the subject, and devoting to it the study and practical attention which it demands, will, with little trouble to himself, securely attain the results which he desires.

I lately visited my wards in Glasgow after an absence of some weeks, and saw, amongst other cases, a compound dislocation of the ankle in a man who had fallen about four feet from the platform at a railway station, and lighted on the outer side of the right foot, which had been forced violently inwards, producing a contused and lacerated wound, about four inches long, crossing the external malleolus, and communicating with the articulation. When I saw the patient the wound had been converted into a superficial sore, cicatrising rapidly; and there had been from first to last no deep-seated suppuration, nor any local or constitutional disturbance. I asked my then house-surgeon, Mr. James Coats, with whom the most critical part of the treatment had rested, whether he could reckon pretty securely upon such results. He replied, "With certainty." I asked the question for the sake of others who were standing by, having little doubt what the answer would be, for when I left him in charge I felt sure that the antiseptic management of the cases would be as satisfactorily conducted as if I were present.

At the same time, it is only right to add, that when

* I hope to bring before the profession the improved antiseptic means above alluded to by publishing from time to time in THE LANCET cases illustrative of their employment.

he entered upon his office, though convinced of the truth of the theory of the antiseptic treatment, he by no means felt the confidence in carrying it out which he has since acquired; and if an able man like Mr. Coats, imbued with the principles which I have striven to establish, required some practical initiation into the subject before he could be regarded as trustworthy, still more must such be the case with those who, educated in the old system, and long habituated to its practice, have to unlearn cherished ideas and instinctive habits.

(To be concluded.)

FURTHER NOTES ON PULSATING TUMOURS OF THE NECK.*

BY JOHN COCKLE, A.M., M.D.,

FELLOW OF THE ROYAL COLLEGE OF PHYSICIANS, AND PHYSICIAN TO THE ROYAL FREE HOSPITAL.

I SUBMIT the details of two additional cases of Dilatation of the Innominate Artery, which, added to those already published by me, may enable some general conclusions to be drawn respecting this affection.

The first case occurred in a patient of Mr. Parrott, of Enfield, and which I saw with him on two occasions during the month of April last. Mr. Parrott informed me that his attention was first directed to the tumour in December, 1868, when called to the case in consequence of several severe attacks of epistaxis, in one of which he was compelled to plug the nostril before the hæmorrhage could be arrested. He considered this circumstance noteworthy, as showing, perhaps, a tendency to disease of the vessels. The artery at that time was pulsating very strongly, from the sternal notch to the origin of the carotid. It was not quite clear to his mind, at this period, whether the aorta was implicated, but he considered that it was. There were no accurate means of knowing how long the tumour had existed, but, in his opinion, it probably originated about that time.

I took the following notes when I saw the case. The patient was a middle-aged widow, somewhat corpulent, and of sallow complexion. A tumour, which had been observed about four months, very large and prominent (but appearing larger than it really was from a large collection of adipose matter in front of it), completely filled the episternal hollow, passing up somewhat in front of the trachea, and from thence obliquely across the right side of the neck. The impulse was very expansive and forcible, but unattended by thrill; the collapse did not feel quite complete, but this might be explained, possibly, from the collection of adipose matter mentioned. The right carotid and right radial pulses (I speak doubtfully) seemed a trifle weaker than those of the opposite side. A double murmur was audible over the tumour, and also down the aorta, to its origin. The heart's impulse was by no means great, nor was its apex lowered. The condition of the pupils could not be noted, as the patient had lost the sight of the right eye for some years.

In a recent communication from Mr. Parrott (Nov. 25th) he states:—"The patient has lately had three attacks of hæmorrhage, always occurring in the night or early in the morning; on awaking, she has blood in her mouth. I do not think the tumour has increased in size since you saw it; she has occasionally some pain in it, but this is always relieved by the application of cold."

I ought, by the way, to mention that this patient was seen in the early stage of the affection by a London surgeon of repute, who suggested the application of instrumental pressure; but the patient either could not or would not persevere in its use.

For the next case I am indebted to the kindness of my colleague, Dr. Rickards. It is a case the more interesting as, in addition to innominate dilatation, there is cirsoid aneurism of the left carotid.

Mrs. G——, admitted under my care at the Royal Free Hospital in July, 1869, is a widow fifty years of age. Her complexion is slightly pallid, but otherwise natural. There is some amount of spinal curvature. She has always been of delicate constitution, and had formerly to work hard. The cause of her father's death she does not know. Her mother died of diseased liver. Her two brothers died of disease of the heart, at the respective ages of fifty and fifty-two. About seven years ago she first felt a beating in the hollow of the throat, and suffered from rheumatism (as she expresses it) of the head and neck. She still suffers much, at times, from this pain, which affects both sides; also from cough in the morning, shortness of breath occasionally, especially on ascending stairs, and from palpitation of the heart on any excitement. On inspection, the left jugular vein is seen distended, but without pulsation. The superficial veins coursing over the left side of the chest are more prominent than those on the corresponding side. The pupils are equal and of natural size. The right radial pulse was stronger than the left when first examined. The swelling of the left carotid artery (the coats of which feel much thickened) involves the upper half of the vessel. Its prominence is very marked about two inches below the ramus of the jaw, as is also the locomotion of the artery, which here advances at each diastole with a rapid and very forcible forward projection alongside the tracheal edge of the left sterno-mastoid muscle, and then as rapidly retreats during the succeeding systole. The tracing of its impulse has been taken by Dr. Hawksley with his stetho-sphygmograph, as also those of both radial pulses. The latter agree in every particular with those taken at the hospital. A pulsating swelling, about the shape and size of a date, is visible, emerging from behind the right sterno-clavicular articulation, and occupying the hollow of the neck. It extends upwards from beneath the inner head of the sterno-mastoid muscle to its outer head, taking a somewhat oblique direction. The impulse is strong, expansive, and liquid during arterial diastole; during systole the swelling perfectly subsides. The heart appears to be displaced horizontally; its apex is situate near the fourth rib, one inch above the left nipple; and there is dilated hypertrophy of the left ventricle. The cardiac impulse is synchronous with that of the tumour and of the radial pulses. No thrill anywhere exists. The right radial pulse, formerly strongest, has appeared of late occasionally to be slightly weaker than the left, but both are perfectly regular, soft, of normal frequency, and without any collapse. The sphygmograph tracing, however, tells plainly of increased arterial resistance. At or just below the right sterno-clavicular junction a double murmur exists, having here a maximum. The first arterial diastolic murmur is soft and somewhat blowing; the second arterial systolic murmur is a little shorter in duration, and of hoarser character. These murmurs, scarcely changed, are audible in the swelling and right carotid artery, but weaker down the aorta. Immediately under the uppermost part of the sternum a musical murmur of intensity is heard at times, and loudest during arterial diastole: it was of remarkable intensity when Dr. Sibson examined this case with me the other day, and we both consider it of venous origin. About one inch above the left nipple, and corresponding to the site of greatest cardiac impulse, exists a second maximum focus of double murmur. The systolic murmur here is most intense, being at intervals of nearly musical *timbre*, and traceable vertically upwards to the right clavicle, and obliquely downwards nearly to the ensiform cartilage. The second murmur is not so loud, neither is it so widely heard. They diminish somewhat as they are traced midway up the aorta, so that, apparently, a minimum point exists between the two maxima foci. At the left axillary line the murmurs lose all their intensity, and are nearly replaced by normal tic tac, except that the first sound remains faintly murmurish. No murmur is audible at the lower angle of the left scapula. On the left side of the neck a closure sound of the sigmoid valves apparently is heard.

Now, are these murmurs of aortic origin? Such murmurs are occasionally well marked at and near the apex of the heart, and, in exceptional cases, the return murmur may weaken upwards in the aorta; the pulse is perfectly regular, and the absence of collapse might be explained by some coexisting contraction. But we should be perplexed in accounting for the absence of a more defined murmur with the upward current. The sphygmographic tracing wants its characteristic crotchet. But our greatest diffi-

* Read before the Medical Society of London, Nov. 30th, 1869.

and wounded soldiers of its own army. From the experience we have had during this war of the various voluntary aid societies, we are not disposed to rank their labours as very efficient. Partly from lack of experience and organisation, partly from the jealousy they excited among military medical men, partly from the abuses to which the "red cross" was subjected, from being assumed by all sorts of people, under all sorts of circumstances, there has been a terrible waste of money and energy. It is a lamentable fact —but fact we fear it is—that all attempts at softening the horrors of wars by neutral powers are liable to misconstruction, and possible mischief. The duty of taking care of the sick must devolve upon the Government employing the troops who have become disabled in its service. The most that can be done is to supplement State aid in various ways, and under circumstances where it would be impossible for the Government to do so, or vain to expect any Government to afford the requisite amount.

Correspondence.

"Audi alteram partem."

SANITATION IN INDIA.

To the Editor of THE LANCET.

SIR,—Miss Nightingale has been so good as to send me the enclosed letter, written, you will observe, for publication in your journal, in reply to what Miss Nightingale is good enough to call my "kind and gentle criticism."

I am glad to find that this very influential writer had no intention or desire to throw cold water on the inquiry in defence of which I wrote. I wish, however, to state that I was not singular in thinking such was likely to be the effect of Miss Nightingale's observations.

In conclusion, I wish your readers to understand that the inquiry in defence of which I took up my pen was not the one instituted by the Sanitary Committee of the War Office, of which Miss Nightingale "was one of the first and strongest advocates," but that more special inquiry suggested by the Senate of the Army Medical School, and now being carried on by Drs. Cunningham and Lewis.

I am, Sir, your obedient servant,
Royal Victoria Hospital, Netley. W. C. MACLEAN.

To the Editor of THE LANCET.

SIR,—In your number of Oct. 29th you inserted a kind and gentle criticism from Professor Maclean on certain parts of my "few words" appended to the last annual India Office Report on sanitary measures.

Since the outbreak of this most terrible of all earth's wars, I have had a hard time of it in defending others, and I have not had the least little moment to defend myself. Still, Sir, if you will allow me, I should wish to say that Professor Maclean seems to have read from a point of view opposite to that which was in my mind when writing these "few words." And I am glad that he has given me an opportunity, with your permission, to explain them.

My object was, as I need scarcely say, purely practical. It was to deprecate a tendency complained of by all of late years (this very complaint came to me from India)—viz., the tendency to base sanitary proceedings on theory. Dr. Maclean appears to think that I question the propriety of the cholera inquiry now proceeding in India. I was one of its first and strongest advocates. I strenuously urged the granting of necessary funds to carry it out; and I consider it one of the most important public Indian inquiries which has been ever undertaken on our subject. The very importance of it lies in this: if a fact is proved, it ceases to be theory. The inquiry in question is to ascertain, as far as may be, what is fact. This was the meaning of the passage which Dr. Maclean interprets as implying "ridicule" on my part.

What I said about the present state of the fungoid theory I learnt from the published report of Drs. Cunningham and Lewis; about the ground water, from Dr. Town-

send's Report on Cholera in the Central Provinces. These statements are not theories, but facts. If they are facts, they cease to be theories. The theories remain just where they were. Of course, if the theories were found on longer inquiry to be true, they too would be no longer theories, but facts; and as such would afford good ground for expending public money in applying the *facts* to save life.

The case of Jenner, cited by Dr. Maclean, is in reality my case. Jenner first started a theory; but the Vaccination Acts, with the costs and penalties, were not enacted until Jenner's theory had become a fact by long experience.

We all have the same object in view—viz., saving human life. This cannot be done without expenditure. And as theories are many and uncertain, all we ask is, that the public should know what we are spending their money for. This, the said cholera inquiry will, perhaps more than anything else, help to tell us.

Also, in what I said about cholera excreta, I simply dealt again with the facts. Dr. Bryden has shown in his Report on Cholera, p. 214, that the dry-earth system, which, in its application, would prevent the dangers of putrid cholera excreta, had not stayed the ravages of cholera. Hence, Dr. Bryden himself calls in question the theory. And I have done no more.

At p. 59, para. 170, of the Report for 1869 by the "Sanitary Commissioner with the Government of India," just received, the results of dealing with cholera excreta are stated as follows:—"With regard to the effect of the careful disinfection and safe disposal of evacuations which seem to have been generally practised, there is no evidence to show that any results can be professedly attributed to them."

Since Professor Maclean's letter appeared in THE LANCET of Oct. 29th, I have received Dr. Lewis's able and most interesting report, the first instalment of the scientific inquiry into cholera which Dr. Maclean fears my remarks may injure. It confirms the former joint reports of Drs. Lewis and Cunningham by a host of microscopic examinations and drawings, from which the following conclusion (No. 3, p. 164, Sanitary Commissioner's Report) is deduced by Dr. Lewis:—"3. That no special fungus has been developed in cholera stools, the fungus described by Hallier being certainly not confined to such stools." But these are the theories which have hitherto occupied the attention of the observers.

Even this information, though most important, we shall not, however, receive as final. We must inquire into objections, and ask further questions. The real inquiry is only about to begin. Mere controversy is here useless.

With many apologies for writing so long a letter, which, had I had more time, I could have made shorter,

Pray believe me, Sir, your faithful servant,
London, Nov. 14th, 1870. FLORENCE NIGHTINGALE.

*** We have been compelled to omit the publication of Professor Maclean's letter (in type), replying to Dr. Morehead's communication of last week, in order to find the necessary space for the insertion of the above.—ED. L.

TORSION OF ARTERIES.

To the Editor of THE LANCET.

SIR,—In the paper by Mr. J. D. Hill, on "Torsion of Arteries as a hæmostatic method" in your impression of the 5th inst., I remark that, in the description he gives of the operation as performed by Amussat, he makes no mention (nor indeed does either Mr. Bryant or Prof. Humphry in their several papers referred to by Mr. Hill) of the special pair of forceps by which the vessel was fixed before being twisted. This instrument, called by Sédillot "pince à rafoulment," and by Malgaigne "pince à baguettes," is figured in the medium operation of the former author. It consisted essentially of a forceps, with branches terminating in smooth cylinders, with which the vessel was seized transversely to its long axis, after being drawn out and freed from the surrounding textures; compression of the arterial coats by its means then led to the division of the two internal ones, whilst their separation and rolling back was facilitated by slight traction on the free end of the artery.

In the modification employed by Mr. Hill, one blade of the forceps is placed within, and the other without, the

ON THE
ANTIPYRETIC ACTION OF SALICYLATE OF SODA.

BY JOHN CAVAFY, M.D., F.R.C.P.,
ASSISTANT-PHYSICIAN TO ST. GEORGE'S HOSPITAL.

PROBABLY few remedies of recent introduction have so rapidly found favour with the profession as salicylic acid. The claims set forth on its behalf by its original introducers may be said to be more than justified, and evidence is daily accumulating to show that a most valuable and active agent has been added to our list. It is in acute rheumatism that it has been chiefly administered, and the numerous cases published leave no doubt as to its beneficial action in this disease. During several months I have had opportunities of watching the results of its administration in many cases of rheumatism with high temperature, and in nearly all great benefit has been derived in a very short time—two or three days at most. The most marked effect is the rapid depression of temperature which ensues, so that fever is practically abolished. I have seen cases in which there was a rise of temperature to 103° or over during the first day after the patient had been put to bed, and salicylate of soda having been then given, there has been a fall of three or four degrees in the next twenty-four or thirty-six hours. This antipyretic action of salicylic acid is, perhaps, its most valuable property, and seems hardly to have attracted the notice it deserves. The case of which I subjoin a very short account shows the action in a very striking manner.

A nurse was warded under my care (during the absence of Dr. Dickinson) suffering from enteric fever. The case was one of considerable severity and of long duration; the evening temperature reaching 104° for many days. In course of time the fever declined considerably, but on the twenty-sixth day of the disease the temperature again began to rise. On this day (Oct. 1st) the morning temperature was 101°; evening 101·8° On Oct. 2nd: morning 102 4°; evening 103 8°. On Oct. 3rd: morning 102 8°. On this day I saw the patient in the afternoon, and for the first time ordered salicylate of soda, half a drachm every four hours. The first dose was given late in the afternoon, and in the evening the temperature was only 100·8° (as against 103 8° on the previous day). One more dose was given at night, but this was followed by vomiting, with cold extremities and very weak pulse. The house-physician, Mr. Blake, who was called to her at 4 A M, found her very low, and at once discontinued the medicine. The temperature was not taken at that time; but at the usual time (8 o'clock) in the morning of Oct. 4th the thermometer marked only 96 9°. No medicine was given during the day, and in the evening the temperature was 103·6°—a rise of nearly seven degrees. During this time there was no diarrhœa, the bowels being opened only once on Oct. 3rd, and not at all on the 4th. There was not the slightest hæmorrhage. Evidently, therefore, the great depression of temperature was due to the salicylate of soda, as is shown also by the enormous rise which ensued on its being withheld.

I am not aware of any published cases in which salicylic acid or its soda salt has been employed in cases of fever, rheumatic or other, in which the temperature has reached or exceeded 107°; but my reason for bringing the above case under the notice of the profession is that it seems to show that we are now in possession of a most valuable remedy for hyperpyrexia, which is usually treated by the cumbrous and tiresome method of cold baths. It shows at any rate that a marked depression of temperature may be produced in some cases of fever, and there is no *primâ facie* reason to believe that hyperpyrexia would prove exceptional. I hope therefore that those who have an opportunity will give the drug a fair trial in cases of this nature, and publish the results. I should feel inclined myself to begin with rather large and frequent doses (say half a drachm of salicylate of soda every hour), and gradually diminish the quantity, and lengthen the intervals of administration, according to the result produced. Salicylate of soda, owing to its free solubility, and consequent ready absorption, is decidedly preferable to the sparingly soluble salicylic acid. It is in all probability, as Binz has stated, decomposed by the nascent carbonic acid in the blood and tissues, the salicylic acid being thus set free throughout the body. The acid, given in powder, is apt to produce gastric and intestinal irritation, and, owing to its very slight solubility, a large quantity no doubt passes off in the fæces unabsorbed.

Upper Berkeley-street, W.

ON VESICO-VAGINAL FISTULA.

BY DR. NATHAN BOZEMAN.

IN the month of November last, Prof. Dolbeau submitted to me for treatment at the Hôpital Beaujon three women with four urinary fistulæ, which he said were incurable by the methods ordinarily employed in France.

Case 1 presented a somewhat elliptical opening extending from the middle of the urethra to the cervix uteri, measuring longitudinally about five centimetres, and transversely between two and three; broad cicatricial bands extended across the rectal wall, which effectually prevented movement of the uterus downwards. This case I did not treat.

Case 2 had a small transverse urethro-vaginal fistula near the bladder, and at the same height a cicatricial contraction of the entire calibre of the vagina to the extent of allowing only the point of the index-finger to pass. This cicatrix involved both edges of the fistula, was thick and unyielding, thus rendering operative procedure upon the latter impossible. Here by preparatory treatment I secured access to the fistula in less than five weeks, and returned the patient to Prof. Dolbeau for completion of the cure, which he then thought could be effected without difficulty.

Case 3 exhibited a urethro-vaginal and a urethro-vesico-vaginal fistula, with a narrow bridge of inodular tissue intervening, and with almost complete atresia of the entire vaginal tract. In this case I converted both fistulæ into one, and dilated the vagina to the extent of four inches in depth and two and a half in width. The fistula then presented an oval form, having its anterior border notched at the urethra, and to the right of this point firmly adherent to the pubic bone; it measured transversely four centimetres and a half, and longitudinally about three and a half. Now, Prof. Dolbeau not wishing to undertake the coaptation of the edges of the fistula, requested me to perform the operation, which I did on the 17th of March. Firm union was effected at the first trial all but two small points separated by the urethra. The left opening, the size of a No. 6 catheter, was caused by the cutting of a corresponding suture, and the right, the size of an ordinary probe, stood directly in the line of union. Both of these little remaining fistulæ can now be easily united, and the whole closed at a second operation, which Prof. Dolbeau will perform soon.

The principle of treatment employed in the third case has been commented upon at length and in a manner highly appreciative* by Dr. Paul Berger, Professor to the Faculty of Medicine of Paris, and to this publication I would respectfully refer all who may feel an interest in the subject. But I may add here that Dr. Berger in his remarks has inadvertently made two or three erroneous statements regarding certain important points of practice, which, in justice to myself, need to be corrected. For this purpose, and in order to call attention to some recent statistical facts regarding obliteration of the vagina, as a means of treating vesico-vaginal fistula, I now ask the use of the columns of THE LANCET. This I deem essential for a better understanding of the subject, not only as regards the result attained in the case in question, but as a principle of general applicability to the cure of a not inconsiderable class of cases, usually regarded amenable only to tentative expedients.

A fistula, whether small or large, complicated with atresia in any form, is, to use a military expression, the stronghold, to be reached only in two ways—namely, by direct attack and by gradual approaches. The first mode,

* La France Médicale, May 13th and 17th.

during the night, but passed off towards morning, when he was better, and the pulse fuller. Brandy was taken readily.

Feb. 13th.—Noon: Pulse 124; temperature 99·4°. Hæmorrhage being observed from the left stump, the stitches were removed, and two bleeding points secured. The cut surface was freely sponged with a tepid solution of boracic acid, and when the flaps were readjusted they were held in position by a fold of lint soaked in the same lotion. Dry cold by means of an ice-bag was applied to repress further bleeding. The right stump was also dressed with the boracic acid solution. Evening pulse 138.

14th.—Noon: Temperature 102·6°; pulse 140; evening pulse 138. Discharge from the stumps slight.

15th.—Noon: Pulse 116; temperature 100·4°. Patient much less feverish than yesterday; looks and feels better; discharge little; same dressing as before, except that the dry cold to left stump is discontinued. Ordered five drops of tincture of perchloride of iron, and ten grains of chlorate of potash, in half an ounce of water, three times a day. Evening pulse 132.

16th.—Noon: Pulse 136; temperature 103·6°. Patient not so well as yesterday; a fold of lint covered with moist charcoal laid along the line of union of the flaps, and lint wrung from boracic acid solution put over this. Ordered internally five grains of sulphate of quinine in an ounce of water, to be taken every four hours, in addition to the iron and chlorate of potash.

17th.—Noon: Pulse 124; temperature 103·8°. The discharge to-day greater in quantity and healthier in appearance.

18th.—Noon: Pulse 118; temperature 102·6°. States that he slept well during the night, and that to-day he feels easier. The wounds continue to look healthier, and to discharge more. Medicines repeated. In the evening patient expressed a desire to be raised in bed, and, immediately on this being done, hæmorrhage commenced from the right thigh. The stitches were taken out, and the origin of the bleeding looked for, but without success. The wound was then closed by silver-wire sutures. About two hours later bleeding from the same stump recurred, and again the stitches were removed, the wound opened, and all clots cleared away. A sponge was then placed in the stump, the flaps laid over it, and tightly bandaged. Dry cold applied by means of ice-bags.

19th.—Pulse 120; temperature 101·2°. Patient delirious during the whole of last night. At noon to-day he was placed under chloroform, when Mr. Spence examined the right thigh, but could find no bleeding vessel to account for the hæmorrhage. He continued delirious all day.

20th.—Noon: Pulse 120; temperature 101·7°. Was ordered last night twenty-five minims of solution of hydrochlorate of morphia and twenty-four grains of bromide of ammonium, but without inducing sleep, which only came on at 6 o'clock this morning. No recurrence of the bleeding.

24th.—Pulse 126; temperature 100·6°. Patient has been suffering since the 22nd from diarrhœa. Complains to-day of pain in the epigastrium. Ordered twenty grains of sulpho-carbolate of potash three times a day.

26th.—Pulse 120; temperature 100·6°. Last night the patient had a little difficulty in passing urine, which, however, was relieved by the application of a hot fomentation over the pubes. This morning he seems better, though he still complains of epigastric pain.

28th.—Pulse 124; temperature 102°. Urine passed easily; diarrhœa stopped.

March 4th.—Pulse 116; temperature 100·3°. The thigh flaps are healing well; those of the leg are somewhat slower, but seem also to be doing fairly.

6th.—Pulse 112; temperature 100°. Wounds continue healthy. Urine alkaline, with deposit of urates and slight amount of phosphates. Ordered ten-minim doses of nitro-muriatic acid three times a day.

13th.—Pulse 108; temperature 98·8°. Urine alkaline, albuminous, phosphatic. Signs of necrosis of bone observable on anterior surface of the tibia and on the head of the fibula.

24th.—Pulse 100; temperature 99°. An abscess which had formed on the inner side of the right thigh was opened by free incision, and a drainage-tube inserted.

April 3rd.—Noon: Pulse 124; temperature 103·8°. Immediately after breakfast this morning the patient complained

of feeling cold; this lasted for an hour, and was followed by heat and fever. He had passed a rather restless night.

4th.—Pulse 96; temperature 99·6°. Slept well. No pain in stumps.

7th.—Pulse 106; temperature 98·8°. Slept well, and has a good appetite. Sulphate of copper applied to correct the weak action in the left stump.

12th.—Pulse 108; temperature 99°. On pressure over the inner side of the right thigh, near the groin, pus can be squeezed out through a sinus near the stump.

May 1st. — Pulse 104; temperature 100·3°. Urine of sp. gr. 1015; contains a little albumen and abundant phosphates.

3rd.—Pulse 102; temperature 99·6°. Mr. Spence opened an abscess in the left stump, and evacuated a quantity of pus.

5th.—Pulse 112; temperature 98·8°. Another abscess in the left stump opened.

7th.—Pulse 82; temperature 98·2°. Albumen in urine one-fourth.

12th.—Temperature and pulse normal. Albumen in urine greatly diminished.

18th.—Temperature and pulse continue normal. Urine of sp. gr. 1012; albumen almost entirely absent, but phosphates abundant.

22nd.—Pulse and temperature normal. Urine of sp. gr. 1015, acid reaction, slightly albuminous, but with the phosphates in normal quantity.

30th.—Pulse 96; temperature 98·5°.

June 5th.—Patient discharged.

Medical Societies.

ROYAL MEDICAL AND CHIRURGICAL SOCIETY.

THERE was an unusually large attendance at the meeting of this Society on the 14th inst., when a paper upon a form of chronic inflammation of bones (osteitis deformans), by Sir James Paget, President, was read and discussed, the speakers being Sir William Gull, Mr. Brudenell Carter, Mr. Barwell, and Dr. Goodhart.

Before the adjournment the medical secretary read a report addressed to the President by the delegates of the Society at the recent Medical Congress at Philadelphia. The report alluded in flattering terms to the management of the Congress, the high character of the communications read there, and to the cordial reception given to all the delegates. The report was signed by Dr. Barnes, Dr. Hare, and Mr. Brudenell Carter.

A paper "On a Form of Chronic Inflammation of Bones (osteitis deformans)," by Sir JAMES PAGET, Bart., D.C.L., LL.D., F.R.S., President, was read by the surgical secretary (Mr. Hulke). It opened with a detailed account of a case which had been for many years under the author's observation. It was that of a gentleman in whose family there was no history of gout or rheumatism, but one of whose sisters had died of chronic cancer of the breast; he was a tall, thin, and well-formed man, and the father of healthy children. When forty-six years of age he began to suffer from pains in the thighs and legs, and at the end of one year he noticed the left shin to be somewhat misshapen. Sir James Paget first saw the patient in 1856, or two years from the commencement of the disease. He was then in good health, prematurely grey, and walked stiffly. There was some enlargement and irregularity of the left tibia and lower half of the left femur, but no tenderness. The urine deposited lithates. The case being regarded as one of chronic periostitis, iodide of potassium was given, but without result. Three years later the author again saw the case, this time in conjunction with Mr. Stanley. The left tibia had become larger and longer, so that it was curved anteriorly; the femur also was more distinctly enlarged, and was arched forwards and outwards. This side of the pelvis appeared widened, and the whole limb was about a quarter of an inch shorter than the right. There was very little suffering, the clumsiness of the limb being the chief trouble. He had taken much iodine and other medicine, without the least effect. For the next seventeen years the disease steadily but slowly progressed. The left tibia continued to enlarge, and became more curved, and the same change taking place on the right side, the two limbs in time became symmetrically affected, and at the same time the knees became gradually bent. The skull also slowly increased in size, the head retaining its natural shape, and the face not being at all affected. The spine became slowly curved and almost rigid, so that the patient's height diminished from 6 feet 1 inch to 5 feet 9 inches; and the chest became narrow, shortened, and deeper from before backwards, and all movement was much restrained. The head was bent forwards, and the neck consequently shortened. The arms, not sharing in the shortening of the trunk, seemed long in proportion (photographs were handed round, showing the condition six months before death), and the angle formed by the shaft with the neck of the femur was diminished. In 1870, the left knee-joint became actively inflamed, and was left more stiff and bent afterwards; at the same time, some insufficience of the mitral valve was detected. In the summer of 1874 the patient suffered partial loss of vision from retinal hæmorrhage, and he also began to be somewhat deaf. He then also suffered from neuralgic pains, chiefly in the upper part of the body. In January, 1876, pain in the left forearm and elbow, followed by swelling in the upper part of the radius, appeared; but he was otherwise in good health, enjoyed a good appetite, and his mind was quite clear. From this time he began to fail, and it was evident that the painful swelling of the forearm was due to a cancerous growth, and on the 24th of March, after suffering from pleural effusion, he died. At the autopsy, the head was retracted to a level with the sternum, and the lower limbs rested upon the nates and heels, from the arching of the bones. The pericranium and dura mater were healthy. The lungs were compressed and contained a few nodules of cancer on their surface. The mitral valve was atheromatous and calcified; the aortic slightly atheromatous. The femur, tibia, and patella, and upper part of the skull were removed for examination. The upper one-third of the left radius was involved in a large pale grey mass of medullary cancer, the rest of that bone being healthy. Some cancerous nodules also occurred in the skull. The spine was shortened, but presented no outgrowths nor anchylosis. All the sutures of the skull were obliterated, the thickness of the bone being about four times the natural. The whole outer surface of the skull-cap was finely porous and reticulated for the passage of bloodvessels, and internally the grooves for the middle meningeal arteries were deepened, and a layer of dense white bone formed the inner table, but in places were intervals where reticulation was marked, in which a quantity of cancerous material was contained. The condition of the long bones was that of fine nodulation of the outer surface without any visible change in the periosteum, the surface being perforated extensively for transmission of vessels. The medulla was natural; the cancellæ had a normal disposition, but the compact substance of the shaft, and especially of the articular ends, was greatly increased in thickness. In places the outer layers of bone appeared to be separating in the form of thin plates, in other parts dense hard patches occurred. Mr. Butlin made a careful microscopical examination of the skull and the tibia, and found a diminution in the number of Haversian canals, which were widened and very confluent, and were occupied by a large amount of fibro-nuclear tissue, leucocytes, and occasionally myeloid cells and fat, around the contained vessels. The lacunæ and canaliculi were numerous, but not different from ordinary bone. A chemical analysis by Dr. Russell showed very little difference in composition to exist between the diseased and normal bone. The disease of which this case is an example is so rare and peculiar in its course that clinically it is not difficult to distinguish it, but specimens of the affection may be met with in museums under the general name of osteo-porosis, hyperostosis, senile rachitis, &c. Case 2. Ten years ago the author saw a gentleman between fifty and sixty years of age, whose general health was good, but who had been suffering for many years from pain in the thighs and legs, attended by progressive increase in the size of the bones. Death took place from medullary cancer, involving the upper end of the humerus. No post-mortem examination was made. Case 3. The author saw, with Dr. Brinton, a gentleman forty to fifty years of age, also in perfect health, with pains, enlargement, and curvature of the tibia; there was some thickening of the periosteum. Iodide of potassium was given without effect. Case 4. A case of this kind is recorded by Dr. Wilks in the Path. Trans., vol. xx. The patient was sixty years of age when he died, and had been under the care of Sir W. Gull. He first suffered pain in the legs fourteen years before death. The tibiæ enlarged, and subsequently the cranium. The thorax also became implicated, the chest gradually becoming contracted and fixed. Sir W. Gull's notes add that the disease was accompanied by weakness, occasional vertigo, lowness of voice, but no pain. The head gradually enlarged, and the stature had decreased. The ribs were thick and immovable, and there was dulness on percussion over the whole chest. Post mortem, in addition to changes in the skeleton, described as "osteo-porosis," or "spongy hypertrophy," there was an epithelioma of the dura mater as large as a chesnut. Case 5 was that of a carpenter sixty years of age, under the care of Mr. Bryant, in Guy's Hospital, with no history of syphilis, but who had for five years been subject to slight attacks of gout. Three years before admission he suffered from pains about the hamstring tendons. When seen by the author, there was marked anterior curvature of the tibiæ, the right being larger than the left; the fibula and patella were also enlarged, as were the bones of the upper limbs, chiefly humeri. The clavicles were thick, and the processes of the scapula enlarged. The ribs of the right side were slightly larger than those of the left. Usually the patient sits with his head bent forward; there is slight thickening about the internal protuberance of the occipital bone. Sir J. Paget had been unable to find recorded any cases precisely similar to these, and he considered the following to be the chief characters of the affection :—It begins in middle age or later, is very slow in progress, may continue for many years without influence on the general health, and give no other trouble than those which are due to the changes of shape, size, and direction of the diseased bones. Even when the skull is largely thickened, and all its bones exceedingly altered in structure, the mind remains unaffected. The disease affects most frequently the long bones of the lower extremities and the skull, and is usually symmetrical. The bones enlarge and soften, and those bearing weight yield and become unnaturally curved and misshapen, suggesting the proposed name, "osteitis deformans." The spine, whether by yielding to the weight of the overgrown skull, or by changes in its own structure, may sink and seem to shorten, with greatly increased dorsal and lumbar curves; the pelvis may become wide, the necks of the femora may become nearly horizontal, but the limbs, however misshapen, remain strong and fit to support the trunk. In its earlier periods, and sometimes through all its course, the disease is attended with pains in the affected bones,—pains widely various in severity, and variously described as rheumatic, gouty, or neuralgic, not especially nocturnal or periodical. It is not attended with fever. No characteristic conditions of urine or of fæces have been found in it. It is not associated with any constitutional disease, unless it be cancer, of which three out of the five cases recorded in the paper were the subjects. The bones examined after death show the consequences of an inflammation affecting, in the skull, the whole thickness, in the long bones chiefly the compact structure of their walls, and not only the walls of their shafts, but, in a very characteristic manner, those of their articular surfaces. The changes of structure produced in the earliest periods of the disease have not yet been observed, but it may be believed that they are inflammatory, for the softening is associated with enlargement, with excessive production of imperfectly developed structure, and with increased blood-supply. Whether inflammation in any degree continues to the last, or whether, after many years of progress, any reparative changes ensue, after the manner of a so-called consecutive hardening, is uncertain. The microscopic characters bear out this view of the nature of the process, and Mr. Butlin, in his report, discussing whether it might be of the nature of new growth, hypertrophy, or chronic inflammation, decides in favour of the latter. The paper goes on to point out the diagnosis from various forms of hyperostosis and osteo-porosis, some of which are dependent upon simple inflammation of bone, others upon strumous, gouty, syphilitic, and other specific inflammatory processes. In such cases it is rare to get the whole length of the bone affected, but the distinction between them and "osteitis deformans" is most evident in the clinical history, and the absolute retention of good general health in the latter. The only parallel in this latter respect is with chronic rheumatic arthritis, which, however, is perfectly distinct, and is never associated with osteitis deformans. Rachitis and osteo-malacia have scarcely a feature in common with osteitis deformans. In rachitis the bones are too short, too small, and have different curves to the elongated and thickened bones of this disease; and in osteo-malacia they are thin and bent in an angular manner. In conclusion, the paper indicated the variety of diseases which have given rise to different examples of the great porous skulls found in museums, mostly without any life history. Some of them are examples doubtless of—(1) osteitis deformans; others (2) of osteo-malacia, as in cases described by Durham and Solly, which are distinguished by their softness and lightness in proportion to their size; (3) of rachitis, where the skull is very light and friable, with a fine felt-like surface; similar skulls from young lions and tigers are to be found in the Museum of the Royal College of Surgeons; (4) from disease in early life, in which both cranial and facial bones become largely thickened, porous, or reticulated, and the cranial cavity diminished; to this group belongs the "leontiasis ossea" of Virchow; lastly (5) enormous, bossed, and nodular outgrowths from the skull, as in the specimen described by Dr. Murchison and Messrs. Hulke and De Morgan in the Pathological Society's Transactions, vol. xvii.

Mr. BRUDENELL CARTER said that three years ago he saw the patient whose case had been described by Sir James Paget. He was suffering from a little cloudiness of vision in one eye, and, speaking from memory, Mr. Carter said that all that could be detected was a number of small hæmorrhages at the periphery of the retina. Dr. Andrew Clark also saw the patient, and considered the heart to be hypertrophied.—Sir JAMES PAGET said that he had vainly tried to discover whom his patient had consulted about his vision, for he was anxious to know whether there was any indication of compression of the optic nerves.—Mr. CARTER replied that, so far as he recollected, there was no change whatever in the disc; the retinal hæmorrhages were attributed to the cardiac hypertrophy.—Mr. BARWELL said that the specimens appeared to show that the bones had lost substance interstitially, with increased deposit in other parts. Was there much increase in weight or in specific gravity? He remarked that the Germans now style the affection known as chronic rheumatic arthritis by the name of "arthritis deformans," but it could equally well be called osteitis deformans, since in it the changes in the bones are as marked as those in the joints. He alluded to the difficulties in distinguishing between dried specimens of osteo-porosis and those of the disease described in the paper.—Sir WILLIAM GULL, referring to the case which had been long under his observation, and which was mentioned in the paper, could not see why it should be considered an osteitis. There was very little pain, but gradual enlargement of the bones; the urine was always normal. If this were an osteitis, he would ask how did it arise? and why were some parts of the skeleton free from it? The clavicles and the hyoid bone were affected, but not the small bones of the hands and feet; the processes of the scapula, but not its blade. The patient died from the effects of thickening of the ribs, and consequent fixation of the chest-walls, and the whole venous system was engorged. This engorgement accounted for his mental confusion as well as for the vascularity of the bones found after death. Was the process represented in comparative anatomy? It had none of the ordinary characters of inflammation, and might be a low physiological process.—Dr. GOODHART said the paper was of great interest in its bearing upon general pathology. He noticed that a large proportion, three out of five, of the subjects of the disease had died from cancer. Was there no link between the two? He ventured to submit the hypothesis that the process was rather of the nature of a generalised tumour—a diffused growth of osseous connective tissue, comparable to the diffused growth of fibrous tissue seen in

molluscum fibrosum. If it were of this nature, and yet inflammatory, the development of cancer at the end of a length of years was very suggestive; it was as if there had been a gradual deterioration of the cells of ordinary inflammation ending in the formation of cancer. — Sir JAMES PAGET, in reply, said that the total weight of the affected bones was much increased, but not their specific gravity. The whole new product was bone, but with altered architecture. He had no doubt as to its being an osteitis, because there was a degeneracy of texture with an increase in its quantity. The gross definition of inflammation was an increased production of imperfect structures. As to its exact pathology, that was certainly doubtful. The name he had given to the disease showed that he knew nothing as to its origin, but in like manner absolutely nothing is known regarding the etiology of chronic rheumatic arthritis. He did not think there was any relation between the disease he had described and chronic rheumatic arthritis. In osteitis deformans the amount of arthritis is trivial, and in not one case of the joint disease was there any such implication of the shafts of bones as in osteitis deformans. In his exhaustive essay on chronic rheumatic arthritis, Dr. Adams, of Dublin, states that in no case does the disease affect the shaft of the bone. To Dr. Goodhart he would say that whilst the changes exhibited were so clearly the result of inflammation, it would be enlarging the field of tumours to include this change under them. He thought the coincidence of cancer in so many of the cases was accidental, and pointed out that in only one case was the cancer developed in connexion with the bone that was the seat of the osteitis; that was the case in which cancer of the dura mater occurred with the affection of the skull. In two other cases not read, one in Leyden and the other in St. Bartholomew's museum, cancer was associated with this condition of bones. At present it was a coincidence which could not be explained.

After the reading of the report of the delegates to Philadelphia, the Society adjourned.

CLINICAL SOCIETY OF LONDON.

AT the meeting of this Society on the 10th inst. (Sir W. Jenner, President, in the chair), a most interesting case of hæmophilia was read by the President, who explained that he had brought forward the case without notice because it enabled him to exhibit the organs in a recent state. After reading the notes in detail, Sir William summed up his experience of the disease in regard to its pathology and treatment. In the brief discussion that followed, some instances of the hæmorrhagic diathesis were related by Mr. Christopher Heath and Dr. Greenhow, and Mr. Howard Marsh made some remarks upon the joint-affections so frequently observed in the subjects of this malady. Dr. Theodore Williams related the sequel of a case of phthisis previously read before the Society, and showed the affected lung; and Mr. Walsham exhibited a patient with fibromatous growth in the scalp. Dr. Broadbent introduced a lad suffering from "leucæmia lymphatica," under treatment by phosphorus. The next meeting will, we believe, be devoted to the discussion of this and analogous cases, contributed by Sir W. Jenner, Dr. Gowers, and Dr. Greenfield.

Sir W. JENNER read the notes of a case of Fatal Hæmophilia. Thomas V——, aged thirteen, a printer's boy, having easy work, good food, and abundant warm clothing, was born in London, where he had lived all his life. When six years old he had scarlet fever mildly, and it was after this that it was noticed that bleeding followed slight cuts out of all proportion to their extent. On one occasion severe hæmorrhage, controlled with difficulty, followed a cut upon the back of the palate. The permanent teeth appeared late, and he had a double row of incisors. He had previously been in the hospital, and during his stay the inner row of incisors was extracted, causing hæmorrhage which was with difficulty checked. From that time to the present—i.e., for six or seven years—he was continually

such excellent results follow on the use of nux vomica and strychnia as medicines.

The really unpromising cases are those where there is emphysema of lung and at the same time a great want of activity about the diaphragm. We observe a distended chest and epigastrium, with very little abdominal movement in respiration, the diaphragm being apparently much depressed and in a semi-paralytic condition. Auscultation shows great feebleness in the air-movement within the chest, prolonged feeble expiration, and marked weakness in the voice. If there be a remedy for such cases it must be sought in careful regulation of diet and the breathing of a pure and tonic air. Another class of cases where bronchial spasm tends ultimately to serious tissue-change may be found in those complicated with atrophous emphysema of the lung. Here the bronchial muscle, worn out by attacks of spasm and inflammation during a course often of many years, becomes thin and wasted, and as this degenerative change progresses bronchial spasm gets less frequent, while dyspnœa of expiratory rhythm becomes constant and abiding. Fibrinous casts of the smaller air-tubes are sometimes expectorated by patients affected with this kind of emphysema, and I have known ulcerative destruction of lung and a true phthisis to lead to a fatal result in more than one instance where these small fibrinous strings have been expectorated. Sometimes the heart participates in the same fibroid or fatty degeneration that affects the lungs; it becomes small and atrophied, and where this change has taken place in the organ it may lead to death by syncope.

The subject of the preventive, palliative, and curative treatment of the various forms of asthma that have now been noticed will form the subject of the next and concluding lecture.

NITRO-GLYCERINE AS A REMEDY FOR ANGINA PECTORIS.

By WILLIAM MURRELL, M.R.C.P.,

LECTURER ON PRACTICAL PHYSIOLOGY AT WESTMINSTER HOSPITAL, AND ASSISTANT-PHYSICIAN TO THE ROYAL HOSPITAL FOR DISEASES OF THE CHEST.

(Continued from p. 81.)

THINKING there might be individual differences of susceptibility to the action of nitro-glycerine, I have laid my friends and others under contribution, and have induced as many as possible to give it a trial. I have notes of thirty-five people to whom I have administered it—twelve males and twenty-three females; their ages varying from twelve to fifty-eight. I find they suffered from much the same symptoms as I did, although it affects some people much more than others. Of the number above quoted, only nine took minim doses without experiencing decided symptoms. Women and those below par are much more susceptible to its action than are the strong and robust. A delicate young lady, to whom, adopting Mr. Field's suggestion, I administered it in drop doses for the relief of neuralgia, experienced very decided effects from it, each dose producing a violent headache lasting from half an hour to three hours. A married woman, aged thirty-five, took one minim with very little inconvenience, but was powerfully affected by two. She was obliged to sit down after each dose, and was positively afraid to move. It made her hot, and caused such a beating in her head that she had to support it with her hands. She experienced a heavy weight on the top of the head, and also a sharp darting pain across the forehead, which for a moment or two was very painful to bear. A friend, who for some days took four drops every three or four hours, informs me that at times it affected his head "most strangely." The pulsation was very distressing, and often lasted an hour or more, being intensified by moving. It has relieved him of an old-standing facial neuralgia, and he is enthusiastic in its praise. A young woman, aged twenty-nine, complained that after every dose of the medicine—one minim—"it seemed as if the top of her head were being lifted off," and this continued sometimes for five minutes, and sometimes longer. The medicine made her bewildered, and she felt sick. A patient with a faint apex systolic murmur was ordered one minim in half an ounce of water four times a day. He took two doses, but it caused "such a beating, thumping, hot pain" in his head that he was unable to continue it. A young man who was given nitro-glycerine in mistake for phosphorus said it made his temples throb, and he could see his pulse beat so distinctly that he was frightened. It caused a burning and flushing in his face, and "took every bit of strength away." This would last for twenty minutes or half an hour after each dose. There was no headache. That alarming symptoms may be produced by large doses, is shown by the following case. A woman, aged fifty-one, was ordered drop-doses of the one per cent. solution every four hours. This was taken well, and at the expiration of a week the dose was doubled. No complaint being made, it was then increased to four minims, and after a time to six. The patient said "the medicine agreed with her," and even leading questions failed to elicit any complaint of headache or the like. After the medicine had been taken continuously for five weeks the dose was increased to ten minims. The patient then stated that the medicine no longer agreed with her; it made her sick after every dose and took her appetite away. She always vomited about five minutes after taking the medicine, the vomiting being immediately followed by headache. The medicine made her "go off in a faint" after each dose. She had three "fainting fits" in one day, and could not venture to take another dose. She became quite insensible, and once remained so for ten minutes. Each fainting-fit was "followed by cold shivers," which "shook her violently all over." Her husband and friends were greatly alarmed, but she thought on the whole it had done her good. She had never noticed that the medicine produced drowsiness. In another case a three-minim dose taken on an empty stomach caused a feeling of faintness; "everything goes dark," the patient said, "just as if I were going to faint." The patient could take the same dose after meals without the production of any unpleasant symptom. Drowsiness is not an uncommon result of taking nitro-glycerine. A woman who was given drop-doses four times a day said that she usually went fast asleep immediately after each dose, sleeping from three to four hours. In my own case the desire for sleep was almost irresistible, although the sleep seldom lasted more than an hour. In exceptional cases none of the ordinary symptoms are exhibited. A man with epispadias—to be presently mentioned—took twenty-five minims of the one per cent. solution without any inconvenience.

From a consideration of the physiological action of the drug, and more especially from the similarity existing between its general action and that of nitrite of amyl, I concluded that it would probably prove of service in the treatment of angina pectoris, and I am happy to say that this anticipation has been realised.

As a preliminary step I was anxious to obtain a comparative series of sphygmographic tracings, and for these I am indebted to the kindness and courtesy of Dr. Fancourt Barnes, whose extensive practical acquaintance with the sphygmograph is a guarantee of their accuracy. During the last three months Dr. Barnes has taken over 150 tracings of my pulse, some showing the influence of nitro-glycerine, in others of nitrite of amyl. It would be tedious to describe the observations in detail, more especially as the tracings speak for themselves, and we consequently give only a summary of our results. Judged by the sphygmographic tracings, the effects of nitrite of amyl and of nitro-glycerine on the pulse are similar. Both drugs produce a marked state of dicrotism, and both accelerate the rapidity of the heart's action. They differ, however, in the time they respectively take to produce these effects. The full action of the nitro-glycerine is not observed in the sphygmographic tracings until six or seven minutes after the dose has been taken. In the case of nitrite of amyl the effect is obtained in from fifteen to twenty seconds after an inhalation or a dose has been taken on sugar. The influence of the nitrite of amyl is extremely transitory, a tracing taken a minute and a half after the exhibition of the drug being perfectly normal. In fact, the full effect of the nitrite of amyl on the pulse is not maintained for more than fifteen seconds. The nitro-glycerine produces its effects much more slowly; they last longer, and disappear gradually, the tracing not resuming its normal condition for nearly half an hour. The effect may be maintained for a much longer time by repeating the dose. Nitro-glycerine is more lasting in its power of producing a dicrotic form of pulse-beat, and consequently in cases where the conditions of relaxation and dicrotism are desired to be maintained for some space of time, its exhibition is to be preferred to that of nitrite of amyl].

Influence of Nitrite of Amyl on the Pulse.

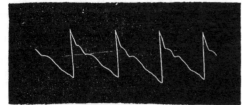

No. 1.—Before inhalation.

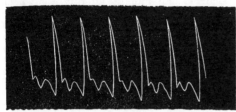

No. 2.—One minute after inhalation.

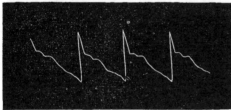

No. 3.—Two minutes after inhalation.

Influence of Nitro-Glycerine on the Pulse.

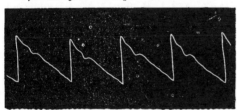

No. 1.—Before dose.

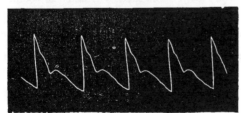

No. 2.—Two minutes after dose.

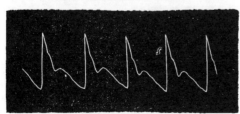

No. 3.—Eight minutes after dose.

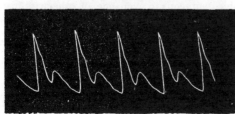

No 4. Nine minutes after dose

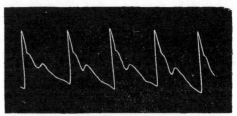

No. 5.—Ten minutes after dose.

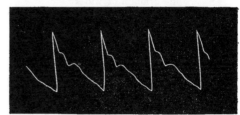

No. 6.—Twenty-two minutes after dose.

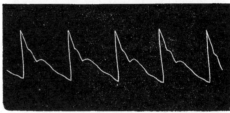

No. 7.—Twenty-six minutes after dose.

Whilst making some observations with nitro-glycerine on a patient suffering from epispadias, he called attention to the fact that the administration of the drug always caused an increased flow of urine. On examination, fifty-three minutes after the administration of a dose of twelve minims of the one per cent. solution, the urine was seen spouting from the extremity of each ureter in a little jet some three or four inches high. Ordinarily the urine dribbles away drop by drop, and never spouts out. The patient was much amazed, and said that in the whole course of his life he had never known it go on in that way. If he took beer or spirits it would increase the flow, but this, to use his own expression, "licked everything." He was made to lie on his face, so that all the urine might be collected. In twelve minutes he secreted 6¾ oz. of urine, the sp. gr. of which was only 1000. He was then given another dose of fifteen minims in a little water, and in the next twelve minutes he secreted 7¾ oz. Three days later, no nitro-glycerine having been given in the mean time, an observation was made with the view of determining the normal rate of secretion. In half an hour he secreted 3½ oz., the sp. gr. of which was 1005. This, he stated, was more than he usually passed, for he had taken three-quarters of a pint of milk about two hours before, and "it was just running through him."

On another occasion a more systematic observation was made. His urine was collected every quarter of an hour for two hours, patient having had nothing to eat or drink for four hours previously. The quantities passed were as follows :—

1st quarter of an hour, 2¾ drachms.
2nd   ,,   ,,   2¾   ,,

He was then given fifteen minims of the one per cent. nitro-glycerine solution in a drachm of water.

3rd quarter of an hour, 12 drachms.
4th   ,,   ,,   16   ,,
5th   ,,   ,,   6¾   ,,
6th   ,,   ,,   8¾   ,,
7th   ,,   ,,   5¾   ,,
8th   ,,   ,,   3   ,,

The times were accurately taken, and in no instance was any of the urine lost. The increased secretion was obviously due to the drug. It is noteworthy that the maximum increase was not till the second quarter. Every specimen was examined as it was passed, and they were all free from sugar and albumen. The quantity was too small to admit of the sp. gr. being taken by the urinometer, except in the case of the fourth quarter, when it was found to be

1003. It should be mentioned that this patient was very insusceptible to the action of the drug, and he experienced none of the ordinary symptoms from this dose.

In another observation on the same patient the results were still more striking. The same method of collecting the urine every quarter of an hour was adopted, and the following figures were obtained :—

			Sp. gr.	Pulse.
1st quarter of an hour,	4 dr.	......	—	 64
2nd ,, ,,	10½ dr.	......	1003	 64

Given twenty minims of one per cent. nitro-glycerine in one drachm of water.

			Sp. gr.	Pulse.
3rd quarter of an hour,	7 oz.	......	1000	 80
4th ,, ,,	7½ oz.	......	1000	 76
5th ,, ,,	1 oz.	......	1002	 72
6th ,, ,,	7 dr.	......	—	 68
7th ,, ,,	4½ dr.	......	—	 64

The acidity of the urine varied inversely as the quantity passed. Thus, before the administration of the drug, it was distinctly acid, during the third and fourth quarters it was almost neutral, the acidity then gradually returned, till, in the seventh quarter, it was as marked as it had been at first. No sugar or albumen was detected either before or after the administration of the drug. The figures given under the head of pulse are averages of several observations made during each quarter of an hour. No subjective symptoms of any kind were produced. The experiment was commenced at ten in the morning, and patient had had nothing to eat or drink since breakfast at six. This epispadiac man was curiously insusceptible to the action of the drug as far as subjective symptoms were concerned. I gave him the one per cent. nitro-glycerine solution on ten different occasions, in doses of 3, 4, 4, 6, 12, 15, 15, 20, and 25 minims, without causing him a moment's pain or uneasiness. He never complained of headache, or beating or throbbing in any way, and yet the influence, both on the pulse and on the secretion of the urine, was well marked. Even the small doses affected the rate of his pulse. Thus, on one occasion, his pulse was taken every minute for eleven minutes, the average being 68. He was then given a little water in a medicine glass—a practice always followed in these observations—to test the effects of expectoration. The pulse remained constant at 68 during the next five minutes, and 6 minims of the one per cent. solution were then given in water. In a minute and a half the pulse had risen to 76, and this increased rate was maintained for the next fifteen minutes, when it sank again to normal. On another occasion his pulse, taken on ten consecutive minutes, was found to be 80. He was then given twenty minims of the one per cent. solution in water. Half a minute after the pulse was still 80, in one and a half minutes after it was 96, and in two and a half minutes after it was 100, the average of the eight minutes following the administration of the drug being 96.

Such were the results of the ten series of observations on this man—negative as regards his own sensations. As a final experiment it was decided that he should take a larger dose. At 11.51 A.M., sitting still in the cool laboratory, and having had nothing since an early breakfast, his pulse was 76. At 11.55′ 30″ he took half a drachm of the one per cent. solution in a little water. At 11.56, pulse 76; at 11.57, 92; at 11.58, 96, soft and regular. At 12.4 he commenced yawning violently, and said he felt very sleepy. At 12.7 the pulse fell to 68, the yawning ceased, and he became very pale and complained of nausea. He was found to be perspiring freely all over the body, and was so hot that he kicked off his boots. The nausea lasted till 12.10, when the colour had returned to his face, and he said he felt all right again ; pulse 76 to 80. There was no headache, and even a sharp run upstairs failed to produce any feeling of pulsation. *(To be continued.)*

ON THE INTRODUCTION OF THE SOUND WHEN IT CANNOT BE PASSED.

A SOLUTION OF THE PARADOX.

BY W. F. TEEVAN, B.A., F.R.C.S.,
SURGEON TO THE WEST LONDON HOSPITAL AND ST. PETER'S HOSPITAL.

IT occasionally happens, on account of a great enlargement of the third lobe of the prostate, or the engorgement of one of its lateral lobes only, or the formation of a valve at the neck of the bladder, or the existence of a tumour of a malignant nature, that, although an elastic catheter may be passed into the bladder, the introduction of the metal sound is an impossibility through the tortuosity of the canal. In such a dilemma English surgery offers no resource ; and, although it may be of the utmost importance to pass a sound to effect a complete exploration of the bladder, that organ would, under such circumstances, remain an unexplored region were it not that a French surgeon has by a simple combination shown how the difficulty may be overcome. A celebrated surgeon being unable, after several attempts, to pass a sound on a gentleman, the patient sought the advice of M. Mercier, who, being equally unsuccessful, put into execution a plan which he had previously devised for such an emergency. The vesical extremity of a large soft catheter having been cut off in such a way as to leave a rounded end (B), a slit (*b a*), about one inch long, was made on the concavity of the tube (A B), and a strong ferrule (C) fixed on the other extremity. Some lard or wax having been put into the slit, so as to make the end smooth, the tube is introduced into the bladder. A long, slender sound, consisting of two portions (B E and F G) respectively thirteen and twelve inches in length, and capable of being screwed together, is now taken. Its beak should be placed at a more obtuse angle to the shaft than usual in order to facilitate the passage of the instrument through the soft tube. A movable handle (H) having been screwed on to the vesical half of the sound, the surgeon holds the ferrule (C) of the soft tube (A B) in his left hand, and passes the sound through the tube till the bulbous extremity of the instrument has fairly emerged from the slit (*b a*). The tube (B A) and the sound (B E) are now to be seen *in situ* as when in the bladder. The next step is to remove the soft tube so as to permit of the free manipulation of the sound and the transmission of sensations unimpaired by the coating of soft tube. This is effected by removing the handle (H) and screwing the long stem (F G)

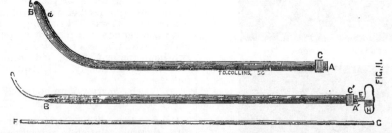

into the vesical portion (E B). The soft tube (B A) can now be retired, and the long stem removed. The handle having been screwed on to the sound again, the instrument is ready for use. Thus by the simple means I have related M. Mercier has enabled surgeons to overcome an otherwise insurmountable difficulty.

Portman-square.

CITY OF DUBLIN HOSPITAL.—Mr. W. Patton has been elected resident surgeon to this institution ; and the appointment has not been made too soon, as the absence of such an officer has caused a good deal of complaint in various quarters. The Corporation of Dublin may on this occasion claim the credit of the appointment, as the suggestion was due to them.

The Lancet,]　　　PROFESSOR PASTEUR ON THE GERM THEORY.　　　[August 13, 1881. 271

TRANSLATION OF AN

Address

ON
THE GERM THEORY.

Delivered at the Meeting of the International Medical Congress,

By PROFESSOR PASTEUR.

GENTLEMEN,—I had no intention of addressing this admirable Congress, which brings together the most eminent medical men in the world, and the great success of which does so much credit to its principal organiser, Mr. Mac Cormac. The goodwill of your esteemed President has decided otherwise. How could one, in fact, resist the sympathetic words of that eminent man whose goodness of heart is associated in no small degree with great oratorical ability? Two motives have brought me to London. The first was to gain instruction, to profit by your learned discussions; and the second was to ascertain the place now occupied in medicine and surgery by the germ theory. Certainly I shall return to Paris well satisfied. During the past week I have learned much. I carry away with me the conviction that the English people are a great people, and as for the influence of the new doctrine, I have been not only struck by the progress it has made, but by its triumph. I should be guilty of ingratitude and of false modesty if I did not accept the welcome I have received among you and in English society as a mark of homage paid to my labours during the past five-and-twenty years upon the nature of ferments—their life and their nutrition, their preparation in a pure state by the introduction of organisms (*ensemencement*) under natural and artificial conditions— labours which have established the principles and the methods of microbie (microbism), if the expression is allowable. Your cordial welcome has revived within me the lively feeling of satisfaction I experienced when your great surgeon Lister declared that my publication in 1857 on milk fermentation had inspired him with his first ideas on his valuable surgical method. You have reawakened the pleasure I felt when our eminent physician Dr. Davaine declared that his labours upon charbon (splenic fever or malignant pustule) had been suggested by my studies on butyric fermentation and the vibrion which is characteristic of it. Gentlemen, I am happy to be able to thank you by bringing to your notice a new advance in the study of microbie as applied to the prevention of transmissible diseases—diseases which for the most part are fraught with terrible consequences, both for man and domestic animals. The subject of my communication is vaccination in relation to chicken cholera and splenic fever, and a statement of the method by which we have arrived at these results—a method the fruitfulness of which inspires me with boundless anticipations. Before discussing the question of splenic fever vaccine, which is the most important, permit me to recall the results of my investigations of chicken cholera. It is through this inquiry that new and highly important principles have been introduced into science concerning the virus or contagious quality of transmissible diseases. More than once in what I am about to say I shall employ the expression virus-culture, as formerly, in my investigations on fermentation, I used the expressions, the culture of milk ferment, the culture of the butyric vibrion, &c. Let us take, then, a fowl which is about to die of chicken cholera, and let us dip the end of a delicate glass rod in the blood of the fowl with the usual precautions, upon which I need not here dwell. Let us then touch with this chaged point some *bouillon de poule*, very clear, but first of all rendered sterile under a temperature of about 115° Centigrade, and under conditions in which neither the outer air nor the vases employed can introduce exterior germs— those germs which are in the air, or on the surface of all objects. In a short time, if the little culture vase is placed in a temperature of 25° to 35°, you will see the liquid become turbid, and full of tiny microbes, shaped like the figure 8, but often so small that under a high magnifying power they appear like points. Take from this vase a drop as small as you please, no more than can be carried on the point of a glass rod as sharp as a needle, and touch with

this point a fresh quantity of sterilised *bouillon de poule* placed in a second vase, and the same phenomenon is produced. You deal in the same way with a third culture vase, with a fourth, and so on to a hundred, or even a thousand, and invariably within a few hours the culture liquid becomes turbid and filled with the same minute organisms. At the end of two or three days' exposure to a temperature of about 30° C. the thickness of the liquid disappears, and a sediment is formed at the bottom of the vase. This signifies that the development of the minute organism has ceased—in other words, all the little points which caused the turbid appearance of the liquid have fallen to the bottom of the vase, and things will remain in this condition for a longer or shorter time, for months even, without either the liquid or the deposit undergoing any visible modification, inasmuch as we have taken care to exclude the germs of the atmosphere. A little stopper of cotton sifts the air which enters or issues from the vase through changes of temperature. Let us take one of our series of culture preparations —the hundredth or the thousandth, for instance—and compare it in respect to its virulence with the blood of a fowl which has died of cholera; in other words, let us inoculate under the skin ten fowls, for instance, each separately with a tiny drop of infectious blood, and ten others with a similar quantity of the liquid in which the deposit has first been shaken up. Strange to say, the latter ten fowls will die as quickly and with the same symptoms as the former ten; the blood of all will be found to contain after death the same minute infectious organisms. This equality, so to speak, in the virulence both of the culture preparation and of the blood is due to an apparently futile circumstance. I have made a hundred culture preparations—at least, I have understood that this was done—without leaving any considerable interval between the impregnations. Well, here we have the cause of the equality in the virulence. Let us now repeat exactly our successive cultures with this single difference, that we pass from one culture, to that which follows it—from the hundredth to, say, the hundred and first, at intervals of a fortnight, a month, two months, three months, or ten months. If, now, we compare the virulence of the successive cultures, a great change will be observed. It will be readily seen from an inoculation of a series of ten fowls that the virulence of one culture differs from that of the blood and from that of a preceding culture when a sufficiently long interval elapses between the impregnation of one culture with the microbe of the preceding. More than that, we may recognise by this mode of observation that it is possible to prepare cultures of varying degrees of virulence. One preparation will kill eight fowls out of ten, another five out of ten, another one out of ten, another none at all, although the microbe may still be cultivated. In fact, what is no less strange, if you take each of these cultures of attenuated virulence as a point of departure in the preparation of successive cultures and without appreciable interval in the impregnation, the whole series of these cultures will reproduce the attenuated virulence of that which has served as the starting point. Similarly, where the virulence is null it produces no effect. How, then, it may be asked, are the effects of these attenuating virulences revealed in the fowls? They are revealed by a local disorder, by a morbid modification more or less profound in a muscle, if it is a muscle which has been inoculated with the virus. The muscle is filled with microbes which are easily recognised because the attenuated microbes have almost the bulk, the form, and the appearance of the most virulent microbes. But why is not the local disorder followed by death? For the moment let us answer by a statement of facts. They are these: the local disorder ceases of itself more or less speedily, the microbe is absorbed and digested, if one may say so, and little by little the muscle regains its normal condition. Then the disease has disappeared. When we inoculate with the microbe the virulence of which is null there is not even local disorder, the *naturæ medicatrix* carries it off at once, and here, indeed, we see the influence of the resistance of life, since this microbe, the virulence of which is null, multiplies itself. A little further, and we touch the principle of vaccination. When the fowls have been rendered sufficiently ill by the attenuated virus which the vital resistance has arrested in its development, they will, when inoculated with virulent virus, suffer no evil effects, or only effects of a passing character. In fact, they no longer die from the mortal virus, and for a time sufficiently long, which in some cases may exceed a year, chicken cholera cannot touch them, especially under the ordinary conditions of contagion which exist in fowl-houses. At this critical point of our manipulation—that is to say, in this interval of time which we have placed between two cultures, and which causes the attenuation—what occurs? I shall show you that in this interval the agent which intervenes is the oxygen of the air. Nothing more easily admits of proof. Let us produce a culture in a tube containing very little air, and close this tube with an enameller's lamp. The microbe in developing itself will speedily take all the oxygen of the tube and of the liquid, after which it will be quite free from contact with oxygen. In this case it does not appear that the microbe becomes appreciably attenuated, even after a great lapse of time. The oxygen of the air, then, would seem to be a possible modifying agent of the virulence of the microbe of chicken cholera—that is to say, it may modify more or less the facility of its development in the body of animals. May we not be here in presence of a general law applicable to all kinds of virus? What benefits may not be the result? We may hope to discover in this way the vaccine of all virulent diseases; and what is more natural than to begin our investigation of the vaccine of what we in French call charbon, what you in England call splenic fever, and what in Russia is known as the Siberian pest, and in Germany as the Milzbrand. In this new investigation I have had the assistance of two devoted young *savants*—MM. Chamberland and Roux. At the outset we were met by a difficulty. Among the inferior organisms, all do not resolve themselves into those corpuscle germs which I was the first to point out as one of the forms of their possible development. Many infectious microbes do not resolve themselves in their cultures into corpuscle germs. Such is equally the case with beer yeast, which we do not see develop itself usually in breweries, for instance, except by a sort of scissiparity. One cell makes two or more, which form themselves in wreaths; the cells become detached, and the process recommences. In these cells real germs are not usually seen. The microbe of chicken cholera and many others behave in this way, so much so that the cultures of this microbe, although they may last for months without losing their power of fresh cultivation, perish finally like beer yeast which has exhausted all its aliments. The anthracoid microbe in artificial cultures behaves very differently. In the blood of animals, as in cultures, it is found in translucid filaments more or less segmented. This blood or these cultures freely exposed to air, instead of continuing according to the first mode of generation, show at the end of forty-eight hours corpuscle germs distributed in series more or less regular along the filaments. All around these corpuscles matter is absorbed, as I have represented it formerly in one of the plates of my work on the diseases of silkworms. Little by little all connexion between them disappears, and presently they are reduced to nothing more than germ dust. If you make these corpuscles germinate, the new culture reproduces the virulence peculiar to the thready form which has produced these corpuscles, and this result is seen even after a long exposure of these germs to contact with air. Recently we discovered them in pits in which animals dead of splenic fever had been buried for twelve years, and their culture was as virulent as that from the blood of an animal recently dead. Here I regret extremely to be obliged to shorten my remarks. I should have had much pleasure in demonstrating that the anthracoid germs in the earth of pits in which animals have been buried are brought to the surface by earthworms, and that in this fact we may find the whole etiology of disease, inasmuch as the animals swallow these germs with their food. A great difficulty presents itself when we attempt to apply our method of attenuation by the oxygen of the air to the anthracoid microbes. The virulence establishing itself very quickly, often after four-and-twenty hours in an anthracoid germ which escapes the action of the air, it was impossible to think of discovering the vaccine of splenic fever in the conditions which had yielded that of chicken cholera. But was there, after all, reason to be discouraged? Certainly not; in fact, if you observe closely, you will find that there is no real difference between the mode of the generation of the anthracoid germ by scission and that of chicken cholera. We had therefore reason to hope that we might overcome the difficulty which stopped us by endeavouring to prevent the anthracoid microbe from producing corpuscle germs and to keep it in this condition in contact with oxygen for days, and weeks, and months. The experiment fortunately succeeded. In the ineffective (*neutre*) *bouillon de poule* the anthracoid microbe is no longer cultivable at 45° C.

Its culture, however, is easy at 42° or 43°, but in these conditions the microbe yields no spores. Consequently it is possible to maintain in contact with the pure air at 42° or 43° a *mycélienne* culture of bacteria entirely free of germs. Then appear the very remarkable results which follow. In a month or six weeks the culture dies—that is to say, if one impregnates with it fresh *bouillon*, the latter is completely sterile. Up till that time life exists in the vase exposed to air and heat. If we examine the virulence of the culture at the end of two days, four days, six days, eight days, &c., it will be found that long before the death of the culture the microbe has lost all virulence, although still cultivable. Before this period it is found that the culture presents a series of attenuated virulences. Everything is similar to what happens in respect to the microbe in chicken cholera. Besides, each of these conditions of attenuated virulence may be reproduced by culture; in fact, since the charbon does not operate a second time (*ne récidive pas*), each of our attenuated anthracoid microbes constitutes for the superior microbe a vaccine—that is to say, a virus capable of producing a milder disease. Here, then, we have a method of preparing the vaccine of splenic fever. You will see presently the practical importance of this result, but what interests us more particularly is to observe that we have here a proof that we are in possession of a general method of preparing virus vaccine based upon the action of the oxygen and the air—that is to say, of a cosmic force existing everywhere on the surface of the globe. I regret to be unable from want of time to show you that all these attenuated forms of virus may very easily, by a physiological artifice, be made to recover their original maximum virulence. The method I have just explained of obtaining the vaccine of splenic fever was no sooner made known than it was very extensively employed to prevent the splenic affection. In France we lose every year by splenic fever animals of the value of 20,000,000f. I was asked to give a public demonstration of the results already mentioned. This experiment I may relate in a few words. Fifty sheep were placed at my disposition, of which twenty-five were vaccinated. A fortnight afterwards the fifty sheep were inoculated with the most virulent anthracoid microbe. The twenty-five vaccinated sheep resisted the infection; the twenty-five unvaccinated died of splenic fever within fifty hours. Since that time my energies have been taxed to meet the demands of farmers for supplies of this vaccine. In the space of fifteen days we have vaccinated in the departments surrounding Paris more than 20,000 sheep and a large number of cattle and horses. If I were not pressed for time I should bring to your notice two other kinds of virus attenuated by similar means. These experiments will be communicated by-and-by to the public. I cannot conclude, gentlemen, without expressing the great pleasure I feel at the thought that it is as a member of an international medical congress assembled in England that I make known the most recent results of vaccination upon a disease more terrible, perhaps, for domestic animals than small-pox is for man. I have given to vaccination an extension which science, I hope, will accept as a homage paid to the merit and to the immense services rendered by one of the greatest men of England, Jenner. What a pleasure for me to do honour to this immortal name in this noble and hospitable city of London!

General Address

ON

THE CONNEXION OF THE BIOLOGICAL SCIENCES WITH MEDICINE.

Delivered at the Meeting of the International Medical Congress.

BY T. H. HUXLEY, LL.D.,
SECRETARY TO THE ROYAL SOCIETY, AND VICE-PRESIDENT OF THE CONGRESS.

THE great body of theoretical and practical knowledge which has been accumulated by the labours of some eighty generations, since the dawn of scientific thought in Europe, has no collective English name to which an objection may not be raised; and I use the term "medicine" as that which

pox. These diseases caused the lowest death-rates in Huddersfield and Bristol, and the highest in Norwich and Wolverhampton. The highest rates of mortality from diarrhœa were recorded in Leicester, Norwich, and Wolverhampton ; from measles in Wolverhampton and Blackburn ; from whooping-cough in Sunderland and Derby ; and from scarlet fever in Wolverhampton and Sheffield. Of the 21 deaths from diphtheria in the twenty-eight towns, as many as 19 were recorded in London. Small-pox caused 9 deaths in London (exclusive of 3 metropolitan cases registered outside Registration London), and 1 in Sheffield. The number of small-pox patients in the metropolitan asylum hospitals situated in and around London, which in the five previous weeks had declined from 1368 to 810, further fell to 640 on Saturday last ; the cases admitted were 64, against 66 and 110 in the two preceding weeks. The Highgate Small-pox Hospital contained 37 patients on Saturday last, 6 new cases having been admitted during the week. The deaths referred to diseases of the respiratory organs in London, which in the two previous weeks had been 198 and 187, further declined to 162, and were 14 below the corrected average. The causes of 92, or 2·3 per cent., of the 4052 deaths last week in the twenty-eight towns were not certified either by a registered medical practitioner or by a coroner. All the causes of death were duly certified in Bristol, Sunderland, Norwich, Derby, and Cardiff. The largest proportions of uncertified deaths were recorded in Blackburn, Oldham, and Huddersfield.

HEALTH OF SCOTCH TOWNS.

The annual rate of mortality in the eight Scotch towns, which had been 20·6 and 20·7 in the two preceding weeks, was again 20·7 in the week ending the 16th inst. ; it was 3·4 below the average rate during the same period in twenty-eight of the largest English towns. The rates in the Scotch towns last week ranged from 13·4 and 13·6 in Paisley and Greenock, to 23·5 in Perth, and 25·9 in Glasgow. The 499 deaths in the eight towns included 51 which resulted from diarrhœal diseases, 29 from whooping-cough, 9 from scarlet fever, 9 from measles, 6 from "fever," 5 from diphtheria, and not one from small-pox ; in all, 109 deaths were referred to these principal zymotic diseases, against 85, 95, and 114 in the three preceding weeks. These 109 deaths were equal to an annual rate of 4·5 per 1000, which was 2·1 below the mean rate from the same diseases last week in the twenty-eight large English towns. The deaths from diarrhœal diseases, which had been 40 and 51 in the two previous weeks, were again 51 last week, and exceeded by 8 the number in the corresponding week of last year ; 27 were returned in Glasgow and 7 in Edinburgh. The rate of mortality from diarrhœa in the Scotch towns did not exceed 2·1 per 1000, while it averaged 4·7 in the large English towns. The 29 fatal cases of whooping-cough were within 2 of the number in the preceding week, and included 20 in Glasgow and 4 in Edinburgh. All the 9 deaths from scarlet fever were recorded in Glasgow, where 6 of the 9 fatal cases of measles were also returned. The deaths from "fever" showed a further increase upon recent weekly numbers, while those from diphtheria showed a decline of 2 from the number in the preceding week. The deaths referred to acute diseases of the respiratory organs in the eight Scotch towns were 64, against 66 and 65 in the two previous weeks, and were 8 below the number returned in the corresponding week of last year. The causes of 77, or more than 15 per cent., of the deaths in the eight Scotch towns last week were not certified.

HEALTH OF DUBLIN.

The rate of mortality in Dublin, which had been 23·0 and 22·4 per 1000 in the two preceding weeks, rose to 24·2 in the week ending the 16th inst. During the first seven weeks of the current quarter the death-rate in the city averaged 22·0 per 1000, the rate during the same period being equal to 23·0 in London and 17·0 in Edinburgh. The 163 deaths in Dublin last week exceeded by 12 the number in the previous week, and included 33 which resulted from the principal zymotic diseases, against 16, 22, and 23 in the three preceding weeks ; of these, 22 were referred to diarrhœal diseases, 6 to scarlet fever, 4 to "fever" (typhus, enteric, or simple), 1 to whooping-cough, and not one either to small-pox, measles, or diphtheria. These 33

deaths were equal to an annual rate of 4·9 per 1000, the rate from the same diseases being 5·1 in London and 2·7 in Edinburgh. The deaths referred to diarrhœa, which had been 11 and 8 in the two previous weeks, rose to 22 last week. The fatal cases of scarlet fever corresponded with the number in the preceding week, while those of "fever" and diphtheria showed a decline. The deaths of infants considerably exceeded the number in the previous week, while those of elderly persons were below the average of recent weeks. The causes of 30, or more than 18 per cent., of the deaths registered during the week were not certified.

THE SERVICES.

Surgeon-Major E. C. Markey, medical officer in charge of the Cambridge Hospital, Aldershot, is held in readiness for immediate embarkation for Egypt. Brigade-Surgeon E. G. McDowell, C.B , has been ordered to Aldershot to assume charge of the Cambridge Hospital.

ADMIRALTY.—Fleet Surgeon Robert Nelson has been appointed to the *Achilles.*

ARTILLERY VOLUNTEERS. — The Tynemouth : Acting Surgeon William Pope Mears, M.D., from the 1st Northumberland and Sunderland Artillery Volunteer Corps, to be Acting Surgeon.

RIFLE VOLUNTEERS.—1st Volunteer Battalion, the Buffs (East Kent Regiment) : Surgeon Charles Holttum is granted the honorary rank of Surgeon-Major.

Correspondence.

"Audi alteram partem."

THE DEMONSTRATION OF THE BACILLUS LEPRÆ.

To the Editor of THE LANCET.

SIR,—The discovery of bacillus lepræ, though made some years before that of bacillus tuberculosis, has not been put to the same very practical use in diagnosis that immediately followed the discovery of the latter bacterium. The reason for this lies in the comparative difficulty hitherto attending the demonstration of the parasite of leprosy. To show it, it has been necessary to excise a portion of affected tissue—an operation naturally objected to even by a leper ; and afterwards the tedious processes of hardening and section-cutting have to be gone through prior to the final staining, washing, and mounting ; and even then, when the preparation, the result of so much labour, is under the microscope, it sometimes, especially to the untrained eye, may require a considerable exercise of faith to recognise in the patches and ill-defined streaks of colour the bacillus. I have shown such specimens to friends, and at times their smiles were more indicative of incredulity than conviction.

By a method I now adopt, the bacillus can be demonstrated as easily, rapidly, and perfectly as can that of tubercle, and the preparations are so clear that on examining them the most thorough sceptic is immediately converted to a belief in the bacillus lepræ. I proceed as follows :—A leper tubercle or infiltrated patch is selected and the whole or part of it included in the jaws of an ordinary thin-bladed pile clamp. The tightening of the clamp has the effect of driving out all the blood from the included tissues, and the tubercle, from being dirty red or purple, becomes like yellow wax. The hold of the clamp is maintained at a degree of tightness sufficient to keep up this state of anæmia, and at the same time the centre of the included mass is pricked with a needle or sharp knife. From the puncture a droplet of perfectly clear fluid exudes, and is to be transferred to one or more cover-glasses, each cover-glass being smeared with rather a thick layer of the leper juice. The cover-glasses are then dried, stained, washed, and mounted in the ordinary way. The Weigert Ehrlich method I have found give good results. Under the microscope slides so prepared show bacilli in prodigious numbers, both free and in dense bundles packing the leper cells. The diagnosis of leprosy from the juice of the leper tubercle is in this way made as easy, expeditious, and reliable as is that of tubercular phthisis from sputum.

Trusting that this hint may be of service to those interested in leprosy and its bacillus,

I am, Sir, yours truly,

Hong-Kong, China, July 9th, 1884.   PATRICK MANSON.

THE CASE OF JOSEPH JAMES DONNELLY.
To the Editor of THE LANCET.

SIR,—Dr. Hughes Bennett finishes a very instructive letter in this day's LANCET upon the case of Joseph James Donnelly by asking a question, which I am very glad to be able to answer if you will grant me space in your columns for the purpose.

Dr. Bennett writes :—"The public have a right to be informed whether this individual is for the future to be considered as a lunatic, and consequently as an innocent man, or whether he is to undergo penal servitude for life as a malefactor." Dr. Bennett will, I am sure, be glad to learn that Donnelly was admitted into the epileptic ward of this asylum on Monday, the 4th inst., where, if Dr. Bennett should ever be in this neighbourhood and should have half an hour to spare, he may, if so inclined, renew his acquaintance with his quondam patient, and at the same time afford me the pleasure of showing him the general arrangements of the asylum.

It is very justly pointed out by Dr. Bennett that, Donnelly being what in his letter to you he describes him to be, two things of a nature to be regretted have happened in his case. The first is, that he was permitted to have the opportunity of killing his sister; and the second is, that he was afterwards tried and sentenced as if he had been a responsible malefactor. Now, although no one would, I think, have the hardihood to hazard the assertion that our statutes relating to lunatics are perfect, or that the resources of civilisation have been exhausted with respect to our modes of procedure in the treatment of these unfortunate persons, still we are, happily, not compelled to own that there is absolutely nothing that could be done, in a similar case in the future, to avert the occurrence of similar unfortunate incidents.

With respect to the means for the possible prevention of the recurrence of similar acts of homicidal violence, I would ask your permission to point out that any medical gentleman who possessed information similar to that which Dr. Bennett possessed as to his patient, at the time of discharging him from hospital, would be taking a legal and justifiable course if he were to address a letter to the relieving officer of the parish to which the patient belonged. stating the circumstances, together with his opinion of the patient's mental condition. Upon the receipt of such a letter every relieving officer of a parish is bound by statute (16 and 17 Vict., chap. 97, sect. 68) to make inquiry into the case.

With respect to the second point, the suggestion that I would venture to make is, that if any medical gentleman should ever be in possession of any facts relating to the mental condition of any person committed for trial upon a charge of murder, and should be in any doubt or difficulty as to the right course to take in the matter, he may. if so disposed, address a letter to me stating the facts, and I will, very gladly, charge myself with the duty of taking steps for bringing before the court and the jury such facts as may reach me in this way. The only stipulations I would make are, that the information should reach me sufficiently long before the trial, and that the facts should either be within the personal cognizance of the writer or be capable of proof by witnesses.

With the view of disarming criticism beforehand, will you permit me to add that I do not offer these suggestions as if I thought that they contained the whole duty of man in the matter, but that I offer them only as possible aids to those in doubt.   I am, Sir, your obedient servant,

W. ORANGE.

Broadmoor Criminal Lunatic Asylum, Aug. 16th, 1884.

To the Editor of THE LANCET.

SIR,—As you do me the honour to refer to a letter of mine in your leading article of the 9th inst. on the above case, I trust you will allow me to state, in as few words as possible, why I find myself unable to agree with some of the remarks in that article.

First of all, you seem to doubt the propriety of interfering to prevent the execution of the capital sentence when once it has been pronounced ; you "think that matters of this sort should be dealt with finally at the time of trial, or rather before it," and although you allow Donnelly's to be one of the exceptional instances which call for inquiry, you state in general terms that you do not "think it expedient, in the interests of public safety, that there should be this last chance of escape open to criminals." My answer is that cases occur not unfrequently in which, from the poverty of the accused and the peculiarities in our English methods of judicial procedure, the arguments in support of the plea of insanity are imperfectly brought out during the trial. Take, for example, this very case. Donnelly's friends were too poor to provide him with any sort of legal assistance, so that had not a member of the Bar kindly undertaken the defence at the request of the presiding judge, the poor fellow would have been left without anyone to plead his cause. As it was, his counsel entered upon his task under every conceivable disadvantage ; no defence had been prepared, no witnesses had been summoned on the prisoner's behalf ; and as the prosecution did not happen to produce the one witness, Dr. Dreschfeld, whose evidence was likely to tell in the man's favour, it was impossible to elicit, in cross-examination, the facts which were necessary in order to sustain the plea. It is perfectly evident, therefore, that the trial could not, in the nature of things, be a satisfactory one ; and to my mind it would be horrible if a decision, arrived at under such circumstances, should be held to be irreversible.

If it be asked why means were not taken to interfere in the matter before or during the trial, I reply that interference by persons not directly concerned in a case that is *sub judice* is generally supposed not only to be impolitic but absolutely reprehensible. It seems to me that I adopted the only course open to me ; I abstained from interference until the trial was over, and until there was imminent danger of a deplorable miscarriage of justice. That the case was one that needed revision is proved by the fact (of which, of course, I was not aware when I wrote to the local papers) that the Government had already sent two medical inspectors to report on the case, and that in consequence of their report the man has been reprieved during Her Majesty's pleasure.

But there is a still more important point in your leading article on which I am compelled to differ from you. You compare the condition of an epileptic maniac with that of a patient rendered irascible and peevish from an attack of gout, or from phthisis in a certain stage, or from the approach of certain changes in the sexual life. In my opinion the two conditions are incomparable. In the case of an epileptic maniac, his acts of violence are done unconsciously, and therefore are uncontrollable ; in all the other cases mentioned, acts of a similar nature would always be done consciously, and would simply be the result of uncontrolled temper. Epileptics like Donnelly have no control over their actions during the maniacal paroxysm, and no recollection of them when it is over. They are therefore legally and morally irresponsible, and no effort can be too great to prevent their being systematically treated as criminals.

I remain, Sir, yours very truly,

CHARLES J. CULLINGWORTH, M.D.. M.R.C.P.,

Lecturer on Medical Jurisprudence at the Owens

August 13th, 1884.   College, Manchester.

P.S.—As my letter happened to be too late for insertion last week, may I be allowed to add a postscript, expressive of the pleasure with which I read Dr. A. Hughes Bennett's letter in THE LANCET of last Saturday ? I entirely concur in the sentiment to which he has given such forcible expression. With regard, however, to the mismanagement of the prisoner's defence, the above letter will show that our system of preparing cases for trial is more to be blamed for the extreme unsatisfactoriness of this inquiry, than the very able advocate who kindly undertook the defence at the last moment, without having received any instructions, and who was consequently at an enormous disadvantage throughout the case.

THE CHOLERA IN FRANCE.
To the Editor of THE LANCET.

SIR,—Before leaving for Paris, I send you a line to say that on visiting the hospitals, both of Toulon and this place, I was agreeably surprised to find all the patients either con-

ON the 10th ult., the death, from fever, occurred at Sierra Leone of Mr. Nathaniel Cameron. The deceased, who was a native of Abernethy, on Speyside, had a distinguished career at college, both in arts and medicine, carrying off high prizes in both departments. In 1876 he graduated at the Aberdeen University with the highest academical honours, and subsequently became Assistant Demonstrator of Anatomy in that University. After acting as resident physician at the Macclesfield Infirmary for a brief period, Mr. Cameron in 1878 entered the Army Medical Department, and went out to Sierra Leone, where, as above stated, he died.

THE salary of Mr. S. W. North, the medical officer of health of the York Urban Sanitary District, has been increased from £150 to £250 per annum. At the meeting of the York City Council, at which the resolution was proposed and carried, a characteristic remark was made by one of the councillors—viz., that "Mr. North had caused the property in that neighbourhood to decrease very much in value." The medical officer could scarcely desire better testimony to the value of his services.

THE polluted state of the river Wey is causing considerable discussion, and several writers in *The Times* have recently called attention to the fact that this river, which used to be a source of delight, not only to those who lived by its borders, but also to the numerous visitors, artists, and others who came to enjoy the lovely scenery, has become little else than an open sewer for the towns of Godalming and Guildford.

DR. ALLARD, physician to the International African Association, who has returned to Brussels after a stay of three years in the Congo territory, has assured a representative of the *Indépendance Belge* that all the stations are in a flourishing condition, that the report that a high rate of mortality prevails amongst Europeans is false, and that the climate is not insupportable, as has been alleged.

AT the competition examination held this week at the London University, Burlington-gardens, for admission into the public medical services, we understand there were seventy-eight candidates for thirty appointments on the Army Medical Staff, twenty-two for seven in the Indian Medical Service, and twenty-two for sixteen in the Royal Navy.

AT a recent meeting of the Finchley Local Board, Dr. Turle, the medical officer, stated that the epidemic of whooping-cough in the district is so severe that he could not give the Board an approximate idea of the number of cases, they being so numerous that the local medical men had been unable to keep an account of them.

MR. A. O. MACKELLAR, M.Ch., F.R.C.S., senior assistant-surgeon to, and lecturer on Practical Surgery at, St. Thomas's Hospital, has been appointed Chief Surgeon to the Metropolitan Police, in the place of Mr. Timothy Holmes, F.R.C.S., resigned.

THE Municipal Council of Marseilles on the 11th inst. voted 100,000 fr. for sanitary improvements. On the same day, at the Paris Academy of Medicine, Dr. Brouardel read a paper on the Bad Sanitary State of Marseilles, severely blaming the negligence of the municipality.

THE *Russkaya Meditsina* says that a medical man recently bought five pounds of camomiles at an apothecary's in Moscow, and on sifting his purchase found a full pound of sand!

THE *Odessa Vestnik* states that a bacterioscopical laboratory has been organised at the town hospital by Dr. Stroganov.

THE Russian medical journal *Vrach* is sending a commission to Spain to study the cholera, consisting of Professor Manassein, the editor, and Drs. Raptschevski and Kurlov.

REPORT
OF
The Lancet Special Commission
ON THE
SANITARY CONDITION OF WINDSOR.

WINDSOR has acquired an unenviable reputation for bad sanitation. This is no new complaint. The grievance rests rather in the fact that the evil, though frequently denounced and of old standing, has never yet been satisfactorily remedied. Even in the time of William IV., when someone was speaking of the approaches to the Castle, the King retorted by qualifying them as the reproach of Windsor. Charles Knight, in 1859, published a humorous denunciation of Windsor, which was his native town. Again, in 1871, some sensation was caused by a detailed technical description given in the columns of the *Builder* of the hotbeds of small-pox that existed in the Royal town; and in 1876 the rector of a parish containing some of the worst slums commenced an agitation, which is still pressed forward with great energy. The authorities have, however, shown exceptional apathy. Public opinion has certainly compelled them to attempt a few slight improvements, but such measures have been taken reluctantly and under protest that there was no cause of complaint. Thus, for nearly fifteen years there has been no revision in the borough bye-laws, though during that time all the more important towns of England have not failed to so recast their sanitary regulations as to make them harmonise with the modern principles of hygiene. Nor is this progress limited to the towns; even the neighbouring rural district of Windsor issued new and admirably conceived bye-laws bearing the recent date of August, 1881, but the town itself is still content to abide by the inferior stipulations enacted by the Windsor Board of Health in 1871. Finally, if we add to these circumstances the fact that the medical officer of health reports the number of deaths during this summer to be above the average, sufficient cause will be found to justify a special inquiry.

Three considerations naturally suggest themselves as reasons why the health of Windsor should be a matter of special solicitude. Firstly, it is a Royal residence and a garrison town; secondly, it is only separated from Eton College by the river; and thirdly, it is visited by a large number of tourists and excursionists. We find, on the contrary, that the town is infected by a poisonous ditch; that the inhabitants are still allowed to drink contaminated well-water; that there are slums within a stone's throw of the Castle gates which are hotbeds of epidemic disease; and that, even in the wealthiest quarters, complaints are constantly made of sewers that smell, and open ditches which receive refuse, soil, and the overflow from cesspools. Further, while so little concern has been shown to prevent epidemics, no steps whatever are taken to cope with them when once they have broken out. There is a sort of hospital consisting of a few private houses strung together, but no fever case would be received into it; and, indeed, it is doubtful if this building possesses the necessary sanitary qualifications for ordinary purposes. At the present moment the wards are vacated, and an investigation is taking place. When fever breaks out the case must be treated at home, however unsuitable the home may be. Thus, in July last year, a case of small-pox occurred in a narrow court immediately opposite the principal entrance to the Castle.

bronchitis, rheumatism, and Bright's disease. The remaining "chill diseases" form a large and rather vague group, for which no very definite cause has been assigned, and which has not yet been divided into definite clinical units. The etiological question to be solved as to these has in consequence not been so stated as to admit of a definite reply. An apparent but needful digression is here intruded and apologised for. The stricter doctrines as to causes which consider them as necessary invariable antecedents—under constant conditions—are not easily applicable in medicine. If they were, we must at once say that these diseases are not caused by cold, although our conclusions become so much the less trustworthy in proportion as we use less stringent tests. The less exact, but still valuable, formula given by Sir Thos. Watson, by which diseases are imputed to certain frequently recurring antecedents with a degree of confidence measured by the uniformity of the conjunction and the rarity of the disjunction of the consecutive events, does not yield certain conclusions, and is, indeed, seldom used with due rigour. More commonly we refer a disease to some apparent outward change, usually held to be competent, such as exposure to cold, and attempt to explain the cases in which no result occurs by assuming a predisposition on the part of those who do suffer. Yet in some simple maladies in which it has been possible to put the question with definiteness the causes have been proved by invariable antecedence, by equality of effect, and by promptitude of action, just as in physical matters. So must the group of chill diseases be dealt with if equally positive conclusions are to be hoped for. They must be divided into defined clinical units, and the etiological question be separately put for each. At present, however, we are taught that the same cause may produce many and very different diseases, and *vice versâ*; or, in other words, that a cause is a variable and inconstant antecedent, and neither measures the intensity nor modifies the quality of the effect. It may be freely granted that where a state of unstable equilibrium exists it may be upset by any one of many diverse and often trivial causes, and that the effects are then determined less by the nature of the disturbing agent than by the kind of relations which subsist between the parts of the mechanism disturbed. Instances of this are common in medical practice. But these cases are not comparable with such diseases as are under consideration, in which we seek the causes of definite diseases in an averagely healthy person. Even where such a state of unstable equilibrium exists, we seek to learn that which brought it about, not so much that which disturbed it, for this may be replaced. We seek what may prevent a malady if it be avoided, or cure if it be removed. It may be as freely granted that disease processes, such as inflammation and fever, are caused by many and different agents; but it does not follow that the various forms of these generic processes are so indifferently caused. The statistical evidence is not a sufficient proof. It tells us not the causes of particular diseases, but some conditions of their action. On such grounds alone we might as well attribute typhus to cold as bronchitis and pneumonia. Moreover, in considering the statistics of disease we must take into account the great variations in nomenclature and diagnosis which exist and impair the value of the data. The topographical distribution of bronchitis and pneumonia in England and Wales, so far as it goes, is in conflict with the current doctrine; and the same may be said of the geographical distribution of rheumatism. Such statistics as exist and are used in support of the doctrine take insufficiently into account contrary instances. These contrary instances which we see in the now frequent therapeutic employment of cold should also be more fully allowed for. The common experience and general acceptance of the doctrine both by the laity and the profession, although difficult to resist, do not amount to proof. The existing prepossessions are, indeed, pitfalls for the investigator, by giving a bias, which is especially shown by patients who continually state their inferences as facts. The common expression "a cold" begs the question, and yet is in almost universal use. My own experience, after nearly thirty years of rather special attention to this question, leads me to say that only in a very small minority of cases can the fact be established that a sufferer from a malady imputed to cold has been exposed to its influence in any unusual degree at an appropriate time prior to the commencement of the malady. So that I would extend Jürgensen's views about pneumonia to many forms of bronchial catarrh, pleurisy, rheumatism, and some other diseases. The cases in which after the action of severe cold serious disease has so promptly followed as to suggest a causal relation are too few in number to materially affect the argument. This doctrine, which refers to cold the production of so many serious and varied diseases of distant viscera, is difficult to reconcile with such notions of pathogeny as are derivable from the study of the simpler maladies, surgical affections, and experimentally produced diseases. These teach us that, conditions being constant, the effect follows the action of the cause with considerable constancy, and is measured by it; so that any variation of the causal agent or of the subject of its action is followed by a corresponding change in the resulting malady. This doctrine conflicts also with our notions of the pathogeny of inflammation as they are shown in triumphs of modern surgery. Conceiving of inflammation as the reaction of a living tissue to an injurious irritation, the rule seems constant that when the irritant is a simple mechanical or physical one the resulting inflammation is in direct proportion to the irritation, limited nearly in extent to the area irritated, as well as in time to a short period beyond that of the action of the irritant. The effects of cold might be expected to follow this rule, and do so as regards those effects about which there is no doubt. But the visceral diseases imputed to it do not; they much more resemble in their clinical aspect some of the infectious diseases. I am, however, inclined to the view that in some at least of these cold may be a factor in the production of the disease. I venture here to suggest that in these visceral inflammations there exists a real and specific distinction—whether clinically recognisable or not—between the forms of bronchitis caused by, say, cold, or by the pollen of certain grasses, or by an overdose of potassium iodide, or by the morbid virus of measles, and so on; and similarly between the pneumonias which are due to diverse causes. Thus I should expect to find almost as many species of inflammation of internal viscera as we now accept for the skin. Although it may not have equal weight with all persons, I attach some importance to a conflict which, to my mind, exists between this doctrine and the idea I have formed of the evolution of the faculty to inflame—in the sense of the power of living things to react against injuries. To me it seems that this faculty to protect by such reaction is more complete as against the more universally prevalent and long-existing injurious agents than against those of more recent and less constant action, and that organisms are thus better protected against mechanical and physical influences than against organic and organised ones.

Its injurious results are a widespread reduction of the average standard of health, brought about by habits which cultivate delicacy, while blindly incurring other and graver risks than those which it is sought to avoid; and a serious hindrance to the rational treatment of disease by abundant aeration, and to a sound hygienic practice.

Summary and conclusion.—I have tried fairly to state the doctrine, the grounds upon which is supposed to rest, its want of definiteness, as well as the weakness of the evidence put forward in its support; and I have ventured to suggest an alternative hypothesis, less indefinite and more open to proof or disproof. Should my views find favour, I should expect that advantages to public health and to both the theory and practice of medicine would result.

FIFTEEN CASES OF
TUMOURS OF THE BLADDER,
DIAGNOSED BY MEANS OF THE ELECTRO-ENDOSCOPIC CYSTOSCOPE.

BY DR. MAX NITZE.

IN the following lines I wish to direct the attention of my English *confrères* to the value of the electro-endoscopic mode of examination of the male urinary bladder, invented by me. I believe I could not have chosen a more suitable theme for that purpose than a short report of the bladder tumours diagnosed by me cystoscopically; for the diagnosis of these new formations offers the greatest difficulty, and in most cases it has been impossible till now to prove their existence with accuracy without digital exploration of the bladder. By the new method of cystoscopical examination the conditions have entirely changed. One look into the bladder, illuminated as if by daylight, is generally sufficient to afford means for forming an opinion of all the questions coming into consideration—viz., size, form, and site of the tumour. The accompanying diagrams (Figs. 1, 2, 3, 4) may give an idea of the appearances which the different forms of bladder tumours present endoscopically. I regret that they cannot show the brightness of the light by which one sees the tumours during examination. The celebrated Vienna specialist, v. Dittel, is right in saying "that they offer sometimes truly charming pictures"; especially certain kinds of villous tumours, whose long slender villi floating in the liquid often present a splendid appearance. The following are the cases cystoscopically diagnosed by me.

CASE 1.—A man, aged fifty-five, under the care of Dr. Ch. Mayer, suffered from attacks of hæmaturia for thirty years. During the last six years he has had dysuria and inability to empty the bladder completely. The patient had been examined by the sound repeatedly by eminent

FIG. 1.

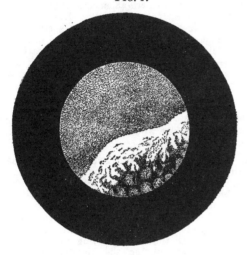

surgeons and specialists, but none could give a certain diagnosis. On Nov. 11th, 1886, I undertook the cystoscopic examination. I found on the anterior wall of the bladder a puffy swelling covered with white masses of mucus. (See Fig. 1.) The trigone was covered by a mass consisting of pointed papillæ. On account of the weakness of the patient extirpation was impossible. The patient became weaker and weaker, and died in June, 1887. The post-mortem examination showed the internal orifice of the urethra surrounded by a swelling representing a continuous tumour as large as a small apple. It was found that the instrument had penetrated through the middle of this swelling, which bled easily on pressure. In spite of this the clearness of the picture was not interfered with in the least.

CASE 2.—A man, aged fifty, was obliged to exert a strong pressure in order to empty the bladder. The flow of urine

FIG. 2.

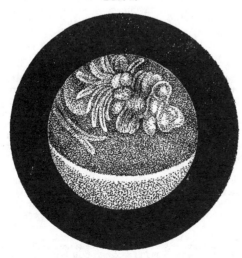

often stopped. He himself introduced a catheter, and on

withdrawing it a piece of villous tissue was found. On Dec. 10th, 1886, I saw, on cystoscopical examination, directly and immediately over the internal orifice of the urethra, a villous swelling hanging from the anterior wall of the bladder. (See Fig. 2.) On Jan. 15th, 1887, extirpation of the tumour by means of the high section was performed by Professor v. Bergmann. The size of the tumour (which was as large as a pigeon's egg) and its position corresponded exactly to the endoscopic picture. The patient recovered.

CASE 3.—A patient under the care of Professor Madelung, aged fifty-five, suffered from attacks of hæmaturia. Examination by sound and rectal palpation had given me negative results. On Feb. 20th, 1887, cystoscopical examination was made. On the left side of the trigone a tumour with a broad base was seen, which resembled somewhat a strawberry in size and form. (See Fig. 3.) On March 1st

FIG. 3.

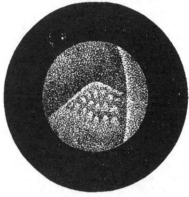

Professor Madelung undertook the extirpation of the tumour. The appearance corresponded exactly to the crystoscopic picture. The patient recovered.

CASE 4.—This was a patient on whom Dr. Israel had performed the high section a long time before, on account of a bladder tumour. The extent was so great that only its most prominent part could be removed. The microscopical examination proved the diagnosis of cancer. Quick healing took place. The patient became free from pain, and the urine became clear. In order to see what had become of the remaining part, the cystoscopical examination was under-

FIG. 4.

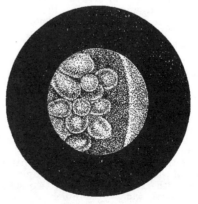

taken on April 3rd. It was easy to see that the right lateral wall was covered to an extent of from three to four centimetres with thick masses of verrucous and fungiform excrescences. (See Fig. 4.)

CASE 5.—A patient of Dr. Boegehold suffered from attacks of hæmaturia for six months. Examination by sound gave negative results. The cystoscopic examination at once showed in the region of the left ureter a tumour consisting of long floating villi. The patient objected to an operation.

CASE 6.—A patient under the care of Dr. Goldschmidt had for seven months repeated attacks of hæmaturia and pain in the region of the bladder. Examination by sound and rectal palpation gave negative results. The cystoscopic examination, on May 7th, 1887, showed the lower half of the right wall of the bladder covered by dense verrucous excrescences. On account of the great extent of the tumour and the probability of malignancy, operation was not deemed advisable.

CASE 7.—This patient, under the care of Dr. Behnke, had for two years and a half, from time to time, attacks of hæmaturia. The cystoscopic examination showed on the left wall of the bladder a large villous tumour. Soon after I showed the patient to the Gesellschaft für Heilkunde. Many members of the profession convinced themselves by inspection of the evident clearness of the appearances. Operation was proposed to the patient, but he refused.

CASE 8.—A patient, aged sixty-three, in the clinique of Professor Leyden, had for a long time profuse hæmaturia. Examination by sound had given negative results. On July 9th, 1887, cystoscopical examination was made, the conditions being particularly unfavourable. The meatus was narrower than normal; the urine contained much blood, and was of a dark, brownish-red colour. In spite of this the cystoscope allowed of a satisfactory view. Many confrères could see the villous tumour hanging from the anterior wall of the bladder. It was as large as a walnut; some of the villi appeared black-coloured in consequence of hæmorrhages. The patient left the hospital soon afterwards.

CASE 9.—A patient, aged sixty, in the clinique of Professor v. Bergmann. For a long time he had had attacks of hæmaturia and difficulty in emptying the bladder. Repeated examinations by sound and rectal palpation had given negative results. On Nov. 14th, 1887, cystoscopic examination was made. I saw on the floor of the bladder a flat button-shaped tumour covered by short villi. The front of the left lateral wall was found covered with similar villi as far as the orifice of the urethra. On Nov. 17th operation (high section) was performed, when the cystoscopical appearances were in every respect confirmed, but at the same time it was observed that the carcinomatous infiltration under the normal mucous membrane was so extensive that a complete removal was impossible. After some time the patient died from the new formation.

CASE 10.—A female patient of Professor Sonnenburg, aged twenty-one, observed for nine months from time to time that the urine was mixed with blood. Lately a well-marked villus was expelled with the urine. The examination by sound showed nothing abnormal. On Nov. 21st cystoscopic examination showed on the outer side of the right ureter a flat coin-shaped tumour consisting of short villi. As the patient was in the fourth month of pregnancy, a radical operation was rejected. Professor Sonnenburg dilated the urethra and scraped the tumour away with his finger-nail. The conditions corresponded exactly to the cystoscopical appearance.

CASE 11.—A man, aged sixty-seven, sent to me by Dr. Behnke, had since January, 1887, attacks of hæmaturia of gradually increasing frequency. On Nov. 30th cystoscopical examination was made. I found on the lowest part of the right wall of the bladder a prominent tumour with a villous surface, as large as a walnut. I removed it by means of the high section on Dec. 9th. Concerning the size, site, and form, the swelling corresponded to the examination. The microscope confirmed the malignant character of the excised swelling. The patient made a good recovery. The wound cicatrised completely, when, in the middle of the new cicatrisation, two suspicious prominences appeared, which grew quickly, and present now a richly proliferating tumour over the symphysis.

CASE 12.—A female patient under the care of Professor Jacobson. For some years she had had intermittent attacks of hæmaturia. Some of the symptoms were in favour of the origin of the blood being from the kidney. On Jan. 21st cystoscopical examination was made. Immediately behind the internal orifice of the urethra, on the floor of the bladder, a tubercular tumour consisting of blunt papillæ was found. Operation was proposed, but refused by the patient.

CASE 13.—A man, aged fifty-three, had suffered since 1885 from intermittent hæmaturia. By degrees the bleeding increased in frequency and quantity. In June, 1887, the patient went into a Berlin hospital, where he was examined

per rectum and by the sound by an eminent surgeon, Nothing abnormal could be detected in the bladder. The examination was followed by fever, which continued for some weeks, the patient at the same time losing strength. The loss of blood ceased for a long time, but there occurred pain on micturition of increasing intensity. In November, 1887, there was a recurrence of hæmaturia. On Dec. 15th I undertook the cystoscopic examination, which was rendered difficult from the fact that on introducing the prism copious hæmorrhage took place. In spite of this, I could distinctly observe on the right wall of the bladder a tumour the size of a small apple. I removed the tumour on Jan. 12th, 1888, by means of the high section. The conditions corresponded exactly to the appearances found on cystoscopic examination. The apple-sized tumour hung from a firm pedicle, of the thickness of two centimetres, with its edges curved in so as to resemble a mushroom. The patient recovered.

CASE 14.—This patient, aged forty-nine, had suffered many years ago from gonorrhœa, accompanied by cystitis, orchitis, and suppurative prostatitis. Eventually these gonorrhœal complications disappeared, but a slight catarrh remained. On account of the presence of blood in the urine, Dr. Marc of Wildungen, under whose care the patient was, suspected the existence of a bladder tumour, and sent the patient to me. On Jan. 14th cystoscopic examination showed a papilloma as large as a walnut, situated on the lower part of the right wall of the bladder. On Jan. 25th I excised the tumour by means of the high section. The conditions confirmed exactly what was observed on endoscopic examination. The wound has now nearly healed, and the patient is otherwise well.

CASE 15.—This patient (a man, aged fifty-seven) was sent to me by Dr. Kreissmann, suffering from repeated attacks of hæmaturia, dating from November, 1887. The cystoscope showed an irregularly shaped tumour covered with short villi on the left wall of the bladder, and also a second one smaller in size and more rounded in form. On March 10th I undertook the extirpation of the tumour, excising the tumour together with the corresponding part of the wall of the bladder, after opening the bladder by means of suprapubic operation. The conditions confirmed the appearances found endoscopically. As yet the patient is free from fever.

The above shortly[1] described fifteen cases of bladder tumours have been diagnosed by me cystoscopically during the last sixteen months. This is a proof, on the one hand, of the value of the cystoscopic examination; on the other hand, of the fact that the new formations in question are not of so rare occurrence as has been hitherto thought. I would like to emphasise that the important results were often obtained under the most difficult circumstances. In several cases the external orifice of the urethra was found abnormally small; in others (Cases 8 and 11) the examination was made during the occurrence of a continuous hæmorrhage from the tumour; in one case (Case 1) I introduced the instrument through the centre of the tumour, which bled on the slightest pressure. In spite of this the appearances were seen satisfactorily. In the first case a post-mortem examination was made; in eight other cases (Cases 2, 3, 9, 10, 11, 13, 14, and 15) the tumour was extirpated, seven times by the high section—in one case, that of a woman, through the dilated urethra. In these nine cases the endoscopic appearances were in every important respect confirmed in the most perfect manner. In every case my opinion regarding the size, position, and form was found to be correct. It is only in those cases where the edges of the tumour overlap the short pedicle that the latter cannot be observed. Besides, the relative good results of the operations undertaken on account of the cystoscopic appearance may be emphasized. Of the eight patients from whom the tumours had been extirpated none died from the result of the operation. Case 9 proved fatal on account of the progressive extension of the growth. In the eleventh case there was a recurrence, but the patient is still alive. Five patients (Cases 2, 3, 10, 13, 14) must be considered entirely cured. Case 15 is still under treatment, and, as the conditions of the patient are at present (ninth

[1] The first eight cases are more fully described in the Arch. für Chirurgie, vol. xxxvi., Part 3 (Dr. Nitze Beiträge zur Endoscopie der männlichen Harnblase). The full account of the last seven cases will be published soon.

day after operation) in every way satisfactory, a complete recovery is anticipated.

Finally, on comparing the above cystoscopic appearances with the results obtained by other methods of examination, it must be observed that the examination of the urine, in most cases carefully made, had only in two cases shown the presence of villous tissue, which in one instance was brought out by the catheter. The rectal palpation, when made, had always given negative results. Further, the examination by means of the sound had been made in nine cases before the cystoscopic examination. In none of the cases had the sound revealed the presence of a tumour (which in two had attained the size of a small apple), although the examination was made by most experienced surgeons and eminent specialists. Those cases show how imperfect an instrument the sound is for the diagnosis of bladder tumours.

FIG. 5.

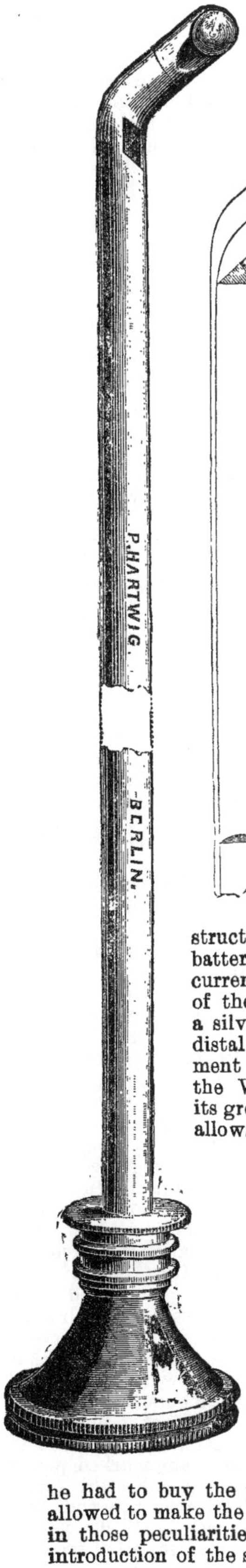

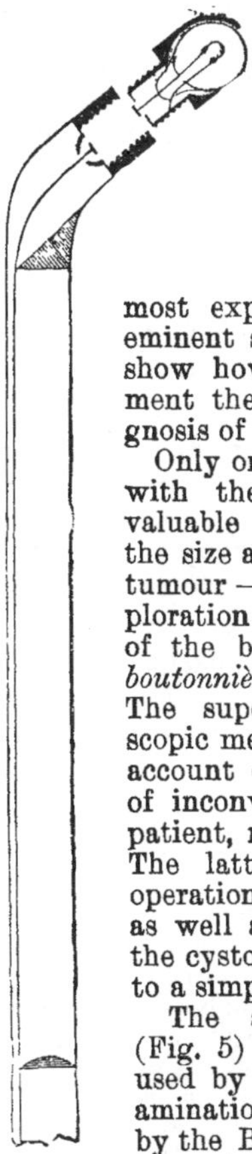

Only one method can compare with the cystoscope in giving valuable information regarding the size and nature of a bladder tumour — viz., the digital exploration of the internal surface of the bladder after a previous *boutonnière*, or the high section. The superiority of the cystoscopic method over the latter, on account of the smaller amount of inconvenience it causes the patient, need not be insisted on. The latter involves a cutting operation not free from danger, as well as deep narcosis, while the cystoscopic method is similar to a simple catheterisation.

The accompanying diagram (Fig. 5) shows the instrument used by me for cystoscopic examination. It has been made by the Berlin instrument maker, Hartwig, according to my instructions. Fig. 6 represents the very simple battery for the production of the electrical current made by the same firm. The source of the light (Mignon lamp) is cemented in a silver capsule, which is screwed into the distal end of the cystoscope. This instrument is superior to that made by Leiter, the Vienna instrument maker, because of its greater simplicity in construction, which allows the lamp to be easily replaced when necessary, and also on account of the greater length of the shaft.

I mention this because it differs from the explanation which Mr. Fenwick gave in his speech concerning my method of examination at the meeting of the Medical Society of London on Jan. 23rd, 1888. I must also strongly contradict Mr. Fenwick's statements concerning the share which he attributed to the Vienna instrument maker in the construction of the instrument. Leiter's connexion with our instrument will be best explained when I say that he had to buy the patent[2] from me first in order to be allowed to make the instrument. Leiter has had no share in those peculiarities which characterise it as new. The introduction of the source of light into the organ had been

practically brought about, the optical apparatus enlarging the view designed, the whole construction perfected, the instrument had proved itself useful in examining patients, and had been demonstrated by me in the Saechsisches Landes Medicinal Collegium before Leiter had any idea of the new invention! Also the eventual replacement of the first source of light (platinum wire) had been

FIG. 6.

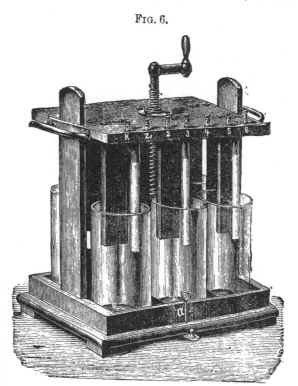

provided for.[3] Leiter has only made a few technical modifications on the finished instrument. I protest most emphatically against the incorrect explanations given by Mr. Fenwick, and against every connexion of Leiter's name with my instruments. I hope to obtain in England the same generous recognition of my labours in this field that has been accorded to me in Germany.

ON THE
MODE OF ACTION OF THE CONTAGIUM AND THE NATURE OF PROPHYLAXIS IN SOME INFECTIVE DISEASES.

BY G. F. DOWDESWELL, M.A.

(Concluded from page 719.)

THOSE who advocate the chemical view of either prophylaxis or the pathogenic action of microbes upon the animal organism overlook the fact that the ultimate action of any chemical substance upon the cells of the tissues is clearly physiological; it does not effect a decomposition of the constituents of those cells, as in the splitting up of the molecule of sugar by the alcoholic ferment; so that this chemical theory merely introduces a third factor in accounting for the action of micro-parasites, and is far from explaining or simplifying it. It has not yet been demonstrated or shown probable that in any case a *pathogenic* microbe acts by the production of or forms a soluble chemical substance, and herein is one distinction between septic and pathogenic or parasitic microbes; but, on the contrary, some of the earliest experiments upon the nature of the contagium—a true pathogenic microbe—in anthrax, by Davaine, Pasteur, Tiegel, Bollinger, and others, were by filtering virulent blood, which, when freed from the living micro-organisms by these (or, in some

---

[2] Deutsche Patentschrifte, No. 6853.

[3] Ibid.

approximates them with great force. The ataxy of all movements is much increased when the eyes are closed. He is unable to hold things, or to perform any delicate action. The sense of posture of the limbs is not affected; he can lift and move his legs best when lying in bed. The muscles are flabby and small from disuse, but not wasted; there are no paralyses of any kind, and no contractures. Muscular actions of all kinds are weak. There is no tremor. Reactions to faradaic and constant currents slightly diminished or normal. Knee-jerks present, about normal. Plantar reflexes very brisk, causing movement of the whole limb. Cremasteric and abdominal reflexes normal. The tendon reflexes in the arms are diminished. Contractions of muscles to direct percussion of their mass not well obtained. No ankle-clonus. Sensation of all kinds quite normal; he has never at any time suffered any pain. Hearing, smell, taste, and sight good. Pupils equal; act well to light and accommodation. No paralysis of any ocular muscle. There is well-marked lateral nystagmus when the eyes are moved to the outer or inner canthus, but not otherwise. The optic discs and fundi are healthy. Speech is slow and rather hesitating, and at times jerky, with elision of syllables. Intelligence good. He can repeat a number of chapters from the Bible, and is very fond of reading. There are no trophic or vaso-motor symptoms. He suffers from constipation; there is no loss of control over the sphincters; the pulse is regular; the muscles seem occasionally to be a little stiff on first being called into action. (See engraving.)

CASE 2.—Isaac A——, aged eleven, is an intelligent boy, and looks healthy. Since the age of four his mother considers that he has been "restless," and that this restlessness increases. He often falls down when walking, and runs in a zig-zag way—i.e., from side to side, like a drunken man. He has had no fits or any bad illness. As he sits he lets his head fall back or from side to side, and keeps his mouth open; this gives him a stupid appearance; at the same time there are rocking movements of head and trunk. Standing with feet together, there is well-marked static ataxia; movements of tendons on dorsum of feet, and slight movements of shoulders, head, and arms, whilst the feet are shifted a little from time to time; when his attention is occupied—as by counting "fifty"—these movements become more marked. He stands by choice with his feet apart. None of the movements at all resemble those of chorea. With his eyes shut there is more general unsteadiness and decided increase in the swaying movements of the trunk and head. There are occasionally slight emotional movements about the mouth, not twitching. There is slight nystagmus on extreme convergence of the eyes. The pupils are equal, and act well to light and accommodation. Sensation and muscular sense normal, muscles firm, and strength fair. Special senses normal. Speech good. The tendon reflexes in the upper limbs were not obtained. The knee-jerk on the left side was about normal; that on the right diminished, but present. Plantar and other superficial reflexes normal. His gait is a little unsteady, and he is quite unable to stand on one leg. The movements of the upper limbs show some ataxy, which becomes more marked when the eyes are shut.

CASE 3.—Caroline, aged eighteen, staymaker. Has had no bad illness; is anæmic, but otherwise appears healthy. She had a fit occasioned by a severe fright when about the age of fourteen. The catamenia appeared at fifteen; since then she has generally had a fit at the onset of a period, but never in the intervals. The fits began with a feeling as if she were turning rapidly round and round; there is then a loud noise in the head, and she becomes unconscious; the period of unconsciousness lasts for half an hour. She is often bruised by the fall, but has never bitten her tongue or passed urine in the fits. In the morning, on first getting up, she suffers from a "jumping" of the muscles and violent spasmodic movements of the limbs or body, so that she drops anything that she may be holding, and, if standing, may be thrown to the ground; she is able, however, to get up again at once. These muscular spasms are more violent during the periods, when they last till midday; on other days they pass off by breakfast-time. I was not able to detect anything abnormal on a careful examination. There was no ataxy of movement. She has been under treatment for about three months without any benefit. I have not seen the patient in any of her fits, and, from the accounts related to me by the mother, could not positively decide that they were purely epileptic in character; on the whole, the evidence went to show that

some were epileptic. The muscular contractions seemed to approximate most closely to the condition known as "myoclonus multiplex." It may be mentioned that, whilst drinking out of a jug one morning, spasmodic closure of the jaws occurred, during which she bit off a piece of the jug and swallowed it.

I examined three other members of the family, and found them healthy in all respects. No evidence could be obtained of any ataxy of movement in the parents or grandparents, or in any of the more distant relatives. It is interesting to note the presence of insanity, diabetes, and croup in the family history, and that the father was addicted to drink. The retention of the knee-jerk in this disease is also unusual; Dr. Griffith[1] states that, of 143 cases, the knee-jerk was reported absent in ninety-one, much diminished in seven, diminished in two, normal in six, normal or exaggerated in one, and exaggerated in six, whilst two of the cases exhibiting exaggeration belong to two of the most typical family groups of the disease.

Clifton.

THE

DISTRIBUTION OF SECONDARY GROWTHS IN CANCER OF THE BREAST.

BY STEPHEN PAGET, F.R.C.S.,
ASSISTANT SURGEON TO THE WEST LONDON HOSPITAL AND THE METROPOLITAN HOSPITAL.

AN attempt is made in this paper to consider "metastasis" in malignant disease, and to show that the distribution of the secondary growths is not a matter of chance. It is urged both by Langenbeck and by Billroth that the question ought to be asked, and, if possible, answered: "What is it that decides what organs shall suffer in a case of disseminated cancer?" If the remote organs in such a case are all alike passive and, so to speak, helpless—all equally ready to receive and nourish any particle of the primary growth which may "slip through the lungs," and so be brought to them,—then the distribution of cancer throughout the body must be a matter of chance. But if we can trace any sort of rule or sequence in the distribution of cancer, any relation between the character of the primary growth and the situation of the secondary growths derived from it, then the remote organs cannot be altogether passive or indifferent as regards embolism.

As regards the relation of the embolus to the tissues which receive it, there is a theory, strengthened by the support of Virchow, that the embolus has a "seminal influence" on the tissues in which it lodges, and that it can make them grow like itself. But there are carefully recorded microscopic observations by Schüppel, Bizzozero, Fuchs, Eberth, Andrée, Langenbeck, and Birch Hirschfeld which go against this theory; and in favour of it I can find only a doubtful case recorded by Brodowski, with a very imaginative picture, and a case, also doubtful, by O. Weber. On the whole, the evidence is against any theory that the embolus and the tissues which receive it may be compared to generative elements acting together. As Langenbeck says, every single cancer cell must be regarded as an organism, alive and capable of development. When a plant goes to seed, its seeds are carried in all directions; but they can only live and grow if they fall on congenial soil. The chief advocate of this theory of the relation between the embolus and the tissues which receive it is Fuchs.[2] He urges that certain organs may be "predisposed" for secondary cancer. He observes that in cases of melanotic sarcoma of the choroid he has sometimes found sarcomatous elements inside the capillary vessels of the retina, but that they do not grow in the retina as they grow in the liver and spleen. He quotes Cohnheim's experiments, who injected fragments of periosteum into the blood of rabbits, and succeeded in getting true tumours of cartilage and bone in their lungs; but these never attained to any marked power of growth. Cohnheim is of opinion that a healthy organ has a certain ability to resist the growth of such an embolus; and he speaks of "diminished resistance" as Fuchs speaks of "predisposition." This theory of predisposition receives

1 Internat. Journ. Med. Sciences, Oct. 1888.
2 Sarkom des Uvealtractus, 1882.

some support from an examination of the statistics of fatal cases of cancer.

I have collected 735 fatal cases of cancer of the breast, in each of which a necropsy was made and recorded. It is true that among them are some cases where death was due to the operation, and some cases where death came early in the disease. But the general results remain unchanged, and are of great interest.

First, is there any associated disease which occurs more often in women who die of cancer of the breast than in other women of the same age? In answer to this, it appears that fibroid tumours of the uterus are found with special frequency in women who die of cancer of the breast. Unfortunately, most of the 750 cases are not recorded with sufficient minuteness to make one sure that the occurrence of such an associated disease would be noted. But Sibley's statistics and the Middlesex Hospital Reports give 243 necropsies, very carefully recorded. No less than 27 had fibroid tumours of the uterus, 4 had polypus of the uterus, 8 had cysts of the ovary, and 3 had dermoid ovarian cysts. Take now, from the same reports, 244 necropsies on cases of cancer of the uterus. Only 7 had fibroid tumours of the uterus, and one of these is doubtful; only 1 had polypus, 9 had ovarian cysts, none had dermoid cysts. Again, take, from the same and similar reports, 75 necropsies on women who died of cancer of some part of the alimentary canal. Only 2 had fibroid tumours of the uterus, 2 had cysts of the ovary, 1 had a dermoid cyst of the ovary, and 1 had a dermoid cyst attached to the appendices epiploicæ. These figures do seem to justify a belief that fibroid tumours of the uterus are more often associated with cancer of the breast than with cancer of the generative organs or of the alimentary canal in women.

Next, there is some reason for thinking that the same holds good for other new growths. In 182 necropsies after cancer of the breast,[3] there were also found bronchocele, rodent ulcer, cavernous growths in the liver, cyst in the cerebellum, and fibrous and warty growths on the body; and one patient had, besides the cancer of the breast, also uterine polypus, dermoid ovarian cyst, molluscum fibrosum, and a fatty tumour on the shoulder. But in 200 necropsies after cancer of the uterus,[4] there was not a single new growth of any kind elsewhere, except the uterine and ovarian growths, which occurred in both sets of cases, and of which I have just spoken. Nor was there one in the 75 necropsies after cancer of the alimentary canal in women, except one blood-cyst of the breast. It is therefore not improbable that with the tendency in women to cancer of the breast there may be associated a tendency to outgrowths of other kinds and in other parts of the body, which is not observed in women who suffer from cancer of the generative organs or of the alimentary canal.

Then as regards "metastasis." Here, too, we shall find evidences of predisposition; we shall see that one remote organ is more prone to be the seat of secondary growth than another. In cases of cancer of the breast, it is strange how often the liver is the seat of secondary cancer. From different sources, I have 735 necropsies after cancer of the breast. Of these, 241 had cancer of the liver, only 17 had cancer of the spleen, and 30 had cancer of the kidneys or suprarenals. The lungs were involved in about 70 cases; but it is sometimes impossible to say whether the lungs or only the pleuræ were attacked, nor can we doubt that in cancer of the breast the lungs often suffer, not as remote organs, but by direct extension from the primary disease.

The same propensity of the liver to become diseased is shown in cases of cancer of the female generative organs. In 244 necropsies after cancer of the uterus, the liver was involved in 35, the spleen in 1 only, the lungs in 8, and the kidneys or suprarenals in 6, one of which was by direct extension. This frequency of secondary disease of the liver is of course a familiar fact; but it acquires fresh interest when we contrast it with the immunity enjoyed by other organs. The spleen has, so to speak, the same chances as the liver; its artery is even larger than the hepatic artery; it cannot avoid embolism. Yet the liver was the seat of cancer in 276 cases; the spleen in 18 only. Such a great disproportion cannot be due to chance. For in pyæmia no such disproportion exists. I have tabulated 340 necropsies after pyæmia, and I find that abscess of the liver occurred

in 66, and abscess of the spleen in 39—a very different proportion from that of 276 to 18.

The disproportion is not so great in melanotic cancer. Taking the record of necropsies by Fuchs,[5] Eiselt,[6] and Pemberton on Melanosis, we find that in 129 necropsies the liver was affected in 77 and the spleen in 17.

Again, if we take the 735 necropsies after cancer of the breast, we find that the ovaries, one or both, were involved in no less than 37 cases; that is to say, twice as often as the spleen, and about as often as the kidneys and spleen put together. This can hardly be chance. And in two of the cases the ovaries alone of all the organs were diseased. It is of one of these two cases that Dr. Coupland says: "To evoke the fact of the physiological sympathy of two such widely removed organs to explain such a case as this is a view perhaps too fanciful to be entertained, but yet it is difficult to put such a consideration entirely out of sight."

Let us now see what is the case as regards the bones in cancer of the breast. If we consider how favourable the lymph glands are to the growth and spread of cancer, and how close the connexion is between the lymph glands and the medulla of the bones, we may look to find something of interest among the cases where the bones were involved. In the first place, there is reason for believing that a general degeneration of the bones sometimes occurs in cases of cancer of the breast, yet without any distinct deposit of cancer in them. Thus Török and Wittelshöfer,[7] in their analysis of 336 necropsies on cases of cancer of the breast, say: "Besides the cases where the bones were manifestly diseased, there were 8 cases of that peculiar brittleness and softness of different bones mentioned by Rokitansky, Lücke, and others, where a cancerous degeneration could not be made out." To these 8 cases we may add the following post-mortem observations from the Middlesex Hospital Reports and from Billroth.[8]

1. Female, aged fifty-six. Cancer of right breast and axillary glands; one nodule in the heart. "Ununited fracture of femur; an associated lesion, not due to cancer."

2. Female, aged fifty-three. Recurrent cancer of right axillary and clavicular glands, pleura, and liver. "Upper part of right thigh, old ununited spontaneous fracture. Left thigh also fractured. In moving the body the right humerus broke just above the elbow. Ribs and sternum very brittle. No sign of cancer in connexion with either of the fractured bones. Skeletal condition like osteomalacia; cortex thinned, medulla diffluent."

3. Female, aged forty-eight. Recurrent cancer in left breast and axillary glands. "Mollities ossium (carcinomatous?)."

4. Female, aged forty-six. Recurrent cancer in breast and liver. "Bones very brittle."

5. Female, aged sixty. Cancer of right breast and glands. Nodules in cranium and dura mater. "Fracture of left humerus; uncertain whether cancerous."

6. Female, aged forty-eight. Cancer of breast, axilla, and liver. "Mollities of cervical spine; lateral curvature."

Here, then, are fourteen cases, besides those noticed by Rokitansky, Lücke, and others, where cancer of the breast was associated with brittleness of the bones, or softness, or ununited fracture. Perhaps this fact may be compared with the extraordinary frequency of malignant disease in cases of osteitis deformans. However this may be, it seems certain that it is not a matter of chance what bone shall be attacked by secondary growth. Who has ever seen the bones of the hands or the feet attacked by secondary cancer? Out of 650 necropsies in cases of cancer of the breast, which give full details as to the distribution of the secondary growths, there is not a single case where the hands or the feet were affected, not one of disease of the radius, ulna, or fibula, and only one of the tibia. In contrast to this, the femur was affected, either by spontaneous fracture or by distinct deposit of cancer, 18 times; the humerus, 10 times; and the cranium, 36.[9] As regards the femur, the deposit of cancer seems generally to affect the medulla of the upper part of the bone; we read of it as occurring "just below the small trochanter," or "at the junction of the shaft with the great trochanter," or "at the junction

---

[3] Middlesex Hospital Reports and Billroth.
[4] Middlesex Hospital Reports.

[5] Das Sarcom des Uvealtractus.   [6] Ueber Pigment Krebs.
[7] Langenbeck's Arch., xxv., 4.   [8] Beiträge z. Stat. der Carcinome.
[9] This high figure for the cranium is due to Török and Wittelshöfer, who say that, in 336 necropsies in cancer of the breast, the cranium was diseased in 33. Probably they include the brain &c

of the upper and middle third."[10] It does not appear that the femur is so often the seat of secondary growth in other forms of cancer. Thus, in 132 necropsies in melanotic cancer, mostly of the choroid or of the skin, reported by Fuchs, Eiselt, Pemberton, and others, though the bones were freely affected, the femur suffered only in one case, and the humerus not at all.

The evidence seems to me irresistible that in cancer of the breast the bones suffer in a special way, which cannot be explained by any theory of embolism alone. Some bones suffer more than others; the disease has its "seats of election." The same thing is seen much more clearly in those cases of cancer of the thyroid body where secondary deposits occur in the bones with astonishing frequency. It is of these that Lücke[11] says: "Secondary tumours occur with striking frequency in the bones, both in the shafts and in the epiphyses. They may attain very considerable size and become much larger than the primary growth." He and Lebert and others have recorded such cases. I have collected notes of about 20; no less than 10 of these had masses of the growth in remote bones; in some cases the disease had attacked half-a-dozen bones at once. A contrast to this involvement of the bones in this form of cancer is found in their freedom from disease in cancer of the stomach and pylorus. In 903 necropsies in this disease, collected by Gussenbauer and von Winiwarter,[12] the bones were not affected in a single case; unless, perhaps, they were affected in some or all of the 11 cases, among the 903, where "general carcinosis" finally took place.

All reasoning from statistics is liable to many errors. But the analogy from other diseases seems to support what these records have suggested. The eruptions of the specific fevers and of syphilis, the inflammations after typhoid, the lesions of tuberculosis, all show the dependence of the seed upon the soil. The best work in the pathology of cancer is now done by those who, like Mr. Ballance and Mr. Shattock, are studying the nature of the seed. They are like scientific botanists; and he who turns over the records of cases of cancer is only a ploughman, but his observation of the properties of the soil may also be useful.

Wimpole-street, W.

EXHAUSTION PARALYSIS.

BY C. W. SUCKLING, M.D. LOND., M.R.C.P.,

PROFESSOR OF MATERIA MEDICA AT THE QUEEN'S COLLEGE, AND PHYSICIAN TO THE QUEEN'S HOSPITAL, BIRMINGHAM.

DR. CH. FÉRÉ, M.D. Paris, recently published an article in *Brain*, Part 42, on "Paralysis by Exhaustion," meaning paralysis produced by excessive and prolonged voluntary movement involving exhaustion of the nerve centres. Hemiplegia after repeated and violent epileptic attacks is an instance of this variety of paralysis. Excessive exercise of one arm may not only produce what is called a professional hyperkinesis, but paralysis also. Hammer palsy was described in 1869 by Frank Smith of Sheffield. It was observed in men who had to work for many hours with a small hammer which had to be rapidly wielded. In these cases the individual was usually anæmic, and the paralysis was hemiplegic in distribution, though more especially affecting the arm; aphasia and sensory disturbances were also occasionally present. In one case, in addition to marked paresis, there was inability to write, and cramp increased when the patient tried to use a hammer. Dr. Féré relates two cases of exhaustion paralysis occurring in his practice. One patient, a blacksmith, after two hours' extra work, noticed that the hammer was unusually heavy and that his hand felt numbed. The next day his right arm was powerless and the right leg weak. Dr. Féré found that he had hemiplegia, the face being affected, and there being considerable anæsthesia on the right side. The patient had almost completely recovered in three weeks. In the second case, a young lady with a neurotic family history, after practising at the piano for nine hours, noticed that her hand was heavy and clumsy; the leg was also weak and both limbs anæsthetic. In a fortnight recovery was almost complete.

I have had the good fortune to meet with a very typical instance of exhaustion paralysis at the Birmingham Workhouse Infirmary. A woman, fifty-one years of age, was admitted into the infirmary on Sept. 22nd suffering from cramp and paralysis of the right leg. She had followed the occupation of cook in a large factory, and had been accustomed to standing for many hours a day, the usual hours being from 6 A.M. to 9 P.M. She would perhaps sit down for a few minutes to her meals, but certainly for not more than half an hour in the day. Besides being constantly on her legs, going up and down stairs, she had to lift and carry heavy weights. She had worked at the factory for some months, and had always left her work completely tired out. Latterly she had noticed that her right leg felt tired towards the end of the day. A few days before her admission, her mistress having been taken ill, she was obliged to stay even later to do overtime, as she called it; and on Sept. 21st, as she was walking home from her work, she was seized with numbness and cramp in the right leg and foot, and was obliged to be carried home, being unable to walk or stand. During the night she was seized every few minutes with violent cramps in the right lower extremity, which occasioned much pain and prevented sleep. When I saw her on the 22nd I found that the right leg was completely paralysed, and observed two or three attacks of violent spasm of the muscles of the thigh and leg. The patient complained of numbness of the whole of the right leg, and of the right side of the body up to the under surface of the right breast. There was distinct but not complete anæsthesia, tactile, thermal, and painful impressions being only slightly perceived in the right lower extremity. The muscular sense was also much impaired, for on the left side she could distinguish between one-ounce and two-ounce weights, while on the right side she could not distinguish between one-ounce and six-ounce weights. The plantar reflex was lost on the right side, but the knee-jerk was excessive. There was no ankle-clonus. There was no bladder or rectal trouble, no retinal changes, no fever, and no albuminuria. There was no neurotic family or personal history, and no trace of hysteria about the woman. She had ceased menstruating for some years, and had enjoyed good health, though she had occasionally noticed numbness in her right hand. The right upper extremity was unaffected, and there was no trace of any facial paresis and no cerebral disturbance. A hypodermic injection of morphia and atropia greatly allayed the attacks of spasm. A mixture of bromide of potassium, chloral, and belladonna was prescribed, and the limb was gently rubbed. On the 23rd the patient was free from cramp, and could lift the leg from the bed, though sensation was still impaired. She improved daily, and in ten days' time was able to walk about, and was discharged perfectly well.

There is no doubt that this was a typical case of functional akinesis or exhaustion paralysis; and it is evident that not only is there a professional hyperkinesis such as writer's cramp, telegraphist's cramp, &c., but also a professional akinesis or exhaustion paralysis, and that there is a close association between them, as shown by their occasionally occurring together in the same subject. A point worthy of notice in the history of the reported cases of exhaustion paralysis is that, though the individual may have worked very hard for years, nothing happens until there is a call for still further effort, when the machinery at once fails. The quick recovery of these cases of exhaustion paralysis contrasts very strongly and favourably with the tedious and slow recovery observed in cases of professional hyperkinesis. Exhaustion paralysis must be added to the list of functional paralyses and its existence borne in mind, for a mistaken diagnosis may readily be made, the paralysis being very complete and often hemiplegic in distribution, with implication of the facial muscles. The functional paralyses described in text-books are (1) hysterical, (2) ideal, (3) reflex, (4) malarial, and (5) anæmic. There were no indications of hysteria in my case, the patient being a hard-working and very matter-of-fact kind of individual, not at all of the neurotic type, and extremely anxious to get out of the infirmary to go to work again. The cramps occasioned very severe pain, and in the intervals between the attacks of cramp the leg was completely paralysed and flaccid. She complained of severe pain round the right side of the body under the right breast

---

[10] See, for four more cases, Ormerod's Clinical Collections, p. 202, and C. Hawkins' Contributions to Pathology, ii., 124.
[11] Krebs der Schilddrüse.   [12] Langenbeck's Arch., xix., 372.

THE LANCET, November 22, 1890.

Further Communications
ON
A REMEDY FOR TUBERCULOSIS.[1]
By PROFESSOR R. KOCH, Berlin.

THE paper opens with a reference to the statement made by the author in his address before the International Medical Congress with respect to his discovery of a method whereby animals could be rendered insusceptible to inoculation with the tubercle bacillus, or in whom tuberculous changes may be arrested. Pursuing this inquiry in regard to human tuberculosis, he had arrived at certain definite results, of which he would have preferred to have had more experience before publishing them, had not the currency of inaccurate and distorted accounts made it imperative on him to give his own account of his work, imperfect as it may be in certain respects. Experiments were carried on under his direction by Drs. Libbertz and E. Pfuhl, and are still in progress; and patients had been furnished by Prof. Brieger from his policlinic, by Dr. W. Levy from his surgical clinic, Drs. Fränkel and Köhler at the Charité Hospital, and Prof. von Bergmann from the University surgical clinic. To these gentlemen and their assistants Prof. Koch tenders his warm thanks for their aid and the lively interest they took in the investigation.

Reserving an account of the nature and preparation of the remedy, he describes it as consisting of a clear brownish fluid, which can be kept without special precautions, and which has to be diluted for use. These dilutions with distilled water are liable to decomposition, becoming turbid from bacterial vegetations, and consequently inefficacious. This change may be avoided by sterilising the solution by heat and preserving it in a vessel closed with a plug of cotton wool, or by the addition of phenol; but as the properties, especially of very dilute solutions, are thereby impaired, he prefers to use freshly prepared solutions.

The remedy does not act when taken into the stomach; it must be injected subcutaneously, for which purpose he uses a syringe provided with a rubber ball instead of a piston, which allows of its being readily kept aseptic by cleansing with absolute alcohol. To this he ascribes the freedom from local abscesses in all the injections— upwards of a thousand—that he has made. After a trial of various spots, the skin of the back between the shoulders and in the lumbar region was selected as the most suitable for the injection, which as a rule produces no local effect and is quite painless. It was soon shown that the action of the remedy on man differed in some important respects from its action on the guinea-pig, the former being far more susceptible to it than the latter. Thus, a healthy guinea-pig may have as much as 2 c.c. injected subcutaneously without being notably affected by it; but in a healthy adult man as little as 0·25 c.c. suffices to excite intense reaction. In other words, regarding the relative body weights, $\frac{1}{1500}$th of the quantity which has no appreciable effect on the guinea-pig is most powerfully active in man. Professor Koch has observed in himself the effects following the injection of 0·25 c.c. into the arm. About three or four hours after the injection he experienced pains in the joints, languor, a tendency to cough, and difficulty in breathing, which rapidly increased; then, at the fifth hour, a very severe rigor, lasting for an hour; then nausea, vomiting, and a rise of temperature to 39·6° C. (103·3° F.). This disturbance ceased at the end of twelve hours, the temperature falling next day to the normal level; the joint pains and lassitude lasted for a few days, and for the same time the site of the injection remained slightly painful and reddened. It was found that the smallest quantity requisite to produce such reaction in healthy individuals was about 0·01 c.c. (or about 1 c.c. of 1 per cent. dilution). This amount produced slight joint pain and transient languor, and sometimes a slight rise of temperature to 38° C. (100·4° F.). Apart from this remarkable difference in the dose the effects in animals and men are apparently similar, the most important being the specific action of the remedy upon tuberculous processes of whatever kind. These latter effects in animals he does not now dwell upon, but proceeds to describe them in the human subject.

First there is the very remarkable fact that whereas in health and in subjects of non-tuberculous disease the injection of 0·01 c.c. has hardly any effect, in the tuberculous this quantity invariably produces a marked general as well as a local reaction.[2] The general reaction consists in an attack of fever, mostly beginning with a rigor, the temperature exceeding 39° C. (102·2° F.), often rising to 40° (104° F.), and even to 41° (105·8° F.), articular pains, cough, great prostration, often nausea and vomiting, sometimes slight icterus, with in some cases a measly eruption on the chest and neck. The attack, as a rule, begins in from four to five hours after the injection, and lasts from twelve to fifteen hours. Exceptionally it may commence later and run a milder course. The patient is but little affected by it, and when it has passed he feels comparatively well or even better than before. The local reaction is best observed in cases where the tubercular disease is visible, as in lupus. Within a few hours after the injection (although at a part remote from that which is diseased) the lupus nodules begin to swell and redden, and this commonly before the rigor occurs. During the fever the swelling and redness increase to such an extent that eventually the lupus tissue becomes in places brownish-red and necrotic. This swollen and discoloured portion is surrounded for the depth of a centimetre by a white zone, outside of which there is a bright-red band. After the fever has declined the swelling gradually diminishes, and in two or three days it has disappeared. The lupus areas become encrusted with dried serum, which changes into scabs, and on their detachment in two or three weeks, and even after only a single injection, a smooth red scar is left behind. Mostly several injections are necessary to completely destroy the lupus tissue. Special importance is attached to the fact that the process is confined to the diseased tissues, so that even a minute patch amid scar tissue may be revealed by its swelling and reddening under the influence of the remedy. Owing to these striking objective effects Professor Koch recommends all who wish to study the action of the remedy to begin by observing its effect in lupus. Less striking but still obvious both to sight and touch are the local changes induced in tuberculosis of lymphatic glands, bones, joints, &c., in which swelling and increased pain, with reddening of the surface, become manifest. The local changes induced in the internal organs—e.g., the lungs—are obviously withdrawn from observation, but the somewhat increased cough and expectoration which follow the first injection may indicate them. Here the general phenomena predominate, but one must infer that changes are taking place similar to those presented to view in lupus. Since these phenomena are produced in the presence of tuberculous processes by a dose of 0·01 c.c., the injection may come to be a valuable aid in the diagnosis of obscure cases of the disease and of commencing phthisis, when neither the test of bacilli or elastic fibres in the sputum nor the physical signs yield positive information. So, too, the tubercular nature of obscure gland affections, bone disease, and skin affections may be established. In cases of apparently cured pulmonary or articular tubercle it may show whether the tubercular process has really come to an end, or whether there still remain isolated foci, which at any time might burst into flame just as a spark which has been left glimmering among the ashes.

Of more importance is its therapeutic action. The effect of the injection upon the lupus tissue is to destroy it more or less thoroughly, and cause it to disappear. In some parts the dose may suffice to effect this forthwith; in others the tissue rather melts or wastes away, requiring the repeated action of the remedy to complete the process. How this occurs cannot yet be stated, since histological facts are wanting; but it is clear that it is not by the killing of tubercle bacilli in the tissue, but rather of the tissue which encloses them. The circulatory disturbance evidenced by the swelling and redness shares in this, showing that there are profound changes in nutrition which kill the tissue in proportion to the degree and manner of action of the remedy. That it

[1] Abstract of a paper published in the Deutsche Medicinische Wochenschrift, Nov. 15th, 1890, and reprinted in the Berliner Klinische Wochenschrift of same date.
No. 3508.

[2] These effects are produced in children from three to five years with one-tenth of this dose, 0·001 c.c.; in very weak children only 0·0005 c.c. produces a marked reaction, but not such as to give rise to anxiety.

destroys the tuberculous tissue and not the bacilli indicates the limits of its activity. It can only affect living tuberculous tissue. It has no action on that which is already dead, as caseous masses, necrosed bone, &c., nor even on that which has been destroyed by the remedy itself. Living bacilli may still exist in such dead portions, and be either expelled with the necrotic tissue, or, under certain conditions, be able to again invade the neighbouring living tissue. This property of the remedy should be carefully borne in mind, and when possible the removal of the dead tissue be effected by surgical means. Where this cannot be done, and the organism has to get rid of it by its own action, the use of the remedy must be continued so as to prevent the reinfection of living tissue. This selection of living tuberculous tissue by the remedy explains the singular fact that it may be given in rapidly increasing doses, so that within three weeks the quantity may be increased to 500 times the original amount. This cannot be due to toleration, for there is no analogy of so powerful a remedy being so rapidly tolerated. It is rather that, whereas at the first there is much tubercular tissue present, so that a small quantity of the active substance suffices to produce marked reaction, with each succeeding injection the amount of tissue that reacts is diminished, and relatively larger doses are needed to produce the same amount of reaction as before. Within limits, too, there may be a certain amount of toleration. So soon as in a tuberculous subject treated with increasing doses there comes to be no more reaction than in the non-tuberculous, then it may be inferred that there is no more tuberculous tissue to be destroyed, and the treatment would have to be continued with slowly increasing doses and at intervals, so long as bacilli are present in the body, in order to protect against a fresh infection. Professor Koch goes on to say that the future must prove whether this idea and the conclusions based on it are correct; at present he is content to show the way in which the remedy must be applied. In the case of lupus the procedure has been to inject the full dose of 0·01 c.c., and after one or two weeks to repeat it, and so on until the reaction weakens and finally ceases to occur. In two cases of lupus of the face so treated, the affected parts were converted into smooth cicatrices after three or four injections; other cases improved in proportion to the duration of the treatment. All these patients had suffered for many years, and had undergone various kinds of treatment without result. It was the same with cases of tuberculosis of glands, bones, and joints, in which, occasionally, larger doses at longer intervals were employed. Rapid healing took place in the milder cases; slowly progressive improvement in the more severe.

The behaviour of phthisical cases, which formed the majority, was somewhat different; such patients being far more susceptible to the remedy than the surgical cases. It was soon found that an initial dose of 0·01 c.c. was too much for the phthisical, and that they would mostly react markedly to a dose of 0·002 c.c. or even of 0·001 c.c.; but that they could bear a very rapid increase of the dose from this minimum. Generally the first injection was with 0·001 c.c., and this dose was repeated on the next and following days if the temperature continued to rise after it; when no reaction followed, the dose was raised to 0·002 c.c., and then by additions of 0·001 or 0·002, until the maximum of 0·01 or more was reached. Such a gradual course is especially needful for those whose strength is feeble. By this plan a patient might be brought to bear considerable doses without fever or without himself being aware of it. In some stronger phthisical subjects the dose was increased more rapidly, with apparently more speedily favourable result. Cough and expectoration commonly increase after the first injection, and then gradually decline or finally quite disappear; the sputa cease to be purulent, and become mucoid. The number of bacilli began to diminish when the sputa became mucoid. Night sweating ceases; the general aspect improves, and there is a gain in weight. Patients in the early stage become free from all symptoms in the course of four to six weeks' treatment, and may be regarded as cured. Even cases with moderately sized cavities are markedly improved and nearly cured. It was only in cases with many and large cavities that no objective signs of improvement take place, although the sputa diminish, and the subjective conditions improve. This experience emboldens Professor Koch to affirm that commencing phthisis may with certainty be cured by this remedy. (In a footnote he points out that this does not imply a definitive cure, for relapses are possible; but it proves that these may be as easily overcome as the original attack. On the other hand, analogy with other infective diseases makes it possible that immunity may be established if cure be once attained, and he reserves this and other questions as open ones.) Advanced cases with large cavities, and mostly complicated by the presence of other micro-organisms in the cavities, and by irremediable morbid lesions in other organs, can only rarely derive permanent benefit from the remedy. But they undergo temporary improvement, showing that even in this class the tuberculous process is influenced as in others, and that failure is attributable to the difficulty of removal of the dead masses of tissue, together with the products of secondary suppuration. It may be found possible to assist in their removal by surgical intervention (similar to that in empyema) or other means. He urgently protests against the indiscriminate application of the remedy to all cases of tuberculosis. The simplest cases are those of commencing phthisis and surgical tubercular affections. But in all other cases there should be careful individual selection and medical treatment used in addition. He therefore pronounces in favour of treating cases in suitable institutions where every care can be taken of the patient in preference to their being treated in their homes. Nor can it be said that the methods hitherto in favour, such as the residence in mountain resorts, fresh air, special dietary, may not well continue to be employed side by side with the new method, particularly in severe and neglected cases and in the convalescence of all. The importance of the earliest possible recognition of phthisis is greatly heightened by the use of this remedy, and should, Professor Koch says, be the aim of every practitioner. For this he lays great stress on the systematic and thorough examination of the sputa for bacilli, a matter which his experience teaches him has been too much neglected. In future such neglect will render the physician responsible for delay in subjecting his patient to a treatment which might save his life, and in doubtful cases recourse might be had to the test-injection, which would establish with certainty the presence or absence of tuberculosis. Then will the new method prove, he says, a blessing to suffering humanity, when every case of tubercular disease is treated as soon as possible, and there are no more neglected cases to form, as hitherto, an inexhaustible source for fresh infection.

The paper concludes by stating that statistics and records of individual cases have been advisedly omitted, the writer leaving their publication to those to whom the patients belonged, and he did not desire to anticipate their descriptions.

Inaugural Address

ON

ANEURYSM, ITS CURE BY INDUCING THE FORMATION OF WHITE THROMBI WITHIN THE SAC.

Delivered before the Midland Medical Society,

By WILLIAM MACEWEN, M.D., C.M., &c.,
SURGEON TO THE ROYAL INFIRMARY, GLASGOW.

MR. PRESIDENT AND GENTLEMEN,—My first duty is to thank you for the honour you have conferred upon me in inviting me to deliver the inaugural address of the Midland Medical Society. If anything can enhance such an honour, it is the knowledge, on the one hand, that the invitation has emanated from such a great centre of surgical activity as Birmingham, from which so many important advances in surgery have taken their origin, and, on the other, the circumstance of which your President in sending me the invitation duly acquainted me, that you have had in former years to inaugurate the opening of your Society a roll of names each highly distinguished in his own sphere, and including men such as Jenner, Lister, Spencer Wells, and Humphry of Cambridge. Having accepted your invitation, I propose to present you with a few facts concerning the cure of aneurysm by inducing the formation of white thrombi within the sac. In certain regions of the body,

INJECTIONS AGAINST CHOLERA.
A LECTURE
BY M. HAFFKINE.

(Specially reported for THE LANCET.)

M. HAFFKINE, who has been on a visit to this country and has made some demonstrations at Netley Hospital of his method of inoculating a modified cholera virus as a protective against cholera, was, prior to his departure to India to study cholera in that country, invited to give at the Laboratories of the Royal College of Physicians and Surgeons a demonstration of his method of procedure.

On Wednesday last, Feb. 8th, a paper which he had prepared was read on his behalf by Dr. Armand Ruffer. There has been very considerable difficulty, arising from many causes, in placing the results of M. Haffkine's researches before the readers of THE LANCET. This difficulty is not in any way attributable to M. Haffkine, and has largely arisen from the excusably imperfect translation into English of his paper, which, however, has been carefully revised in the following report.

Dr. Pavy having briefly introduced M. Haffkine to the large audience, Dr. Ruffer proceeded to read the paper, which was as follows :—

"The discovery that microbes may change their characters and are capable of transformation by artificial means into vaccines of fixed and ascertained power is without doubt the greatest step which has been taken in medical science since disease-producing microbes were first studied. The task which then presented itself to investigators was that of discovering the germs of contagion which were recognised as being the cause of disease and of elaborating substances protective against them.

"M. Pasteur, after having discovered the first principles of this method by experiments in 'fowl cholera,' developed them greatly by his studies on anthrax; he then turned his attention to hydrophobia, which, being a disease common to both men and animals, was an appropriate one in which to employ the methods previously applied to animals in the treatment of human diseases.

"The experience acquired in the endeavour to prevent hydrophobia by inoculation—the first human disease treated according to the new method—led to the formation of a perfectly clear programme, to be followed by investigators in the direction in question. It was shown that success was to be arrived at through the preparation of a virus gradually increasing in strength according to a fixed scale until it reached a degree of virulence above that of the ordinary virus, which would allow of the organism becoming accustomed to the poison with which it was infected. The *traitement intensif* of hydrophobia, based upon the acquisition of a virus of maximum strength, has shown the true *rôle* of the virus kept in a fixed state of 'exaltation' by specially appropriate experiments. The acquisition of virus of this kind and the establishment of a method suitable for keeping it in a fixed state are the ultimate aims of the research for a vaccine, since it is essential gradually to accustom the organism under treatment to this fixed virus. It is known that this task may be accomplished by the transference of infective organisms through a series of animals and that it is by cultivating it through a long series of such living animals that the microbe acquires the maximum of its infective power.

"In the case of cholera the first attempts towards the solution of this problem began with the infection of animals through the digestive canal. In this way the culture of the microbe took place in a part in which other microbes existed, which fact from the first rendered the means employed uncertain. The result of the introduction of a microbe into such parts depends upon the nature of the microbe. The purification of the microbe by intermediate artificial culture made in transmission between two animals is a source of diminution of virulence which counterbalances the 'exaltation' obtained. This explains how MM. Pfeiffer and Nocht in seeking to strengthen the cholera microbe by passing it alternately through animals and cultures were not able to obtain a microbe capable of overcoming the natural resistance of birds; and this is the reason why M. Roux and myself (M. Haffkine), in trying to transfer the intestinal contents from one animal directly to another, according to the method used by Gamaleia, have seen our series broken after the third or fourth transference.

"The idea which M. Gamaleia had in 1888 of cultivating the microbe in the thoracic cavity of animals gave rise to considerable hope, and at one time the task was regarded as accomplished. Unhappily this method, perfectly applicable to the microbe which M. Gamaleia used—the 'vibrio Metchnikovi'—was found to be defective when it was applied to the Asiatic cholera microbe, as M. Roux and myself ascertained in the series of trials which we have made in this direction. M. Hueppe in 1888 conceived the idea of producing infection of animals by the introduction of the cholera microbe into the peritoneal cavity; this has since been revived by M. Pfeiffer, who stated that in the case of the cholera microbe a change was produced similar to that seen in diphtheria, tetanus and other diseases which are characterised by a local development of the living organism without an invasion of the blood or of the visceral organs. This change is simply that the infective agent itself disappears in the animal killed by the microbe; and if it were possible to again find the remains of the culture injected, and to transfer them to a second animal, this second animal would retain no further trace of the microbes, and the further passage would be interrupted. In the work carried out in the Pasteur Institute with regard to inoculation against Asiatic cholera the infection of the animal by the peritoneal cavity was chosen as the starting point, from which point a method has been worked out which permits of the culture of the microbe in the animal organism in a state of purity during an infinite series of generations, the exaltation of it to an ascertained maximum strength, and the possibility of keeping it at the same degree of virulence for an unlimited period of time. This method is exemplified by three series of experiments which were the subject of a publication in the *Comptes-rendus de la Société de Biologie* of Paris. These are as follows :—

"(*a*) Giving the first animal a dose larger than the fatal dose and killing this animal in a sufficiently short space of time to be able easily to find the more resisting microbes.

"(*b*) Exposing the discharge taken from the peritoneal cavity to the air for several hours.

"(*c*) Then transferring this discharge to the next animal, of large or small size, according to the concentration of the discharge.

'The method has been verified by other experimenters with satisfactory results. The properties of the virus which is obtained in this way may be ascertained by observing that upon intra-peritoneal inoculation it always kills guinea-pigs in about eight hours, and the fatal dose for this animal is reduced to about twenty times less than that which it would have been necessary to administer for the microbe with which the experiment began. With the same inoculation it kills rabbits and pigeons by a dose which would have been harmless at the beginning of the infection experiments. It kills guinea-pigs when it is injected into the muscular tissue. Inoculation under the skin causes the formation of a large swelling, which produces sloughing of that part of the skin and the formation of a gaping wound which is curable in two or three weeks. This is the basis of my researches.

"The virus when injected under the skin of a healthy animal gives the creature, after several days, immunity from the poison of cholera, however it may be conveyed to it. If an attempt be made to infect an animal which has been so treated, either by Koch's method through the alimentary canal, by neutralisation of the gastric juice and the injection of opium into the peritoneum, by the introduction of the microbe into the intestines by the method of Nicati and Rietsch, through the muscles, or by (the most fatal of all) intra-peritoneal injection, the animal resists, whilst the control animals are killed. Inoculation of animals against cholera in this manner has been definitely established. But the operation thus described cannot be applied to man. The wound following on the injection under the skin is alarming to look at, and is in all probability painful. Besides, although it does not in itself present any danger to the health of the individual, it subjects him to all the dangers arising from an open wound. By growing it at a temperature of 39° C. and in an atmosphere freely exposed to the air this corrosive action is removed from the microbe. Under these conditions the first crop of the cholera microbes die rapidly, say in from two to three days; but others are sown again in new centres immediately before the death of the first. After a series of generations of this kind a culture is obtained which, if injected under the skin of animals even in very large doses, produces merely a temporary œdema and so prepares the inoculated organism that the injection of this modified virus of fixed exalted vaccine produces only a local reaction of the slightest kind. Thus the method of inoculation deals with two vaccines—a mild one obtained by weakening the 'fixed virus,' and a 'strengthened vaccine' which is really the exalted virus itself. The reason an ordinary virus is not used to obtain the weakened vaccine, but one the nature of which has been previously ascertained in the laboratory, is that the viruses in their natural state, especially when they have reached a saprophytic stage of development, present such great differences that there is no certainty in their application. This recalls to mind the story of inoculation for small-pox. The mildness or the severity of an infection does not depend merely on the real strength of the contagious substance, but upon the resistance of the individual from whom the poison has been taken. Thus in taking vaccine for use as vaccine lymph from a subject slightly affected a very weak substance was sometimes obtained incapable of causing protection, but still able to kill individuals less resistant. The great point of Jenner's discovery lay in the fact that it indicated a substance fixed by successive passages through animals at a virulence above that which is fatal to human beings. Another example is given in the old method of inoculation against anthrax by Toussaint, the first of its kind, which has had to give way to the method of M. Pasteur simply because Pasteur's method was based upon a virus of fixed strength and produced results with certainty, conditions which were wanting in the former method. In 1885 Dr. Ferran of Barcelona, with the object of preserving the population of the Peninsula from cholera, injected his patients with the ordinary virus taken from dead bodies and cultivated in the laboratory. The statistics of the results obtained by him were so uncertain that it could not be recommended. The fundamental feature of the Pasteurian method was the possibility of treating the animal organism by vaccines of an absolutely fixed nature by means of special operations. That was the whole secret and the sole guarantee of the success of its application.

"The method of inoculation against cholera worked out by experiments on guinea-pigs was afterwards tried upon rabbits and pigeons before it was applied to man. These animals were chosen in order to secure very differently organised subjects, and to obtain the power of generalising the conclusions before extending the experiments to human beings. The same results were obtained on all these animals and it was decided to apply the operation to man. The symptoms produced by this operation have been described in several scientific publications. The method has been tried at Paris, at Cherbourg and at Moscow on about fifty persons of both sexes, between the ages of nineteen and sixty-three, of French, Swiss, Russian, English and American nationalities. [M. Haffkine was the first to be inoculated with his own virus. He has undergone the operation three times.]

"In all cases the method has proved to be absolutely harmless to health. The symptoms consisted merely of a rise of temperature, a local sensitiveness at the place of inoculation and the formation of a temporary swelling at the same place. The symptoms appear about two or three hours after inoculation—viz., fever and general indisposition, which disappear in from twenty-four to thirty-six hours, and sensitiveness and œdema lasting three or four days. The symptoms following the second inoculation are usually more marked but of shorter duration; the whole giving rise to a feeling as of a bad cold in the head, lasting from one to two days. The microbes which are introduced under the skin do not propagate, but die and disappear after a certain time. It is the substances which they contain which being set free on the death of the animals act upon the animal organism and confer immunity upon it. It is found that the same result can be obtained if the microbes be killed before inoculation. Thus vaccines have been preserved in weak solutions of carbolic acid in which the microbes die at the end of several hours, and the vaccine preserved in this way has been found to be still efficacious six months after its preparation. There is evidently considerable advantage in preserving the microbes in this way. It enables them to be used by persons having no bacteriological training, and the absence of living germs makes the vaccines perfectly safe. The carbolic acid that they contain preserves them against any invasion of other microbes, and as they can be kept for several months

their preparation may be carried out at a central laboratory whence the vaccine *ampoules* can be sent out to operators. But it is probable that the immunity given by these preserved vaccines does not equal in persistency that produced by living germs, and as the method is not yet supported by verified statistics it is better that inoculations should be made as much as possible with living virus, so as to secure the most reliable results.

"As to the length of time that immunity so produced will last, there were no animals at the laboratory of the Pasteur Institute that had been inoculated for a period longer than four months and a half. At the end of that time their immunity was found to be perfect and was likely to last much longer. The experiments upon man, added to the hundreds of experiments which had been made upon animals, testify to the absolutely harmless nature of these operations, and there is no difficulty in proving their efficacy by experiment, independently of the species of animal which may be employed.

"On Wednesday last Dr. Woodhead inoculated six animals with the first vaccine. The second inoculation was made two days ago. Yesterday, in presence of Dr. Woodhead and several other gentlemen, these six animals were inoculated with 6 c.c. of virus of the cholera culture into the peritoneum. At the same time six other animals, which had not been inoculated before, were injected with half the dose which the first set of animals had received. The result is that the inoculated animals are to-day perfectly well. To any one accustomed to the clinical appearance of guinea-pigs after inoculation the animals you see before you have a perfectly normal appearance. On the other hand, of the six animals which were inoculated with half of the dose, two are already dead, two are very ill, and there is not the slightest doubt that the two others will be dead to-morrow.

"It is unnecessary to say that we cannot perform a similar experiment on man, although this would be the only means by which a definite experimental demonstration could be given. This being the case, evidently the objection might be raised that, although this vaccination renders guinea-pigs, rabbits and pigeons very resistant, yet it might be possible that man might escape this law. That, indeed, is not impossible, and—we lay stress, much stress, upon the fact—it is by experiment that our method must be established. It is by direct application and experiment that we must verify to ourselves and others the true value of the means extolled. Yet, after the experience already acquired, we think there is little probability that a negative result will be obtained. The difference between a mammal like the rabbit or the guinea-pig and a bird like the pigeon, from an anatomical and physiological point of view, is much greater than between rodents and man. Hence, when the same law is proved to exist amongst animals so different, there is little probability that man is not also subject to it. The symptoms following on inoculation of our vaccines are analogous in all the animals experimented on, including man. The same changes of temperature take place in all. In the animals which have been rendered resistant against cholera immunity is evidenced by the fact that every subcutaneous inoculation, made even with weakened virus, induces a rise of temperature greater than the preceding. The same thing takes place in man. We hope that the parallel will extend to this modification of the organism which produces the resistance against an infective agent. But the sole and definitive confirmation of this hope can be obtained only by the application of the method where cholera makes ravages amongst the human race."

Guinea-pigs were exhibited to show the effects on the animals when inoculated under the skin and when inoculated into the peritoneal cavity. The difference between the effects of the strong virus and the weak virus was also demonstrated. One of the animals was inoculated on Saturday last with one-tenth part of the tube of the weak vaccine. If they would examine it, they would find that it had, at the point of inoculation, a small localised œdema, but there was nothing resembling abscess or anything of the sort. It would disappear in a very few days. On the other hand, another animal was inoculated on Saturday at the same time, subcutaneously also, with the stronger vaccine, and they found that a very definite little abscess was formed, that the skin was necrosed over its surface, and that it would take some time to heal. Another animal inoculated with the same quantity of virus into the peritoneal cavity died within from sixteen to twenty-four hours. The experiment on the one which had re ceived the weak vaccine would be continued. The result would be that when it was inoculated again the abscess as shown in the other animal would not form. That was the reason why these two vaccines were used in inoculating man. The first produced a slight œdema, but it did not produce an abscess, and when they used the strong virus after the weak one, instead of producing an abscess, they simply got a small swelling which disappeared in a few days. Since M. Haffkine had been in England two gentlemen, one of whom had proceeded into a dangerous part of Persia, the other being a medical officer of health near London, had been inoculated by him. The following is a clinical report on one of these gentlemen, taken by his son, who is a medical man and a pathologist. The notes were as follows :—"The first inoculation was made on Feb. 4th, 1893. The gentleman in question is fifty-six years old. Temperature at the time of inoculation 97° F. under the axilla. After three hours slight lassitude set in. At 5 P.M. slight pain in the side ; temperature 98° F. in the mouth ; seat of inoculation red, indurated, two inches by two. At 7 P.M., temperature 99° F. At 9 P.M. lassitude increased ; took a slight dinner. The son notices that his father looks markedly febrile, feels tired and goes to bed ; temperature 99° ; pulse increased to about 80 ; feels slightly cold and there is slight pain in the limbs. At 10.30 slept well since going to bed ; temperature 99° ; respiration above normal. Soon went to sleep again and passed very good night. Feb. 6th, 9 A.M., temperature 98° ; appetite not so good as usual ; was quite able to resume usual duties ; symptoms by no means severe ; the most remarkable phenomena are the onset and the feeling of lassitude and sleepiness. At 11.40, temperature 99°. Feb. 6th, morning temperature 98°, evening 97°. Feb. 8th, morning temperature 97° ; evening 97·5°. Feb. 8th, morning temperature 97·5°. The second inoculation was made to-day." The notes in the case of the other gentleman had unfortunately been lost, but practically the same result ensued. This gentleman summed up his experience by declaring that he would rather be inoculated against cholera than be vaccinated again. M. Haffkine made a post-mortem examination of one of these inoculated animals that had succumbed to the intraperitoneal injection of the exalted virus, and the pathological appearances as shown in guinea-pigs were demonstrated. There was a red injected spot showing that a portion of the inoculation had entered the muscular tissue. The abdomen was distinctly distended and contained serous fluid. The bowels were red and injected much more than is usual in guinea-pigs. All the other organs were normal. On the liver, between the diaphragm and that organ, slight traces of lymph could be seen. The spleen, if the animal lives for a certain length of time, is slightly enlarged ; in this case the spleen was distinctly enlarged, the animal having lived twenty-four hours. The cultures from which all these experiments were made were from a case of cholera which occurred in Cochin China, and were forwarded direct to M. Haffkine.

M. Haffkine then made a cover-glass preparation of the œdematous fluid from the peritoneal cavity to show that it contained a pure culture of the cholera bacillus, and this was examined with much interest by many who were present.

Dr. Pavy at the termination of the proceedings expressed the thanks of the audience to M. Haffkine for the demonstration, characterising it as an act of courtesy and kindness in him to remain in England solely for the purpose of giving this demonstration. It was sincerely to be hoped that the promise afforded by his observations which were now being conducted would be realised, and that we might have an illustration of the power of knowledge in the bringing under subjection of one of those diseases which formed a great terror to mankind. Turning to M. Haffkine, he said : "We desire to express our gratitude to you for having remained here in England to afford us an opportunity of witnessing this demonstration, and I would ask Dr. Ruffer, who has served us so well as a medium between yourself and us, to play the opposite part and serve as a medium between us and M. Haffkine by conveying to him the thanks of the meeting." This Dr. Ruffer did in felicitous terms, and the demonstration then concluded.

LITERARY INTELLIGENCE. — Mr. H. K. Lewis announces the issue at an early date of a second edition of Dr. Radcliffe Crocker's work on Diseases of the Skin, which has been greatly enlarged and brought up to date. A new volume of Lewis's Practical Series is also nearly ready, and is entitled "Public Health Laboratory Work," by H. R. Kenwood, M.B., D.P.H.

The Lancet Special Commission
ON
SEAMEN'S DIETARIES.

CONSIDERABLE attention has been drawn during the past three or four months to the food of British merchant seamen and a committee consisting of the representatives of many of the shipowners' associations has been investigating the question with the object of ascertaining in what respects a revision of the scales now in vogue is advisable. We have independently made many inquiries from representative seamen themselves, and have thought it well to lay their views before the profession when comparing the present dietaries and that proposed for future adoption in the merchant service with some dietaries laid down for representative bodies of landsmen, so that the question may be studied from as many sides as possible. We may say at once that very few complaints have been made to us as to the quality of the articles supplied to sailors, with the exception of tea and coffee, which were often stated to be of very inferior quality. There is an almost unanimous opinion that the quality of the staple articles of beef, pork, bread and flour has immensely improved in late years. The quantities fixed by the minimum scale are said to be not too great for protracted and arduous work, and to be far too small in the special long voyage sailing ship scale. It is generally supposed that the Board of Trade fixes the amount and examines into the quality of the food supplied to the sailor, but this is not the case, for in the form of agreement issued by the Board of Trade no detailed scheme of dieting is given: there is only found a skeleton scale of the provisions to be allowed and served out to the men during the voyage for which the agreement is made.

This skeleton scale (Table I.) must be filled in before the agreement is signed, and the quantity and quality of provisions supplied are therefore solely a matter of contract between the owner and the crew. But practically a regular scale is inserted into the articles, and when the sailor signs these with the "usual" diet scale filled in, he clearly understands by that term that the minimum scale of 1854 (Table II.) is intended, and this is deemed a sufficient one by the authorities. It is stated by the shipowners that this scale is rarely adhered to, and this is quite true in many cases, but from our inquiries amongst the sailors it is clear that it is sometimes most rigidly followed ; and it is obvious that if it is compulsorily adhered to nothing in addition can be insisted on, and that no objection can be taken by the sailor after he has signed articles. We must therefore take it into consideration as being the actual basis on which alone the seaman can insist, and which in many ships is all that he will get during a voyage.

The absence of any preserved meats or vegetables and the monotony of a diet practically limited to bread, salt beef and pork, with soup once and dough three times a week, at once shows that such a scale is only fitted for short voyages or for voyages in which the ship is not too long from port to port where the substitutes of fresh meat and vegetables can be often made use of. The supplying of these substitutes should not be optional at the master's discretion ; they should be compulsory whenever the ship arrived at a port. The shipowners clearly recognise that this diet is deficient in fresh provisions, for a special long-voyage scale (Table III.) is also in use, and in this preserved meats, potatoes and vegetables, raisins, preserves and molasses are included. This scale is agreed to by the sailor also when he signs his agreement, and he is quite conversant with its particulars before he starts on a long voyage.

A comparison of the two dietaries shows that in the long voyage scale the seaman loses per week 1¾ lb. of bread, 2½ lb. of beef and 1¾ lb. of pork, and gains 2 lb. of preserved meat, a quarter of a pint of soup and half a pound of flour. The preserved potatoes (6 oz.), preserved vegetables (1 lb.), coffee (1¾ oz.), raisins (3 oz.), suet (2 oz.), butter (½ oz.), preserves (1 lb.) and molasses (half a pint), although excellent varieties in a dietary and most useful as aids in the prevention of scurvy, can hardly be considered as efficient substitutes for the above-mentioned loss of the more nutritious articles—biscuits, beef and pork. In fact, instead of being called substitutes, all these antiscorbutics should

As regards small-pox and vaccination we can measure results far more accurately, for although the intensity changes and climatic conditions are inconstant the course of events under the old and new order of things can be observed concurrently year by year and day by day ; and it is this fact which makes the protective influence of vaccination perhaps the most clearly established of all points in preventive medicine. In every epidemic the two classes, the unprotected and the artificially protected, can be observed side by side, under like conditions. But even in regard to small-pox the change of type has led to fallacy. At Leicester it has been alleged that with speedy isolation of persons attacked, and quarantine of those exposed to infection, small-pox may be held in check, and that vaccination is unnecessary even if beneficial. The proof advanced is that small-pox has not succeeded until lately in spreading amongst the imperfectly vaccinated population of Leicester. Many fallacies in this line of reasoning have long ago been pointed out. It ignores the assistance rendered by vaccination, even in Leicester. It presupposes early knowledge of all cases, however slight, compulsory isolation and quarantine, and the observance of a like thorough policy in all other localities, rural as well as urban. And further, if Leicester escaped because it had and used means of isolation and quarantine, how are we to account for the temporary escape of Keighley ? A more probable explanation seems to be that the Leicester experiment with isolation and the Keighley experiment without it have only been tried during years of low intensity when small-pox has scarcely been able to hold its ground in any part of England. Epidemic centres have been few, the chances of repeated importation comparatively small, and the power of diffusion slight. The real test has still to come, when the conditions are altered, as they seem likely to be within the next few years. It is not enough to introduce small-pox amongst a population imperfectly protected by vaccination. That the recently vaccinated will not take small-pox is certain, but it is not equally certain that the unprotected will at once be attacked. Something depends upon the quality of the small-pox itself, and it cannot safely be assumed that its power of epidemic spread is always the same, even if equal facilities be afforded.

Underlying all that mere death-rates or even mere attack-rates can teach us there is a variable type of disease, only imperfectly shown by such records.

SUMMARY.

1. Epidemic prevalence may be brought about either by increased potency of the disease itself or by increased mechanical facilities for diffusion.

2. Epidemics of the latter class, including water epidemics, milk epidemics and, as a rule, seasonal prevalence, are attended with lowered case mortality, because the conditions under which they occur imply a lessened average susceptibility and therefore a less severe average attack.

3. Underlying all great epidemics there is a change of epidemic type, a change in the quality of the disease itself.

4. There is evidence of a like change on a smaller scale in most, if not all, epidemic diseases, the intensity rising and falling at intervals which are not necessarily uniform for the same disease and are very different in different diseases.

5. Whether on the larger or smaller scale, the intensification is marked by greater severity of attack, greater power of overcoming comparative insusceptibility, and greater power of epidemic diffusion.

6. Whilst some diseases are capable of rapid or even abrupt changes in intensity, others are not ; and this distinction serves to mark off broadly two principal groups, those which are mobile and those which are comparatively constant in type.

7. The first group, that of diseases which are capable of most rapid change in type, includes those which are most nearly allied to saprophytic life, most readily cultivated in artificial media, most dependent upon filth conditions, most able to infect soil, water, milk and lower animals, most liable to relapses, and least protective.

8. Diseases of this class may be highly modified, and some of them may assume and maintain a form so slight that their true character is unrecognised.

9. Under favourable conditions their intensity may slowly or suddenly increase, giving rise to epidemics of severer type.

10. Amongst diseases of this class an epidemic normally begins and ends with the milder forms, the more severe attacks occurring at the time of greatest prevalence. The severity and prevalence rise and fall together.

11. In the second group, amongst diseases of more fixed character, extreme modification of epidemic type does not occur ; but individual attacks may be extremely mild owing to high resistance.

12. Amongst such diseases there is evidence of a rise and fall of intensity if the epidemic course be traced for a term of years, perhaps covering several minor epidemics.

13. In these brief outbursts of diseases of more constant type there is little if any change of intensity comparable to that of the mobile class, the prevalence being determined and controlled mainly by external conditions, but the type being that of the prevailing phase of a broad cycle.

CRETINISM TREATED BY THE HYPODERMIC INJECTION OF THYROID EXTRACT AND BY FEEDING.

BY EDWARD CARMICHAEL, M.D. Edin. &c.

ALTHOUGH several cases of myxœdema treated by thyroid extract and feeding have been reported, as also a case or two of cretinism by transplantation of the thyroid, few, if any, cases of the latter disease have been recorded as treated by the hypodermic injection of thyroid extract and feeding ; I therefore desire to state briefly the following regarding a case which has been under my care. When first asked to see the patient some three years ago I found her very much as the engraving from the first photograph represents. Although between five and six years of age, she was like an infant ; her features were broad and massive, her skin was dry and harsh, her abdomen prominent, the umbilicus protruding

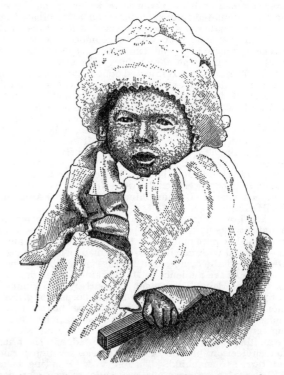

or rather kept in position by plaster, the supra-clavicular pads of fat well marked, and the hair sparse, dry and unhealthy— as was remarked, "she had no hair at all." She made no attempt to walk. Her intelligence was very feeble, although she recognised faces and was capable of showing affection towards her parents. Her appetite was extremely capricious, and if the nurse tried to give her a meal she did not care for it was immediately vomited. Obstinate constipation was present, relieved, however, by massage with castor oil. The temperature was always low, but on account of the difficulty of taking it I can give no consecutive table ; on several occasions it was about 96° F., sometimes lower.

History.—The child from birth had been slow in action and in vital powers—e.g., vaccination was particularly long in developing. There was a history of a fall from a perambulator when some months old, but I do not think much importance is to be attached to this. Her rate of growth had been about one inch annually. As regards the history of former treatment, the parents had seen several consultants. No medicines, of course, had caused any improvement, but general massage seemed to have brought about some amelioration. Up till April, 1892, any treatment I employed was on account of some special symptom—e.g., eczema, which was very troublesome, or constipation or other complication.

Treatment.—In April, 1892, I got the parents to consent to try the effect of the hypodermic injection of thyroid extract. I began with ten minims twice a week, but after about twelve injections the mother found that the child was restless, irritable and sleepless, and apparently worse after the injections. Accordingly I reduced the injection to ten minims weekly, thereafter every second week, and on three occasions left four weeks between the injections. This brings us down to October, when I began the feeding with the raw gland, giving half a lobe per week at first, then, after two weeks, one lobe per week, when I tried two lobes one week, and by this time found the temperature normal; but the child was evidently "out of sorts," so the amount was reduced to one

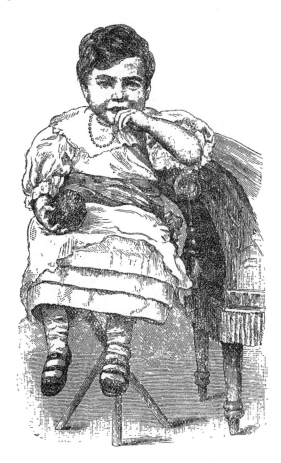

lobe a week and was continued at this till recently, when one lobe and a half were given. It was administered in cool beef-tea.

The result of the thyroid treatment was continuous improvement. After the first few injections the appearance of the child had completely changed; there was a marked diminution in the size of the abdomen, so that a bodice which fitted before the commencement of this treatment now overlapped by four or five inches. The thick lips and alæ nasi were now of normal size, the skin was pliant and soft, the temperature to touch improved, and the hair apparently more healthy, though still sparse. As week by week passed some mark of improvement was always seen. In October the child began to walk, and soon was running about and even walking long distances. The head, smaller to appearance, became covered with a fine crop of healthy hair. Marked improvement in intelligence was seen in many little actions. The engraving from the second photograph shows the patient's

appearance after nine months' treatment, six months by hypodermic injection and three months by feeding with raw gland. During the nine months the child has grown fully four inches; the supra-clavicular pads have quite disappeared; the appetite has improved amazingly, her dietary being a much larger one now; the constipation is gone, the umbilicus no longer protrudes, and there is no tendency to eczema. The temperature remains at about 97° F. The improvement is such that a friend and regular visitor at the house, who had been absent for some weeks, on seeing the child, did not recognise her, and thinking she was a stranger asked whose child she was. One point I may mention—namely, that prior to the thyroid treatment there frequently appeared a dark, almost black, part on the scalp, which after increasing in depth of colour came away in scales. I judged it to be a coloured sebaceous secretion.

I have also had two cases of myxœdema in adults which I treated with extract and feeding, with markedly beneficial results, but many such cases have already been reported.

Loudon-street, Edinburgh.

THE CHOLERA EPIDEMIC IN RUSSIA.

BY FRANK CLEMOW, M.D. EDIN. &C.

No. I.

IN CENTRAL ASIA AND SIBERIA.

(Continued from p. 516.)

IN marked contrast with the comparative intensity of the epidemic in Uralsk was its mildness in the province of Turgai, lying immediately adjacent on the east. The first cases were reported from there on July 24th, and the whole province escaped with the small loss of 296 cases with 167 deaths. The inhabitants of both these provinces are mostly Kirghiz and Kalmuck Tartars, living a more or less nomadic life. Their water-supply is derived from rivers and wells; the river water is said to be of satisfactory quality, but the well water is less so; whilst in the dry season the tribes drink extremely polluted water from lakes, not, however, without a rough process of filtration or, rather, straining. As early as July 14th cases were reported from Omsk and the large district of which it is the principal town. This district contains the three provinces of Akmolinsk, Semipalatinsk and Semiretchinsk, and is known officially as the General Governorship of the Steppes. The numbers of cases and deaths were at no time very high from any of these provinces, of which Akmolinsk was the greatest sufferer. The totals for the whole of this immense district were only 2133 cases with 1124 deaths, representing a case-rate of 118 and a death-rate of 62 per 100,000. These figures sink into insignificance when compared with those of the neighbouring province on the north. In this province, the government of Tobolsk, the epidemic raged with great violence. The first cases occurred on July 17th, and the total number reported was 26,301, of which 12,729 proved fatal; the proportion of cases and deaths to the population being expressed by the figures 1865 and 903 respectively. In the middle of July cases of cholera were reported amongst exile prisoners in the town of Tomsk, and from this distant government there were, in all, 4697 cases and 2272 deaths. Finally, the disease was reported from Irkutsk on Aug. 2nd and from Yeniseisk on the 4th, but in neither of these northerly governments did it attain any hold.

The following table gives the numbers of cases and deaths, the proportion of both to the population, and the ratio of deaths to cases in each division of Asiatic Russia beyond the Caspian Sea during the whole course of the epidemic. For these figures, as well as for much valuable material and information, I am indebted to Dr. Ragozin, the Director of the Medical Department of the Ministry of the Interior; whilst for kindly revising and verifying all the statistics given in this paper my thanks are due to Dr. Grebentschikoff, the head of the statistical division of the same Department.

PUERPERAL SEPTICÆMIA: USE OF STREPTO-COCCUS ANTITOXIN.

By ANGUS E. KENNEDY, L.R.C.P. LOND.,
M.R.C.S. ENG., L.S.A.

A PRIMIPARA aged twenty-eight years was confined on Aug. 28th, 1895. The presentation was left occipito-posterior, and a child weighing ten pounds was delivered with forceps, the occiput not rotating and the perineum being torn to the sphincter. The labour lasted twelve hours. She recovered fairly well and progressed till the evening of the fourth day, when her temperature rose to 103° F. and she had a shivering fit; but after a copious motion—the bowels had not been open since the confinement—the temperature became normal, and she went on without regaining strength till Sept. 11th, when the temperature rose to 101° in the evening. On Sept. 12th she was carried to a sofa, but soon asked to go back again. On Sept. 13th she was not well enough to be moved. On Sept. 14th, seventeen days after labour, she had a slight rigor in the morning, followed by a more severe one in the afternoon, when the temperature rose to 104°. On Sept. 15th her temperature was 104°, the pulse 130 and very feeble. The abdomen was somewhat distended and tympanitic, the tongue being fairly clean. There was no uterine tenderness. After a copious evacuation of the bowels her temperature fell, and she remained very exhausted and feeble, but with a normal temperature till the evening of Sept. 17th, when it rose to 103° and her pulse to 120. There were no local symptoms whatever, and the distension of the abdomen had disappeared, but her pulse was so bad and her general condition so very much worse that I gave her 40 c.c. of the antitoxin at once. In six hours her temperature had fallen to 100°, and the pulse to 112, and she said her head felt much clearer; but fourteen hours after the first injection her temperature had risen to 102°, and the pulse to 120, and I then gave her 45 c.c. of antitoxin. Her temperature reached 99° in six hours, and in twenty-four hours was normal, and since then there has been constant improvement, though she remained so exhausted that it was seven weeks before she was able to walk across the room alone, and she is as thin as a convalescent from typhoid fever. The child was of course weaned before the first injection. My idea of the case is that there was a septic thrombus in a vein, which was loosened and carried into the general circulation when she was taken out of bed; but the actual cause of the symptoms is very obscure, though no one seeing her would have doubted its being septic.

Being the first time that streptococcus antitoxin has been used in England the case seemed worth publishing, and I am indebted to Dr. Ruffer for his kindness in getting me the antitoxin.

Plaistow.

A CASE OF COMPLETE SEPARATION OF THE UPPER JAW.

By G. HERBERT HOPKINS, F.R.C.S. ENG.,
SURGEON TO THE SWANSEA GENERAL HOSPITAL.

A MAN aged forty-nine years was admitted to Swansea Hospital on Aug. 7th, 1895. He had been struck on the back of the head by a wooden beam and knocked forward on to a coal truck, the sharp edge of which had caught him at the root of the nose. On examination the whole of the upper jaw was found to be detached from the skull, the nasal processes of the superior maxillary bones and the zygomatic processes of the malar bones being fractured. There was over an inch of separation in the middle line. The frontal sinus and anterior ethmoidal cells were opened up. The eyes were quite uninjured. The parts were cleaned and stitched up, free drainage being provided for by the nose. A Smith's gag was used, which kept the parts in very good position. The patient wore this continuously for a fortnight. He is now quite well with the exception of slight ptosis of the right eye.

Swansea.

A **Mirror**
OF
HOSPITAL PRACTICE,
BRITISH AND FOREIGN.

Nulla autem est alia pro certo noscendi via, nisi quamplurimas et morborum et dissectionum historias, tum aliorum tum proprias collectas habere, et inter se comparare.—MORGAGNI *De Sed. et Caus. Morb.* lib. iv. Proœmium.

LIVERPOOL ROYAL INFIRMARY.

CASE OF HYDROCEPHALUS; TREPHINING; OPENING OF THE FOURTH VENTRICLE; RECOVERY.[1]

(Under the care of Dr. GLYNN, and Mr. THELWALL THOMAS).

THIS case is a brilliant example of the good results obtained by modern surgery in a disease which has hitherto, with very few exceptions, proved fatal. It is only necessary to read the subjoined notes to understand how desperate the condition was in this patient. The methods formerly adopted by surgeons for the relief of hydrocephalus—tapping the lateral ventricles of the brain through the anterior fontanelle or after trephining when the skull had already closed—were but palliative in their effects, and death was only postponed for a time. Drainage of cerebro-spinal fluid from the spinal canal has been unsuccessfully tried, and until Mr. Parkin, following out some suggestions made by Mr. A. C. Morton, trephined a child aged four years and a half on April 4th, 1893,[2] we were without proof that the operation could be done on the living subject. It is true that this first case was unsuccessful, but great temporary relief was afforded to the patient, and when the case alluded to by Mr. Thelwall Thomas in his remarks came under treatment operation with slow drainage for eighteen days was followed by complete success. It is very evident from this brief abstract that the number of cases in which it is possible to do any good by operation is very few, for it may be taken for granted that if such came under the observation of physicians they would eagerly avail themselves of this chance of effecting a cure. The operation is only in its infancy as yet, and therefore it behoves those with any experience to give the profession the benefit of it. For the notes of this case we are indebted to Mr. Thelwall Thomas, senior surgeon to the infirmary.

The patient, a young man aged eighteen, was admitted into the Royal Infirmary, Liverpool, on March 15th, 1895, with the following history. Eighteen months previously, when a steward on an Atlantic steamer, he began to suffer from occasional attacks of severe headache and giddiness, which lasted for a few hours at a time. The pain was most marked in the back of the head. The attacks increased in severity and frequency, so that for the last six months he had hardly been free from pain. Latterly the attacks of giddiness had been so severe that he fell during them, always towards the right, although surrounding objects appeared to revolve to the left. For five minutes before an attack he felt very sick (he had only vomited once, three months previously, when an iron hook struck the back of his head and determined a fit); his head felt very hot, but he experienced a sensation of coldness and numbness in the trunk and limbs and a buzzing noise in both ears. If he closed his eyes the giddiness was not so troublesome, and he could avoid falling if he clutched at a railing or some article of furniture. When he fell he had remained on the floor as long as half an hour, conscious, but unable to rise or speak, although he understood what was said to him. Memory, sight, and hearing had been gradually failing. For six months he had suffered from insomnia, occasionally getting a few hours' sleep only to wake up with intense headache. For the last three weeks he had been afraid to leave his bed on account of the giddiness. On admission he was found to be a well-nourished thick-set youth with a very dull look and a large head twenty-five inches in circumference. His temperature was 97.6° F. and the pulse was 66. Severe headache was referred to the right occipital region; the head was tender

---

[1] This case formed the subject of a paper read before the Medical Institution, Liverpool, on Oct. 17th, 1895, the patient being exhibited.
[2] THE LANCET, Nov. 18th, 1893.

She had been taking two-minim doses of tincture of digitalis in iced water with a few drops of brandy every half hour since the previous day. On the 22nd she had another bad night with decided increase of delirium and awful dyspnœa and some wandering during the day. The face, if possible, was more dusky. When seen at 9 P.M. she appeared to be moribund. The breathing consisted of a succession of short jerky sighs, the hands were icy cold, and the legs cold up to the knees. The radial pulse was fluttering and barely perceptible and there was whispering delirium. She was ordered one-tenth of a grain of morphine and stimulants with local application of warmth. She slept well after this and on the 23rd had rallied surprisingly in all directions. The improvement was maintained throughout the day, but towards evening the unfavourable symptoms returned. At midnight the patient awoke from a restless sleep and asked the nurse for some water, but before this could be given her she had fallen back dead.

It is matter for regret that an account of the post-mortem appearances is not available. The grouping of symptoms, however, and the character and development of the physical signs leave little doubt as to the nature of the case—blocking in the first instance of one of the branches of the pulmonary artery in the right lung with subsequent extension of the thrombus to other branches, pulmonary apoplexy, and death from cardiac failure. The chief interest of the case lies in the occurrence of this well-known series of events in a young girl who was apparently in perfect health. A diligent inquiry into the cause of the accident has been entirely negative in its results, and we have had to fall back on the hypothesis that the seeds of the mischief had been sown during the severe illness above referred to, possibly in the form of adherent thrombi in the right cavities of the heart, one of which became detached on June 16th.

Chandos-street, W.

NOTE ON THE PICRIC ACID TEST FOR SUGAR.

By MARK McDONALD, M.B. DUB.

WHILE carrying out some work on the urine some time since I came across certain reactions with the picric acid reduction test with which it is not generally credited. The importance which this test has acquired in the estimation, both qualitatively and quantitatively, of sugar in urine is sufficient excuse for bringing forward any points bearing on the subject.

When to a drachm of urine there are added a drachm of a saturated solution of picric acid, half a drachm of liquor potassæ, and one and a half drachms of water (as recommended by Sir George Johnson in the quantitative estimation of sugar), an orange-red colour is produced in the cold, due to the kreatinin present in the urine reducing the yellow potassium picrate to red picramate. On heating, this colour becomes more intense. Should the urine contain sugar in any quantity the effect of its presence will not be observed until the temperature reaches nearly 100° C., at which point the colouration is evidently much intensified. If, however, before heating the mixture it be largely diluted—the addition of two ounces of water produces the effect most typically as a rule—the liquid is seen to gradually darken as it is heated, until it boils. Should the urine be normal it will be observed after a few seconds' boiling that the colouration has disappeared, and prolonged boiling does not bring it back; but if the liquid be cooled the colour gradually reappears, and this reaction may be repeated with the same solution any number of times. Should the urine contain sugar in any quantity the solution as before gradually darkens as heat is applied until it boils, when the colour (due to kreatinin) disappears, but if the boiling be prolonged in this case the solution again becomes coloured. This paradoxical reaction depends on the weakness of the solution in potassium picrate. Solutions of the latter when very weak are only with great difficulty partially reduced. The picramate produced by the action of kreatinin in the cold is on boiling reoxidised to picrate; sugar, on the other hand, reduces the weak picrate solutions only on prolonged boiling. A solution of pure urinary kreatinin (prepared by Mr. S. Johnson's method) acts in a manner similar to a normal urine, more liquor potassæ being,

of course, required, as Sir George Johnson pointed out. A dextrose solution on similar treatment caused reduction of the picrate only on very prolonged boiling.

It appears, then, that under certain conditions potassium picramate, when boiled in the presence of the substances by whose oxidation it has been produced from picrate, undergoes reoxidation at the expense of these oxidised bodies. The conditions necessary are weakness of the picrate solution and capability of the oxidised bodies to easily undergo reduction. The latter condition is met with in the case of kreatinin. Other substances, as for example the alkaline sulphides, though they reduce in the cold, nevertheless do not reoxidise the picramate on boiling, as the products of their oxidation are very stable bodies. Dilution of the kreatinin solution also assists the reaction. Corresponding results are obtained if, instead of diluting the solutions before boiling, they are first boiled at the usual strength and then diluted with two ounces of water. In the case of normal urines and kreatinin solutions boiling removes the colour, while with sugar and alkaline sulphides no diminution takes place however prolonged the boiling may be. It is noteworthy in all these cases that when heat is applied after dilution the liquid assumes a distinctly darker colour before the boiling point is reached, showing that in the process of dilution and cooling some reoxidation of the picramate had taken place.

If the behaviour of normal urines and kreatinin solutions, on the one hand, and saccharine urines and dextrose solutions, on the other hand, be compared, their reducing power being equal, it is found that after prolonged boiling of the diluted solutions those which contain dextrose have a distinctly darker colour. The intensity of this final colour is proportional, too, to the quantity of dextrose present. It is possible by means of the different actions of kreatinin and sugar to determine whether the reducing effect of a urine is in part due to sugar. This can usually be effected by heating the diluted solution to nearly the boiling point in a long test-tube of small diameter, and then boiling the upper half of the liquid. The colour due to kreatinin disappears, and on boiling for a minute or two the upper part of the solution again darkens if sugar is present. It is important to remember that if the diluted liquid contains less than 1 part of dextrose in 10,000 no sugar reaction takes place, since, as Sir George Johnson noticed, its effect on alkaline picrate vanishes with higher degrees of dilution. This disturbance may be obviated by adding less water, or a dilute solution of potassium picrate may be prepared by mixing a drachm of saturated picric acid solution with half a drachm of liquor potassæ and adding eight and a half drachms of water. To one drachm of this solution one drachm of a twice or four times diluted and neutralised urine is added and the mixture treated as usual. In some cases it is necessary to compare the final colouration with that given by a kreatinin solution of equal reducing power.

Though I have occasionally during the last few months found this reaction of picric acid useful in deciding a diagnosis of glycosuria, I bring it forward less as a practical test than as a warning against a possible disturbance of the usual test for sugar.

Waterloo, Liverpool.

THE DISCOVERY OF A BULLET LOST IN THE WRIST BY MEANS OF THE ROENTGEN RAYS.

By ROBERT JONES, F.R.C.S. EDIN.,
HONORARY SURGEON TO THE ROYAL SOUTHERN HOSPITAL, LIVERPOOL;

AND

OLIVER LODGE, F.R.S.,
PROFESSOR OF PHYSICS, UNIVERSITY COLLEGE, LIVERPOOL.

A BOY aged about twelve years was brought to me by Dr. Simpson of Waterloo, Liverpool, having shot himself in the left hand just above the deep palmar arch. The wound was enlarged, but the bullet could not be found, and it was thought injudicious to prolong the search in view of the important structures in the vicinity unless one possessed a clue to its position. Professor Lodge kindly consented to take a photograph and the position of the bullet was very clearly outlined. It lies against the base of the third metacarpal bone over its articulation with the os magnum. This is, I think, the first photograph taken of a bullet embedded in a wrist—in this case considerably thickened as a result of inflammation. It will now be quite easy to extract it but it is thought better to await subsidence of inflammatory action. The photograph was taken in the presence of Mr. Houlgrave, who succeeded Dr. Simpson in the treatment of the case. Arrangements are being competed for fitting up a department for the employment of Roentgen's rays at the Royal Southern Hospital.

Note by Professor OLIVER LODGE.—The patient was brought to my laboratory by Mr. Robert Jones, with a pellet of lead lost in his left hand or forearm. Two

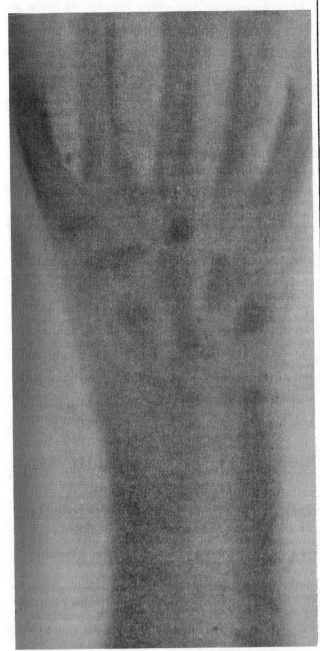

Roentgen radiograph of the left wrist of a lad aged twelve years, showing a small bullet which had been lost in it. The bullet is located between the base of the middle metacarpal bone and the os magnum. Taken by Professor Oliver Lodge, F.R.S., after two hours' exposure to a well exhausted home-made vacuum tube excited by a small ordinary coil. The sensitive plate was an Edwards's isochromatic, nine inches distant from the vacuum tube, screened from light by sheet aluminium.

preliminary short exposures to Roentgen rays indicated that the metal was not in a fleshy part readily penetrable by those rays, but was probably embedded among the bones of the wrist. The difficulty consisted in the opacity of those bones. I therefore took a tube with large electrodes made and

exhausted by my assistant, Mr. E. E. Robinson, containing potash, so that its vacuum could be adjusted to the best value, and arranged a magnet to concentrate the inside cathode-rays on a definite part of the glass, which phosphoresces and acts as the source of the rays. the rays spreading from each point of the glass in all directions. The boy was comfortably seated at a table with his palm down on an aluminium-protected Edwards' isochromatic half-plate, nine inches vertically below the vacuum tube, and rather more than two hours' exposure was given. The coil used was an ordinary Ruhmkorff, giving about two inches spark at most, and it was excited by five storage cells. The vacuum was such that a one-inch spark in air was usually preferred to the tube. The result was to bring out the wrist-bones clearly and to show the position of the pellet.

Liverpool.

LATENCY IN SYPHILIS.

By ARTHUR H. WARD, F.R.C.S. ENG.,
SURGEON TO OUT-PATIENTS, LONDON LOCK HOSPITAL, AND SURGICAL
REGISTRAR TO ST. GEORGE'S HOSPITAL.

IN the admirable paper read by Mr. Ernest Lane before the Royal Medical and Chirurgical Society on Dec. 10th, 1895, many cases were brought forward in proof of the fact of latency in syphilis; but neither in the paper nor in the discussion which followed was much said as to the causation of that latency which all admitted. I believe that some reasons may be brought forward to account for both the apparent and real latency of syphilis. By apparent latency I mean a period during which there are no visible lesions although the microbes are "doing their work," as Mr. Hutchinson put it, more or less actively. Real latency, however, I take to mean a period during which the microbes are absolutely inactive. In a former paper[1] I ventured to state a working hypothesis to account for the causation of syphilis and now state it thus: (1) Syphilis is associated with the growth of a microbe in the organism; (2) this microbe produces a toxine, which is the active cause of the phenomena of syphilis; and (3) this toxine when entering the human body in small and slowly increasing quantities establishes immunity. It would seem to be hardly necessary at the present time to adduce arguments in favour of the existence of such a microbe and consequent active toxine, since the microbe is generally admitted, while the activity of so many other microbes has been shown to be due to the formation of toxines. However, a somewhat striking evidence of its presence is furnished by the experiments of Straus and Tessier, who found that strong reactions occurred in cases of secondary syphilis when tuberculin injections were made; and that in a case of rupia an inflammatory areola formed round the lesions "identical with that occurring in cases of lupus" when injected.[2] It will be admitted that reaction following tuberculin injection certainly indicates the presence of the tubercle bacillus and its toxine, consequently a similar reaction in a case of syphilis indicates the presence of an analogous microbe and toxine in that disease.

The incubation period of syphilis is one of apparent latency. I think it is due to the circumstance that the microbe is a slow-growing one, as the course of the disease indicates, and also to the fact that only a few microbes can possibly be implanted at the moment of infection. Consequently these take time to grow into a colony large enough to produce an appreciable amount of toxine. Induration, the result of the chemiotaxic action of the toxine, can, therefore, not occur at once; but when a growth of three weeks or so has taken place toxine enough to attract round cells into the colony can well be formed. These cells when they have accumulated sufficiently distend the inter-cellular spaces and cause the indurated papule, which grows steadily with the peripheral growth of the colony and generally breaks down in the centre forming the indurated sore. It is to be noted that primary tuberculous inoculations also produce indurated lesions. The next period of apparent latency in the course of syphilis is the so-called second incubation period between the formation of the primary sore and the outbreak of secondaries. This period, I think, must have been in Mr. Hutchinson's mind when he spoke of microbic activity being

[1] THE LANCET, Sept. 10th, 1892.   [2] Medical Week, 1893, p. 399.

another thirty years it would then have entirely disappeared. The first great drop in its rate took place in the decade 1840–50, about the time that serious attention began to be given to sanitary reforms and especially to land drainage. It then remained scarcely reduced for about seventeen years; but from 1867 to 1894 it has been steadily on the decline. It is in this period that most of the great sanitary works have been carried out in this country. Can we doubt that it is to them that we owe so substantial a diminution of the disease? And need we despair of carrying it on to its fitting close? Let it be remembered that this improvement has taken place in spite of the increasing aggregation of the population in towns and without any special measures of repression having been attempted. It is, indeed, only recently that tubercle has been reckoned amongst preventable diseases, and although some slight efforts at the disinfection of sputum and the cleansing of rooms occupied by phthisical patients have been made we certainly cannot ascribe any part of the improvement that has taken place to these causes.[10] What may we not hope for when these measures come to be recognised as a part of the duty of every sanitary authority throughout the kingdom?[11] It is interesting to note that the other tuberculous diseases—such as scrofula, mesenteric disease, and tuberculous meningitis—have not diminished in like proportion.

Dr. Tatham has kindly sent me the following table from his decennial supplement, not yet published, from which it will be seen how slight a change has taken place in the rates of these diseases in the last thirty years. I have marked on the chart the annual rates per 10,000 for the last twenty years, as given in the Registrar-General's report for 1894. The difference between the first and last decennial periods per million is only 69, or rather less than 9 per cent. The rates under the heading of scrofula have, in fact, considerably increased—a fact difficult to account for if the causes of phthisis and scrofula are the same.

Annual Mortality per Million Living from Tuberculous Diseases, other than Phthisis.

Decennia.							Rates per million.
1861–70	...	...	...	...	...	...	765
1871–80	...	...	...	...	...	...	747
1881–90	...	...	...	...	...	...	696

The only possible sources of fallacy that can be discovered in these figures are (1) the uncertainty of diagnosis in the earlier periods of the registration of the causes of death, and (2) the acknowledged longer duration of phthisis in the later years. If in former days more cases of bronchitis or broncho-pneumonia were mistaken for phthisis, then these mistaken cases might have raised the apparent rates of mortality of this disease. Again, in more recent years the extension of the average duration of its progress before it ended in death would for a time postpone the appearance of these deaths in the register and would by so much lessen the phthisis rate without necessarily diminishing the real prevalence of the disease throughout the country. It is probable, however, that neither of these intrusive faults would account for the remarkably steady fall in the rate. Phthisis is a disease so easily recognised in its later stages that it has probably been reported with a fair degree of accuracy all through the period in question, and sooner or later most of the chronic cases of phthisis would have found their way into the death-roll. There is thus no important bar to our hope of a speedy extinction of phthisis if not of other tuberculous diseases, and the prophecy drawn from the analogy of leprosy is already in process of being fulfilled.

Bournemouth.

[10] A talented writer, Mr. G. Archdall Reid, in a recent work on The Present Evolution of Man (Chapman and Hall, 1896, pp. 279–286) ascribes the lower rate of mortality from tuberculosis amongst the British races to an increased resistance to the microbe, a power due to "the accumulation of inborn variations"; but this explanation will surely not apply to so rapid a decline as the diminution of from 60 to 70 per cent. in the course of sixty years. It is far more likely to be due to the causes to which we have assigned it: to the sanitary measures, including improved diet, which have at once and directly diminished the infecting power of the bacillus and increased the bodily powers of resistance in the mass of the population.

[11] We may, perhaps, find an additional feature of likeness between leprosy and tubercle in the fact that they have both given way, not to intentional measures of repression, but to general reforms in sanitation, by which the whole physical welfare of the nation has been raised.

SUPERANNUATION ALLOWANCE. — Mr. Thomas Francis, L.R.C.P. Edin., M.R.C.S. Eng., late medical officer for the first district of the Bradford Union, has been granted a superannuation allowance of £107 13s. 4d. per annum.

ON THE TREATMENT OF INOPERABLE CASES OF CARCINOMA OF THE MAMMA: SUGGESTIONS FOR A NEW METHOD OF TREATMENT, WITH ILLUSTRATIVE CASES.[1]

BY GEORGE THOMAS BEATSON, M.D. EDIN., SURGEON TO THE GLASGOW CANCER HOSPITAL; ASSISTANT SURGEON, GLASGOW WESTERN INFIRMARY; AND EXAMINER IN SURGERY TO THE UNIVERSITY OF EDINBURGH.

I HAVE no doubt it has fallen to the lot of nearly every medical man to have been consulted from time to time by patients suffering from carcinoma so widely spread or so situated that it has been quite apparent that nothing in the way of operative measures could be recommended. Such cases naturally excite our sympathy, but they also bring home to us the fact that once a case of cancer has passed beyond the reach of the surgeon's knife our curative measures are practically *nil*, and "that whether the case advance with giant strides or with slow and measured steps the result is equally sure and fatal." Of late, owing to my taking up the work of surgeon to the Glasgow Cancer Hospital, I have seen a considerable number of such cases, and an opportunity has been furnished me of working out a line of treatment which I am not aware has been as yet tried by others and which is founded on a view of the etiology and nature of cancer which is entirely opposed to the local parasitic theory of the disease and which seems to me to offer a more reasonable explanation of it. As these inoperable cases of cancer may be arranged into two groups— first, those which have been operated on, but in which, sooner or later, there has been a recurrence, or, as it should perhaps be better expressed, a re-appearance of the disease; and, secondly, those in which no operation has been attempted, but in which, when they first present themselves, the disease has progressed so far that no local removal could be attempted—I shall bring forward three cases, one of which is illustrative of the first group and the other two of the second.

The first case, then, that I wish to bring under notice is that of a woman who consulted me on May 11th, 1895, at the Glasgow Cancer Hospital, bringing me the following letter:—

"Apsley-place, May 6th, 1895.
"DEAR DR. BEATSON,—The bearer is, and has been, suffering, I fear, from a malignant breast. She has been in the Royal Infirmary before she came to me. My own opinion is that nothing can be done for her, but as she is a woman of great courage you might have a look at it for my sake, and perhaps you can order her something in the way of dressing. Even this little will be accepted by her as a great deal.
"With kindest regards, yours very truly,
"JAMES W. WALLACE."

The history she gave me was that she was thirty-three years of age, married, and the mother of two children, the oldest three years of age and the youngest fifteen months. She nursed both her children for from ten to twelve months, chiefly on the left breast, the first child entirely so, as the right breast suppurated for two or three weeks. While nursing her first baby she observed a small, hard lump at the outside of her left breast, and as it was painless and did not increase in size she took no further notice of it. It was only when her second baby was born twenty months later that she became aware it was increasing. She nursed the child on both breasts notwithstanding, and it was not for ten months, by which time the tumour had grown a good deal, that she weaned the child and sought advice at the Glasgow Royal Infirmary. In January of 1895 she was admitted to that institution, and the journal report states that an examination showed the left mammary gland to be a little more swollen than the right one and to present a hard and nodular appearance. In its centre was felt a large mass, measuring 5 in. across and 3½ in. in vertical diameter, while small nodules from this infiltrated the skin around. About 2 in. upwards and to the left of the nipple was seen an ulcer 1 in. in size, two nodules about the size of beans bordering on the extreme left of this ulcer. The patient

[1] A paper read before the Edinburgh Medico-Chirurgical Society on May 20th, 1896. Microscopic sections, kindly prepared by Dr. K. M. Buchanan, were shown of the growths in the cases described in the paper.

appeared to be strong, healthy, active, and robust. On Jan. 25th, 1895, she was operated upon. The hospital journal says that the left breast was excised, a large area of skin free of tumour being taken away. The axillary glands were removed, also a considerable part of the pectoral muscle which appeared to be implicated. A plastic incision was made parallel to the trunk to allow of the edges of the wound being approximated. The patient seemed to have made a good recovery and to have left the Infirmary towards the beginning of March with the wound almost healed. About a month after she had gone home—that is, within three months of the operation—she noticed that the wound had opened, that a little discharge was coming away, and that pain of a shooting character had developed. She observed also that some hardness was developing at the side of the scar, and so she returned to the Infirmary for advice. She was there told that she should come into the hospital again. She was readmitted for a few days and then discharged, as it was thought that an operation would be useless. The journal report is as follows : "April 28th, 1895: Dismissed. General involvement of whole scar by large tumours, cancerous in nature, to remove which entirely was thought impossible. Adherent axilla and chest walls. One of the wounds from the recurring secondary tumours has given way and there is now an ulcerated surface." Such, briefly, was the outline of her personal history as detailed to me. On questioning her nothing could be elicited in her family history that showed any hereditary tendency to cancerous disease. On May 11th, at the time she presented herself to me, the local condition for which she sought advice was as follows. On the left side of the thorax there was seen a very extensive cicatrix in the situation of the left mamma, which had apparently been entirely removed. The scar extended from the middle of the axilla to within $1\frac{1}{2}$ in. of the xiphi-sternum. It was irregularly curved in aspect. Above the centre of the scar was a cicatrising area, which had broken out after the operation in January last. This was now granulating and seemed healthy, but immediately below and arching over the centre of the long scar was a mass of recurrent tumour, hard and nodular, with much thinning and discolouration of skin. This mass was curved in shape, about $2\frac{1}{2}$ in. broad at its broadest part, and about $3\frac{1}{2}$ in. in length. There were other nodules in the cicatrix as far back as the axilla. Four inches lower down there was the linear cicatrix of a plastic operation, made apparently to allow of the sliding together of the edges of the operation wound. No enlarged glands could be felt in the axilla or above the clavicle, but there was a distinct tumour of the left lobe of the thyroid gland, with some enlargement of the isthmus. This, however, she said had been present as long as she could remember. The right breast and axilla were free from any disease. The patient's weight was 9st. 9lb. She looked pale and careworn, and when questioned admitted she felt ill and was quite unable to perform her household duties. From the clinical history she had given me and from the local condition present I had no doubt that the case was one of carcinoma—a diagnosis that was subsequently confirmed by our pathologist, Dr. R. M Buchanan, who reported as follows on a portion of tissue taken from the ulcerated surface above the line of the cicatrix : "The portion of tissue ...... is typically cancerous. The cellular elements predominate over the stroma very largely."

The question that had to be decided was whether anything further could be done for the case. As regards local removal I was quite at one with the opinion already expressed at the Royal Infirmary that it was unjustifiable, because the prospects of complete eradication of the cancerous material were not good, and previous experience had shown me that in young patients such as the present the attempt is seldom successful and, indeed, sometimes seems to hasten the progress of the disease, which assumes an acute and fulminating form, most disappointing and disastrous. Failing, then, local measures, could the disease be attacked in any other way and by any other channels ? To answer this it is necessary that I should put before you views that I have for some time held as to the etiology or cause of cancer generally, but more particularly of that of the female mamma. Before, however, doing so I think it will be advantageous that I should very briefly lay down what I consider is the present state of our knowledge of carcinoma or cancer, so that I may make it quite clear what I mean by that term and that there may be no difference of opinion as to what it is we are discussing. Well, I think I put the case fairly when I say

that there are certain points in carcinoma on which we are all agreed and others on which there is great diversity of opinion. I think we are all at one on the following : 1. That carcinoma is a tumour taking origin in epithelium and having an epithelial structure. 2. That the essential feature of the disease is the continuous and excessive growth of this epithelium, which invades the surrounding tissues, spreads along the lymphatic vessels, passes from one set of glands to another, and eventually forms deposits in distant organs and parts of the body. 3. That once this proliferation of epithelium has begun nothing that we know of has the power of arresting it. 4. That if a microscopic section of a carcinoma is made sufficiently thin and stained certain special cells are observed, which cells, although not fulfilling the *rôle* of Lebert's specific cancer-cell, are yet sufficiently characteristic of the disease and are now known as "cancer-bodies." 5. That clinically it is a matter of common observation that the younger the patient the more rapid the cell proliferation and the more quickly fatal the disease; while in many old persons cancer assumes the atrophic or withering form from fatty degeneration and absorption of the epithelial cells, little more being left than a mass of fibrous tissue with here and there a few cells surrounded by granular débris. 6. That cancer kills either by septicæmia from absorption of unhealthy products, or by hæmorrhage, or by interference with the function of some important organ. 7. That in our present state of knowledge of the nature and etiology of cancer the best treatment we can offer our patients is the complete removal of the disease by the surgeon's knife, and that the aseptic surgery of the present day allows this to be done more freely than heretofore, so that very extensive operations are performed nowadays.

There is, however, not the same unanimity of opinion on the two following points in connexion with cancer : (1) as to the purely local origin of the disease ; and (2) as to the interpretation to be put upon the structures known as cancer-bodies.

Taking the first point, we find that some hold that the carcinomatous growth has a purely *local* origin—starts, in fact, from an irritation developed locally, and that if that irritation and its effects are freely removed the patient is cured. Others, again, teach that carcinoma, though an affection of the solid tissues, as shown in the local cell proliferation it causes, is really a blood disease and that the tumour is only a local manifestation of a blood affection. Lastly, there is what I may term a third school, who hold that there is a certain state of the system or of the tissues in which a local injury, such as a blow, will start a carcinoma of the part, and without this local irritation a cancer will not develop. Coming next to the interpretation to be put upon the cancer-bodies, a large number of observers, and amongst them men of the highest standing, look upon them as intra-cellular organisms of the nature of coccidia, or psorosperms, as French writers call them, and they regard them as the cause of the cell activity and proliferation characteristic of cancer. One distinguished member of the Edinburgh Medico-Chirurgical Society, Dr. Russell, has brought out the fact that these cancer-bodies can be particularly well displayed by fuchsin staining, but, if I remember correctly, he looks on them as closely related to the yeasts. Others, however, are not satisfied as to the parasitic nature of these cancer-bodies. They explain them as arising from the embedding of leucocytes within certain of the cells, or, as Klebs puts it, from the fructifying influence of the leucocytes upon them ; while others, again, think that they are simply epithelial cells undergoing vacuolation in the course of what is evidently a mucoid degeneration. I confess that of late this latter has been my own feeling.

I must now be allowed briefly to mention what has led me to modify still further my views about these cancer-bodies, and also to lean to an explanation of the exciting cause of cancer that is quite opposed to the parasitic theory of the disease. I shall do so as shortly as I can. It is just twenty years ago that I was asked to take medical charge of a man whose mind was affected, and I went to reside with him at one of his estates in the west of Scotland. My duties were at times exciting, but never onerous, and I had a good deal of leisure to myself. I thought it would be a good opportunity of writing my M.D. thesis, and after consideration I decided I would take up the subject of lactation. What suggested it to me was the weaning of the lambs on a large adjoining sheep farm soon after I went down to my patient. Accordingly I commenced to work at it, getting all the practical information I could about it from the farmers and shepherds round. At that time, however (1876), cerebral localisation was being much talked about, and I took up the disease study in sheep instead, as there were a good many cases of it just then. I yet, however, elicited the following points in connexion with lactation that struck me as of great interest. 1. I found that the secretion of milk, though undoubtedly affected by the general nervous system, had no special nerve-supply of its own to control it. Neither section of the sympathetic nor of the spinal nerves seems to influence it. The erectility of the nipple is affected by cutting the latter, but nothing more. 2 It was clear to me that the changes that take place in the mammary gland in the process of lactation are almost identical, up to a certain point, with what takes place in a cancerous mamma. We have, under both these conditions, the same proliferation of generations of epithelial cells which block the ducts and fill the acini of the gland; but in the case of lactation they rapidly vacuolate, undergo fatty degeneration, and form milk, while in the carcinoma they stop short of that process, and, to make room for themselves, they penetrate the walls of the ducts and the acini and invade the surrounding tissues. In short, lactation is at one point perilously near becoming a cancerous process if it is at all arrested. 3. I learnt this very remarkable fact, that it is the custom in certain countries to remove the ovaries of the cow after calving if it is wished to keep up the supply of milk, and that if this is done the cow will go on giving milk indefinitely. This fact seemed to me of great interest, for it pointed to one organ holding the control over the secretion of another and separate organ, and thus explained the absence of that distinct nervous control that I pointed out as characteristic of the mamma. Of course, the close intimacy between the ovary and the mamma is well known to all of us, as seen in the absence, as a rule, of the menstrual function during lactation, but I certainly was not aware until then that it was of the nature that it would seem to be and almost of a distinct control. In our country farmers have not gone the length of spaying cows as in Australia, but they attain the same end of having a continuous supply of milk by getting rid of all ovarian influence in another way. We know that during pregnancy the ovary is, as a rule, functionless—that is to say, we have not the indications of its activity in the shape of the menses, and it would seem to be in its turn brought under the control of the pregnant uterus. Farmers knew that their cows after calving usually begin to menstruate every three weeks and that with the establishment of this function the mammary secretion gradually lessened. They also knew that during the nine months the cow carried her calf she did not menstruate, so to prevent menstruation and lessened milk they put the bull to the cow usually two or three months after the calf is born and when the milk secretion is becoming lessened, the result being that with pregnancy the secretion ceases to lessen and remains copious. I need hardly say that though I temporarily abandoned the subject of lactation for my thesis I did not lose sight of the facts above mentioned, for they seemed to me to point to influences at work in the human system that had not as yet been generally reckoned with or recognised. Above all, I was struck with the local proliferation of epithelium seen in lactation. Here was the very thing characteristic of carcinoma of the breast, and, indeed, of the cancerous process everywhere, but differing from it in that it was held in control by another organ, and could either be arrested by that organ altogether or continued to a further stage, where the cells became fatty and passed out of the system not only in an innocuous but nourishing fluid—milk.

Now I think I am correct in saying that the spirit of modern pathology is this—that all pathological changes are merely modified physiological ones, that there is no essential difference between the two, and that a knowledge of the forces controlling the one may sometimes give us a clue to the other. I often asked myself, Is cancer of the mamma due to some ovarian irritation, as from some defective steps in the cycle of ovarian changes; and, if so, would the cell proliferation be brought to a standstill, or would the cells go on to the fatty degeneration seen in lactation were the ovaries to be removed? For an answer to these questions I felt I must wait; but on settling in practice in Glasgow in 1878 I determined to look further into this point of the control the ovaries seemed to have over the function of lactation. Accordingly I obtained at the end of 1878 a licence for performing the experiment of removing the ovaries from

suckling rabbits. Through the kindness of Professor M'Kendrick I was able to carry my experiments out at the University laboratory. Space will not allow me to go into them in detail, but I may say that the three cases I tried all confirmed the fact. As long as the young ones were at the breast the milk-supply continued, and when eventually they were taken away the milk-supply ceased; but the creatures increased very much in size, and post-mortem examination revealed that this was due to large deposits of fat around the various organs, and, above all, in the lumbar region, where there were masses of pure adipose tissue, showing that the secretion of milk was still going on, but, not being discharged by the usual channels, was deposited in the various tissues of the body as fat.

In the year 1882 a case of uterine cancer, unsuitable for local removal, came under my care, and I thought I would try on it the effect of removal of the tubes and ovaries, as the patient was willing to submit to any operation. I found, however, on performing abdominal section that the disease had extended so much into the broad ligaments that a satisfactory removal of the appendages could not be accomplished and I abandoned the operation. She made a good recovery from the laparotomy, but died some months later from her disease. With this single attempt to put my views to the test I was for a time content, as I was very unwilling to do anything of the nature of experiments on my fellow creatures. Further, with the rise and progress of bacteriology I began to share in the hope that in this quarter a solution of the true nature of cancer would be found, and, with the announcement of the so-called cancer bodies, now generally recognised, I began to think less and less of my ovarian theory of the origin of cancer.

On taking up my work at the Glasgow Cancer Hospital, which I may say has been established not only for the treatment of cancer in all its stages but also for the pathological study of the disease, I felt that the position of matters was that our present state of knowledge has nothing better to offer than the surgeon's knife for the cases where the tumour was limited and could be thoroughly removed; but that in inoperable cases, if the so-called cancer-bodies were not parasites at all but merely cells undergoing mucoid degeneration, it was possible a free administration of thyroid extract might influence the growth and work through time a cure. Failing this, I thought I might follow up my old line of reasoning, and in cases of advanced carcinoma of the breast in young patients see what effects the removal of the tubes and ovaries would have on the progress of the cancerous growth in the way of arresting the cell proliferation and converting the cells into fatty matter. Although the breast had been removed, this was the line of procedure I decided to adopt with the case under notice, and accordingly on May 11th she was put upon the thyroid tabloids. They were pushed until their physiological action was made apparent; but as no appreciable change was seen in the diseased condition at the end of a month I put it to her husband and herself as to whether she should have performed the operation of removal of the tubes and ovaries. Its nature was fully explained to them both, and also that it was a purely experimental one, but that it could be done without risk to life; and that, if it should have no effect on the cancerous process, it would cause her no increase of suffering. She readily consented that I should do anything that held out any prospect of cure, as she knew and felt her case was hopeless. On June 15th I operated and removed the tubes and ovaries on both sides. The right ovary seemed healthy; the left one was somewhat cystic. Subsequently there was some little trouble with the action of her bowels; but she made a good recovery and on June 28th was sitting up. No local application was made to the diseased areas on the thorax. They were simply kept clean with boric lotion and dressed with protective and boric lint. On July 12th the administration of the thyroid tabloids, three daily, was resumed, as I felt that though I hoped by my oöphorectomy to arrest the cell proliferation and favour, perhaps, fatty degeneration of the cells, there was present such a large amount of cancerous material that a powerful lymphatic stimulant such as thyroid extract might be useful. On July 19th, in about five weeks after operation, an examination of the diseased areas on the left side of the thorax showed, as the hospital report states, undoubtedly a marked change compared with their condition some weeks ago. The larger mass of disease was much less vascular. It was also smaller, flatter, and altogether less prominent, and the same may be said of all the other secondary foci of disease. The tissues around were also softer and more pliable. On Aug. 1st it was noted that the local improvement continued and that the measurements of the largest area of disease were— length, $2\frac{3}{4}$ in.; breadth, $1\frac{1}{4}$ in.; while the depth was hardly appreciable. The colour was a dull yellowish-white and the vascularity slight. There were five small nodules in the axillary region, which were also diminishing in size and vascularity, though perhaps not so much as the larger growth. The patient's general health and nourishment were satisfactory; and as she was an intelligent and reliable woman, and interested in her own case, I allowed her to go to Bridge of Allan for a change, and asked her to report herself from time to time. This she did, and without going into a detailed account of her condition on each visit that she made I may say that the local improvement continued, and my note on Oct. 12th, just four months after the operation of oöphorectomy, was as follows: "On examination of the left breast the condition of the tissues is favourable. The most remarkable feature of the case is the yellow fatty look that the former thick bar of cancerous tissue above the scar of the incision for removal of the breast presents. It is to my mind the most striking feature of the case. The cancerous tissue has been reduced to a very thin layer and is in no way raised above the surrounding skin. In fact, the whole surface is smooth and level, and to the naked eye it seems as if the skin at this part had a yellow look. So distinct is this that one could easily trace out the outline of this yellow-coloured tissue. At places the surrounding skin seems pushing its way into the yellow mass and the processes of bluish cicatricial tissue are to be noted. The yellowish nodules at the axillary end of the incision are still apparent from their colour, but they seem thinning out. The whole of the tissues on the chest wall are more movable and the surrounding skin has a clear and healthy look. The scar of the former ulcer above the mammary excision cicatrix is sound and no new nodules are at present observable. The patient expresses herself as feeling very well and looks so. She is taking four 5-gr. tabloids of thyroid extract daily." I need not trouble with any further detailed account of this patient than to say that eight months after my operation all vestiges of her previous cancerous disease had disappeared, and that I am able to show her with a sound cicatrix and healthy thoracic tissues, and that she is apparently in excellent health.

(To be concluded.)

NOTE ON EUCAINE AS A LOCAL ANÆSTHETIC.

BY ROBERT BRUDENELL CARTER, F.R.C.S. ENG.,
CONSULTING OPHTHALMIC SURGEON TO ST. GEORGE'S HOSPITAL.

THE *Medizinische Novitäten* for June quotes from the *Aerztlicher Central-Anzeiger* a condensed account of a paper read before the Hufeland Society of Berlin by Dr. Gaetano, of Vinci, Messina, on the properties of "eucaine" as a local anæsthetic, and this account induced me to make further inquiry into the subject. I have since seen an English summary of the paper in which the author is described as "Dr. G. Vinci," and I do not know which of the two versions of his name is correct.

I am informed that eucaine is not derived from the vegetable kingdom, but that it is a laboratory product which can be prepared in any quantity at moderate cost. I am also informed that its proper designation is "methyl-benzoyl-tetramethyl-oxypiperidine-carboxylic-acid-methyl-ester," a combination which seems to open a door, either in speech or writing, for infinite possibilities of error. The trivial name "eucaine" is comparatively free from this objection; but I neither know by whom it was invented nor what idea, if any, it is intended to convey. It is apparently compounded of the prefix "eu" and of the last syllable of "cocaine," and if so may perhaps be regarded as a first cousin of "chlorodyne." But "eucaine" seems to have no meaning, while "green pain" has, at least, the semblance of one.

Dr. Gaetano, or "Dr. G. Vinci," whichever it may be, described eucaine as possessing the properties of cocaine as a local anæsthetic, but as being less toxic and as having no effect upon the pupil. The last statement seemed to me to be of practical importance, because a dilated pupil is an impediment to the performance of many operations upon the eye. It has long been my practice to neutralise the dilating effect of cocaine by a preliminary application of eserine, but this course is not entirely satisfactory. It is difficult to secure the precise degree of effect which is desired, while the eserine dilates the vessels of the iris and occasions free bleeding when they are incised. It also renders the iris tissue comparatively rigid, so that it is less easily drawn out of the anterior chamber.

I obtained a supply of a 5 per cent, watery solution of eucaine hydrochloride from Mr. Rogers, of 327, Oxford-street, and used it last week for a cataract extraction, the patient being a woman. Before my arrival the nurse had applied a drop of the solution within the lower lid every five minutes for six times, and I found the eye perfectly insensitive. The pupil was unaffected and acted readily to light. There was scarcely any bleeding from the cut iris; there was perfect quiescence of the muscles and there was no pain. I asked the patient whether she had felt anything and she replied. "I felt something moving about my eye but it did not hurt me." There was no pain afterwards and healing was uninterrupted. I have since successfully used a single application of the same solution as a preliminary to the removal of a foreign body embedded in the cornea.

In the original paper it is said that eucaine has been successfully used in dentistry and laryngology, and that solutions may be injected hypodermically without injury. My first experiments will certainly induce me to use it again, and for tenotomies as well as for iridectomy or extraction. It is said that the solution above mentioned may be sterilised by boiling, again and again if necessary, without undergoing decomposition or suffering any deterioration of quality.

Harley-street, W.

ON THE ORGANIC MEMBRANES AS INSULATORS.

BY SIR BENJAMIN WARD RICHARDSON, M.D., F.R.S.

UP to the present time we have been content to look upon a membrane of the body, the pericardium, the periosteum, the capsule of the kidneys, and any structure of the kind, as a covering of the organ wrapped up in it, that holds the organ, as it were, in a mould, supports it in its place, allows it to glide, and by virtue of the fluid secreted keeps it distinct and separate. There can be no question that these grand functions belong to the membranes, which have ever been to us structures of the utmost moment. I have watched the influence of many substances upon them; have noted their conditions during the various stages of life, and have examined their degenerations during disease and after death. But I have recently made observations on these structures—membranes—which, if I am right, give them a new value, or rather a value that has not before been appreciated. It seems to me they are *electrical insulators*, and by their presence confine and render useful the vital force that is developed in the organs they surround. My first observations leading to this conclusion were conducted on the nervous membranes—those that envelop the cerebral convolutions and the spinal cord; from these I passed on to the other membranous envelopes to find that they all have a common quality.

I obtained an electrical battery consisting of twenty-four small cells, so arranged that one cell could be put on at a time, or the whole or part of the whole as might be required. I commissioned Messrs. Faraday of Berners-street to construct for me a delicate galvanometer, the needle of which moved in a millimetre circle and certified, with accuracy, the force of the current transmitted. I fixed to one pole of the battery a conductor which was connected to the galvanometer, and from the opposite pole of the battery attached a platinum conductor of the same length and carried it also to the galvanometer. This last conductor I divided in the centre and joined the end of the portion from the galvanometer to a platinum disc that was secured by its under surface to a porcelain slab. The other half of the conductor (from the battery) was allowed to remain free with a probe-like end which could be used at any moment to touch the platinum disc and complete the circuit or to touch any substance laid

REPORT OF

The Lancet Special Commission

ON THE

RELATIVE STRENGTHS OF DIPHTHERIA ANTITOXIC SERUMS.

THE discovery by Behring of the existence of antitoxin in the blood of animals rendered immune to diphtheria, and his application of this antitoxin to the cure of the disease, must be regarded as the most important advance of the century in the medical treatment of acute infective disease. On the Continent the advantages of the new treatment have been fully recognised alike by the specialist and the practitioner, and the results obtained have approximated in some cases even to the prophecy of its discoverer—that the death-rate from diphtheria would eventually be reduced to 5 per cent. In this country, however, no such unanimity of opinion prevails, and the detractors of the treatment, who deny its efficacy and even affirm that its use is accompanied by increased risk, are at any rate as numerous as are those who believe in its therapeutic value. In consequence of this conflict of opinion, and perhaps also because striking results were not obtained in the first cases which were subjected to the new treatment, medical practitioners as a body, in this country, have not used the new remedy in the very general and extended way in which it has come into operation abroad. Inasmuch as the introduction of the serum treatment on an extended scale elsewhere has been immediately followed by a most marked and unmistakeable decrease in the mortality from diphtheria it is absolutely necessary to make full inquiry into those causes which have tended to interfere with its general adoption in this country. This must no doubt be ascribed in part to the conservative instincts of our countrymen, and in part to a certain distrust of the application of the results of bacteriological investigation to the treatment of disease which originated in the failure of the tuberculin treatment of phthisis to justify the high claims put forward for it by Koch and certain other bacteriologists. It must, however, be recognised that still other causes have operated in this direction, since many practitioners who made a trial of the antitoxic serum treatment on its first introduction into this country were so dissatisfied by the absence of the striking results described in France and Germany that they soon abandoned it, and we now have the remarkable fact that there are at the present time large districts, both in England and in Scotland, where the serum treatment has practically passed out of use. For some time it has been suggested by those intimately acquainted with the question that this neglect of the remedy must be ascribed in great part at any rate to the quality of the serum manufactured and distributed in this country. In support of this contention they have pointed out that those who have obtained the most satisfactory results and who have been the warmest supporters of the serum treatment have been those who have been able to treat cases of diphtheria during the very early stages of the disease where even a small dose of weak serum is sufficient to check the course of the disease. In this connexion it has been shown on the Continent that the death-rate may be almost abolished among those cases treated during the second or third day of the disease ; whilst the experiments, as regards the quantity of antitoxin necessary to save animals at different stages of the disease, afford still more striking evidence on this point.

Thus it has been shown by Wernicke and Behring [1] that it is necessary to inject ten times as much antitoxin into a guinea-pig that has received subcutaneously a lethal dose of diphtheria toxin eight hours previously. as when it is treated immediately after the injection of the toxin, whilst after twenty-four hours fifty times the initial quantity is

necessary to effect a cure. That the importance of this fact is fully recognised is indicated quite clearly by Behring in the directions sent out with the serum prepared under his supervision. Thus he recommends as sufficient a dose of 600 normal antitoxin units (No. 1 phial, green label) " in cases where the serum treatment is commenced on the appearance of the first symptoms of the disease," whilst at a more advanced stage doses of 1000 (No. 2 phial, white label) or 1500 (No. 3 phial, red label) normal units are required. In the appended table (Table I.) the quantities of the English and foreign serums (purchased in this country in August, 1895) which it would be necessary to inject in order to ensure this dose of 1500 units being given. It will be observed that the table contains, in the case of Behring, a record of only the minimum dose of antitoxin sent out under his supervision. This was due to the fact that the English agents appeared at this time to stock only this quality, owing, perhaps, to the absence of demand for the more concentrated forms, some of which contain 1500 normal units in 6–7 c.c. of serum.

TABLE No. 1.

Source of serum.	Estimated number of units in bottle.	Quantity required for dose of 1500 units.
British Institute of Preventive Medicine (Sample No. 1)	600	75 c.c.
Burroughs, Wellcome, and Co. (Sample No. 2)... ...	240	187 c.c.
Bacteriological Institute, Leicester (Sample No. 1)...	100	300 c.c.
Behring, Höechst, Germany (Sample No. 1)	600	15 c.c.
Schering, Berlin (Sample No. 2)	500	15 c.c.
Pasteur Institute, France (Sample No. 1)	450	33 c.c.

It is evident from the low antitoxic value of the English serums at this period that only such a dose as could be expected to be effective at the early stage of the disease could under ordinary circumstances be injected into a child, as it can readily be understood that in private practice, where no doubt the parents would regard the treatment as more or less of an experimental nature, the practitioner would hesitate to inject large quantities of the fluid. That this is the case is shown in the following table, in which a few of the cases recorded about this period are given.

TABLE No. 2.

Date of Illness.	Source of serum.	Dose injected and day of month.
April 18th, 1895.	British Institute of Preventive Medicine.	10 c.c., 21st.
May 3rd, ,,	Burroughs, Wellcome, and Co.	20 c.c , 5th + 20 c.c., 7th.
May 8th. ,,	Schering.	3 5 c.c. (1 drachm), 12th.
May 14th, ,.	Schering.	1·75 c.c. (½ drachm), 17th.
May 18th, ,,	Burroughs, Wellcome, and Co.	15 c.c., 20th + 10 c.c., 21st.
May 23rd. ,,	Schering.	1 c.c. (20 minims), 25th + 0·75 c.c. (15 minims. 28th + 0 5 c.c. (10 minims), 30th.
May 26th, ,,	British Institute of Preventive Medicine.	10 c.c., 30th.
May 27th, ,.	Burroughs, Wellcome, and Co.	15 c.c., June 2nd + 7·5 c.c. + 7·5 c.c., 3rd.
July 12th, ,.	British Institute of Preventive Medicine.	10 c.c. + 10 c.c., 14th + 10 c.c., 15th.

It has already been stated that serum of low antitoxic power, such as those on the market at this period, may have been very effective if given at a sufficiently early period of the disease. It must be remembered, however, that such serum could not be expected to exert a sufficiently marked influence on a case in a more advanced stage, and therefore a medical man who was testing the efficacy of

---

[1] Physiologische Gesellschaft, Berlin, 1893.

488 THE LANCET,] NEW INVENTIONS. [AUGUST 20, 1898.

New Inventions.

A NEW PATTERN OF UTERINE REPLACER.

THE instrument figured below was the outcome of difficulties occasioned by a case of uterine displacement caused some months previously by a severe fall which occurred abroad in a place some three or four weeks' journey removed from the help of any instrument maker. The patient, a married nullipara, had cessation of the menses without any symptoms pointing to pregnancy. Digital examination revealed the uterus completely anteverted. By curving an ordinary uterine sound to a right angle it was introduced to the fundus after much difficulty, but the angle to which the sound was bent prevented its being rotated, nor could any form of stem be introduced to help to replace the uterus, and chloroform was steadily refused. The instrument figured was devised and made in two weeks entirely by myself and has one or two important points. It is made entirely of metal—German silver; its parts are fixed together by screws, so that it can be readily

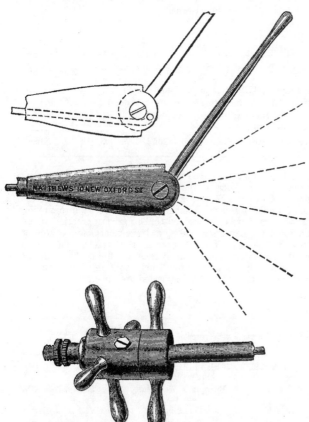

The upper figure is a plan showing the screw rod which works the probe through different angles. The middle figure shows the instrument itself. The lower figure shows the handle for working the screw rod.

taken to pieces, if necessary, for thorough disinfection; and also during its use, while the right forefinger retains its position at the os externum, it can readily be manipulated backwards or forwards by the left hand turning the screw nut, the length of the end of the screw projecting beyond the nut serving as an index to the position of the probe end of the sound. It is sufficient to say that in a week or two after its employment the uterus in this case was restored to its natural position, menstruation was re-established, and a month after all treatment had been suspended the uterus still in its normal position. There is nothing new under the sun, but I do not know of any instrument which possesses the useful points of the above, and having served me well I trust it may be of use to others. Messrs. Matthews Bros., of 10, New Oxford-street, have undertaken its manufacture.

Madeira.   F. J. HICKS.

THE *RÔLE* OF THE MOSQUITO IN THE EVOLUTION OF THE MALARIAL PARASITE.

THE RECENT RESEARCHES OF SURGEON-MAJOR RONALD ROSS, I.M.S.

AT the meeting of the British Medical Association in Edinburgh Dr. Patrick Manson, the President of the Section of Tropical Diseases, gave by special request and with the permission of the Secretary of State for India and of Surgeon-Major Ronald Ross, I.M.S., a lecture and exposition of the work done lately by the latter in the investigation of this subject. Surgeon-Major Ross has also sent us an advance copy of his recent report on the cultivation of Proteosoma, Labbé, in grey mosquitos. From this report we make the following extracts :—

"*A discovery of pigmented cells in grey mosquitos fed on larks with proteosoma.*—In February, 1898, I was placed by the Government of India on special duty to prosecute these researches and was given the use of Surgeon-Lieutenant-Colonel D. D. Cunningham's laboratory in Calcutta for the purpose. Steps were immediately taken to find again, if possible, the pigmented cells by feeding different species of mosquitos on blood containing different species of gymnosporidia. It was found that Calcutta abounded in the grey or barred-back species of mosquito, which is the filaria-bearing species, and with which I had already experimented. These had uniformly yielded negative results in Secunderabad when fed on blood containing crescents. Nevertheless, owing to difficulties in the way of obtaining other varieties, both of mosquitos and of malaria cases, numbers of this kind were again fed on a patient infected with crescents. Out of forty-one of these searched exhaustively for pigmented cells not one contained them. An unrecorded number, say fifty more, examined unfed, or, after feeding on healthy persons, gave similar negative results. As it was not the malarious season of the year, and as cases of hæmamœbiasis suitable for these experiments were not at all easy to procure, it was thought advisable to commence work on the so-called malaria parasites of birds. Accordingly a crow (*Corvus splendens*) and two tame pigeons infected with halteridium were obtained; and on the night of March 11th and 12th these, with four short-toed larks (*Calandretta dukhunensis*) and six sparrows (*Passer Indica*), whose blood had not yet been carefully examined, were placed in their cages, all within the same mosquito netting, and a number of grey mosquitos of the species I had lately been experimenting with were released within the net. Next morning numbers of these insects were found gorged with blood and were caught in test-tubes in which they were kept alive for two or three days.

"On March 13th I commenced to examine them. Out of fourteen of them pigmented cells were at last found in one. Believing as I did that these cells are derived from the gymnosporidia I judged from this experiment that the grey mosquito which now contained them had fed itself on one of the birds which happened to be infected by a parasite capable of transference to the grey species of mosquito. As all the birds had been placed together in the same net the question now was which of them had the mosquito fed herself upon. This could be easily ascertained. A number of mosquitos of the same species had meanwhile been fed separately on the crow and two pigeons with halteridium; but out of thirty-four of these examined not one contained pigmented cells. Hence I came to the conclusion that the mosquito with pigmented cells had not derived them from the crow and the two pigeons. The larks and sparrows remained. The blood of these had not yet been carefully searched. I now found that three of the larks and one of the sparrows contained proteosoma (Labbé) and therefore thought it possible that the mosquito had been infected from one of these. Accordingly, on the night of March 17th and 18th a number of grey mosquitos were released on the three larks with proteosoma and next morning it was found that nine of these had fed themselves. On the morning of March 20th—that is, from forty-eight to sixty hours after feeding—these nine insects were examined. Pigmented cells were found in no less than five of them. After the long-continued negative experiments with this kind of mosquito (and, indeed, I may say, after three years' doubtful attempts to cultivate these parasites) this result was almost conclusive. It indicated, as was surmised before, that when a certain species of mosquito is fed on blood containing a certain species of gymnosporidia pigmented cells are developed. Hence it would follow, as an easy corollary, that the cells are a stage in the life-history of the gymnosporidium in the mosquito.

"It was now necessary, however, to confirm and amplify this observation and obtain formal proofs of the theorem by repeating these experiments and by studying the pigmented cells themselves. Accordingly from March 18th to the present date (May 21st, 1898) many differential experiments have been completed by feeding grey mosquitos as follows : (a) on larks, sparrows, and a crow with proteosoma; (b) on crows, pigeons, and other birds with halteridium only ; (c) on a lark and a sparrow with immature proteosoma only ; (d) on a healthy sparrow. Only the insects fed on group (a) have contained pigmented cells.

"MacCullum had previously shown that in the case of the analogous parasite—the halteridium—the flagellum, of the flagellated phase, after breaking away entered certain spherical, pigmented halteridia, causing them to be transformed into little travelling pigmented vermicules, which, in virtue of their sharp beak and mechanical power, traverse freely red and white corpuscles. Analogy suggests that

namely, the body cavity of the host—there appear to be no means by which they can escape from that host during its life to undergo sporulation in external nature, as is the case with coccidium oviforme. It would appear then that sporulation should occur either within the living host, as with eimeria, or within the dead host. The first would point to a completion of the life cycle by a direct infection of men and birds by the coccidium spores in the mosquito ; the second to a more circuitous infection, perhaps by a second generation living free in water."

In the paper read by Dr. Patrick Manson at the Edinburgh meeting of the British Medical Association the speaker was able to quote from telegraphic communications with Surgeon-Major Ross which showed that the further researches spoken of have been undertaken. The next stage seems to be that the coccidia now burst and what Surgeon-Major Ross calls germinal vermicules which had formed in its interior are set free in the body, blood and tissues of the mosquito. Then came a step in the investigation of great consequence : it was no other than the discovery of these vermicules in the venemo-salivary glands of the mosquito. Surgeon-Major Ross during dissection of the mosquito found a couple of head glands with a duct leading towards the proboscis of the animal and traced the parasite vermicules into these glands. The climax of the discovery was now within his grasp and

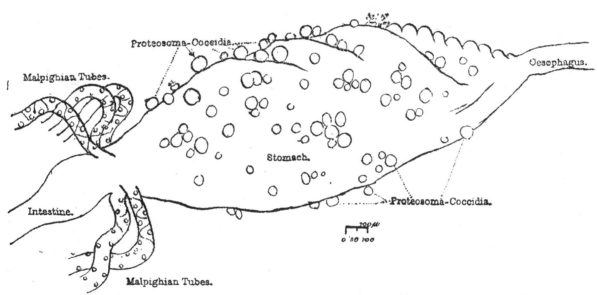

Figure reproduced from Surgeon-Major Ross's report and showing appearance of coccidia on the sixth and seventh day.

a similar thing occurs in proteosoma and that the travelling pigmented proteosoma vermicule enters the tissue of the mosquito's stomach and becomes Ross's pigmented bodies, in the same way as Manson has shown took place in the case of the filaria sanguinis hominis. Arrived in the stomach wall of the mosquito, the proteosoma increases rapidly in size until it projects beyond the stomach walls into the coelom or body cavity of the mosquito as a rounded body, which he styles the proteosoma-coccidia. During its progress and growth various changes take place in size and in the appearance of the contents of the coccidia. Pigment diminishes and then disappears and as the parasite protrudes into the coelom it is seen that the contents have a more or less granular appearance.

"I have said that after this point I have witnessed no further growth of the coccidia, even in mosquitos kept alive to the twelfth day. Hence we may perhaps expect that they have become ripe for sporulation. No such thing has, however, been observed ; and we may therefore conjecture, unless I happened to have overlooked it, that it may occur either (a) in the living insect after twelve days, or (b) some time after the insect's death. Further research is therefore required on this which now becomes the most important and interesting period of the life-history of the gymnosporidia, because on it depend our chances of future progress. To plunge into hypothesis for a moment we may remark that since the mature coccidia find themselves in a closed cavity—

he elucidated it thus : He allowed mosquitos to feed on birds infected with proteosoma ; after a few days he fed the mosquitos on birds whose blood was void of any parasite infection. He found in due course that the parasite-bearing mosquito had infected the healthy birds and that their blood was charged with proteosoma.

Thus the analogy between bird and human infection has only to be proved to establish that the mosquito is a carrier of malaria and an infector of man. Much has yet to be done, however, before the full significance of the mosquito in malaria is worked out. Malaria, we know, multiplies without the intermediary of any vertebrate. Does it do so solely in mosquitos? If so, we have yet to learn how it passes from mosquito to mosquito. Does it multiply in other media? If so, what are they? There is here given merely the outline of Surgeon-Major Ross's work. Doubtless he or others will soon grapple with the other problems it suggests and show how to solve them. It is impossible in a short space to give in detail the multitudinous experiments and observations which he has carried out. Suffice it to say that they have been done in a masterly way. The practical applications of the discovery are immeasurable and the establishment of the fact that as the bite of the snake or the rabid dog inoculates the blood of the victims of these creatures so the mosquito conveys malaria, would open up a new and hopeful phase as regards the prevention of disease in the tropics.

from 204 cases of new growth, such as carcinoma of the ovary, cancer of the rectum, carcinoma of the body of the uterus, epithelioma of the tongue, epithelioma of the cervix uteri, carcinoma of the parotid gland, sarcoma of the maxilla, and carcinoma of the breast. From all these cultures M. Bra has been able to isolate without fail a fungus bearing a strong resemblance to the family of the ascomycetes. It appears in the form of round cells which form spherules, which give rise to spores shaped like cylinders which in turn produce hyphæ. The spherules are yellow in colour, round or ovoid, possessing a hyaline membrane, and furnished with a pore through which the spores escape.

New Hospital Buildings.

A new block has been opened at the Hôpital St. Antoine. It is to be devoted to the *clinique médicale* of Professor Hayem. Dr. Brouardel, Dr. Napias, director of the Assistance Publique, and M. Liard, head of the Education Department, have officially taken over the buildings which they have handed over to Professor Hayem who gave an address on the occasion of his receiving them and who also drew up the plans for them. The new block looks on to the large gardens of the hospital. In it is realised the utmost perfection of modern hospital architecture and it possesses a theatre, examination halls, a large chemical laboratory, a laboratory for pathological anatomy, a bacteriological laboratory with three culture stoves and three autoclaves. There are also a lift, a room for electro-therapeutics, and rooms for gynæcology and other subjects. The building is admirably ventilated and lighted. The theatre may be darkened instantaneously for lantern shows and radiographic experiments, and galleries from the wards communicate directly with this theatre, so that patients may be at once transferred when necessary from the one to the other. —The town of Havre has just decided to build a new sanatorium for isolating and treating cases of tuberculosis, in accordance with the report of Dr. Sorel. The sanatorium will be in the form of a villa on the shore, and a committee composed of three members, in addition to M. Sorel, have gone to study the organisation and construction of the sanatoria on the banks of the Rhine.—A new hospital at Tunis has just been opened, and the head physician, Dr. Bari, has been awarded the Legion of Honour.

The late Dr. Grubi.

Dr. Grubi recently died in Paris at the age of eighty-nine years. Although a Hungarian by birth, he came very early in life to Paris, where he devoted himself to laboratory work. His microscopical researches led him amongst other discoveries to that of the special fungus of tinea tonsurans. He then gave up strictly scientific work and devoted himself entirely to his patients, among whom his success was brilliant. He had for patients many of the men of letters of the Second Empire, such as Alexandre Dumas and Heine. He was remarkable for his extraordinary prescriptions which made his *confrères* consider him as somewhat of a charlatan or else as a facile employer of suggestion. For instance, he would frequently prescribe to a patient to live in a room entirely green and to this end to have all the window-panes, the wall-paper, the curtains, and all the furniture entirely new. Sometimes, too, he would order his patients to wear nothing but clothes of a certain colour and a certain cut and only to walk in certain streets and on a certain side of the pavement; the position (*orientation*) of the bed was also rigidly laid down according to his ruling. As he suffered from morbus cordis he gave out a long time ago that he was perfectly determined to die alone and for many months he never quitted his room where he lived practically a prisoner, only being seen by one servant and locking the door whenever this man took his departure. Under these circumstances he died, and the police commissary, called by the servants, forced open the door and found that he had been dead for some days. Before he died he had taken care to blow out the candle.

Nov. 28th.

BERLIN.

(FROM OUR OWN CORRESPONDENT.)

A New Hypnotic.

A NEW hypnotic, to which the name of "heroïn" has been given, has been tried in the medical clinic of Professor Gerhardt in Berlin. According to a communication made by Dr. Strube to the *Berliner Klinische Wochenschrift* it is a product of the di-acetic ester of morphia, and it was discovered by Professor Dreser, chief of the chemical department of the Elberfeld Farben Fabriken. Large doses given to animals were followed by narcosis attended by disappearance of reflex movements and a diminished rate of respiration. In cats tetanic convulsions developed. Smaller doses reduced the number of respirations in a given time but caused an increase in the respiratory force. No paralysis of the respiratory centre was ever observed and the circulation was unaffected. The action of heroïn is very like that of codeia, but smaller doses of the former are required. It is especially useful in dyspnœa, where a decrease of the number of respirations is indicated. Heroïn is a fine white powder of slightly bitter taste; it is practically insoluble in water but its solubility is increased when a few drops of acetic acid are added. Dr. Strube administered it in cases of pulmonary affection and in tuberculosis in place of morphia and codeia, the dose being ½ centigramme ($\frac{1}{14}$ grain) given either in pills or in powder or even in the form of drops. The limits of 1 centigramme (⅙ grain) for a dose or 25 centigrammes (3¾ grains) in twenty-four hours were not exceeded. The effect was satisfactory in nearly every instance. The patients had no objection to the remedy; after taking ½ centigramme or 1 centigramme they fell asleep, their dyspnœa was relieved, and the cough was stopped. The action of the drug began in about half an hour and lasted from two to four hours, after which another dose was given the effect of which continued till next morning. In a few instances, however, heroïn proved useless and subcutaneous injections of morphine had to be resorted to. Dr. Strube also tried this substance for the relief of neuralgic pains. In two cases of brachial neuralgia and sciatica respectively a centigramme was injected subcutaneously but proved to be without any effect. No undesirable complications were observed and the respiration continued to be regular, the pulse was strong and full, and the temperature was not influenced.

Long Retention of a Pessary.

A remarkable case was lately under observation in the midwives training school in Strasburg. A woman, aged sixty-five years, came to the out-patients' department there to have a pessary removed which she had worn for five years. The pessary had not been withdrawn for the last two years and a midwife consulted by the patient before coming to the hospital had not been able to dislodge it. Dr. Frank, writing in the *Münchener Medicinische Wochenschrift*, stated that the woman could neither stand nor walk without severe pain. The pessary proved to be as it were imprisoned in the vagina, for it could be rotated but not moved to or fro. When it was pulled with some force there was profuse hæmorrhage from the cicatricial formations which retained it in its position. As these structures bled freely when incised and as the woman was rather weak Dr. Frank endeavoured to subdivide the pessary and remove it piecemeal. It was therefore cut up with a saw into portions which were withdrawn without difficulty and without any serious hæmorrhage. When the vagina was at last cleared it was ascertained that the prolapse for which the pessary had been applied was overcome by the extensive cicatrisation, so that the woman's self-neglect had turned out to her advantage.

The Prophylaxis of Puerperal Fever.

Professor Hofmeier of Würzburg has recommended the prophylactic disinfection of the vagina and cervix uteri at the beginning of labour in order to avoid puerperal complications. He uses for this purpose irrigations with solution of corrosive sublimate. To his already published list of 3000 cases treated in this way he now adds in the *Berliner Klinische Wochenschrift* a new series of 1000 cases treated in the obstetrical clinic of Würzburg. The results obtained by him were excellent. In the last series only 7 women died; there was no case of puerperal infection following normal delivery. In all the 4000 cases already published there were only 6 cases of puerperal infection, of which 4 may have arisen within the hospital. Among the last 1000 cases there were 106 in which the temperature rose to over 38° C. (100·4° F.) during the puerperium; in 50 of these 106 cases the elevation of temperature was not due to puerperal infection but to other causes—especially to mastitis. Among the remaining 56 cases there were 10 in which the temperature rose above 39° C. (102·2° F.) and in 2 cases a severe complication (septic

Public Health and by the reproduction of a letter from the chairman of the council of the Institute to the First Lord of the Treasury urging the appointment of a medical officer to the Education Department.

In the August number of the *Pall Mall Magazine* Mr. G.·S. Street discourses from his London Attic upon that curse of modern cities the "newspaper boy fiend." Mr. Street says of the curse: "He is a happy instance of the atrocious results of our half-and-half individualism which allows a man to be an unmitigated nuisance to his neighbours and at the same time debars his neighbours from their natural remedy of killing him." It is only the halfpenny "evening" papers which publish a "second edition" at about 10 A.M. which appeal to the boy-fiend's heart, and as the penny papers get on quite well without torturing inoffensive citizens we implore the London County Council to pass that long-waited-for Street Noises By-law.

Analytical Records

FROM

THE LANCET LABORATORY.

ASPIRIN.

(THE BAYER COMPANY, LIMITED, 19, ST. DUNSTAN'S-HILL, E.C.)

ASPIRIN is the acetic derivative of salicylic acid which presents certain clinical advantages when substituted for the salicylates or salicylic acid. It is a white crystalline powder not dissolving appreciably in water but easily in alcohol. It disappears, however, in weak potash solution, the addition of acid to this alkaline solution leading to the reappearance of a crystalline substance. This fact is of clinical importance, since aspirin would pass through the stomach unchanged until it reached the alkaline digestive juices in which it would be decomposed and the salicylic acid would be appropriated. On this account the irritation in the stomach caused in some cases by salicylic acid and its salts is prevented. Further, it is said that owing to aspirin decomposing gradually the singing in the ears sometimes produced by ordinary salicylates is to some extent avoided. Aspirin is almost free from taste but is slightly acid; it is not sweet like the salicylates. Clinical cases are recorded indicating the advantages of aspirin over salicylic acid and its salts. It may be conveniently administered by combining 15 grains of the derivative with from 50 to 60 grains of sugar dissolved in half an ounce of water.

VERY OLD PALE COGNAC.

(J. AND F. MARTELL, COGNAC.)

This brandy shows excellent features on analysis while the evidence of taste is distinctly in favour of the description that it is an old and matured grape spirit. It possesses that etherial fragrance due to the peculiar ethers of wine. Our analysis yielded the following results: Alcohol, by weight 41·00 per cent., by volume 48·43 per cent., equal to proof spirit 84·87 per cent.; acidity expressed as acetic acid, 0·033 per cent.; extractives, 0·69 per cent.; mineral matter, *nil;* alcohol in volatile ethers, two grammes per 10 litres. The flavour is soft and mellow and the aroma is characteristic of a sound and mature wine-derived spirit. In view of these analytical and general evidences this brandy may be described as particularly suitable for medicinal purposes.

JOHANNIS POTASH WATER.

(THE APOLLINARIS CO., 4, STRATFORD-PLACE, OXFORD-STREET, W.)

The addition of a definite amount of bicarbonate of potash to a natural mineral water affords an agreeable and effective way of exhibiting an alkaline draught. Johannis potash water possesses a taste distinctly superior to and more satisfactory than the ordinary potash water made with artificial gas. It is smooth and soft to the palate and affords an excellent beverage with milk or with lemon juice. We found on analysis that the water possessed an alkalinity per bottle equal to 7·9 grains of bicarbonate of potash. Allowing for the normal alkalinity of the natural water this accords with the statement that seven and a half grains of the potash salt are added to each bottle. Johannis potash water offers the advantage where alkaline treatment is indicated of presenting a constant amount of the potash salt, which as is well known is useful as a diuretic and in preserving the alkalinity of the blood. The efficacy of the waters of certain continental spas in the treatment of gout have been referred to the definite though small quantities of potassium salts—chiefly bicarbonates—contained in these waters.

SANDRONS'S IRON TONIC.

(SANDRONS, LIMITED, 34, DEVONSHIRE-STREET, PORTLAND-PLACE, W.)

This somewhat viscous fluid is described as an assimilable iron tonic of vegetable origin, but according to our analysis there is very little iron in the preparation available for assimilation. We found only 0·042 grain of iron in each fluid ounce. There was evidence of some fermentative change having taken place in the fluid for it was frothy and evolved bubbles of gas. On evaporation a treacly residue amounting to 7·36 per cent. was obtained. The ash from this residue proved to contain an abundance of mineral salts of the class commonly yielded by vegetables and plants. Possibly by exerting a favourable influence on the processes of nutrition the exhibition of this fluid may have a tonic effect, but any such effect due to iron must be inappreciable in view of the very small quantity of iron present. There would be much more iron contained in an average dietary, especially when this comprises a fair proportion of fruit or vegetable.

VASOGENS.

(VASOGEN FABRIK, PEARSON & CO., LIMITED, HAMBURG. LONDON AGENT: E. J. REID, 11, DUNEDIN HOUSE, BASINGHALL-STREET, E.C.)

We have called attention to the interesting substance known as vasogen on a previous occasion in our analytical columns. Briefly, vasogen is a partly oxidised hydrocarbon with properties resembling vaseline but more suitable than that substance for medicinal purposes, as for inunction or internal use. Applied to the skin it is readily absorbed and carries with it certain medicaments which it may contain. Thus when iodine vasogen is rubbed on the skin there is very soon evidence of iodine in the urine or saliva. Further vasogen has the peculiar property of rendering drugs which may be incorporated with it soluble in water or at least emulsifiable with it and thus it readily forms emulsions with the secretions of the body. The liquid vasogen compounds comprise camphor vasogen chloroform, creasote vasogen, ichthyol vasogen, iodine vasogen, iodoform vasogen, guaiacol vasogen, beta-naphthol vasogen, menthol vasogen, sulphur vasogen, and tar vasogen. A vasogen ointment base is also prepared and with this mercury salts are combined. Lastly, several vasogens are contained in capsules for internal use. The clinical evidence in favour of the administration of vasogen compounds published chiefly in the German medical journals ought to encourage more extended application of this interesting compound and its combinations in this country.

SCOTCH WHISKY.

(EDWARD ARCHER AND CO., GREAT MALVERN.)

Two specimens of Scotch whisky were analytically examined, known respectively as "the Bowman blend" and "the Balmoral blend," the former being said to be seven years old and the latter 10 years old. The evidence both of taste and analysis was perfectly in

"We all sat without moving or trying to escape. The foot of the ladder was close by, yet none of us made any effort to go to it and ascend even a single rung. We none of us tried to walk a dozen steps which would have led us to the other side of the shaft partition where we all knew there was a current of better air." The same paper alludes to the remarkably fresh and life-like appearance of the corpses as they were brought to the surface, and what is still more interesting, as it bears somewhat on the treatment, we read that as soon as a warning was given that there was foul air about there was a rush among the men for the ladders and a general climbing commenced. It was soon observed that of these men, who were really poisoned before they knew it, only the elder ones got up to the top, and nearly all those "well under 30" fell down and were recovered afterwards only when they were dead. This Dr. Miller ascribed to cardiac failure consequent on the greater exertion made by the younger men to escape, it being conjectured that the elder ones took matters more leisurely and so put less strain on their heart muscles. It appears to me that, though this explanation may not appeal to all, its important bearing upon treatment seems to lie in the consideration as to whether continued vigorous efforts at artificial respiration may not by exhausting a semi-exposed patient do more harm than good.

The symptom of convulsive rigidity which was present in the only one of these two women who was found alive is so commonly stated to be present that it calls for a little remark. These spasms have been supposed to be asphyxial in their nature. They have been mostly observed to affect the extensors of the trunk and the flexors of the limbs, for in asphyxia, as Sir T. Lauder Brunton has shown, these groups of muscles overcome their antagonists and thus opisthotonos and flexion of the limbs are produced.[7] It will be remembered that the arms of the younger woman were described by the nurse as "stiff and drawn up." Whether this be the correct interpretation of the symptom or not it is well to recollect that at least two gases are present in poisoning by coke or charcoal vapour, and it is quite possible that some of the symptoms we find may be produced by either gas acting separately.

I have only been able to find one case of poisoning by the pure gas carbonic oxide. This is recorded in an old edition of Beck's Medical Jurisprudence.[8] A man at Dublin inhaled the gas for an experiment and was nearly killed. In him the poison certainly acted promptly on the central nervous system and the heart, for total insensibility and lifelessness came on at once and lasted half an hour. On introducing oxygen gas into the lungs he recovered with convulsive agitation and quick and irregular pulsation, and for some time after recovery total blindness, sickness, and vertigo were present.

One would imagine from à priori reasoning that as carbonic oxide forms such a stable compound with hæmoglobin there is but little chance of setting free this combined hæmoglobin, and that the only method of treatment would be to remove some of it and inject fresh into the system. And this experience fully proves to be the case. A case is related where a man was saved by this means after being in an apparently hopeless state for 48 hours.[9] He was bled to 800 grammes, and 110 grammes of defibrinated blood were injected. The record of successes is certainly not so large as one would hope. In 1885, 23 cases were collected in which transfusion had been resorted to. Recovery had ensued in eight.[10] We are not told, however, whether the blood was defibrinated in every case, nor even whether blood was used in every instance; for I note that Halstead of New York[11] has stated that saline injections are equally serviceable in the case of animals poisoned by carbonic oxide. Although he quotes Kühne as an authority for his statement, one is at a loss to understand by what means such a proceeding would be likely to do good.

I have already alluded to the possible harm that might result from the prolonged use of artificial respiration. Alone it certainly seems to be but of little use, but with the aid of such adjuncts as the inhalation of oxygen, slapping and friction over the cardiac region, and faradaisation of the phrenics it has proved of great service. The fall of temperature has suggested the use of the hot bath, and certainly the

external application of warmth and the avoidance of undue exposure of the body while artificial respiration is being carried on are things to be most carefully attended to.

It has been kindly pointed out to me by Dr. E. Casey that no allusion to this subject of carbonic oxide poisoning is complete without a reference to the growing use of so-called "water-gas" as an illuminant. True water-gas, or the gas produced by the action of steam upon carbon, consists of about equal volumes of hydrogen and carbonic oxide with small quantities of nitrogen and carbonic acid.[12] This, of course, would not be of much use for illuminating purposes. The term, however, is very loosely applied and generally includes gaseous mixtures used for illumination which are distinguished from coal gas by the large quantity of carbonic oxide they contain. The main point is that the high percentage of carbonic oxide usually entails a loss of the characteristic odour of illuminating gas and hence the great danger arising from an escape of water-gas into a bedroom during the night. Water-gas as used for illuminating is said usually to contain about 30 per cent. of carbonic oxide while ordinary coal gas contains only 7 per cent. of carbonic oxide.[13] Since the introduction of water-gas into New York the deaths from burner escapes are said to have increased tenfold and in one State of America a law has been introduced limiting the percentage of carbonic oxide to 10 per cent.[14]

Windsor.

GENERAL NERVOUS SHOCK, IMMEDIATE AND REMOTE, AFTER GUNSHOT AND SHELL INJURIES IN THE SOUTH AFRICAN CAMPAIGN.

BY MORGAN I. FINUCANE, M.R.C.S. ENG., L.S.A.,

CIVIL SURGEON ATTACHED TO THE CONNAUGHT HOSPITAL,
NORTH CAMP, ALDERSHOT.

THE following notes of nine cases—out of a total of over 60 cases seen during the past two and a half months—with similar symptoms affecting the nervous system sufficiently illustrate some of the results, immediate and remote, which have been noticed as occurring in soldiers invalided home from the front. It is likely that in the near future the country will be deprived of a large number of our most capable and experienced men if the cases continue to occur in such frequency.

CASE 1.—At Colenso on Dec. 15th, 1899, Corporal —— was in the firing line when a bullet struck him in the left ear, entering the external auditory canal, rupturing the membrana tympana, and lodging in the mastoid process. A Mauser bullet was extracted from behind the ear at Pietermaritzburg Hospital, it being deeply imbedded in the bone, six days later. The patient was unconscious for six hours after the injury; he vomited, and blood escaped from the ear, the nose, and the mouth. Some loss of power down the left side was experienced for a month after. The wound healed well, the patient recovering power of the left side, but he still remains deaf in the left ear, with continual noises.

Present condition.—The patient is a thin and pale man with an anxious, careworn expression; he is only 32 years of age but looks older. His movements are slow and laboured. His body surface is cold and there is want of general muscular tone. There is a small, almost imperceptible, scar behind the left ear, over the mastoid process. The external auditory canal is normal in appearance; the membrana tympanum is gone, but no other abnormal appearance can be detected in the middle ear. He is somewhat deaf in this ear, but nothing very marked. He complains of giddiness, languor, and inability for sustained exertion of body or mind. His memory is bad and is getting worse; he is nervous and shaky, easily upset and put out, he suffers from sleeplessness at times, and his vision is dim with constant noises and lightness of head. The muscle movements are slow and impaired and he has continuously suffered with headache since the injury and in spite of every care is steadily losing weight.

7 THE LANCET, Jan. 25th, 1896, p. 217.
8 T. K. Beck and J. B. Beck: Elements of Medical Jurisprudence, London, 1836, p. 90.
9 Annales d'Hygiène, tome ii., 1843, p. 1155.
10 Brit. Med. Jour., vol. i., 1888, p. 1185.
11 Medical Times and Gazette, vol. i., 1884, p. 508.

12 Thorpe's Dictionary of Applied Chemistry.
13 Asclepiad, 1885, p. 287.
14 Ibid.

Case 2.—At Spion Kop a private of the 2nd Battalion King's Own Royal Lancashire Regiment, aged 24 years, was wounded in the left ankle, injuring the fibula and traversing the limb, and making its exit behind the tendo-Achillis. The aperture of entry was larger than that of exit. The injury was sustained whilst reinforcing the firing line. A comrade removed his boot and sock and applied the first and final dressing. The patient made an uninterrupted recovery after one month of the local injury.

Present condition.—Beyond some impairment of muscle movements on the plantar surface of the foot and slight stiffness around the ankle the local symptoms around the seat of injury are *nil;* there is wasting of muscles of both legs and impaired movements. There are areas of hyperæsthesia and anæsthesia and muscle reflexes are much exaggerated in both limbs; there are tremors of muscles and night twitchings of muscles of the chest and upper extremity. The patient feels very unsteady and shaky, with noises in the head and giddiness. His memory is bad and failing. The patient suffered from nerve shock and panic at Spion Kop before being wounded owing to the alarming character of the surroundings.

Case 3.—At Colenso on Dec. 15th a private of the 2nd Queen's Regiment was wounded in the left groin with a Mauser bullet over the kidney, traversing the abdominal cavity, causing subsequent hæmaturia and peritonitis, and travelling along the inside of the right thigh and becoming lodged on the under and inner surface of the right patella, whence the bullet was removed 14 days later. The loin wound healed in 10 days and the incised wound near the patella healed rapidly after extraction of the bullet. The injury was sustained while lying down with the right leg raised.

Present condition.—The patient complains of abdominal pain and pain in the legs and general weakness; he is incapable of continued exertion, bodily or mental. Formerly he was a smart soldier. The pains do not follow the course of any nerve trunks, and a general nervousness and weakness are noted of the upper as of the lower extremities. The patient is pale and thin with general vaso-motor impairment, and his circulation is sluggish. His age is 27 years.

Case 4.—At Colenso on Dec. 15th a private of the 2nd Royal West Surrey Regiment whilst in the firing line was knocked senseless by the explosion in close proximity of a nine-inch shell. The patient was not actually hit by a portion of the shell, but by the turning up of the ground. Subsequently the patient had partial loss of power down the right side in South Africa, which afterwards got better, but since coming home on July 7th he has had another attack of unconsciousness accompanied with some loss of power more noticeable on the right side.

Present condition.—There is distinct loss of power on both sides of the body. The patient is very nervous and shaky, suffering from twitching and especially over the right side, giddiness, noises in the head, dimness of sight, and some deafness. The skin is cold and the muscles are soft and flabby; the reflexes are exaggerated with tremors of the hands and tongue. A general condition of neurasthenia is noted.

Case 5.—At Spion Kop on Jan. 21st a private was in the firing line when he was shot in the left temporal bone, rupturing the tympanum and passing through the mastoid process. He was unconscious, but made a good recovery from the immediate effects.

Present condition.—The patient is now thin and nervous, with distinct loss of power in the upper part of the body. This is general evidence of vaso-motor impairment of the skin, muscles, and subcutaneous tissues. He has vertigo, headaches, flushing, and periods of stupidness and unconsciousness. His memory is bad and is getting worse. The patient describes his nerve break-down as due to shock and panic at Spion Kop, even before receiving his wound, as the result of heavy shell-fire and rifle-fire from the Boers, who were invisible and well under cover whilst the English troops were freely exposed. The patient is only 28 years old.

Case 6.—At Spion Kop a private was wounded in the right thigh with a Mauser bullet. The wound occluded by a first and final dressing and the patient made a rapid recovery from the local wound.

Present condition.—The patient has weakness, pain, and tremors in the muscles of the back and both lower limbs. His gait is unsteady and he is incapable of sustained or arduous exertion. There is no apparent loss of power. The apertures of entry and exit have healed, showing only small scars. The body-surface is cold and there is want of muscular tone. He is in a dull, lethargic mental state.

Case 7.—A private was wounded at Colenso on Dec. 15th in the abdomen and thigh with a Mauser bullet, escaping the abdominal cavity, since which date he has had constant lightning pains in the legs and shooting into the loins and he is now quite unable to do duty.

Present condition.—The patient has pain, hyperæsthesia, and tenderness over the superficial and deep nerve trunks. His movements are impaired and painful. The gait is unsteady. The scars of the bullet wounds are quite healed. There is general unsteadiness of speech with restlessness. The patient's age is 27 years.

Case 8.—A private was wounded at Slingersfontein on Feb. 12th in eight places—the hip and back, the right leg and the left arm—the bullets traversing structures and the wounds healing rapidly, since which date he has suffered from general weakness.

Present condition.—The patient has general tremors of most muscles of the trunk and loss of muscle tone. Shake surface of the body is cold. The patient's speech is slow and hesitating and he is very nervous and shaky, and unfit for long-continued mental or bodily exertion.

Case 9.—At Spion Kop on Jan. 24th a private was wounded in the right foot with a Mauser bullet and sprained his left ankle in falling. The bullet wound did well.

Present condition—The patient has loss of power and general tremors of both legs and lightning pains shooting up both legs and into the spine, especially the left leg. The patient is scarcely able to walk. There are twitchings and tremors about the face, which has an anxious and pinched appearance. He sleeps little owing to night pain. The muscles of the lower extremities are wasted and reaction of degeneration is noticed. There is some tenderness along the course of the great nerves.

Remarks.—The most noticeable features in our large military hospitals at present to be seen amongst South African invalids sent home for gunshot injuries are the almost total want of further surgical interference required, or any marked deformity, and the trivial nature of the entrance and exit apertures produced by the Mauser rifle bullet. In all the cases coming under my care I have had none in which the bullet-wounds were not healed, and although in many cases these were very numerous they have produced little or no deformity. The number of cases of injury from shell-wounds have been proportionately very small. The apertures of entry and exit of bullet-wounds in most cases are of a similar size and the scar is markedly small with no evidence of previous laceration or contusion of surrounding parts. The history of most of these patients immediately after the wounds is that of rapid healing by first intention with little or no suppuration; from inquiries made of patients the practice of antiseptic occlusion by first and final field dressings—whether that be on the field or in the field hospital—being responsible for the rapid healing and entirely successful results of the wounds themselves. Nearly all the cases observed had been subcutaneous flesh wounds, escaping or uninjuring bones and joints in the most marvellous way, although traversing tissues and cavities in close proximity to both. The lodgment of bullets in the soft or bony parts or in the cavities, necessitating removal, is an extremely rare occurrence, due, I take it, to the high velocity and shape of the projectile. The only cases I have seen here were lodged fragments from an exploded shell.

The clinical fact of most interest undoubtedly is the large number of cases of functional impairment of nerve sense and motor power, associated with psychical symptoms akin to nervous shock or those observed after railway accidents. These nerve symptoms do not bear any ratio to the extent or size of the wounds inflicted, but have been noted by me as being more common in injuries of the lower extremities and the head, and in cases that look originally to be not severe. The implication of nerves or their sheaths is not a marked feature and in most instances there is no local evidence of the bullet or its course having been near the track of a nerve. The effects are of sufficient importance to the military authorities and to the profession generally by reason of the necessity there is at present, and probably will be in the future, before the campaign in South Africa is concluded, of invaliding a large body of our best and most seasoned and experienced soldiers out of the service as unfitted for future service as soldiers, thus denuding our army of these experienced and gallant men. A large number of such cases have come before me, where after six months' or shorter periods of complete rest and every care, the patient's nervous system shows no signs of recovering its former steadiness and there is nothing for it but to invalid them out of the service as permanently unfit.

Again, the prognosis in such cases is extremely unsatisfactory and no definite one can properly be given under a year, whereas the military authorities require it much earlier. The surrounding circumstances of modern gunshot wounds have apparently lost much of the seriousness recorded of these injuries in most text-books, and it would appear that the resulting nerve shock and injury to the nervous system are the most frequent sequelæ and at the same time difficult to prevent and treat, but those towards which, in my opinion, our efforts must be directed. The absence of local nerve lesion or injury producing the nerve change is significant, and the number of cases observed would not support the theory of these symptoms occurring in nervous persons only. It would be interesting to ascertain the actual numbers of men who have been invalided out of the service as the result of the South African campaign after bullet wounds and shell injuries whose permanent disability is purely shattered nerves. If possible the engagement in which the patient was wounded should be ascertained. Badly conceived projects by generals and commanding officers causing panic and disaster may then be found to be largely responsible for the development of such nervous cases quite apart from surgical injuries.

Aldershot.

A Mirror

OF

HOSPITAL PRACTICE,
BRITISH AND FOREIGN.

Nulla autem est alia pro certo noscendi via, nisi quamplurimas et morborum et dissectionum historias, tum aliorum tum proprias collectas habere, et inter se comparare.—MORGAGNI *De Sed. et Caus. Morb.*, lib. iv. Proœmium.

FRENCH HOSPITAL AND DISPENSARY.

A CASE OF PLASTIC BRONCHITIS WITH ITS POST-MORTEM APPEARANCES.

(Under the care of Dr. A. VINTRAS.)

PLASTIC bronchitis is an exceedingly rare disease, but it has been recognised from very early times and Galen has mentioned that solid masses of fibrin may be expectorated.[1] In 1897[2] Clarke and Lister explained the real method of formation of the casts and showed that they were not due to the coagulation of blood. Up to the present time more than 100 cases have been recorded, even if allowance be made for some which were probably not instances of true plastic bronchitis. The case recorded below is almost typical of the disease. Hæmoptysis is a very frequent symptom, for it occurs in about one-third of the cases, and epistaxis has also been observed.[3] The treatment by inhalations of lime-water appears to have been suggested[4] by Kuchenmeister's observation of the solubility of diphtheritic membrane in lime-water,[5] though Dixon[6] had pointed it out long before. For the notes of the case we are indebted to Dr. Henry Dardenne, physician to the French Hospital.

The patient was a man, aged 68 years. He had been for seven years a soldier in the French army and had served all his time in Africa. Since then he had had no regular occupation. He was admitted into the French Hospital on August 18th, 1894, under the care of Dr. Vintras. He complained of cough, shortness of breath, hæmoptysis, and pains across the chest both in front and behind between the shoulder-blades. His illness began three months previously after allowing his clothes, which had been soaked through with the rain, to dry on him. He remained after this for two days in bed. Since that time he had been troubled with fits of coughing which were now and again very severe. A month previously to admission he noticed for the first time

that after one of these fits his expectoration was tinged with blood, very thick, and almost gelatinous in consistence. He used to feel better for a day or two and then he would have another attack of coughing. These also became more severe. A week before admission he spat about three ounces of dark coagulated blood. He had for 12 hours a very severe pain across the chest in front, and this, together with a most distressing cough, lasted until he had expectorated some very thick and dark matter. His breathing then became much easier. He had before this always enjoyed good health. His habits had always been regular and he never drank to excess. There was nothing particular in his family history. His father died at the age of 78 years from cerebral hæmorrhage, his mother at 50 years of age from pneumonia. He remembered nothing about his grandparents. An uncle of his suffered from asthma and died from kidney disease. The patient was 5 feet 11 inches in height and was very emaciated. His weight six years before was 12 st. and on his admission it was only 10 st. His features were sharp and his complexion was sallow and pasty. His lips and ears were slightly cyanotic. His conjunctivæ were slightly jaundiced. The alæ nasi moved freely with each inspiration. The veins of the cheeks were dilated. His expression at times was very anxious and careworn. His temperature was normal. On examination his chest was found to be barrel-shaped. Its mobility was deficient. The sterno-mastoids stood in bold relief and could be seen to contract on inspiration. The vocal fremitus and resonance were normal. The chest was tympanitic in front. The right base behind was somewhat dull. On auscultation rhonchi and sonorous and sibilant râles were present over the whole chest both in front and behind. At the right base behind there was a respiratory murmur very indistinct and the vocal fremitus here was slightly impaired. The pulse was regular, full, incompressible, and beating at the rate of 100 per minute. The arteries were tortuous and indurated. The apex beat could be felt and seen in the sixth left intercostal space, half an inch outside the mamillary line. The heart-sounds could not be distinctly heard and neither the superficial nor the deep cardiac dulness could be detected owing to the emphysematous condition of the lungs. The teeth were decayed. The tongue was large and flabby, the papillæ were very prominent, and there were here and there a few superficial fissures. It was coated with a white fur except at the tip and edges. He had at times some difficulty in swallowing his solid food and this had increased within the last fortnight. He complained of no morbid sensations either before or after food. His appetite was good. His bowels were regular. The other systems appeared to be normal. On August 22nd, four days after the patient's admission, Dr. Dardenne was hastily summoned to the patient. He found him suffering from intense dyspnœa and he seemed to be on the verge of suffocation. His face was livid and covered with a cold perspiration. His eyes were bloodshot and looked as if they would come out of their sockets. The muscles of forced inspiration were acting powerfully and both hypochondriacal regions receded during inspiration. His breathing was about 60 per minute. His voice could scarcely be heard and the patient complained of pain and of a sense of pressure in the epigastrium and between the shoulder-blades. He had an incessant and harassing cough, and this would at times be relieved by the expectoration of a thick, sanguinolent fluid. Suddenly his face became quite black and he gasped for breath. His body was shaken with a severe fit of coughing. Tracheotomy appeared to be inevitable. However, with considerable effort he succeeded in expectorating a dark mass of the size of a cherry-stone, and this was followed by about two ounces of dark, semi-clotted blood. He felt instantly relieved and sank back exhausted. On floating the little black mass into water it turned out to be a perfect cast of a middle-sized bronchus with its ramifications. It was yellowish in colour and three and a half inches in length. For the next two or three days he spat some muco-purulent fluid and felt much easier. The respiratory murmurs were more distinct at the right base behind. The pains had disappeared and he expectorated no casts, only some dark blood and mucus. On the 26th he had another attack of dyspnœa, not so severe as the previous one, but he complained of the same severe pain in the epigastrium and between the shoulder-blades. On this occasion he expectorated about 15 casts. They were this time very soft and friable and much whiter than the first one. Peculiar adventitious sounds were to be

[1] De Locis Affectis, Book i., chapter i.
[2] Philosophical Transactions, vol. xiv.
[3] S. West: Practitioner, August, 1889.
[4] Wilson Fox: Diseases of the Lung and Pleura, 1891, p. 51.
[5] Oestreichische Zeitschrift für Praktische Heilkunde, 1863.
[6] Medical Commentaries, 1785, vol. ix.

rather than my own, as they give the records of an independent observer. He writes under date Feb. 26th, 1901 :—

Only five cases of rheumatism came into hospital free from cardiac trouble. Of these five, three developed cardiac symptoms, and in each of them the sign of which you told me was well marked.

No. 1, Mrs. ——, admitted Oct. 20th, 1900. Heart normal ; expansion of chest normal. Oct. 21st: deficient expansion on left side. Oct. 24th : systolic murmur heard in mitral and pulmonary areas. Subsequently disappeared.

No. 2, ———, aged 18 years, admitted Nov. 26th, 1900. Heart sounds and chest expansion normal. Nov. 29th : deficient expansion on left side of chest. Nov. 30th: systolic murmur in pulmonary area. Jan. 15th, 1901 : systolic murmur in pulmonary and mitral areas.

No. 3, ———, aged 19 years, admitted Jan. 28th, 1901 : heart sounds and chest expansion normal. Jan. 31st: deficient expansion of left chest. Feb. 2nd : heart sounds faint, no murmur (myocarditis). Feb. 5th : well-marked pericardial friction. This patient died and pericarditis, endocarditis, and myocarditis were found post mortem.

It seems to me incredible that this sign should not have been previously recorded, but I know of no such record. I advance it for the consideration of the profession in the belief that it will prove true and useful.

Guernsey.

Clinical Notes :
MEDICAL, SURGICAL, OBSTETRICAL, AND THERAPEUTICAL.

—

NOTE ON THE RESULTS OBTAINED BY THE ANTI-TYPHOID INOCULATIONS IN EGYPT AND CYPRUS DURING THE YEAR 1900.

BY A. E. WRIGHT, M.D. DUB.,
PROFESSOR OF PATHOLOGY, ARMY MEDICAL SCHOOL, NETLEY.

I AM indebted to the kindness of Colonel W. J. Fawcett, R.A.M.C., Principal Medical Officer in Egypt, for the following statistics dealing with the incidence of enteric fever and the mortality from the disease for the year 1900 in the inoculated and uninoculated among the British troops in Egypt and Cyprus.

—	Average annual strength.	Number of cases of enteric fever.	Number of deaths from enteric fever.	Percentage of cases calculated on average annual strength.	Percentage of deaths calculated on the same basis.
Uninoculated ...	2669	68	10	2 5	0·4
Inoculated... ...	720	1	1	0·14	0·14

These figures testify to a nineteen-fold reduction in the number of attacks of enteric fever and to a threefold reduction in the number of deaths from that disease among the inoculated.

In a note appended to the statistical table printed above Colonel Fawcett observes that the measure of protection resulting from the inoculation is not fully disclosed by a comparison of the figures of cases and deaths given in the table. Owing to the circumstance that soldiers inoculated in previous years are in the statistics included among the uninoculated, the number of the uninoculated was in reality less, and the number of the inoculated was in reality greater, than the figures set down for these groups in the first column of the above table. The figures in the second and third columns, on the other hand, accurately represent the number of cases and deaths in the inoculated and uninoculated, inasmuch as none of those inoculated in previous years contracted enteric fever.

A further point adverted to by Colonel Fawcett is that the only case which occurred among the inoculated occurred in the case of a patient admitted to hospital on the thirty-third day after inoculation. It would seem that the disease was in this case contracted before anything in the nature of protection had been established by the inoculation.

Netley

PRIMARY LARYNGEAL DIPHTHERIA.
BY E. M. SPENCER, L.R.C.P. & S. EDIN., M.D. TORONTO.

THE case of suspected laryngeal diphtheria published in THE LANCET of April 6th, p. 1009, by Mr. A. De Winter Baker induces me to send a short note of a very similar case, but one in which laryngoscopy was available leading to a positive diagnosis. On March 17th, 1901, I was called in to see a boy, aged 14 years, who was said to have a "cold." I found the patient dressed and, with the exception of slight hoarseness, seemingly not very unwell, with a pulse of 104 and of good volume, and complaining merely of slight sore-throat. A careful survey of the pharynx revealed nothing but a little hyperæmia of the fauces, and I made a diagnosis of slight laryngitis and expected the patient to mend soon. On the following day, however, I received a message that the boy seemed very "bad in his throat," and on my second visit he was suffering from constant slight dyspnœa with occasional exacerbations of urgent distress, accompanied by great excitement and cyanosis. There was now complete aphonia. Inspection of the pharynx revealed nothing but the slight redness noticed before. There was marked stridor on auscultating the trachea which became very loud on the accession of an attack of "suffocation" which was doubtless partly spasmodic. I inquired as to the possibility of lodgment of a foreign body, but this was negatived. Seeing that the case was urgent and rapidly growing worse I had the patient removed to my house for purposes of examination. Laryngoscopy revealed firstly great redness and swelling of the arytenoids, and then a larynx and a trachea literally full of typical diphtheritic membrane, the trachea being reduced, as far as I could judge, to about one-third of its normal diameter. The boy returned home and I followed immediately and injected 2000 units of anti-diphtheritic serum. The patient has made a steady recovery and is now practically well. At no time was a trace of membrane visible to ordinary examination. The aphonia was complete for a week, but the voice has now regained considerable volume.

Modbury, Devon.

FOREIGN BODY IN THE EAR.
BY L. K. HENCHEL, M.D. VIENNA.

THE following short account of a case in which a foreign body was impacted in the ear may, I think, be of interest.

The patient was a girl who, when five years old, had a bead of a rosary put into her ear in sport by a playfellow. This fact was kept secret from her parents and teachers (nuns) for two and a half years. After that time the ear was so troublesome that the child was taken to a specialist and then the story came out. The second time this specialist syringed the ear a white bead was found in the basin, but the girl remarked that the rosary from which the bead had become detached was a black one. No attention was paid to this remark at the time. For two and a half years the child suffered more or less from irritation in, discharges from, and pains in, the ear with loss of hearing. The case came to me on Feb. 15th, 1901, with a well-developed furunculosis. As the swelling in the meatus subsided under treatment I saw a black object partially obscuring the membrana tympani, and on syringing with moderate force a shell of japan lacquer came out. The meatus was very much reddened where the foreign body had lain so long—namely, for five years. When the little patient came to me the next day she had a rather severe hæmorrhage from her ear. I could plainly see blood oozing out from the reddened surface. I moistened some pure cotton with liquor ferri sesquichloridi, twisted it firmly over a fine boxwood stick, such as is commonly used on the continent for a toothpick, and under the guidance of the light applied it to the bleeding surface. The further history of the case was quite uneventful. The blood-clot formed by the styptic came away in two portions several days afterwards and the girl, who had been unable to hear a watch quite close to the affected ear, can now hear it as well as with the other ear, and a tuning fork is heard better now with the affected ear than with the other one. Neither the rosary nor the white bead is now to be found, a thing not to be wondered at after a lapse of several years.

Villa Carlotta, Bordighera.

resume their normal appearance gradually. This production of pseudo-parasites during each paroxysm of an intermittent fever and disappearance during the apyretic interval would of course render more difficult the differentiation of parasitic from non-parasitic ague except by experts. The establishment of the theory that there is an intermittent fever due to environment would, however, relieve Laveran's supporters from the difficulty of explaining how those cases in which no parasites can be discovered in the blood can possibly be caused by parasites. Moreover, the presence of pseudo-parasites in the blood of such cases would enable us to understand the assertion of those who maintained that the bodies they found in malarial blood were not parasites at all but simply altered blood corpuscles. Manson says that the staining process for diagnosing malaria is not to be depended on unless carried out by those with great experience.

IX.—INCREASE OF WATER IN THE BLOOD WILL PRODUCE ENLARGEMENT OF THE SPLEEN.

As we have seen, increase of water in the blood increases hæmolysis or the destruction of red blood corpuscles. But the taking up and disposal of the fragments of disintegrating red blood corpuscles is the normal function of the spleen. Hence when increase of water in the blood produces increased destruction of these corpuscles increased functional activity of the organ and therefore increase of its size or bulk follows. Moreover, the increase of water by increasing the volume of the blood will of itself also directly tend to enlarge the spleen.

When critical elimination of water (sweat) occurs there is, of course, diminished volume of the blood, diminished destruction of red blood corpuscles, and consequently diminished functional activity and size of the organ which is normally called on to dispose of the disintegrated corpuscles. Hence in the apyretic intervals the spleen resumes normal size. But if this intermittent increase of water in the blood is frequently repeated the organ will become permanently enlarged, for it is known that transitory but repeated hyperæmia of any organ leads to a permanent enlargement of the organ, such as is found in ague cake, in those suffering from chronic malaria.

Now this view that the enlargement of the spleen is in some cases of intermittent fever at all events due to the intermittent excess of water produced by meteorological environment receives some support from a consideration of the periodical change in size of the organ that takes place in health. In health it is known that the spleen enlarges to some extent after every meal, reaching its maximum after some hours and then returning to its normal size. When food is taken into the stomach the first portion of it to be absorbed is its water, which enters the blood directly through the gastric vessels. This addition of water, of course, increases the volume of blood, and also destruction of blood corpuscles, thus leading, as described above, to the enlargement of the organ. This rapid absorption of water of the food by disintegrating and so getting rid of the old and useless blood corpuscles prepares the blood for the pouring into it some hours later of the other constituents of the food *viâ* the longer route of the intestinal lacteals and thoracic duct.

Another point which supports this view of the cause of enlargement of the spleen is that whatever other medicines, &c., we may also employ, a free use of hydragogue purgatives is indispensable for the reduction of the organ to its normal size. Is not this an indication that in the first instance its enlargement is due to increase of water in the blood?

The spleen is enlarged in ague, then, because in this disease there is increased destruction of red blood corpuscles, the disposal of which in ague, as in health, is the normal function of the organ, and the increased destruction of corpuscles is produced by increase of water in the blood.

X.—THE MEASURES FOUND MOST USEFUL IN THE PREVENTION AND TREATMENT OF AGUE REDUCE CONSIDERABLY THE AMOUNT OF WATER IN THE BLOOD.

Prevention.—Drainage of the soil in paludal districts undoubtedly eradicates or at least considerably reduces the prevalence of ague. The most obvious effect of drainage is, however, that it dries the soil and therefore the superincumbent atmosphere. Drainage removes or at least reduces one factor (atmospheric humidity) of the environment that produces increase of water in the blood. In well-built, well-raised houses the humidity of the air is less than in the open, and those occupying such houses are therefore less likely to contract the fevers to which I am referring than those who are liable to exposure at night. The same may also be said of residence in huts, tents, or even within mosquito curtains.

Treatment.—All effective treatment of ague reduces the amount of water in the blood. Diaphoretics, diuretics, and purgatives certainly do so. And it is to this that I attribute the curative and, indeed, preventive action of quinine When ague becomes chronic a course of Turkish or *dry*-air baths is most beneficial; and what so obviously reduces the amount of water in the blood? Removal from the influence of the meteorological environment that produces increase of water in the blood usually cures ague.

XI.—SUMMARY.

What I have written above may be shortly summarised as follows : 1. Cases of fever, clinically identical with malaria, occur in the blood of which parasites could not be found after repeated search before quinine had been given. 2. The meteorological environment found where such cases occur, and indeed in all malarial climates, increases the amount of water in the blood of those exposed to its influence by impeding elimination through the skin and lungs (evaporation—heat loss) and through the kidneys. 3. There is known to be increase of water in the blood of those suffering from ague (Liebermeister). 4. Increase of water in the blood increases metabolism—i.e., heat production—and produces a rise of body temperature (Payne). 5. As environment thus causes diminished heat loss from the body and increased heat production within the body it is plain that it causes pyrexia. 6. This pyrexia must be of intermittent variety as the environment which produces it is of intermittent intensity—i.e., undergoes diurnal variation. 7. Elimination of water from the blood (sweat) in ague reduces the temperature to normal. 8. Increase of water in the blood produces poikilocytosis, pseudo-parasites, liberation of hæmoglobin, extensive destruction of red blood corpuscles, and melanæmia. 9. An extreme degree of these changes obviously leads to hæmoglobinuria. 10. Increase of water in the blood produces enlargement of the spleen. 11. Removal from the environment that produces increase of water in the blood usually cures ague. 12. All treatment of ague which is efficacious reduces the amount of water in the blood. 13. From these facts I think it is not unreasonable to conclude that those cases of ague or intermittent fever in which no parasites can be found are demonstrably due to the environment under which they arise.

If my view is correct it is only one more illustration of the truth of the old saying that pathology in many instances seems to be but physiology in distress.

RESULTS IN HAVANA DURING THE YEAR 1901 OF DISINFECTION FOR YELLOW FEVER,

UNDER THE HYPOTHESIS THAT THE STEGOMYIA MOSQUITO IS THE ONLY MEANS OF TRANSMITTING THE DISEASE.[1]

BY W. C. GORGAS,

MAJOR, MEDICAL CORPS, UNITED STATES ARMY; CHIEF SANITARY OFFICER OF HAVANA.

IN order clearly to show the results of our work in Havana it may be well to go over the ground and to point out what the conditions were before we commenced work, and to look into some general considerations with regard to the habitat of yellow fever. When we attribute the results of the work here to our methods of destroying infected mosquitoes it has been objected that yellow fever has disappeared from many other cities under other methods of disinfection and when no particular effort was made to stamp out the disease ; and instances are cited of cities of the United States, such as Boston, Philadelphia, New York, and New Orleans, and some of the smaller towns in the West Indies, Mexico, and South America.

Havana is unique in being the only city in the Western

1 A paper read before the International Sanitary Congress held at Havana, Cuba, on Feb. 15th, 1902.

Continent where yellow fever has really always been endemic during historic times, and when we come to look into the matter the reasons are obvious. In any community where frost occurs yellow fever will always disappear during the winter. Even in our Southern ports, such as New Orleans, Mobile, and Pensacola, yellow fever habitually disappears at that period. Incidents might be adduced of its persisting through the winter, but such instances are rare. The natural tendency of these cities would be to free themselves of yellow fever if re-introduction from the outside is prevented. In the smaller towns within the tropics, those having a non-immune population of, say, 50, the same tendency is observed from other causes. While yellow fever would not die out from climatic conditions, in the course of a year or two these few non-immunes would disappear as non-immunes either from death or by becoming immune from having had yellow fever, and the tendency would be for this disease to disappear and to re-appear when the population had again become non-immune to a considerable extent. This is really the history of the disease as observed. Of course, the larger the non-immune population in the tropics the longer the epidemic period lasts, sometimes many years. Even cities of the size of Vera Cruz and Santiago de Cuba are not truly endemic foci in the same sense that Havana is. Looking back over the history of these cities many years at a time can be found in which there was no yellow fever, and if introduction from the outside could have been prevented they would have freed themselves from yellow fever from the above causes. In Havana the conditions have been different: it is the principal port of entry for Cuba and there has been a considerable influx of non-immune Spaniards—from 4000 to 30,000 annually. Theoretically, from the existing conditions we would expect that yellow fever would be endemic in Havana, and as a matter of fact as far back as the records go from which any at all reliable history of the statistics of the city can be obtained a month has never passed until the American occupation without a death from yellow fever. And there has probably in all this time never been a day on which there was not a case of this disease in Havana. This is the only city in the world of which that can be said. Probably Rio de Janeiro can in future be placed in the same category. Its large population, large immigration, and latitude would seem to make the conditions very similar to those of Havana.

I go over this ground to show that the causes which have made yellow fever disappear from other cities in all latitudes of the Western Hemisphere cannot occur in Havana. The statistics of yellow fever for Havana, as far back as we have official record, are given in the appended table and show the deaths from this disease month by month.

When we commenced work in Havana the island had been suffering for five years from an exhausting civil war and during the few months preceding the city had undergone a blockade by the American fleet. The hygienic conditions of the city were therefore at that time considerably worse than they were in normal times. But the non-immune population was small; immigration had dwindled during the war and had practically stopped for the year preceding. We went to work on the usual sanitary lines with our efforts directed more particularly toward yellow fever. I will not attempt any description of the general sanitary work but will enumerate the methods adopted towards yellow fever.

Up to July of the first year of American occupation there was little yellow fever in the city. Then immigrants began to pour in and some 16,000 reached Havana between July and Dec. 31st in the year 1899. From July to Dec. 31st we had quite an epidemic of yellow fever, and the December of 1899 was the severest December as regards yellow fever that had occurred for years. In February, 1900, I was appointed the Chief Sanitary Officer of Havana and I know from personal observation that from that time the regulations with regard to yellow fever were carefully carried out.

The reporting of yellow fever was compulsory. Upon the report of a case it was promptly isolated and quarantined by guards employed by the Sanitary Department. No communication whatever was allowed within the quarantined area except that of the visiting physicians and the sanitary inspector. All supplies had to pass through the sanitary guard. The isolation was as complete as military authority and liberal expenditure could make it. The case was then referred to a board of experienced physicians who visited the patient and made the diagnosis. If the case terminated in death the body was buried with the usual sanitary precaution adopted in highly dangerous diseases. In all cases the quarantined area was disinfected. First, by carefully wiping down everything with a bichloride solution and then

TABLE SHOWING DEATHS FROM YELLOW FEVER IN THE CITY OF HAVANA.

Months	1901	1900	1899	1898	1897	1896	1895	1894	1893	1892	1891	1890	1889	1888	1887	1886	1885	1884	1883	1882	1881	1880	1879	1878	1877	1876	1875	1874	1873	1872	1871	1870	1869	1868	1867	1866	1865	1864	1863	1862	1861	1860	1859	1858	1857	1856
January	7	8	1	7	69	10	15	7	15	15	10	10	17	8	5	4	4	26	14	9	7	16	11	26	8	24	16	7	32	20	18	—	—	—	—	—	—	—	—	—	—	—	—	—	—	—
February	5	9	0	1	24	7	4	4	6	10	3	4	5	8	6	0	3	16	9	11	3	9	13	13	9	24	16	4	23	13	23	—	—	—	—	—	—	—	—	—	—	—	—	—	—	—
March	1	4	1	2	30	3	2	2	4	1	4	4	5	14	8	0	1	8	21	14	3	20	6	5	11	29	32	18	27	4	12	—	—	—	—	—	—	—	—	—	—	—	—	—	—	—
April	0	0	2	1	71	14	6	4	8	8	5	13	8	24	22	1	2	32	34	18	6	44	13	28	8	33	34	22	37	4	54	—	—	—	—	—	—	—	—	—	—	—	—	—	—	—
May	0	2	0	4	88	27	10	16	23	7	7	23	17	26	84	1	3	55	75	84	6	40	40	53	16	103	32	85	127	13	91	—	—	—	—	—	—	—	—	—	—	—	—	—	—	—
June	0	8	1	3	174	46	16	31	69	13	41	38	37	36	128	14	4	66	162	176	37	50	237	184	143	292	142	172	378	68	201	—	—	—	—	—	—	—	—	—	—	—	—	—	—	—
July	1	30	2	16	168	116	88	77	118	27	66	67	48	74	102	33	13	131	177	195	90	179	475	504	249	675	187	361	416	68	234	—	—	—	—	—	—	—	—	—	—	—	—	—	—	—
August	2	49	13	16	102	262	120	73	100	67	66	60	73	113	73	39	34	97	148	73	127	148	417	374	285	250	144	416	127	70	138	—	—	—	—	—	—	—	—	—	—	—	—	—	—	—
September	2	52	18	34	56	166	135	76	68	70	65	33	37	63	36	37	32	41	50	56	94	75	148	179	234	97	102	186	35	59	72	—	—	—	—	—	—	—	—	—	—	—	—	—	—	—
October	0	74	25	26	42	240	102	40	46	54	48	32	21	48	33	16	41	24	72	33	39	32	44	106	185	42	109	91	28	38	55	—	—	—	—	—	—	—	—	—	—	—	—	—	—	—
November	0	54	18	13	26	244	35	23	28	52	24	15	21	33	20	13	22	8	45	36	38	21	31	53	150	31	105	42	5	85	51	—	—	—	—	—	—	—	—	—	—	—	—	—	—	—
December	0	20	22	13	8	147	20	29	11	33	17	9	14	21	15	9	6	7	42	24	35	11	9	34	76	19	82	21	9	73	42	—	—	—	—	—	—	—	—	—	—	—	—	—	—	—
Totals	18	310	103	136	858	1282	553	382	496	357	356	308	303	468	532	167	165	511	849	729	485	645	1444	1559	1374	1619	1001	1425	1284	515	991	572	1000	290	591	51	238	555	590	1386	1020	439	1193	1396	2058	1309

by filling all rooms with formalin gas, using a litre of the 40 per cent. solution to each 1000 feet of space disinfected. Fabrics of all kinds were taken to the steam disinfecting plant and there disinfected. Under this system we hoped to decrease yellow fever greatly and in the course of a few years to eradicate it from the city.

The general sanitary measures adopted appeared to be rapidly decreasing the general death-rate. The general death-rate in 1898 was 91·03 per 1000, in 1899 it fell to 33·67, and in 1900 continued to decrease to 24·40. But our work apparently had no effect upon yellow fever. The winter epidemic of 1899 continued through the spring and summer, reaching in the fall the proportions of a sharp epidemic, even for Havana. We had during the year 1900 1244 cases of yellow fever, with 310 deaths. All classes suffered, particularly the higher officials on the military governor's staff. The chief quartermaster of the island, the chief commissary for the island, and one of the aides of the military governor died from yellow fever.

The Sanitary Department was much discouraged at the result of the work. It seemed to me that general sanitary measures could not be more extensively carried out than we had done during this year. We had all the power of the military authority behind us and ample means. During this year, on the internal sanitation of houses, exclusive of street-cleaning, disposal of garbage, &c., we spent about $25,000 per month and employed some 300 men daily. The general sanitary conditions were improving in the most satisfactory manner but we evidently had not produced the slightest effect upon yellow fever. We commenced 1901 much discouraged, with the most unfavourable outlook as far as yellow fever was concerned. The non-immune population was larger probably than it had ever been before. 26,000 immigrants had come into Havana during the year 1900. Yellow fever was in every part of the city. The deaths from yellow fever in January and February were large and the probabilities all pointed to our having a more severe epidemic in 1901 than in 1900.

The results of the investigations by the Army Board of the theory that the stegomyia mosquito was the only carrier of yellow fever, first advanced by Dr. Charles Finlay, were published about this time. This work was so brilliant in its execution and so positive in its results that, as I look back now, I am surprised that I was not at once convinced. But many years of contact with men engaged in the practical work of managing yellow fever and my own personal experience with this disease had so impressed me with the belief that fomites were the principal, and practically the only, carrier of the disease that I had scant belief in the mosquito theory. But General Wood was determined that every possible measure should be taken for the reduction of the disease and he authorised me to go to any reasonable expense in providing for the destruction of mosquitoes, which I then considered only a possible and exceptional means of transmitting yellow fever. But having undertaken it the department bent every energy to carrying it out thoroughly, and as I look back I have the satisfaction of believing that we could not have carried it out more thoroughly even if we had known that the results would be what they have been.

In looking over the ground beforehand we concluded that for practical operations three fields of work had to be considered. In the first place, to destroy all the stegomyia we could, so as to limit the number of insects capable of conveying the disease. For it seems obvious that if we had no stegomyia we would have no yellow fever. In the second place, to prevent the stegomyia from biting the yellow fever patient ; because, if we could prevent the mosquito from becoming diseased we would also prevent yellow fever. And in the third place, to destroy all mosquitoes that had bitten yellow fever patients and thus become infected ; because if these are destroyed it is evident that the disease would be stopped.

With the object of reducing the number of mosquitoes an ordinance was issued requiring all people within the city limits to keep receptacles containing water mosquito proof. The city was divided up into districts and an inspector was appointed for each district who kept up a constant inspection, with the view of enforcing these ordinances. He was accompanied by men with oil-cans to pour oil into all puddles, cess-pools, &c., about the dwellings, and after sufficient notice had been given all receptacles in which larvæ were found were destroyed. All persons having larvæ on their premises were fined under the municipal ordinances.

50 men were employed in this work. 100 men during most of the summer were employed under proper superintendence in the suburbs, draining all pools and low ground and pouring oil into such places as could not be drained—that is, during most of the past summer 150 men devoted their attention to killing mosquitoes in the larval stage.

To meet the second proposition—that is, to keep the stegomyia from biting the infected man—all hospitals where yellow fever was received were ordered to be thoroughly screened, and this was at first enforced. In cases of yellow fever occurring in private houses the sanitary department screened them at public expense. Ordinarily, within two hours after the report of a case of yellow fever the quarantined area was thoroughly screened. We kept a sufficient number of ready-made screens on hand for the purpose and 30 men were employed in this work.

To meet the third proposition—that is, killing the infected mosquitoes—the infected building and all adjacent buildings were gone over from top to bottom with pyrethrum powder ; 150 pounds, on the average, were used in each case. This work was done in addition to the disinfection as carried out the preceding year. While pyrethrum powder is not as good a mosquitocide as some other substances it is the least objectionable to the people whose dwellings are being fumigated. It causes no injury to fabrics and within four or five hours the room can be again occupied without discomfort. It, however, does not kill all mosquitoes. A good many of them are simply intoxicated and will revive if exposed to fresh air. For this reason the mosquitoes have to be carefully swept up and destroyed. The houses contiguous to the infected house were gone over in the same way on the possibility of infected mosquitoes having escaped to neighbouring houses. Every room was carefully sealed and pasted just as we had done in using formalin. In this work some 40 men were employed during the summer. We used a pound of pyrethrum powder to each 1000 cubic feet of air space.

In January, 1901, we had 24 cases of fever with seven deaths—a large number for that month ; in February there were eight cases and five deaths.

The mosquito work was inaugurated on Feb. 27th. We went through March with only two cases, which occurred on the 2nd and 8th. I was much pleased with this but not particularly impressed, knowing that it might be a coincidence. We then went to April 20th without another case. This was unexpected, particularly as the year had commenced so badly and as there was plenty of non-immune material around. The table will show that this condition of affairs had never been approximated before in Havana. On April 21st and 22nd there were two more cases, but under our system of disinfection the disease did not spread. I began to feel pretty certain by this time that the results were due to our mosquito work. On May 6th and 7th we had four more cases, but this focus was promptly controlled. We then went through the whole month of June up to July 21st before we had another case.

It was exceedingly important to have all cases reported so as not to let a focus get started and spread. A great element in the reporting of cases was to have as little opposition as possible on the part of the people. The fumigation for the mosquito caused very little inconvenience compared with the disinfection of fomites and after much discussion and deliberation with the officers in charge of the disinfecting work I determined, the latter part of June, to do away with all sanitary measures against yellow fever, except those directed towards the mosquito, as the only means of the transmission of the disease.

These measures went into effect on July 1st and after that time nothing was sent to the disinfecting plant in yellow fever cases and at the infected point only measures looking to the destruction of mosquitoes were taken. The guard was still kept at the infected house, but the physician was allowed to specify a reasonable number of immunes who might go to and from the quarantined area. The guard was directed to see that the screen doors were kept closed and that the ordinary sick-room hygiene was carried out.

About the middle of June a pronounced focus of yellow fever developed in Santiago de las Vegas, a town about 12 miles from Havana. The successful management of this focus was another evidence of the efficacy of the methods adopted in Havana, but the length of this paper does not allow me to go into details of these cases. Santiago de las Vegas is a town of 5000 inhabitants, with a non-immune population of 475. It is really a suburb of Havana and considerable numbers of people come and go every day. Besides Santiago de las Vegas there were three or four other towns with direct communication that were having yellow fever about this time. We discovered nine cases that came into the city of Havana from Santiago de las Vegas during June, July, and August. As Havana had been entirely free from yellow fever during June I am inclined to think that Santiago de las Vegas was the point from which we became reinfected. During July we had four cases in Havana, with one death ; during August we had six cases with two deaths. Becoming satisfied that we were being reinfected from outside towns I obtained authority from the Military Governor to place inspectors on all railroads coming into Havana from infected points. These took the names of all the non-immunes coming into the city and kept them under observation for a week. This worked very well in practice. All the cases known to have come into the city were reported by these inspectors.

As the infection was severe in Santiago de las Vegas an appropriation of $4000 was made for the purpose. We adopted the same methods there as in Havana and at once controlled the disease. The last case occurred in Santiago de las Vegas on August 31st. A case from this point was reported on Oct. 14th, but I, personally, do not think it was a case of yellow fever. It was an exceedingly mild and doubtful case, though diagnosed as yellow fever by the board. On Sept. 28th we had our last case in Havana. During October, December, and January we had none.

The whole year has been very unusual in its yellow fever conditions and is far below any preceding year of which we have record in the number of cases which have occurred. October and November have always been months when yellow fever was rife in Havana, and to have had none at all in these months in 1901 is remarkable. During 1900 the general death-rate had been greatly lowered by the sanitary work done, but yellow fever had not been much affected and we had a sharp epidemic. In 1901 all the conditions were unchanged, except that work for the destruction of mosquitoes was carried out, with the result that yellow fever at once almost disappeared and really did disappear in the last three months of the year.

I submit that this is evidence of the practical demonstration of the mosquito theory.

Havana.

CASE OF RIGHT AORTIC ARCH WITH ABNORMAL DISPOSITION OF THE LEFT INNOMINATE VEIN AND THORACIC DUCT.

BY S. CAMERON,
JUNIOR DEMONSTRATOR OF ANATOMY, GLASGOW UNIVERSITY.

FEW parts of the human body are subject to such interesting abnormalities as are the pulmonary artery, the aorta, and its branches, and since the researches of Rathke, Allen Thomson, and others it has been possible to account for and to classify the vast majority of these abnormalities on embryological grounds. It will be remembered that in the early fœtus the dorsal aorta is formed by the junction of the fourth arches on the right and left sides, and that a great portion of the fourth right arch afterwards disappears, the remnant forming the right subclavian artery, while the fourth left arch becomes the arch of the aorta. The fifth right arch also disappears, whilst the fifth left arch is represented in the adult by the pulmonary artery and by the ductus arteriosus connecting that artery with the aorta. The causes of variation from the normal are obscure, but it is a natural supposition that when inflammation or obstruction affects those vessels which should normally persist and causes them to atrophy compensation will be brought about by an increase in the size of the corresponding vessel on the opposite side. A certain degree of inherent instability in the development of the fœtal vessels must also be considered as existing apart from pathological causes.

The subject of the present irregularity was an adult male. The position of the heart was quite normal and there were no irregularities of its valves, septa, arteries, or veins. The ascending aorta, which was somewhat large, arose from the base of the left ventricle and took a course upwards and to the right, passing behind the sternum, crossing the trachea

until it reached the level of the second dorsal vertebra on the right side. It here bent acutely backwards on itself, thus coming in contact with the right side of the third dorsal vertebra. The vessel was now directed gradually towards the middle line, but when it reached the level of the upper border of the seventh dorsal vertebra it described a gentle curve with the convexity towards the right side, till it reached the middle line between the twelfth dorsal and first lumbar vertebræ. It will thus be observed that the vessel in its course arched over the root of the right lung. The main arterial trunks were given off in the following order :— (1) left common carotid ; (2) right common carotid ; (3) right subclavian ; and (4) left subclavian. It will be observed that the innominate artery was absent. The left common carotid was somewhat larger than usual and measured 14 centimetres from its origin to its bifurcation. The right common carotid measured 11 centimetres. These vessels pursued a normal course, as did also the right subclavian artery. The

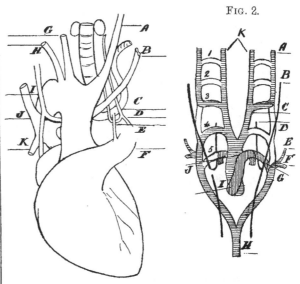

FIG. 1.

FIG. 2.

FIG. 1.—Diagram of case recorded. A, Left common carotid. B, Left innominate vein. C, Left subclavian artery. D, Left vagus nerve with recurrent laryngeal. E, Ductus arteriosus. F, Pulmonary artery. G, Right common carotid. H, Right subclavian artery. I, Right vagus nerve with recurrent laryngeal. J, Right innominate vein. K, Vena azygos major.

FIG. 2.—Diagram from Quain showing the mode of development of the great arteries in the present case. 1, 2, 3, 4, 5, The primitive vascular arches. A, Internal carotid. B, Vagus nerve. C, Common carotid. D, Recurrent laryngeal nerve. E, Vertebral artery. F, Subclavian artery. G, Ductus arteriosus. H, Descending aorta. I, Pulmonary trunk. J, Ascending aorta. K, External carotid.

left subclavian presented some points, however, which are of much interest ; as noted above it was the last of these vessels arising from the aorta. Its origin was from a pouch-like process projecting from the left side of the descending aorta. This pouch measured one and a half centimetres in length and equalled a normal common iliac in diameter. It ran to the left side at right angles to the aorta, having the third dorsal vertebra behind it, while the posterior surface of the œsophagus rested on its anterior wall. This pouch presented several undulations on its posterior and under wall. At the point where the subclavian took its origin from this pouch the ductus arteriosus, which was very well marked and of large size, joined the pouch, thus connecting it with the left pulmonary artery. The ductus arteriosus measured four centimetres in length. It was quite impervious and lay to the left of the œsophagus. The pulmonary arteries were normal both in their relations and distribution. The subclavian after arising from the pouch ascended to gain the inner margin of the scalenus anticus. There were two left bronchial arteries arising from the dorsal aorta, the left (upper) arising by almost a common origin with the fourth left intercostal artery. There was one right bronchial artery which also arose from the front part of the descending aorta. The left innominate vein was of large size and began behind the inner part of the clavicle. In its descent it passed forwards and inwards and came to lie immediately in front of the origin of the left subclavian artery from the

INOCULATION WITH HAFFKINE'S PLAGUE PROPHYLACTIC: A REVIEW OF 30,609 CASES.

BY CHARLES E. P. FORSYTH, M.B. ABERD., M.R.C.P. LOND.,

LATE INOCULATING MEDICAL OFFICER TO THE PUNJAB GOVERNMENT; LATE ASSISTANT MEDICAL OFFICER, EASTERN FEVER HOSPITAL, HOMERTON, N.E.

HAFFKINE'S plague prophylactic has been in use now for some years and a goodly number of reports exist as to its efficacy in reducing both the attack-rate and the case mortality of the disease. The scheme instituted last season, 1902-03, by the Punjab Government for the carrying out of inoculation against plague on a grand scale was not by any means the success which had been hoped for or anticipated. But even in its limited success it will doubtless afford further evidence of the value of the prophylactic when the whole mass of accumulated statistics comes to be officially published. The figures given here are arranged from a total of 30,609 inoculations with Haffkine's prophylactic performed by me while acting as one of the medical officers appointed with reference to the above-mentioned scheme. Deductions from them would seem to point a very strong case in favour of inoculation as an agent in stemming the disease which works such havoc throughout India. Actually the figures may fairly be said to do so, though for a variety of reasons the deductions drawn can only be imperfect. Absolutely reliable statistics are very hard to obtain and this is not surprising when one considers the way in which the plague returns are compiled. The primary agent in the matter is the "*patwari*" or village registrar. With him rests the question of diagnosis, and he also reports as to the fact of inoculation in each individual plague case or death from plague which he returns from his village. The question of diagnosis must necessarily be obscure, not so much perhaps in the bubonic form of the disease (fortunately the most common), but certainly so in the other types, yet it is fair to suppose that this rights itself to some extent—actual cases of plague that have been missed making up for those wrongly notified as such.

As to the fact of inoculation a good degree of accuracy can be reached. This is checked by the comparison of the *patwari's* return with the inoculating officer's register. Every person at the time of his inoculation receives a certificate with his full description as to name, caste, &c. A duplicate of this is retained and entered in a register. A plague return being verified, an additional entry is made stating the date and type of attack with its result, whether recovery or death. The figures under notice will have some disadvantages which will be mentioned as they present themselves.

TABLE I.—*Giving the Plague Statistics in the whole Number of Inoculations performed—30,609.*

Number attacked by plague.	Deaths.	Case mortality (per cent.).
329	50	15·1

Attacks or deaths returned after the closure of the figures (May, 1903) should be allowed for, but these must be few, if indeed any, as the epidemic in the district dealt with had then undergone its usual seasonal decline.

The reduction in the case mortality—a reduction to 15·1 per cent. in a disease in which it may reach 70, 80, or 90 per cent. and is usually about 50 per cent.—is worthy of note. Determination of the attack-rate is here of no value owing to the distribution of the population with the varying conditions of surroundings and exposure to infection. Included in these 329 are some cases which obviously had been inoculated whilst in the incubation stage of the disease, as will be seen in Table II. which gives particulars of the attacks occurring from one to 30 days after inoculation.

TABLE II.—*Time after Inoculation in 76 Cases with 16 Deaths.*

Time after inoculation.	Number of cases.	Deaths.	Case mortality (per cent.).
1 to 7 days	19	6	31·5
7 ,, 14 ,, ...	9	1	11·1
14 ,, 21 ,, ...	14	2	14·2
21 ,, 30 ,, ...	34	7	20·5

The average case mortality here—21 per cent.—is somewhat higher than in the whole number of cases, yet it is still comparatively low—a fact going to confirm the present belief that the prophylactic, far from doing harm, really tends to do good when given after infection, a belief contrary to that expressed by the Indian Plague Commission (1898–1900). An important question is the length of time for which protection is conferred by the inoculation of the prophylactic. It seems very uncertain, but the minimum period has been given on good evidence [1] as about three months. Its determination is difficult indeed in dealing with large numbers and the present figures, as will be seen in Table III., unfortunately can throw no light on the matter.

TABLE III.—*Time of Attack after Inoculation in 329 Cases with 50 Deaths.*

Time of incidence of attack of plague after inoculation.	Cases.	Percentage of cases to total.	Deaths.	Case mortality (per cent.).
1 month and under... ...	76	23·1	16	21·0
1 to 2 months	92	27·9	14	15·2
2 ,, 3 ,, ...	83	25·2	13	15·6
3 ,, 4 ,, ...	35	10·6	4	11·4
4 months and over... ...	43	13·0	3	6·9

To obtain proper data in this respect it would seem necessary to observe a proportion of inoculated individuals living in a small community under constant conditions of infection for a lengthy period, and this circumstances rendered impossible. From the figures given it might almost appear as if the nearer the time of inoculation the greater the liability to attack. The apparent contradiction to accepted views may perhaps be explained to a large extent by reference to Table IV., where it will be seen that the height of the epidemic (cf. Table V. for number of villages declared infected) corresponded in time to the period when the proportion of inoculated persons was at a maximum.

TABLE IV.—*Inoculations (30,609) and Attacks (329) arranged as to Months.*

Month.	Number of cases of plague amongst inoculated.	Number of inoculations performed.
October	*Nil.*	2380
November	2	2604
December	4	1525
January	6	8367
February	27	8209
March	122	6839
April	168	685

The nearer the figures can be confined to a limited population living under the same conditions the greater the value of the inferences that may be drawn from them. Thus in Tables V. and VI. an attempt at further accuracy has been made. The statistics have here been fined down to those obtained from a group of 50 villages, all situated in the Garhshankar Tahsil of the Hoshiarpur district of the Punjab. These villages were declared infected at varying times from October, 1902, to March, 1903, and inoculation was carried on in the group immediately prior to and during

---

[1] Report on Inoculation in the Punjab, 1899–1900: Wilkinson.

the worst state of the epidemic. These points are shown in Table V. :—

TABLE V.—*Showing in the 50 Villages the Period of the Epidemic when Inoculations were Performed.*

Months.	Number of villages declared infected.	Number of villages inoculated for the first time.	Number of inoculations performed.
October	5	0	0
November... ...	5	2	2386
December... ...	6	2	166
January	4	19	5363
February	17	22	3630
March	13	5	1341
Totals... ...	50	50	12,886

None of these villages had been declared to be free from infection at the end of March, 1903. They have a total population according to the latest census returns of 44,760 and in them from November, 1902, to March, 1903, inclusive 12,886 inoculations were performed, distributed as to time as shown in Table V.

Thus the total population may be divided into the two classes of uninoculated, numbering 31,874, and inoculated numbering 12,886, both classes living approximately under the same conditions as regards surroundings and risk of infection.

In Table VI. the relative behaviour of these two classes towards plague is set down.

TABLE VI.—*Showing the Relative Behaviour of Uninoculated and Inoculated Persons towards Plague.*

Classes.	Number in each.	Cases of plague.	Attack-rate per cent.	Deaths.	Death-rate per cent.	Case mortality per cent.
A. Uninoculated	31,874	1457	4·5	659	2·06	45·2
B. Inoculated ...	12,886	171	1·3	29	0·22	16·9

The percentage of the inoculated to the total population was 28·7. A slight error lies in the fact that some few persons were inoculated twice; these were certainly under 1 per cent. of the whole. From this it is evident that Class B (the inoculated) have a decided advantage over Class A (the uninoculated). In Class B the attack-rate of plague is over one-third—nearly one-fourth—of the attack-rate in Class A, the death-rate is one-tenth, and the case mortality is reduced by nearly 30 per cent. In this series of cases the usefulness of the measure would appear to be established and as to its freedom from ill-effects it may be stated that in the whole number of 30,609 inoculations no serious consequences came to light. To speak more exactly abscesses developed in 16 cases at the site of inoculation. 15 of these were traced to one particular bottle of the prophylactic which had become contaminated in some unknown way. The remaining abscess was the only accidental one reported. It may be said with some safety that there were no others, as the people are not at all backward in reporting anything of the kind, and beyond these few septic complications, none of which were ever serious, there were no ill-effects known. The technique recommended by M. Haffkine was adopted throughout, with some little variations suggested by local circumstances, and the almost complete absence of communicated sepsis is, indeed, surprising as well as satisfactory when one considers the very unclean habits of the majority of the people dealt with. In estimating the amount of good done by the prophylactic it must always be assumed that a dose had been given sufficient to insure a good reaction. The utmost importance of this is a matter of firm belief with the writer. The mere inoculation of a number of people exposed to plague with an uncertain small dose of prophylactic gives no criterion of its usefulness. It must be given in a dose that may be reasonably expected to protect against possible infection. The only test of this is the production of a distinct reaction with

a temperature of probably at least 102° F. in each individual inoculated. Stress is laid upon this owing to the small attention actually paid to it in the carrying out of the Punjab scheme. The systematic taking of temperatures was indeed recommended in the official instructions and strongly urged personally by M. Haffkine that it should be done in as large a percentage of cases as possible—10, 20, and 30 hours after inoculation—with a preference to the ten-hour record and the future dose modified accordingly. This is undoubtedly the right course and all the more important in that the prophylactic itself can be only imperfectly standardised, but in my experience at least it was found impossible to carry it out except in a very limited way. This was always a matter of regret, but it was not possible to do more than was done with the allotted staff owing in large part to the number of inoculations performed and to the distance that had to be covered daily.

The plan followed by me to obtain approximate results for future guidance was to get personal reports from each village as to the general state of the people after inoculation. This method, though scientifically useless, was practically of great value in aiding the determination of a dose satisfactory in its reaction but still not powerful enough to make the people afraid of coming forward. It should be recognised how very important it is to educate the people not only to accept inoculation, but also to be dissatisfied with it unless it produces a pronounced reaction. Though the first point is being surely gained—true, in the writer's experience at least—the second is scarcely understood at all. The people come for inoculation, but naturally, in their ignorance, are glad to escape with the minimum of discomfort. This being so, and so long as the individual dose remains uncertain, just so long will Haffkine's prophylactic fail to give the very great protection against plague which it undoubtedly does give under proper circumstances. With perseverance in inoculation and common-sense methods of disinfection and segregation properly and correctly carried out the disease in India would be stayed. The curiously spasmodic and half-hearted measures unfortunately so common can accomplish nothing and can only mean failure. Acknowledgment is due to Captain M. Corry, I.M.S., for access to his registers. In this way it was possible to obtain the plague figures in Table VI.

Albion-road, N.

SOME OBSERVATIONS ON OVER 6000 INOCULATIONS AGAINST PLAGUE.

BY J. W. MILLER, M.D. VICT., D.P.H. CANTAB.,
LATE PLAGUE MEDICAL OFFICER, PUNJAB, INDIA.

THE above inoculations were done in the Punjab during 1902 and 1903. Haffkine's prophylactic was used throughout and was supplied in bottles containing 30 cubic centimetres, the maximum dose being from 5 to 7·5 cubic centimetres. A 20 cubic centimetre syringe was used and this as well as the needles used were first sterilised by drawing up oil heated to a temperature of 160° F. into the syringe and leaving the heated oil in contact for a few minutes; the oil was heated by a spirit lamp and this method of sterilisation was found to be very useful as it was rapid and did not take as long as disinfection by boiling. The needles were left in a vessel containing the heated oil for a few minutes; a little of the prophylactic was drawn up into the syringe to wash the oil away before filling it.

The left arm was chosen for inoculation for the sake of convenience and as causing less pain and inconvenience afterwards to the person inoculated. The arm could easily be kept at rest and did not necessitate the patient being kept in the recumbent position, which would have been the case had inoculation been performed in the abdomen or the groin. In some cases inoculation was performed in other situations at the request of the person to be inoculated, a common site being in the situation of the knee, the hip-joint, and shoulder-joint, the idea being that rheumatism and other pains would be cured, and there is no doubt that the counter-irritation produced by the inoculation does in many cases relieve pain. Before inoculation the upper and outer parts of the arm were washed with soap-and-water. This was especially necessary, as a large number of individuals came straight from their work in the fields to be

periods of intense depression, phases of despair giving place to the elaboration of plans for a distant future, fits of hypochondria, relief from which is sought in intense application to work, a reckless indulgence in sensual pleasures and exaggerated idealism with a tendency to sentimentality and generalisation ; in other words, there is a well-marked intensification of cerebral function, the manifestations whereof are subject to the temperamental peculiarities of the individual. During the stage of invasion a certain tendency to refinement is noticeable, both physical and mental, and under its influence the artistic and imaginative faculties are often stimulated to unprecedented feats, doomed but too often to failure by abrupt collapse of physical energy.

The tendency to take a sanguine view of things becomes more marked as the disease advances. When a patient first learns that his lungs are affected he usually displays great anxiety and is depressed. The mental depression, however, gradually subsides until at the terminal period, in spite of overwhelming evidence that his days are numbered, the victim obstinately make plans or initiates enterprises incapable of achievement in the brief space of life that remains. Patients are buoyed up by a hope that knows no contradiction and display impatience or even anger when attempts are made to get them to realise the seriousness of their plight. This holds good of most cases of pulmonary phthisis, though of course it varies in degree according to the fundamental temperament of the subject and the degree of impairment of nutrition. This tendency to take a sanguine view of things manifests itself in other directions. Although their constitution is being slowly undermined the phthisical are often of exuberant spirits and prone to exertions far in excess of their physical powers. The reproductive function is peculiarly active and the fertility of tuberculous couples is almost proverbial. These subjects throw themselves into "life" with a zest which is often assumed to be the cause, instead of the result, of the tuberculous process. These features are specially well marked in cases characterised by a short, acute terminal period. Up to a certain point the exaggerated metabolism appears to provide the necessary supply of nervous energy until the final breakdown comes and the impoverished organism falls an unresisting prey to the tuberculous invasion.

Far more interesting are the changes that occur as the result of mechanical interference with the cerebral functions due to the presence of tuberculous deposits on the meninges or in the brain. I can best illustrate my meaning by relating two cases in the same family in which an initial localised pulmonary lesion was followed by a marked deterioration in the moral being of the victims.

CASE 1.—A lad, aged 15 years, whose father was healthy but whose mother was alcoholic, had an attack of pleurisy with effusion which kept him in bed for a month. Previously a highly intelligent, well-conducted youth, it was noted soon after the attack that he had become untruthful and in many respects untrustworthy—in fact, the perception of right and wrong seemed to have been blurred. He suffered from cough and lost weight considerably, but under suitable treatment he recovered to a certain extent. His mental condition, however, steadily became worse and he became morally irresponsible, though probably not to a degree that would be recognised by a court of law as exempting from punishment. He was ultimately sent to sea but in the course of his first voyage he developed tuberculous meningitis and returned home to die. Post-mortem examination revealed old-standing tuberculous lesions on the meninges and fresh foci at the base of the brain. The tuberculous nature of the pleurisy was evidenced by the spread of the process into the adjacent lung substance.

CASE 2.—The sister of the previous patient had an attack of what was diagnosed to be influenza followed by bronchopneumonia at the age of seven years. This ran a protracted course and after her recovery she began to manifest the same loss of moral tone, was untruthful, eccentric, and addicted to coarseness of language and behaviour. These changes coincided with the development of internal strabismus which was not improved when a moderate degree of hypermetropia was corrected by the use of spectacles. Formerly lively, playful, and fond of lessons, she became listless, indifferent, and would, if left undisturbed, remain motionless for hours immersed in a "brown study." Her intellectual powers were greatly impaired. She could not be taught to tell the time by the clock until she was 15 years

of age, and the simplest problems in arithmetic quite baffled her. At 16 she suffered for some months from goitre which attained such dimensions as to press upon the trachea causing stertor on slight exertion, but this subsided under appropriate treatment. In this case the conclusive proof of the tuberculous causation of the mental disturbance is wanting since she is still living and enjoys fairly good health, so far as the bodily functions are concerned.

Some time ago in an article by M. Camille Mauclair,[1] entitled "Watteau et la Phtisie," I found unexpected confirmation of my ideas on the subject. The author ascribes Watteau's transcendental delicacy of perception and execution to the exaltation begotten of tuberculous intoxication and he instances a number of great men whose death was due to pulmonary phthisis in whom the tuberculous infection seemed to have developed their faculties to a previously unattained brilliancy. He describes them as suffering from an intellectual affection which he calls "*la maladie de l'infini.*" It is seen, he says, in Schubert ; in Novellis, who died when only 29 years of age ; in Frederick Chopin, who died at 39 years of age ; in Verlaine, Henri Heine, Mozart, &c. Though he uses the term malady he is careful to explain that he does not wish it to be inferred that there was anything morbid in their achievements, the physiological influence of phthisis merely accentuating a natural predisposition to idealism. Dr. Mott tells me that melancholia is nearly always met with in insane patients suffering from tuberculosis and that the onset of the mental symptoms often appears to coincide with the development of the tubercle. It is noteworthy that general paralytics are very free from tubercle in contrast with imbeciles, idiots, and the subjects of primary dementia of adolescence who are particularly prone thereto. I am conscious that my contribution can have but a limited value if for no other reason than my inability to adduce sufficient anatomical evidence of the co-relation of meningeal and cerebral tubercle with mental deterioration. The subject, however, is one of considerable interest.

Mustapha Supérieur, Algiers.

Clinical Notes:
MEDICAL, SURGICAL, OBSTETRICAL AND THERAPEUTICAL.

A PRACTICAL EXPERIENCE WITH ADRENALIN AS A CARDIAC AND VASO-MOTOR STIMULANT.

BY H. O. BUTLER, M.B. CANTAB.

THE use of adrenalin as a local vaso-motor constrictor is well enough known but I do not think that its general action on the circulatory mechanism is sufficiently recognised. That this action in suitable cases may be of the utmost practical value the following case will show.

The patient, a child aged ten years, was taken ill with measles on Jan. 2nd. She was attended by a most competent nurse and beyond diagnosing the affection I paid no visits. On the 14th without having left her bed the patient contracted pneumonia. The general course of the disease was of interest from three points : (1) the only physical signs during the whole duration were a few crepitations at the left base, a slight accentuation of the stomach sounds, and for two days a small pleuritic rub—a central left-sided and basal pneumonia obviously accounting for this ; (2) the high range of temperature, this remaining steadily between 106° and 107° F. except when lowered by sponging and ice packs ; and (3) the toxæmic and not local character of the disease. The treatment was symptomatic throughout. The crisis occurred on the seventh day and stimulants were indicated and freely given. 24 hours later I was called and was told that the temperature was 96·8°, the pulse was 60, the colour was bad, and the respirations were inclined to be of Cheyne Stokes type. The child looked when I saw her as if her temperature were decidedly raised, the face being very flushed, but the pulse was of extremely low tension. This appeared to be due to exhaustion of the vaso-motor controlling centre. Stimulants and strychnine, hypodermically as

[1] Revue Bleue, August, 1904.

well as by the mouth, were pushed, but as the tension steadily became less I infused one pint of normal saline solution subcutaneously. The pulse improved promptly but fell back again in a quarter of an hour. Five pints of the solution were then slowly infused, two hours being taken altogether, but the general condition became steadily worse. At 3 P.M. the pulse was 50, the vessel walls were completely relaxed, and the child was to all appearance dying rapidly. In desperation I thought of the theoretical effect of adrenalin and injected 15 minims. By this time the pulse was imperceptible and the child, I thought, at the point of death. The immediate effect of the injection was that the child to all appearance died, but in about five minutes a nurse came to tell me that the child had spoken and that the pulse had improved wonderfully. The change I noticed was extraordinary ; the child's face was flushed, her pulse was 100 and of good tension, and she was talking about ordinary affairs. In about 15 minutes the pulse weakened again and 10 minims were given by the mouth and in another quarter of an hour eight minims hypodermically. The pulse for the next five hours remained of fair tension and strychnine and stimulants were pushed to the utmost. Signs of the pulse weakening again appearing, three injections of five minims of adrenalin were given at two-hour intervals as the condition of the pulse demanded. Each time, however, it was noticed what was most apparent after the initial large injection—namely, that the immediate effect was an increase of pallor and a weakening of the pulse, followed by great and rapid improvement. This with each injection becoming more apparent, five minims by the mouth were substituted for the injection, but was only once necessary. All this time the child was in a perfect bath of perspiration, due, I suppose, to the large amount of fluid injected *plus* the return of vaso-motor tone. Convalescence from this point was uninterrupted except that a post-critical rise in temperature to 103° occurred.

No words of mine can express the absolutely marvellous nature of the change in the child's condition due to the drug, and I trust that this note may be the means of calling the usefulness of adrenalin in suitable cases to the attention of others. Probably if it had been infused with the normal saline solution the result would have been still better. The preparation I used was Messrs. Parke, Davis, and Co.'s 1 in 1000 solution.

Chiswick.

A CASE OF MARKED INTOLERANCE OF BELLADONNA.

BY T. R. WEBSTER ATKINS, L.R.C.P., L.R.C.S. EDIN., L.F.P.S. GLASG.

THE following case is remarkable as showing a very marked idiosyncrasy with respect to belladonna. The patient, who was a nurse suffering from cellulitis of the leg unattended with any abrasion of the skin, was ordered an application of "glycerine and belladonna." 40 minims of this mixture, that is approximately 20 grains of extract of belladonna, were applied to the inner side of the foot. Within half an hour the patient complained of great swelling of the leg and a sensation as if the skin would burst. Dryness of the throat and lips, a feeling as if the nipples were being forcibly retracted, and difficulty of speech quickly followed. The patient now became delirious, the pupils were widely dilated and insensible to light, the hands were kept in perpetual motion groping for imaginary objects, and efforts were made to tear the bedclothes. This delirium lasted for some hours, after which she gradually became more composed but felt as if she had passed through a severe illness. In 48 hours the dryness of the throat and the pain in the breasts had disappeared, though the pupils remained dilated and only resumed their normal condition on the fourth day. The treatment consisted in the administration of hot coffee and a quarter of a grain of morphine, together with the use of continuous hot applications.

Shepherd's Bush-road, W.

A CASE OF INTUSSUSCEPTION IN AN INFANT.

BY BERTRAM ADDENBROOKE, M.D. DURH.

THE following case seems to be worth recording on account of the rarity of the recovery of an infant of six months after extensive intussusception which was relieved by abdominal section. The history of the case is shortly as follows. The child was taken suddenly ill about 8 A.M. on Jan. 11th last with convulsions and vomiting. The medical man who was called in ordered the usual hot bath and castor oil, and saw the child again the following morning. By that time the convulsions had ceased, but as the child was obviously worse and per rectum a mass could be felt he was immediately sent into the Kidderminster Infirmary under my care for operation. Having to come from some distance in the country I could not operate till 8.30 P.M., about 36 hours after the probable commencement of the intussusception. After abdominal section, with the aid of an assistant's finger in the rectum, I was enabled to reduce the bowel and found the foremost part of the intussuscipiens to be the ileo-cæcal valve with the vermiform appendix ; the whole operation from the commencement of the anæsthetic to the finish took 25 minutes ; the child was very collapsed and ill for the next few days, though he had a good motion within 14 hours of the operation and I believe that a great help towards his recovery were the night and morning injections of $\frac{1}{200}$th of a grain of digitalin combined with $\frac{1}{120}$th of a grain of strychnine. The child returned home a month after the operation quite well and with the wound soundly healed.

Kidderminster.

THE OPERATION OF APPENDICOSTOMY.

BY H. M. W. GRAY, M.B. ABERD., F.R.C.S. EDIN., SURGEON TO THE ABERDEEN ROYAL INFIRMARY.

WITH reference to the recent communications on appendicostomy it may be interesting to place on record two cases which were operated on by me about 20 months ago (in the summer of 1904).

CASE 1.—The patient was a man, aged 30 years, with ulcerative colitis causing profuse bloody and mucous stools. He had never been abroad. The disease had resisted all treatment by the mouth and rectum and as the patient was evidently in a desperate condition I performed appendicostomy and washed out the colon through the opening—as described first by Weir—with various antiseptic and astringent lotions. He improved markedly for three weeks but then went downhill and died a week later. Post mortem there was found advanced ulceration of the colon and lower part of the ileum. This case was Mr. J. Marnoch's and came under my care as Mr. Marnoch was off duty for the time being.

CASE 2.—The patient was a young woman, aged 22 years, who discharged extensive casts of the colon and had frequent calls to stool. The condition was more annoying than detrimental to her health, but was quite sufficient to make her welcome any prospect of relief by operation, as it had resisted all other forms of treatment. Appendicostomy was performed and a weak solution of argyrol was used to flush out the colon. In three weeks cure had apparently resulted and the stump of the appendix was allowed to close, which it did very readily. Recently there has been a tendency of the colitis to relapse. If this becomes serious or is persistent I have advised her medical attendant to open the stump of the appendix (now level with the skin) and to wash out the bowel as before.

Aberdeen.

AUTOMOBILE EXHIBITION.—The eleventh annual International Automobile Exhibition will be held at the Royal Agricultural Hall, London, from March 24th to 31st. The latest types of British as well as Continental cars will be on view and prominence will be given to Italian cars and to some cars at popular prices. Further information in reference to the exhibition can be obtained from Messrs. Cordingley and Co., 27 to 33, Charing Cross-road, W.C.

TAUNTON ISOLATION HOSPITAL.—At the meeting of the Taunton town council held on Feb. 13th the subject of the joint management of the isolation hospital by the town council and the rural council was again discussed. The matter has been already alluded to in THE LANCET. Eventually it was decided, as a means of putting an end to the present deadlock, to advertise for a medical attendant for the institution. Dr. H. J. Alford, the medical officer of health, was in entire agreement with this decision.

THE LANCET, May 19, 1906.

Three Lectures

ON

THE PRESERVATION OF HEALTH AMONGST THE PERSONNEL OF THE JAPANESE NAVY AND ARMY.

Delivered at St. Thomas's Hospital, London, on May 7th 9th, and 11th, 1906,

By BARON TAKAKI, F.R.C.S. Eng., D.C.L.,

LATE DIRECTOR-GENERAL OF THE MEDICAL DEPARTMENT OF THE IMPERIAL JAPANESE NAVY.

LECTURE I.

Delivered on May 7th.

Mr. Treasurer and Gentlemen,—I am here to-day owing to an invitation from the staff of St. Thomas's Hospital and Medical College. I feel that it is a great honour to me personally and also a great compliment paid to the medical profession of the Japanese empire, and I thank you all on their behalf for your cordial and friendly feeling towards us.

I think some of you are already aware that I was invited by Cartwright's Lecture Committee of the Alumni Association of the College of Physicians and Surgeons of Columbia University of New York to deliver the Cartwright lecture and I chose the Sanitation of the Japanese Navy and Army as the subject of my lecture. At that time I had no idea and never thought that I should be asked to speak before such a large and distinguished assembly as is present here to-day. But when I was in America I was requested by the staffs of this hospital and St. Thomas's Medical College to tell them some of my experiences and I could not resist accepting such an honour from this hospital, with which I may claim very close relation, in so much as I am one of the graduates of this ancient institution and have worked under this roof as house officer. The subject of my address here is the same as in the Cartwright lecture, the reason being that on this subject I may claim to having had some practical experience and knowledge on account of my long service in the navy.

number of sailors lost through death and made invalid owing to general diseases was 24·09 per 1000 and those lost through death and invaliding from beri-beri 10·43 per 1000. If we now subtract 10·43 from 24·09 only 13·66 remain. Therefore it was clear that if beri-beri could be wholly exterminated the number of losses from illness would decrease to 13·66.

From 1881 to 1883 the number of cases of illness slightly decreased. In 1884 the general aspect of the health of the navy suddenly changed for the better and the number of general diseases as well as cases of beri-beri markedly decreased. The number of general diseases was 1865·02 per 1000—that is, one person became ill 1·8 times a year. Deaths per 1000 decreased to 7·98 and invalids to 7·80. The number of beri-beri cases averaged 127·35 per 1000. Deaths from it decreased to 1·42. Therefore, the average of deaths and invalids from general diseases decreased to 15·78 and that of beri-beri to 1·60 per 1000. Similarly in 1885 the number of general diseases decreased to 992·48 per 1000 and deaths to 7·08 per 1000. Beri-beri decreased to 5·93 per 1000 without death. So the number of deaths and invalids decreased to 12·14. In 1886 general diseases per 1000 averaged 577·46, deaths 7·43, and beri-beri 0·35, without death or invaliding. In 1887 general diseases per 1000 were 434·22, deaths 6·04, and invalids 6·15. In 1888 general diseases per 1000 averaged 400·59, deaths 7·08, and invalids 9·15. In short, the number of losses through deaths and invalids per 1000 in 1884 was 15·78, in 1885 12·14, in 1886 12·57, in 1887 12·19, and in 1888 16·33. If we now compare these five years with three years from 1878 to 1880 we find a marked decrease of general diseases and disappearance of beri-beri with corresponding decrease in the loss of sailors year by year. These good results must depend upon certain causes and in order to explain them I will first of all try to describe various important facts since the establishment of the Naval Medical Bureau in 1872.

The Establishment of the Naval Medical Bureau.

The Naval Medical Bureau of the Japanese Empire was established for the first time in 1872. At that time there was no one who had a thorough idea of naval hygiene because up to that time there was no special sanitary work carried out by medical officers in our navy, and other officers thought that the necessity of medical men in the Navy was simply for treating diseases and wounded. Even the medical officers thought in the same way. They never had the

TABLE I.—SHOWING THE GENERAL HEALTH OF THE NAVY.

Year.	Strength.	All diseases and injuries.								Cases of kak'ke or beri-beri.					
		Cases of disease or injury.	Ratio of cases per 1000 of strength.	Average ratio of cases per person per annum.	Died.	Ratio of deaths per 1000 of strength.	Invalided.	Ratio of invalided per 1000 of strength.	Cases of kak'ke.	Ratio of cases of kak'ke per 1000 of strength.	Died.	Ratio of deaths per 1000 of strength.	Invalided.	Ratio of invalided per 1000 of strength.
1878	4528	17,788	3928·45	3·93	56	12·37	44	9·72	1485	327·96	32	7·07	19	4·20
1879	5031	22,426	4413·70	4·41	119	23·42	39	7·68	1978	389·29	57	11·20	8	1·57
1880	4956	22,819	4604·32	4·60	63	12·71	43	8·68	1725	348·06	27	5·45	9	1·82
1881	4641	15,766	3397·12	3·40	81	17·45	29	6·25	1163	250·59	30	6·46	16	3·45
1882	4769	12,074	2531·77	2·53	103	21·60	30	6·29	1929	404·49	51	10·69	17	3·56
1883	5346	16,380	3063·97	2·90	85	15·90	28	5·24	1236	251·20	49	9·17	4	0·75
1884	5638	10,515	1865·02	1·81	45	7·98	44	7·80	718	127·35	8	1·42	1	0·18
1885	6918	6,866	992·48	0·91	49	7·08	33	4·77	41	5·93	—	—	1	0·14
1886	8475	4,874	577·46	0·52	63	7·43	52	6·14	3	0·35	—	—	—	—
1887	9016	3,954	434·22	0·40	55	6·04	56	6·15	—	—	—	—	—	—
1888	9184	3,679	400·59	0·40	65	7·08	48	9·15	—	—	—	—	—	—

Here I have Table I. showing various details from 1878–1888 and I am now going to explain all the details. From 1888 to the present day there have been no important changes. In looking over this table we find the average number of general diseases during 1878, 1879, and 1880 to be just over 4327 per 1000—that is, one sailor suffered 4·32 times every year. The death-rate averaged 16·34 per 1000 and the invaliding-rate 8·75. The number of beri-beri (kak'ke) patients was 349·33 per 1000. Those who died from it averaged 7·96 and those invalided 2·45. Therefore, the

slightest idea of doing anything in preventing disease or in general hygiene. Accordingly, the only medical record left from 1872 to 1877 was limited to the description of results of treatment, name of diseases, and names of patients taken into hospitals. Between 1878 and 1883 the record gradually began to include facts about hospital and non-hospital patients and some hygienic affairs. Finally, from 1884 the records became more and more complete, giving various tables illustrating hygienic conditions by the issue of instructions relating to the duties of the medical officers.

THE LANCET, May 26, 1906.

The Nobel Lecture

ON

HOW THE FIGHT AGAINST TUBERCULOSIS NOW STANDS.[1]

By Professor ROBERT KOCH.

Only 20 years ago tuberculosis, even in its most dangerous form, pulmonary phthisis, was not considered infectious. By the labours of Villemin and the experimental investigations of Cohnheim and Salomonsen, indeed, certain proofs had already been given that this view was erroneous. But it was not till the tubercle bacillus was discovered that the etiology of tuberculosis was placed on a sure foundation and the conviction gained that it is not only a parasitic —i.e., an infectious—but also an avoidable disease. Even in my first publications on the etiology of tuberculosis I pointed to the dangers which arise from the dissemination of the secretions of those suffering from pulmonary phthisis containing bacilli and called for prophylactic measures against the pestilence. But my words were not attended to. The reason was that it was still too early and they therefore could not yet meet with full understanding. On this, as on so many similar occasions in the history of medicine, it happened that a long time had to elapse before old prejudices were overcome and the new facts recognised by medical men as correct. But then the recognition of the infectious nature of tuberculosis gradually spread and struck ever deeper root, and the more the conviction of the dangerous nature of tuberculosis made its way the more the necessity for protection against it forced itself upon mankind. The efforts made in this direction first made themselves noticeable in instructive and warning publications. Soon after arose sanatoriums for consumptives suggested by the success of Brehmer's dietetic and hygienic treatment of pulmonary diseases, and these sanatoriums were followed by convalescent homes, seaside homes, dispensaries, and similar institutions. A vast activity on the part of societies developed. International congresses were held. Notification, optional or obligatory, was introduced here and there. In many states and cities completely elaborated laws against the danger of tuberculosis were enacted. I suppose there is hardly any country now in which the conflict against tuberculosis has not been begun in one way or another, and it is exceedingly satisfactory to see how universally and how energetically the dangerous enemy is now being attacked. But, on the whole, all these efforts have borne a decidedly unequal character ; the goal, indeed, was the same for all, but they chose quite different ways to it. In one country all was to be attained by instruction, in another it was hoped that tuberculosis could be got rid of by therapeutic measures, and in a third efforts were directed almost exclusively against the dangers with which bovine tuberculosis is said to threaten us. Quite lately, it is true, a certain equalisation has set in, inasmuch as the several countries no longer proceed quite so independently as before, and the one adopts from the other those means of conflict which seem to have stood the test of experience. Considering, however, how great a variety still exists in the ways in which tuberculosis is combated, it is nevertheless necessary to inquire what measures are most consonant with the demands of science and with the general experience that has been gained in the combating of pestilences.

Before addressing ourselves, however, to the answering of this question we must attain to absolute clearness as to the manner in which infection in tuberculosis takes place— i.e., as to how the tubercle bacilli get into the human organism, for the sole purpose of all prophylactic measures against a pestilence must be to prevent the entrance of the germs of disease into man. Now, as regards infection with tuberculosis only two possibilities have hitherto presented themselves—namely, infection by tubercle bacilli emanating from tuberculous human beings and infection by tubercle bacilli contained in the flesh and milk of tuberculous cattle. After the investigations which I have made hand-in-hand with Schütz as to the relation between human and bovine tuberculosis we may dismiss this second possibility, or at least regard it as so slight that this source of infection as compared with the other falls quite into the background. We arrived, namely, at the result that human tuberculosis and bovine tuberculosis are different from one another and that bovine tuberculosis is not transmissible to man. With reference to this latter point, however, I wish, in order to prevent misunderstandings, to add that in saying this I mean only those forms of tuberculosis that have to be taken into account in connexion with the combating of tuberculosis as an epidemic disease—namely, generalised tuberculosis and above all pulmonary phthisis. It would lead us too far if I were to go deeper into the very lively discussion this question has given rise to ; I must reserve this for another occasion. On this head I wish only to add that the testing of our investigations which has been carried out with the utmost care and on a broad basis in the Imperial Office of Health in Berlin has led to a confirmation of my opinion, and that, moreover, the harmlessness of the bacilli of bovine tuberculosis to man has been directly proved by the repeated inoculating of human beings with the material of bovine tuberculosis by Spengler and Klemperer. In connexion with the combating of tuberculosis, then, only the tubercle bacilli emanating from human beings have to be taken into account.

But now the disease does not in all cases assume such forms that tubercle bacilli are expelled in a manner deserving of attention. Strictly speaking, it is only those who suffer from laryngeal and pulmonary tuberculosis that produce considerable quantities of tubercle bacilli and disseminate them in a dangerous manner. At the same time, however, attention must be paid to the fact that it is not only the secretion of the lungs called sputum that is dangerous as containing bacilli, but that according to Flügge's investigations the minutest droplets of phlegm that are flung into the air by the patients when they cough and clear their throats and even when they speak also contain bacilli and can thereby cause infection. We therefore arrive at the quite sharply defined limitation that only those tuberculous patients who suffer from laryngeal or pulmonary tuberculosis and whose sputa contain bacilli are dangerous to those around them in a noteworthy degree. This form of tuberculosis is called "open" in contrast to the "closed" form, in which no tubercle bacilli are given off to those around. But among patients with open tuberculosis also distinctions are to be made as regards the degree of dangerousness to be ascribed to them. It is matter of common observation that such patients live for years in their families without infecting anyone. In hospitals for pulmonary phthisis it is in certain circumstances possible that no cases of infection occur among the attendants, or at any rate so few that in former times it was thought necessary to regard this as a proof of the non-contagiousness of tuberculosis. But if one examines such cases more carefully it is found that there are good reasons for the apparent non-contagiousness. It then appears that the patients in question are people who are very cautious about their sputum, see to the cleanliness of their dwellings and clothing, and live in copiously aired and lighted rooms, so that the germs that get into the air can be swiftly swept away by the current or killed by the light. If these conditions are not fulfilled there is no lack of infection even in hospitals and the dwellings of the well-to-do, as experience teaches daily. And it becomes the more frequent the more uncleanly the patients are as regards their sputum, the more lack there is of light and air, and the more closely crowded together the sick live with the hale. The danger of infection becomes especially great when healthy people have to sleep in the same rooms with sick people and even, as unfortunately still frequently happens among the poor, in the same bed. This kind of infection has struck attentive observers as so important that tuberculosis has been frankly and justly called a dwelling disease.

To recapitulate briefly, the essential facts regarding infection in tuberculosis are these. Patients with closed tuberculosis are to be regarded as quite harmless. Even those who suffer from open tuberculosis are harmless so long as the tubercle bacilli expelled by them are prevented by cleanliness, airing, &c., from infecting. The patient becomes dangerous only when he is personally uncleanly or becomes so helpless in consequence of the far-advanced disease that

[1] This lecture was delivered at Stockholm on Dec. 12th, 1905, but is now published for the first time in English.

No. 4317.

he can no longer see to the suitable removal of the sputa. For the healthy the danger of infection increases with the impossibility of avoiding the immediate neighbourhood of a dangerous patient—i.e., in densely inhabited rooms, and quite specially if the latter are not only overcrowded but also badly ventilated and inadequately lighted.

I now address myself to the task of testing the measures now in force as to the degree in which they take the etiological facts just stated into account. If, in doing this, I confine myself mainly to German circumstances the reason is that they are best known to me and that it would not be practicable to go into the circumstances of other countries in a single lecture.

The starting-point for the combating of all pestilences is *notification*, because without it most cases of disease would remain unknown. So we must demand it for tuberculosis too. But in the case of this disease the competent parties have, out of consideration for the patients, scrupled to prescribe notification to the medical men or those on whom the obligation lies in other cases. Justly recognising, however, that not only consideration for the sick but also protection for the healthy is in question here, the authorities have in not a few places introduced notification, first optional, and then, when it was found that the dreaded disadvantages did not occur, obligatory. As, therefore, experience has already proved the practicability of notification in the case of tuberculosis it ought to be introduced everywhere. Its purpose, however, can be fully attained if it is limited to cases that are dangerous to those around the patients—i.e., to patients with open tuberculosis under hygienically unfavourable circumstances. If we make notification obligatory on medical men we must at the same time take care that they are able to judge of the cases in question correctly, especially as regards the existence of open tuberculosis. This can be done only by establishing institutions in which the sputum of the patients is examined for tubercle bacilli gratis. They may be independent or, better perhaps, in connexion with hospitals, ambulatory clinics, or the care-stations which I shall mention later. Such establishments for the examination of sputum already exist in some countries but their number is far too small. This necessity will have to be adequately provided for. But now, once they are known, what is to be done with the patients who are to be regarded as dangerous? If it were possible to lodge them all in hospitals and thus to render them comparatively harmless tuberculosis would diminish very rapidly. But for the present, at least, this is absolutely out of the question. The number of tuberculous patients in Germany, for instance, for whom hospital treatment would be requisite is reckoned at more than 200,000. It would require more means than can be got to lodge such a number of patients in hospitals. But it is also not at all necessary to lodge all tuberculous patients at once in hospitals. We may count upon a decrease of tuberculosis, though a slower one, if a considerable fraction of these patients are admitted to suitable establishments. Let me remind you, in this connexion, of the exceedingly instructive example of the combating of leprosy in Norway. There, too, they have not isolated all the lepers but only a fraction of them, including, however, just the most dangerous, and the result has been that the number of the lepers, which in 1856 still amounted to nearly 3000, has now gone down to about 500. This is the example to be followed in the combating of tuberculosis and if all cases of pulmonary phthisis cannot be provided for, at least as many as possible, including the most dangerous—i.e., those in the last stage of the disease—ought to be lodged in hospitals.

In this respect, however, more is already done in many places than is generally supposed. In Berlin during the last decade more than 40 per cent. of the cases of pulmonary phthisis died in hospitals. In Stockholm, too, the state of affairs must be very favourable in this respect, for Carlsson states in his publication on the combating of tuberculosis in Sweden that 410 cases of pulmonary phthisis are being cared for in the hospitals of this city, no small number for a city of 300,000 inhabitants. The number of patients that are thus placed in circumstances under which they can no longer infect is very considerable and cannot fail to influence the course of the pestilence. In connexion with this I wish to draw your attention to a phenomenon which deserves the greatest consideration—I mean the equable and very considerable decrease of the consumption death-rate in some countries. In England this decrease has been going on for about 40 years. Strange to say, it is less in Scotland, and in Ireland there is no decrease at all. In Prussia the decrease of tuberculosis is very marked. During the ten years from 1876 to 1886 the pulmonary phthisis death-rate still stood equally high. Since 1886, however, it has fallen from year to year and the decrease is now more than 30 per cent.—i.e., about one-third. It has been calculated that, though the population has meanwhile increased, the number of people who die every year from pulmonary phthisis in Prussia is now about 20,000 less than it was 20 years ago. In other countries, Austria and Hungary, for instance, the pulmonary phthisis death-rate has remained at the former very considerable height. It is hard to give reasons for this singular behaviour of tuberculosis in the said countries. Probably several factors have coöperated. The improvement of the situation of the lower classes and the better knowledge of the danger of infection, the consequence of which is that people no longer unwittingly expose themselves to it, have certainly helped to reduce tuberculosis. But I am firmly convinced that the better provision for patients in the last stage of pulmonary phthisis—namely, the lodging of them in hospitals, which is done in England and in Prussia to a comparatively large extent—has contributed most to the improvement. I am specially confirmed in this opinion by the behaviour of tuberculosis in Stockholm where, as already mentioned, comparatively many cases of phthisis are tended in hospitals and where also in the course of the last decades the death-rate from phthisis has gone down 38 per cent. From this, however, we are to derive the lesson that the greatest stress is to be laid on this measure—namely, *the placing of cases of pulmonary phthisis in suitable establishments*, and far more care should be taken than hitherto that such patients do not die in their dwellings, where, moreover, they are for the most part in a helpless situation and inadequately nursed. If cases of pulmonary phthisis are no longer, as hitherto, rejected by the hospitals as incurable; if, on the contrary, we offer them the best imaginable nursing gratis and can even in some cases hold forth the hope of cure; if, moreover, their families are cared for during their illness, not the slightest compulsion will be necessary to induce a still much greater number of these unfortunate patients to go to hospitals than at present.

I now pass to the discussion of a measure the purpose of which is to combat tuberculosis in quite a different way—I mean the sanatoriums. They were founded in the expectation that in them a large number, perhaps even the majority, of tuberculous patients might be cured. If this supposition were correct sanatoriums would decidedly be among the best weapons in the battle against tuberculosis. But the results obtained by the sanatoriums have been the theme of much debate. Some people maintained that they cured up to 70 per cent. of their patients: others that they did no good at all. Now it must be admitted that the figure "70 per cent." has reference not to real cures but only to cases in which patients had been enabled once more to earn a livelihood. From the prophylactic standpoint, however, that is no gain, for a patient who is not perfectly cured but only so far bettered that he can earn again for awhile, afterwards falls into the condition of open tuberculosis and suffers all the consequences already described. The reason of the comparative fewness of the real cures effected in sanatoriums evidently is that the duration of the treatment in them is much too short and that very many of the patients they receive are in so far advanced a stage that the dietetic and hygienic treatment no longer suffices. Many sanatorium medical officers have already recognised this. They therefore take care that only patients who are in an early stage of tuberculosis are received, and besides the sanatorium treatment they apply the preparation of tuberculin in order to effect more rapid, and especially more lasting, cures. In this way considerably better results than formerly have already been obtained in several sanatoriums and it is probable that, if the sanatoriums adopt this course and hold to it, they will do quite essential service in the combating of tuberculosis, at least in Germany, where in more than a hundred sanatoriums about 30,000 patients are already treated every year.

If thus provision is made for as great a number of patients in an advanced stage of phthisis as possible by their admission to hospitals and for first-stage patients by the sanatoriums, a great number of patients still remain whom also it is absolutely necessary to take into account. These are the advanced-stage patients who remain in their dwellings and those who are already too far gone for the sanatorium treatment but not yet so far that they are unfit for work and must go to a hospital. Should these tuberculous patients, whose number, as already said, is very considerable, be left to their fate, a great gap would be made thereby in the line of battle. The merit of having filled this gap belongs to Calmette, to whom occurred the happy idea of providing for this class of patients by the *dispensaries* organised by him. Calmette's suggestion has met with approval everywhere, especially in Germany, where more than 50 such dispensaries already exist and where many cities are about to provide themselves with such. It was in Germany, too, that the dispensaries, which were originally intended only to give working people gratuitous advice, medicinal treatment, and at the same time material support, were widened and completed in an important manner under the guidance of Pütter and Kayserling. In their present form they are intended to serve not one particular class only but all helpless tuberculous patients in every way. The patient is visited in his dwelling and instruction and advice as to cleanliness and the treatment of the sputum are given to him and his family. If the domiciliary conditions are bad, money is granted in order to render the separation of the patient from the healthy members of his family possible and thus to convert a dangerous patient into a comparatively harmless one by hiring a suitable room or even another dwelling. In other respects also poor families are supported by gifts of suitable provisions, fuel, &c. The dispensary itself does not undertake the treatment of the patients, in order not to get into conflict with practitioners, but it takes care that they are placed under medical treatment and, if advisable, admitted to a hospital, a sanatorium, or a health-recruiting home. One specially important part of their work is that they supervise the family, and especially the children, and have them examined from time to time to see whether infection has taken place in order to be able to bring help as early as possible. In this way these dispensaries really take care of poor consumptives and they have therefore with perfect justice been named " care-stations." I regard them as one of the most powerful means of combating tuberculosis, if not the most powerful of all, and I believe that when, as we may hope, a dense net of care-stations overspreads the land they are destined to do a most blessed work.

The measures hitherto discussed—namely, notification, hospitals, sanatoriums, and care-stations, are the heavy artillery in the battle against tuberculosis. But there are lighter weapons, too, which cannot themselves exercise so incisive an effect, but the coöperative help of which we cannot dispense with. Among these I reckon in the first place all efforts to *instruct the people as to the danger of tuberculosis* and to keep the interest of the masses in the combating of tuberculosis awake by popular publications, lectures, exhibitions, and other such means. Later, when there are care-stations enough, the said instruction will emanate from them so copiously that we shall hardly need special arrangements for that any more, but for the present we cannot dispense with them. Very valuable help is also given by the numerous associations which take part in the combating of tuberculosis by collecting money in order to found sanatoriums and health recruiting homes, endow free beds, support the families of poor phthisical patients, &c. We must not shut our eyes to the fact that the combating of tuberculosis demands a great deal of money. It is at bottom only a money question. The more free beds are endowed for cases of pulmonary phthisis in well organised and conducted establishments for the cure and care of the sick, the more adequately the families of tuberculous patients are supported, so that the latter may not be deterred from going to such establishments by anxiety on behalf of those belonging to them, and the more care-stations are established, the more rapidly will tuberculosis as an epidemic disease decrease. As, however, it is hardly to be expected that the municipalities, many of which already make very large sacrifices for the tuberculous patients, will be able in the immediate future to do justice to all requirements in this respect, private help is greatly to be desired. Care must be taken, however, that the means collected by the associations or placed at disposal by individual benefactors be not applied to minor matters, but accrue to the benefit of the most effective measures, above

all the establishments for the accommodation of the sick and the care-stations.

In the conflict against tuberculosis hardly anything remains for the State to do, and yet it, too, can take an effective part in it. It can by legislation introduce *obligatory notification*, which already exists for all other important epidemic diseases, for tuberculosis too. In several States this has already been done, and it is to be hoped that the other civilised States will soon follow this example. Many demand also a legal basis for the compulsory isolation of patients who are a special source of danger to those around them. My experience in the combating of pestilences, however, teaches that we can dispense with this hard measure. If only we as far as possible facilitate the admission of consumptives to suitable establishments for the sick in the manner already indicated, we shall attain all we need. In one respect, however, the State can render aid of extraordinary utility with a view, namely, to *bettering the unfavourable domiciliary conditions*. Against this evil private activity is almost powerless, whereas the State can easily provide a remedy by suitable laws. If we look back on what has been done in the last few years in the combating of tuberculosis as an epidemic disease we cannot but get the impression that a truly important beginning has been made. The fight against tuberculosis was not dictated from above and has not always developed in accordance with the rules of science. No ; it emanated from the people itself who have rightly recognised its deadly enemy at last. It is pressing forward with elementary force, sometimes in a rather wild and disorderly manner but gradually striking more and more into the right paths. The fight is kindled all along the line and the enthusiasm for the lofty purpose is so general that flagging is not to be feared. If it goes on in this vigorous style victory is sure.

Three Lectures

ON

THE PRESERVATION OF HEALTH AMONGST THE PERSONNEL OF THE JAPANESE NAVY AND ARMY.

Delivered at St. Thomas's Hospital, London, on May 7th, 9th, and 11th, 1906,

By BARON TAKAKI, F.R.C.S. ENG., D.C.L.,

LATE DIRECTOR-GENERAL OF THE MEDICAL DEPARTMENT OF THE IMPERIAL JAPANESE NAVY.

LECTURE II.[1]

Delivered on May 9th.

MR. PRESIDENT AND GENTLEMEN,—On Nov. 29th, 1883, I had the honour of being presented to his Imperial Majesty at Akasaka Palace, and on this occasion explained my views as regards the cause of, and preventive measures for, beri-beri.

THE METHODS FOR INVESTIGATING THE CAUSE OF BERI-BERI.

1. As we could not discover the true origin of beri-beri in spite of examination of symptoms, pathology, &c., we must use some other means. 2. In order to examine the food necessary for nourishing the human body it is important to know the comparative scale of nutritive elements—that is, proteids, fat, carbohydrates and salts, and of carbon and nitrogen. 3. On examining the food taken by those suffering from beri-beri it is found that the proportion of these elements is not correct. 4. The causes of this disease are due to the loss of equilibrium in the proportion of nutritive elements and also to the deficiency of a certain element—that is, the composition of food is not correct. 5. The occurrence of beri-beri due to the deficiency of a certain element—that is, proteids—is shown in the examples of the long voyages of the *Asama, Tsukuba, Ryujo,* &c. The disease does not occur if the food is well supplied ; for example, it does not occur among men having a sufficient

---

[1] Lecture I. was published in THE LANCET of May 19th, 1906, p. 1369

THE LANCET, August 11, 1906.

A Clinical Lecture

ON

THE HANDS OF SURGEONS AND ASSISTANTS IN OPERATIONS.

Delivered at University College Hospital,

By ARTHUR E. J. BARKER, F.R.C.S. Eng.,

SURGEON TO THE HOSPITAL, ETC.

GENTLEMEN,—We have now arrived at an era in which we may claim to know a good deal about septic processes. We also know something at least about the life-history of most of the organisms upon which these processes depend, thanks to the patient labours of countless bacteriologists. It is also now pretty well understood how the various septic fungi may be destroyed by heat or chemical agents. But it is only comparatively recently that the several avenues by which the dreaded microbes gain access to the living tissues have been more or less clearly recognised and their relative dangers apportioned. And only more recently still has this knowledge led to fairly practical efforts —first, towards the reduction in their numbers in all localities where operations are undertaken, and, secondly, to their exclusion from the field of operation during the procedure itself. But notwithstanding this advance much remains to be done in the direction of utilising the knowledge gained.

The avenues of infection may be thus summarised. 1. Access to injured surfaces from within the patient's own body—e.g., lungs, alimentary and genito-urinary tract. 2. Access to injured surfaces from without. Under this last heading, with which we are alone concerned to-day, the possible sources of infection of a recent wound are : (*a*) the surrounding air and solids ; (*b*) the object which has made the wound ; (*c*) the instruments employed in treatment; (*d*) the ligatures, swabs, and dressings employed and the clothing of operator and assistant which may come in contact with the wound ; (*e*) the patient's own skin and hair; and (*f*) the surgeon's and assistants' hands.

Now these half-dozen possible avenues of infection are not all of the same importance. This has been proved by a long series of original bacteriological investigations of the most laborious and ingenious nature ; and if I were to give you the mere titles of only those of them which I have myself carefully studied the list might be so long as to discourage some of you. But the following conclusions may be drawn from all this work—theoretical, experimental, and practical.

(*a*) First, that the air of most rooms devoted to surgical operations, if the usual precautions as to general cleanliness are adopted and if they are not too crowded and if rapid currents of air are avoided, is not such a danger to open wounds as was formerly supposed in the days of the carbolic spray. This is not to say that the influence of the air as a germ carrier can be ignored as a *quantité négligeable* in all cases and under all conditions. It means simply that with ordinary commonsense precautions as to cleanliness, especially of the floor, and stillness of the air of a room we can operate in it without undue anxiety. That the absence of common sense is conspicuous in the arrangements with regard to some operating rooms is quite another matter. Rooms are dangerous to wounds in proportion to the numbers of people in them and to the activity of the movements of these persons to and fro. In a well-known clinical lecture room the following averages were established by a long series of bacteriological observations. When occupied by the usual audience the exposure for an hour of a four-inch Petri dish with sterilised agar showed on cultivation 155 colonies of organisms. On the other hand, when the same room was empty and the air at rest a similar exposure only showed 37. In contrast to this the aseptic operation theatre of the same institution in use and at rest only showed 60 and three colonies respectively after an hour's exposure.

(*b*) As to a wound made by an instrument or other object which is dirty, it need only be said that if seen early and it is possible the area involved should be cleanly *excised* and then the resulting wound treated as aseptic. If seen too late for this it should be thoroughly scrubbed and treated with antiseptics and left open.

(*c*) Speaking generally, the instruments employed in surgical operations can nearly all be rendered sterile by careful washing and boiling in soda solution. There are, however, some which are spoiled by boiling and the common antiseptics, and among these the most important are knives, scissors, and needles. Fortunately, washing with hot water and soap, followed by immersion for a quarter of an hour in methylated spirit, is quite adequate to render their plane surfaces aseptic. It may be said, then, that infection from an instrument can easily be prevented.

(*d*) The same may be said of the overalls, swabs, dressings, and bandages employed in most cases if saturated steam be employed. The last three, as you know, are in my own technique the same thing. For the sake of simplification of procedure my swabs are merely eight-inch lengths cut off the four-fold gauze rollers also to be used as bandages and dressings and all come out of the same sterilising drum in most cases. Simplification of procedure is to my mind one of the most important desiderata in aseptic surgery and is very sadly neglected at present. It eliminates many opportunities of confusion and of accidental contamination and saves much time and thought in preparation and manipulation as well as much expense.

On the subject of ligatures and sutures much might be said. The amount of investigation as to the best material to employ and the modes of its preparation is simply enormous. But it must not be forgotten that almost any material used for ligatures may be left in any tissue of the body, if *sterile*, without hurt if in small quantity. It becomes, then, a question what ligature can be best sterilised and what material is so strong that its thread can be very fine and yet very strong, so that the smallest foreign body is left in a wound. But that some materials are not easily sterilised is clear. As for my own work, after giving an extended trial to many substances—catgut, tendon, horse-hair, silkworm gut, pure twist silk, and linen thread—I have for years exclusively used the last for ligatures and sutures.

But beyond all this there is the possibility of restricting the use of ligatures in a great many operations almost to zero by the use of hæmostatic forceps. This gets over a great difficulty. But we know that the extent to which forceps may supersede ligatures is not realised by many operators, especially abroad. In my own work ligatures are but rarely used. I do not think, for instance, that in the last 50 amputations of the breast ten have been employed, perhaps not five. The forceps of Péan and Spencer Wells have been all that was necessary.

(*e*) If you wish to realise the abundance and variety of the flora of the human skin you have only to repeat for yourself one of the many careful and extended observations made years ago on this point by several investigators abroad as follows. After one or more rigorous hot baths, with plenty of soap, put on a vest previously sterilised by steam. But before doing so stitch on various spots of its inner surface small, one centimetre, patches of some woven substance, say in the axillæ and groins, the abdomen, and the back. When this vest has been worn for the day separate these patches with sterile scissors and forceps and place each in a tube of sterile agar. After shaking and stirring them up in the fluid pour the latter into Petri dishes and place these in an incubator. After 48 hours an inspection of the results will convince you of the omnipresence of septic organisms even on a clean skin where it is not exposed to the air and will give you an idea of their relative abundance on the various parts of the body over which the little patches have been worn. If these results are obtained from a well-washed skin a surgeon may well be uneasy in the case of the average patient. And if this is true, how much more so must it be of the skin of the head, hands, and feet which are constantly exposed. If any further proof is necessary read the reports of some bacteriological tests of the number of organisms found in a cubic centimetre of water taken from the Seine in Paris first above and then below the laundry stations on its shores. The difference runs into millions. After this you will need no proof that the whole skin of a patient to be operated on requires the most careful cleansing not once but many times before an operation is undertaken. (Many other proofs might be given.) And why many times? Simply because though one washing with or without germicides may render the surface of the skin *relatively* pure it does not reach the hair, sweat, and sebaceous follicles which are constantly the hosts of countless microbes and these latter only come to the surface in the course of natural secretion. Individuals vary,

F

may with advantage be tilted slightly by placing blocks under the lower end of the table. Should the circulatory shock be associated with shallow breathing the withdrawal of the anæsthetic may be coupled with chest pressure during expiration. In acute cases in which respiratory arrest quickly follows pulselessness the operation must be temporarily suspended, the patient's body drawn towards the anæsthetist, so that the head hangs over the end of the table, and rhythmic chest compression commenced. By alternately forcibly compressing the sides of the chest with the flat hands and relaxing the pressure air may generally be made to pass out of and into the lungs, but if there be the slightest difficulty in securing this end systematic artificial respiration must be practised. As already mentioned, recovery almost invariably takes place within a minute or two. If it be delayed the artificial respiration must be combined with more or less complete inversion of the body. Although the state we are considering is essentially a circulatory one care must be taken to avoid the slightest obstruction in respiration. Personally, I am not a believer in the use of drugs in this condition: lung ventilation and proper posture are the two cardinal remedies. In one of the most acute cases of surgical shock that I ever witnessed the pulse at both wrists disappeared for 20 minutes, but no remedial measures beyond keeping the legs high and the head low and maintaining free respiration were adopted: at the conclusion of the operation (the first stage of Kraske's operation) the pulse and colour had returned and the patient's condition became quite satisfactory. The patient made such a good recovery, indeed, that the second half of the operation was performed in two or three days' time. In exceptionally bad cases in which the patient's condition does not rapidly improve it may perhaps be advisable to administer a saline injection or infusion.

CONCLUSIONS.

1. Two distinct varieties of surgical shock are met with during general anæsthesia: (1) respiratory and (2) circulatory. In pure respiratory shock the respiration is primarily affected (reflexly), the circulation only failing secondarily. In pure circulatory shock the circulation is primarily affected (reflexly), the respiration only failing secondarily.

2. When respiratory shock becomes complicated by circulatory, or circulatory by respiratory, a state of mixed or composite surgical shock is produced.

3. Respiratory surgical shock, which may occur under all anæsthetics, is most common during *light* or *moderate* anæsthesia—i.e., before the corneal reflex has vanished; whilst circulatory shock, which is far more common under chloroform than under other agents, is met with during *profound* narcosis.

4. The risk of preparing patients or commencing operations before full anæsthesia has been secured is from the *respiratory* and not from the *circulatory* side, as is generally believed.

5. Respiratory shock may arise during any operation, but it seems specially liable to complicate operations upon the rectum, urethra, abdominal organs, uterus, perineum, and kidney. The immediate cause of the respiratory arrest is usually a reflex spasm affecting either (*a*) the tongue, fauces, palate, and adjacent parts, and having stertor as its audible expression; (*b*) the larynx, and producing stridor; or (*c*) the respiratory muscles, and bringing about respiratory spasm.

6. Circulatory shock is chiefly, if not exclusively met with during operations upon parts which possess important nerves or are rich in nerve supply. The immediate cause of the circulatory phenomena is usually a more or less sudden relaxation or paralysis of the vaso-motor system, generally associated with some cardiac inhibition. In some cases the effect produced by the nerve injury is chiefly one of cardiac inhibition.

7. The most favourable conditions for the occurrence of acute and threatening respiratory shock are: (1) partially established anæsthesia; (2) manipulations or operations upon sensitive parts; and (3) the presence of an airway liable to become occluded.

8. The most favourable conditions for the occurrence of acute and threatening circulatory shock are (1) deep chloroform anæsthesia; (2) the horizontal, semi-recumbent, or sitting posture; and (3) intestinal, omental, uterine, or renal traction.

9. Certain subjects, by reason of the conformation of their upper air passages, seem specially liable to respiratory shock, whilst others, possibly from some abnormal instability of their vaso-motor systems, may perhaps be prone to circulatory shock. The state of the heart itself seems to have little or no influence.

10. There may be such a close resemblance between simple chloroform overdosage and circulatory shock under chloroform that the latter condition may be readily mistaken for the former.

11. Whilst surgical shock may undoubtedly be largely prevented by gentleness on the part of the surgeon, its prevention is also largely in the hands of the anæsthetist. The respiratory variety may usually be avoided by securing full anæsthesia before the patient is moved or the operation is begun, and by so adjusting the degree of anæsthesia that reflex modifications in respiration are as far as possible eliminated. As circulatory shock is very rare under ether it may generally be prevented by employing this anæsthetic. Should chloroform or a chloroform mixture be used there are only two ways in which to prevent circulatory shock during certain operations—viz., (1) to avoid too deep an anæsthesia, or if the patient be deeply anæsthetised to lessen the depth of anæsthesia so that the corneal reflex returns; or (2) to place the patient in the Trendelenburg posture. With the rarest exceptions, circulatory shock is never seen in the Trendelenburg posture.

12. The treatment of respiratory shock is to re-establish respiration as quickly as possible by such procedures as separating the clenched teeth, sponging out the fauces, pushing the lower jaw forwards, tongue traction, artificial respiration, and if need be, laryngotomy and direct lung inflation.

13. The treatment of circulatory shock in its milder form is simply to lessen the depth of anæsthesia and to substitute the C.E. mixture or ether for chloroform. In its acute form circulatory shock must be treated by withholding the anæsthetic, lowering the head, raising the feet, and, should respiration show signs of failure or actually cease, by performing artificial respiration. Unless the patient be so deeply anæsthetised by chloroform as to be in peril from this additional quarter recovery from circulatory shock may generally be effected very rapidly—within a minute or two—and the operation may then be proceeded with. Drugs are of little or no value as compared to the lines of treatment here indicated.

THE CARRIAGE OF INFECTION BY FLIES.[1]

BY R. M. BUCHANAN, M.B. GLASG., F.F.P.S. GLASG.,
BACTERIOLOGIST TO THE CORPORATION OF GLASGOW.

I PURPOSE to present a few experiments in demonstration of the part which flies are capable of playing as agents in carrying and spreading infection. The experiments were undertaken as opportunity offered to test the value to be attached to the opinion frequently expressed of late years and emphasised by observations in the Cuban and South African campaigns that flies convey on their bodies infective material and contribute to the spread of certain diseases.

The flies used in the experiments were the common housefly (*Musca domestica*) and the bluebottle (*Musca vomitoria*). The latter is referred to hereafter in this paper as the blue fly. The flies were allowed a limited contact with infective material and then transferred directly to the surface of a solidified nutrient medium in a Petri capsule, and in some instances to a succession of such surfaces. By rotating the capsule, held at an angle, it was frequently possible to make the insect traverse the greater part of the surface of the nutrient medium, and when its transference to another capsule was desired this was accomplished without injury by means of a pair of curved sterilised forceps.

It may be remarked that the form and structure of the fly's foot (tarsus) are such as render it capable of carrying a large amount of infective material. It consists of five segments or "joints" which are clothed with short hairs and armed with numerous bristles and spines. The terminal segment is also provided at its tip with a pair of moveable claws and a pair of membranous flaps (pulvilli)—the latter coming into action on smooth surfaces (Fig. 1).

The diseases which were made the subject of the experiments were typhoid fever, swine fever, staphylococcal abscess, pulmonary tuberculosis, and anthrax.

---

[1] A paper read before the Glasgow Medico-Chirurgical Society on Nov. 16th, 1906.

Typhoid Fever.

Experiment I.—Six house-flies were caught by means of a net in three enteric wards of the Glasgow fever hospital (September, 1903) and placed in Petri capsules containing a layer of bile salt, lactose agar, with neutral-red and crystal-violet—i.e., the medium of MacConkey[2] modified by

FIG. 1.

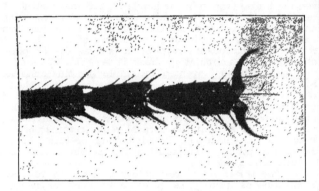

Part of a fly's foot showing the claws and pulvilli of the terminal segment and the general armature of bristles and spines. The clothing of short hairs is not visible in the illustration. × 70.

Grünbaum and Hume.[3] This medium favours the growth of bacilli of the colon and typhoid groups, and inhibits most other species. For the sake of convenience and brevity this medium will hereinafter be designated L-R-V-B agar. The flies were allowed to walk over the surface of the medium for a short time and were then withdrawn. A few colonies of coliform organisms appeared on three of the nutrient surfaces but no trace of bacillus typhosus was found. It will be observed that a possible fallacy entered into this experiment inasmuch as the flies were caught in a fly net, the fabric of which would tend to remove any infective material clinging to their feet.

Experiment II.—To obviate the possible fallacy mentioned in the previous experiment seven flies were caught by means of sterilised forceps in the enteric wards of the fever hospital and each fly was immediately placed in a Petri capsule containing L-R-V-B agar over which it was allowed to walk for at least five minutes. No growths resulted in any of the capsules.

Experiment III.—It was therefore decided to make the test in a more direct manner by bringing flies (collected in the kitchen of a restaurant) into direct contact with the dejecta of typhoid patients—one patient being in the eighth day of illness, two in the eighteenth, and one in the twenty-fifth. This object was attained by placing each fly in a Petri capsule, having in the bottom half a thin film made from a typhoid stool by means of a sterilised swab. The fly was introduced within the Petri capsule before the film had time to become dry, and after walking over the surface for a few minutes it was transferred to the culture medium and allowed similarly to traverse its surface for a few minutes. Thereafter the fly was transferred to a second and in most instances to a third capsule holding a similar layer of L-R-V-B agar or ordinary agar. Many bacteria were deposited on the nutrient surface from the insect's feet in each case and they were numerous in some instances, even on the third surface. From two of the fæcal films the flies were found to have carried typhoid bacilli to the surface of the nutrient medium, but the number of these bacilli was relatively very small. Thus in the case of B—— (eighteenth day of illness) there was only one colony of bacillus typhosus amongst 22 colonies of other species and in the case of L—— (twenty-fifth day of illness) two colonies of bacillus typhosus amongst 60 of other species. No typhoid bacilli appeared on the second and third surfaces traversed by the flies.

Swine Fever.

Experiment IV.—An opportunity offered itself in an outbreak of swine fever in September, 1905, to test flies alighting upon pigs which had died from the disease and which had

2 THE LANCET, July 7th, 1900, p. 20.
3 Brit. Med. Jour., 1902, vol. i., p. 138.

been subjected to post-mortem examination. The flies (*Musca vomitoria*) were caught by placing over them when quite still a wide tube of about one inch diameter (a Buchner tube). They at once rose into the inverted tube and were secured by a pledget of cotton wool which was pressed into the tube sufficiently to fix the insects so that they were prevented from moving about and removing any matter from their feet. In this way nine flies were collected from two carcasses and transferred to the laboratory. Each fly was placed in a Petri capsule containing a layer of ordinary agar and allowed to traverse the surface of the medium for about a minute. A very rich bacterial flora appeared on incubation, so much so that the agar was covered by a mixed confluent growth in most of the capsules. The bacillus of swine fever was isolated from one of the capsules. The flies were swarming on these carcasses and on other infective material, and were frequently seen to pass directly therefrom to the feeding troughs.

Staphylococcal Abscess.

Experiment V. (November, 1905).—Pus from an abscess containing staphylococcus aureus was spread in a thin film in the lower half of a Petri capsule by means of a sterilised swab. A house-fly was caused to walk over this slightly moist purulent film and was then transferred to another Petri capsule containing a layer of agar. After incubation at 37° C. for 48 hours the agar showed a profuse mixed growth in which staphylococcus aureus predominated.

Pulmonary Tuberculosis.

Experiment VI. (November, 1905).—To test the carrying power of flies in the same way in relation to expectoration a specimen of tuberculous sputum rich in bacillus tuberculosis was spread in a thin film in the bottom half of a Petri capsule. A house-fly was introduced into this capsule and caused to walk over the film for a few minutes. It was then transferred to another Petri capsule containing a layer of agar. On washing the surface of the agar with one cubic centimetre of bouillon and inoculating a guinea-pig intraperitoneally therewith, tuberculosis was induced which killed the guinea-pig in 36 days.

Anthrax.

Experiment VII.—In the course of the examination of a guinea-pig dead from anthrax (October, 1903) it was observed that a blue fly had gained entrance to the laboratory and it

FIG. 2.

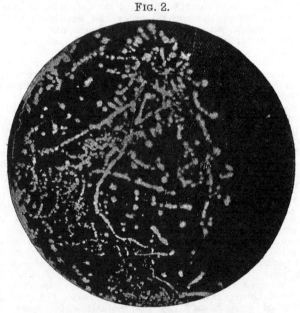

Growth of bacillus anthracis (24 hours) resulting from inoculation of agar surface in a Petri capsule by a blue fly which had just previously alighted on, and walked over, the skinned carcass of a guinea-pig dead from anthrax (Oct. 26th, 1903).

was forthwith decided to make the intruder serve the purpose of an experiment. The fly was accordingly placed under a bell-jar. The carcass of the guinea pig, deprived of the skin and internal organs, was then placed under the same bell-jar. After alighting upon the moist surface of the carcass several times, the fly was transferred to a surface of agar in a Petri capsule and was allowed to walk thereon for a short time. A second agar surface was provided on which it was also allowed to walk for the same time. Incubation for 24 hours at 37° C. brought forth on both agar surfaces a very profuse growth of bacillus anthracis (Figs. 2 and 3).[4] It was

FIG. 3.

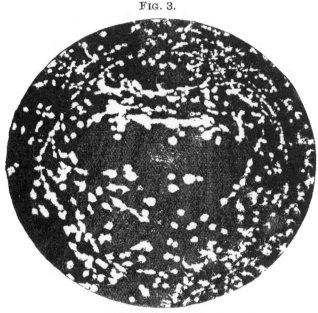

The second agar surface traversed by the same blue fly, showing by the profuse growth of bacillus anthracis (24 hours) the large amount of infection which still remained on the insect's feet after contact with the first agar surface.

not anticipated that the second surface would show so much growth, and it would have been of interest and importance had the cultures been extended in a longer series to determine how many fresh surfaces such a fly was capable of infecting. Its potentialities in the direction were altogether underestimated.

Experiment VIII.—With the view of testing the value of these results under conditions of ordinary experience an anthrax carcass (ox) which had been seized by the veterinary

FIG. 4.

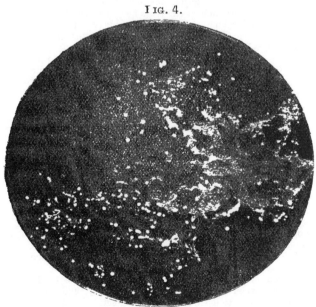

Growth of several species of bacteria (24 hours), including seven colonies of bacillus anthracis, resulting from inoculation of agar surface in a Petri capsule by a house-fly which had just previously alighted on, and walked over, a part of the hind quarter of an imported anthrax carcass (ox) seized in the Glasgow Dead Meat Market (Nov. 15th, 1905).

[4] The photographs illustrating this paper were taken by Mr. W. R. Ogilvie.

surgeon in the Glasgow Dead Meat Market (November, 1905) was made the subject of experiment. A house-fly was placed under a bell-jar resting on one of the hind quarters of the carcass, the surface of the part being quite firm and dry. When the fly had alighted on and walked over the part several times it was transferred to a Petri capsule and caused to traverse the surface of the nutrient medium. After 24 hours' incubation at 37° C. a growth of various species appeared, including seven colonies of bacillus anthracis (Fig. 4). A second fly, held by the wing by means of forceps, was directed across the cut surface of the kidney and gave rise to a profuse growth of bacillus anthracis, amongst other species, on solidified agar (Fig. 5). A third

FIG. 5.

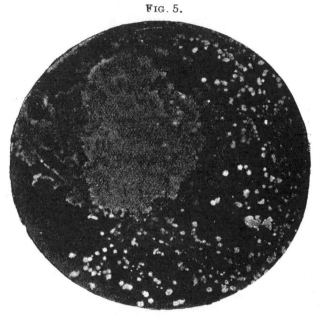

Profuse growth of bacillus anthracis amongst other species (24 hours) resulting from inoculation of agar surface in a Petri capsule by a house-fly which had just previously been allowed to walk over the cut surface of the kidney in the same carcass.

fly, directed in like manner over the cut surface of the thigh muscles, produced a profuse growth of several species, amongst which were found two colonies of bacillus anthracis.

The experiments conclusively show that flies alighting on any substance containing pathogenic organisms are capable of carrying away these organisms in large numbers on their feet and of depositing them in gradually diminishing number on surface after surface with which they come in contact. They further serve to demonstrate the necessity for the exercise of stringent measures to prevent the access of flies to all sources of infection and to protect food of all kinds against flies alighting on it.

Glasgow.

THE ROYAL NATIONAL ORTHOPÆDIC HOSPITAL. —Arrangements for the amalgamation of the Royal National and City Orthopædic Hospitals have now been completed and the patients of both hospitals are being seen in the temporary premises of the amalgamated institution, Nos. 45–47, Bolsover-street, immediately behind the old hospital in Great Portland-street. Dr. J. Hughlings Jackson has been elected honorary consulting physician to the Royal National Orthopædic Hospital and Dr. G. A. Sutherland, Mr. John Poland, and Mr. J Jackson Clarke have been elected honorary physician, honorary surgeon, and honorary surgeon respectively. The new building operations have been begun and a hospital for 213 in-patients is being built on the site of the old hospital and the adjoining premises. The new out-patient department is to be separated from the hospital and will be on the opposite side of the road, on the east side of Bolsover-street, the hospital and the out-patient department being connected by a subway beneath Bolsover-street. Temporary accommodation for in-patients is provided in three of the vacant wards at Charing Cross Hospital which have been rented by the Royal National Orthopædic Hospital.

THE LANCET, July 4, 1908.

𝕿𝖍𝖊 𝕮𝖗𝖔𝖔𝖓𝖎𝖆𝖓 𝕷𝖊𝖈𝖙𝖚𝖗𝖊𝖘

ON

INBORN ERRORS OF METABOLISM.

Delivered before the Royal College of Physicians of London on June 18th, 23rd, 25th, and 30th, 1908,

By ARCHIBALD E. GARROD, M.A., M.D.
Oxon., F.R.C.P. Lond.,

ASSISTANT PHYSICIAN TO, AND LECTURER ON CHEMICAL PATHOLOGY AT, ST. BARTHOLOMEW'S HOSPITAL; SENIOR PHYSICIAN, HOSPITAL FOR SICK CHILDREN, GREAT ORMOND STREET.

LECTURE I.

Delivered on June 18th, 1908.

GENERAL AND INTRODUCTORY.

MR. PRESIDENT AND FELLOWS,—It is my first agreeable duty to offer my sincere thanks for the honour conferred upon me in the invitation to deliver the Croonian lectures of the current year before this College. I trust that the subject which I have selected will be found to conform closely to the instructions to the lecturer, for it is one which lies upon the very border-line of physiology and pathology and pertains to both sciences alike; nor is it without bearing upon the control and cure of disease, in so far as no study which helps to throw light upon the complex chemical processes which are carried out in the human organism can fail in the long run to strengthen our hands in the combat with the pathogenic influences which make for its destruction.

The differences of structure and form which serve to distinguish the various genera and species of animals and plants are among the most obvious facts of nature. For their detection no scientific training is needed, seeing that they cannot escape the notice of even the least cultivated intelligence. Yet with the growth of knowledge we have learned to recognise the uniformity which underlies this so apparent diversity and the genetic relationship of form to form. With regard to the chemical composition of the tissues of living organisms and the metabolic processes by which those tissues are built up and broken down, the advance of knowledge has been in the opposite direction, and the progress of chemical physiology is teaching us that behind a superficial uniformity there exists a diversity which is no less real than that of structure, although it is far less obvious. The differences of ultimate composition and crystalline form which distinguish the hæmoglobins of animals of distinct genera have long been known. That the fats of animals are not alike in composition is well recognised, as also are the differences of their bile acids, to quote only a few of the most conspicuous examples. As instances of distinctive end-products of metabolism may be mentioned kynurenic acid, which is present in the urine of animals of the canine tribe and which bears witness to a generic peculiarity in the manner of dealing with the tryptophane fraction of proteins, and the excretion by birds and reptiles of the bulk of their nitrogenous waste in the form of uric acid, whereas in the urine of mammals urea is the chief nitrogenous constituent.

A more extended study even by strictly chemical methods will doubtless serve to reveal innumerable minor differences, such as are foreshadowed by Przibram's[1] work on muscle proteins. The delicate ultra-chemical methods which the researches of recent years have brought to light, such as the precipitin test, reveal differences still more subtle, and teach the lesson that the members of each individual species are built up of their own specific proteins which resemble each other the more closely the more nearly the species are allied. Obviously it is among the highly complex proteins that such specific differences are to be looked for rather than in the simple end-products of their disintegration. The many amino-acids which enter into the structure of the protein molecules are capable of almost innumerable groupings and proportional representations, and each fresh grouping will produce a distinct protein; but all alike in their breaking down will yield the same simple end-products, urea, carbon dioxide, and others.

Nor can it be supposed that the diversity of chemical structure and process stops at the boundary of the species, and that within that boundary, which has no real finality, rigid uniformity reigns. Such a conception is at variance with any evolutionary conception of the nature and origin of species. The existence of chemical individuality follows of necessity from that of chemical specificity, but we should expect the differences between individuals to be still more subtle and difficult of detection. Indications of their existence are seen, even in man, in the various tints of skin, hair, and eyes, and in the quantitative differences in those portions of the end-products of metabolism which are endogenous and are not affected by diet, such as recent researches have revealed in increasing numbers. Even those idiosyncrasies with regard to drugs and articles of food which are summed up in the proverbial saying that what is one man's meat is another man's poison presumably have a chemical basis.

Upon chemical as upon structural variations the factors which make for evolution have worked and are working. Evidences of this are to be detected in many directions, as, for example, in the delicate selective power of the kidneys, in virtue of which they are enabled to hold back in the circulation the essential proteins of the blood but at the same time allow free passage to other proteins which are foreign to the plasma, such as hæmoglobin, egg albumin, and the Bence-Jones protein, when these are present in any but quite small amounts. The working of these factors is also seen in the various protective mechanisms against chemical poisons, such as that which averts the depletion of the fixed alkalies of the organism by the neutralisation of abnormal supplies of acids by ammonia. This mechanism is well developed in the carnivora and in man, but in vegetivorous animals which from the nature of their diet are little exposed to acidosis it appears to be wanting.

Even in the normal metabolic processes the working of such influences may be traced, as in the power which the organism possesses of destroying the benzene ring of those aromatic amino-acids which enter into the composition of proteins and cannot therefore be regarded as substances foreign to the body; whereas the benzene ring of foreign aromatic compounds, with very few exceptions, are left intact, and such compounds require to be rendered innocuous by being combined with sulphuric acid to form aromatic sulphates, or with glycocoll to form the acids of the hippuric group and so combined are excreted in the urine and got rid of. The few exceptions referred to are compounds which so closely resemble the protein fractions in their structure that they fall victims with these to the normal destructive processes.

The great strides which recent years have witnessed in the sciences of chemical physiology and pathology, the newly-acquired knowledge of the constitution of proteins and of the part played by enzymes in connexion with the chemical changes brought about within the organism, have profoundly modified our conceptions of the nature of the metabolic processes and have made it easier to understand how these changes may differ in the various genera and species. It was formerly widely held that many derangements of metabolism which result from disease were due to a general slackening of the process of oxidation in the tissues. The whole series of catabolic changes was looked upon as a simple combustion and according as the metabolic fires burnt brightly or burnt low the destruction of the products of the breaking down of food and tissues was supposed to be complete or imperfect. A very clear setting forth of such views will be found in the lectures of Bence Jones[2] on Diseases of Suboxidation, delivered and published in 1855, but the thesis in question is chiefly associated with the name of Bouchard,[3] who expounded it in his well-known lectures on Maladies par Ralentissement de la Nutrition, published in 1882. The so frequent clinical association of such maladies as gout, obesity, and diabetes was involved in its support, nor was it regarded as a serious obstacle to the acceptance of such views that there is but scanty evidence to show that failure to burn any particular metabolic product, such as glucose, is associated with inability to deal with others.'

Nowadays, very different ideas are in the ascendant. The conception of metabolism in block is giving place to that of metabolism in compartments. The view is daily gaining ground that each successive step in the building up and

---

[1] Hofmeister's Beiträge, 1902, Band ii., p. 143.

[2] Medical Times and Gazette, 1865, vol. ii., pp. 29–83.
[3] Maladies par Ralentissement de la Nutrition, Paris, 1882.

THE LANCET,]   DR. H. FRASER & DR. A. T. STANTON: THE ETIOLOGY OF BERI-BERI.   [FEB. 13, 1909.   451

a high hæmomanometer reading, and that if you relax the arteries with the one hand you must encourage and help the heart with the other. You require a fairly strong heart to send the blood on after the vessels are relaxed. You will often prevent cerebral softening by properly appreciating these relations and often rapidly cure your hemiplegias. I have no hesitation in claiming that I have done that for people over and over again and we can all do it.

The subject I have brought before you is one full of interest. I have merely given you an outline sketch of it, but one I hope which will arouse your interest sufficiently to lead you to look into it further and satisfy yourselves that these things are true—that this action of the blood upon the vessel wall is a truth which we have ignored—why, it is not my business to inquire—and that the muscle-movement of the vessel wall has also been practically ignored. In these two observations lies the explanation of the production of arterio-sclerosis, confining that term to the medial and intimal changes which are the common anatomical changes in the thickened radial and other arteries so well known to the clinician. In conclusion, I have indicated to you that the hæmomanometer is of clinical value as giving you a record of the contraction and relaxation of the arterial wall rather than of the blood pressure. This interpretation will, I believe, soon come to be recognised as much more practically and clinically useful than the other.

AN INQUIRY CONCERNING THE ETIOLOGY OF BERI-BERI.

A PRELIMINARY COMMUNICATION.

BY HENRY FRASER, M.D. ABERD., D.P.H.,

AND

A. T. STANTON, M.D., C.M. TORONTO, M.R.C.S. ENG., L.R.C.P. LOND.

(From the Institute for Medical Research, Kuala Lumpur, Federated Malay States.)

THE etiology of beri-beri has long been recognised as one of the most difficult problems in medicine and many hypotheses have been put forward to account for the obscure features in its epidemiology. Certain features of beri-beri long ago led observers to direct attention to rice as a possible source of the disease-producing agent. Professor Hirsch wrote of this suggestion in his "Handbuch der Historisch-geographischen Pathologie" (1883), quoting Malcolmsen (1835) and Kearney (1872).

An investigation carried out by Vorderman in 1895 and 1896 in the prisons of Java and Madoera, based on the conclusions of Eijkman from experimental work on fowls, showed that the incidence of beri-beri among the prisoners varied directly as did the amount of white rice in the diet. Among those dieted on red rice the incidence of beri-beri was 0·01 per 1000, among those on a mixture of red rice and white rice 2·4 per 1000, and among those on white rice 28 per 1000. The distinction between red and white rice is that in the case of the former but little of the spermoderm and perisperm is removed, whilst in the case of the latter the spermoderm and most of the perisperm are removed.

Braddon, from observations on the disease in the Federated Malay States, has drawn attention to the curious discrepancy in the incidence of beri-beri among the immigrant peoples of the Peninsula, the Chinese suffering severely and the Tamils very slightly. He believes that the disease is due to the consumption of stale white rice, the staple article of diet among the Chinese immigrants, and that the Tamils remain free from the disease so long as they consume only rice prepared in the Indian manner—that is, by parboiling before husking. A similar immunity from the disease enjoyed by Malays under primitive conditions he believes to be due to the fact that they consume only rice prepared from padi newly husked. Braddon has given the names "uncured," "cured," and "fresh" respectively to these forms of rice. He concludes that beri-beri is due to a specific fungus which, like that of toxic rye and lolium, is probably a parasite affecting the surface of the seed. This view of the etiology of beri-beri enunciated by Braddon constitutes, if correct, an important advance upon any of the hypotheses hitherto formulated which seek for the origin of the disease in food.

He has dealt with the whole question in some detail in a recent publication, "The Cause and prevention of Beri-Beri."

The rice consumed by immigrant labourers in the Malay Peninsula is grown mainly in Siam, Burma, the Siamese Malay States, French Indo-China, and Province Wellesley. All classes, except the Tamils, prefer white rice; this is the "stale uncured rice" of Braddon and is the variety believed by him to be the source of the causative agent of beri-beri. White rice is imported as such from Siam and Burma or is prepared in the mills of Singapore and Penang from padi imported mainly from Siam, the Western Siamese States, and French Indo-China. In the preparation of this form of rice no preliminary treatment of the padi (unhusked rice) is required; it is milled by machinery and the husk, together with the pericarp and the surface layers of the seed, is removed. This rice is sold under the trade names of Siamese, Rangoon, and Saigon rice, terms which may indicate the country of origin of the grain but which, generally speaking, are only of commercial significance. All such rices are here referred to as "white rice"; we avoid the descriptive terms employed by Braddon as it has been held by some authorities that the use of these tends to prejudice the issues involved.

The Tamil labourer prefers a form of rice similar to that consumed by him in India and for its production a process analogous to the one in use in that country is employed in the mills here. Large concrete tanks are used in which the padi is placed and soaked in water for a period of from 24 to 48 hours. After this the padi is transferred to lightly covered cylinders and steamed for from five to ten minutes. Subsequently it is removed to open paved courts and dried by exposure to the sun. It is thereafter stored as padi or milled at once. This rice is of a yellowish colour, more or less translucent, and is here called parboiled rice (the "cured rice" of Braddon). Parboiled rice is imported from India and to a small extent from Sumatra (Asahan) but the bulk of that consumed in this country is prepared in the mills of Penang and Singapore from padi imported from Siam, the Western Siamese States, and French Indo-China. As compared with similar rices imported from India and Sumatra the local product has a peculiar disagreeable musty odour, the exact cause of which has not been determined.

The investigation hereinafter described was undertaken primarily to determine if, when other factors were excluded or controlled, people fed on white rice did develop beri-beri, and if people under exactly similar conditions but fed on parboiled rice did not develop the disease. It was hoped, also, that opportunity would be forthcoming for the investigation of other aspects of the question. At the outset it is necessary to state that the disease under investigation is that form of multiple peripheral neuritis known as beri-beri, which occurs endemically in this peninsula and the neighbouring islands. As much confusion has been caused by assigning this name to classes of cases differing widely in their clinical manifestations, it is desirable to make it clear that we seek only for an explanation of this disease as met with here.

For the purpose of the inquiry it was necessary to observe two parties of men under similar conditions as to environment, &c., and whose food-supply was definitely known. In view of the suggestion made by numerous observers that the disease may be bacterial or protozoal in origin, it was desirable that the places chosen should have been hitherto uninhabited or that no case of beri-beri should have occurred there for some time previously; further, the places should be in an isolated district sufficiently remote from towns or villages to exclude as far as possible the entrance of a supposed infection. Such a situation would also have the advantage, on account of the absence of shops, that the men under observation could not readily obtain food other than that supplied to them. It is obvious that the conditions required for such an investigation could not be secured in a public institution, as in all such in these States beri-beri is known to be endemic.

Various places were visited with a view to securing satisfactory conditions, and it was finally decided to carry on observations with regard to some 300 Javanese indentured labourers employed in the work of road construction in a remote part of the Jelebu district in the State of Negri Sembilan. The places in which they were at this time located, the fifty-first mile and the fifty-eighth mile from Seremban, were sufficiently remote from the nearest village or town for the purpose, and Malay villages in the district were few in number and small in size. In connexion with these latter it should be remembered that abundant evidence exists to show that Malays in such situations do not suffer from beri-beri. Under the terms of the contract the rice issued to these labourers was supplied by the employer. It may be added that the Javanese prefer white rice, which is the kind consumed by them in their own country. In the early months of 1906 cases of beri-beri had occurred among these labourers, and in May, June, and July of that year it was a serious source of invaliding and mortality. From August 2nd, 1906, the employer, adopting the suggestion of Dr. Braddon, issued only parboiled instead of the white rice hitherto issued and thenceforward it is stated, and this statement is confirmed by the hospital records, no case of beri-beri appeared.

Here, then, the conditions seemed to be in every way suitable for an inquiry into the part played by rice in the causation of beri-beri, because these labourers without exception still desired to return to a white rice diet, and at this time the evidence of a connexion between the consumption of white rice and beri-beri was by no means convincing either to the general body of medical and scientific workers or to ourselves. The importance of reaching some conclusion regarding the origin of the disease cannot be over-estimated, as the number of its victims in this peninsula alone runs into many thousands annually. Throughout these States no labourers other than Tamils will consume parboiled rice unless compelled to do so, and while there was any doubt as to the harmful influence of white rice no effective measures could be taken for the suppression of beri-beri. By acceding to the wishes of the group of labourers comprised in this investigation opportunity would be afforded for a thorough testing of the position of dietary factors as causative agents. The labourers were therefore given the option of returning to a white rice diet after it had been fully explained to them that by so doing they ran the risk of contracting beri-beri. Without exception they chose the white rice, but as for the purpose of comparison two parties were required, half the number only were allowed this diet. It was hoped also that by continuous observation of a large party of men on a parboiled rice diet it might be determined whether, apart from its disagreeable musty odour, any grounds existed for the objections made to the consumption of this rice.

At the time the investigation was commenced, April, 1907, the labourers, about 300 in number, were divided into two parties of approximately equal numbers, the one party at the fifty-first mile and the other at the fifty-eighth mile. The clearings for the quarters had been made in virgin jungle and no case of beri-beri had occurred at either place. The quarters were well raised from the ground, the floors being made of split bamboo, the walls of bark, and the roof of light ataps; thus they were well ventilated. In all cases the lines were well drained and near running water. The sanitary conditions were good.

In April all the labourers were examined and found to be free from any sign of existing or recent beri-beri. The results of the physical examination of each person were recorded for future reference and an arrangement made that any person subsequently joining the parties should be carefully examined previously. An interval was allowed to elapse during which any latent case might be expected to develop and as all remained healthy white rice was issued to the party at the fifty-eighth mile for the first time on May 12th, the party at the fifty-first mile remaining on parboiled rice as before The daily ration was as follows: rice,

21·3 ounces; dried fish, 4·25 ounces; onions, 1·75 ounces; potatoes, 1·75 ounces; cocoanut oil, 0·85 ounce; cocoanut 1·50 ounces; tea, 0·12 ounce; and salt, 0·1 ounce.

The parties as originally formed are designated Party No. 1 at the fifty-eighth mile, Party No. 2 at the fifty-first mile, and Party No. 3 a small party at Pertang. On July 1st the requirements of the work necessitated the division of Party No. 1 into two groups. One group of approximately 50 (Party No. 1A) remained at the fifty-eighth mile, and the other group, about 100 in number (Party No. 1B), was transferred to the fifty-sixth mile. The quarters at this latter place had been newly erected in a fresh clearing. The conditions as regards food remained unchanged. The persons in these two groups, being under similar dietary conditions, were for the purpose of this investigation regarded as one party and were moved freely from one place to the other. The distribution of the parties, the sort of rice consumed, and the results obtained in each case are indicated in the sketch map.

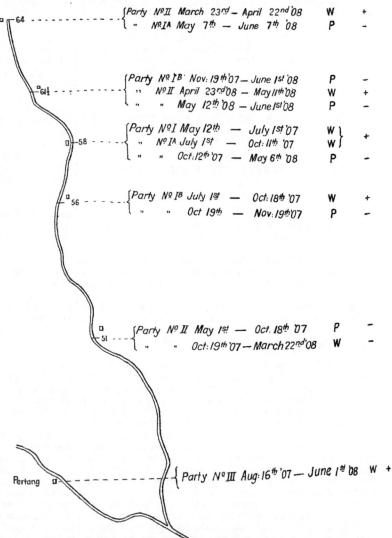

Sketch showing arrangement of parties, rice consumed, and results obtained.
W, White rice. P, Parboiled rice.

PARTY No. 1.

Party No. 1 comprised those individuals who were or white rice at the fifty-eighth mile from May 12th unti July 1st, when the party was divided into two groups The history of Party No. 1 calls for no special comment No case of beri-beri occurred during the period May 12tl to July 1st.

PARTY No. 1A.

This party was formed on July 1st of those members o Party No. 1 who remained at the fifty-eighth mile. Th members of it had for the most part been on white ric since May 12th; a few had joined after that date. Th first case of beri-beri occurred at the fifty-eighth mile on August 7th, the second case on August 19th, 12 days after the first case, and the third case on Sept. 3rd. These dates indicate the time of commencement of an indisposition which terminated in, or was followed by, definite signs of beri-beri ; in nearly all cases this date is antecedent to the loss of the knee-jerk.

It is necessary to deal with these cases in the first instance from the point of view of infection. The first patient had been from May 12th continuously in residence at the fifty-eighth mile, as had also the second case. The third patient had been transferred from Party No. 1B (fifty-sixth mile) on August 23rd, and the peculiar manner in which he came in contact with the first two cases of beri-beri at the fifty-eighth mile, to which reference will presently be made, suggested the likelihood of his having acquired the disease by infection. The fourth case which developed on Sept. 6th had also been intimately associated with the first two patients.

Assuming an infection, the period of incubation from these cases may be fixed at from 10 to 15 days. While there is nothing in the histories of the first two cases to suggest any intimate association the third and fourth cases to develop were known to have been in intimate contact with the first two patients. The third patient on his transference to this party was inadvertently assigned quarters in the hospital, a partitioned-off part of the quarters, and the fourth patient had been in this hospital under treatment for malaria since August 23rd. As the first patient had been continuously in residence the question naturally arises as to how he acquired the infection. He is believed to have suffered from beri-beri about two years previously in Java, but no residual paralysis or sign other than diminished knee-jerks remained to support this history. Still, it might reasonably be suggested that he may either have had a relapse or have acquired an infection from without. In regard to the second of these possibilities it is necessary to consider the conditions in this party for 15 days preceding the development of the disease—that is, from July 22nd to August 7th. On July 22nd there were present in this party 28 individuals. *During* the interval under review three left the party and 10 joined, five of these from Party No. 1B at the fifty-sixth mile, four from Party No. 2 at the fifty-first mile, and one from hospital at Kuala Klawang, where he had been under treatment for pulmonary tuberculosis. Neither in Party No. 1B nor in Party No. 2 did any cases of beri-beri exist at this time. There is no evidence that the man from the hospital had ever had beri-beri previously and he had no signs of the disease on joining the party nor did he develop any signs later. He died some months afterwards from pulmonary tuberculosis. There is little doubt that while in hospital this man would be in contact with cases of beri-beri, and the only remaining explanation is that this person may have been the means of conveying the hypothetical infection though he did not himself suffer from the disease, or only suffered from it in such mild form as to be impossible of recognition clinically.

Granting that the deduction as to the period of incubation is erroneous and that this period is really longer, we shall deal with those who joined this party earlier than July 22nd and exclude the individuals joining from Parties No. 1B and No. 2, which were known to be free from beri-beri. One man joined the party from hospital on June 7th. He developed no signs of beri-beri. Another joined the party from hospital on May 20th and after a stay at the fifty-eighth mile subsequently joined Party No. 1B, returning to the fifty-eighth mile, and developed beri-beri there on Sept. 3rd. If he acquired the infection in hospital the period of incubation must be fixed at some four months. In any case we can scarcely accuse this man of having introduced the disease, as he did not develop it until a month after the first case. Another joined from hospital on May 20th and did not develop the disease. Another joined from Pertang on July 5th and more than three months later developed beri-beri. He had no signs of the disease when he joined. Another joined from hospital on June 7th and after a stay at the fifty-eighth mile joined Party No. 1B, afterwards returning to the fifty-eighth mile, from which place he was sent to hospital on Oct. 5th for treatment of an eye affection. Another joined the party from gaol on June 20th and shortly afterwards was transferred to Party No. 1B. He did not develop signs of beri-beri.

Thus in seeking for an origin of the hypothetical infection in this place we must conclude that it was conveyed by some person from without and who himself showed no signs, or that the period of incubation is more than three months. Any discussion as to the disease having originated *de novo* in the first case or that it was a relapse after two years' interval would be futile. The chances of infection having been introduced by persons not under observation, such as Malays or Chinamen passing along the road, are very remote indeed.

Dealing now with the question of food as a source of the disease, Party No. 1A was on white rice from May 12th until Oct. 11th. During this period 30 members of the party were on white rice for three months or longer and amongst these seven cases of beri-beri occurred. During the time that beri-beri was present at the fifty-eighth mile, August 7th to Oct. 11th, seven individuals joined the party, either from Party No. 2 or from hospital ; there was no white rice issued at these places and none of these seven developed beri-beri, though they were exposed to the chances of an infection equally with the other members of the party. Of 13 individuals who came from Party No. 1B where white rice was being issued two subsequently contracted beri-beri. The results in this party therefore suggested the possibility that a diet of which white rice formed the staple was in some way concerned in the production of beri-beri.

PARTY No. 1B.

The first case of beri-beri to develop in this party was in a patient who was taken ill on Sept. 29th. He had been in the party since its formation on July 1st and had been on white rice in all 141 days. The second case developed on Oct. 10th. This man had been on white rice for 152 days. The third, fourth, and fifth cases followed rapidly, the dates being Oct. 12th, 16th, and 18th. These cases had been on white rice for 154, 158, and 160 days respectively.

From the view-point of infection there is little to be said regarding this party. Such may easily have been introduced from Party No. 1A at the fifty-eighth mile, where the disease had broken out seven weeks previously. These two parties were located only two miles apart and on holidays, which occurred twice a month, very slight restraint was placed upon their movements, as for the primary purpose of this inquiry they were regarded as one party. The introductions from outside into this party were one man who returned from hospital on July 12th ; another who joined Party No. 1 from gaol on June 22nd and was transferred to Party No. 1B on its formation on July 1st ; five individuals who were transferred to this party from Party No. 1A on July 23rd, after which date no other transfers were made ; and six people who were moved from Party No. 2 to this party. None of the individuals here referred to developed beri-beri.

It is proper to mention here that in determining whether a given case was to be admitted as a case of beri-beri the most rigid exclusion was practised. Only such cases as presented unequivocal signs of the disease were admitted. In every instance the diagnosis was based on the opinion of at least two medical men, in most instances on that of four. Where any doubt was cast upon the accuracy of the diagnosis such case was rejected. The result, therefore, is that, apart from the cases here recorded, there were many others which, in our opinion as well as in that of those associated with us in this inquiry, were really mild or obscure cases of the disease. The difficulties in this respect will be appreciated by those who have had to deal with the disease clinically. No such doubtful case was at any time observed among the people on parboiled rice and the inclusion of cases of this type occurring in the white rice parties in no way strengthens the case for an infectious origin of the disease.

By Oct. 11th seven cases had occurred in Party No. 1A and by Oct. 18th five cases in Party No. 1B. As there was apparently nothing further to be gained from a continuance of the white rice diet it was thought that the time was suitable by a change to parboiled rice to observe the effect of this alteration of diet upon the course of the outbreak. Accordingly parboiled rice was substituted for white rice in the diet of Party No. 1A on Oct. 12th and in that of Party No. 1B on Oct. 19th. After this change no case of beri-beri occurred in either party and such cases as showed signs suspicious of beri-beri rapidly got well. This abrupt cessation of the outbreak constitutes important evidence of a causative relationship between the consumption of white

Correspondence.

"Audi alteram partem."

"A VICTIM TO SCIENCE": X RAY MARTYR.

To the Editor of THE LANCET.

SIR,—The whole medical profession will, without doubt, greatly appreciate the exceedingly kindly action of Sir William Treloar in bringing to public notice the lamentable condition of Mr. Cox, one of the most truly pathetic cases of scientific martyrdom the world has ever known, and will, I am sure, show considerable practical sympathy with this suffering "victim to science" by a hearty and generous response to Sir William Treloar's appeal.

Early in December last it was my painful experience to visit Mr. Cox, three weeks after his right arm had been amputated, and a more pitiable case I have never witnessed in any human being during my 32 years' professional career.

Sir William Treloar in his letter of Jan. 11th to the *Daily Telegraph* truly describes the excruciating agony Mr. Cox has endured for the past six years, which must have been borne with a fortitude beyond conception, and the many very serious and soul-wearing operations he has been compelled to undergo even to maintain the life that must be almost bereft of human consolation, but words cannot depict the awful condition of the man who has sacrificed his living and shortened and distorted his life for the benefit not only of his country but of the whole human race. His suffering, his martyrdom to the sacred cause of science means the alleviation of pain and sickness in the future of countless thousands of suffering and tortured human beings throughout the world.

This "Victim to Science" has indeed made the English nation his debtor by the extreme efforts he put forth during the dark period of the South African War, as mentioned in Sir William Treloar's communication to the *Daily Telegraph* in the following words : "Working day and night testing the appliances to ensure the utmost value of the X ray apparatus for the use of the English surgeons at the front in the South African War."

To Mr. Cox is also largely due the important invention he worked out with Mr. Hall-Edwards by means of which not only is the position of a bullet located but also its depth, so that a surgeon can now remove an obstacle with a minimum amount of suffering to the patient. Mr. Hall-Edwards, Mr. Cox's co-worker, who lost both his hands, and who, I am pleased to say, has recovered in health and, I understand, is pursuing his profession, was rightly shown his country's gratitude by being granted a pension from the Civil List, but poor Cox, whose shattered health is beyond all doubt irrecoverable, has not only lost his right arm and the middle finger of his left hand, which left hand is withered, but he is totally incapacitated and precluded from earning his living in consequence of his devotion to duty which culminated in contracting the terrible and painful malady of rodent ulcer and a most serious cancerous condition attacking his face, chin, and jaw.

Mr. Donnithorne, in his letter to the *Daily Telegraph* of Jan. 12th, undoubtedly strengthens Sir William Treloar's appeal by the statement that, "Thanks largely to the improvements originated by Mr. Cox cases of martyrdom such as his will be unheard of among future X-ray workers."

Mr. Cox was always ready to give the treatment freely to poor people who could not afford to pay. On the occasion of my visit Mrs. Cox had been occupied for two hours dressing her husband's terribly affected face, and I agree with the Reverend T. Rippon's statement in his letter to the *Daily Telegraph* of Jan. 13th: "I know not who to admire more, the patient sufferer in his agony or the brave wife who nurses him."—I am, Sir, yours faithfully,

FREDK. WM. ALEXANDER, M.R.C.S. Eng., &c.
Hardy-road, Blackheath, S.E., Jan. 18th, 1910.

PS.—Any subscriptions with a view to alleviating his most piteous sufferings will be gladly received and gratefully acknowledged by Sir William Treloar, if sent to the "Cox Fund," 69, Ludgate-hill, London, E.C. Cheques to be crossed London, City, and Midland Bank, Ludgate-hill.

ASEPSIS AND ANTISEPSIS.

To the Editor of THE LANCET.

SIR,—Sir Watson Cheyne contends that there are only three answers to the facts which he has brought forward. The second answer is to show that results as good, if not better, can be obtained by methods other than the antiseptic method. In our paper of November last we attempted to show that at the same hospital, with the same surgeons, seven in number, working during 1906 under "antiseptic," and during 1908 under "aseptic" conditions, and with their results tabulated by the same individuals making the same inclusions and exclusions of cases, the figures, so far as they went, seemed to point in favour of the "aseptic" method. Our figures may not be good, but it is possible that they do include individual results which are as good as those of Sir Watson Cheyne. But this personal equation, which, to our regret, Sir Watson Cheyne introduced into his remarks on our paper, was the very thing we wished to avoid, and it does not come within our province to extract these personal statistics out of our figures. The only really fair method of comparison would be for an independent surgeon to collect from all the London hospitals the results (1) of those surgeons using the "antiseptic" method; (2) of those surgeons using the "aseptic" method, and to exhibit them side by side. We are, Sir, yours faithfully,

HERBERT S. PENDLEBURY.
IVOR BACK.
Brook-street, Grosvenor-square, W., Jan. 17th, 1910.

To the Editor of THE LANCET.

SIR,—Sir Watson Cheyne says "there are only three answers to the facts which I brought forward in my paper of Jan. 1st : (1) to admit their importance, and look into the methods by which they were obtained ; (2) to show that results as good, if not better, can be obtained by other methods ; and (3) to throw doubt on the accuracy of the observations and the judicial care which had been exercised in classifying them."

To deal with the third and least important point first. I am sorry that Sir Watson Cheyne should have thought that I intended to throw doubt upon the accuracy of his observations. In assuming this to be my attitude he has missed the point of my remarks, which was to ascertain whether his criterion of wound infection was the same as my own. Since that criterion is the same—namely, the clinical observation of even the slightest trace of pus visible to the naked eye—I am satisfied that the comparison of the sets of figures given below is a fair one.

The first point can be as readily dealt with. It was, of course, the recognition of the importance of Sir Watson Cheyne's statements which led me to look into the methods by which they were obtained. Those methods include not only the details of his technique but also the criteria upon which the results were judged.

Having obtained answers to both these points from his letter and from the Bradshaw lecture to which he referred me, I am now in a position to gratify his desire to be answered according to the conditions of his second postulate. I think that the comparison which I am able to make is a fairer one than that which Sir Watson Cheyne took in his somewhat exultant paper on the subject of the St. George's statistics. As I pointed out in my previous letter, it was unfair to compare the figures of an individual surgeon with the collected statistics of a number of different operators. Moreover, as I read it, Mr. Pendlebury and Mr. Back were not putting forward their figures as the best possible results of the aseptic system, but in order to show the superiority of that system in the hands of the same operators.

I am well aware of the fallacies which attend the drawing of general conclusions from small numbers of cases. In this connexion the thousand odd cases tabulated by Sir Watson Cheyne was a small number, and those of my own of which I have accurate records—namely, of the two years during which I was resident assistant surgeon at St Thomas's Hospital, and of the years 1908 and 1909—are still smaller. I have, however, been able to balance this drawback by tabulating the results of the last seven years of the late Mr. Clutton's personal cases at St. Thomas's. I do this because the details of my own methods are founded upon,

·results from its use. Dr. Cohen mentions cactus grandiflorus as an instance of a drug which has been pronounced to be pharmacologically inert by some writers as the result of experimental tests, while, on the other hand, another good authority maintains that it possesses high clinical value when carefully prepared and properly used in suitable cases. In deciding on the inclusion of a new drug or the exclusion of an old one a general consensus of opinion among practising physicians must be the criterion. It has been urged ·that when a drug is fairly well represented by an active constituent the latter should be retained to the exclusion of the crude drug and its galenical preparations. Complaint has also been made against the inclusion of too many remedies of one therapeutic class. Dr. Cohen holds the opinion that it would be unsafe for physicians to limit their official armamentarium. Thus, strophanthus and adonis should find a place equally with digitalis; opium, morphine, and codeine should all be officially recognised, and the useful salts of cinchona side by side with the drug itself. There are cases in which continued medication is necessary for a long period when it is desirable to vary that medication. In order to be ·of use to the whole profession it is permissible and even ·necessary to include in a pharmacopœia many drugs of similar action and many preparations of one drug. Active ·principles should not displace crude drugs and their galenical ·preparations, unless physicians in general agree that the active ·principle is the only necessary or desirable preparation.

Mr. Charters J. Symonds will deliver the opening address ·on "The Treatment of Chronic Abscess of Bone by Means of Metal Drains," illustrated by patients, preparations, and ·radiograms, at the Medical Society of London, on Monday, ·Oct. 10th, at 8 P.M. A discussion, to be opened by Sir ·W. Watson Cheyne and Mr. A. E. Barker, will follow.

THE first Hunterian Society's lecture will be delivered at ·the London Institution, Finsbury Circus, E.C., on Wednesday, ·Oct. 12th, at 8.30 P.M., by Dr. H. D. Rolleston, on "Acute ·Arthritis of Doubtful Origin."

THE Harveian Oration will be delivered by Dr. H. B. ·Donkin at the Royal College of Physicians of London, at ·4 o'clock precisely, on Tuesday, Oct. 18th.

THE annual dinner of the London School of Tropical Medicine will be held on Friday, Oct. 14th, at the Hotel Savoy, under the presidency of Mr. James Cantlie.

PRESENTATIONS TO MEDICAL MEN. — On Sept. 26th Mr. J. H. Marsh, medical officer of health of Macclesfield, was the recipient of a silver-mounted walking-stick and leather letter case from the children of Prestbury, ·Lancashire. A short time ago a severe epidemic of scarlet ·fever passed through Prestbury, and under an arrangement between the rural sanitary authorities of Prestbury and the Macclesfield corporation the cases were removed for treatment to the borough isolation hospital at Macclesfield. So ·impressed were the children with the kind treatment which ·they received at the hospital under the direction of Mr. Marsh that on their return home they decided to show their ·love for their medical attendant by making him a presentation. To Mrs. Marsh they gave a handbag and a basket of flowers.—Dr. J. R. Kaye, county medical officer of health for the West Riding of Yorks, and honorary secretary and treasurer for the past 17 years of the Yorkshire branch of the Incorporated Society of Medical Officers of Health, was on Sept. 30th presented with a silver epergne for fruits and flowers by the members of the society. The presentation, which was in connexion with the silver wedding of Dr. Kaye, was made by Dr. J. S. Cameron (Leeds) at the County Hall, Wakefield.

EHRLICH-HATA "606."

BY FLEET-SURGEON W. E. HOME, R.N.

A NOTE by the Berlin correspondent of THE LANCET last July[1] gave an account of the historic meeting of the Berlin Medical Society on June 22nd, when Dr. Wechselmann and the others announced the wonderful results they had been obtaining with Ehrlich's "Hata preparation" in the treatment of syphilis. Being a naval surgeon I was deeply interested, and as I could get to Germany, and was, by the kindness of the Editor of THE LANCET, provided with an introduction to Dr. Wechselmann, I went to see him. He is the head of the division for skin diseases (which includes venereal diseases) in the great (3000 beds) Rudolph Virchow Hospital in Berlin. *Inter alia*, he has long been known for research work done on the protozoa. Before detailing what I managed to pick up about the astonishing effectiveness of this medicine, I think it will be well for the benefit of other general practitioners like myself, who learnt their pathology a good while ago and do not know how the Hata-preparation was discovered nor how it acts, to briefly abstract a paper on this subject by Professor Ehrlich. He gave me a copy when I was in Frankfort, and I hope he will forgive the use to which I put it. It is termed "The Chemotherapy of Infectious Diseases," and was read, I suppose, about August, 1909.[2]

Professor Ehrlich on the Exact Treatment of Infectious Diseases.

"There are two ways of treating disease, one by immunising the patient, immuno-therapy, the other by curing with drugs, chemotherapy. These methods are at certain important points the same; thus the production of antibodies is of the greatest value in each system; still, their differences are more important. Immuno-therapy concerns itself only with the antibodies, which owe their strongly marked specificity to their individual origins. These antibodies direct themselves exclusively against the bacteria and their poisons, to the protoplasm of the patient they do no harm; that is why immuno-therapy is the ideal, the perfect treatment. Without damage to the body it attacks the parasites only. Every sensible man will try to secure for his patient an immunity, active or passive, if immunity be attainable. But in the class of diseases caused by protozoa, malaria, tick fever, and the others, the desired production of antibodies does not occur. Their clinical course shows that this curative reaction of the organism is hindered by the nature of the parasites themselves, so we have to go on killing them with chemical substances, just as we have been doing in the past with quinine, mercury, iodides, and atoxyl. All such chemical substances are poisons; unlike the antibodies, they attack also the patient's organs and tissues and may do him harm even in the doses required to produce their therapeutic effect. Such considerations urged me to make the thorough and systematic examination of this department of therapeutics to which in the last few years I have devoted myself.

In ordinary chemistry the first principle is, *Corpora non agunt nisi soluta;* on the contrary, in chemotherapy, the first principle is, *Corpora non agunt nisi fixata.* That is to say, that unless a drug can combine with the bacteria it cannot kill them; such drugs are called parasitotropic, they attack the parasites. But being poisonous, they also attack the organs of the body, and so are termed organotropic The practical utility of the drug depends on the relation which these activities bear to one another. The organotropic effect should be low, the parasitotropic high, if the drug is to be of any use to us.

The next thing was to find out how the drugs became fixed to the cells, and the most significant ideas came from the study of drug-resisting strains of trypanosomata. Thousands of drugs had been tried against trypanosomes, and those that had curative results fell into three groups:—1. Arsenic group, arsenious acid, then atoxyl, and later the other substitution products of arsenobenzol—viz., arsacetin, and arsenophenylglycol. 2. Azo-stains, trypan red, blue, and violet. 3. Basic stains, parafuchsin, methyl violet, pyronin.

1 THE LANCET, July 9th, 1910, p. 136.
2 Chemotherapie von Infektionskrankheiten v. Professor Ehrlich, Zeitschrift für Aerztliche Fortbildung, No. 23, 1909. Jena, Fischer.

Strains of trypanosomes can be grown to resist either of these groups. When I examined this more exactly (and it was convenient to work with a strain resistant to atoxyl and arsacetin) I began to see there· must be some special arrangements with affinity for particular chemical groups to fix them to the cell. These special arrangements, these bonds, I name chemoceptors. The chemoceptors of the parasite which fix arsenic, and which I call arsenoceptors, unite trivalent arsenic (arsenic as in arsenious acid) to the cell. They do not disappear from an arsenic resisting strain, but only become chemically altered so as to have less affinity for arsenic. And now the arsenic must be present in relatively considerable excess before it can unite with the parasites in such quantity as ultimately to destroy them. Under the microscope these drugs are seen to affect the parasites, causing paralyses, slower movements, or swelling, and in testing the drugs we have to employ them in very various concentrations, and we must also try them on infected animals. In the laboratory examination of each drug there are four possible events.

1. No effect *in vitro*, none *in vivo*. Then neither the parasite nor the body has chemoceptors with affinity for this drug, which is therefore neither parasitotropic nor organotropic.

2. Marked effect *in vitro*, none or little *in vivo*. (This is the action of sublimate on anthrax.) Methylene blue 1/6,000,000 is effective against the spirillum of relapsing fever *in vitro;* used 500 times as strong it produces no effect *in vivo* (Hata). This substance is markedly parasitotropic, but its organotropy [its affinity for the body cells] is so marked that *in vivo* none gets away to attack the parasites.

3. This is called the indirect effect. Nothing *in vitro*, good effect *in vivo*. (*a*) The drug inactive outside is within the body changed into a very active substance. Thus atoxyl, containing five-valent arsenic as arsenic acid, is in the body reduced to para-amido-phenylarsenious acid, trivalent, and that is readily fixed by the arsenoceptors. (*b*) The drug may have no evident effect on the life of the parasite, but may quite prevent its reproduction by some action on its chromatic substance. This race-sterilisation is of the utmost importance when it is with short-lived organisms like trypanosomes we are dealing.

4. Marked effect *in vitro*, even greater *in vivo*. Those parasites killed early, just after the injection, when dead awake an active formation of antibodies, which assist the action of the drug.

Four kinds of effect are also to be noted in the therapeutic results produced by these drugs on infected animals :—

1. No influence—no parasitotropy or organotropy markedly in excess.

2. Exacerbation of the disease. The substance is very little parasitotropic ; indeed, as is usual in small doses, it stimulates the parasites. This occurs with methylene blue, not with arsenic. This result is often met by people working at cancer growth. It is called a contrary effect or Hata's phenomenon.

3. Therapia sterilisans convergens. This is a very common effect, that at which we aim. The parasites gradually decrease in geometrical progression.

4. Therapia sterilisans divergens (Browning's phenomenon). The parasites first increase before finally they disappear.

Now we return to our pharmacology and to the arsenic-resisting strains of trypanosomes. A race of trypanosomes resistant to atoxyl was not affected by the ordinary arseno-benzol derivatives, but we found arseno-phenylglycin which overcame their resistance, and in time we immunised them against this too. We had now two strains immune to arsenic, but each proved still susceptible to arsenobenzol derivatives, provided these had acetic acid in their molecules. So, besides their arsenoceptors, trypanosomes had aceticoceptors, by whose help they could be fixed to more arsenic and so destroyed. The drug was then attached to the trypanosome, not by one, but by several of its receptors (like a butterfly to a setting board by papers), and so I learned there were primary and secondary haptophores. The aceticoceptor is the primary haptophore which fixes the arsenic to the cell. If, then, we wish to use the arsenic group against a class of parasites by the methods of chemotherapy we can only succeed if we find the special suitable attachment, associate therewith the effective chemical group, and in this way make the specific attachment possible.

For the trypanosomata this is achieved through the aceticoceptors. Now the iodide of arsenobenzol which Bertheim

prepared has no effect on trypanosomes in mice, but, as Rohl and Hata have shown, it kills spirilla in mice. Iodising the arsenobenzol nucleus has so reduced its power of fixing itself to trypanosomes that it reaches them in too small quantity to be deadly. But as for spirilla, the iodine enables the arsenobenzol to attach itself to them doubly, with increased effect. And so anyone who busies himself with chemo-therapy must endeavour to find a chemoceptor which shall enable him to force his drug on the parasite concerned.

These advances should lead to great results. Already Hata, Kitasato's sterling pupil, has succeeded after long endeavour in finding amongst a great number of substances two preparations of Dr. Bertheim, No. 599 and No. 606, which are specially fatal to spirilla, and has cured mice of relapsing fever, and fowls of fowl-spirillosis. Rabbit syphilis also gives encouraging results. A large chancre full of spirilla yielded none the day after injection of the animal, and in two or three weeks was well, only a slight scar remaining.

So far I have dealt only with the first stage of the research, which decides whether a substance has therapeutic value and how it may be safely administered. Next, with great expense of time and material, from amongst all these we must choose the best. We may not be able to use a drug though it can cure ; it may be too dangerous. The efficient dose may be 8/10ths or 9/10ths of the poisonous dose ; 1/4th is as near as we dare go. [The fraction for "606" in rabbit syphilis is 1/7th to 1/10th. In man about 1/12th.—Trans.]

I have now completed my account of the labours of the school of chemical therapy. We had set ourselves exclusively to devise substances which we have sifted through innumerable experiments on animals. People feared we would flood the·world with new remedies, but, after all, we have only recommended four—arsacetin, arsenophenylglycin, tryparosan, and the new "606," which Hata investigated.

Now that the work of the laboratory students is ended, a new and at least as difficult a study begins—the introduction of the new remedy into medical practice. Our first difficulty is that in man we cannot directly determine the maximum dose, but only learn it by slow and patient observation. Then men have idiosyncrasies towards about half the drugs we already know. From these animals are free. In relation to these strange and powerful drugs these susceptibilities of men may well be heightened. So the new drugs must only at first be used in well-managed hospitals and under the most patient, thorough, and continuous observation : with the person kept in bed, and all his organs and systems carefully examined. We must exclude all doubtful cases, people of extreme age, people with advanced disease, positive or doubtful history of previous arsenical treatment, special susceptibility to arsenic (which should be tested), retinal changes, and so on. Only after a great number of cases have been so scrutinised and reported on can the remedy be put at the disposal of the profession."

Clinical Employment of the Remedy.

The drug was first tested on man at Uchtspringe, under the direction of Dr. Alt, by two of his assistants, who in October or November, 1909, had 0·1 gramme (1½ grains) injected into themselves. The drug has been used continually ever since in increasing quantity and without disaster. This is largely due to Professor Ehrlich's preliminary work. Dr. Alt said in Berlin, on June 22nd, that the foundation work done by Ehrlich went so deep down there was nothing more required but care and to transfer to man with forethought what was known of its effects on animals. I could not hear in Germany of any disappointments. I was told in England—the story came from Aix—that the new preparation was so dangerous that its use had been forbidden in Germany. This was quite untrue, there never was such an order ; there never was need for such an order. Every case is most exhaustively examined before treatment, special attention being given to the conditions of heart, urine, and retinæ. Retinitis and albuminuria are not absolute contra-indications. That depends on etiology. "606" has cured them when due to syphilis. The blood must be examined by the Wassermann reaction so that recovery may be gauged.[3] Every precaution is taken that no unwished result may occur, or that, occurring, it may give guidance so we may prevent it in future. Unwished results have, in fact, not occurred, so careful and complete were the rules Professor Ehrlich drew up for the first transfer

---

[3] The practitioner may do the Wassermann reaction with von Dungern's bedside apparatus (Merck).

to men of the experience gained by experiments with "606" on many kinds of animals. Besides, he trusted the remedy at first only to most expert and loyal physicians. It is urged that some new-born children succumbed after treatment. True, but their death is not the important thing to remember. Eight newborn children were in the hospital (Wechselmann), all obviously dying from pemphigus neonatorum. Three were treated by the old methods and all died, as had been forecast. With great anxiety, for the drug was new, the other five were injected. Of them, three indeed did die, but the astonishing, outstanding, illuminating fact is that the other two of these doomed infants, injected with the new remedy, contrary to any possible chance there would have been for them three months before, did recover.

As I saw the injection done it was prepared a little differently from that so well described by Mr. J. E. R. McDonagh.[4] But the technique varies between Frankfort and Berlin. I saw it done thus. In the first place everything is sterilised. The pale yellow "606" is shaken out of its glass capsule into a sterilised agate mortar and there rubbed up with some 10 to 15 minims of a 15 per cent. solution of caustic soda till it is all dissolved; a drop of phenolphthalein indicator is added, and next glacial acetic acid to neutralisation. This brings down a bright yellow fine precipitate, and all the contents of the mortar are washed into a test-tube which is centrifuged, the supernatant liquid is poured off, the precipitate mixed with 5 c.c. (ʒi.) or so of normal saline solution and injected in suspension with a sterile syringe. The needle must have a large bore and must be particularly carefully wiped clean with sterile muslin before being used, to diminish the risk of skin necrosis. Women get 0·5 gramme or less, men 0·6 gramme or more. Women are now injected usually under the right mamma; men about the scapular angle. I should think the anterior injection more comfortable, as the patient does not want to lie on the place. The skin, clean already, is painted just before the injection with, I suppose from the colour, liquor iodi fortis half strength. The injection is subcutaneous, but intravenous injection is being considered more effective. The whole dose is able to attack the spirilla at once without the delay of waiting for absorption. The great fear is that the spirilla may, if slowly attacked, develop immunity. Hata found in rabbits that a fourth injection produced no additional effect. Further, intravenous injection causes no pain. The subcutaneous injection causes no trouble worth mentioning at the time; a few hours later pain and swelling begin, and quite often there may be an unimportant rise of temperature of 2° F. for a couple of days. Sometimes there is a necrosis, but that is rare. It is unimportant; I saw the positions of many injections with only two necroses, never an ulcer. The tendency is to increase the dose. If it be too small the Jarisch-Herxheimer reaction is noted—i e., the exanthem deepens or brightens in colour before it disappears. If the roseola develops in two or three days that matters not, but if it appears a fortnight after injection the dose must be repeated. It is difficult for me, who was merely "walking the hospitals," to report on cases; besides, so many have been completely published it is almost unnecessary.

Case shown. "This man had a chancre here, two days ago he was injected. You see the chancre has healed." When a chancre occurs on the skin, if possible I, in my practice, always excise it, and, with luck, it heals by first intention. This saves the patient and his attendants trouble and time; but here is the sore healed, the glands are reduced and no roseola will follow, all by an injection of 9 grains of "606," a vastly superior therapeusis.

I saw an infant about August 23rd that to my inexperienced eye appeared ordinarily healthy. It had been dying a month before from congenital syphilis. July 20th, 0·02 gramme was injected. July 21st, Wassermann positive. August 3rd, repeated 0·02 gramme. August 18th, Wassermann negative. This treatment has only been in use ten months, but relapses do not seem to occur. We hope it kills all the spirilla, but malarial parasites do seem sometimes to hide in the spleen and escape quinine. It may be so here, we cannot know yet.

A woman was injected during pregnancy and her child showed no sign of syphilitic infection. Perhaps we shall be be able to do without the two years' quarantine before marriage. A man walked in. "This man was dying last April

with ulcers of tonsils, uvula, and legs. He was injected and began at once to recover." Probably he got too small a dose as he was so weak, for he had been injected since, in June and August. He had lost nearly all the soft palate, but everything was healed up and he very grateful. So was a woman who appeared another day, having been injected five weeks before. Dr. Wechselmann demonstrated her chest now free of rash, though then quite covered. "Yes," she burst in, "blue-red spots all over it." She was delightedly grateful to her healer. Another case had beside him a painted model of his lesion as it was before his injection ten days ago. There was an ulcer on the palm of the left hand of the size of a crown-piece at the base of the second and third fingers, going deep at the edges. Now all was smooth and on one level, the scar being much the same colour it had been on the cast. Three days later I saw him again. The colour of the scar had faded; it was now shading off into the surrounding epidermis. A remarkable recovery in a fortnight.

A very bad lupus case was shown, injected four days previously; the crusts had now all fallen off without other treatment, and this in four days! Ulcers, too, due to breaking-down of gummata were unusually clean and flat. Their repair is said to be accelerated astonishingly. Local treatment consisted only of acetate of alumina compresses.

Staff-Surgeon Dr. Gennerich of the German Navy showed me two interesting recoveries from paralysis in his wards in the Naval Hospital at Kiel. One man with complete paralysis of the left side of the head and right side of the body, from gumma in the brain, injected yesterday could to-day move his leg and foot and also slightly his hand and fingers. Staff-Surgeon Gennerich had treated 30 cases, all with satisfactory results and with no undesirable complications. He finds larger doses up to 0·7 and 0·75 gramme suitable for young healthy men (Professor Ehrlich subsequently approved this). He also took the greatest trouble in the kindest way to make me thoroughly understand the principles and practice of "606" administration, for which I am very grateful.[5]

In Professor Ehrlich's waiting-room at Frankfort I found a dozen other doctors from Brazil, Holland, Belgium, and elsewhere. (In Dr. Wechselmann's clinique I had met others from Russia, Austria, and Hungary.) Professor Ehrlich's janitor told me that they had been besieged by people wanting the new remedy. I only noted one English name in the visitors' book, that of an Oxford professor. Some were much vexed when they found that there was none of the preparation to be had at the moment. I was the last to see the Professor, and only after an hour's wait. What a tax on his time! He allowed that the discovery of the new remedy was a direct outcome of the side-chain theory of immunity; confirmed what Dr. Gennerich had told me, that the amido group in the "606" molecule took, in curing, the place of complement, which was interesting; recommended intravenous injection; kindly gave me copies of some valuable papers by Hata and himself; and said that supplies at present were scanty, but it was hoped that by November the Höchst Farbwerke would be able to supply the popular demand for the Hata preparation. I then bowed myself out.

I see that it has been used in the Hamburg Tropical Disease School in the treatment of that other obstinate protozoal infection malarial fever from Mamory, in South America, by Dr. Nocht and Dr. Werner.[6] To each of five cases they gave 4½ grains, a very small dose. One case appeared to be cured; in three cases the parasites and fever disappeared for the time, but returned; while in the fifth case the number of the parasites only decreased. A speaker at the Berlin Medical Society on June 22nd stated that the drug had great effect in the healing of wounds. That I have not seen again stated since. Everyone who has any of the remedy wants it for his worst cases of syphilis, especially for those which resist mercury and iodides. It is thought too valuable for that purpose to be employed out of curiosity for anything else yet.

This seeking information about the new preparation was a memorable experience. And again it is a great pleasure to me to acknowledge the courtesy, the warmth of the welcome one gets from our German colleagues. The origin of Ehrlich-Hata "606" is a striking story of a research definitely planned to find a drug which should kill protozoal parasites without injuring their human host. That Ehrlich directed

4 THE LANCET, Sept. 3rd, 1910, p. 711.

5 His paper appeared in Berliner Klinische Wochenschrift, No. 38, Sept. 12th, 1910.
6 Deutsche Medizinische Wochenschrift, 1910, No. 34.

his fellow-workers' efforts successfully in this task demands praise ; that he then got it safely introduced into clinical medicine without disasters arousing suspicion demands our gratitude as well as wonder.

MEDICINE AND THE LAW.

Deaths after Operations and the Jurisdiction of the Coroner.

A QUESTION which may be described as being of some antiquity, but one not often discussed, was raised recently at an inquest held at the Royal Infirmary, Preston, upon the dead body of a man who had died after an operation had been performed upon him.[1] The evidence of the house surgeon, who had been for three years on the staff of the infirmary, was to the effect that the deceased was admitted suffering from intestinal obstruction ; that an operation, if successfully performed, offered the only means possible by which life might be saved ; that one was performed but did not save life, the man dying so soon after the operation that in the witness's opinion the death must be described as having been "accelerated" by it. Without the operation the man would have only survived for a few hours. Upon the replies thus apparently the question was raised as to how far deaths following operations were, or should be, reported to the coroner from the infirmary, and the house surgeon very reasonably pointed out that if an inquest were to be held whenever a patient's death ensued within a few hours of an operation surgeons would naturally be deterred sometimes from performing operations which might, or might not, save life. The coroner and jury unfortunately seem to have resented a statement which for some reason they regarded as a threat, and the reason for which the coroner professed himself unable to understand, but the house surgeon pointed out the probable ill effects of publicity in such a case in causing the public to blame the surgeon for his lack of success and to regard operations with alarm. The coroner, in spite of this, expressed his own opinion that it was compulsory upon him to hold inquests upon persons dying in the circumstances described, owing to their deaths being "unnatural" within the meaning of the Coroners Act, 1887. In this we believe him to have been mistaken, and he would hardly have expressed such an opinion with confidence if he had considered some of the recent pronouncements upon a subject which, as we have said, is by no means a new one. We may point, for example, to the first or general report of the recent Departmental Committee upon the law relating to coroners, in paragraph 16 of which the question of deaths under anæsthetics is dealt with briefly. A recommendation is made that in such cases the death should be reported, but the coroner after inquiry should be enabled to dispense with an inquest when satisfied that due care and skill have been used. The committee does not seem to have thought it necessary to refer in its report to cases of death following recovery from the anæsthetic but accelerated, or suspected of being accelerated, by the operation itself. As to this the committee had before it the evidence of Mr. J. Brooke Little, a barrister of 30 years' standing, and a high authority upon the subject of coroners' law, upon which he was called to speak as an expert. He had it put to him definitely by Sir Horatio Shephard that under the words of the Coroners Act, 1887, a man who dies under an operation dies a violent death. The Act, as all will remember, refers to "either a violent or an unnatural death," but the word violent sufficiently brought the section to the mind of Mr. Brooke Little, who made no suggestion whatever that there was a legal obligation to inform the coroner on such occasions. His answer was, "I do not think that comes within the meaning of a violent death. The usual death certificate of a doctor is 'death from shock.' I think that is the general formula when an operation is being done and the patient dies," and he added as an example when asked whether it was not the unnatural form of stimulus which produced the shock, "You give the symptom, appendicitis, and the immediate cause of death you give as syncope from shock or heart failure, so that it would not be a violent death." The question relating to deaths under anæsthetics, as distinct from those accelerated by the operation, frequently recurred in the evidence of other witnesses before the committee, and

we may refer to the opinion expressed by one of these, Mr. R. Henslowe Wellington, who spoke of the undesirable tendency of reports of inquests to cause alarm in the minds of the public as a reason for not holding them when patients die under an anæsthetic. This gentleman, whose experience as a coroner and writer upon coroners' law is considerable, had no such confidence as that of his colleague at Preston, even where deaths under anæsthetics were concerned. He gave it as his opinion that the law required an inquest, but he said that there was a difference of opinion among coroners on the subject, some holding inquests whenever such deaths were reported to them, and others not doing so if satisfied by inquiry that all care had been exercised. We have, however, cited enough authority to show that the coroner at Preston is almost certainly wrong in an interpretation of the law which differs from that of the great majority of his colleagues. The matter would have been settled long ago if coroners were liable to have their decisions on points of law submitted to the consideration of the High Court, and it might have desirable results if this were in some way to be provided for by statute. As it is, we do not understand that the Bill for amending the law relating to coroners introduced by Sir William Collins in the House of Commons touches the topic which we have discussed above. Clause 9 is designed to enable a coroner to dispense with an inquest if, after the inquiry for which the Bill affords facilities, "he is satisfied that the deceased died a natural death," but this would not affect the decision of a coroner who considered that all deaths accelerated by surgical operations were unnatural.

Another Fatal Case of " Christian Science Healing."

At Urmston, near Manchester, recently an inquest was held upon the body of Walter Statham, a cashier, 53 years of age, who in May of the present year had been attended by a medical practitioner owing to the condition of one of his legs, and at that time had been willing to seek the advice of a surgeon. The surgeon in consultation, with the assent of Mr. Statham's medical adviser, had recommended amputation as necessary, but to this the patient refused to submit and subsequently discontinued all treatment and had recourse to " Christian Science " until his death, which took place on Sept. 25th. A " healer," William Pitfield by name, undertook the case for a consideration of 10s. per week for three visits, at which he offered prayers, accompanied by readings from " Christian Science " text-books and from the Bible. This gentleman declined at the inquest to admit that his "treatment" had been a failure, and was told by the foreman of the jury that he had juggled away the man's life. The coroner, however, pointed out that although if the deceased had been a child a verdict of manslaughter might have been returned against someone, as he was of full age he must be held to have been responsible for his own actions, and a verdict of " Death from septic poisoning " was returned.

The Case of an Unregistered Woman Practising as a Midwife at Leeds.

Three cases at Leeds, heard in the courts upon two consecutive days, recently called attention to the practice as a midwife of a woman named Johnson described as the wife of a miner. An inquest was held on Sept. 22nd on the ground that a child had been buried upon a medical certificate that it was still-born, whereas in fact it had been born alive and had died about three hours afterwards. Johnson had apparently attended the mother when she was confined, and had recommended the father to send for a medical practitioner as the child was " right bad." A medical student at the Leeds Infirmary proceeded to the house on the summons being received at the infirmary, but the child died a few minutes after his arrival in spite of his efforts to restore respiration. The resident obstetric officer at the infirmary, who was informed by the student that the child had given two gasps after his arrival, and that his attempt to induce artificial respiration had failed, after inspecting the body gave the certificate upon which the child was buried, and which stated that it was not born alive. This, he stated in evidence, was because it was prematurely born and could not have lived. In this case the jury returned a verdict of " Death from natural causes," and the coroner referred to the possibility of further inquiry being made with which the jury was not concerned. In that event, no doubt, an explanation of the giving of a certificate in the circumstances described or of

[1] THE LANCET, Oct. 1st, 1910, p. 1046.

THE LANCET,]   THE FORCIBLE FEEDING OF SUFFRAGE PRISONERS.   [AUGUST 24, 1912. 549

PRELIMINARY REPORT ON

THE FORCIBLE FEEDING OF SUFFRAGE PRISONERS.

By AGNES F. SAVILL, M.D. GLASG. ;

C. W. MANSELL MOULLIN, F.R.C.S. ENG. ;

AND

SIR VICTOR HORSLEY, F.R.S., F.R.C.S. ENG.

Danger and Pain.

IT has been stated by the Home Secretary that the practice of forcible feeding is unattended by danger or pain. We have carefully considered the written statements of 102 of the suffrage prisoners, of whom 90 have been subjected to the operation of forcible feeding; we have personally examined a large number of these prisoners after their release, and we have communicated with the physicians who have attended those prisoners whose condition on release necessitated medical care. The facts thus elicited give the direct negative to the Home Secretary's assertion that forcible feeding as carried out in H.M.'s prisons is neither dangerous nor painful. We are confident that were the details of the statements we have read and cases we have examined fully known to the profession, this practice, which consists in fact of a severe physical and mental torture, could no longer be carried out in prisons of the twentieth century.

Forcible feeding has been carried out by nasal and by œsophageal tubes, and by the feeding-cup. The feeding-cup method is frequently forcibly administered solely by the wardresses, without the supervision of a qualified medical practitioner. In the majority of cases the feeding has, on principle, been resisted to such a degree that two doctors and four to six wardresses are required for each operation, and in several instances the officials were held at bay for periods varying from ten minutes to over an hour. But it is to be observed that even in many cases where no resistance was offered, great pain was experienced under the operation. In these circumstances it is not surprising that many prisoners state that after one operation of forcible feeding they experienced more serious symptoms and pain than after several days' starvation. One prisoner we examined (K. M.), a strong woman of fine physique, was so seriously injured by only one feeding that she had to be removed to hospital after it, and she is but typical of a considerable number.

The suffrage prisoners, it should be noted in passing, have never hunger-struck to shorten their sentences, but only to obtain equality of prison treatment for prisoners convicted of like offences, and for justice in observance by the prison officers of the prison rules, especially 234a granted by Mr. Churchill when Home Secretary, but withheld for some time or in part by Mr. McKenna.

According to the Home Secretary, forcible feeding was instituted by him to keep the suffrage prisoners in health and also to prevent them bringing about remission of their sentences, for which, however, they have never hunger-struck. But in the large majority of the cases it has had precisely the opposite effect. Mr. Ellis Griffith admitted in the House of Commons that on one day (June 26th, 1912) from three prisons (Holloway, Maidstone, and Winson Green, Birmingham) no fewer than 22 prisoners had to be released and placed under the care of their friends in order to save their lives. Again, at the commencement of the hunger-strike 12 prisoners were immediately released upon whom forcible feeding was never attempted because the doctors of the prison were afraid to risk the operation upon them. Further, out of a total of 102 cases of prisoners who joined in the hunger-strike we have investigated, 46 were released long before the termination of their sentences because their health had been so rapidly reduced as to alarm the medical officers. In many cases the forcible feeding with the nasal or œsophageal tubes had been carried so far that the condition of the prisoners was so enfeebled thereby as to compel the authorities to release them under the care of a special attendant who accompanied them to their homes and remained with them until the assistance of their friends could be obtained. It is, therefore, not correct to say, as the Home Secretary did in the House of Commons, that he ordered this forcible feeding in order to preserve the health of his prisoners.

No Danger to Life or Health when Prisoner does not Resist.

The Home Secretary, further, has repeatedly stated (see especially Hansard, May 20th, 1912): "There is no danger to life or health from the process of feeding by tube. Where there is any danger it arises from the violent resistance sometimes offered by the prisoners." And Mr. Ellis Griffith stated in reference to a particular case: "If she suffered any pain it was due entirely to the violent resistance she offered to what was necessary medical treatment."

These statements are not borne out by our investigations. One example out of several will suffice to illustrate this point :—

M. F., a skilled trained nurse, never resisted the operation. At Easter she was fed twice daily for eight days. The pain endured surpassed that of any nasal operations she had undergone in previous years, and she lost 13 lb. in weight. The "privileges" of the prison rules demanded being granted by the Home Secretary, the hunger-strike ended. She regained her health, and felt quite strong and well when a second hunger-strike began in June. On the second day of the forcible feeding she had to be discharged on "medical grounds." The pain caused by the forcible passage of the tube through her nose caused a collapse after each feed, and on account of the palpitation and cardiac irregularity set up, the doctors considered further feeding too "dangerous to health" to be persisted in.

This also is a type of many similar cases.

Physical Injuries Inflicted on Prisoners.

During the struggle before the feeding prisoners were held down by force, flung on the floor, tied to chairs and iron bedsteads. As might be expected, severe bruises were thus inflicted. The prisoners, however, did not complain of these. They regarded them as the inevitable consequences of political war.

Forcible feeding by the œsophageal or nasal tube cannot be performed without risk of mechanical injury to the nose and throat. Injuries to the nose were especially common owing chiefly to the lack of previous examination and skill in operating. Though the medical officers were informed in several cases that the nasal passage was known to be blocked and narrowed by previous injury, no examination was made. The prisoners were usually flung down, or tied and held while the tube was pushed up the nostrils. The intense pain so produced often forced uncontrollable screams from the prisoners. In most cases local frontal headache, earache, and trigeminal neuralgia supervened besides severe gastric pain which lasted throughout the forcible feeding, preventing sleep.

One says : "After each feeding it (the nasal pain) gets worse, so that it becomes the refinement of torture to have the tube forced through." The nasal mucous membrane was frequently lacerated, as evidenced by bleeding of the nose and swallowing of blood from the back of the nose. Sometimes the tube had to be pushed up the nostrils three to five times before a passage could be forced. In several such cases bleeding continued for some days ; in one case it recurred for ten days. In another case an abscess followed, with intense pain over the frontal region, which lasted for weeks after release. Swelling of the mucous membrane of the nose and pharynx developed almost invariably ; it was accompanied by Eustachian pain, and frequently this was succeeded by severe pain over the entire area of distribution of the fifth nerve. This trigeminal pain continued as long as the forcible feeding was continued. The equally invariable pharyngitis, which was obviously of septic origin, lasted in certain cases for some time after the release of the prisoner. When the œsophageal tube was employed the mouth was wrenched open by pulling the head back by the hair over the edge of a chair, forcing down the chin, and inserting the gag between the teeth. Naturally, in this process the lips, inside of the cheeks, and gums were frequently bruised, sometimes bleeding and sore to touch for days after. In a number of cases when the wardresses attempted to forcibly feed with a cup, they endeavoured to make the prisoner open her mouth by sawing the edge of the cup along the gums. In one case a cup with a broken edge was used and caused laceration and severe pain.

Accidents.

The danger of forcible feeding is increased by the accidents liable to accompany the passage of tubes down the nose or throat. In several instances the œsophageal tube was passed into the larynx. Even in cases who did not offer resistance great pain and suffocation was caused by the clumsy use of the nasal tube when it coiled up in the back of the throat or came out of the mouth, and then had to be re-inserted several times. The severe choking and vomiting which sometimes accompanied the passage of the tube led to danger from the entrance of food into the larynx.

The injection of food into the lung actually occurred in the case of one unresisting prisoner in whom the operation immediately caused severe choking, and vomiting was followed by persistent coughing. All night the patient could not sleep or lie down on account of great pain in the side of the chest. She was hurriedly released next day, so ill that the authorities discharging her obliged her to sign a statement that she left the prison at her own risk. On her arrival at home she was found to be very ill, suffering from pneumonia and pleurisy due to the food passed into the lung, Being fortunately a young and strong woman, she escaped with her life.

Effects on the Circulatory System.

In a large number of the written statements we find that after the feeding violent palpitation occurred, frequently so severe as to prevent sleep. In certain cases it would appear that the cardiac nerve mechanism was profoundly affected, for a degree of irregularity of the cardiac rhythm is reported even by the physicians attending released prisoners. In some cases who had never previously suffered from any heart trouble this irregularity continued to occur for some weeks after release, in spite of rest in bed under medical care. Giddiness, faintness, and weakness were frequent symptoms. Collapse took place in many cases after but few (2–4) attempts at forcible feeding. The prisoner became icy cold and had to be removed to the hospital cells and surrounded with hot bottles. In most of the cases which came under our personal observation and under the care of other physicians the temperature remained subnormal ($96\cdot4°$ to $97\cdot4°$) for some weeks after release, even although the time was spent in bed with careful feeding and other medical treatment.

Effects of Forcible Feeding on the Stomach and Alimentary System.

The well-known principles and precautions for correct artificial feeding were not observed in the prison forcible feeding. Into the completely empty and contracted stomachs of patients who had fasted for variable periods (usually 24 to 48 hours) the officials (a) rapidly poured (b) large quantities of (c) often cold liquid. Such a procedure, as is well recognised in hospital practice, inevitably causes pain, often agonising, with distension and ballooning of the stomach, as well as spasm of the muscular wall of the organ. As a necessary consequence, regurgitation and vomiting followed in by far the large majority of the cases. The following statement may be quoted as a typical example :—

In Birmingham (May 29th) I was fed by nasal tube. Knowing what to expect I braced up my nerves and sat quietly in the chair instead of struggling and fighting against it as I had done in Newcastle. The passage of the tube through the nose caused me but little inconvenience this time, but its further passage caused me to retch, vomit, shake, and suffocate to such an extent that in the struggle for air I raised my body till I stood upright in spite of three or four wardresses holding me down, after which I sank back in the chair exhausted. When the tube was withdrawn I seemed to be afflicted with chronic asthma and could only breathe in short gasps. To take a deep breath caused me excruciating pain. Two wardresses helped me back to my cell where I lay in agony, the pain becoming worse every moment. I vomited milk which eventually became tinged with blood, &c.

When vomiting did not occur the majority of prisoners suffered acutely from the severe pain of the sudden distension of the stomach. Every prisoner has suffered from indigestion—pain, distension, heartburn, nausea, and sickness. All the medical certificates we have before us from practitioners who have examined prisoners after release include these facts. The following certificate is typical : "At midnight on July 1st I was called to see Miss R. and found her just recovering from an attack of pain, so severe as to collapse her, after attempting to take food on her return from Holloway. I put her on the very lightest nourishment in very small quantities, and otherwise found it necessary to treat her as a complete invalid for some days."

Vomiting often continued for hours after the operation of forcible feeding. The nutritive value of such "ordinary medical treatment," as it has been termed by the Home Secretary, was, of course, in the majority of cases nil, and in many cases life had to be saved, not by forcible feeding, but by the prompt release and restoration of the prisoner to her friends and to legitimate medical treatment. Vomiting was not, as has been alleged in Ministerial statements, brought on by resistance. One of the worst cases was that of a married woman beyond middle life, who made no resistance at all. The following is an abbreviation of her statement :—

After the first feeding by the nasal tube she was locked in her cell and felt as if she would go mad with pain in the ears, running of the nose, and vomiting all through a sleepless night. On the following day she was gagged (though not resisting) and fed by the œsophageal tube, which caused her extreme pain and faintness. The throat bled and she vomited profusely. She fell exhausted on the bed, and was left alone in her cell, where she vomited at intervals all the morning. In the afternoon the feeding process was actually again begun, when suddenly the heart appeared to stop beating. The tube was immediately pulled out, but the patient fainted. She vomited incessantly during the night, feeling intensely ill with a swollen sore throat. In the morning she was released by urgent order of the Home Secretary, and was removed to a nursing home where she slowly recovered strength, until after some days she could be removed to her home.

In this, as in many others, no respite of the feeding or any medical treatment were given. That such malpractices and torture could be meted out to prisoners by medical officers we should have believed impossible at the present day had we not numerous cases of the kind before us. As may be readily understood, the severe indigestion set up by forcible feeding led to other troubles of the bowel. However incredible it may seem, it is a fact that in Holloway Prison the prisoners were locked up in their cells for three to four hours consecutively, by order, it is stated, of the prison doctors, thus being prevented from access to the lavatories at a time when most required. In very many cases dyspepsia has continued for weeks or months after release.

General Inanition.

Medical practitioners who knew certain prisoners before their imprisonment and examined them after release report the supervention of anæmia with considerable loss of weight. One lost 13 lb. in eight days of forcible feeding ; another 9 lb. in five days, another 8 lb. in a fortnight, while others report a loss of 9 lb., of 1 stone, and 2 stone during the term of imprisonment. This is not surprising when one remembers what has been already pointed out in the description of the effects upon the alimentary canal. As the majority of the prisoners vomited up so much of the liquid administered to them, anæmia and decrease in weight were necessary consequences. This result of prison forcible feeding is directly contrary to the results of tube-feeding when used as a form of medical treatment in asylum and hospital practice.

Effects on the Nervous System.

Every physician who has examined the released suffrage prisoners agree that in the majority of cases by far the most serious effects of the treatment by forcible feeding fall upon the nervous system. The younger prisoners escape with the least serious effects, but in those over thirty years of age the nervous symptoms are more marked and more lasting. Before enumerating the symptoms, we desire to point out that the suffrage prisoners enter prison in a totally different state of mind to that which is met with in asylum practice to which the condition of treatment has been compared. These women are normal individuals who go to prison as political offenders ; they are protesting against what is, to them, an unjust anomoly, and they assert in consequence that they should not be treated as common felons. With the keen sense of suffering political injustice rankling in their minds, they determine on the hunger-strike not to obtain release, as has been asserted, but to obtain equal treatment in prison during the term of their sentences for prisoners convicted of like offences, or to obtain from the authorities the due observance of the prison rules.

We are not here concerned to discuss the right or wrong of the political methods of the militant suffragist. We merely point out that on admission the prisoners are in a normal mental condition, which cannot be said of the patients who refuse food in the asylums. We have personally examined a number of the released prisoners, we have obtained medical certificates from the physicians who have attended others immediately on release, we have questioned the friends, and we have carefully considered the statements of those who have not come under medical care until some time after their release. In the evidence we have personally examined, and in the certificates afforded us by other physicians, there is certainly no evidence of "hysteria" —using that much-abused word in the sense of exaggerated or excessive display of emotion. On the contrary, the suffrage prisoners have invariably described their experiences with precision and restraint, deprecating their own share of suffering, and minimising what they have themselves endured. They only expressed themselves with feeling when relating the sufferings of their friends and the repulsive conditions of the prison.

We may group the effects on the nervous system under the following headings : (*a*) Symptoms on release from prison ; (*b*) mental condition during imprisonment.

(*a*) *Symptoms on release from prison.*—Undoubtedly the strain on the nervous system was in every case extremely severe. In general terms, the younger and stronger the physique of the prisoner the less the torture told on the general condition. On the other hand, the better the physique of the patient, the longer she was compelled to endure the feeding, and hence it happened that in several women a state of acute delirium set in, after a long period of courageous endurance, ended only by a hurried release. They can remember nothing of the last 12 hours in prison, the mind being a blank except for the recollection of a sudden consciousness that the doctor and wardresses were surrounding the bed and promising immediate release. For weeks afterwards sleep was broken and disturbed by horrible nightmares and dreams. These patients were on the verge of acute neurasthenia, apathetic and indifferent to matters of interest and importance. In the older patients who had been released at an earlier stage of the forcible feeding, there was a constant feeling of apprehension, with the same symptoms of broken sleep and painful dreams. In others, the characteristic symptoms of neurasthenia were present—inability to concentrate the attention on the simplest matter, loss of memory, hyper-sensitiveness to sounds, great fatigue, and general muscular weakness. In others, again, the following physical signs predominated—weak pulse, irregular at intervals, dyspepsia, pruritus, and vaso-motor instability, all indicating profound disturbance of the system generally. In many cases, under efficient medical care, the nervous system recuperated by means of a maximum of sleep. The patient would be drowsy all day and sleep for 14 to 16 hours out of the 24 during the first week after release was not uncommon. In none of the cases seen by us or by other physicians, nor in the written statements, have we found any mental condition resembling the introspective or irrelevant ramblings met with so constantly in the average self-centred neurasthenic of the text-books and the consulting-room. These patients, without in any way exalting their experiences, regarded them as horrors which must be borne for the sake of the political and moral principle for which they were undergone.

Further physical signs of cerebro-spinal neurasthenia were present in the large majority of the cases examined. The knee reflexes were exaggerated. The patients were readily startled and easily fatigued. In some cases the extreme pain, headache and neuralgia, which had been started by the passage of the tubes, remained as troublesome symptoms. Most were unable to concentrate their attention on professional work for months after. Many patients were kept in bed for a month ; some had tremors, and for several weeks were scarcely able to walk. In one case an attack of functional paralysis of the upper part of the body on the right side followed the sixth attempt at forcible feeding. The patient describes it thus : "The whole of my face and the upper part of my body became rigid, and though I was quite unable to move, or speak, it was fearfully painful to be touched. I had great difficulty in breathing. Later in the evening the doctor told me that he could not stop feeding me on account of this attack. They attempted to feed me next morning, but after several attempts, found it impossible to get the tube down my throat. The same symptoms of paralysis occurred. I was released later in the same day."

Severe retching occurred in every case. In a large number of cases there was frequent vomiting, even when the patient felt too weak to resist the operation, and was suffering only from nervous exhaustion. A few prisoners describe a condition of nervous prostration, with breathlessness, lasting from a few hours to several days. In one case, although the patient took her food in the ordinary way after the first attempt at forcible feeding, the horror of the recollection of the operation, combined with the effects of the shock and pain, reduced her to this condition.

(*b*) *Mental condition during prison.*—To the physical torture of forcible feeding the prison officials in many cases added the intellectual torture of solitary confinement, and to this was added the mental anguish caused by hearing the cries, choking, and struggles of their friends. When there were many cases selected by the medical officers or the Home Secretary for forcible feeding, this mental torture was hours twice and sometimes three times daily. With a nervous system already overwrought by this ordeal, each prisoner faced her own struggle. On an average the resistance could only be overcome by the united services of four to six wardresses and two doctors. After the insertion of the tube the patient often fell into a state of collapse, from which she had scarcely emerged before the terrible noise and cries of the next feeding time began again. Many robust and healthy-minded women whom no one could term neurotic, state that they feared they were going mad ; they could not sleep, and many felt that suicide would be preferable. The terror was accentuated by the fact that in most of the prisons for the greater part of the time of imprisonment they were locked up in their cells of solitary confinement, and left all day and night with the thought of the past and the dread of the future ordeal always before them.

One prisoner whom we interviewed, and whom we can certify as possessing a normal mental condition, writes : "As the hour for forced feeding drew near I could not help being deeply agitated, and I used to stand, or sit, or walk about in a state of horrible suspense, with my heart thumping against my ribs, and listening to the footsteps of the doctors and wardresses as they walked to and fro and passed from cell to cell, and the groans and cries of those who were being fed, until at last the steps paused at my door. ...... My turn had come."

A skilled trained nurse writes : "I will say nothing of the mental misery which accompanies such experiences, because this in indescribable."

Another writes thus : "From 4.30 until 8.30 I heard the most awful screams and yells coming from the cells. I had never heard human beings being tortured before, and I shall never forget it. I sat on my chair with my fingers in my ears for the greater part of that endless four hours. My heart was going like a hammer and the suspense of it all was terrible."

One prisoner had to be dismissed to her home immediately after only a single feeeing because the acute nervous symptoms which followed the operation led the prison officials to fear a complete mental breakdown and to release her immediately in charge of two attendants, although she had only served 12 days of a four months' sentence. The wonder is that so many of the prisoners retained their sanity. Neurologists, however, will understand what consequences may develop in the future.

Many points in this matter of forcible feeding of political prisoners and prison discipline and prison hygiene have a direct medical bearing, but cannot be now considered. In the present one of forcible feeding the importance of sterilisation of the tubes after each case is obvious, and where a number of patients with septic conditions of the nose, throat and mouth, phthisis, &c., are herded together in a prison the danger of infection cannot be exaggerated. Full details of what steps were sometimes taken by the officials in the different prisons cannot be ascertained, but that many prisoners were forcibly fed, one after another, with tubes not sterilised between each case, and by doctors and assistants with unwashed hands was observed by eye-witnesses, as well as by those forcibly fed. Naturally a great deal of infection of the nose and throat occurred.

In the light of the facts enumerated in this briefly summarised paper the position of the medical profession in regard to forcible feeding of suffrage prisoners must be considered anew. We cannot believe that any of our colleagues will agree that this form of prison torture is justly described in Mr. McKenna's words as "necessary medical treatment" or "ordinary medical practice."

VITAL STATISTICS.

HEALTH OF ENGLISH TOWNS.

IN the 95 largest English towns, with an aggregate population estimated at 17,639,881 persons at the middle of this year, 8794 births and 3942 deaths were registered during the week ending August 17th. The annual rate of mortality in these towns, which had been 11·3, 11·0, and 11·5 per 1000 in the three preceding weeks, rose again to 11·7 per 1000 in the week under notice. During the first seven weeks of the current quarter the mean annual death-rate in these 95 towns averaged 11·3 per 1000, and was equal to the average rate recorded in London during the same period. The annual death-rates in the several towns last week ranged from 6·1 in Swindon, 6·3 in Ilford and in Northampton, 6·4 in Wallasey, 6·6 in Rotherham, and 6·7 in Derby, to 16·8 in Bury, 17·2 in Oldham, 17·3 in Liverpool, 17·6 in Plymouth, and 19·1 in Wigan.

The 3942 deaths from all causes in the 95 towns last week showed an excess of 52 compared with the number in the previous week, and included 423 which were referred to the principal epidemic diseases, against numbers steadily rising from 342 to 495 in the six preceding weeks. Of these 423 deaths, 199 resulted from infantile diarrhœal diseases, 109 from measles, 49 from whooping-cough, 30 from diphtheria, 20 from enteric fever, and 16 from scarlet fever, but not one from small-pox. The mean annual death-rate from these epidemic diseases last week was equal to 1·3 per 1000, against 1·3 and 1·5 in the two preceding weeks. The deaths of infants under 2 years of age attributed to diarrhœa and enteritis, which had increased from 72 to 239 in the six preceding weeks, declined to 199 last week, and included 89 in London and its suburban districts, 12 in Manchester, 10 in Birmingham, 10 in Liverpool, 9 in Leeds, and 7 in Sheffield. The deaths referred to measles, which had declined from 156 to 115 in the four preceding weeks, further fell to 109 last week, and caused the highest annual death-rates of 1·3 in Gateshead, 1·5 in Bootle, 2·0 in Wakefield and in Hull, 2·5 in Merthyr Tydfil, and 3·4 in Middlesbrough. The fatal cases of whooping-cough, which had been 44, 54, and 66 in the three preceding weeks, declined to 49 last week ; 13 deaths were recorded in London, 6 in Liverpool, and 2 each in Ipswich, Manchester, Burnley, and Sunderland. The deaths attributed to diphtheria, which had been 40, 31, and 36 in the three preceding weeks, declined to 30 last week, and included 8 in London, and 2 each in Portsmouth, Bolton, Huddersfield, and Hull. The deaths referred to enteric fever, which had been 10, 15, and 10 in the three preceding weeks, rose to 20 last week, of which number 3 were recorded in Bradford, 2 in Portsmouth, and 2 in Rhondda. The fatal cases of scarlet fever, which had

in a paper referred to above, was soon afterwards rediscovered and elaborated in so far as it applies to the sigmoid flexure and the descending colon by Cavaillor and Chalier.[18] The principle applies equally to the operation upon the right side. When carried out thoroughly it results in the colon having as great freedom of movement as the small intestine.

The choice between the two methods of anastomosis—side-to-side or end-to-end—has exercised the minds of surgeons for some years. There are advantages in both. If the peritoneal investments are complete in both ends to be united, then end-to-end anastomosis seems to me an excellent method. It is, however, far more difficult to do with accuracy, neatness, and precision; if done in a slipshod manner disaster is bound to follow, leakage will occur from the suture line, and a general peritoneal infection or a localised abscess will be the result. If the serous covering is incomplete in one or other segment of the bowel, then I think it more prudent to close the two cut-ends and to approximate their serous surfaces in a side-to-side anastomosis, which should always be of ample size. Healing in such an attachment occurs readily, and the union is sound and firm within a few hours. It has been supposed, and the supposition receives undoubted support from experimental observation, that an end-to-end anastomosis allows a more easy onward progression of the intestinal contents. It may be so, but I have never seen any difficulty arise in my own cases when the anastomosis has been made laterally. And as Dr. W. J. Mayo, whose experience is unrivalled, points out, the side-to-side anastomosis seen a few months after its formation differs from the end-to-end very slightly in appearance; a small elbow alone marks the point at which the junction has been made.[19]

THE KINETIC THEORY OF SHOCK AND ITS PREVENTION THROUGH ANOCI-ASSOCIATION (SHOCKLESS OPERATION).

BY GEORGE W. CRILE, M.D.

Introduction.

WHEN a barefoot boy steps on a sharp stone there is an immediate discharge of nervous energy in his effort to escape from the wounding stone. This is not a voluntary act. It is not due to his own personal experience (i.e., his ontogeny), but is due to the experience of his progenitors during the vast periods of time required for the evolution of the species to which he belongs—i.e., his phylogeny. The wounding stone made an impression upon the nerve receptors in the foot similar to the innumerable injuries which gave origin to this nerve mechanism itself during the boy's vast phylogenetic or ancestral experience. The stone supplied the phylogenetic association, and the appropriate discharge of nervous energy automatically followed. If the stone be only lightly applied there is a discharge of nervous energy from the sensation of tickling, but if the sole of the foot is repeatedly bruised or crushed by the stone shock may be produced. The body has had implanted within it other similar mechanisms of ancestral or phylogenetic origin, the purpose of which is the discharge of energy for the good of the individual.

According to my kinetic theory of shock it is one of these mechanisms—the motor mechanism in particular—which, through its phylogenetic association with injury of the individual, is responsible for the discharge of energy represented by shock. According to this theory, the essential lesions of shock are in the brain cells, and are caused by the conversion of potential energy in the brain cells into kinetic energy at the expense of certain chemical compounds stored in the cells.

There is strong evidence that animals capable of being shocked are animals whose self preservation originally depended upon some form of motor activity. In man and other animals this motor activity expressed itself in running and fighting; hence the motor mechanism comprises the muscles and all the organs that contribute to their activity.

Motor activity is excited by the adequate stimulation of the nerve ceptors, both of the *contact* ceptors in the skin and in other tissues, and of the *distance* ceptors or special senses. I assume that stimulation of the distance ceptors (special senses) is as potent as stimulation of the contact ceptors in producing a discharge of energy. I assume, further, that the environment of the past (phylogeny), through the experience of adaptation to environment, predetermines the environmental reactions of the present. In each individual at a given time there is a limited amount of potential energy stored in the brain cells. Motor activity, expressed as action or emotion, following upon each stimulus, whether traumatic or psychic, diminishes by so much the amount of potential energy left in the brain cells. Stimuli of sufficient number or intensity inevitably cause exhaustion or death. If this motor activity, resulting from response to stimuli, takes the form of obvious work performed, such as running, the phenomena expressing the depletion of the vital force are termed *physical exhaustion*. If the expenditure of vital force is due to traumatic or to psychic stimuli which lead to no obvious work performed, especially if the stimuli are strong and the expenditure of energy is rapid—the condition is designated "shock." Shock may, of course, be produced by physical injury without anæsthesia. The first question then is:

Does Inhalation Anæsthesia Prevent Shock?

The word anæsthesia—meaning without feeling—describes accurately the effect of inhalation anæsthetics. Although no pain is felt in operations under inhalation anæsthesia, the nerve impulses set up by a surgical operation reach the brain. We know that not every portion of the brain is fully anæsthetised, since surgical anæsthesia does not kill. The question then is, What effect has trauma under surgical anæsthesia upon that portion of the brain that remains awake? If in surgical anæsthesia the traumatic impulses of operation cause an excitation of the wide-awake cells, are the remainder of the cells of the brain, despite anæsthesia, influenced in any way? If influenced, they are at least prevented by anæsthesia from expression through conscious perceptions or muscular action.

We determined whether or not the "anæsthetised" cells are influenced by trauma under inhalation anæsthesia by noting in patients the physiological functions after recovery from anæsthesia and by examining the brain cells of animals which had been subjected to shock-producing trauma. It has long been known that the vaso-motor, the cardiac, and the respiratory centres discharge energy in response to traumatic stimuli applied to various sensitive regions of the body during surgical anæsthesia. Our experiments have shown that if the trauma is sufficient, exhaustion of the entire brain may be observed after the effects of anæsthesia have disappeared; that is to say, despite the complete paralysis of voluntary motion and the loss of consciousness due to inhalation anæsthesia, the traumatic impulses do reach and influence every other portion of the brain. We observed also that in every instance the changes in the brain cells of the cortex and of the cerebellum were more marked than in those of the medulla and the cord. (Fig. 2.)

There is also strong negative evidence that traumatic impulses are not excluded by ether anæsthesia from that part of the brain that is apparently asleep. For if the factor of fear be excluded, and if in addition traumatic impulses are prevented from reaching the brain by blocking the nerve trunks by local anæsthesia, then, despite the intensity or the duration of the trauma, within the zone so blocked no exhaustion follows after the effect of the anæsthetic disappears, and no morphologic changes are noted in the brain cells. Still further negative evidence that inhalation anæsthesia offers to the brain cells little or no protection from trauma is derived from the following experiments. Dogs whose spinal cords have been divided at the level of the first dorsal segment and that have then been kept in good condition for two months show a recovery of the spinal reflexes, such as the scratch reflex. Animals so treated are known as "spinal dogs." Now in a "spinal dog" the abdomen and the hind extremities have no direct nerve connexion with the brain. For four hours at a time we submitted such dogs to a continuous severe trauma of the abdominal viscera and of the hind extremities. There resulted but slight change in either the circulation or the respiration, and no microscopical alteration of the brain cells

18 Lyon Chirurgical, 1908, vol. i., p. 379.
19 Annals of Surgery, 1910, vol. l., p. 200.

was noted. (Fig. 3.) Judging from a large number of experiments on normal dogs under ether, such an amount of trauma would have caused, not only a complete physical exhaustion, but also a morphologic alteration of all the brain cells and the physical destruction of many; indeed, it would quite surely have killed the animal. We must, therefore, conclude that, although ether anæsthesia produces unconsciousness, it is in reality only a veneer, as it protects none of the brain cells against exhaustion from the trauma of surgical operations.

The Cause of the Exhaustion of the Brain Cells from Trauma of Various Parts of the Body under Inhalation Anæsthesia.

First, Are the brain cell changes due to anæsthetics *per se?* Numerous experiments on animals to determine the effect of ether anæsthesia *per se*—that is, ether anæsthesia without trauma—showed neither the characteristic physiologic exhaustion after the anæsthesia had worn off nor characteristic changes in the brain cells. Observation of the behaviour of individuals under deep and under light anæsthesia during physical injury at once gave the cue to the cause of the discharge of energy, the consequent physiologic exhaustion, and the morphologic changes in the brain cells. Under surgical anæsthesia, if rough handling of sensitive tissues is made, there is observed usually a marked increase in the respiratory rate and an alteration in blood pressure. Under light anæsthesia severe manipulation of the peritoneum often causes such vigorous contractions of the abdominal muscles that the operator may be greatly hindered in his work. Muscular response to trauma under inhalation anæsthesia may be only purposeless moving, but if the anæsthesia is sufficiently light and the trauma is sufficiently strong, movements, unmistakably purposive, may be produced. To injury under inhalation anæsthesia every grade of response may be seen, varying from the slightest change in the respiration or change in the blood pressure to a vigorous defensive struggle. As to the purpose of these subconscious movements there can be no doubt—*they are efforts to escape from injury.* The respiratory centres and the circulatory centres are doing their part in crying out—in trying to escape. So, too, all the rest of the brain cells are doing their part in crying out, in trying to escape, but because of the anæsthetic paralysis the voluntary muscles cannot express themselves. Were it not for the muscular paralysis the patient's face would without doubt express motor activity as strongly as in the accompanying picture of the athlete (Fig. 4) whose motor mechanism is driven by voluntary impulses only. The motor mechanism of a patient under inhalation anæsthesia may be driven even more powerfully, though in silence, throughout the course of a surgical operation.

The result is the same as it would be if a major surgical operation were to be performed under curare alone. Curare completely paralyses all voluntary muscles, but produces no anæsthesia. It gives, therefore, complete muscular relaxation—a dead paralysis that would satisfy the roughest surgeon. During such an operation there would be absolute stillness, but after the paralysing effect of the curare had worn off and the patient had become again able to express himself what would he say? What would the surgeon think? Yet this is just the punishment the surgeon inflicts daily on the subconscious brain, and this explains why a patient in the flood of health and with composed face may emerge broken and shattered and with the facies of the tortured from a severe, perhaps rough, operation under inhalation anæsthesia.

If the trauma under inhalation anæsthesia be sufficiently strong and if it be repeated with sufficient frequency, the brain cells will finally be deprived of so much of their potential energy that they will become exhausted. The resulting exhaustion is the same as that which follows a strenuous and too prolonged muscular exertion, such, for example, as running a Marathon. (Fig. 4.) Whether the nerve energy of the brain is discharged by injury under anæsthesia, by normal physical exertion, or by emotion, identical morphologic changes are seen in the brain cells. The impairment of function in shock from injury, in exhaustion from overwork, and in exhaustion from pure fear is the same. In each a certain length of time is required to effect recovery, and in each morphologic changes in the brain cells are produced. (Compare Fig. 3 and Fig. 10.)

The next questions are these: Is shock produced with equal facility under ether and under nitrous oxide? and What effect has local anæsthesia?

The Anæsthetic Factor in Shock.

Assuming that the morphologic changes in the brain cells are due to the fact that nervous energy is produced by the conversion of certain chemical compounds in the brain cells into simpler compounds, and that this conversion of potential energy into kinetic energy is due to oxidation, then one would expect to find that a given amount of trauma under an anæsthetic like nitrous oxide would produce less change than an equal amount of trauma in an animal under ether; for nitrous oxide, more than ether, owes its anæsthetic property to its interference with the use of oxygen by the brain cells. Testing this point experimentally, we found that under approximately equal trauma the changes in the brain cells were approximately three times as great under ether anæsthesia as under nitrous oxide anæsthesia; that the fall in the blood pressure was on the average two and a half times greater under ether than under nitrous oxide (Fig. 5); and finally, that the condition of the animal was better after trauma under nitrous oxide than after equal trauma under ether. In the course of operations on the human body one observes constantly the same protective effect of nitrous oxide. This, however, is what one should expect if the kinetic theory of shock is true. Then, too, the mere excitation due to the feeling of suffocation while inhaling ether causes a certain amount of exhaustion. On the kinetic theory no shock could be produced by traumatising a territory infiltrated with local anæsthetics—a territory whose nerve connexion with the brain has been broken by nerve blocking, thus reproducing the condition of a "spinal" dog whose cord has been divided in the upper dorsal region. Our experiments showed that neither brain cell changes nor physical exhaustion were produced by any trauma, however severe or prolonged, inflicted upon a "blocked" territory. We concluded, therefore, that the traumatic impulses must reach the brain to cause shock. (See Fig. 3.)

We have not yet shown, however, that the brain cell changes are not due to some secondary factor, such as internal secretions, altered gases in the blood, or other metabolic changes.

Are the Brain Cell Changes due to Internal Secretions or to Altered Gases in the Blood?

If the kinetic theory of shock be correct, then if the circulation of two dogs be so anastomosed that the blood streams of both animals freely intermingle and if only one animal be traumatised, the functional impairment and the brain cell changes will be limited to the animal receiving the injury; but if shock be due to the production of some noxious secretion, to some poisonous product of metabolism thrown into the blood stream, secondarily affecting the brain, or if shock be due to gaseous changes in the blood caused by trauma, then both dogs should suffer equally.

Our experiments were as follows. The proximal end of one carotid artery of Dog A was anastomosed with the distal end of the corresponding carotid artery of Dog B, and one jugular vein of Dog A was then anastomosed with the corresponding vein of Dog B, so that the blood streams of both animals intermingled with entire freedom and in large volume. (Fig. 6.) The dogs were approximately of equal weight and physical condition. For two hours Dog A was traumatised. The animals were killed simultaneously, and their brain cells were studied by parallel technique. The experiment showed brain cell changes—typical shock changes—only in Dog A, the dog whose body had been traumatised, and no brain cell changes in Dog B, whose body had not been traumatised, but through whose brain the blood of the traumatised dog flowed freely during the two hours. This result strongly supports the kinetic theory, and with equal strength opposes any theory which implies that internal secretions, gaseous changes in the blood, or the production of noxious products may secondarily cause brain cell changes. (Fig. 7.)

Does Anæmia Alone Cause Brain Cell Changes?

There remains also the possibility that low blood pressure —anæmia alone—may cause the brain cell changes. We have shown elsewhere the destructive effects of anæmia on the brain cells; that in resuscitation experiments a total anæmia of seven minutes caused fatal brain cell changes; and that brain cell changes are also produced by low blood

FIG. 1.—*Classification.*

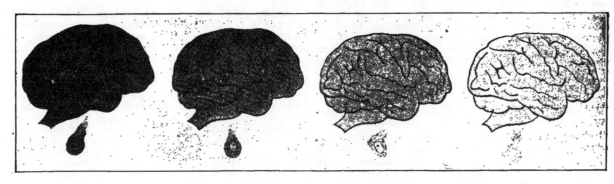

Hyperchromatic.   Normal.   Fatigued.   Exhausted.

FIG. 3.—*Areas from Cerebellum.*

FIG. 2.

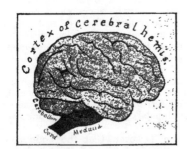

Changes more marked in cortex and cerebellum than in medulla and cord.

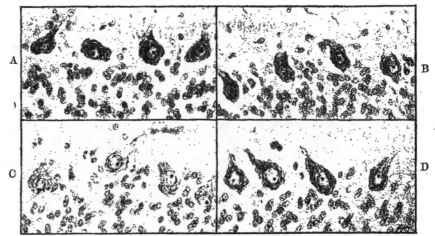

A, Normal dog.   B, Shocked "spinal" dog.   C, Shocked dog (ether anæsthesia).
D, Shocked dog (N₂O anæsthesia.)

FIG. 5.

FIG. 4.

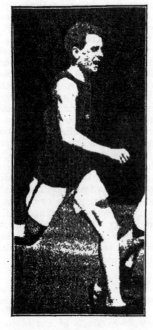

A Marathon runner.

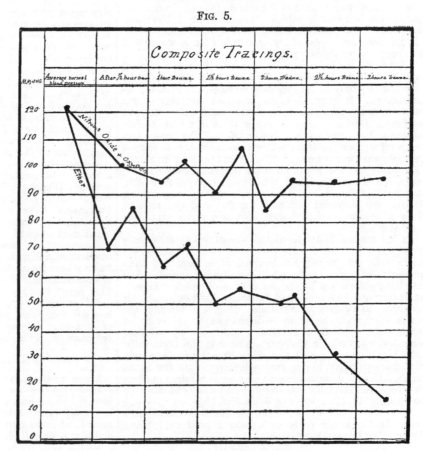

injection of the guinea-pig with anti-rabbit-plate serum, and *vice versâ*. Recently, being in possession of a supply of anti-guinea-pig-plate, anti-rabbit-plate, and anti-rat-plate sera, one of us has carried out the following experiment, which shows clearly that a heterologous anti-plate serum has no purpura-producing property.

TABLE V.

Rat A, 150 gm., received 7/12/1914, 3 c.c. anti-rat-plate serum.
„ B, 90 „   „   „   3 „ anti-guinea-pig-plate serum.
„ C, 140 „   „   „   4 „ anti-rabbit-plate serum.
(All inoculated subcutaneously.)

Guinea-pig A, 230 gm., received 7/12/1914, 3 c.c. anti-guinea-pig-plate serum.
„   B, 230 „   „   „   3 „ anti-rat-plate serum.
„   C, 230 „   „   „   4 „ anti-rabbit-plate serum.
(All inoculated subcutaneously.)

Rabbit A, 400 gm., received 7/12/1914, 4 c.c. anti-rabbit-plate serum.
„   B, 380 „   „   „   4 „ anti-guinea-pig-plate serum.
„   C, 380 „   „   „   4 „ anti-rat-plate serum.
(All inoculated intraperitoneally.)

On Dec. 8th Rat A showed several purpuric spots near tail and also on legs. Other two rats showed nothing and appeared quite lively. Guinea-pig A had an extensive hæmorrhagic infiltrate over the whole of the abdomen and did not appear well. The other two animals showed no purpura and were quite lively. Rabbit A had numerous purpuric spots all over its skin and was obviously ill. The other rabbits were quite lively and showed no purpura. On Dec. 9th the animals inoculated with the homologous sera were still more drowsy and listless. Other animals appeared quite well. On Dec. 10th Guinea-pig A and Rabbit A dead.

Post mortem: Guinea-pig A showed beautiful skin purpura, extensive œdematous and hæmorrhagic infiltrate spreading over abdomen from seat of injection and extending deeply into the thigh muscles, and miliary purpura of stomach. There was no cataract, and the urine was quite clear. Rabbit A showed a large œdematous and hæmorrhagic subcutaneous area over upper thorax, neck, and fore limbs, also a larger hæmorrhage under skin of left cheek. Miliary purpura of stomach and slight purpura of intestine. Liver yellow and mottled. No cataract. Urine quite clear.

The other animals remained well and put on weight.

Dec. 11th: Rat A dead. Post mortem: Purpura of skin particularly marked over skull and cheek. A few spots in pyloric portion of stomach and a few in small intestine. Urine was blood-stained (hæmoglobinuria).

The other animals, which received the heterologous plate sera, remained well and put on weight.

Summary and Conclusions.

1. Data have been recorded on the blood changes in guinea-pigs after inoculation with anti-guinea-pig-plate serum. The early fall in the number of platelets simultaneously with the outburst of skin purpura is found to be a marked feature.

2. Purpura has also been produced in rabbits and rats by inoculation with the respective anti-plate serum. The blood changes in rabbits have been followed with results similar to those obtained in guinea-pigs.

3. Anti-plate serum, in addition to its purpura-producing properties, possesses in common with other cytolytic sera considerable lytic powers, which in all probability contribute largely towards the fatal issue in small animals. Death, however, may occur as the result of extensive hæmorrhages alone without any obvious lytic changes as evidenced by hæmoglobinuria.

4. Sera obtained by immunisation with red cells or leucocytes do not produce purpura.

5. Purpura is not produced by inoculating animals with heterologous anti-plate sera.

The histology of the purpuric lesions will form the subject of a later communication.

A CONTRIBUTION TO THE STUDY OF SHELL SHOCK.

BEING AN ACCOUNT OF THREE CASES OF LOSS OF MEMORY, VISION, SMELL, AND TASTE, ADMITTED INTO THE DUCHESS OF WESTMINSTER'S WAR HOSPITAL, LE TOUQUET.

BY CHARLES S. MYERS, M.D., SC.D. CAMB.,
CAPTAIN, ROYAL ARMY MEDICAL CORPS.

THE remarkably close similarity of the three cases which are described in this paper is shown in the following synopsis:—

—	Case 1.	Case 2.	Case 3.
Cause... ...	Shells bursting about him when hooked by barbed wire.	Shell blowing trench in.	Shell blew him off a wall.
	Preceding period of sleeplessness.	As in Case 1.	?
Vision ...	Amblyopia. Reduced visual fields.	„	As in Case 1.
Hearing ...	Slightly affected for a brief time.	Not affected.	As in Case 2.
Smell... ...	Reduced acuity.	Total anosmia.	Unilateral anosmia and parosmia.
Taste	Almost absent.	Reduced acuity.	As in Case 2.
Other sensations ...	Not affected.	As in Case 1.	As in Case 1.
Volitional movements	„	„	„
Defæcation	Bowels not opened for five days following shock.	„	„
Micturition	Urine not passed for 48 hours.	Not affected.	As in Case 2.
Memory ...	Apparently slightly affected.	Very distinct amnesia.	„
Result of treatment	Gradual improvement by rest and suggestion.	As in Case 1, supplemented by hypnosis	As in Case 1.

CASE 1.—Private, aged 20. Admitted on Nov. 5th, 1914. On the nights of Oct. 28th and 29th he slept in the booking hall of X station; "not much sleep there." On the 30th he motored in a 'bus from X to Y, arriving there at 7.30 P.M.; billets found at 8 P.M.; on guard from 10–11.30 P.M., and from 1.45–3.45 A.M. At 11 A.M. on the 31st for the first time he went to the firing line. His platoon advanced to one set of trenches and then crossed the road to another, only to find it filled with cavalry and to be told that there was no room for them. During the retirement from this trench, at 1.30 P.M., they were "found" by the German artillery. Up to that time he had not been feeling afraid; he had "rather been enjoying it," and was in the best of spirits until the shells burst about him.

He was now retiring over open ground, kneeling on both knees and trying to creep under wire entanglements, when two or three shells burst near him. As he was struggling to disentangle himself from the wire three more shells burst behind and one in front of him. (An eye-witness in this hospital says that his escape was a sheer miracle.) After the shells had burst he succeeded in getting back under the wire entanglements; all his comrades had retired already. He managed to get into a trench, and as the firing slackened he rejoined his company. Immediately after the shell burst in front of him his sight became blurred. It hurt him to open his eyes, and they "burned" when closed. The right eye seemed to have "caught it" more than the left. At the same moment he was seized with shivering, and cold sweat broke out especially round the loins. He thinks the shell behind him gave him the greater shock—"like a punch on the head, without any pain after it." The shell in front cut his haversack clean away and bruised his side, and apparently it burned his little finger. It was this shell, he says, which "caused his blindness."

Falling in with two comrades, he was led by them, one on either side, to the dressing station. He opened his eyes occasionally to see where he was going, but everything

928 THE LANCET,]   NEW INVENTIONS.   [OCT. 23, 1915

combination. The total amount of iron found in four oysters was 0˙0054 gramme (Fe). Of this a notable proportion occurred in the gills, which is consistent with the view that the green pigment is due to vegetable matter (e.g., sea algæ or sporules of the seaweed called crowsilk) containing, of course, chlorophyll with its complement of iron.

It is well established that the blood of molluscs contains hæmocyanin, which is identical with the hæmoglobin of mammals except that instead of iron combined with protein it is copper, and therefore it is not surprising to find traces of copper in the oyster, but the quantity is so minute as to place it beyond any suspicion of harmful action. It is interesting to remember, also, that hæmocyanin is not a copper salt in the ordinary sense, as it does not give the reactions of copper ions until decomposed. At all events, we have found decidedly more copper in the ordinary oyster or the white-beard than in the greenbeard, and so the theory of the green pigment in the latter being due to copper receives practically no support in the light of these results. Copper is, we find, an invariable constituent of oysters, but by far the largest proportion of it occurs in the fleshy part of the oyster, chiefly liver, and not in the beard even of the greenbeard. It was unfortunate that this oyster was ever called the greenbeard. Such a name as the "crow-silk" oyster would perhaps have forestalled prejudice altogether.

Objection against the greenbeard on account of its colouring cannot be sustained, and such a prejudice does not only an injustice to an important and deserving industry but leaves neglected a source of wholesome food-supply at a time when every available food-stuff should be employed. The war has very seriously handicapped our fisherfolk chiefly by restricting their operations within narrow limits round our coasts, so that much of the usual harvest of the sea is lost. Many of them are turning their attention perforce, therefore, to in-shore fishing. Our trade with the continent has necessarily declined in such matters as oysters, and oysters were exported in large quantity before the war. In the narrow channels or "fleets" running up between the extensive areas of practically uninhabited walled marshes which lie between the south-west portion of Mersea island and the estuary of the Blackwater, there exists an extensive system of oyster cultivation, conducted on the small holding system by working dredgermen. Each man cultivates one or more layings, usually about 100 yards long, and the width of the "fleet" varies from, say, 30 to 100 yards. The men have now formed a coöperative society with the view of establishing a home retail trade so that the public can obtain oysters and other fish direct from the fishermen. This enterprise claims support, for its development would help a worthy group of fisherfolk to secure subsistence during very anxious times, while the public would have the assurance of getting a fresh and wholesome supply of fish food.

New Inventions.

A NEW FOLDING STRETCHER.

AN improved form of folding stretcher for bringing the wounded back from the firing line has been designed by Messrs. A B. and F. Willis, of 25, St Mary Axe, London, E.C. When fully extended it has precisely the dimensions of the standard type of stretcher and fits into ambulance wagon

FIG. 1.

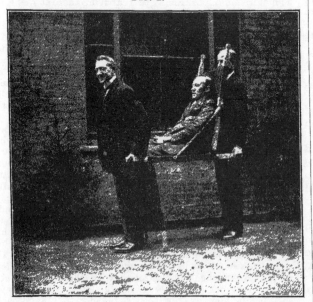

or train ; but it can instantly be folded so that the patient takes up a sitting posture when there is not room in the trench for a long stretcher. (Fig. 1.) The makers believe that all the wounded who can be picked up could be taken along the communication trenches to the hospitals by means of their patent stretcher, and that without delay or exposure to fire in places where the length of the ordinary stretcher has necessitated either removal from the stretcher or tilting to negotiate the sharp corners or passing over the parapet of traverses, &c. It can also when folded be easily carried strapped on to the back (Fig. 2) as the weight is only about 28 lb., but for this purpose the addition of shoulder straps is desirable. We have tested the stretcher, carrying a member of the staff along a tortuous communicating passage, and can confirm the claims made on its behalf. The illustrations show the general features ; the construction is strong and simple, and the difficulty of connecting the folding bars so that they shall be sufficiently rigid when straightened has been successfully overcome The design is a further development of the short Fusilier trench stretcher, in which the patient's feet hang down and his back rests against the hinder bearer, described by Captain G. K. Aubrey, R.A.M.C., in THE LANCET of Dec. 26th, 1914, p. 1488, and appears to us a distinct improvement on this in its ready convertibility We are informed that ten of these stretchers are now being tried in France.

FIG. 2.

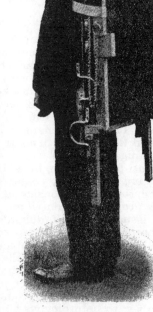

Correspondence.

"Audi alteram partem."

COLD-BITE + MUSCLE-INERTIA = TRENCH-FOOT.

To the Editor of THE LANCET.

SIR,—Venous stasis, the anatomical basis of the trench-foot, is not simply an effect of cold or of wet, or of both. The feet may be aglow after a ten-mile snowshoe tramp with the thermometer 20° below zero. The men actively at work on the big timber rafts in Canada have wet and cold feet for weeks without any ill-effects. So long as the muscles of the legs work freely the circulation in the feet is good. It is not the cold, nor the wet, nor the puttees, nor the type of boot; the damaging factor is the comparative inertia of the leg muscles. To keep the trenches dry will help, to shorten the time spent in them will help, special socks may help, but the disabling effects of cold-bite are inevitable in feet attached to legs whose muscles have not play enough to maintain a circulation hampered by gravity and cold and wet.

I am, Sir, yours faithfully,

Oxford, Dec. 12th, 1915.   WILLIAM OSLER.

"TRENCH FEVER."

To the Editor of THE LANCET.

SIR,—Captain G. H. Hunt and Major A. C. Rankin give in THE LANCET of Nov. 20th a most interesting description of their research to ascertain the cause of the intermittent pyrexia known as trench fever. Although they have not so far arrived at any positive conclusion as to its cause, they have at all events excluded micro-organisms, protozoal or bacterial, as a possible cause of the fever.

It did not, apparently, occur to them to investigate the atmospheric environment of the men in the trenches as a possible cause of this fever, for I am unable to find any reference to it in their paper, with the exception that nearly all their patients suffering from this fever had been exposed to cold and damp from sleeping on wet ground or from rain. Cold and damp are, however, very indefinite terms unless supplemented by actual readings of the dry and wet bulb thermometers. A patient in the initial, chilly stage of pyrexia may feel the air cold, although the thermometer shows it is warm, 14·6° C. (58·0° F.) to 22·2° C. (72·0° F.) or even hot, i.e., above 22·2° C. (72·0° F.). So also a patient in the hot stage of pyrexia may feel the air dry when the hygrometer shows it to be damp, i.e., having a relative humidity of from 66 per cent. to 80 per cent., or even very damp, i.e., above 80 per cent. of saturation. In Ravenstein's classification of climates he confines the term cold to those climates having a mean atmospheric temperature of 0·0° C. (32·0° F.) or lower, and the term damp to those climates which have a mean atmospheric humidity between 66 per cent. and 80 per cent. of saturation.

In order to appreciate the impediment to loss of heat from the body by radiation, by evaporation, and by conduction and convection, presented by the atmospheric conditions in the trenches it would be necessary to have hourly records of the dry and wet bulb temperature, and the rate of movement of the air for a continuous period of 24 hours. If such records were available then it would, within certain limits, be a simple matter to show whether the physical atmospheric conditions in the trenches are such as would raise the body temperature of those immersed therein above normal, i.e., cause fever, and also whether the fever so caused would be of intermittent, remittent, or continued type. For we have a standard of physical atmospheric conditions which are known to raise the body temperature of many of those immersed therein to 37·7°C. (100·0° F.) and even higher in less than four hours. This standard is to be found in the valuable reports of the Departmental Committee on Humidity and Ventilation in the spinning and weaving sheds in Lancashire and in Ireland. In these reports are recorded certain definite combinations of atmospheric temperature, humidity, and stagnancy which were found by observation to raise the body temperature of many of the operatives above normal, and also the degree to which the body temperature was raised thereby. By comparing the atmospheric conditions in the trenches with these it would be possible to see whether the former are such as would cause fever and also whether the type of such fever would be intermittent, remittent, or continued.

The trenches are apparently deep, narrow, sinuous ditches, excavated from the soil and partly covered, in which the air does not circulate very freely, and often having wet floor and sides. When such trenches are crowded with men, each having a body temperature of 36·6°C. (98·4°F.) and giving off water vapour freely from his skin and lungs, the air in the trenches must rapidly become warm or even hot, damp, and stagnant, especially in the warm or hot seasons, similar to the atmosphere which raised the body temperature of the operatives in the spinning and weaving sheds to 37·7°C. (100·0° F.) or even higher in less than four hours. If the physical atmospheric conditions are recorded as I have suggested, then by comparing the details of temperature, &c., with those of the atmosphere which raised body temperature in the spinning and weaving sheds it could be seen whether the atmospheric conditions in the trenches are such as would cause fever.

If any medical officer or meteorologist going into the trenches desires it I will be glad to furnish him with a list of 56 different combinations of atmospheric heat (between 69·0° F. and 90·0° F.), humidity, and stagnancy which were found to raise body temperature to 37·7° C. (100·0° F.) and even higher in less than four hours. Then with the aid of dry and wet bulb thermometers and a delicately constructed anemometer he could easily prove whether the atmospheric conditions in the trenches are such, especially in the summer and autumn, as would cause fever or not.

I am, Sir, yours faithfully,

MATHEW D. O'CONNELL, M.D.

Harrogate, Dec. 8th, 1915.

To the Editor of THE LANCET.

SIR,—In his letter of Nov. 27th Dr. Henry Robinson suggests that some, if not all the reported cases of trench fever were examples of paratyphoid fever. The following points would go to disprove this supposition :—

1. The temperature chart, with its characteristic fall to normal about the fifth day, is very unlike that of paratyphoid fever.

2. The pulse is not slowed.

3. No rash, although repeatedly looked for, has ever been found.

9. The theory of "acidosis" is still incomplete. The modes of origin of "acetonuria" are complex, and are largely influenced by the amount of carbohydrate food assimilated.

10. For the solution of such difficult problems the coöperation of clinical physicians and experts in organic chemistry is essential.

Appendix.

Examples of errors and inaccuracies culled from text-books on medicine and on urinary analysis.

1. Acetone gives a red colour with ferric chloride. This error occurs in Fagge, "Practice of Medicine," edited by Pye-Smith, 1888; and also in Roberts's "Treatise on Urinary and Renal Diseases," fourth edition, 1885. Gerhardt's test for acetoacetic acid was described in 1865.

2. Other substances (than acetoacetic acid)—e.g., formic, carbolic, and salicylic acids—give the *same* reaction in both fresh and previously boiled urine. For *same* read *somewhat similar*. No practised eye would confound the colours.

3. Both oxybutyric acid and acetoacetic acid react similarly with the ferric chloride test. This is not the case.

4. "Fehling's solution is reduced by acetone, but this test should be applied to the distillate from the urine." Acetone does not reduce the copper solution.

5. Rothera's nitroprusside test is true for acetone only. It is a much more sensitive test for acetoacetic acid.

6. Many drugs produce temporary diabetes. For *diabetes* read *glycosuria*.

7. "Large quantities of water are required (by the patient) to keep the sugar in solution, and for its excretion in the urine." Glucose is soluble in its own weight of water. The quantity of glucose in the blood of a severe case of diabetes is a fraction of 1 per cent.

Dublin.

TREATMENT OF SEPTIC WOUNDS, WITH SPECIAL REFERENCE TO THE USE OF SALICYLIC ACID.

NOTES BASED ON CASES AT THE MILITARY HOSPITAL, ENDELL STREET.

BY LOUISA GARRETT ANDERSON, M.D., B.S. LOND.,

CHIEF SURGEON;

HELEN CHAMBERS, M.D., B.S. LOND.,

PATHOLOGIST;

AND

MARGARET LACEY, B.Sc.,

RESEARCH ASSISTANT UNDER THE MEDICAL RESEARCH COMMITTEE.

THIS paper is based upon observations made upon approximately 1000 cases of septic wounds treated in the wards and operating theatres of the Military Hospital, Endell-street, during the period of six months from May to October, 1915. With the exception of a few cases from Gallipoli, all the men belonged to the British Expeditionary Force in France, and the majority were admitted to the hospital a few days after they were wounded.

While anaerobic infection was comparatively rare, septic infection was present to a varying degree in all the wounds. In order to test the effect of treatment on the bacterial growth in the wounds numerous agar cultures were made. The usual procedure has been to take cultures from the surface of the wounds, before and immediately after the dressings, each morning on successive days. After overnight incubation at 37° C. the relative number of colonies which developed on these cultures was noted. When wounds are irrigated with reagents such as hydrogen peroxide, weak solutions of perchloride of mercury, carbolic or boric acid lotion. there is often little difference to be noted in the number of colonies which develop on the cultures taken before and after the dressing or from day to day. For this reason the efficiency of many antiseptics when applied to wounds has been questioned, and it is evident that with reagents such as these the action of the lotion is often largely mechanical.

Many of the cases on admission were treated with hypertonic saline solution, either with continuous irrigation or with wet applications repeated two or three times a day. A preliminary test was made to determine the extent of bacterial growth which occurs in a nutrient medium containing varying quantities of salt. The organisms used were the staphylococcus pyogenes aureus and the bacillus coli communis, and cultures were grown in a series of broth tubes containing from 0·5 to 12 per cent. sodium chloride. Quantitative estimations were made of the number of living bacteria added to the culture tubes and the number present after varying periods of incubation. With both micro-organisms proliferation occurred in 5 per cent. salt broth—i.e., in the strength of saline usually employed for surgical purposes; this was, however, much less rapid than in the lower salt dilutions. For example, in broth containing 5 per cent. saline staphylococcus pyogenes aureus increased after 24 hours incubation at 37° C. from 9 millions to 77 millions, and after three days to 708 millions. In broth containing 0·5 per cent. saline staphylococcus pyogenes aureus increased in 24 hours from 9 millions to 435 millions, and in three days to 1012 millions. In the 7 per cent. and 8 per cent. salt media multiplication was still further delayed. In the 10 per cent. and 12 per cent. salt cultures no proliferation occurred; the cultures of staphylococcus pyogenes aureus were still alive after 24 hours, but those of bacillus coli communis were sterile. It follows that when 5 per cent. hypertonic saline is applied to a wound the inhibition of growth due to the salt alone can only be very slight.

The majority of septic wounds heal rapidly if good drainage is provided and frequent dressings are applied. The choice of lotion seems immaterial provided the one selected is non-irritating and fresh infection is prevented. The ultimate recovery of the patient depends upon physiological processes, and if preference is given to any of the above reagents for routine treatment it would be to that which reinforces the physiological processes in the tissues of the wounds—viz., hypertonic saline solution.

In certain cases treatment with the so-called antiseptic lotions and hypertonic saline was not successful, and it was recognised that some improved method was required. The plan adopted was to select a few wounds which did not yield to ordinary treatment. These cases were made the object of a special investigation. Two antiseptic reagents were tried: (1) Eusol, as introduced by Professor Lorrain Smith and his collaborators [1]; and (2) salicylic acid.

Treatment with eusol.—In eusol we possess a valuable and cheap antiseptic. In our experience the immediate effect of eusol is to sterilise the surface of the wound with which it comes in contact. Cultures taken directly after irrigation remain sterile. Numerous colonies, however, will develop on cultures taken after an overnight interval, and there is often no reduction of bacterial growth from day to day. The effect of the eusol is temporary only, because of the infection of the deep tissues. This is well recognised, and to meet the difficulty frequent application or continuous irrigation has been advised. In some cases, however, it is not easy to arrange for continuous irrigation, and whatever contrivance is adopted there is a tendency for the lotion to flow through certain channels to its exit, with the result that large areas of the wound do not get irrigated. In spite of these disadvantages, the clinical results obtained from eusol are very encouraging, and some cases have responded more rapidly to it than to other reagents. The following case illustrates its use :—

CASE 1.—Private, aged 19. A large abscess of the calf of the leg was opened; the pus grew staphylococcus pyogenes aureus. The cavity was irrigated with eusol and packed loosely with gauze soaked in eusol. Irrigation and the dressing were repeated twice daily, and each morning cultures were taken from the wound immediately before the irrigation. A series of cultures were thus obtained. From the first to the sixth day numerous colonies grew, and the cultures were indistinguishable from one another. On the seventh day there was a marked reduction in the number of colonies. On the eighth day only two or three colonies developed, and the subsequent healing of the wound was rapid. This series can be explained by the fact that free exudation from the abscess during the first six days diluted the eusol and washed it away from contact with the tissues. It was only when the exudation ceased that the antiseptic remained in contact sufficiently long for its action to be evident after an overnight interval.

In cases where eusol has not been a success the failure was apparently due to the fact that continuous treatment was impossible, and the effect of the antiseptic was transitory. Very little reagent is left in contact with the

---

[1] Brit. Med. Jour., July 24th, 1915; THE LANCET, Feb. 5th and 12th, 1916.

surface of a well-drained wound after irrigation with a watery solution. Treatment with salicylic acid in various forms was therefore tried, in some cases with conspicuous success.

Treatment with salicylic acid.—The examination of healing wounds shows that the presence of a certain number of bacteria need not be detrimental. In many instances rapid healing occurs in spite of their presence. Healing is usually not delayed unless exudation collects or the bacterial growth becomes sufficiently plentiful to liberate toxin or to produce ferments which digest the tissues. A continuous inhibition of bacterial growth may be more effective than the action of a powerful but transitory reagent. Salicylic acid is not such a powerful antiseptic as the hypochlorites, but it lends itself to continuous administration. Its properties as an antiseptic are well known, and it has recently been recommended by Sir William Watson Cheyne and his collaborators for use as a powder mixed with boric acid for a first field dressing. It is a light powder, feebly soluble in saline solution. If applied to a wound in a crystalline form it does not dissolve sufficiently freely to cause necrosis. Tested with a Ponder's film, salicylic acid is a positive chemiotactic agent. It is also a lymphagogue.

The method has been to keep a saturated solution of salicylic acid in alcohol and to add a little of this to the last funnelful of saline solution with which the wound is irrigated in a proportion of 2-3 drachms to a pint. If applied in this way suspended in saline solution the crystals can be deposited over the surface and reach every part of the wound. They pass into solution slowly and exert a continuous bactericidal action. This method has the advantage that drainage-tubes can be used and free exit for discharge maintained. Dusting the wound with the dry powder has the disadvantage that the crystals float and do not reach deep crevices.

If the crystalline deposit reaches all parts of the wound where exudation is being discharged an immediate diminution occurs in the number of living bacteria on the surface of the wound. This decrease in the number of colonies occurs even when the cultures are made 24 hours after the last dressing, and this change in the bacterial flora is associated with a diminution in the amount of pus and usually with an improvement in the patient's general condition.

Salicylic acid may cause smarting, which usually subsides quickly, and in contact with blood it produces dark-brown acid hæmatin, which has an unpleasant appearance. These slight disadvantages do not, however, detract from its value as an antiseptic.

A thick paste of salicylic acid in sterile saline (1 gm. acid, 9 c.c. saline) has been used for the cut surfaces of long bones in septic amputations. In some cases the stumps have healed by first intention. In others slight sepsis occurred in the muscular flaps. In every case no infection of the bone marrow occurred.

The following cases illustrate the use of salicylic acid as an antiseptic dressing :—

CASE 2.—Private, aged 19. Admitted with septic wound of right knee-joint. The bullet had penetrated the joint and lodged in the outer condyle of the femur. The patient had been in hospitals in France for some weeks previously, and was in a very septic condition. The bullet had not been removed. The knee-joint was drained thoroughly and washed out twice daily with eusol. His condition improved, and sepsis subsided except in the neighbourhood of the outer condyle of the femur in which the bullet was embedded. At a second operation for removal of the bullet it was found that rarefactive changes had occurred leading to the formation of a considerable cavity in the bone, in the centre of which the shrapnel bullet lay. The walls of the cavity were scraped and cleaned with dry gauze and the space then filled with thick salicylic paste, and the external wound closed except for a small drainage-tube which was left in for 24 hours. Dry gauze dressing was applied externally. For the next three weeks no irrigation was employed, the gauze dressings only being changed. The temperature remained normal, and six weeks after the operation an X ray examination failed to show any trace of the cavity in the bone. He made an uninterrupted recovery.

CASE 3.—Private, aged 23. Was admitted with a compound fracture of the neck of the femur and necrosis of the separated head. After weeks of sepsis excision of the head of the femur was undertaken. For ten days following the operation the joint cavity, which was exceedingly septic, was treated with eusol twice daily. The pain and position of the wound prevented more frequent dressing. As the sepsis did not improve eusol was discontinued and the cavity of the joint was filled with a mixture of salicylic acid and saline. Immediate diminution in the discharge and number of bacteria took place, and the patient entered on a slow but steady convalescence.

Salicylic gelatin.—Treatment with salicylic acid in a crystalline form has only been adopted for acute cases and for a short time. In the case of large wounds where the treatment was prolonged, it was thought desirable to diminish the quantity of the drug used. A gelatin medium was therefore made containing salicylic acid 2-4 per cent., in the hope that the viscosity of the mass would help to retain the reagent in the wound. This medium has been used for a large number of cases with considerable success.

The gelatin is prepared in the following way : 300 gm. of gelatin are added to 600 c.c. of freshly made normal saline solution. After melting in the steamer the medium is cleared with egg-albumin and filtered. It is divided into quantities of 100 c.c. and put into glass-stoppered bottles, which are then sterilised at 100° C. for three successive days. Special care must be taken with sterilisation as gelatin is liable to contain tetanus spores. When required for use a bottle is placed in warm water until the gelatin has melted and 2-4 gm. of pure salicylic acid are added. The acid must be added after sterilisation is complete and when the temperature is below 40° C. If the medium is subjected to prolonged heat after the acid is added the viscosity is lost. In 2 per cent. solution the salicylic acid dissolves completely and combines with the gelatin. In 4 per cent. solution some of the crystals remain in suspension. The fluid gelatin is poured into the crevices of the wound either through an irrigating funnel or directly from the bottle, and requires to be repeated daily.

In cases where the medium is retained in the wound it has often been noted that the bacterial flora will change when the treatment commences, pure cultures of streptococci being obtained, after an overnight interval, in wounds which previously grew a variety of organisms. The following cases illustrate the value of this treatment.

CASE 4.—Private, aged 32. Was admitted from a base hospital in France, where a flapless amputation had been performed through the lower third of the left thigh. The wound was very septic. Treatment with saline irrigation and later with strong solution of permanganate of potassium was employed for six weeks. He lost ground. Pus tracked up the muscles of the thigh. Operations were performed for opening sinuses, &c. He became emaciated and cachectic, and finally it was decided that further surgical interference could not be undertaken. At this stage treatment with salicylic acid gelatin was commenced and was applied twice daily. Local reaction was immediate. In a few days the pain ceased, the discharge diminished, and the temperature gradually subsided. Some days later an abscess was opened in the thigh, and after this he made an uninterrupted slow recovery.

CASE 5.—Private, aged 24. Admitted from a base hospital in France, where a flapless amputation had been performed through the middle of the left thigh. The bone was projecting and the wound was extremely septic. After six weeks' treatment with hypertonic saline solution a secondary amputation was done and large drainage-tubes inserted. Three days later the flaps became inflamed and septic. The trouble subsided rapidly under irrigation with peroxide of hydrogen and the application of salicylic gelatin introduced by means of an irrigating funnel.

Conclusions.—The conclusions to be drawn from these observations are :—1. The bactericidal action of many of the so-called antiseptics when applied to septic wounds is negligible. 2. The majority of wounds heal without the application of an antiseptic, provided free drainage is supplied and dressings are changed frequently. Hypertonic saline, in so far as it aids physiological processes, is preferable to many so-called antiseptics. 3. A strong antiseptic, such as eusol, can sterilise the surface of a wound with which it comes in contact, and, if applied continuously, gives excellent results. 4. Salicylic acid applied in a suitable form can often save cases when other methods have failed. It is particularly useful when dressings cannot be repeated at frequent intervals. 5. In all cases where recovery is delayed and the effect of the reagents of doubtful value the treatment should be controlled by making repeated cultures from the wound surfaces.

special destructive action on the infecting parasite. But vaccines are only active against bacteria mediately in that they stimulate the production of bodies which possess special destructive powers toward particular organisms. Vaccines are, therefore, in a sense only specific at second-hand.

As the action of vaccines is merely stimulative of certain natural powers of the body, it is clear that if the body is already exhausted, if it is no longer able to produce the substances, the vaccine fails. Moreover, in cases where it does not fail, its success is proportional to the power of the tissues to respond to its call. To expect uniform success from vaccines is therefore as unreasonable as to suppose that the body can never fail in its defence against attack.

It follows that the cases in which we may expect the best results of vaccine treatment are those in which (1) the body has not yet lost its natural power of resisting infection, and (2) in which there has not been great tissue change. If the body has no power of resisting infection the vaccine is quite inert. It is as useless as a trumpet-call in a deserted barrack-square. It is not possible to tell whether such cases really occur, nor how to recognise them if they do. We must, however, be prepared to meet them and not to be disappointed if the inevitable happens.

The second qualification is of more practical interest. When grave tissue changes have taken place we cannot hope by any method of treatment either to restore lost tissue or to cause the absorption of masses of new tissue of a degenerate order. Vaccines can only produce a resistance to an infective process—they have no effect in dealing with the results of that process after the process has ceased. I do not suggest that there are not other agencies in the body at work to restore damaged tissue to the normal, but these agencies are neither helped nor hindered by vaccines. Let me take one example :—

A Fallopian tube becomes infected by, let us say, the gonococcus and suppuration follows. While the infection lasts, its progress may be hampered or prevented by vaccine treatment. But once the gonococcus loses its vitality, vaccines give no help to the tissues in their struggle to return to the normal. Neither will vaccines cure a stricture of the urethra consequent on gonorrhœa. This is so obvious as to appear commonplace. But let us supply the same reasoning to the effects of rheumatic infection, whether on the joints or on the valves of the heart. We may reasonably hope to hamper the progress of rheumatic injury or to arrest it altogether. But if gross tissue changes have occurred, they cannot be repaired by vaccines. It would be as reasonable to suppose that, if the invaders were to-morrow driven from the fields of Flanders, those fields would be restored forthwith to the condition in which they were three years ago. The battle may be over, and the invaders destroyed, but many of the traces of battle are ineradicable, while others will persist for years. Louvain and Ypres will never be again what they were three years ago. Neither will the heart valves that have been eroded and fibrosed in the battle between the infecting cocci and the protective agencies of the body be the same again.

SCOPE OF VACCINE TREATMENT.

The question is not infrequently asked, What class of diseases should vaccines be employed in? The answer, bearing in mind the limitations I have already suggested, is, Every infective disease due to bacterial origin in which the bacterial cause can be discovered. The acuteness or chronicity of the condition is beside the point, though it may have much to do with the method of administration. A similar remark applies to the question whether the disease is general or local. In every case where a fight is going on between the body and an invading bacterium there is reasonable hope that the defensive forces will be strengthened by the administration of a vaccine. But, as vaccines are specific, a correct bacteriological diagnosis is necessary. In this vaccines are at a distinct disadvantage if contrasted with other methods of treatment. By rest, suitable food, good nursing, and relief of unpleasant symptoms we cure, or rather assist nature to cure, many of our patients. If before treating them an accurate diagnosis were necessary how many successes would we have? But if vaccines are to have any effect at all their use must be preceded by correct diagnosis. We must be sure that we are treating with the infecting organism. Of course, if the infection be mixed, as is so often the case, we must often be content to treat with a group of organisms—i.e., with a mixed vaccine—being assured that at least one element in our vaccine is specific for the infection, and that the others, if not helpful, are at least harmless.

No greater misconception can exist than the notion that vaccine treatment is incompatible with the use of other methods of treatment. On the contrary, one rarely gets the best results from vaccine treatment unless one makes full use of whatever concomitant measures his own experience or the accumulated experience of others may suggest. Few drugs are in any way inimical to the action of vaccines, and those that are, are depressant to the natural resistive powers of the body, and are therefore contra-indicated in the class of diseases in which vaccines are employed. Of these the only drug in common use is alcohol, the employment of which in septic diseases should by now be obsolete except under rare conditions. Vaccine treatment, therefore, goes side by side with treatment by drugs.

In surgical conditions, operative measures, or anything else that surgical knowledge suggests should, of course, be practised when required. The only precaution to be observed is to withhold inoculations in immediate proximity to any manipulative proceeding which may gives rise to auto-inoculation. Otherwise vaccines, of course, act in their normal manner of increasing the protective power of the body.

I said at the beginning that much misjudgment of vaccine treatment by the profession has been due to the treatment being so largely committed to men unaccustomed to clinical work. It cannot, however, remain in the hands of a special class. As an important branch of therapeutics it must become familiar to every practitioner. No student can be considered to have gained a sufficient knowledge of therapeutics who has not become familiar with both the doctrine of immunity and the practice of immunisation. In this way vaccine treatment will come to take its proper place—not as something peculiar and special, but as an essential part of the treatment of infective disorders of bacterial origin.

Dublin.

A VARIETY OF

WAR HEART

WHICH CALLS FOR TREATMENT BY COMPLETE REST.

BY ARCHIBALD E. GARROD, C.M.G.,
M.D. OXON., F.R.S.,
COLONEL, A.M.S.; CONSULTING PHYSICIAN, BRITISH MEDITERRANEAN FORCES.

TWO chief factors are concerned in bringing about the heart troubles of soldiers. One of these, the physical and emotional strain of military life, has attracted much attention since the war began, and the group of symptoms named by Dr. T. Lewis and his fellow-workers the "effort syndrome" has been treated of by many medical writers. The second factor, the temporary weakening of the heart muscle by campaign diseases, has received much less notice.

Among soldiers of the Mediterranean Forces the effort syndrome has been as much in evidence as on the Western front, but we have also seen very many cases in which malaria and some in which other epidemic diseases, such as dysentery and trench fever, have left the myocardium damaged for a time.

It is the aim of this note to call attention to these cases and to emphasise the fact that treatment by graduated exercises, which has proved so useful in the differentiation and cure of the functional cases, is unsuitable and *does actual harm* in the organic cases, so long as the physical signs of damage to the heart muscle persist.

The symptoms described by the patients are shortness of breath on exertion, inability to walk any distance, and, in some cases, præcordial pain. The physical sign is an extension of the cardiac dullness towards the right, often to $1\frac{1}{2}$ or 2 inches beyond the mid-sternal line. Only in extreme cases is there any conspicuous extension towards the left. The dull area has a clearly defined outline, and yields a sense of resistance on percussion. The resistance can also be appreciated by dipping with the pads of the fingers along the course of the ribs or intercostal spaces. This method of palpation was taught me, years ago, at the Hospital for Sick Children, by an American friend and pupil, Dr. T. Wood Clark, and I am convinced that, as a means of marking out the cardiac area, it supplies a valuable control to percussion. It is better to mark out the area by palpation first, and to check the findings by percussion.

I am well aware that some physicians, whose opinions are entitled to all respect, deny the possibility of determining the right border of the cardiac area by percussion, let alone by palpation, but this is wholly at variance with my experience. Many of us working in association here (as previously in England) have examined cases and have checked each other's findings, with open eyes and blindfold. We have agreed in our markings, have watched the drawing-in of the area of dullness under treatment, and its re-expansion after renewed strain or relapses of malaria, and are confident of the correctness of our observations. My colleague, Colonel H. H. Tooth, allows me to quote him as endorsing this statement. Murmurs are not often heard in the cases under discussion, and when present are of the functional kinds, so common in soldiers. The patients are many of them anæmic, but there is no obvious relation between the degree of anæmia and the increase of the cardiac area. Their blood pressure is often above the normal for their ages, as is usual in soldiers who have recently been on active service, and often fluctuates widely with position, emotion, or exercise. The great majority are of the younger military ages.

The signs described are such as my late colleague, Dr. D. B. Lees, taught us to look out for in rheumatic children, in whom the enlargement of the cardiac area, ascribed to myocarditis, often precedes any indication of endocardial lesion.

The X ray shadow of a normal heart extends some way beyond the right border of the sternum, and the right auricle, to which this shadow is mainly due, is covered by the edge of the lung. Extension of the cardiac dullness to the right must indicate a pushing aside of the lung and the bringing of a larger area of the heart's surface into direct contact with the chest wall. My assistant, Major G. Graham, has pointed out that the abnormal dullness is abolished when the patient draws and holds a deep breath. Presumably the dullness results from dilatation of the auricles, especially of the right auricle, and it does not necessarily follow that such dilatation will cause a conspicuous extension of the cardiac shadow. Major Graham is making a series of accurate measurements of the shadows of such hearts and of normal controls. His results, which are as yet incomplete, will be recorded by him in due course.

We have had opportunities of watching the effects of various treatments in these cases of post-malarial dilatation, and in one of our military hospitals wards have been set apart for them under the care of Dr. Prudence Gaffikin. It is to be hoped that she will publish an account of her results later on, and it is only necessary to give a few general conclusions in this note.

Our experience has convinced us that the fitting treatment for such patients is complete rest until the cardiac dullness has returned to its normal limits and for at least a week afterwards. The hearts of many patients which have not responded to modified rest have come in after complete rest has been imposed. The patient is not allowed to rise from his bed for any purpose, nor even to sit up in bed for his meals, nor is he permitted to smoke. We have seen patients who have been treated by exercises *ab initio*, and others who have been allowed up after a short period of rest, although their hearts were still dilated. Neither plan has anything to recommend it, and the results have been wholly unsatisfactory. When the dilatation is recent the cardiac area may return to its normal limits within as short a period as a week. In cases of longer standing, in which rest has not been imposed at the outset, longer periods, up to six or eight weeks, have been required. In no case has the heart failed to come in sooner or later.

In Dr. Gaffikin's wards the patients have begun gentle resistance exercises in bed 10 days after the cardiac dullness has come in. Then follow graduated exercises in the erect posture, and, if all goes well, they are sent to a convalescent camp, where the exercises are continued, under careful medical supervision, in an organised heart clinic.

As a rule, under such treatment, the heart does not re-dilate. If the area of dullness should again spread to the right a further period of rest is imposed. In some cases a relapse of malaria has caused a return of the signs, even

during the period of complete rest. A few patients show a great liability to repeated re-dilatations under very slight provocations—a condition for which the apt nickname of "concertina heart" has been coined. Drugs play a comparatively small part in the treatment. Some of us advocate digitalis, and others nux vomica, but I am not convinced of the efficacy of either. Major Graham believes that digitalis lessens the chance of re-dilatation.

To sum up, the "soldier's heart" is not a clinical entity, but includes a variety of morbid states. Even amongst those patients who exhibit what is called the "effort syndrome," some respond well to exercises and others do not, and it is one of the chief claims of the exercises that by their means we are able to sort out the fit from the unfit. Again, as I have tried to show, we meet, in the course of our military work, with cardiac troubles in the treatment of which the most important factor is rest.

Malta.

AN ANALYSIS OF CASES OF TETANUS TREATED IN HOME MILITARY HOSPITALS

DURING AUGUST, SEPTEMBER, AND PART OF OCTOBER, 1916.

BY SIR DAVID BRUCE, C.B., F.R.S., F.R.C.P.,
SURGEON-GENERAL, ARMY MEDICAL SERVICE.

TWO analyses of cases of tetanus treated in home hospitals have been published in THE LANCET—one on Oct. 23rd, 1915, the other on Dec. 2nd, 1916. This paper continues the subject, and gives an analysis of the cases which occurred in August, September, and part of October, 1916. During this time reports on 200 cases have been received ; of these, 127 recovered and 73 died—a mortality of 36·5 per cent.

In the first analysis there were 231 cases, with a mortality of 57·7 per cent.; and in the second 195 cases, with a mortality of 49·2 per cent. This shows a regular and satisfactory fall in the rate of mortality, which it is hoped will continue until the 20 per cent. aimed at is attained. This fall is probably due to the introduction of the primary prophylactic injection of antitoxin, and also to the earlier diagnosis and earlier specific treatment of the disease. If the fall continues it will depend on the introduction of multiple prophylactic doses, the vigilance of nursing sisters in detecting early symptoms, and the prompt and thorough treatment by medical officers by means of antitoxin.

It had been intended to give an analysis of cases of tetanus treated in home hospitals at the end of each year of the war. Now it is thought better to give one at more frequent intervals. This is due to the great interest taken in the subject by medical officers in charge of wounded at home. It ought to conduce to the keeping up of this interest if the results of new recommendations made by the Tetanus Committee be reported on at more frequent intervals than one year. In fact, the intention at present is that in future each series of 100 cases as they are completed will be shortly reported on.

During the same time two analyses have been published by Colonel Sir William Leishman on the cases of tetanus occurring among the British troops in France. In the first, 179 cases were dealt with, with a case mortality of 78·2 per cent. In the second, in collaboration with Major A. B. Smallman, 160 cases were analysed and gave a case mortality of 72·7 per cent. The cases dealt with in France are naturally more acute and severe than the cases which arise in England.

DIAGRAM 1.

1916	Aug.ᵗ	Sep.ʳ	Oct.ᵗ
No. of cases	53	76	67

THE DISTRIBUTION OF CASES OF TETANUS DURING AUGUST, SEPTEMBER, AND OCTOBER, 1916.

Diagram 1 represents the number of cases which occurred in each month. Sixteen of the cases which occurred at the end of October do not come into this analysis. The diagram

border-line of good family, who most vaunt themselves regarding their descent. They do not realise that in these days it is a man's ascent that ennobles him, not his descent, even if, paradoxically, ascent is not possible without good rich blood : it is the progressive accretion of properties, not the progressive loss. But, suggests Professor Bateson, in nature it is the opposite : it is by the progressive loss of properties that from being an amorphous mass of protoplasm man has become man. Life, according to him, first appeared upon earth enshrined in matter of maximum complexity, so complex that it was without form and void, and only as through the vast æons of geological time, this matter fell into order and simplified itself, and successive species developed, did we eventually in these latter days arrive at that simplest and least complex of all creatures, man—simple man.

Does it not appear to you that this is topsy-turvydom ? Is it not, on the face of it, more probable that the reverse has been the case—that the earliest matter that could be recognised as living was the simplest. It is not that the earliest living matter possessed all the determinants of all the organised parts of all future forms of life, but that its constitution was such that it possessed, in consequence of its metabolic activities, the potentiality to undergo progressive modifications of that constitution, which modifications manifested themselves, as an outcome, in progressive changes of structure. *The potentiality was there, not the determinants.*

CONCLUSION.

One last word. I feel that, as one on active service, some apology may be required from me for having taken your time and, it may be said, my country's time, in dealing in the course of these four lectures with a matter so wholly foreign to the war, to military medicine, and military duties. Were what I have placed before you wholly new, had I collected, thought out, and elaborated the material of these lectures during the two years since I received the invitation to deliver the course, an apology would, I think, rightly be in place. As a matter of fact, these lectures are little beyond what I have taught and written in the 15 years and more preceding the war ; they are a digest and compend of those earlier writings and conclusions, brought up to date by means of an occasional modern instance confirmatory of that earlier work. Fours hours ago, at lunch time, in order to complete my bibliography, I went to the library in Wimpole-street and took out the volume of the *British Medical Journal* for 1901, containing an address delivered by me at Brooklyn, New York, in May of that year.[12] That address I had not looked up for a decade or so, and it was not with a little surprise that I found laid down there the physico-chemical conception of inheritance here given, and the doctrine of direct inheritance of metabolic conditions, such as gout and of disturbances of the internal secretions. Rather, therefore, the apology should be that I have plagiarised myself in so wholesale a manner. I shall, however, be satisfied if in these Croonian lectures it is demonstrated that the work of medical men of this generation, of pathologists and bacteriologists, work founded upon the observations and methods of the great biologists of the past, is repaying the debt to biology by establishing principles which are basal for general biological advance.

12 Brit. Med. Jour., 1901, i., 1317.

AN INDIAN CIVIL MEDICAL SERVICE.—The desirability of a separately recruited Indian Civil Medical Service, lately considered by the Royal Commission on the Public Services in India, has been decided in the negative, at all events, for the present. The general feeling in India appears to be that the question will arise in an acute form after the war. Numbers of civilian medical officers are now employed in important if not very lucrative civil surgeoncies.

A SCHOOL OF MASSAGE.—University College Hospital, Gower-street, W.C., and the National Hospital for the Paralysed and Epileptic, Queen-square, W.C., have appointed a joint committee to manage a school of massage and allied treatment on behalf of the two hospitals. The school is situated in Queen-square, Bloomsbury, and has been named the National Hospital and University College Hospital School of Massage and Electrical Treatment. The curriculum will include the teaching of massage, remedial exercises, and medical electricity, and it is expected that the first term will commence early in October. There is a comfortable hostel in connexion with the school for the use of students who desire to be resident.

PURULENT BRONCHITIS.

A STUDY OF CASES OCCURRING AMONGST THE BRITISH TROOPS AT A BASE IN FRANCE.

BY J. A. B. HAMMOND, M.B. LOND.,
LIEUTENANT, R.A.M.C. ; MEDICAL OFFICER, —— GENERAL HOSPITAL ;

WILLIAM ROLLAND, M.D. GLASG.,
CAPTAIN, R.A.M.C. ; PATHOLOGIST, —— GENERAL HOSPITAL ;

AND

T. H. G. SHORE, M.B. CANTAB., M.R.C.P. LOND.,
LIEUTENANT, R.A.M.C. ; OFFICER IN CHARGE, MORTUARY,
—— ADMINISTRATIVE AREA.

THE numerous cases of purulent bronchitis which have arisen at one of the bases in Northern France during the winter of 1916–17 have presented features of marked clinical and pathological interest. Patients suffering from this unusually fatal disease present a symptom complex so distinctive as to constitute a definite clinical entity. The results of bacteriological and post-mortem examinations tend also to support this belief. The earlier cases were admitted during December, 1916, but it was not until the end of the following January, when exceptional cold prevailed, that the disease assumed such proportions as to constitute almost a small epidemic. Later, when the frost abated, there was a very striking diminution in the number of cases.

The disease has been very fatal. This is shown most readily by post-mortem records referring to this period. During February and early March, while the outbreak was at its height 45 per cent. of the necropsies in this area showed the presence of purulent bronchitis.

It is proposed to discuss this condition from three standpoints : (1) that of the clinician ; (2) that of the bacteriologist ; and (3) that of the morbid anatomist.

1. THE CLINICAL ASPECT.

Clinical types.—The cases which came under our notice can be divided broadly into two types.

The first and more acute presents a clinical picture which closely simulates ordinary lobar pneumonia with a sustained temperature of about 103°, and expectoration at first bloodstreaked—rather than rusty—which, however, rapidly becomes quite purulent. The pulse-rate in these cases is out of all proportion to the temperature in its rapidity. Dyspnœa and cyanosis are prominent features. The patient usually dies from "luug block," resulting in embarrassment of the right side of the heart on the fifth or sixth day. For the last day or two there is often incontinence of the fæces, due, no doubt, to the condition of partial asphyxia. The mental state is one of torpor ; delirium is the exception.

The second and less acute type is marked by a more swinging temperature with a range of 2° or 3°. The expectoration at first may be frothy and muco-purulent, but it very soon assumes the typically purulent character. This form may run a long course of from three to six weeks, during which time the patient wastes a great deal and has frequent and profuse sweats ; indeed, at a certain stage the illness is most suggestive of acute tubercular infection, and it is only by repeated examination of the expectoration that the clinician can satisfy himself he is not really overlooking a case of acute pulmonary tuberculosis. The majority of our cases conforming to this type have ultimately recovered, but the convalescence is slow and tedious.

Detailed Symptomatology.

Onset.—Whilst a history of a previous catarrhal condition lasting for a few days is often obtained, the disease quickly assumes an acute character ; we have been able to observe this in patients admitted in the first instance for a surgical condition. Taking the average readings from the charts of patients admitted into this hospital with purulent bronchitis, we find the temperature is between 102° and 103°, the pulse 120 or over, and the respiration about 35. The patient frequently complains of shivering and looks pathetically miserable, but we have not seen an actual rigor. Despite his obvious shortness of breath, the sisters have noticed that, at any rate at first, he prefers a lateral position low down in the bed, and resents any attempt to prop him up.

Cough.—This for the first day or two may be irritable and distressing with a little frothy expectoration, but as the latter becomes more purulent the cough is less troublesome, and soon the patient is expectorating easily and frequently until the latter stages are reached; when owing to increasing asphyxia the patient becomes more and more torpid, the cough subsides, and hardly any secretion is brought up. This failure becomes an added factor in bringing about a rapidly fatal termination.

Expectoration.—The sputum, with its yellowish-green purulent masses, is very characteristic, and may be one of the first indications of the serious nature of the illness the patient is suffering from. A fuller description follows in the bacteriological section.

Temperature.—The fever of this complaint does not follow any very constant type. In nearly all our cases the pyrexia was of sudden onset, and for the first few days was more or less sustained at about 103°. Later it conformed more to the swinging type with a range of several degrees. In a few cases a curious gradual ante-mortem drop has been observed. The accompanying charts demonstrate this point. (See Charts 1, 2, and 3.)

Pulse.—Tachycardia is a very constant feature throughout the illness. The rate is frequently well over 120, though the volume may remain surprisingly good until immediately before death.

Some degree of dyspnœa is always present, and is usually progressive, though towards the end in the fatal cases when the mental acuteness is dulled by the increasing asphyxia the patient is not distressed by its presence. In some cases there have been paroxysmal exacerbations of the breathlessness, accompanied by a state of panic, in which the patient struggles wildly and tries to get out of bed in order to obtain relief. Cyanosis is another prominent feature throughout the illness. At first it may not be more than duskiness, but in the later stages it becomes very evident. It is only slightly relieved by oxygen; this, no doubt, is partly explained by the difficulty in giving the oxygen efficiently owing to the patient's objection to any mouth-piece that fits at all tightly and partly by the blocked condition of the bronchioles interfering with the absorption of the oxygen.

Physical Signs.

The condition usually begins with the presence of a moderate number of sharp crepitant râles, often first heard in the region of the root of the lung; these quickly become generalised. In the majority of the cases signs of broncho-pneumonic patches can be made out; these are generally situated near the root of the lungs. In a certain number of cases these patches spread and become confluent, giving practically all the physical signs of a lobar pneumonia. As the disease progresses the air entry is diminished; on listening one is often struck by the small volume of sound heard. The resonance of the lungs may also be lessened. A slight pleuritic rub was heard in a few of our cases, but this was soon masked by the bronchitic signs.

Treatment.

The treatment of this condition is not satisfactory. So far, in the worst cases, we have been unable to find anything that has any real influence on the course of the disease.

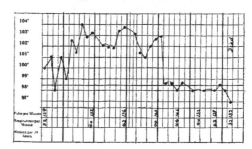

CHART 1 (Private M.).

Shows the temperature course in the more acute type of case. The temperature ends by crisis, but the pulse-rate remains high and the symptoms (cough, dyspnœa, &c.) persist. Death occurred in this case two days after the crisis. *Bacillus influenzæ* isolated in this case.

Inhalations of steam with eucalyptus, tinct. benzoin. co., &c., seemed to give considerable relief, and in order to make this as continuous as possible we have recently treated our more urgent cases in a steam tent with encouraging results. The cough is rendered less troublesome, and the expectoration being kept less tenacious is more easily expelled, a most important point, for once the patient ceases to bring up the purulent secretion he quickly goes downhill, becoming more and more cyanosed with right-sided failure of the heart.

The results obtained from oxygen are disappointing, the relief being slight and very transitory. We have already mentioned our explanation of this observation.

Venesection has likewise failed to benefit the patient for more than a very short time, though possibly we have not resorted to this treatment sufficiently early.

For drugs we have chiefly relied on digitalis and iodides with other expectorants. In the last stages, when the patient has ceased to expectorate, atropine given hypodermically has given temporary relief. Adrenalin has also assisted to prolong life. Pituitary extract increased the incontinence so many of our patients suffered from towards the end, and for this reason probably did more harm than good. Strychnine and camphor in oil were also tried, but without any marked benefit. A suitable vaccine may be shortly forthcoming, but up to the present we have not been able to give this line of treatment a fair trial.

2. BACTERIOLOGY.

Since the outbreak of the epidemic of purulent bronchitis with which this investigation is concerned 20 specimens of sputum have been submitted to the laboratory for bacteriological examination. These have all been taken from cases which in their clinical aspect differed from cases of ordinary bronchitis, and most of which presented many of the signs and symptoms described in another part of this paper. In 4 of the cases the sputum examination was supplemented by an examination of pus taken post mortem from one of the

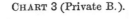

CHART 2 (Private C.).

A less acute case than the preceding. Note the prolonged, rather swinging temperature and the fall by lysis without diminution of pulse-rate just before death. *Bacillus influenzæ* isolated.

CHART 3 (Private B.).

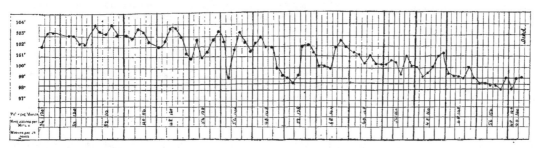

his shows a course similar to that of the preceding case but of longer duration. The ante-mortem fall of temperature is again very marked. A Gram-negative bacillus resembling *Bacillus influenzæ* present in large numbers in films, but *B. influenzæ* was not isolated.

smaller bronchi. In most of the fatal cases a histological examination of the lungs and other organs was made, while in 3 of them an unsuccessful attempt was made to obtain a growth from the enlarged bronchial glands. Certain animal experiments were also made in 3 of the cases ; these will be described later.

Sputum Examination.

In each case, after noting the naked-eye appearance of the sputum, films were made and stained by Gram's method and a portion was afterwards plated out on blood-agar or trypsin-broth-legumin-agar.

Character of sputum.—This is in nearly every case markedly purulent. Usually no mucus is present, but in some cases the sputum is muco-purulent. The colour is yellow or greenish-yellow and the consistence thick. Usually it has a nummular character. No blood has been observed in any of the specimens submitted. There has been no appreciable odour.

Examination of films.—In all but three of the cases direct examination of films of the sputum showed the presence of more than one organism. In 18 of the 20 cases there was present a small Gram-negative cocco-bacillus, which was afterwards identified as the *Bacillus influenzæ*. This occurred as a rule in typical clumps consisting of large numbers of bacilli. The individual organisms appeared sometimes as minute elongated cocci, often arranged in pairs, and in other cases were less coccoid and more definitely bacillary. In 10 of the cases in which it was found it was the predominating organism, being present in some in enormous numbers. In 3 of the cases no other organisms could be seen in the films, but *B. influenzæ* was abundant.

Cultural examination.—The method employed was to remove a small piece of sputum by means of sterilised forceps from the sterile bottle in which it had been collected. The sputum was then thoroughly washed by shaking in sterile saline, and a piece of the washed sputum was plated out on blood-agar or trypsin-broth-legumin-agar. The latter, on account of its transparency and the relative ease with which *B. influenzæ* grows on it, gave the better results. In this way the influenza bacillus was isolated in 10 of the 18 cases in which an organism resembling it was seen in direct films.

In the investigation of the other organisms present many were diagnosed both from their morphological and cultural characters. But in some of the cases, owing to lack of time, the appearance of the organism as seen in direct films was alone noted. With this proviso it may be stated that in the cases here shown the following organisms other than *B. influenzæ* were found :—

	Cases.		Cases.
Pneumococcus	13	*M. tetragenus*	2
Streptococcus	5	A Gram-positive diplococcus	1
A Gram-negative diplococcus resembling *D. catarrhalis*	5	A large Gram-negative bacillus	1
Staphylococcus	3	*B. tuberculosis*	1

From the following table it will be seen that in most of the cases in which *B. influenzæ* was present in large numbers the pneumococcus also occurred.

Characters of the Bacillus Influenzæ Isolated.

The microscopical appearances are usually those of a minute, slightly elongated coccus with a tendency to grow in pairs end to end. Some longer and more definitely bacillary forms are also, as a rule, present. The organism stains somewhat slowly with ordinary stains and is always definitely Gram-negative.

On " trypagar " growth does not usually appear until 36 hours at least have elapsed. Very small translucent colonies can then be seen which have a convex surface and regular rounded edges. In primary cultures from sputum the influenza bacillus appears to grow more luxuriantly in the vicinity of colonies of other organisms. The colonies are very easily emulsified in water. Attempts at subculture on legumin-agar nearly always failed. On blood-agar growth appears within 24 hours in the form of small transparent colonies. The organism can be repeatedly subcultured on this medium, and though it ultimately tends to die out one strain has at the time of writing been kept going on it for over a month, subcultures being made about once a week. With ordinary agar, glycerine-agar, solidified blood serum, broth and gelatin no growth is obtained. Nor could the organism be cultivated anaerobically on any of the media used.

Table Showing that in Most of the Cases in which B. Influenzæ *was Present in Large Numbers the Pneumococcus also Occurred.*

Serial No.	Name, &c.	Examination of films.	Result of culture.	Other organisms present.	Death or recovery.	Remarks.
1	Pte. C.	+++	+	...	D	Case of bacillary dysentery with septic bronchitis.
2	Pte. H.	+	—	D. catarrhalis.	D	Had broncho-pneumonia, right pleural effusion and toxic nephritis.
3	Pte. K.	++	+	None.	D	Had broncho-pneumonia
4	Pte. M.	++	+	D. catarrhalis.	D	No pneumonia.
5	Pte. G.	++	—	Streptococcus. Pneumococcus. D. catarrhalis.	D	Broncho-pneumonia and toxic nephritis also.
6	Pte. C.	+++	+	Streptococcus. Pneumococcus. D. catarrhalis.	D	...
7	Pte. A.	+++	+	Pneumococcus (scanty).	D	Marked emaciation.
8	Pte. U.	+	+	Pneumococcus. D. catarrhalis. A Gram-positive diplococcus.	D	Widespread broncho-pneumonia.
9	Pte. G.	++	—	Pneumococcus. Numerous others.	R	...
10	Pte. W.	++	—	Many others.	R	...
11	Pte. W.	++	—	Pneumococcus. Streptococcus.	D	Broncho-pneumonia.
12	L/C. S.	++	—	Pneumococcus.	R	...
13	Pte. D.	—	—	Pneumococcus.	R	...
14	Pte. V.	++	—	B. tuberculosis. Staphylococcus. Pneumococcus.	D	Acute tubercular broncho-pneumonia.
15	Pte. H.	+++	+	Staphylococcus. Streptococcus. M. tetragenus.	D	Broncho-pneumonia and emphysema.
16	Rev. G.	—	—	Pneumococcus. Streptococcus. M. tetragenus.	R	...
17	Pte. T.	—	+	Pneumococcus.	R	...
18	L/C. H.	++	—	Pneumococcus.	D	Double lobar pneumonia.
19	Pte. F.	++	+	Pneumococcus. Large Gram-negative bacillus.	R	Lobar pneumonia.
20	Pte. C.	+++	+	None.	D	No pneumonia. Ante-mortem fall in temp.

Col. 3: +, *B. influenzæ* present in small numbers; ++, in moderate numbers; +++, in large numbers; —, not found.
Col. 4: +, *B. influenzæ* isolated ; —, not isolated.

Animal experiments.—Two strains of the organism isolated were injected into mice intraperitoneally and into rabbits intravenously. In another case in which the *B. influenzæ* was present in the sputum in large numbers and was practically the only organism found, a suspension of the sputum in saline was similarly injected into a rabbit and a mouse. In all cases the animals survived and showed no signs of illness.

Vaccine therapy.—A vaccine was prepared from the organism isolated from one of the later cases, but by the time this was ready the epidemic was almost over, and up to the time of writing there has not been a suitable opportunity of using it. It is not, however, likely, if one may judge from the blocked state of the bronchioles, that vaccine therapy will be of any value except in the early stages.

3. MORBID ANATOMY.

The prevalence of bronchitis of a purulent type is seen from a study of 156 consecutive necropsies made during February and early March, 1917, in which it occurs as a primary condition in 45 and as a secondary condition in 26 of the cases examined. Altogether purulent bronchitis was found in 45·5 per cent. of the total cases. In the cases examined bronchitis is more than five times as numerous as lobar pneumonia, which is the other prominent pulmonary disease. Tuberculosis in the form of obsolete foci in lungs or glands was present in 8 of the total 71 cases. In the whole 156 cases tuberculosis was noted in 14. In none of the cases of bronchitis did tuberculosis appear to be active. It occurred in 3 which are regarded as primary, and in 5 secondary cases. It would appear not to bear any definite relation to the incidence of the condition.

Appearances which might be regarded as typical are as follows.

The face is more often than not cyanosed, and often a considerable degree of wasting is present, though in the more rapidly fatal cases this is not so apparent.

The lungs show three prominent features. They are almost always bulky on account of a great amount of emphysema which affects chiefly their anterior margins. The heart is often greatly obscured by bulky lung when the chest is opened.

Some degree of pleurisy is generally present; more often this is plastic in type, though occasionally small collections of fluid are found in the pleural cavities; clear yellow fluid was found in 8 of the cases examined, 5 of these being primary. In only 2 cases did the effusion exceed a few ounces; both of these were cases of primary bronchitis. Empyemata are not often found.

The third feature is the constant appearance of a thick yellowish pus in the bronchi. In the larger bronchi it is mixed with air, and often is discoloured by altered blood; but in the small tubes cut in section the pus exudes spontaneously as a rule, with little or no admixture of air. A lung cut in the ordinary way may show large numbers of small yellow points from which pus is exuding.

Considerable œdema is commonly associated with the above appearances, and a greater or less degree of collapse, generally at the vertebral borders of the lower lobes, was found in 15 of the cases examined.

A certain number of cases pass on to a condition of broncho-pneumonia, and when this occurs it usually shows itself in the form of small solid nodules, in the centre of which are pus-containing bronchioles. Consolidation has been first observed near to the roots of the lungs, and in a few has been so extensive as to simulate lobar pneumonia at the necropsy. Broncho-pneumonia was recorded in 32 of the 71 cases examined, of which 22 occurred in cases primary from the start.

In 34 of the cases of primary bronchitis lymphatic glands in the root of the lung, the bronchial group, and the tracheal glands were noted as greatly enlarged, and on section they were grey or pinkish-grey in colour. Not uncommonly the mesenteric and retroperitoneal and even inguinal and axillary glands were found affected.

The spleen in many cases was found engorged and not soft. On cutting the organ the corpuscles were often found to stand out prominently as if sharing in the disorder of the lymphatic glands.

Some degree of derangement of the kidneys was noted in 25 out of the 45 primary cases, taking the form of some swelling and pallor of the cortex. Often the kidneys had lost their firm consistence and were flabby and in a few cases soft. Engorgement, on the other hand, was noted in a few, generally accompanied by engorgement of the spleen. The liver very often showed evidence of fatty change.

The right side of the heart was almost always dilated and the myocardium commonly pale and friable. No evidence of endocarditis was found in any case. A few ounces of pericardial fluid, always pale yellow and clear, were found in 10 cases, but this was not associated with any roughening of the pericardium or cohesion of its surfaces. Broadly speaking, these findings fall into two groups. In one the organs are congested, the heart dilated, though fairly healthy, and the patient cyanosed; in the other the organs are flabby or soft, the heart muscle pale and friable, and the patient pallid. The first group corresponds with a suffocative and the second with a toxic death.

Histology.

An examination of portions of lung, bronchial gland, and kidney taken from eight of the fatal cases was made. The following is a summary of the histology of these organs.

Lungs.—The most striking changes are in the smaller bronchi. Their walls are thickened and the vessels engorged; the lining epithelium, which is at first intact, is later detached in parts from its basement membrane, and the epithelial cells can be seen lying free in the lumen. In a still more advanced stage the bronchiole is entirely denuded of mucous membrane, and its wall consists of granulation tissue which greatly diminishes its calibre. The bronchi are in the less advanced stages almost completely filled with pus, in which, in some cases, the influenza bacillus was found in appropriately stained sections. Later on columnar epithelial cells in small masses are mixed with the polymorphonuclear pus cells, and by the time the epithelium is entirely shed the amount of pus in the bronchus is greatly diminished. Many of the specimens show marked broncho-pneumonia, but in some there is no great extension of the inflammatory process to the surrounding lung tissue. Indeed, the small extent to which catarrhal pneumonia is often present in the vicinity of markedly involved bronchi would

suggest that the pneumonia is due to a local toxic effect rather than to an infection of the corresponding area of lung tissue.

Bronchial glands.—There is extreme congestion and enlargement of lymph nodes. In one specimen one of the larger arteries was thrombosed, but no suppurative change was present in any of the cases.

Kidneys.—In almost all there is degenerative change in the tubular epithelium due to toxic action. This varies in degree, and in the most marked cases there is desquamation of epithelium, round-cell infiltration, and congestion, the condition being indistinguishable from an acute tubular nephritis.

CONCLUSIONS.

1. We are here dealing with an epidemic of a variety of purulent bronchitis.

2. For the following reasons we consider the cause of the disease to be the influenza bacillus : (*a*) The almost constant occurrence of this organism in the sputum ; (*b*) its presence in the pus of the affected bronchioles ; (*o*) in some typical cases it occurs apart from the presence of any other organism ; (*d*) the outbreak of the disease in epidemic form at the time of year when influenza epidemics are most common and whilst one was actually in progress ; (*e*) the marked signs of toxic poisoning which are found during life and post mortem.

3. There are well-marked clinical features which distinguish these cases from ordinary cases of bronchitis. The most prominent are the characteristic sputum, the extreme tachycardia, the cyanosis, the course of the temperature (notably the ante-mortem fall), and the extremely high mortality.

4. Treatment has so far been unsatisfactory. The most encouraging results have been obtained by use of a steam tent. Vaccines have not yet had a trial, but it is unlikely, in view of the blocked condition of the bronchioles, that they would be of great benefit.

5. The morbid anatomy consists of three groups of changes. (*a*) The lung condition : Marked purulent bronchitis, the smaller bronchi being filled with thick pus, from which air is notably absent. In some cases secondary broncho-pneumonia and œdema, pleurisy, and emphysema are common. (*b*) Evidence of toxæmia : Especially seen in kidneys, spleen, liver, lymphatic glands, and heart muscle. (*o*) Signs of right side heart failure and passive congestion. Some cases die of the toxæmia and others of the cardiac failure.

6. The histological changes are those of an acute purulent bronchitis affecting the smaller bronchi with or without some surrounding catarrhal pneumonia. Degenerative changes are seen in other organs, notably in the kidneys, where the appearances of a toxic nephritis may be found.

We are indebted to Colonel Sir John Rose Bradford, K.C.M.G., who originally pointed out to us the distinctive nature of these cases and who has given us much kind assistance throughout the investigation. Our thanks are also due to Professor J. H. Teacher, of Glasgow, for his kindness in preparing the photo-micrographs.

DESCRIPTIONS OF FIGS. 1 TO 6.

FIG. 1 (Case 7).—Marked congestion of bronchial wall with polymorph infiltration. Mucous membrane well preserved except at one part. Lumen almost completely filled with pus. No peri-bronchial pneumonia. (Same size as original.)

FIG. 2 (Case 7).—Part of the wall of a large bronchus showing congestion of submucosa, emigration of leucocytes through the swollen mucous) membrane, and the purulent collection in the bronchial lumen. (× 120.

FIG. 3 (Case 4).—A moderately large bronchus with muscular and cartilaginous wall. There is free desquamation of epithelium which is seen lying among the pus in the lumen. The adjacent lung tissue (of which very little is here shown) is markedly congested, but not consolidated. (× 60.)

FIG. 4 (Case 6).—A bronchiole almost full of pus. Only here and there can the remains of mucous membrane be detected. There is a pneumonic condition in the surrounding air vesicles, large pigmented catarrhal cells being present. (× 60.)

FIG. 5 (Case 6).—A high-power view of part of the preceding specimen. It shows the purulent bronchial contents. the remains of mucous membrane, and the surrounding catarrhal pneumonia. (× 120.)

FIG. 6 (Case 3).—A small bronchus showing a later stage than the other photographs. Epithelium completely shed and the much-thickened mass consisting entirely of young granulation tissue. Surrounding lung tissue congested, but no pneumonia present. (× 60.)

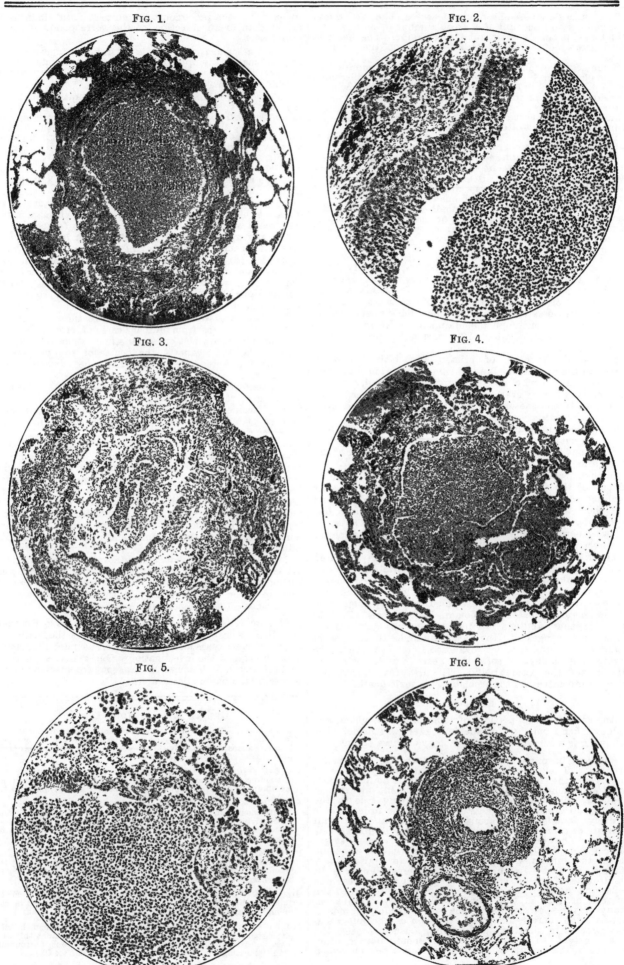

Fig. 1.   Fig. 2.

Fig. 3.   Fig. 4.

Fig. 5.   Fig. 6.

THE LANCET,]   CAPT. W. H. R. RIVERS : THE REPRESSION OF WAR EX. 'ERIENCE,   [FEB. 2. 1918   173

An Address
ON
THE REPRESSION OF WAR EXPERIENCE.

Delivered before the Section of Psychiatry, Royal Society of Medicine, on Dec. 4th, 1917,

BY W. H. R. RIVERS, M.D. LOND., F.R.C.P. LOND., F.R.S.,
LATE MEDICAL OFFICER, CRAIGLOCKHART WAR HOSPITAL.

MR. PRESIDENT AND GENTLEMEN,—I do not attempt to deal in this paper with the whole problem of the part taken by repression in the production and maintenance of the war neuroses. Repression is so closely bound up with the pathology and treatment of these states that the full consideration of its rôle would amount to a complete study of neurosis in relation to the war.

THE PROCESS OF REPRESSION.

It is necessary at the outset to consider an ambiguity in the term "repression," as it is now used by writers on the pathology of the mind and nervous system. The term is currently used in two senses which should be carefully distinguished from one another. It is used for the *process* whereby a person endeavours to thrust out of his memory some part of his mental content, and it is also used for the *state* which ensues when, either through this process or by some other means, part of the mental content has become inaccessible to manifest consciousness. In the second sense the word is used for a state which corresponds closely with that known as dissociation, but it is useful to distinguish mere inaccessibility to memory from the special kind of separation from the rest of the mental content which is denoted by the term "dissociation." The state of inaccessibility may therefore be called suppression in distinction from the process of repression. In this paper I use repression for the active or voluntary process by which it is attempted to remove some part of the mental content out of the field of attention with the aim of making it inaccessible to memory and producing the state of suppression.

Using the word in this sense, repression is not in itself a pathological process, nor is it necessarily the cause of pathological states. On the contrary, it is a necessary element in education and in all social progress. It is not repression in itself which is harmful, but repression under conditions in which it fails to adapt the individual to his environment.

It is in times of special stress that these failures of adaptation are especially liable to occur, and it is not difficult to see why disorders due to this lack of adaptation should be so frequent at the present time. There are few, if any, aspects of life in which repression plays so prominent and so necessary a part as in the preparation for war. The training of a soldier is designed to adapt him to act calmly and methodically in the presence of events naturally calculated to arouse disturbing emotions. His training should be such that the energy arising out of these emotions is partly damped by familiarity, partly diverted into other channels. The most important feature of the present war in its relation to the production of neurosis is that the training in repression normally spread over years has had to be carried out in short spaces of time, while those thus incompletely trained have had to face strains such as have never previously been known in the history of mankind. Small wonder that the failures of adaptation should have been so numerous and so severe.

I do not now propose to consider this primary and fundamental problem of the part played by repression in the original production of the war neuroses. The process of repression does not cease when some shock or strain has removed the soldier from the scene of warfare, but it may take an active part in the maintenance of the neurosis. New symptoms often arise in hospital or at home which are not the immediate and necessary consequence of war experience, but are due to repression of painful memories and thoughts, or of unpleasant affective states arising out of reflection concerning this experience. It is with the repression of the hospital and of the home rather than with the repression of the trenches that I deal in this paper. I propose to illustrate by a few sample cases some of the effects which may be produced by repression and the line of action by which these effects may be remedied. I hope to show that many of the most trying and distressing symptoms from which the subjects of war neurosis suffer are not the necessary result of the strains and shocks to which they have been exposed in warfare, but are due to the attempt to banish from the mind distressing memories of warfare or painful affective states which have come into being as the result of their war experience.

THE ATTITUDE OF PATIENTS TO WAR MEMORIES.

Everyone who has had to treat cases of war neurosis, and especially that form of neurosis dependent on anxiety, must have been faced by the problem what advice to give concerning the attitude the patient should adopt towards his war experience.

It is natural to thrust aside painful memories just as it is natural to avoid dangerous or horrible scenes in actuality, and this natural tendency to banish the distressing or the horrible is especially pronounced in those whose powers of resistance have been lowered by the long-continued strains of trench-life, the shock of shell-explosion, or other catastrophe of warfare. Even if patients were left to themselves most would naturally strive to forget distressing memories and thoughts. They are, however, very far from being left to themselves, the natural tendency to repress being in my experience almost universally fostered by their relatives and friends, as well as by their medical advisers. Even when patients have themselves realised the impossibility of forgetting their war experiences and have recognised the hopeless and enervating character of the treatment by repression, they are often induced to attempt the task in obedience to medical orders. The advice which has usually been given to my patients in other hospitals is that they should endeavour to banish all thoughts of war from their minds. In some cases all conversation between patients or with visitors about the war is strictly forbidden, and the patients are instructed to lead their thoughts to other topics, to beautiful scenery and other pleasant aspects of experience.

To a certain extent this policy is perfectly sound. Nothing annoys a nervous patient more than the continual inquiries of his relatives and friends about his experiences of the front, not only because it awakens painful memories, but also because of the obvious futility of most of the questions and the hopelessness of bringing the realities home to his hearers. Moreover, the assemblage together in a hospital of a number of men with little in common except their war experiences naturally leads their conversation far too frequently to this topic, and even among those whose memories are not especially distressing it tends to enhance the state for which the term "fed up" seems to be the universal designation.

It is, however, one thing that those who are suffering from the shocks and strains of warfare should dwell continually on their war experience or be subjected to importunate inquiries ; it is quite another matter to attempt to banish such experience from their minds altogether. The cases I am about to record illustrate the evil influence of this latter course of action and the good effects which follow its cessation.

RECORDS OF ILLUSTRATIVE CASES.

Straightforward Example of Anxiety Neurosis.

The first case is that of a young officer who was sent home from France on account of a wound received just as he was extricating himself from a mass of earth in which he had been buried. When he reached hospital in England he was nervous and suffered from disturbed sleep and loss of appetite. When his wound had healed he was sent home on leave where his nervous symptoms became more pronounced, so that at his next board his leave was extended. He was for a time an out-patient at a London hospital and was then sent to a convalescent home in the country. Here he continued to sleep badly, with disturbing dreams of warfare, and became very anxious about himself and his prospects of recovery. Thinking he might improve if he rejoined his battalion, he made so light of his condition at his next medical board that he was on the point of being returned to duty when special inquiries about his sleep led to his being sent to Craiglockhart War Hospital for further observation and treatment.

On admission he reported that it always took him long to get to sleep at night and that when he succeeded he had vivid dreams of warfare. He could not sleep without a light in his room because in the dark his attention was attracted by every sound. He had been advised by everyone he had consulted, whether medical or lay, that he ought to banish all unpleasant and disturbing thoughts from his mind. He had been occupying himself for every hour of the day in order to follow this advice and had succeeded in restraining his memories and anxieties during the day, but as soon as he went to bed they would crowd upon him and race through his mind hour after hour, so that every night he dreaded to go to bed.

When he had recounted his symptoms and told me about his method of dealing with his disturbing thoughts I asked him to tell me candidly his own opinion concerning the possibility of keeping these obtrusive visitors from his mind. He said at once that it was obvious to him that memories such as those he had brought with him from the war could never be forgotten. Nevertheless, since he had been told by everyone that it was his duty to forget them he had done his utmost in this direction. I then told the patient my own views concerning the nature and treatment of his state. I agreed with him that such memories could not be expected to disappear from the mind and advised him no longer to try to banish them but that he should see whether it was not possible to make them into tolerable, if not even pleasant, companions instead of evil influences which forced themselves upon his mind whenever the silence and inactivity of the night came round. The possibility of such a line of treatment had never previously occurred to him, but my plan seemed reasonable and he promised to give it a trial. We talked about his war experiences and his anxieties, and following this he had the best night he had had for five months.

During the following week he had a good deal of difficulty in sleeping, but his sleeplessness no longer had the painful and distressing quality which had been previously given to it by the intrusion of painful thoughts of warfare. In so far as unpleasant thoughts came to him, these were concerned with domestic anxieties rather than with the memories of war, and even these no longer gave rise to the dread which had previously troubled him. His general health improved; his power of sleeping gradually increased and he was able after a time to return to duty, not in the hope that this duty might help him to forget, but with some degree of confidence that he was really fit for it.

The case I have just narrated is a straightforward example of anxiety neurosis, which made no real progress as long as the patient tried to keep out of his mind the painful memories and anxieties which had been aroused in his mind by reflection on his past experience. his present state, and the chance of his fitness for duty in the future. When in place of running away from these unpleasant thoughts he faced them boldly and allowed his mind to dwell upon them in the day they no longer raced through his thoughts at night and disturbed his sleep by terrifying dreams of warfare.

Another Case of Improvement after Cessation of Repression.

The next case is that of an officer, whose burial as the result of a shell explosion had been followed by symptoms pointing to some degree of cerebral concussion. In spite of severe headache, vomiting, and disorder of micturition, he remained on duty for more than two months. He then collapsed altogether after a very trying experience, in which he had gone out to seek a fellow officer and had found his body blown into pieces, with head and limbs lying separated from the trunk.

From that time he had been haunted at night by the vision of his dead and mutilated friend. When he slept he had nightmares in which his friend appeared, sometimes as he had seen him mangled on the field, sometimes in the still more terrifying aspect of one whose limbs and features had been eaten away by leprosy. The mutilated or leprous officer of the dream would come nearer and nearer until the patient suddenly awoke pouring with sweat and in a state of the utmost terror. He dreaded to go to sleep, and spent each day looking forward in painful anticipation of the night. He had been advised to keep all thoughts of war from his mind, but the experience which recurred so often at night was so insistent that he could not keep it wholly from his thoughts, much as he tried to do so. Nevertheless, there is no question but that he was striving by day to dispel memories only to bring them upon him with redoubled force and horror when he slept.

The problem before me in this case was to find some aspect of the painful experience which would allow the patient to dwell upon it in such a way as to relieve its horrible and terrifying character. The aspect to which I drew his attention was that the mangled state of the body of his friend was conclusive evidence that he had been killed outright and had been spared the long and lingering illness and

suffering which is too often the fate of those who sustain mortal wounds. He brightened at once and said that this aspect of the case had never occurred to him, nor had it been suggested by any of those to whom he had previously related his story. He saw at once that this was an aspect of his experience upon which he could allow his thoughts to dwell. He said he would no longer attempt to banish thoughts and memories of his friend from his mind, but would think of the pain and suffering he had been spared.

For several nights he had no dreams at all, and then came a night in which he dreamt that he went out into No Man's Land to seek his friend and saw his mangled body just as in other dreams, but without the horror which had always previously been present. He knelt beside his friend to save for the relatives any objects of value which were upon the body, a pious duty he had fulfilled in the actual scene, and as he was taking off the Sam Browne belt he woke with none of the horror and terror of the past, but weeping gently, feeling only grief for the loss of a friend.

Some nights later he had another dream in which he met his friend, still mangled, but no longer terrifying. They talked together and the patient told the history of his illness and how he was now able to speak to him in comfort and without horror or undue distress. Once only during his stay in hospital did he again experience horror in connexion with any dream of his friend. During the few days following his discharge from hospital the dream recurred once or twice with some degree of its former terrifying quality, but in his last report to me he had only had one unpleasant dream with a different content, and was regaining his normal health and strength.

Case in which Method was not Applicable.

In the two cases I have described there can be little question that the most distressing symptoms were being produced or kept in activity by reason of repression. The cessation of the repression was followed by the disappearance of the most distressing symptoms and great improvement in the general health. It is not always, however, that the line of treatment adopted in these cases is so successful. Sometimes the experience which a patient is striving to forget is so utterly horrible or disgusting, so wholly free from any redeeming feature which can be used as a means of readjusting the attention, that it is difficult or impossible to find an aspect which will make its contemplation endurable.

Such a case is that of a young officer who was flung down by the explosion of a shell so that his face struck the distended abdomen of a German several days dead, the impact of his fall rupturing the swollen corpse. Before he lost consciousness the patient had clearly realised his situation and knew that the substance which filled his mouth and produced the most horrible sensations of taste and smell was derived from the decomposed entrails of an enemy. When he came to himself he vomited profusely and was much shaken, but carried on for several days, vomiting frequently and haunted by persistent images of taste and smell.

When he came under my care several months later, suffering from horrible dreams in which the events I have narrated were faithfully reproduced, he was striving by every means in his power to keep the disgusting and painful memory from his mind. His only period of relief had occurred when he had gone into the country far from all that could remind him of the war, and this experience, combined with the utterly horrible nature of his memory and images, not only made it difficult for him to discontinue the repression, but also made me hesitate to advise this measure with any confidence. The dream became less frequent and less terrible, but it still recurred, and it was thought best that he should leave the Army and seek the conditions which had previously given him relief.

Effect of Long-continued Repression.

A more frequent cause of failure or slight extent of improvement is met with in cases in which the repression has been allowed to continue for so long that it has become a habit.

Such a case is that of an officer above the average age who, while looking at the destruction wrought by a shell explosion lost consciousness, probably as the result of a shock caused by a second shell. He was so ill in France that he could tell little about his state there.

When admitted to hospital in England he had lost power and sensation in his legs and was suffering from severe headache, sleeplessness, and terrifying dreams. He was treated by hypnotism and hypnotic drugs and was advised neither to read the papers nor talk with anyone about the war. After being about two months in hospital he was given three months' leave. On going home he was so disturbed by remarks about the war that he left his relatives and buried himself in the heart of the country, where he saw no one, read no papers, and resolutely kept his mind from all thoughts of war. With the aid of aspirin and bromides he slept better and had less headache, but when at the end of his period of leave he appeared before a medical board and the president asked a question about the trenches he broke down completely and wept. He was given another two months' leave, and again repaired to the country to continue the treatment by isolation and repression.

This went on till the order that all officers must be in hospital or on duty led to his being sent to an inland watering-place, where no inquiries were made about his anxieties or memories; but he was treated by baths, electricity, and massage. He rapidly became worse ; his sleep, which had improved, became as bad as ever, and he was transferred to Craiglockhart War Hospital. He was then very emaciated, with a constant expression of anxiety and dread. His legs were still weak, and he was able to take very little exercise or occupy his mind for any time. His chief complaint was of sleeplessness and frequent dreams in which war scenes were reproduced, while all kinds of distressing thoughts connected with the war would crowd into his mind as he was trying to get to sleep.

He was advised to give up the practice of repression, to read the papers, talk occasionally about the war, and gradually accustom himself to thinking of, and hearing about, war experience. He did so, but in a half-hearted manner, being convinced that the ideal treatment was that he had so long followed. He was reluctant to admit that the success of a mode of treatment which led him to break down and weep when the war was mentioned was of a very superficial kind. Nevertheless he improved distinctly and slept better. The reproduction of scenes of war in his dreams became less frequent and were replaced by images the material of which was provided by scenes of home life. He became able to read the papers without disturbance, but was loth to acknowledge that his improvement was connected with this ability to face thoughts of war, saying that he had been as well when following his own treatment by isolation, and he evidently believed that he would have recovered if he had not been taken from his retreat and sent into hospital. It soon became obvious that the patient would be of no further service in the Army, and he relinquished his commission.

I cite this case not so much as an example of failure or relative failure of the treatment by removal of repression, for it is probable that such relaxation of repression as occurred was a definite factor in his improvement. I cite it rather as an example of the state produced by long continued repression and of the difficulties which arise when the repression has had such apparent success as to make the patient believe in it.

Dissociation.

In the cases I have just narrated there was no evidence that the process of repression had produced the state of suppression or dissociation. The memories or other painful experience were at hand ready to be recalled or even to obtrude themselves upon consciousness at any moment. A state in which repressed elements of the mental content find their expression in dreams may perhaps be regarded as the first step towards suppression or dissociation, but, if so, it forms a very early stage of the process.

There is no question that some people are more liable to become the subjects of dissociation or splitting of consciousness than others. In some persons there is probably an innate tendency in this direction ; in others the liability arises through some shock or illness ; while other persons become especially susceptible as the result of having been hypnotised.

Not only do shock and illness produce a liability to dissociation, but these factors may also act as its immediate precursors and exciting causes. How far the process of voluntary repression can produce this state is more doubtful. It is probable that it only has this effect in persons who are especially prone to the occurrence of dissociation. The great frequency of the process of voluntary repression in cases of war neurosis might be expected to provide us with definite evidence on this head, and there is little doubt that such evidence is present.

As an example I may cite the case of a young officer who had done well in France until he had been deprived of consciousness by a shell explosion. The next thing he remembered was being conducted by his servant towards the base, thoroughly broken down. On admission into hospital he suffered from fearful headaches and had hardly any sleep, and when he slept he had terrifying dreams of warfare. When he came under my care two months later his chief complaint was that, whereas ordinarily he felt cheerful and

keen on life, there would come upon him at times, with absolute suddenness, the most terrible depression, a state of a kind absolutely different from an ordinary fit of the blues, having a quality which he could only describe as "something quite on its own."

For some time he had no attack and seemed as if he had not a care in the world. Ten days after admission he came to me one evening pale and with a tense anxious expression which wholly altered his appearance. A few minutes earlier he had been writing a letter in his usual mood when there descended upon him a state of deep depression and despair which seemed to have no reason. He had had a pleasant and not too tiring afternoon on some neighbouring hills, and there was nothing in the letter he was writing which could be supposed to have suggested anything painful or depressing. As we talked the depression cleared off and in about ten minutes he was nearly himself again.

He had no further attack of depression for nine days, and then one afternoon, as he was standing idly looking from a window, there suddenly descended upon him the state of horrible dread. I happened to be away from the hospital and he had to fight it out alone. The attack was more severe than usual and lasted for several hours. It was so severe that he believed he would have shot himself if his revolver had been accessible. On my return to the hospital some hours after the onset of the attack he was better, but still looked pale and anxious. His state of reasonless dread had passed into one of depression and anxiety natural to one who recognises that he has been through an experience which has put his life in danger and is liable to recur.

The gusts of depression to which this patient was subject were of the kind which I was then inclined to ascribe to the hidden working of some forgotten yet active experience, and it seemed natural at first to think of some incident during the time which elapsed between the shell explosion which deprived him of consciousness and the moment when he came to himself walking back from the trenches. I considered whether this was not a case in which the lost memory might be recovered by means of hypnotism, but in the presence of the definite tendency to dissociation I did not like to employ this means of diagnosis, and less drastic methods of recovering any forgotten incident were without avail.

It occurred to me that the soldier who was accompanying the patient on his walk from the trenches might be able to supply a clue to some lost memory. While waiting for an answer to an inquiry I discovered that behind his apparent cheerfulness at ordinary times the patient was the subject of grave apprehensions about his fitness for further service in France, which he was not allowing himself to entertain owing to the idea that such thoughts were equivalent to cowardice, or might, at any rate, be so interpreted by others. It became evident that he had been practising a systematic process of repression of these thoughts and apprehensions, and the question arose whether this repression might not be the source of his attacks of depression rather than some forgotten experience.

The patient had already become familiar with the idea that his gusts of depression might be due to the activity of some submerged experience, and it was only necessary to consider whether we had not hitherto mistaken the repressed object. Disagreeable as was the situation in which he found himself, I advised him that it was one which it was best to face, and that it was of no avail to pretend that it did not exist. I pointed out that this procedure might produce some discomfort and unhappiness, but that it was far better to suffer so than continue in a course whereby painful thoughts were pushed into hidden recesses of his mind only to accumulate such force as to make them well up and produce attacks of depression so severe as to put his life in danger from suicide.* He agreed to face the situation and no longer to continue his attempt to banish his apprehensions.

From this time he had only one transient attack of morbid depression following a minor surgical operation. He became less cheerful generally and his state acquired more closely the usual characters of anxiety neurosis, and this was so persistent that he was finally passed by a medical board as unfit for military service.

Variety of Experiences leading to Repression.

In the cases I have recorded the elements of the mental content which were the object of repression were chiefly distressing memories. In the case just quoted painful anticipations were prominent, and probably had a place among the objects of repression in other cases. Many other kinds of mental experience may be similarly repressed. Thus, after one of my patients had for long baffled all attempts to discover the source of his trouble, it finally appeared that he was attempting to banish from his mind feelings of shame due to his having broken down. Great improvement rapidly followed a line of action in which he faced this shame, and thereby came to see how little cause there was for this emotion. In another case an officer had carried the repression of grief concerning the general loss of life and happiness through the war to the point of suppression, the suppressed emotion finding vent in attacks of weeping, which came on suddenly with no apparent cause. In this case the treatment was less successful, and I cite it only to illustrate the variety of experience which may become the object of repression.

I will conclude my record of cases by a brief account which is interesting in that it might well have occurred in civil practice.

A young officer after more than two years' service had failed to get to France, in spite of his urgent desires in that direction. Repeated disappointments in this respect, combined with anxieties connected with his work, had led to the development of a state in which he suffered from troubled sleep with attacks of somnambulism by night and "fainting fits" by day. Some time after he came under my care I found that, acting under the advice of every doctor he had met, he had been systematically thrusting all thought of his work out of his mind, with the result that when he went to bed battalion orders and other features of his work as an adjutant raced in endless succession through his mind and kept him from sleeping. I advised him to think of his work by day, even to plan what he would do when he returned to his military duties. The troublesome night thoughts soon went, he rapidly improved, and returned to duty. When last he wrote he had improved so much that his hopes of general service had at last been realised.

CAUSATION AND TREATMENT.

In the cases recorded in this paper the patients had been repressing certain painful elements of their mental content. They had been deliberately practising what we must regard as a definite course of treatment, in nearly every case adopted on medical advice, in which they were either deliberately thrusting certain unpleasant memories or thoughts from their minds, or were occupying every moment of the day in some activity in order that these thoughts might not come into the focus of attention. At the same time they were suffering from certain highly distressing symptoms which disappeared or altered in character when the process of repression ceased. Moreover, the symptoms by which they had been troubled were such as receive a natural, if not obvious, explanation as the result of the repression they had been practising.

If a person voluntarily represses unpleasant thoughts during the day it is natural that they should rise into activity when the control of the waking state is removed by sleep or lessened in the state which precedes or follows sleep or occupies its intervals. If the painful thoughts have been kept from the attention throughout the day by means of occupation, it is again natural that they should come into activity when the silence and isolation of the night make occupation no longer possible. It seems as if the thoughts repressed by day assume a painful quality when they come to the surface at night, far more intense than is ever attained if they are allowed to occupy the attention during the day. It is as if the process of repression keeps the painful memories or thoughts under a kind of pressure during the day, accumulating such energy by night that they race through the mind with abnormal speed and violence when the patient is wakeful, or take the most vivid and painful forms when expressed by the imagery of dreams.

When such distressing, if not terrible, symptoms disappear or alter in character as soon as repression ceases, it is natural to conclude that the two processes stand to one another in the relation of cause and effect, but so great is the complexity of the conditions with which we are dealing in the medicine of the mind that it is necessary to consider certain alternative explanations.

Catharsis.

The disappearance or improvement of symptoms on the cessation of voluntary repression may be regarded as due to the action of one form of the principle of catharsis. This term is generally used for the agency which is operative when a suppressed or dissociated body of experience is brought to the surface so that it again becomes re-integrated with the ordinary personality. It is no great step from this to the mode of action recorded in this paper, in which experience on its way towards suppression has undergone a similar, though necessarily less extensive, process of re-integration.

There is, however, another form of catharsis which may have been operative in some of the cases I have described. It often happens in cases of war neurosis, as in neurosis in general, that the sufferers do not repress their painful thoughts, but brood over them constantly until their experience assumes vastly exaggerated and often distorted importance and significance. In such cases the greatest relief is afforded by the mere communication of these troubles to another. This form of catharsis may have been operative in relation to certain kinds of experience in some of my cases, and this complicates our estimation of the therapeutic value of the cessation of repression. I have, however, carefully chosen for record on this occasion cases in which the second form of catharsis, if present at all, formed an agency altogether subsidiary to that afforded by the cessation of repression.

Re-education.

Another complicating factor which may have entered into the therapeutic process in some of the cases is re-education. This certainly came into play in the case of the patient who had the terrifying dreams of his mangled friend. In his case the cessation of repression was accompanied by the direction of the attention of the patient to an aspect of his painful memories which he had hitherto completely ignored. The process by which his attention was thus directed to a neglected aspect of his experience introduced a factor which must be distinguished from the removal of repression itself. The two processes are intimately associated, for it was largely, if not altogether, the new view of his experience which made it possible for the patient to dwell upon his painful memories.

In some of the other cases this factor of re-education undoubtedly played a part, not merely in making possible the cessation of repression, but also in helping the patient to adjust himself to the situation with which he was faced, thus contributing positively to the recovery or improvement which followed the cessation of repression.

Faith and Suggestion.

A more difficult and more contentious problem arises when we consider how far the success which attended the cessation of repression may have been, wholly or in part, due to faith and suggestion. Here, as in every branch of therapeutics, whether it be treatment by drugs, diet, baths, electricity, persuasion, re-education, or psycho-analysis, we come up against the difficulty raised by the pervasive and subtle influence of these agencies working behind the scenes.

In the case before us, as in every other kind of medical treatment, we have to consider whether the changes which occurred may have been due, not to the agency which lay on the surface and was the motive of the treatment, but at any rate in part to the influence, so difficult to exclude, of faith and suggestion. In my later work I have come to believe so thoroughly in the injurious action of repression and have acquired so lively a faith in the efficacy of my mode of treatment that this agency cannot be excluded as a factor in any success I may have. In my earlier work, however, I certainly had no such faith and advised the discontinuance of repression with the utmost diffidence. Faith on the part of the patient may, however, be present even when the physician is diffident. It is of more importance that several of the patients had been under my care for some time without improvement until it was discovered that they were repressing painful experiences. It was only when the repression ceased that improvement began.

Definite evidence against the influence of suggestion is provided by the case in which the dream of the mangled friend came to lose its horror, this state being replaced by the far more bearable emotion of grief. The change which followed the cessation of repression in this case could not have been suggested, for its possibility had not, so far as I am aware, entered my mind. So far as suggestions, witting or unwitting, were given, these would have had the form that the nightmares would cease altogether, and the change in the affective character of the dream, not having been anticipated by myself, can hardly have been communicated to the patient. It is, of course, possible that my own belief in the improvement which would follow the adoption of my advice acted in a general manner by bringing the agencies of faith and suggestion into action, but these agencies can hardly have produced the specific and definite form which the improvement took. In other of the cases I have recorded faith and suggestion probably played their part, that of the officer with the sudden and overwhelming attacks of depression being especially open to the possibility of these influences.

Such complicating factors as I have just considered can no more be excluded in this than in any other branch of therapeutics, but I am confident that their part is small beside that due to stopping a course of action whereby patients were striving to carry out an impossible task. In some cases faith and suggestion, re-education, and sharing troubles with another undoubtedly form the chief agents in the removal or amendment of symptoms of neurosis, but in the cases I have recorded there can be little doubt that they contributed only in a minor degree to the success which attended the giving up of repression.

FITNESS FOR MILITARY SERVICE.

Before I conclude a few words must be said about an aspect of my subject to which I have not so far referred. When treating officers or men suffering from war neurosis we have not only to think of the restoration of the patient to health; we have also to consider the question of fitness for military service. It is necessary to consider briefly the relation of the prescription of repression to this aspect of military medical practice.

When I find that a soldier is definitely practising repression I am accustomed to ask him what he thinks is likely to happen if one who has sedulously kept his mind from all thoughts of war, or from special memories of warfare, should be confronted with the reality, or even with such continual reminders of its existence as must inevitably accompany any form of military service at home. If, as often happens in the case of officers, the patient is keenly anxious to remain in the Army, the question at once brings home to him the futility of the course of action he has been pursuing. The deliberate and systematic repression of all thoughts and memories of war by a soldier can have but one result when he is again faced by the realities of warfare.

Several of the officers whose cases I have described or mentioned in this paper were able to return to some form of military duty, with a degree of success very unlikely if they had persisted in the process of repression. In other cases, either because the repression had been so long continued or for some other reason, return to military duty was deemed inexpedient. Except in one of these cases no other result could have been expected with any form of treatment. The exception to which I refer is that of the patient who had the sudden attacks of reasonless depression. This officer had a healthy appearance and would have made light of his disabilities at a medical board. He would certainly have been returned to duty and sent to France. The result of my line of treatment was to produce a state of anxiety which led to his leaving the Army. This result, regrettable though it be, is far better than that which would have followed his return to active service, for he would inevitably have broken down under the first stress of warfare, and might have produced some disaster by failure in a critical situation or lowered the morale of his unit by committing suicide.

NECESSITY OF ADOPTING A MIDDLE COURSE.

In conclusion, I must again mention a point to which reference was made at the beginning of this paper. Because I advocate the facing of painful memories and deprecate the ostrich-like policy of attempting to banish them from the mind, it must not be thought that I recommend the concentration of the thoughts on such memories. On the contrary, in my opinion it is just as harmful to dwell persistently upon painful memories or anticipations and brood upon feelings of regret and shame as to attempt to banish them wholly from the mind.

It is necessary to be explicit on this matter when dealing with patients. In a recent case in which I neglected to do so, the absence of any improvement led me to inquire into the patient's method of following my advice. I found that, thinking he could not have too much of a good thing, he had substituted for the system of repression he had followed before coming under my care one in which he spent the whole day talking, reading, and thinking of war. He even spent the interval between dinner and going to bed in reading a book dealing with warfare. There are also some victims of neurosis, especially the very young, for whom the horrors of warfare seem to have a peculiar fascination, so that when the opportunity presents itself they cannot refrain from talking by the hour about war experiences, although they know quite well that it is bad for them to do so.

Here, as in so many other aspects of the treatment of neurosis, we have to steer a middle course. Just as we prescribe moderation in exercise, moderation at work and play, moderation in eating, drinking, and smoking, so is moderation necessary in talking, reading, and thinking about war experience. Moreover, we must not be content merely to advise our patients to give up repression; we must help them by every means in our power to put this advice into practice. We must show them how to overcome the difficulties which are put in their way by enfeebled volition and by the distortion of experience when it has long been seen exclusively from some one point of view. It is often only by a process of prolonged re-education that it becomes possible for the patient to give up the practice of repressing war experience.

I am indebted to Major W. H. Bryce, R.A.M.C., for permission to publish the cases recorded in this paper, and for his never-failing support and interest while working under his command in Craiglockhart War Hospital.

THE PREDISPOSING FACTORS OF WAR PSYCHO-NEUROSES.

BY CAPTAIN JULIAN M. WOLFSOHN, M.S., M.D., M.R.C.,

ASSISTANT PROFESSOR NERVOUS DISEASES, LELAND STANFORD JR. UNIVERSITY, CALIFORNIA.

(*The Maudsley Extension, 4th London General Hospital, Denmark Hill.*)

THROUGHOUT the massive literature which has sprung up within the past three years one reads passing references mostly to the relation of the symptoms of war psycho-neuroses to a previous neuro-potentially unsound soldier; most authors have elicited an inherited or acquired neuropathy in the majority of their patients afflicted with shell shock, neurasthenia, or any of the neuroses resulting from the strain of the war. But enough actual specific data on the inherited and acquired neurotic factors in these cases have not been published. To Lieutenant-Colonel F. W. Mott, R.A.M.C. (T.), I wish at this time to express my sincere thanks for suggesting this investigation, for his kindly advice, and for the free access to his wards at the Maudsley Extension, 4th London General Hospital.

Scope of Investigation.

In previous publications Mott has laid considerable stress on the former temperament of the soldiers suffering from war neuroses. He writes:—

" A large majority of shell-shock cases occur in persons with a nervous temperament, or persons who were the victims of an acquired, or inherited, neuropathy; also a neuro-potentially sound soldier in this trench warfare may, from stress of prolonged active service, acquire a neurasthenic condition. If in a soldier there is an inborn timidity or neuropathic disposition, or an inborn germinal or acquired neuropathic or psychopathic taint causing a *locus minoris resistentiæ*, it necessarily follows that he will be less able to withstand the terrifying effects of shell fire and the stress of trench warfare."

Pierre Marie, Charcot, Nonne and others have come to similar conclusions. Thus, in order to evaluate properly the effects of environment on an individual either in peace time or during the war, it is necessary to study the forces inherent in that individual.

Before drawing generalisations on this subject, one should try to answer some of the following pertinent questions: 1. Of what kind of forbears is the patient a representative? 2. What is the personal temperament of the patient? 3. What was his former calling, and how has he shouldered his responsibilities during active war service? 4. Do acquired war psycho-neuroses occur, and what are the causes thereof? 5. What is the relation of the last "shock" to the production of the war neurosis? 6. Why do not all soldiers suffer from war neurosis?

Before answering any of these questions one must examine all available data, up to the time of active service, and also the actual causes and circumstances exciting the outbreak

EPIDEMIC STUPOR IN CHILDREN.

By FREDERICK E. BATTEN, M.D. Cantab., F.R.C.P.,

PHYSICIAN TO THE HOSPITAL FOR SICK CHILDREN AND TO THE
NATIONAL HOSPITAL, QUEEN-SQUARE;

AND

GEORGE F. STILL, M.D. Cantab., F.R.C.P.,

PHYSICIAN TO THE HOSPITAL FOR SICK CHILDREN, GREAT ORMOND-
STREET, AND TO KING'S COLLEGE HOSPITAL.

DURING the months of March and April, 1918, there have come under our observation a series of cases in children exhibiting an unusual condition of stupor. Three of these children have been admitted to the Children's Hospital, Great Ormond-street, aged 11, 7, and 4 years respectively, and one into King's College Hospital, aged 3½ months, in a condition of stupor which at first sight suggested the diagnosis tuberculous meningitis. The children were taken ill on Feb. 27th and March 9th, 22nd, and 25th.

The stupor is said to have developed rapidly, without convulsions—in one case it was preceded by listlessness, a dreamy state, and inability to do his work at school; in another case, although the boy had been ailing and had had headache for 2-3 months, yet his stupor dated from one week before admission to the hospital. The children were brought to the hospital in a stuporose condition and lay on their backs with the eyes closed, the legs extended, the arms sometimes flexed, sometimes extended.

There was general rigidity of the muscles, but the limbs could be moved passively in any direction and tended to remain in whatever position they were placed, a cataleptic condition being present. A rhythmic tremor of the hands and forearms has also been observed. The rigidity has the character of "plastic tone," described by Sherrington, and the face has a peculiar mask-like appearance. Although apparently unconscious, the children could be roused, would on command put out the tongue, open the eyes and follow a light or the finger, but without showing any sign of recognition of the object. When the children are asked to open the eyes a flickering movement occurs before the eyes open. If the eyelids are raised passively the eyes may be seen to be divergent. Irregular nystagmoid movements occur, the eyes moving in all directions in an incoördinate manner. In addition to the divergent squint, there was in one case upturning of the eyes so that the cornea was only half seen, and in two cases less movement of one side of the face than the other when the child cried.

Swallowing was usually good. The child aged 4 years, even when most stuporose, would eat solids, and the infant, when in similar condition, sucked the breast well; in one case, however, the feeding-tube had to be used. The children do not speak, but emit a peculiar cry which may persist for hours. There is no retraction of the head or neck, but the neck and trunk show the same rigidity as is exhibited by the limbs. If the children are placed on their legs they will balance and will walk slowly forward if encouraged to do so, but take no apparent notice of their surroundings. Urine and fæces are passed incontinently into bed.

On physical examination no sign of organic disease of the systemic or nervous system can be found. The temperature may be slightly raised for a few days at the onset, but after this is usually normal throughout. The pulse remains slow; in one case it was irregular, the respirations normal. The children may perspire profusely, especially about the head and upper extremities. In one case the feet were in a position resembling tetany, and the veins over the feet were dilated. In this case the child would, if the forefinger of one's hand were placed in the palm, grasp it so tightly that she could be raised off the bed just as with the prehensile grasp of the new-born infant. All the deep and superficial reflexes are normal. The fundus oculi is normal. The cerebro-spinal fluid on lumbar puncture flows out under normal pressure and shows no cytological or chemical change. The Wassermann reaction of the cerebro-spinal fluid and blood is negative. The blood shows no change, no malarial parasite, trypanosome, or other organisms being present; blood culture is negative. The fæces contain no parasitic ova and the urine is normal.

On the physical side every method of investigation so far adopted has resulted in a negative. On the psychological side the cases have been investigated by Dr. John MacCurdy and he has gone fully into the attitude of two of the children to air raids. The younger child, aged 4, has never shown any fear of them; the elder child has always been a nervous boy, and has great terror immediately the warning sounds. Dr. MacCurdy is inclined to regard the condition as a "defence reaction to a terrifying experience."

Course of the disease.—The course of the disease has been towards recovery. After lying for 3-5 weeks in the stuporose condition the children slowly recover, open their eyes, take notice of their surroundings, begin to speak in a slow and hesitating manner and often indistinctly. It is striking that although these children have been in an apparently unconscious condition, yet they are conscious of their surroundings, for in one case, that of the boy aged 11, he was able to say that he was brought to the hospital in a taxi-cab, and that he had been fed with a tube and a white fluid (milk). He could tell the day of the week from the fact that his mother visited him on Sunday. Although the children have so far recovered, yet they are still far from normal. One boy, aged 7, remains very thin and nervous, with a good deal of irregular fidgety movements of the face and limbs. Another boy, aged 11, stands with the body bent, the arms flexed in a position resembling that adopted by a patient with paralysis agitans. This boy also has the fixed expression, the short shuffling gait, and retropulsion often seen in that disease. In this connexion it is interesting to note that Dr. Farquhar Buzzard, in THE LANCET, April 27th, p. 616, in a letter headed "Toxic Encephalitis," emphasises the "paralysis agitans" appearance of the patient described. The younger child, aged 4, when stood up and making an attempt to walk, crosses the legs like a cerebral diplegia. The intelligence does not seem to be impaired. The interference with nutrition is remarkably little; indeed, the infant gained some weight during the illness, and the child aged 4, though not actually weighed, was thought to have gained flesh during the period of stupor. The boy aged 7 was thin on admission and has undoubtedly wasted since his illness.

Date of onset of illness.—The boys were at school till the onset of their illness—viz., Feb. 27th and March 22nd. The child aged 4 was taken ill on March 9th and the infant on the 25th.

Locality.—The three children in the children's hospital came from the same district in the north of London. The other child in King's College Hospital from Peckham.

Family history.—No other members of the families of these children have been affected. The mother of the infant aged 3½ months states that she and her husband have been perfectly well; she has suckled her infant and she is quite sure that it has had no other food of any sort.

Remarks.—A note in THE LANCET of April 27th, p. 611, describes an epidemic of obscure origin occurring in children in Paris, the prominent symptoms of which were headache and lethargy. M. Netter describes the condition provisionally as a form of encephalitis. It seems this condition may be similar to that here described. So far it has not been possible to ascertain the cause of this condition of stupor in children. We have carried out such methods of investigation as were open to us with negative results, and we would acknowledge our indebtedness to our co-workers—to Miss M. A. Blandy and Miss R. Jobson for the clinical records; to Dr. David Nabarro and Dr. C. W. Daniels for the various investigations of the blood, cerebro-spinal fluids, and stools; to Dr. John MacCurdy for his psychological investigation; and to Dr. A.F. Voelcker for permission to refer to the case under his care.

Conclusions.—From these cases, all having their onset within a period of about four weeks, and particularly from the case occurring in an infant entirely breast-fed, it seems justifiable to draw the following conclusions :—

1. That a new disease having an epidemic distribution has appeared which, whilst it may affect adults, with whom we are here not concerned, affects children and even infants at the breast.

2. That the disease, which we have called "epidemic stupor" from its most characteristic symptom, is probably of infective character. Any supposition that it might be due to nervous shock from air raids seems to us to be negatived by its affecting an infant only 3 months old, and also by the fact that the onset of illness in this case, as in another, was at least three weeks later than any air raid.

3. That it is not due to any inflammatory disease of the meninges, for the cerebro-spinal fluid is normal.

4. That it is not essentially dependent upon the ingestion of sausage, ham, or tinned foods, or any other supposed source of so-called botulism, for it has occurred in an exclusively breast-fed infant.

5. That if due to bacterial cause the infection can be conveyed by means other than food.

TOWARDS the memorial to the late Captain P. Levick, R.A.M.C., medical officer to the Guards Division, who was thrown from his horse and killed, the officers, non-commissioned officers, and men at the front have sent a cheque for £77 to the treasurer of the Royal Surrey County Hospital, Guildford, "in token of the honour and esteem in which he was held."

GALVANOMETRIC OBSERVATION OF THE EMOTIVITY OF A NORMAL SUBJECT (ENGLISH)

DURING THE GERMAN AIR-RAID OF WHIT-SUNDAY, MAY 19TH, 1918.

BY A. D. WALLER, M.D., F.R.S.

A. M. W., a lady of middle age, of an equable temperament, with whose degree of emotive excitability I have become familiar by many previous observations, was the subject of the following observation during the afternoon and evening of Whit-Sunday, May 19th, inclusive of the period from 11 P.M. to 1.30 A.M., which was the time occupied by the raid on London by a considerable fleet of German aeroplanes.

A. M. W. was connected with a recording galvanometer during the day, so that her state of emotivity at the time was well ascertained. She remained on the wires during the evening from 10 P.M. to 2 A.M.; warning (by maroons) occurred at 11 P.M. and the end of the raid was sharply indicated by a second warning (by siren) at 1.30 A.M.

The experimental conditions of observation were therefore as perfect as possible, the subject sitting at rest in an arm-chair connected with a recording galvanometer reading a quiet book, with a key fixed to the arm of the chair by which she could signal any remarkable occurrence.

The reactions of A. M. W., taken at 4 P.M., were as follows :—

Conductivity = 14 γ (R = 70,000).

Response to threatened pin-prick	...	...	...	...	...	...	+1·4 γ
„ real „	...	...	...	...	...	...	3·6
„ threatened burn	...	...	...	...	...	...	2·0
„ real „	...	...	...	...	...	...	6·0

Her emotivity during the air-raid period—from 11 P.M., first warning (M.), to 1.30 A.M., second warning (S.)—is shown in the following graph, in which her conductivity

Emotivity of A. M. W. during the Air-raid on Whit-Sunday, 1918.

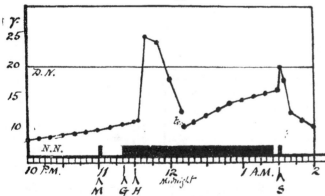

M indicates the time of the first warning by maroons at 11 P.M. G indicates the commencement of gun-fire. The duration of the disturbance was from 11.20 P.M. to 1.30 A.M. H marks the moment of maximum alarm, when the swelling hum of approaching aeroplanes was most audible. S indicates the second warning by siren at the termination of the disturbance. The electrodes were transferred from the left to the right hand at 12.5. The horizontal lines D.N –N.N. indicate the average normal day and night conductance of A. M. W., ascertained from other observations.

readings at ten-minutes' intervals have been plotted from the records. The most interesting portion of the period between 11 and 11.30 is herewith reproduced ; it shows, firstly, the effect (slight) of the warning maroons ; secondly, that (also not considerable) of our anti-aircraft guns ; and thirdly, the relatively considerable effect of the increasing humming sound made by presumably approaching German aero-planes. As can be seen on the record, the intermittent noise of our guns, noise made by a presumably defensive agent, gave little response. The growing hum caused by a presumably offensive agent produced a rela-tively large effect with a delay of about three minutes, during which the humming grew to its maximum intensity. This period was punctuated by two distinct explosions that shook the ground, inclusive, of course, of the galvanometer, the spot being shaken off scale ; but these brief interrup-tions did not interfere with the regularity of the record nor produce any reaction of the subject beyond her general response.

Remarks.

The observation is instructive in several respects.

The mental attitude of A. M. W. affords in my judgment a very fair illustration of the sane and sound attitude of an English population in presence of this latest develop-ment of German mentality which is calculated (" mis-calculated " from our standpoint) to produce terror. The subject was, in fact, alarmed but remained completely self-possessed, showing none of the ordinary external signs of emotion. She reacted only by the palms of her hands, which exhibited by the galvanometer a normal physiological response significant of fully controlled emotion. She under-stood the meaning of the various noises heard, and reacted only to such noises as indicated real possibility of injury, such as the increasing hum of aeroplanes ; she also reacted to some extent to the second warning signal by siren, which excited surprise and therefore some degree of apprehension associated with novelty ; there was no appreciable response to the first warning signal by maroons, nor even to noises that were accompanied with evident earth tremor and there-fore attributed to exploding bombs. (N.B.—A. M. W. does not share the fear of thunder and lightning experienced by many over-excitable persons. The fact that she remained perfectly quiet and self-possessed during two hours of con-siderable noise may in itself be taken as a satisfactory proof of equanimity. The electrodes were transferred from left to right hand just after midnight by reason of normal physical fatigue.)

My previous knowledge of the normal responses of A. M. W. and of her normal diurnal waxing and waning of excitability has enabled me to mark upon her chart what I regard as being the normal levels of her palmar resistance during the day and during the night. The full discussion of this diurnal phasing is reserved for a future occasion, when I hope to give the results of systematic observations of this periodicity on various persons. I allude to the fact itself now in order to call attention to the actual values of these normal levels in terms of the electrical resistance of the palm of the hand. These are for A. M. W. approximately 5 and 20 γ, or 200,000 and 50,000 ohms respectively— i.e., the values are enormously in excess of the values usually assumed to exist in clinical tests of the human subject by constant currents. In this case the testing current is supplied by two Leclanché cells only (= 2·8 volts), whereas in a clinical examination the resistance when taken is taken with voltages that produce considerable electrolysis and indefinitely falling resistance. In my own case the day and night levels (maximum and minimum) as a result of systematic observations for 10 day and night periods are 8 and 90 γ respectively, or approximately 125,000 and 11,000 ohms.

By reason of this diurnal variation of resistance I have adopted the practice of making first tests as far as possible during the afternoon ; in any case the time of day when a test is taken should be noted.

The principal practical advantage of the palmar test of emotivity is that the results are entirely uncontrollable by voluntary effort. They are independent of the ordinary signs of emotion, which may or may not be suppressed. The galvanometric signs of palmar change are especially well marked in the case of suppressed emotion.

THE BELGIAN DOCTORS' AND PHARMACISTS' RELIEF FUND.

SUBSCRIPTIONS TO THE SECOND APPEAL.

THE following subscriptions and donations to the Fund have been received during the week ending June 22nd :—

	£	s.	d.		£	s.	d.
Dr. James Craig	2	2	0	Mrs. de Meray*	0	5	0
Dr. C C. Easterbrook ...	1	0	0	Dr. T. M. Cuthbert ...	1	1	0
Dr. Thomas Guthrie ...	2	2	0	Dr. W. A. Bond	2	2	0
Mr. Percy Hoar*	200	0	0	Anon	0	17	6
Mrs. Harrison†	5	0	0				

* Per Dr. Des Vœux. † Per Sir Rickman Godlee.

Subscriptions to the Fund should be sent to the treasurer of the Fund, Dr. H. A. Des Vœux, at 14, Buckingham Gate, London, S W. 1, and should be made payable to the Belgian Doctors' and Pharmacists' Relief Fund, crossed Lloyds Bank, Limited.

were slight, but the pharyngitis appeared to cause considerable discomfort. Laryngitis was not uncommon, and cough was frequent and troublesome. The pulse-rate was not rapid, considering the temperatures, and usually fell, when the temperature became normal, to about 80 per min. The tongue in nearly every case was heavily furred. In 11 cases labial herpes was severe.

The age of men affected was very interesting. At first the younger men went down, while as time went on it was the older ones who succumbed.

The figures were as follows :—

No. in camp under 19 ...	157
Over 19 and under 20 ...	72
,, 20	287
Total	516

No. of influenza cases :—

Under 19	83 or 53%
Over 19 & under 20	16 ,, 22·2%
,, 20	50 ,, 17·4%
Total ...	149 28·9%*

* Of number in camp.

Symptoms.	No.	Per-centage of cases.
Subjective { Headache ...	140 ...	94·0
Frontal ...	88 ...	59·0
Occipital..	11 ...	7·4
General ...	41 ...	27·5
Pains in back or limbs	99 ...	66·5
Sore throat..	39 ...	26·2
Pain in eyes	40 ...	26·9
(No pains in back or limbs)	14 ...	9·4
Objective { Conjunctivitis ...	57 ...	38·2
Pharyngitis .	29 ...	19·5
Laryngitis ...	21 ...	14·1
Herpes... ...	8 ...	5·3
Tonsillitis ...	2 ...	1·3
Bronchitis ...	1 ...	0·6
Epistaxis ...	2 ...	1·3
Diarrhœa ...	3 ...	2·0

Treatment of symptoms by drugs was unavailing. Rest in bed till the temperature subsided was the only thing that could be done.

As to methods of prophylaxis, avoidance of confined atmospheres, as far as possible, was insisted upon; morning and evening nasal lavage and gargling with normal saline was carried out. Coughing, spitting, and cigarette-smoking were discouraged.

Tents were struck frequently and bedding put out in the sun daily.

The graphs attached show : (1) total daily admissions ; (2) admissions by age, daily ; and (3) per cent. admissions by age, daily.

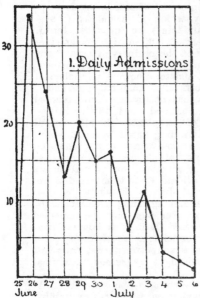

1. Daily Admissions

2. Age Incidence of Daily Admissions
— under 19.
×—×—× 19-20
○—○—○ over 20

3. Percentage Admissions by Age daily.
— under 19
×—×—× 19-20
○—○—○ over 20

SHORTAGE OF NURSES.—The Queen's Hospital for Children (Hackney-road, London, E. 2) is appealing, with the support of the Bishop of London, for the nursing service at the hospital. The number of beds lying vacant for want of nurses is now 24, with a prospect of further reduction in the near future. The weekly attendances at the hospital number about 2000.

THE SUCCESSFUL USE OF ANTIMONY IN BILHARZIOSIS

ADMINISTERED AS INTRAVENOUS INJECTIONS OF ANTIMONIUM TARTARATUM (TARTAR EMETIC).

BY J. B. CHRISTOPHERSON, M.A., M.D. CANTAB., F.R.C.P. LOND., F.R.C.S. ENG., DIRECTOR OF THE CIVIL HOSPITALS, KHARTOUM AND OMDURMAN.

AFTER trying and confirming the conclusions of previous workers on the use of intravenous injection of antimonium tartaratum (tartar emetic) in cases of Oriental sore, internal leishmaniasis, and naso-oral leishmaniasis (espundia) as found in the Sudan,[1] in May, 1917, I commenced at the Khartoum Civil Hospital to treat bilharziosis (vesical and rectal) by the same drug. Amongst the natives of the Sudan bilharziosis is not so frequent as amongst Egyptians ; still, in the clinic of a hospital such as Khartoum Civil Hospital there are sufficient cases to give the treatment a very fair trial.

The treatment of bilharziosis up to the present has been altogether palliative and unsatisfactory. It has baffled all attempts to find a satisfactory remedy. Time was the sole hope of cure, but as time takes years (a considerable number, perhaps 10)* to effect a cure, and in the meanwhile the patient is running no small risk, to say nothing of the pain and inconvenience of repeated attacks of cystitis and the debilitating effect of loss of blood, anything which promises even alleviation is to be welcomed.

There is no doubt that antimony given as intravenous injections of tartar emetic considerably interferes with the bilharzia and suspends its activities, even when it does not actually kill. My own opinion, based on the cases treated during the last year, is that antimony (antimony tartrate) is a definite cure for bilharziosis, and that the intravenous injections of tartar emetic kill the *Schistosomum hæmatobium* in the blood and render it harmless.

List of Cases.

No.	Age.	Nationality.	Date.	Quantity injected.	No.	Age.	Nationality.	Date.	Quan'ity injected.
				gr.					gr.
1	21	Egyptian.	5/6 17	15 *	7	15	Sudanese.	14/11 17	27
2	21	,,	5/6/17	15 †	8	17	,,	3/3/18	25½
3	20	Sudanese.	10/6 17	22 †	9	17	,,	5/3/18	29¾ †
			12/3/18	11	10	17	,,	5/3/18	33½
4	25	Egyptian.	23/10/17	22¾ ‡	11	12	Egyptian.	6/4/18	30
5	17	Sudanese.	4/11/17	20½	12	19	Arab.	17/4/18	— §
6	13	,,	6/11/17	18½	13	11	Shagii.	20/4/18	22

* Treatment suspended.   † Relapse.   ‡ Treatment not completed.   § Details mislaid.

Record of Cases.

These observations are based on 13 cases of *Schistosomum hæmatobium* (see Table) ; more than 13, however, were treated by the method.

Three of the cases were 13 years of age or under, the remainder from 15 to 21. Three were Egyptians, the others natives of the Sudan. Three had relapses ; the total amount of tartar emetic injected in these cases was :—
(1) 15 gr. in 6 injections in 10 days, relapse after 25 days.
(2) 10 gr. in 10 days, relapse after 8 months.
(3) Had 7 injections, relapse in one month.

Two patients were discharged before completion of treatment, being "time-expired" soldiers.

The case (No. 2) which relapsed in 25 days was an Egyptian soldier who had a heavy infection of bilharzia of rectum and bladder, and injections had to be suspended after six had been given in ten days (15 gr.) owing to phlebitis. He was one of the time-expired soldiers who would not remain in hospital after their time had expired.

In Case 4, Egyptian, the injections were suspended owing to the patient being weak, but they were resumed again after ten days. He had 22¾ gr. of antimony tartrate in 13 injections in 30 days. He was 44 days in hospital ; discharged at own request, being a "time-expired" soldier. The ova were very scanty, if present at all, on discharge, but as ova had only been absent a few days previous to discharge, this case can at most be put down as improved.

---

* Loos says the worms only live three to five years, while the eggs remain, and are the real cause of the disease.

THE LANCET,]   LIEUT. G. BOUSFIELD: ANGINA PECTORIS.   [OCT. 5, 1918   457

dentine is but thinly and unequally covered. The cutting edges may present sharp points, giving a very characteristic appearance. The defect usually extends from the cutting edge, and may, in severe cases, involve the whole crown. The teeth affected are the central and lateral incisors, the tips of the canines, and the crowns of the first molars of the permanent dentition. Usually the depth of the defect is greater in the enamel of the central incisors than of the lateral incisors, and the enamel as a rule affected is the enamel laid down in the first two years of the child's life. This condition is almost pathognomonic of rickets.

2. *Honeycombed teeth.*—This condition is much the same as the first, except that the deficiency in the enamel leads to the formation of small depressed pits scattered over the surface of the teeth, giving a very characteristic appearance.

3. *Horizontal bands of thickened enamel and transverse grooves in the enamel*, indicating acute illnesses of a more or less prolonged nature. Short acute illnesses seem less likely to produce this condition than prolonged debilitating conditions such as measles, especially when followed by whooping-cough.

4. *Chalky appearance of the enamel*, varying from white patches or transverse bands on the surface of the enamel to a general opacity affecting its whole surface. This is a very well-marked defect, and the contrast which this condition gives with the clear semi-transparency of healthy enamel is one of the chief things that strike the observer in the teeth of poorly nourished children. As will be seen, it is the commonest defect found in malnutrition.

5. *Brown lines of Retzius* or brown staining of the enamel is a common and well-marked defect found in cases of malnutrition. This defect may be found as a brown line running as a rule across the incisors, and it may be the canines or it may be a brown patch of varying size and intensity of colouring, though it is usually a rusty brown. Very commonly it is associated with marked opacity of the enamel, and it seems to indicate a somewhat severe degree of disturbance of the nutrition.

Placing the frequency of occurrence in the poor-class and the better-class children side by side, the following is the result given in percentages :—

	In 281 poor-class children.	In 122 good-class children.
Opaque chalky enamel	28·5%	9%
Brown line of Retzius	13·0%	1 case.
Hypoplasia	8·5%	5%
Honeycombed teeth	2·5%	0

As already shown, out of 281 poor children, 114, or 40 per cent., had defective enamel, as compared with 13 per cent. amongst the better-class children. Taking the 114 cases with defective enamel among the poorer-class children there was found—

Chalky enamel	80 = 70%	Typical hypoplasia ...	24 = 21%
Brown lines of Retzius	38 = 33%	Honeycombed teeth...	7 = 6%

It is of great importance to note the teeth most commonly affected. In the children where the enamel was opaque and chalky the teeth were affected in the following order of frequency.

Central incisors...	78%	Premolars	20%
Lateral incisors...	55%	First molars	10%
Canines	30%	Second molars	5%

These figures are accurate except in the case of the first and second molars. The first molars were frequently badly decayed or the tooth had been extracted. The second molars in many of these cases had not yet been erupted.

In 38 cases when the teeth showed the brown lines of Retzius—

Central incisors affected in 36 = 95%	Canines affected in 5 = 13%
Lateral „ „ 11 = 29%	First molars, 1 case.

It is important to note that in hypoplasia and in cases where the chalky patches and the brown lines of Retzius were found the teeth which suffered chiefly were, first, the central incisors ; secondly, the lateral incisors ; and, thirdly, the canines in this order of frequency. Reference to the diagram will show that the calcification of the enamel of the crowns of these teeth goes on during the first two years of the child's life. So that these defects are due to errors of nutrition affecting the child at this early period when the rate of growth, and notably that of the brain, is relatively enormous. Rickety conditions are especially operative at this period. Hypoplasia, as we have seen, affects the incisors, canines, and first molars. Much more rarely the premolars and the second molars are affected by hypoplastic changes. White patches in the enamel, one of the commonest signs of malnutrition, are, however, fairly commonly found in the premolars and second molars, which must be due to conditions operating on the child between the second and the sixth year.

ANGINA PECTORIS:

CHANGES IN ELECTROCARDIOGRAM DURING PAROXYSM.

BY GUY BOUSFIELD, M.B., B.S. LOND.,
LIEUTENANT, R.A.F.

THE accompanying curves were taken from a patient who had aortic disease. There was an old history of syphilis, scarlet fever, and several attacks of rheumatism. The typical diastolic murmur and water-hammer pulse were present.

As I was about to photograph the first lead the patient had an attack of angina pectoris, to seizures of which he had

FIG. 1.

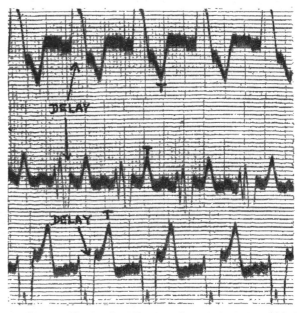

been subject. Having hastily sent for amyl nitrite capsules, I felt justified in proceeding with the cardiogram until the remedy arrived. Under these conditions Plate 1 was taken. Plate 2 was obtained from the same patient when the attack had completely subsided.

FIG. 2.

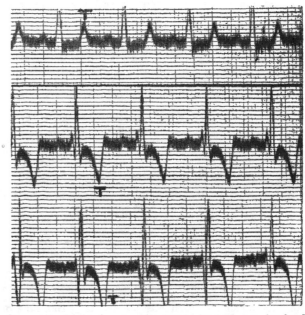

Curves in Plate 1 are quite typical of those obtained in severe cases of aortic disease, showing marked delay in the transmission of the nervous impulse through the right branch of the auriculo-ventricular bundle. It is quite clear,

THE LANCET, March 15, 1919.

AN

Experimental Investigation

ON

RICKETS.

Two Lectures Delivered at the Royal College of Surgeons of England

By EDWARD MELLANBY, M.A., M.D. Cantab.,

ACTING SUPERINTENDENT OF THE BROWN INSTITUTE,
LONDON UNIVERSITY.

LECTURE I.

HAVING described in the first two lectures of this course the experimental results obtained in a Research on Alcohol for the Central Control Board (Liquor Traffic), I propose in the next lectures to deal with another social evil—rickets—and to give an account of an experimental investigation made for the Medical Research Committee with the object of finding the essential cause of this disease.

THE SERIOUS RESULTS OF RICKETS.

It is but little realised how great and how widespread is the part played by rickets in civilised communities. If the matter ended with bony deformities obvious to the eye it would be bad enough, but investigations have demonstrated that such deformities only represent a small part of the cases affected. Schmorl's histological investigations on children dying before the age of 4 years showed that 90 per cent. had had rickets. Again, Lawson Dick's examination of the children in London County Council schools, and more particularly the examination of their teeth, led him to state that 80 per cent. of such children had had rickets. The relation between rickets and defective teeth has been placed on an experimental basis recently by the work of my wife,[1] and there can be little doubt that any remedy which would exclude the one would almost certainly improve and might eradicate the other. The rachitic child, in fact, carries the stigma of the disease throughout life in the form of defective teeth.

Nor is this the most serious part of the evil, for the reduced resistance to other diseases of the rachitic child and animal is so marked that the causative factor of rickets may be the secret of immunity and non-immunity to many of the children's diseases which result in the high death-rate associated with urban conditions. It is a striking fact to remember that in the West of Ireland, where the death-rate is only 30 per 1000, rickets is an unknown disease, whereas in poor urban districts of this country where rickets is rife the death-rate in children varies from 100 to 300 per 1000. It is at least suggestive that there may be some relation between rickets and the enormous death-rate of towns, even although the disease in itself does not kill.

The experimental work I wish to describe in these lectures has shown that the rachitic condition need not be at all advanced before the animal's whole behaviour is transformed. It becomes lethargic and is far more liable to be affected by distemper and broncho-pneumonia and is very susceptible to mange. The low resistance of animals which develops as the result of conditions which ultimately lead, under favourable circumstances, to rickets is impressive.

So many of the conclusions regarding the aetiology of rickets have been based on a small number of experiments that it may not be out of place to record that this investigation, undertaken for the Medical Research Committee, has already involved the use of 200 puppies and is still incomplete.

On referring to the literature at the beginning of the research it was soon obvious that the number of hypotheses put forward to explain the aetiology of rickets was legion, while discussion on the subject with those having clinical knowledge only emphasised the completely speculative nature of the ideas held by those whose business it is to deal with the disease.

A considerable number of experiments were first made in an attempt to see whether the aetiology of rickets was to be sought along non-dietetic lines and it was only after failure that the dietetic solution was resorted to. This type of work has continued and has clearly shown that, however important other factors may be, and that there are other

factors is not denied. the dietetic problem is the primary key to the situation. In the next lecture some of the more commonly held hypotheses of rickets will be mentioned and discussed in relation to the results obtained in this work.

EXPERIMENTAL METHODS.

Although it is well recognised that different breeds of dogs vary considerably in their susceptibility to rickets, no special type has been used in this work. In some ways this may be disadvantageous; but, on the other hand, to be driven to associate rickets with a particular breed is in itself unsatisfactory and obviously leads the investigator into a blind alley if the ultimate object is to extend the results to children.

The experimental methods used to detect rickets have depended on (1) X ray examination of the bones; (2) calcium estimation of the bones after death; (3) histological preparations of the bones.

The calcium estimation of the bones has been made by Cahen and Hurtley's modification of the oxalate method. In comparative estimations it is useful; but, since it is well recognised that the calcium content of bones varies considerably and independently of the rachitic condition, this method can never be used alone and must always be controlled by histological examination. [In the lecture further details of the methods were described and X ray photographs and histological specimens were demonstrated by means of the epidiascope].

In these lectures I propose to illustrate the normality and degree of rickets obtained by means of the calcium oxide content of the bones. Histological preparations can be seen if desired and also the X ray photographs of many of the dogs. In all cases histological preparations of the bones were made and corresponded, in comparative experiments, with the CaO results given.

[A series of puppies with and without rickets was then shown]. In the puppies exhibited it will be observed that the differences between normal and rachitic puppies are similar to the differences between normal and rachitic children. Like the rachitic child, the puppy shows abnormally large swellings at the epiphyseal ends of the bones; it has a marked rickety rosary, its tendons and ligaments are loose, the bones tend to bend, and thereby help to exaggerate the leg deformity. The amount of deformity often depends on the weight of the animal. Again, the rachitic puppy is lethargic and does not jump about; its power to run, apart from the leg deformity and before this develops, is comparatively limited; there is, in fact, a general loss of tone of the musculature. Similarly, just as the rachitic baby is a good baby and does not cry much, so also the dog in this condition seldom barks or makes the superfluous efforts practised by the normal healthy puppy.

The puppies were started on their diets after leaving the mother, the ages varying between 5 and 8 weeks, the latter being the more usual. They were kept for varying periods according to the type of experiments. In the earlier periods they were usually killed after five to six months, but as the work progressed and the diets became more rachitic this time was considerably shortened.

DETERMINATION OF RACHITIC DIET.

Having determined to see what part diet played as a causative factor in rickets, it was necessary to get a standard diet which would always produce this condition in the experimental animals. The first diet used consisted of whole milk (175 c.cm. per diem) and porridge made up of equal parts oatmeal and rice, together with 1-2 g. NaCl. The oatmeal and rice was later replaced by bread and found to be as effective and easier to use. This second diet was afterwards modified as the experimental results were obtained. The following four diets (Table I.) have therefore been used

TABLE I.—*Rachitic Diets.*

Diet I.	Diet II.	Diet III.	Diet IV.
Whole milk, 175 c.cm.	Whole milk, 175 c.cm.	Separated milk, 175 c.cm.	Separated milk, 250–350 c.cm.
Oatmeal, rice. 1-2 g. NaCl.	Bread ad lib.	Bread (70 per cent. wheaten) ad lib.	Bread (70 per cent. wheaten) ad lib.
		Linseed oil, 10 c.cm.	Linseed oil, 5–15 c.cm.
		Yeast, 10 g.	Yeast, 5–10 g.
		NaCl, 1-2 g.	Orange juice, 3 c.cm.
			NaCl, 1-2 g.

[1] THE LANCET, 1918, ii., 767.

occupied Luderitzbucht (now Bothaland) in 1914, the dust of that remarkable sandy, diamond-strewn desert, blown by the prevailing wind, proved so troublesome that the eyes of the transport mules required protection by goggles.

In lizards a long slender tendon fixed to the roof of the orbit passes in the usual fashion to the lower corner of the nictitating membrane. (Fig. 5.) At the level of the optic nerve this tendon threads a sling in the bursalis muscle, which muscle represents the retractor bulbi of mammals ; it

FIG. 6.

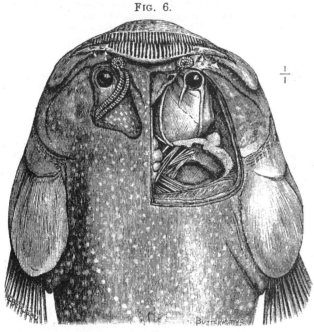

Orbit of the Stargazer, dissected to show the electric muscle.

arises from the back of the orbit, runs parallel with the optic nerve, and is inserted into the sclerotic coat of the eye. When the bursalis contracts it acts on the tendon and draws the nictitating membrane across the eye. It is a rare arrangement for a muscle to be inserted into the tendon of another muscle. There is an example in man in his foot : the muscle is called accessorius.

The pyramidalis is curiously modified. In crocodiles it is relatively big and muscular throughout. In birds it is one-fourth muscle and three-fourths tendon. In lizards the pyramidalis, entirely represented by a tendon, is activated by the retractor (bursalis) muscle. In sheep and many mammals the retractor works the nictitating membrane indirectly by acting on the globe. In man it is represented by a fibrous funnel that serves as the wall of a lymph-channel. In a fish, *Astroscopus*, some of the orbital muscles become electric organs.

ELECTRIC MUSCLES IN THE ORBIT.

The contractile substance of muscles is structureless and enclosed in a husk, called the sarcolemma. The jelly in each muscle husk receives the terminal of a motor nerve and serves as a means for the discharge of the force developed in nerve cells. Embryologists have discovered that in spite of the differences in structure of muscle cells and nerve cells they have the same origin but nerve cells are modified to originate impulses which are conducted by the nerves and discharged by the muscles.

Organs are not strictly adapted to one purpose ; they have a main function and subsidiary functions. Changes may gradually affect an organ and a secondary function become dominant. This happens to a surprising degree in some fishes, for definite tracts of muscle are so modified that the electric property predominates. In such fishes the electrical muscles, like ordinary muscles, are under voluntary control and become exhausted by use.

Electric muscles exist in several fishes—torpedo, skate. electric eel (which is not an eel), the stargazer, and the mormyr, a fish of peculiar shape living in the Nile. It was venerated by the ancient Egyptians and depicted on monuments. The proof that electric organs are modified muscles is furnished by the skate. In this fish the electric

muscles lie in the tail. When the skate is young and like a big tadpole its electric organs are muscles, and **Ewart** succeeded in tracing the transformation of the muscle cells into electric cells.

The eyes of the stargazer are on the top of its head and the mouth is in such a position that, without knowledge of the cunning contrivance in the orbits, it would not be easy to understand how this fish secures food. Each orbit is roofed with a patch of soft skin, and this covers an electric organ. (Fig. 6.) The fish lies in the sand, and small fishes passing over it, paralysed by an electric shock, tumble into its open mouth. In an example dissected by Dahlgren the stomach contained a number of small swiftly swimming fishes, such as young herring and mackerel. The electric organ lies in the midst of the orbital muscles, and receives a large branch from the third nerve and branches from the trigeminus (Sylvester).

Progress in the acquisition of reliable knowledge concerning life depends on accurate instruments. For example, the minute structure of muscle was unknown before the invention of the microscope, and the elucidation of the physics of muscular contraction required the assistance of delicate measuring apparatus. An accurate knowledge of animal heat was obtained by the use of a reliable and delicate heat measurer, the thermometer, an instrument which proved that animals have within themselves a source of heat. To-day clinical thermometers are as common in nurseries as the toy called Noah's Ark. John Hunter, when he laid by experiments controlled by Ramsden's reliable thermometers, the foundations of modern knowledge on this important matter, never imagined that muscles are the chief source of animal heat.

The study of the muscles concerned in the movements of the third eyelid may cause you to reflect deeply on the absorbing subject of the physiology of muscles. Such a study may lead some of you to make discoveries in physics and neurology that will one day make the world gape with astonishment.

References.
Dahlgren and Sylvester: Anat. Anzeiger, 1906. xxix.
Lockwood C. B.: Journ. of Anat. and Phys., 1883, xx., 1.
Tenon : Mémoires et Observations sur L'Anatomie, Paris, 1806.
Weber, M.: Arch. f. Naturgesch., 1877, xlviii., 261.

SEROLOGICAL DIFFERENCES BETWEEN THE BLOOD OF DIFFERENT RACES.

THE RESULT OF RESEARCHES ON THE MACEDONIAN FRONT.[*]

BY DR. LUDWIK HIRSCHFELD,
DOZENT AT THE UNIVERSITY OF ZURICH ;

AND

DR. HANKA HIRSCHFELD,
OF THE CENTRAL BACTERIOLOGICAL LABORATORY, ROYAL SERBIAN ARMY.

Race Problems and Researches in Immunisation.

IT is a well-known fact that it is possible to produce antibodies by injecting an animal of one species with the red blood corpuscles of an animal of a different species. These antibodies, which we call hetero-antibodies are capable of reacting with the erythrocytes of all representatives of the species used for immunising. A rabbit immunised with the blood of a man of any race will produce agglutinins or hæmolysins which can influence to a greater or lesser degree the blood corpuscles of men of any race. The hetero-antibodies are thus specific for a species and cannot bring us nearer to the solution of the race problem.

But, as Ehrlich showed in goats and von Dungern and Hirschfeld [1] in dogs, we do possess a means of finding serological differences within a species. This is effected by immunisation *in the species.* The reason for this can be explained in a few words. These antigen properties which are common to the giver and receiver of blood cannot give rise to any antibodies, since they are not felt as foreign by the immunised animal. The

* Paper read before the Salonika Medical Society, June 5th, 1918, and submitted to us for publication in September 1919.
[1] Von Dungern : Münchener medizinische Wochenschrift, 1911. Von Dungern and Hirschfeld: Zeitschrift für Immunitätsforschungen, 1911, Comm. I., II., III.

676 THE LANCET,]   DRS. L. & H. HIRSCHFELD : SEROLOGICAL RACIAL DIFFERENCES.   [OCT. 18, 1919

antibodies produced within the species which we call iso-antibodies do not, therefore, act against the whole of the antigen properties of the species, but only against the differences between the blood of the animal which provides the blood for injection and that of the recipient. The iso-antibodies thus do not influence all representatives of the species, but only the blood used for injection and other kinds of blood similar to it. If we inject into dogs the blood of other dogs it is in many cases possible to produce antibodies. By means of these antibodies we have been able to show that there are in dogs two antigen types. These antigen types, which we recognise by means of the iso-antibodies, we may designate biochemical races.

It was, therefore, clear to us from the beginning that we could only attack the human race problem on serological lines if we could succeed in making use of antibodies of this kind, for the iso-antibodies alone are capable of selecting from the whole of the biochemical elements which serologically characterise human blood as such those elements that are characteristic of the blood of only a part of the human species.[2]

Such a differentiation of the human species is now possible by means of the iso-agglutinins first analysed by Landsteiner. If the serum and the blood corpuscles of different pairs of human beings are brought together agglutination sometimes occurs. Accurate analysis of the agglutinable properties of the blood and of the agglutinating properties of the serum showed that this phenomenon has nothing to do with disease. It depends on the following physiological facts. There are present in human blood two agglutinable properties, which, however, are not equally marked in all individuals. In the serum there is never present an agglutinin reacting with its own blood, but always an agglutinin which reacts with that property which is absent in that particular blood. As has often been pointed out in the literature of the subject, these properties are of great importance in blood transfusion, for a blood must never be injected which can be agglutinated by the recipient. Either of the two agglutinable properties may be present or both together, or both may be absent, and we can therefore distinguish four different combinations in man. In the literature of the subject we therefore most often find the statement that there are in the human species four different groups. But since we have, indeed, four groups but only two agglutinable properties, von Dungern and Hirschfeld[1] introduced another definition which is shown in the accompanying table. (Table I.) They

Group O. In accordance with Landsteiner's rule that in the blood there are always agglutinins against the qualities lacking in the corpuscles we have here both the shaded anti-A and the black anti-B arrows. Finally, in the fourth square are represented the red corpuscles, which have both A and B properties, and accordingly no agglutinins. Below our diagram we have given the classification used by English writers on the subject. The English Group I. corresponds to our A B, Group II. is our A, and Group III. our B. As against Mosse, we wish to point out that Group I. does not represent any special individuality, but merely, as can easily be proved by absorption experiments, the combination of the properties A and B. For the differentiation of the groups, therefore, we require not three, but only two sera, A and B.

Results of Experiments.

What biological significance, then, has this peculiar differentiation of the blood within the human species, and how are these marks of the biochemical race inherited? Von Dungern and Hirschfeld first undertook experiments on the inheritance of these characteristics in dogs, and found that the biochemical properties of the blood are sometimes inherited and sometimes disappear in the off-spring. They established, further, that the anatomical and biochemical characteristics are inherited independently of one another. Young dogs which had the general structure and colour of the mother showed the agglutinable properties of the father and vice versa.

Researches on the inheritance of the bio-chemical group properties in man as differentiated by means of Landsteiner's iso-antibodies permitted von Dungern and Hirschfeld to come to an important conclusion as to the nature of these properties. We succeeded in showing that the A and B properties are generally inherited, but sometimes may disappear in the offspring. When the parents had A or B we found sometimes the Group O occurring in the children. On the other hand, we never found either A or B property in a child when it was absent in the parents. This observation will permit under certain circumstances of medico-legal decisions being made in order to find the real father of a child. If we find in a child either A or B property when it is absent in the mother it must be present in the real father.

The analysis of our numerical results proved that we can apply Mendel's law to the inheritance of the biochemical properties A and B. Since the A and B properties may disappear but never appear spontaneously, we can regard them according to Mendel's law as those properties which once present in the germ-plasm must also be outwardly visible. Mendel, as we know, named such a property or quality, which always gives the species its outward appearance, the dominant, while the absence of the property (which property may appear in children although absent in the parents) is considered as latent or recessive, and is set in contra-distinction to the dominant. If, for example, the dominant is *red* the Mendelian quality or property antagonistic to it—e.g., *white*—is described as *non-red*. If we introduce the Mendelian terminology we can in our cases speak of non-A

TABLE I.—*Landsteiner's Law of Iso-agglutinins.*

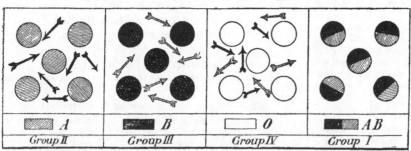

A	B	O	A B
Group II	Group III	Group IV	Group I

called the agglutinable property, which is common in Central Europe, A, the other, which is rare in Central Europe, B. In the figure the blood corpuscles possessing the A property are shown shaded, those with the B property are black. Landsteiner's rule lays down that there are always present in the serum agglutinins against the agglutinable property which is absent in the blood corpuscles of the same blood. If the individual has in the blood corpuscles the A property, he has in his serum agglutinin anti-B, and vice versa. These agglutinins are represented diagrammatically by arrows corresponding with the agglutinable property, the anti-A being shaded, the anti-B black. We see in the first square of the figure the shaded red blood corpuscles A surrounded by the black arrows anti-B, while in the second square are the black blood corpuscles B with the shaded anti-A agglutinins. In the third square we see the non-agglutinable red blood corpuscles which possess neither A nor B property, called by von Dungern and Hirschfeld the

and non-B. With certain premises, which are discussed in the second part of von Dungern and Hirschfeld's paper, the figures showing the frequency of occurrence of A and B in central Europe can be brought into harmony with Mendel's law, the properties A and B being recognised as dominant, the properties non-A and non-B (the combination of which gives Group O) as recessive. A and non-A thus may be regarded as Mendelian pairs and similarly B and non-B.

What are the laws, then, governing the relationships of A and B with each other. The calculation showed that they simply fit in with the calculation of probability according to which A and B can come together when they do not influence each other. When A, for instance, occurs in half of all cases and B in one-tenth, A B will be found together in about one-twentieth—i.e., in 5 per cent. Experience has shown that the occurrence of Group I. (our Group A B) approximates to this figure. If, therefore, Landsteiner's rule is regarded from the broad biological point of view it can be stated as follows: There are within the human species four properties of blood, A, non-A, B, and non-B.

---

[2] This only applies to non-absorbed sera.

1920s–1950s
From **IRON LUNGS** to **ULTRASOUND**

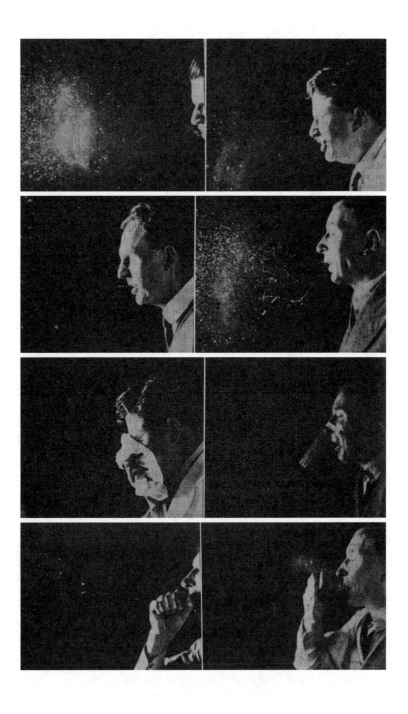

1920s–1950s

1938   **Brain *et al*.: Our colleagues in Austria.**   263
26.3.1938: 749
Eighteen eminent members of the British medical profession express serious alarm about Nazi victimisation of colleagues on the continent.
The protest was courageously published in prime position by *The Lancet*.

1938   ***The Lancet*: Editorial – Family allowances.**   264
1.10.1938: 784
The Lancet was an influential voice in the development of 'family allowances' in Britain. This editorial provides a flavour of its successful campaign, which stressed comfort, decency and subsistence, after a long period of suffering during the Great Depression of the 1930s.

1939   **Maclean, Rogers and Fleming: M. & B. 693 and pneumococci.**   265
11.3.1939: 562–568   (Extract: last page only)
Eve: A new tiltable bed: its medical uses.   265
11.3.1939: 568–569
Charming article on a 'cheap and simple' manoeuvreable hospital bed devised by a clinician, accompanied by an excellent photograph. The text reminded readers that the word 'clinician' derives from the greek word for a bed, but that this important 'clinical implement' was often overlooked by clinicians themselves.
Alexander Fleming was a co-author of the paper preceding Eve's, of which only the final summary is seen here, reporting on a systematic study of the treatment of pneumococci with the most widely used of the sulphonamide drugs, 'M&B 693' (now known as sulphapyridine). The paper expressed serious concern about resistant strains of these bacteria, and more worryingly, about their ability to establish tolerance while treatment with the drug was in process. The danger of the drug's toxic effects, and the authors' concern that doctors might be using it without justification, led to their recommendation of appropriate testing where possible and the use of combination therapy – vaccines and sulphapyridine – to help boost the patient's immune system.

1939   **Devenish and Miles: Control of *Staphylococcus aureus* in an operating-theatre.**   267
13.5.1939: 1088–1094
This ubiquitous pathogen was a problem then, too. A really fine paper, showing the ways in which infection-spread was understood and dealt with just before the arrival of penicillin.

1939   **Murray: Heparin in the prevention of thrombosis.**   274
15.7.1939: 133–134
Murray had pioneered the use of heparin for embolectomy, in Canada. This is an account of a talk he gave on a visit to the Royal Society of Medicine, London (on 6.7.1939), and the ensuing discussion.

1940   **Young and Medawar: Fibrin suture of peripheral nerves. Measurement of the rate of regeneration.**   276
3.8.1940: 126–128   (Extract: first two pages only)
Fine paper from these two brilliant scientists working together on animal models to knit severed sciatic nerves using concentrated blood plasma, coagulated to form a temporary firm medium in which nerve ends knit. Medawar, working with Seddon, later showed this method worked sufficiently well to permit sensory recovery in the human hand: *Lancet* 25.7.1942: 87–88. Important work, especially in wartime.

1940   **Chain *et al*.: Penicillin as a chemotherapeutic agent.**   278
24.8.1940: 226–228
Penicillin had been shown by Fleming (in 1929) to inhibit growth of staphylococci, streptococci, gonococci, meningococci, and the bacterium causing diphtheria (corynebacterium diphtheriae). But the prevailing preoccupation with the chemical-based anti-bacterials, the sulphonamides, probably served to delay interest in this naturally occurring bactericide. Chain and Florey thought it seemed promising, and were able to demonstrate both its low toxicity and its remarkable effect in counteracting killer diseases. The sense of something momentous is conveyed here in the simplest terms.

1947   **Platt: Two essays on the practice of medicine.**   294
30.8.1947: 305–307
This double essay (on History-Taking and on Therapeutics) is a fine instance of Platt, and *The Lancet*, taking time out of the clinic to think about the practice of the discipline.

1948   **Alwall, Norviit and Steins: Clinical extracorporeal dialysis of blood with artificial kidney.**   297
10.1.1948: 60–62
The development of dialysis for kidney failure, successfully using cellophane as the osmotic filter. An intriguing article by Voureka on the re-sensitisation of penicillin-resistant bacteria follows.

1948   **Gibson: Salicylic acid for coronary thrombosis?**   300
19.6.1948: 965
Intelligent suggestion in a *Lancet* letter which may have prompted significant later findings (see *1968*).

1948   ***The Lancet*: Editorials – Our Service, and History at Geneva.**   301
3.7.1948: 17–18
Two *Lancet* editorials, the first on the arrival of the National Health Service (the Appointed Day for its inception was July 5th), followed on the same page by another on the establishment of the post-Second World War World Health Organisation. Both editorials are good, and, showing a typical *Lancet* mix, the next item is on the surgical physiology of the stomach.

1949   **Bradford Hill and Galloway: Maternal rubella and congenital defects – data from National Health Insurance records.**   303
19.2.1949: 299–301   (Extract: first page only)
Support for the recent Australian finding of an association between rubella during pregnancy and birth defects. This was a trial attempt to use records deriving from UK National Health Insurance to trace individuals for health studies.

1949   **Medical Research Council and British Tuberculosis Association: Para-aminosalicylic acid and streptomycin in pulmonary tuberculosis.**   304
31.12.1949: 1237
Preliminary report of results of a joint MRC+BTA trial of tuberculosis treatment using a blend of drugs, demonstrating that the combination of 'PAS' (see *1946* above) and streptomycin considerably reduced the risk of resistant strains of tuberculosis.

1950   **Learoyd: The Carnage on the roads.**   305
25.2.1950: 367–369
Opinion piece in *The Lancet*'s 'Points of view' column, attacking complacency about death on the roads. Makes a convincing argument for seeing road accidents as an urgent matter of public health. Learoyd's opening salvo is noteworthy: "Children in this country are robbed of some fifty thousand years of life each year by motor traffic".

1950   **Collings: General practice in England today – a reconnaissance.**   308
25.3.1950: 555–585   (Extract: first page only)
The Lancet knew that the profession would find a 30 page report of this kind unpalatable, but, true to the Wakley tradition published it nevertheless. Sadly it is too long to include here in full. The Collings Report was an analysis of the state of general practice in Britain by an observant outsider. It provided a word-picture of the Dickensian standards of general practice inherited from the private sector by the new publicly-funded National Health Service. Collings noted patchy improvement, indeed, in some places what we might call 'centres of excellence', but in general the standards of premises and care were unimpressive. The reverberations of this report were felt over the next 30 years; the government appointed a royal commission to investigate, general practice professionalised itself and organised itself into a Royal College, and group practice in decent premises became established as the norm.

1956   **Stewart *et al*.: Malignant disease in childhood and diagnostic irradiation in utero.**   330
1.9.1956: 447
Exposure to X-rays *in utero* shown here to be related to later childhood cancers. This was a preliminary finding announced early as a result of a survey of 1500 children who had died of leukaemia or malignant disease between 1953 and 1955.

1956   **Medical Research Council: Poliomyelitis and prophylactic inoculation against diphtheria, whooping-cough, and smallpox.**   331
15.12.1956: 1223–1231   (Extract: first page only)
Report of an investigation looking at a suspected relationship between polio and childhood immunisation for other diseases. An estimate of 13% of patients between the ages of 6 months and 2 years were found to have been affected by paralysis causally related to inoculation for diphtheria and whooping-cough (but not for smallpox). A clear relationship was demonstrated and confirmed between the site of inoculation and the site of paralysis.

1958   **Donald, MacVicar and Brown: Investigation of abdominal masses by pulsed ultrasound.**   332
7.6.1958: 1188–1195   (Extract: first page and page 1192 only)
Ultrasound, developed during the Second World War, was being used in industry in the 1950s, and it is clear from this lengthy report (eight pages, only two of which can appear here) that there was a race on to investigate its medical potential. Wild and Neal had shown in 1951 that ultrasound waves could be used to detect changes in biological tissues, differentiating for example waves deriving from normal and tumour tissue in brain and breast (*Lancet* 24.3.1951: 655–657).
Donald, MacVicar and Brown demonstrated its value especially in gynaecology, showing ovarian cysts, tumours, fibroids, lumps and bumps of all sorts, and on page 1192, the beautiful arc of a baby's head. This last was a wondrous event, since the patient had been diagnosed with a recurrence of fibroids and was due for an operation to remove them. The excitement in the ultrasound room when this image emerged is described as 'considerable'. The pregnancy went on to term and the mother delivered safely. The authors took time to address the matter of the safety of this new method of medical imaging, and also stated that the technique required refinement to improve image quality: the images reproduced in *The Lancet* were the best of 450 taken.

1958   **Abrams *et al*.: Total cardiopulmonary bypass in the laboratory – a preliminary to open heart surgery.**   334
2.8.1958: 239–243   (Extract: first page only)
The technology of life support. "We outline here the work done by a team anxious to gain the knowledge necessary to carry out safe total cardiopulmonary bypass."
Good illustration of a heart–lung machine, too.

1958   **College of General Practitioners, SE Scotland: Cytological screening of 1000 women for cervical cancer.**   335
25.10.1958: 895–896
Collaborative research in general practice (a new phenomenon) which found 1.5% of women given cervical smears on an opportunistic basis had positive indications of pre-cancer. The test was easily done and not resented by patients.

1959   **Ford *et al*.: The chromosomes in a patient showing both mongolism and the Klinefelter syndrome.**   337
4.4.1959: 709–710
Jacobs *et al*.: The somatic chromosomes in mongolism.   338
4.4.1959: 710
Two papers simultaneously reporting the discovery of an extra chromosome in Down syndrome.

purposes, a normal-looking skin. I find in these cases that before the itching is relieved the pH value of the urine has to be pushed up to 7·5 or 8.

The Urine and the Action of Alkalis in Other Diseases.

It is with diffidence that I write on the high pH value of the urine in other diseases than those of the skin, and it is really to suggest the lines that research workers might follow that I state my limited experiences. In gout and rheumatism the pH value is high and alkalis give marked relief. Neurologists might test out the acidic value in their cases. Epilepsy, neurasthenia, and hysteria are examples of diseases in which I have found a high percentage of abnormal acidic urines. It would be of great interest if independent observers would record their researches in the large group of psychic and other ailments of the central nervous system, many of them involving a derangement of the autonomic system, vago- and sympathicotonic, and which in many cases exhibit cutaneous manifestations. It would seem worth while if the pH value of the urine of all patients admitted to hospital was ascertained, as alkalis are of such remarkable value in diseases as far apart as blackwater fever and broncho-pneumonia. It may account for the benefit some people derive from taking proprietary salts, and attendance at alkaline spas.

I have recently examined the urine in the cases that have shown a marked reaction to vaccination, injections of T.A.B. vaccine and serums. They all show a pH value of from 5 to 5·6, even when they were well again. If alkalis are given to cases that have a high hydrogen-ion concentration to their urine, I find that when their urine is approaching the normal limit the patient generally volunteers the statement that any symptom of stiffness after exercise, headache or heavy feeling, previously complained of, has gone, and that he wakes up fresh in the morning, and getting up is no longer any trouble to him. Chronic dyspepsia is greatly relieved or has absolutely disappeared, also, in some instances, certain articles of diet which before caused inconvenience or even rashes or other toxic symptoms, can now be eaten with no bad after-effects. Strawberries and bananas are two instances.

Treatment with Alkalis.

In each case it is necessary to experiment before the exact dose can be gauged. Dr. Barber and Dr. Semon, in the article quoted above,[1] state how difficult it often is to bring the urine to the normal limit. Here my experience in the treatment of gonorrhœa was useful, especially that gained when I was experimenting with acriflavine, which has to be given with the patient's urine alkaline. The mixture which I now always start with, and which I call mist. acidosis (for want of a better name), is a modification of Dr. Langdon Brown's mixture for the treatment of the acidosis in diabetes. It consists of :—

℞	Sod. bicarb.	..	..	..	gr. 30
	Pot. bicarb.	..	..	..	gr. 25
	Pot. cit.	..	..	..	gr. 20
	Tinct. card. co.	..	..	min. 30
	Aquam menth. pip.	..	.. ad oz.	1

This is given three times a day, between meals, increasing or decreasing the dose according to the pH value of the urine.

My best thanks are due to Dr. Barber for his advice and help, to Dr. Lyn Dimond for his interest in my work and for his skill in carrying out the pathological side of the investigations, and also to Major R. E. Todd, M.B., R.A.M.C., for many useful suggestions and his help and encouragement.

References.

1. Barber and Semon : Jour. Roy. Army Med. Corps, 1919, xxxiii., 244.
2. Sutton, Richard L. : Diseases of the Skin, fourth edition, London : Henry Kimpton, 1921, p. 910.
3. Sweiter and Michelson : Arch. f. Dermat. and Syph., Chicago, 1920, ii., 61.

THE PREVENTION OF A HIGH MATERNAL MORTALITY FROM PUERPERAL SEPSIS.

BY ETHEL CASSIE, M.D. EDIN., D.P.H. EDIN. & GLASG., CHIEF MEDICAL OFFICER FOR CHILD WELFARE, BIRMINGHAM.

MUCH attention has been directed recently to the fact that maternal mortality in childbirth remains almost unaffected by the general fall in the deathrate, and that the most important single factor in maintaining this high mortality is puerperal sepsis. In spite of the attention directed to the subject and its importance, a certain vagueness and lack of focus appear to prevail in the attitude adopted to the condition. There still seems to be considerable disagreement as to its nature, its evidence, and as to the methods of prevention.

The history of our knowledge of the condition has been retailed so frequently of late that no further recapitulation is required. It is unnecessary to go further than Dame Janet Campbell's recent report on Maternal Mortality, in which a brief and admirable historical summary is given. It is rather surprising, however, to find a little further in the report the statement "we have not as yet exact knowledge as to the causation of the infection." As long ago as 1910 Dr. A. W. W. Lea, in his valuable book "Puerperal Infection," set forth what is the accepted modern view, which simply considers puerperal sepsis as a wound infection, and therefore due to any organism capable of producing a septic infection. The variation in the organisms found is therefore what one would expect. Unfortunately, there still appears to be a widespread idea that puerperal sepsis must be a specific infection. This belief is, I believe, a mischievous one, since it affects the attitude of the attendants on the patient, and leads to mistakes in both preventive and curative methods. Considering the condition then as a wound infection, the points of interest are how far infection depends on the varying factors involved : on environment, on injury, on hæmatogenous infection, on insufficient drainage, and finally, how much it is influenced by the resistance of the patient. These are important points and have been much debated ; it is possible, however, that there may be some interest in considering them afresh in the light of a special and close investigation carried out in every case of puerperal sepsis notified in Birmingham during a period of 12 months. The whole interest of the inquiry centred on the question of prevention, methods of treatment were noted, but their relative value was not contrasted.

It is first necessary to consider the position in Birmingham as regards the midwifery service. There are 196 certified midwives in practice, whose work is closely supervised by the public health authorities. These women undertake a large proportion of the midwifery. During 1922 they attended 13,128 women in childbirth, representing 66 per cent. of the total births in the city. The larger proportion of the remaining cases were attended by medical practitioners assisted by the midwives or handywomen. Unfortunately, a very large proportion of women are still permitted by the medical practitioners to engage these handywomen to assist actively at the confinement and in the nursing during the puerperium. In addition the maternity hospital dealt with 787 cases ; these were either primiparæ or cases where some abnormality was present or suspected, while a rather larger number were confined in the Poor-law hospitals, there being no restriction as to admission. There are several small maternity homes, including a municipal maternity home. Puerperal sepsis cases are treated at the Women's Hospital in a special ward. Cases are also treated in the Poor-law Hospitals. The patients in all three institutions are under the care of skilled obstetricians, and no case is refused admission. In consequence of this excellent provision for treatment the number of puerperal sepsis cases notified in Birmingham per 1000 of the population is higher than in other cities—e.g., Leeds and Liverpool—where the only provision is a ward in the infectious disease hospital; while in Nottingham, where no special provision appears to have been made, the case incidence was at a minimum. The mortality per 1000 births from puerperal sepsis is a more reliable figure than the case-incidence, and in this Birmingham is below all the larger cities except Bristol. (Table I.)

TABLE I.

—	Case-incidence. Per 1000 of population.	Mortality. Per 1000 births.
England and Wales ..	0·06	1·38
London	0·08	1·42
Birmingham	0·11	1·21
Manchester	0·23	1·94
Liverpool	0·07	1·83
Leeds	0·07	1·28
Sheffield	0·12	1·68
Bristol	0·08	0·60
Nottingham	0·03	1·30

The number of cases notified during the period of 12 months (October, 1921, to October, 1922) amounted to 129. Of these 129, 35 were abortions, and the remaining 94 pregnancies in which the period was over seven months. Of these 94, five were not cases of puerperal sepsis. These five were of some interest from the point of view of diagnosis and are given below: 1. Pyelitis (chronic). 2. Scarlet fever (previous case in house). 3. Mammary abscess (pyrexia on the fifteenth day). 4. Acute bronchitis. 5. Chronic nervous disease (probably disseminated sclerosis, though a final diagnosis was not made. It was taken for a cerebral embolus, with puerperal sepsis, owing to the incomplete history).

Incidence.

In 1922, 19,850 births were notified in Birmingham, and the number of cases of notified puerperal sepsis was 137; this gives a percentage of 0·69, which is, of course, a very low incidence, but may be taken as an average. Consideration of this figure raises the question, "What is the true incidence of puerperal sepsis?"

Obviously the notified cases give no real indication of the condition, since only the severe cases requiring hospital treatment, or those who cannot well be treated at home for other reasons, are notified. Some indication can be obtained from the number of midwives' cases in which medical help was called for pyrexia. This is not, of course, an absolute guide, but the figures are very suggestive as shown by subsequent inquiry. It should be noted that only a small proportion of these cases are included among the notified cases of puerperal sepsis. The midwives sent for medical help for rise of temperature alone in 111 cases during 1922.

In 30 of the midwives' cases investigated in this inquiry medical help was called for during the puerperium; this may be taken as an average figure, for though the period does not absolutely coincide it is near enough for the purpose. It may then be taken that roughly two-thirds of the cases in which midwives summon medical help during the puerperium for rise of temperature are not notified as cases of puerperal sepsis. The majority of these cases are undoubtedly cases of mild sepsis. In addition it is probable that many rises of temperature are overlooked by the midwives, owing to their habit of visiting once a day only, and that in the morning. Taking everything into consideration, it would probably be fairly correct to state that at least three times as many cases of puerperal sepsis actually occur as are notified. The majority of these are undoubtedly mild cases, but a proportion are certified as dying of pneumonia or some other secondary complication. In addition many cases of phlegmasia alba dolens are known to occur, and are never notified, although these are, of course, cases of puerperal sepsis. Many practitioners who write of having delivered so many hundreds of women without a single case of puerperal sepsis have been extraordinarily lucky, or have failed to consider any case septic unless the condition was a severe general septicæmia or pyæmia. The whole question is one of definition. A clear and authoritative pronouncement is needed, and has not yet been made.

Environment: (a) Attendance at Labour.

TABLE II.

Doctor and handywomen	..	..	14
Doctor and midwife	..	..	10
Doctor and midwife (hospital)	..	..	11
Doctor and relative	..	..	3
Midwife alone	..	..	30
Midwife and doctor (called during labour)			12
Midwife (institution)	..	..	5
Medical students and midwife	..	..	4

Doctors' cases .. 38
Midwives' cases .. 51

From the figures in Table II. it will be seen that omitting the institutional cases and those attended by medical students, doctors were primarily in attendance in 27 cases, or 30 per cent., and midwives in 42 cases, or 48 per cent. This must be taken with the fact that the midwives normally attend 65 per cent. of all confinements, so that the percentage of puerperal sepsis in midwives' cases is not unduly high.

Nature of Labour.

Normal (no interference beyond vaginal examination)	52
Instrumental	29
Version, manual removal of placenta, &c.	8
Total	89

These figures show that the presence of the doctor does not under present conditions in any way safeguard the patient. Dame Janet Campbell has drawn a picture of the methods employed by the medical practitioner which is absolutely accurate for working-class practice as a whole, and which has been confirmed in this inquiry. The use of gloves and sterilised gowns is quite exceptional, while the preparation of the bed and of the dressings, &c., is primitive, when considered in the light of modern surgical procedure. As a rule, too, all swabbing and cleansing of the patient is left to the nurse, who is frequently an untrained handywoman. The methods of the midwife leave much to be desired, but a higher standard could be obtained from her if a better example were set. The attendance during the puerperium is equally important with the attendance at labour, and here again both doctor and midwife are inclined to do too little. The doctor in a large proportion of cases leaves all the nursing to the handywomen, frequently not even taking the temperature. The midwife in her turn, though more efficient than the handywomen, is inclined to visit only in the morning and to omit Sunday. There is no suggestion here of the need for careful dressing, and the securing of efficient drainage for an open wound or wounds. No change in procedure is attempted even with a severe perineal or cervical laceration. After the ministration once in 24 hours of the midwife, the woman is allowed to change her own dressings and do what she can with the help of a neighbour.

The importance of careful nursing in the puerperium is well illustrated in the cases studied in this inquiry. In 52 of the 89 cases labour was normal, with no interference beyond the usual vaginal examinations, yet in 36 of these normal labours there was injury, incomplete evacuation, or both. Where the cervical injury occurred alone, as it did in nine cases, its presence was not even suspected, while the presence of placental and membranous fragments in utero was not considered possible, even in cases where considerable quantities were subsequently evacuated. The importance of careful dressing and observation during the puerperium, with early and energetic treatment, is obvious. The attendance and nursing in domestic midwifery practice are far below the hospital standard, and taking this into consideration the actual amount of sepsis is very low.

(b) *Home Conditions.*—The small influence of the general environment of the patient on the incidence of puerperal sepsis is at first sight somewhat remarkable, but it is after all only another illustration of the greater liability to infection from a personal agent which is being so widely recognised in infective conditions generally. Probably the only important influence of environment on the incidence of puerperal sepsis is through the effect on the general health with a consequently lowered resistance, but even here the effect is seen less on the incidence than on the death-rate. Thus :—

Health of mother in all cases (total 89)—
   Good, 64 (71%) .. .. Poor, 15 .. .. Bad, 10
Health of mother where death followed (total 19)—
   Good, 11 (59%) .. .. Poor, 3 .. .. Bad, 5

The home conditions appear to be in themselves an almost negligible factor apart from the type of attendance and nursing available. In only three instances in this inquiry was it possible to account for the infection by the environment alone.

Local Conditions.

(a) *Injury.*—It is not easy to exaggerate the importance of this factor in the liability to puerperal infection. It is the most frequent cause of phlegmasia alba dolens and cellulitis. Very many cases of prolonged disability follow both these conditions, while no one can overlook the disability resulting from a badly torn and unrepaired perineum. The great majority of these cases are not notified as puerperal sepsis. It is only the more severe and generalised infection which is notified, yet among the 89 cases under consideration injuries were present in 44, or 49 per cent., and in 11 the injury appeared to be the only cause of the infection, there having been no undue interference or incomplete evacuation. The *nature* of the injuries was as follows :—

Perineal tear alone   11
Cervical injury alone   9
Cervical and vaginal injury   5
Vaginal injury   2
More than one injury including perineal tear 17
Severity.—Very extensive, 4; very severe, 12; severe, 15; slight, 13.

Such injuries are in a majority of instances inevitable, but their presence should be ascertained, and when ascertained suitable treatment applied. The point is that no special care is employed to obviate or minimise infection with the result indicated. At the same time, there can be no doubt that with adequate antenatal care, including careful abdominal examinations, the larger proportion of the severe injuries could be eliminated, and with them the gravest risks to the patients.

(b) *Imperfect Drainage and Incomplete Evacuation.*—In this inquiry 49 cases, or 52 per cent., showed incomplete drainage or evacuation. This varied in degree, but in 25 cases considerable placental fragments were subsequently removed. It appears certain that in far the largest proportion of cases injury and imperfect emptying of the uterus play a predominant part. In fact, in only 25 of the 89 cases were neither present—i.e., in only 28 per cent.

While injury of a severe type was naturally found to a predominant extent in instrumental labours, it must be emphasised that such labours form only a proportion of those in which the two factors under consideration play a part in the onset of sepsis. The number in which both or one occurred was 65, or 73 per cent., and in 36 of these cases the labours were apparently normal without interference of any kind beyond the usual vaginal examinations.

(c) *Presence of Tumours.*—This is a comparatively rare complication, but it is one that should not be overlooked. Two cases with fibroids occurred in this series, and in both the tumours became infected, leading in one case to death. Both women were elderly multiparæ, and this serves to indicate the importance of antenatal examination even in this class of patient, since this would have obviated much of the risks.

General Health and Hæmatogenous Infection.

Reference has already been made to this under "Environment," and it is obvious that a lowered resistance must result from any condition leading to general debility. Rather unexpectedly, however, the effect appears as making the prognosis worse after infection has occurred, rather than increasing the risk of sepsis. These women if they escape sepsis suffer from post-puerperal anæmia and debility, but no evidence is available that *in the absence of other factors* they suffer from a greater liability to sepsis. This modifies one's views as to the part played in hæmatogenous infection in puerperal sepsis. Probably with a local factor the presence of an infective nidus elsewhere increases the liability to, and the severity of, a puerperal infection, but without a local factor its occurrence appears problematical, since septic foci of one kind or another, especially of the mouth, exist in such a high proportion of mothers with no ill-effects. In this series one case was very suggestive. The patient suffered from a whitlow at the onset of labour, and subsequently died with a definite septic endometritis and thrombosis in the left broad ligament. There was, however, placenta prævia, and a bipolar version was performed, considerable hæmorrhage occurring.

Epidemic Form of Puerperal Sepsis and the Rôle of the Carrier.

Undoubtedly the part played by the carrier in puerperal sepsis is now of considerably less importance than in the past. Owing to the general recognition of the danger and the strict supervision of midwives, outbreaks are less frequent, but they still occur. The danger of carrying infection through an attendant from patient to patient is, of course, a very real one, and is constantly being illustrated in small and inefficiently run maternity homes. There is, however, another type of carrier infection which is in a sense even more dangerous since it is not so clearly recognised—viz., where the attendant suffers from an infective condition, such as a septic throat, a nasal catarrh or a sinusitis, and produces septic infection among her patients. These may be mild cases or the reverse. In this series such an outbreak occurred. A probationer nurse doing her district training attended, while suffering from a cold and sore-throat, several confinements which subsequently developed symptoms of mild sepsis. One of these cases was notified. The patient suffered from marked parametritis and phlegmasia alba dolens with considerable pyrexia. Medical officers whose duty it is to supervise the work of midwives are familiar with this type of puerperal sepsis; it is difficult to guard against, as the possibility of its occurrence is not sufficiently emphasised in midwifery training.

Early Diagnosis and Treatment.

The above may be taken as the main factors concerned in the onset of puerperal sepsis. Sepsis having actually occurred, however, the important thing is the prevention of death, disability, and spread. Of the last nothing more need be said, but the importance of early recognition and treatment is so paramount that insistence on any point bearing on them cannot be omitted. In this connexion the time of onset is of interest. In the cases investigated in this inquiry the onset in 79 of the 89 cases was in the first week, while in 52 cases, or 57 per cent., the onset was within the first three days. Yet of the 72 cases sent to hospital only 32 were sent in the first week. There is undoubted delay in many cases. On the other hand, in eight cases the onset definitely occurred after the eighth day, and these late cases are important, since an impression appears to be prevalent among midwives that puerperal sepsis does not occur after the eighth day. The death-rate in this series was 21 per cent. Nineteen women lost their lives. Contrasted with the death-rate of other

THE LANCET,]   DR. P. K. McCOWAN : POST-ENCEPHALITIC PSYCHOSES.   [FEB. 7, 1925   277

infections this is very high. Among these deaths, the points which call for special comment are the high proportion of normal labours, 49 per cent., and the high proportion of women in bad health, 42 per cent. ; 25 per cent. of the deaths were in primiparæ. The actual cause of death was general peritonitis in 42 per cent. of the cases. In all but one case there was delay in securing hospital treatment, which certainly in a proportion of the cases was apparently responsible for the fatal result.

Antenatal Care.—In no case was any antenatal examination made by a private medical practitioner nor was the urine examined. In 19 cases the patients had attended clinics at hospitals and child welfare centres, and in four cases midwives had examined the urine. This was the extent of antenatal care in this series.

Abortions.

During the period of the inquiry 35 abortions were notified as puerperal sepsis ; of these 25 were septic cases, and four deaths occurred. Abortions, however, present rather a different aspect of the problem and should be considered separately. One point requires emphasis, however—the need for early and skilled treatment.

Conclusions.

It is clear that the prevention of puerperal sepsis and a diminution in its mortality are dependent upon an improvement in (a) management of and attendance at childbirth ; (b) nursing in the puerperium ; (c) provision for treatment ; (d) antenatal care.

(a) *Improved Management of and Attendance at Childbirth.*—A normal labour is a physiological event and so the presence of the medical attendant is not required. It borders, however, on the pathological, and for this reason a skilled and highly trained midwife should be in attendance, capable not only of using surgical cleanliness during labour but of readily diagnosing any untoward happening requiring medical intervention. Such medical intervention, when required, should be given by an obstetrical surgeon specially trained for the work, since his aid is sought only when the case is already pathological. It has recently been suggested by Prof. Louise McIlroy that the situation should be met by appointing whole-time obstetricians in the public health service who could be called in by the midwife. While agreeing with Prof. McIlroy that it is only the obstetrical surgeon who can suitably deal with these cases, one cannot agree with her as to the method of supplying the need. The public health service, as at present constituted, is not a national service, all its activities depending on local authorities, whose views diverge widely on every medical question, and few of whom can be relied on to take long views. We already have a national medical service which is uniform throughout the country, and which is centrally controlled and guided—viz., the National Insurance Medical Service. Under the insurance scheme something is already being done for maternity, in the form of maternity benefit. Additional benefits—e.g., dental benefit—are being included in the scheme. There appears to be no sound reason why an approved maternity service should not be provided, replacing if need be the present maternity benefit. Under such a scheme a panel of midwives could be arranged whose work would require to conform to a definite standard, and at the same time a panel of obstetrical surgeons with special training and experience could be arranged, not only to attend the difficult cases but to undertake antenatal care in every case. Antenatal care should not be left to the midwife. She can do a limited amount, and should be expected to do that amount, but a thorough medical examination is required in every case in the later months of pregnancy. There appears to be no reason why public health authorities should not when possible allow suitable child welfare centres to be used for such antenatal work where such an arrangement is considered convenient. Such a service would put midwifery practice on an entirely new basis. While encouraging younger medical men

and women to specialise in obstetrical work, it would be no hardship as far as those doctors are concerned who are already specially interested in this work. It need not be a condition that other forms of practice are necessarily given up, but it should be clearly understood that a general panel of more than 500 is not allowed. It is not possible to combine specialised obstetrical work with a large panel practice. In rural areas some modification of such a rule may be required, but there should be no serious difficulty in cities. The need for more maternity beds is constantly being emphasised, and is an obvious and urgent feature of any scheme for an improved midwifery service. The cost of such a scheme need not be prohibitive, while its influence not only on maternal mortality in childbirth but on the incidence of neonatal deaths among infants should be considerable.

(b) *Improved Nursing in the Puerperium.*—A detailed consideration of a series of cases must impress the importance of this factor on any observer. The proportion of normal labours is so high that some other factor must come into play apart from the mismanagement of labour. It is a point on which sufficient stress does not appear to have been laid. Probably medical opinion has failed to realise the actual circumstances, not so much from lack of knowledge as from lack of visualising the conditions. This has already been dealt with, however. Under present conditions no midwife can give adequate attention in the puerperium. In order to earn her living she must take an excessive number of cases. If improved nursing is to be secured improved payment is essential. It becomes once again a financial question.

(c) *Improved Provision for Treatment.*—The provision made by many local authorities for the treatment of puerperal sepsis is inadequate and unsuitable. It is not possible for the medical attendant to insist on his patient consenting to removal unless he feels that such removal will lead to satisfactory treatment by skilled obstetricians. The mortality of the condition cannot be lowered without improvement in this direction.

(d) *Improved Antenatal Care.*—While antenatal care is probably of less importance than the previous factors, there is no doubt that a considerable percentage of cases could be prevented by ascertaining the likelihood of a difficult labour and making suitable preparations. The importance of antenatal care is seen even more markedly in the other causes of our high maternal mortality. A better training in midwifery for both doctors and midwives is being urged in every direction, and it is undoubtedly the first and most important step. But in this paper an attempt has been made to consider other aspects of the problem.

OBSERVATIONS ON SOME CASES OF POST-ENCEPHALITIC PSYCHOSES.

BY P. K. McCOWAN, M.D. EDIN., M.R.C.P. LOND., D.P.M.,

ASSISTANT MEDICAL OFFICER, WEST PARK MENTAL HOSPITAL, EPSOM.

UNDER an arrangement originally emanating from the Board of Control the majority of cases of post-encephalitis in L.C.C. mental hospitals have been transferred to West Park Mental Hospital. A study of these cases has been made in the hope that some new light might be cast on the intricate problem of mental sequelæ in this disease. The number of cases collected is surprisingly small, even allowing for the fact that not all cases have so far been sent to West Park. Nine male and three female cases comprise the total number. In the case of three of the males the diagnosis is very doubtful, and in another, a man of 63 years of age, paralysis agitans is present, but unless the theory is held that this and encephalitis lethargica

THE DOG AS TEST OBJECT.
To the Editor of The Lancet.

SIR,—In the experimental work which led to the isolation of the internal secretion of the pancreas in a form suitable for repeated subcutaneous administration to patients suffering from diabetes mellitus diabetic dogs were used as test objects for extracts made from the degenerated pancreas of the dog. The dog was greatly superior to other animals as a test object because the frequent samples of blood necessary in order to follow the blood-sugar level could be easily obtained by vena puncture by the same painless technique as is used to secure blood samples from patients. Secondly, the pancreas of the dog can be completely removed and a severe diabetes produced. The pancreas of the cat can also be removed, but it is extremely difficult to obtain blood samples from this animal. Blood samples can be easily obtained from the rabbit, but the pancreas is so diffuse that an investigator is never certain if removal has been complete. Thirdly, the signs and symptoms of diabetes in the dog have been more completely recorded than for any other species so that the beneficial effects of an antidiabetic substance could be more easily detected and more accurately estimated in this animal than in any other. It is quite probable that the anti-diabetic effect of the first extracts prepared in Toronto would have been missed if a less satisfactory test animal had been used.

Since the dog was the largest laboratory animal in which it had been shown that ligation of the pancreatic ducts was followed by disappearance of the acinous tissue more pancreas was available in this species, in which to seek the elusive antidiabetic substance than in any other. Furthermore, since the most advantageous test animal was the dog it seemed probable that unnecessary difficulties would be encountered if extracts made from the tissue of a foreign species were used.

I am, Sir, yours faithfully,
C. H. BEST.

Department of Physiology, University College,
Gower-street, W.C., Nov. 30th, 1926.

** Dr. Best's letter brings up to date the memorandum issued by the Medical Research Council in 1919 and is dealt with in a leading article.—ED. L.

MEDICINE OR SURGERY FOR THE OCULIST ?
To the Editor of The Lancet.

SIR,—Mr. Ernest Clarke, in his presidential address to the Section of Ophthalmology of the Royal Society of Medicine (THE LANCET, Nov. 20th, p. 1052), has raised a topic of some general interest by his remarks on the advance in the education of the intending oculist. The facts are admirably crystallised in the paragraph :—

"In the early days the only eye work was surgical, and when the various hospitals established eye departments one of the surgeons on the staff was selected as head of that department. Naturally, the younger men who aimed at specialising in eye work concentrated on surgery, and took the Fellowship of the Royal College of Surgeons, the study for which occupied all their time to the exclusion of any deep knowledge of medicine ; consequently the proportion of oculists without a special medical degree at this time was 4 to 1. As the knowledge of ophthalmology increased it became apparent that medicine was as important, or even more important, than surgery, so that now almost all the younger oculists possess a medical degree and the proportion is reversed."

While everyone will agree with this, the F.R.C.S. remains the indispensable key to hospital appointments, and the waste-paper basket is the receptacle for any application from a Member of the Royal College of Physicians. No doubt the possession of both these diplomas is the ideal, but if one alone is to constitute eligibility, perhaps the "Membership" might be considered more appropriate than the "Fellowship." The much closer relationship of the subject matter of ophthalmology with general medicine than with general surgery is obvious, and it seems unfortunate that Mr. Clarke should have followed up the statement I have quoted above by recalling a paper of seven years past in which it was hinted that "the time might come when some *conscious of not being good at surgery* (my italics) would concentrate on the medical side and call themselves medical ophthalmologists, with the prefix of 'Dr.' which (in London) is not considered to be our correct designation." In the spirit of this remark Mr. Clarke appears to ally himself with the regulations—obsolescent on his own showing—of the hospitals, and, indeed, to impute (which he can hardly wish to do) a motive other than a desire for efficiency to those oculists who have neglected the "Fellowship" for other qualifications.

No one will deny the status of the work done by ophthalmic surgeons in the past, but this has nothing to do with the point ; to argue on this would be to confuse *post* and *propter* once more. Nor is the tremendous educational value of the primary examination for the Fellowship in question.

Shorn of irrelevancies, the question is that of "Medicine or Surgery for the Oculist." I do not propose any lowering of standards, but rather a widening of them. The advance is now chiefly in the direction of medicine. Will this be recognised by the equalisation of surgical and medical diplomas ? It is to be noted, in passing, that a gynæcologist can be appointed on a medical diploma. I hope that some oculists of experience will think the subject worthy of an expression of their views. I ought to state that I have neither of the diplomas mentioned.

I am, Sir, yours faithfully,
Nov. 22nd, 1926.　　　　　　　INCIPIENS.

AN APPEAL.
To the Editor of The Lancet.

SIR,—A medical man, aged 70, who has no knowledge of this appeal, is sorely pressed. Twenty years ago he was advised on medical grounds to leave his general practice. His health recovered, and for many years he has been able to act as locum tenens, doing work which has kept him alive, but which has prevented him putting by. His wife, who is in indifferent health, does what she can by dressmaking. Of four sons who would now all be helping, three died at the age of 21 ; one, my friend, in the *Queen Mary* at Jutland ; one of cerebro-spinal meningitis at St. Omer ; and the other elsewhere abroad. The remaining boy is in the air branch of the Navy, and he sends home the little he can afford.

Recently a prolonged illness, lasting over four months and necessitating several operations, has prevented the doctor from earning a penny, and his financial state is critical. A friend has opened a subscription list with £50 ; and I, who know the facts, shall be very glad to receive, acknowledge, and forward subscriptions from sympathetic professional colleagues. Perhaps someone may know of an opening for the doctor, preferably in London, on the clerical side of a hospital or its appeal department, or of a medical or other society. He aspires only to a small living wage, and for this he would do first-rate work.—I am, Sir, yours faithfully,

HILDRED CARLILL, M.D. Camb.,
Physician to Westminster Hospital, &c.
146, Harley-street, W., Nov. 29th, 1926.

BULB DERMATITIS.
To the Editor of The Lancet.

SIR,—In your issue of Nov. 13th you published a paper by me on the occurrence and features of dermatitis from handling flower bulbs. This article attracted the attention of the lay press, and extracts subsequently appeared in several of the daily papers. As a result, numerous requests from all parts of the country have reached me, either directly or through you, asking for details of prevention and cure.

The prevention of the distinctive peri- and hyponychial dermatitis from handling flower bulbs is

THE LANCET,]   DRS. W. B. WOOD AND S. R. GLOYNE : PULMONARY ASBESTOSIS.   [MARCH 1, 1930 445

pneumonia " of congenital syphilis. There is much gelatinous œdema, but no purulent exudation and no softening. The trachea and bronchi are injected. The bronchial glands are not enlarged. The spleen in both cases is slightly enlarged ; congested but not soft. The other viscera show cloudy swelling and congestion. An intramuscular hæmorrhage of recent origin is present in the abdominal wall of Case 9. It is not at the site of a serum injection. The bowel contents are fluid, and in the cæcum are four small shallow acute ulcers, the peritoneum over which is natural.

The *histological study* of the changes in the lungs demands more detailed investigation. Yet the preliminary stage in the examination already shows certain peculiar features.

In both cases the main condition may be described as a broncho-pneumonia, the cytology of the alveoli in the actual areas of consolidation showing no unusual characters. Neighbouring areas of lung are œdematous. In addition there are small foci of suppuration and in some places there are areas of complete necrosis. In Case 3 (Figs. III. and IV.) one of these areas is at the periphery of the lung and the presence of a thrombosed artery at its apex suggests that it may be an infarct. However, thrombosed vessels are seen in other parts of the lung, without adjacent necrosis. A further peculiarity in this case (3) is the presence in the lung of plugs of coagulated material in many of the alveoli. These are of regular, circular, or oval shape, and contain no cells except shed alveolar epithelium bordering them. No structures exactly comparable with these have yet been seen in the second case.

General Remarks.

The study of the cases hitherto reported under the provisional name of psittacosis, together with these here recorded, makes the conclusion almost irresistible that there is a septicæmic form of disease in human beings closely associated in causative fashion with disease in parrots and kindred birds. This conclusion is borne out alike by the clinical features of the disease, by the peculiar morbid anatomical findings—especially in the lungs—in fatal cases, and by the evidence of contact, direct or indirect, with sick or dead parrots.

Amongst the clinical features in the series of cases here noted the prevalence of epistaxis during the early stage of the disease, the tendency to diarrhœa with collapse, and the special liability to pulmonary complications towards the end of the first week are noteworthy. If the cases are to be accepted as a group in which the infection is of the same order throughout, it is clear that the disease may be in some instances extremely severe, carrying a very grave prognosis, and in others quite mild. There is also some suggestion that age is a factor in prognosis, in that the severest cases have been in patients over 30 years of age. There appears to be no recorded case of a severe illness in a patient under 20 years of age. Case 8 in the present group, a boy of 11 years, was very mild, as was the case in a boy of 7 years, the youngest in Dr. A. P. Thomson's series of 21 cases.[1]

In considering the *differential diagnosis* the acuteness of the onset with headache, general pains, anorexia, and insomnia very naturally suggest influenza. In neither disease have we any diagnostic criterion either as regards physical signs, clinico-pathological findings, or bacteriological tests. Absence of leucocytosis marks both diseases, at all events in their early stage. Epistaxis or delirium occurring during the first few days should raise suspicion that the case is not influenza. The similarity between the diseases may obviously be so close that further knowledge can alone help us to decide how many cases labelled " influenza " properly belong to this more recently studied infection. Although it is no doubt true to say with Dr. Thomson that the

outstanding features of psittacosis are consequent on the pulmonary involvement, it must be remembered that this is also true of the more severe cases of influenza. If, however, in a doubtful case, pulmonary signs appear during the first three days the diagnosis of influenza is the more probable. On the other hand, an influenza-like disease which persists for more than five days without pulmonary complications should lead to inquiries, *inter alia*, concerning sick birds. From the enteric group psittacosis is marked off in the main by its more abrupt onset, negative blood culture in the early days, the absence of an agglutination reaction in the second week, and the rarity in typhoid nowadays of pulmonary complications other than signs of slight bronchial catarrh. General tuberculosis will sometimes present a difficulty, but here again the onset is likely to be less acute, the pulse frequency raised more in proportion to the temperature, and the appearance of toxæmia, as expressed by the facies, anorexia, and delirium, less marked than in psittacosis.

In the matter of the incubation period of psittacosis no reliable evidence is afforded by a study of the cases here reported. They do suggest, however, that it is not less than ten days.

We desire to express our thanks to several of our colleagues—to Drs. James Maxwell, R. S. Johnson, and L. P. Garrod for pathological investigations ; to Dr. E. R. Cullinan for his preliminary report on the histological appearances in the lungs ; to Dr. E. L. Sturdee (of the Ministry of Health) for sundry communications ; and especially to Dr. Desmond Urwick for his careful analysis of the group of eight cases recorded in the text, and his permission to make use of his notes.

PULMONARY ASBESTOSIS.

BY W. BURTON WOOD, M.D. CAMB.,
M.R.C.P. LOND., D.P.H.,
PHYSICIAN TO OUT-PATIENTS, CITY OF LONDON HOSPITAL FOR DISEASES OF THE HEART AND LUNGS, VICTORIA PARK, E. ;

AND

S. ROODHOUSE GLOYNE, M.D. LEEDS, D.P.H.,
PATHOLOGIST TO THE HOSPITAL.

ALTHOUGH asbestos and asbestos products have been used in industry for a long time, it is only during the last few years that pulmonary asbestosis has been recognised as a serious industrial disease.

Asbestos, which was known to the ancient world, is a silicate occurring in minerals in combination with iron, copper, calcium, or magnesium. It is quarried or mined in various parts of the world, Italy and the Mediterranean, South Africa, Rhodesia, Canada. In its natural state it occurs in strands of long silky fibres which are highly resistant to heat, strong acids, and alkalis. These masses are usually broken up into short lengths before exportation into this country. In this country the lengths are crushed and disintegrated and then either mixed with various substances for hardening into slabs, pipes, boards, &c., or carded, spun, and woven into various products like mats and mattresses, or used as an inert diluent or filling of a heat-resisting character. At certain stages in these industrial processes dust consisting of fine asbestos fibres is generated. When examined microscopically by dark-ground illumination the asbestos fibre gives the impression of a sharp, brittle metallic wire broken off at various angles and in different lengths, and, being highly refractile, has the appearance of the glowing filament of an electric bulb. These fibres can be found in the nose and mouth, and in the asbestos corns and minute skin lesions of the workers. On reaching the lung the fibres set up a pneumonokoniosis of a characteristic variety.

[1] THE LANCET, Feb. 22nd, p. 396.

in this property, but it is common to them all in a greater or lesser degree ; moreover, the reactive capacity of the inoculated animals varies widely with the same specimen. Derrick and Swift [21][22] have shown further that the hyperergy or allergy produced is not strain-specific and depends more on the method of inoculation than on the streptococcus used, and that in animals states varying from a high degree of immunity to a high degree of hypersensitivity may be produced, and moreover the hypersensitivity may be local.

The conclusion to which one is forced, both from experimental and clinical observation, is that the important factor in chronic streptococcal illnesses depends not so much on the infecting streptococcus as upon its mode of entry into the host, upon the host itself, and its previous experiences with the indifferent streptococci. Such a theory holds out a hope that one day we may be able to deal effectively with the chronic streptococcal illnesses. It is obvious that it is useless to try to deal with such infections on the same lines as those which are effective in dealing with diseases like typhoid or plague. In these infections we are able to a large extent to eradicate the infecting organism, but the streptococci are unfortunately ubiquitous. The solution of the problem lies in a better understanding of bacterial allergy and immunity. When we have discovered the difference between complete immunity, which makes the patient safe, and the dangerous state of allergy or hypersensitiveness, which is apparently a partial or perverted immunity, we shall have discovered the key to the practical treatment of the chronic streptococcal illnesses.

References.

1. Birch-Hirschfeld, F. V.: Wiesbaden Medical Congress, 1888.
2. Poynton, F. J., and Paine, A : THE LANCET, 1900, ii., 861.
3. Horder, T. J.: The Practitioner, 1908, lxxx., 714.
4. Swift, H. F., and Kinsella, R. A.: Arch. Int. Med., 1917, xix., 381.
5. Small, J. C.: Amer. Jour. Med. Sci., 1927, clxxiii., 101.
6. Birkhaug, K. E.: Jour. Infect. Dis., 1927, xl., 549.
7. Irvine-Jones, E. I. M.: Arch. Int. Med., 1928, xlii., 784.
8. Kaiser, A. D.: Jour. Infect. Dis., 1928, xlii., 25.
9. Hart, A. P.: Can. Med. Assoc. Jour., 1929, xx., 159.
10. Hitchcock, C. H., and Swift, H. F.: Jour. Exp. Med., 1929, xlix., 637.
11. Faber, H. K.: Ibid., 1915, xxii., 615.
12. Coombs, C. F., and Poynton, F. J.: Brit. Med. Assoc. Report, 1926.
13. Schottmüller, H.: Munch. Med. Woch., 1903, i., 849.
14. Andrewes, F. W., and Horder, T. J.: THE LANCET, 1906, ii., 708.
15. Gordon, M. H.: Report of Medical Officer (Local Govt. Board), Lond., 1903-04.
16. Grant, R. T., Wood, J E., and Jones, T. D.: Heart, 1928, xiv., 247.
17. Kurtz, C. M., and White, P. D.: New Eng. Jour. Med., 1929, cc., 479.
18. Holman: Arch. Path., 1928, v., 68.
19. Douthwaite, A. H.: Treatment of Rheumatoid Arthritis, H. K. Lewis, 1929.
20. Wilkie, A. L.: Brit. Jour. Surg., 1927-28, xv., 450.
21. Derick, C. L., and Swift, H. F.: Proc. Soc. Exp. Biol. and Med., 1927, xxv., 222.
22. Clawson, B. J.: Amer. Jour. Path., 1928, vi., 565.
23. Derick, C. L., and Swift, H. F.: Jour. Exp. Med., 1929, xlix., 883.

PRINCE ALFRED HOSPITAL, SYDNEY.—The in-patients admitted during the year ended on June 30th, 1929, numbered 9526, of whom 5916 contributed towards the cost of their maintenance. This number is a record for any general hospital in the Australian Commonwealth. In the year the out-patients rose from 49,386 to 56,657, an increase partly due to the opening of the radium clinic— 916 patients presented themselves at this special department. The average residence of in-patients was 20·70 days. At 9902 the number of operations has much more than doubled since 1913. The congestion in the out-patient department is such " that the situation is daily becoming quite intolerable," and the hope is expressed that the new State Hospital Commission will speedily provide the means for erecting new admission and casualty departments. The financial situation is " very much in the nature of a continuous nightmare." The year closed with a deficiency exceeding £53,000, besides an overdraft, guaranteed by the Government, of almost £112,000. The State subsidy for the year was £66,400.

MICRO-ORGANISMS IN PSITTACOSIS.

BY ALFRED C. COLES, M.D., D.Sc., F.R.S. EDIN., M.R.C.P. LOND.,

PHYSICIAN TO THE ROYAL NATIONAL SANATORIUM AND CONSULTING PHYSICIAN TO THE ROYAL VICTORIA HOSPITAL, BOURNEMOUTH.

HAVING regard to the interest shown in and the numbers of workers engaged on the small and probably short-lived outbreak of psittacosis in this country, I venture to record my findings in this preliminary note. Thanks to the kindness of my friend Dr. G. T. Western, of the Inoculation Department of the London Hospital, I have been able to examine a few films of blood from this disease. Dr. Western at first sent me two air-dried blood films from a woman suffering from psittacosis, dated Feb. 18th, 1930. These I fixed in alcohol and stained in Giemsa for 9 and 30 hours respectively, the stain in the latter case being renewed two or three times. With an entirely open mind I carefully examined these films, step by step, using a one-tenth inch oil immersion objective and compensating ocular 6—i.e., with a magnification of about 600 diameters, looking for the unknown, whether protozoa, bacteria, or virus bodies. After a very exhaustive, and even more exhausting, search of one of these films, extending over 28 hours, I found a few organisms which were definite enough to be suggestive. On examining the second film and looking more particularly for similar organisms, I found a very few quite definite specimens. Subsequently Dr. Western was good enough to send me the following :—

1. Air-dried films made from the blood, spleen, and liver of a hen successfully inoculated with human material on Feb. 25th.
2. Two air-dried films made from citrated blood from a case at Eastleigh, dated March 1st.
3. A small tube of citrated blood from a case at Guy's Hospital dated March 4th. The resident medical officer at Guy's Hospital later kindly sent me blood films from this case, a woman aged 19, on the twentieth day of disease, dated March 12th.
4. Films from heart blood and spleen of a mouse, M.12, inoculated on March 14th from a parrot which died of the disease on the 20th.
5. A small quantity of the filtrate from the spleen of a mouse, M.28, which died, four days after the inoculation, on March 26th. Subsequently Dr. Western informed me that this filtrate was virulent and produced the disease in a mouse.

In all these cases the method adopted was the same. The air-dried films were fixed in alcohol and stained in Giemsa. The citrated blood was centrifuged and films made from the deposit, whilst a small drop of the filtrate was spread on a perfectly clean slide, and when dry these were stained in exactly the same way.

The Organisms Found.

Very similar if not identical organisms were found in all these specimens—viz., minute diplococcoid and coccoid bodies, and in most cases a very few small bacilli or diplobacilli. The most characteristic were the diplococcoid bodies, which consisted of two minute well-defined dots, varying slightly in size and usually staining red with Giemsa. In a few films, especially in preparations made from citrated blood, they stained a pale blue. The average measurement of these paired cocci is about 0·6 to 0·7 μ in length, and about 0·3 to 0·4 μ in diameter. In one of the human blood films two or three ordinary cocci and diplococci were seen, and the contrast in the size and the deep-blue staining of these with the minute, generally red-staining diplococcoid bodies found in this disease was very striking. Isolated coccoid bodies were also seen, but of course they were not as conspicuous as the paired bodies.

The bacilli were very thin rods measuring on an average about 2 μ, very sharply defined, and

1012 THE LANCET,] MR. J. W. BURNS: CÆSAREAN SECTION UNDER SPINAL ANÆSTHESIA. [MAY 10, 1930

usually staining a red colour with Giemsa, but in a few films having a blue tint. On very careful examination of typical examples they are seen to have a division in the centre, so that they apparently consist of two minute bacilli. A few bacilli stained red were found to be somewhat longer, reaching 3 or even 4 μ in length, and some of these showed a beaded appearance. The diplococcoid forms were found in very small numbers in all the cases, but the bacilli were extremely scanty, only three to five being found in a film.

The coccoid and paired coccoid bodies were more numerous in the blood and especially the spleen of

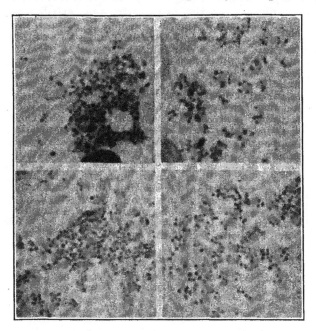

Film from the spleen of an inoculated mouse showing free and intracellular groups of the coccoid *x* bodies of psittacosis.

the hen, whilst in the liver of the hen they were not much more numerous than in the blood. The filtrate from the infected mouse was examined in Giemsa-stained films, in preparations made with Indian ink, and with nigrosin as in Burri's method, and by dark-ground illumination. A very large number of minute coccoid bodies was shown by all these methods, but, as was anticipated, considerably fewer diplococci were present.

Distinctive Bodies in the Spleen of the Inoculated Mouse.

Films of the blood of the inoculated mouse showed relatively numerous coccoid and diplococcoid bodies, and two or three red-stained bacilli were also found. But the films made from the spleen of the same mouse showed the most important and suggestive structures. Here I found not only isolated and scattered coccoid and paired coccoid bodies but, on prolonged search, I came across several groups or clusters of these structures. These agglomerations, which were for the most part lying free, varied in size according to the compactness or otherwise of the granules, and generally measured about 6 to 10 μ in diameter. They stained a peculiar bluish-red colour with Giemsa, and were quite readily distinguished from the very numerous cell granules present. When one-half of a Giemsa-stained film was treated with a drop or two of orange tannin (orange G 1, tannin 5, water 100) for a minute or two and then washed, these small masses were exceedingly well differentiated, and were totally unlike other granules. The groups consisted of fairly closely packed coccoid bodies, single, in pairs, or three or four together. Their outline is remarkably definite, and I find, from photomicrographs taken at a magnification of 2000 diameters, that they measure about 0·25 to 0·45 μ. Mr. Eliot Merlin, by very exact measurements, says that

he finds that the smallest range from 0·24 to 0·3 μ, but that many are somewhat larger. Not only are these clusters found free, but some are also seen in the interior of greatly swollen endothelial cells, and their sharp outline, somewhat regular size, and the peculiar staining reaction prevents confusion with the normal cell contents.

To my mind they very closely resemble some of the rickettsia bodies. I compared them with a slide of *Rickettsia prowazeki* of typhus fever in the louse, and they bore a striking similarity to the coccoid and paired coccoid stage of these bodies, but the colour was somewhat different, the rickettsias being bright red (possibly from the fading of the blue of the Giemsa stain, as the film was made in 1922).

The photomicrographs (see Figure) taken at a magnification of 1500 diameters are here reproduced at a magnification of about 2200, and show the distinctive features of the coccoid bodies in clusters from the spleen.

The question which naturally arises is: What is the nature of these organisms; are they accidental, commensal, or secondary invaders, or are they causal? Any speculation about their nature or relationship must be premature at this time, with such limited material at hand, and much more work must be undertaken before a definite expression of any opinion can be given as to the part they play in the causation of psittacosis. I am of the opinion that the small bacilli will prove to be secondary invaders, but that the coccoid and diplococcoid bodies found in the blood of man and infected animals are probably identical with the very characteristic and suggestive groups or masses of these bodies in the spleen of the inoculated mouse. The coccoid bodies are small enough to pass the Seitz filters and have been very definitely found in the filtrate, and these may prove to be the causal organisms of this obscure disease. They might provisionally be termed the coccoid X bodies of psittacosis.

I would here like to express my sincere thanks to Dr. Western for his kindness in sending me specimens.

CÆSAREAN SECTION UNDER SPINAL ANÆSTHESIA.*

BY JOHN WILLIAM BURNS, M.D. DUB..
F.R.C.S. EDIN., F.B.C.O.G.,
HON. SURGEON TO THE LIVERPOOL MATERNITY HOSPITAL, AND TO THE LIVERPOOL AND SAMARITAN HOSPITAL FOR WOMEN.

THE obstetrician is always faced with a very difficult problem when called upon to deal with pregnancy and labour complicated by a serious cardiac lesion and weak or failing compensation. There is another type of case which causes considerable anxiety—the patient faced with a complicated labour, who is at the same time suffering from bronchitis or some other respiratory difficulty which would render a general anæsthetic risky. During the past two years I have performed Cæsarean section under spinal anæsthesia on ten patients; seven of these were suffering from advanced cardiac disease with failing compensation, one had severe bronchitis and malpresentation (flying fœtus), and two were cases of contracted pelvis. It is extremely doubtful that any of the cardiac cases would have survived even a simple straightforward labour.

Technique.

No morphia or other sedative is given before the operation. The patient is placed upon the operating table lying on the right side with the knees drawn up and the back arched forwards. One of the lumbar spaces is chosen just above the level of the iliac

* Read before the North of England Obstetrical and Gynæcological Society, April 11th, 1930.

summary of what patients and friends have told me for many years. The severe winters are bracing for the strong, but highly dangerous to the weak. There is an absence of home comforts, home interests, home employment. It is difficult often to exercise in the open because of hills and snow, and graded exercise and work are specially difficult to arrange. It must be admitted that our own climate is superior to that of Switzerland in most respects. Dr. Harrison's final sentence is worthy of quotation : " It is a reproach to medical men that so many of these unfortunates should be allowed to die in a foreign land."

I am, Sir, yours faithfully,
R. S. McCLELLAND.
Llwynwern, Dowlais, July 28th, 1930.

THE USUAL VICTIM.

To the Editor of THE LANCET.

SIR,—It has recently been impressed on me that the gentle art of bilking the doctor can be applied with such finesse as to extort a reluctant admiration even from the victim.

Most practitioners of a few years' standing have discovered that among the growing army of the hard-up, the doctor is recognised as the person whose bills can safely be paid last, and who is the easiest to bilk—he is the usual victim. I was not aware until recently, however, how far the latter process can be carried out with the aid of expert backing from the law.

Last summer I undertook the care for a month of a colleague's case while he went on holiday. The patient's family insisted on specialist supervision, and the fees were agreed upon. After a respectable interval I sent in my bill, and as no notice was taken, repeated the process on several occasions. My last two communications were returned marked by the postal authorities " Gone away."

After a period for meditation I placed the matter in the hands of my solicitors. They were informed by the opposing solicitors that trade was in a very bad state, and that their clients could not possibly pay the amount (although they had been able to reside for the season in an expensive part of London). Encouraging my solicitors to persevere, they were successful in obtaining £10 on account. There was a lull after this for a time, and then hostilities recommenced on a grand scale by the taking out of a writ in the High Court of Justice by my solicitors for payment of the balance. The enemy countered by paying into Court the amount of the debt *less one-third* of the original total. That was a polite intimation that they challenged the amount of the fees. I was then left with the alternative of accepting the reduced amount or proving my case in Court—that the fees were reasonable, &c., which would have required the appearance of medical witnesses to speak of my standing, professional ability, and so on.

The technique was described by my solicitors' clerk as a " dirty trick," but is evidently quite legitimate in the eyes of the law. I may mention, in conclusion, that my colleague's bill was considerably larger than mine, and as he is a Fellow of the Royal College of Physicians, his chances of recovering his fees are somewhat tenuous. We may depend upon it that such experts in the gentle art are aware of the College's prohibition.

I am, Sir, yours faithfully,
FREDERICK DILLON, M.D.
Wimpole-street, W., July 22nd, 1930.

HYPOGLYCÆMIA AND SUPRARENAL TUMOUR.

To the Editor of THE LANCET.

SIR,—Your annotation on this subject (July 26th, p. 200) prompts me to say that quite recently I saw a case of Addison's disease with cerebral seizures remarkably like those due to overdosage with insulin, which I attributed to hypoglycæmia. I then came across a paper by G. Maranon (*Presse Méd.*, 1929, xxxvii , 1021), recording a low blood-sugar in 71 per cent. of his cases of Addison's disease, in which acidosis was also frequent. Cerebral seizures occurred in a number of the cases. He, too, attributes a large part, but not the whole of this to hypoglycæmia. It is interesting in view of the failure of intravenous injections of glucose to benefit the case described in your annotation, that Maranon found this procedure positively dangerous, producing a febrile reaction with serious collapse, and even death. Glucose by the mouth in doses of 25 g., three or four times a day, on the other hand, was distinctly helpful. The reason for this difference is not clear, but it is important to bear it in mind in the treatment of the hypoglycæmia of Addison's disease.

I might add, as you mention the occurrence of hypoglycæmia in necrosis of the liver, that Maranon has shown the existence of hepatic insufficiency in Addison's disease, and that I have seen striking improvement follow the administration of liver extract in this condition.

I am, Sir, yours faithfully,
W. LANGDON BROWN.
Cavendish-square, W., July 26th, 1930.

CONGENITAL ATRESIA OF THE ŒSOPHAGUS.

To the Editor of THE LANCET.

SIR,—I have lately had under observation a case resembling the one described by Dr. Polson in your issue of July 19th (p. 135).

A female child, a few hours old, was admitted to the Queen's Hospital for Children, Hackney-road, on July 16th, under the care of Dr. Helen Mackay. It was born at full term after an easy labour lasting two hours, weighed 8 lb., and appeared to be a strong healthy infant. On attempting to feed the child it became cyanosed and vomited. On admission to hospital it was dyspnœic, and was vomiting mucus ; there was marked retraction of the intercostal spaces. The air passages were cleared as much as possible with a mucus catheter, and the general condition improved. The child became cyanosed and vomited whenever attempts were made to feed it. A radiogram showed an œsophageal pouch.

At autopsy atresia of the œsophagus was found at the level of the upper border of the sternum. The upper segment was dilated to form a sac, the lower was narrowed to form a cord, and was not patent. There was an opening ¼ in. in diameter in the trachea at the level of the bifurcation connecting with the lower segment of the œsophagus. There was complete absence of the septum ventriculorum, but no other congenital abnormality was found.

I am, Sir, yours faithfully,
C. B. SMITH, M.R.C.S.
Queen's Hospital for Children, London, E., July 23rd, 1930.

EOSINOPHILIA IN ASTHMA.

To the Editor of THE LANCET.

SIR,—In a report of the scientific meeting of the Asthma Research Council (THE LANCET, 1930, i., 1293) Dr. Marjorie Gillespie, in describing the eosinophil count in asthma, stated that the highest

should or should not be included in a small manual of this size is undoubtedly a problem. And the subject is an integral part of midwifery and in so intimate a relation with its whole practice that it is difficult to determine those portions that can be separated out as being, to use the authors' words in the preface to the second edition, within " the province of the title of the book." But one matter, clearly within its province, and indeed essential to an adequate presentation of its title, is that it should give a proper perspective of all that is comprised in antenatal supervision, and that cannot be done if the social and educational aspects are left out of the picture. Drs. Haultain and Fahmy have written from the standpoint of the obstetric specialist and from that of the hospital or consultative clinic. Thus they have devoted several pages to the intra-natal and curative treatment of developed eclampsia, placenta prævia, and other conditions that belong rather to the labour ward than to the antenatal clinic and ward. If an authoritative ruling on this matter is required, reference may be made to Memo. 156/M.C.W., recently issued by the Ministry of Health, where there is a ministerial pronouncement that the antenatal clinic has a two-fold function : (a) medical and nursing, and (b) educational and social. We make this suggestion because it is probable that another edition will soon be called for ; the teaching in the book is otherwise sound, and it seems unfortunate that it should represent but a one-sided view of antenatal care.

The Materials of Life : A Simple Presentation of the Science of Biochemistry.

By T. R. PARSONS, M.A., B.Sc. London : G. Routledge and Sons, Ltd. 1930. Pp. 288. 10s. 6d.

Mr. Parsons has attempted a difficult task. He aims, as he says, " to give an account that everybody shall be able to understand of the materials of which living things are made, and of the complex but fascinating changes that these materials undergo during life." He has succeeded but moderately well. We can imagine very few laymen who would work their way through such a detailed narrative. The serious student, on the other hand, will need something more solid. The book might be useful to medical men whose physiology is long out of date, though they must not expect to find anything about stomach-ache in the chapter headed " Digestion and Indigestion " which is simply an account of the normal process. As one would expect from the author, the information given is accurate and up to date, though there is a first-rate howler on page 100 where bread and butter is called a protein-free diet.

Pleasure and Instinct.

By A. H. BOULTON ALLEN. London : Kegan Paul, Trench, Trübner and Co., Ltd. 1930. Pp. 336. 12s. 6d.

THIS volume bears a title which does not do it full justice. It contains a careful and thoughtful analysis of the major instincts—reproduction, curiosity, gregariousness, and the impulse to power. All the outstanding theories of pleasure-pain are described and discussed, and the relationship of the psychology of feeling to sensation and instinct is argued with considerable skill, and much illumination of an obscure subject is the result. In so far as any discussion on feeling is incomplete without a consideration of the nature of æsthetics and values, these somewhat philosophical subjects are dealt with also in an up-to-date and succinct manner. From the point of view of psychological medicine, the chapters on instincts and their relationship to feeling will reward reading and study.

The Formenkreis Theory
and the Progress of the Organic World.

By O. KLEINSCHMIDT. Translated by F. C. R. JOURDAIN. London : Witherby. 1930. Pp. 192. 10s. 6d.

THIS book ought not, we feel, to have been translated without clarification and condensation. It is a confused statement of the author's belief that " real species " of animals date much further back in evolution than has been supposed, though it is not clear whether he is prepared to go the length of multicentric origins. There are many querulous complaints that everyone does not agree with him.

NEW INVENTIONS

A SIMPLE FACE-MASK FOR ACCOUCHEURS.

THE belief that many cases of puerperal sepsis result, either directly or indirectly, from infection from the throats and noses of those who are in attendance upon the cases and who are " carriers " of virulent organisms has been growing in strength during the last few years. Therefore it has become necessary that some efficient means should be devised for protection from droplet infection. A good maternity mask should conform to the following requirements : (a) it should be cheap ; (b) comfortable to wear ; (c) it must be efficient to prevent the passage of organisms through it ; and (d) it should be easy to sterilise.

The mask here illustrated has been submitted to Dr. Leonard Colebrook, of the Inoculation Department of St. Mary's Hospital, to Prof. Miles Phillips, of Sheffield, and to Prof. Beckwith Whitehouse, of Birmingham,

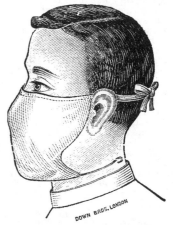

and on their advice and criticism it is submitted for general trial. The mask consists of a piece of jaconet attached to a strip of flexible aluminium, to the ends of which tapes are attached, which are tied round the back of the head. The strip is moulded by the wearer to the shape of his nose and face. To the lower side of the jaconet is attached a light, open, metal neck-spring, which serves to prevent the mask from flapping forward when the wearer bends forward. The mask can be sterilised by simple washing in a strong antiseptic solution. It is germ proof, does not fog the glasses, can be worn in any place, and is reasonably comfortable to wear. The price is modest.

Messrs. Down Bros. Ltd., St. Thomas's-street, S.E., are the manufacturers.

HOWARD E. COLLIER, M.B., Ch.B. Edin.

superimposed on a brain with an existing porencephalic defect, the latter acting as a locus minoris resistentiæ.

The following is an illustrative case of the traumatic group.

A female, aged 32, was admitted to Derby Mental Hospital in March, 1929, as a case of imbecility with epilepsy.

History.—Since infancy she had suffered from occasional epileptiform convulsions. In August, 1927, she had a serious fit and was comatose for two days. Her fits were not frequent, numbering about three or four a year. She had always had slight difficulty in walking, and had also suffered from a squint since infancy. Mental backwardness showed itself early, and at the age of 14 she had only reached Standard IV. She had never been able to earn her own living and was subject to frequent attacks of headache.

Her birth was abnormal. A fortnight before term her mother had a bad fall which brought about a premature

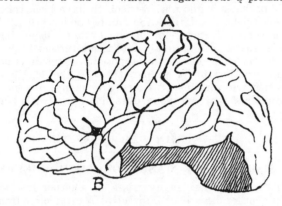

labour; this was prolonged, but not instrumental. The patient was the twelfth child. No obvious abnormality was discovered after the birth. The fits began about a year later.

On admission she was an under-developed, but well-nourished female. No stigmata of degeneration were present, but there was a mild degree of right-sided pes cavus. In the heart, lungs, and alimentary system no abnormality was detected. The urine contained no albumin or sugar. The Kahn reaction of the blood was negative.

The pupils were equal and regular in outline and reacted to light and accommodation. There was right external strabismus. Marked nystagmus was present, most noticeable when the patient looked to the left. The sight of the right eye was greatly impaired, though probably the condition was a right-sided homonymous hemianopia as, owing to her mental state, very little coöperation could be obtained from her. The tendon reflexes were abnormally brisk in the right lower limb, which was slightly spastic and showed a certain loss of coördination. The right upper limb was normal in all respects except for a rather weakened grip. A Babinski sign was obtainable on the right side at times. No anæsthesia could be detected.

The patient was hesitating and slurring in speech, dull and retarded in thought, and had little educated intelligence. Her memory was impaired and she was unable to do the simplest calculations. She could give no connected account of herself and was childish in her ways.

During her stay in hospital she had only one fit, which was of an epileptiform nature. She was able to get about the ward and did some useful light work. In December, 1929, she developed pulmonary tuberculosis, and she died in June, 1930.

Autopsy findings.—The calvarium showed increased thickness in its left posterior quadrant. The meninges and vessels appeared normal. The brain weighed 32½ oz. The right hemisphere appeared normal and weighed 16 oz. The left hemisphere was the seat of a large porencephalic cyst in its posterior half and weighed only 10 oz.

In the diagram the porencephalic area is represented as situated to the right of the line A–B, and the shaded area represents the porus covered with membrane.

The cavity was found to be in direct continuity with the lateral ventricle and to contain cerebro-spinal fluid. It measured 8¼ cm. × 6½ cm. × 3½ cm. and extended from the occipital pole almost to the apex of the temporal lobe, undermining the central white matter beneath the Rolandic area. The lining of the cavity was smooth. The unaffected cortex at the edges gradually thinned out to form the cyst wall. This thinned cortex had lost its normal configuration, and no definite gyri or sulci could be identified. It had a uniform thickness of 2–3 mm. except on the medial surface, where it measured 11–12 mm. with the configuration retained. Inferiorly the thinned cortex merged into the

membrane roofing over the gap. This membrane consisted of two layers, the outer layer being continuous with the pia-arachnoid, the inner with the lining of the cyst and the lateral ventricle. A curious feature presented itself: an offshoot of the choroid plexus was attached to the inner surface of the membrane and formed a conspicuous band of choroid tissue stretching across the cavity.

On section the corpus callosum was found to be greatly thinned, especially in its posterior half. The internal capsule, too, was much wasted, though the basal ganglia appeared normal, and in the medulla a marked diminution in the size of the pyramid was evident on the left side.

Microscopic section of the pre- and post-central gyri showed paucity in the number of pyramidal cells and disturbance of lamination, with exaggerated gliosis, especially towards the surface. No trace of any inflammatory exudate or perivascular round-celled infiltration could be seen. The thinned cortical cyst wall consisted of a dense network of neuroglia and degenerated nerve fibres with total absence of nerve cells. The membrane consisted of an outer layer of pia-arachnoid carrying blood-vessels and an inner composed of flat or low cubical epithelium, identical in structure with ependyma: interposed between the two were strands of neuroglia fibres.

Porencephaly may be suspected, but cannot often be diagnosed during life for, as Tredgold says, the hemiplegia in some cases of pronounced porencephaly discovered post mortem is often astonishingly insignificant. This can only be explained by the faculty of the contra-lateral hemisphere to undergo relative compensatory hypertrophy and thus to assume functions of the atrophied half. Diagnostically, besides the history, the only suggestive features are the occurrence in a mental defective of epileptiform convulsions, headache, hemiplegia, and a flattening of one side of the skull. The latter sign, however, is frequently absent, as in the case related above. Here the history of a difficult premature labour following an injury to the mother again illustrates the importance of trauma at birth in the ætiology of this rare condition.

I am indebted to Dr. J. Bain, medical superintendent, for permission to publish this case.

REFERENCES.

Kundrat, H.: Die Porencephalie, Graz, 1882.
Schultze, F.: Beiträge zur Lehre v. d. angeborenen Hirndefekten, Strassburg, 1885.
Strümpell, A. von: Jahrb. f. Kinderh., 1884, xxii.
Globus, J. H.: Arch. Neurol. and Psychiat., 1921, vi., 654.
Jaffé, R. H.: Arch. Pathol. and Lab. Med., 1929, viii., 787.
Tredgold, A. F.: Mental Deficiency, 4th ed., London, 1922.

PROLONGED ADMINISTRATION OF ARTIFICIAL RESPIRATION.

BY PHILIP DRINKER, S.B., CH.E.,

ASSOCIATE PROFESSOR OF INDUSTRIAL HYGIENE, HARVARD SCHOOL OF PUBLIC HEALTH, BOSTON, MASS.

IN a series of papers published elsewhere there have been presented physiological[1] and clinical[2] data obtained by the use of a mechanically operated device for administering artificial respiration over long periods.

The device used is known as a respirator and consists of a sheet metal tank equipped with a comfortable bed and mattress (Fig. 1). The patient's head protrudes through a flat soft rubber diaphragm or collar attached to the body of the respirator, the rubber collar making an air-tight seal about the patient's neck. The diameter of the collar is adjustable, and thus excessive tension on the neck of the patient is avoided.

By means of electrically driven blowers and an appropriate valve arrangement, the air pressure within the tank is changed alternately from a few centimetre of water negative pressure to normal atmospheric pressure. The negative pressure induces inspiration —the chest and diaphragm of the patient expand and air is inhaled. The return to atmospheric pressure allows the recoil of the thorax and the respiratory muscles, together with the elasticity of the lungs, to cause expiration. Both the depth and the rate of breathing are under the control of the attendant and can be measured (or recorded) by means of a suitable U-tube manometer, filled with coloured water and connected by rubber tubing to the body of the respirator.

In general, a negative pressure of about 12 to 18 cm. of water suffices to maintain adequate ventilation in an adult or child with complete respiratory paralysis. In the case of new-born babies in which respiration does not begin within a few minutes after birth, smaller negative pressures (from 8 to 10 cm.) have been found adequate.[3] Our experience indicates that the negative pressure used should just be sufficient to prevent cyanosis or obvious respiratory distress; nothing is gained by using excessive negative pressures for long periods, while we have reason to believe that such pressures actually do harm to the lung tissue, particularly in the case of infants whose lungs may be atelectatic.[4]

Without having the pump stopped, the patients can eat, drink, and sleep while in the respirator. A bed-pan can be passed through one of the portholes, enemas can be given, and rectal drips can be administered in deglutition cases. The noise of the machinery, although not excessive, is sufficient to prevent the use of a stethoscope in chest and heart examinations. We have taken rontgenograms of patients' chests both while the respirator was running and when the bed was pulled out and the pump stopped.

Of possible interest to physiologists is the fact that such slight negative pressures—equivalent to

FIG. 2.

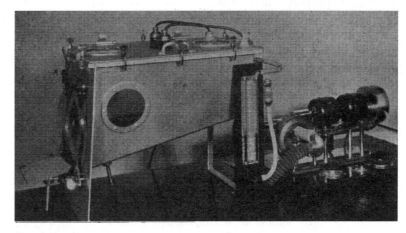

Respirator for infants. The chamber is heated, when necessary, by two electric bulbs on the inside.

12 to 18 cm. of water—are sufficient to induce inspiration in a person whose respiration has ceased, and that it has been found unnecessary to use positive pressures inside the respirator. In the case of an animal deeply anæsthetised or curarised still smaller negative pressures suffice. The method offers the advantage, over intratracheal insufflation, that it imitates normal breathing fairly accurately.

Severe apnœa can be produced on normal humans by intentional over-ventilation of the subject. In clinical practice the severely paralysed patient may be over-ventilated by increasing the depth of the respirations just prior to being withdrawn from the apparatus for a few minutes, in order that he may be bathed and changed. Without such over-ventilation he may become cyanotic too quickly to permit reasonable nursing care or medication.

This apparatus has had two years' trial in the United States and Canada and has been used in some 100 cases of respiratory failure from acute poliomyelitis, over 50 cases of unusually severe carbon monoxide poisoning, about 10 cases of alcoholic coma, 7 of drowning, 1 of post-diphtheritic paralysis, and over 30 of asphyxia of the new-born. In general the intercostal paralysis of poliomyelitis can be treated with immediate relief and comfort to the patient, the length of treatment varying from a few hours to several months, according to the severity of the disease. Cases of gas-poisoning, alcoholic coma, and drug poisoning seldom require more than 24 hours' treatment, while new-born babies rarely require over one to two hours' continuous treatment.

With the exception of those with poliomyelitis the patients usually recover completely. Numerous cases of both children and adults with severe intercostal paralysis from poliomyelitis have made gratifying recoveries, although we have several who have recovered the use of their intercostals but are otherwise crippled.

In view of the fact that over 70 of the adult machines and 12 of the infant size (Fig. 2) are in successful use in America, the

FIG. 1.

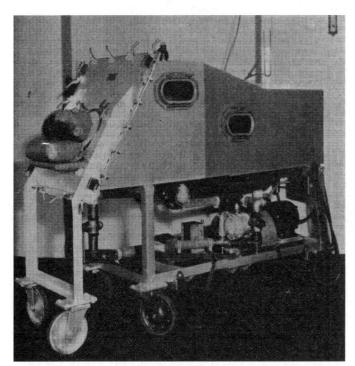

Respirator (for adults) showing patient in the apparatus. (Photographs by courtesy of Messrs. Siebe, Gorman and Co.,

manufacturing details have been entrusted to Messrs. Siebe, Gorman and Co., of London, and the apparatus will be made here as desired by the medical profession. No profits will accrue to any person in any way concerned with the development or sale of the apparatus in America.

This apparatus was developed and subsequently made available through the generosity of the Consolidated Gas Co., of New York City, who gave the funds to the Harvard School of Public Health to cover the expenses of the original research, and later bought and presented 14 adult-sized respirators to various hospitals in New York City.

REFERENCES.

1. Drinker, P., and Shaw, L. A.: Jour. Clin. Invest., 1929, vii., 229 ; Ibid., 1929, viii., 33.
2. Drinker, P., and McKhann, C. F.: Jour. Amer. Med. Assoc., 1929, xcii., 1658 ; Wightman, H. B., and Shaughnessy, T. J.: Ibid., 1929, xciii., 456 ; Shambaugh, G. E., jr., Harrison, W. G., jr., and Farrell, J. I.: Ibid., 1930, xciv., 1371 ; Drinker, P., Shaughnessy, T. J., and Murphy, D. P.: Ibid., 1930, xcv., 1249.
3. Murphy, D. P., and Coyne, J. A.: Ibid., 1930, xcv., 335.
4. Murphy, D. P., Drinker, C. K., and Drinker, P.: Arch. Internal Med., March, 1931, p. 424.

CLINICAL AND LABORATORY NOTES

A CASE OF APLASTIC ANÆMIA.

BY W. J. FENTON, M.D. CAMB., F.R.C.P. LOND.,

CONSULTING PHYSICIAN TO CHARING CROSS HOSPITAL ; PHYSICIAN TO THE HOSPITAL FOR CONSUMPTION, BROMPTON ;

AND

A. TURNER, M.D. DURH.

A MAN, aged 52, complained of acute pain in the epigastrium, mainly dependent upon the taking of food and frequently appearing during the night. It had first been noticed some six months previously. Pallor and dyspnœa appeared three months later. There was nothing noteworthy in his previous medical history and no history of venereal disease. He had noticed a tendency to "bleed" from small wounds, and four years before had had an attack of epistaxis, for which his nostrils had been plugged. He thought that his family, especially on the male side, was more than usually liable to bleed.

He was very abstemious and smoked little. His normal weight was 14 st. 7 lb. ; when first seen it was 14 st. His appetite was good, but he suffered from considerable pain and discomfort after meals, with occasional pyrosis. The bowels were regular, and no blood had been noticed in the motions. Vomiting had not occurred. The urine contained a trace of albumin but nothing otherwise noteworthy. On physical examination he was remarkably anæmic but without a lemon tint. A few purpuric spots were noticed on the mucous surfaces of the lips, but not elsewhere. The pulse-rate was 92 and the pulse was regular and of medium force ; the radial wall was healthy. The systolic blood pressure was 146 and the diastolic 66 mm. Hg. There was nothing discoverable in the viscera of the chest or abdomen except such as might be directly associated with the anæmia. The teeth were poor and the tongue slightly furred. There was no œdema, no history of sweating, and no evidence suggesting associated disease of the central nervous system. The diagnosis appeared to lie between duodenal ulcer, gastric neoplasm, and pernicious anæmia.

An X ray examination after an opaque meal was made by Dr. Stanley Melville and the conclusion reached that, although the behaviour of the stomach was not typical of duodenal irritation, a definite residue at two and six hours made it impossible to exclude ulceration in this region. The result was thus inconclusive as regards the presence of ulceration but appeared to negative malignant disease. Examination of the stools for occult blood showed that this was present in moderate amount. The blood count made at the time was as follows : white blood corpuscles, 3200 per c.mm. ; red blood corpuscles, 2,500,000 per c.mm. ; hæmoglobin, 22 per cent. ; colour-index, 0·44 ; polymorphonuclear leucocytes, 63·0 per cent. ; eosinophils, 1·5 per cent. ; basophils, 0·5 per cent. ; large hyalines, 6·0 per cent. ; small lymphocytes, 29·0 per cent. ; poikilocytosis, anisocytosis, and polychromatophilia were present, but no nucleated red cells were seen. The coagulation time was not altered. The result of the blood examination was thus not specially indicative of pernicious anæmia, but rather suggested an anæmia secondary to hæmorrhage from duodenal ulceration. The patient was accordingly put to bed and treated upon this supposition. No improvement was obtained ; the occult blood persisted in spite of all forms of treatment, including injections of horse serum, and no marked change was noticed in the general condition.

A consultation was held with Mr. G. Gordon Taylor and, while the difficulties of the case were fully appreciated, it was felt that, with the history of gastric symptoms already detailed, the persistence of occult blood in the stools and the absence of any other form of bleeding, together with the obviously serious condition of the patient, it would be advisable to open the abdomen and search for ulceration. This was accordingly done, but nothing was found to throw light upon the symptoms. The patient made a successful recovery from the operation, no special tendency to bleed having been noted, and his general condition remained in statu quo. The teeth meanwhile had received attention. A course of treatment by liver was tried and he was subsequently transfused, but without success.

Blood examinations were made from time to time and, while some of the counts had features suggestive of pernicious anæmia, none was typical, and nucleated red cells were never found. It now became apparent that the case was a true blood disease to which the anæmia and hæmorrhages were secondary, and the diagnosis of aplastic anæmia was made. The patient returned home and died about nine months after our first consultation, all forms of treatment having proved unavailing. The final count made three months before his death was as follows : white blood corpuscles, 6200 per c.mm. red blood corpuscles, 1,750,000 per c.mm. ; hæmoglobin, 25 per cent. ; colour-index, 0·7 ; polymorphonuclears, 62·5 per cent. ; eosinophils, 6 per cent. ; lymphocytes, 30·5 per cent. ; mononuclears, 6 per cent. The stained film showed marked poikilocytosis and anisocytosis was very evident ; there was a considerable number of megalocytes. A few cells showed polychromasia, but there were no nucleated forms. The report added the suggestion that despite the low colour-index, this count had several of the features of a true pernicious anæmia.

POST-MORTEM EXAMINATION.

The body was that of a well-nourished middle-aged man with pronounced pallor of the skin. Post-mortem staining was absent. There was a comparatively thick layer of yellow subcutaneous fat and the pericardial fat was increased. There was extensive and advanced fatty degeneration of the myocardium with fatty striation of the musculature of the walls of both ventricles as well as of the papillary muscles. There was an excessive deposit of fat in the omentum and mesentery, but no enlargement of the mesenteric glands. The intestines were normal ; ulceration and neoplasm were both absent. The liver was enlarged and very soft, rusty brown in colour with deeper coloured areas suggestive of chronic passive congestion. The macroscopic appearances were consistent with widespread fatty change and some atrophy. The ferrocyanide reaction was only very slight. The spleen was a little enlarged, its pulp soft, and the normal markings lost. The cut surface presented a uniform appearance which might have been due to post-mortem changes. The kidneys were pale and apparently fatty, but showed nothing otherwise noteworthy. No special changes were observed in the pancreas and suprarenals. The bone-marrow of the femur was very pale and appeared to be mostly fatty, with the exception of a pinkish streak about 5 mm. in diameter. It was evident that erythrogenetic activity was inconsiderable.

HISTOLOGICAL REPORT.

Liver.—No changes of special importance beyond passive congestion and areas of central atrophy and fatty degeneration.
Lungs.—Œdematous.
Spleen.—The most striking feature was the comparative absence of red corpuscles. The Malpighian corpuscles were very poorly represented and appeared to be inactive. The reticulum cells were also apparently diminished in number and the connective tissue reticulum of the organ was very evident, although no new formation of fibrous tissue had occurred. A very fine fatty infiltration of the reticulum was present. The ferrocyanide reaction was negative.

THE LANCET]   THE NECESSITY FOR A SAFE MILK-SUPPLY   [OCT. 7, 1933 829

revolution in the patient's living and circumstances, something quite outside our therapeutic armamentarium, may be necessary to distract his attention from his viscera. Some faulty habits of hygiene we may correct, especially irregularity and carelessness of meals and of eating. Perhaps we insist unduly upon exercise, but its absence generally means a badly ordered life with insufficient recreation, so that our solicitude benefits indirectly.

In respect to diet we are often too fussy and ceremonial. This is really the fault of our patients in their insistence upon the provision of a " diet sheet." This request it is easy to understand. A patient not unnaturally resents mass production therapy ; he likes to regard himself as an individual problem and expects a dietary which has been elaborated for his particular requirements. Moreover, he succeeds in this way in transferring the responsibility for his recovery to his doctor and exonerates himself from personal effort. Yet diet should play a very small part in the therapy of " nervous indigestion." Idiosyncrasies must of course be respected, but these it is impossible for us to deduce or guess. Apart from these a dyspeptic should be encouraged to accept as a principle that what has once agreed with him may in future be permitted notwithstanding his impression of its unsuitability on subsequent occasions. The alternative of excluding everything which has disagreed will eventually lead to the elimination of everything edible and even cold water. Dyspepsia from relative starvation is probably more frequently encountered than dyspepsia from over-eating unless chronic gastritis is present. The really serious disturbances of the nervous system responsible for gastro-intestinal symptoms bring the patient within the province of the psychotherapist or even the alienist.

SPECIAL ARTICLES

THE NECESSITY FOR A SAFE MILK-SUPPLY *

By G. S. WILSON, M.D., F.R.C.P., D.P.H.

PROFESSOR OF BACTERIOLOGY AS APPLIED TO HYGIENE, LONDON SCHOOL OF HYGIENE AND TROPICAL MEDICINE

MILK is a valuable food, and so far as its nutritive properties are concerned it is not an expensive food. Its importance in infant feeding, its power to stimulate the growth of under-nourished school-children, its easy assimilability by the sick and convalescent, and its provision of a wholesome source of energy to the normal population, amply justify for it a very special place in the human dietary. It is therefore all the more surprising to consider that, while rigid control is exercised over the purity of water-supplies, of meat, and of certain other foods, there are no public health regulations that ensure in practice the cleanliness and safety of our milk-supplies.

Cleanliness and Safety

Before proceeding further, it is important to define our terms. It is often assumed that " cleanliness " and " safety " are synonymous. This is a mistake. By " cleanliness " I understand the freedom of milk from extraneous matter, from pus, from blood, and from an undue number of micro-organisms, especially those of the putrefactive type—using this term in its broadest sense. By " safety " I mean the freedom of milk from pathogenic or potentially pathogenic micro-organisms and its consequent liability to give rise to infective disease in human beings consuming it. Many unclean milks, though æsthetically undesirable, are perfectly safe to drink, while very clean milks may, as the literature of milk epidemics shows, be highly dangerous.

It is perhaps desirable to elaborate this point in order to render it clear. The commonest pathogenic organisms that have been found in milk are : the tubercle bacillus responsible for tuberculosis ; the bacillus of contagious abortion responsible for undulant fever ; the typhoid, paratyphoid, food-poisoning, and dysentery bacilli responsible for enteric fever, acute gastro-enteritis, and dysentery ; hæmolytic streptococci, responsible for scarlet fever and septic sore-throat ; and the diphtheria bacillus, responsible for diphtheria. Of these, the first two gain access to the milk from the cow's udder, while the remainder are usually introduced by human beings who are either carriers of these organisms or are suffering from an actual attack of the disease caused by them. With the exception of the tubercle bacillus, milk that is produced under the most cleanly conditions from tuberculin-tested herds is almost as subject to contamination with the remaining organisms as is milk that has been produced without any special regard to sanitary precautions. The reason for this is that contamination with pathogenic bacteria of human origin takes place quite unconsciously, a few organisms finding their way into the milk from the fingers or throat of the milker or other person handling the milk. Once the organisms have been introduced, even in very small numbers, multiplication is liable to occur, since milk, clean or unclean, is an excellent nutrient medium for the growth of bacteria. To avoid contamination from human sources medical inspection of the personnel, combined with bacteriological examination of the secretions and excreta, is sometimes recommended, and is in fact practised in many parts of the United States of America ; but while occasional long-standing carriers of pathogenic micro-organisms may be detected by this method, it is quite incapable, short of daily examination of every member of the milk personnel, of bringing to light the early clinical cases, the subclinical infections, and most of the purely latent infections in healthy carriers, which constitute so grave a menace to the safety of the milk-supply.

Milk-borne Disease

At present a great deal of the raw milk sold in this country is neither clean nor safe. Much of it, besides having a high bacterial count, contains manure, pus, and even blood, the latter two coming from animals with diseased udders. Such a condition excites no protest, because these substances are conveniently obscured by the suspended fat globules in the milk. One wonders how many people would accept bread or sugar that was soiled with such products !

The frequency of tuberculous infection of the milk-supply has recently been the subject of a special inquiry, and the figures show that a proportion of raw market milk samples, varying in different parts of the country from 2 to 13 per cent., with an average figure of 6·7 per cent., contains living virulent tubercle bacilli (Report, 1932).

The presence of *Brucella abortus*, an organism

---

* Being the substance of a paper read before the Agricultural Section of the British Association at Leicester on Sept. 12th, 1933.

1·5, to give a rate of secretion per hour. This should reduce the errors of volume estimation to one quarter.

Some opposite conclusions of Comfort and Osterberg [20] must be noted here. These workers made a direct comparison of the Ewald and histamine tests on 120 patients, and could find no advantage in the use of histamine. Their results with histamine were, however, strikingly different from those of Polland in several respects, noticeably in the greater overlapping of cancer and ulcer cases and in the difference between gastric and duodenal ulcers. Since Polland's series contains a much larger number of cases it would seem that we must accept it in preference pending further confirmation by others.

In conclusion, some obvious criticisms of the methods of calculation may be anticipated. It must be freely admitted that a number of assumptions have been made which are not strictly accurate, and that a number of relevant facts have been ignored owing to poverty of data. The inquiry may perhaps be considered to have served a useful purpose if only to expose the lack of existing knowledge on these points. The fact that the same assumptions were applied to each of the three tests still leaves some justification for drawing conclusions as to their relative value.

The principal flaws in the method lie in the following considerations :—

(1) Age and sex have been largely neglected. We now know, thanks to the work of Vanzant et al.[11] and of Bloomfield and Polland,[12] that gastric acidity decreases with age and is higher in the male sex. What are required, therefore, are detailed standards for each sex and for each decade, to include ulcer and cancer as well as normal persons. When these become available the accuracy of test-meal diagnosis will be materially increased. Polland's normal standards fulfil a long-felt want but he has not tabulated in detail the volumes of acid secreted. Since it is hardly likely that any one clinic will have sufficient material to establish satisfactory pathological standards, it is to be hoped that future publications will give full details of the age and sex of their patients so that their results may eventually be pooled.

(2) We have assumed the same distribution of acidity in doubtful carcinomas and ulcers as in carcinomas and ulcers in general. Further data are certainly necessary on this point. It has previously been supposed that the test-meal failed in just these cases, for malignant ulcers are frequently accompanied by the presence of free hydrochloric acid, and, as we have seen, the older test-meals cannot then give any additional information (unless of course characteristic signs are present in the resting juice). Bloomfield and Polland,[1] however, claimed to find a low output of acid in such cases by the histamine test, and certainly they have recorded many cases of carcinoma with free acid present but yet well outside their ulcer range. If this finding be confirmed the histamine test should prove of the greatest value in these cases.

The question of malignant degeneration in a simple ulcer is not so hopeful, and we can hardly hope at present that any assistance will be forthcoming in these cases, which are likely to show an acidity within the ulcer range.

(3) Only in one case has the attempt been made to allow for errors of random sampling, and this can only represent a first approximation owing to the inadequacy of the available data.

Conclusions

(1) A new method has been developed by means of which the efficacy of the test-meal in the differential diagnosis of ulcer and cancer of the stomach may be tested. This has been applied to typical data from the Ewald, fractional, and histamine tests with the results given below.

(2) The test-meal is of little value in cases of suspected ulcer.

(3) In the differential diagnosis of doubtful gastric lesions demonstrated by X rays, the test-meal may be of considerable value in a proportion of cases. This proportion is much the highest in the histamine test.

(4) The histamine test is superior to the other two. The Ewald and fractional tests are about equal except that the examination of the resting juice gives an advantage to the fractional test.

(5) The limitations and possibilities of this method of calculation are discussed, and the need for further data is emphasised.

It is a pleasure to express my thanks to Prof. E. C. Dodds for his advice and criticism.

REFERENCES

1. Bloomfield, A. L., and Polland, W. S. : Jour. Amer. Med. Assoc., 1929, xcii., 1508.
2. Vanzant, F. R., Alvarez, W. C., Berkson, J., and Eusterman, G. B. : Arch. Internal Med., 1933, lii., 616.
3. Comfort, M. W., and Vanzant, F. R. : Proc. Staff Meet. Mayo Clinic, 1933, viii., 271.
4. Bennett, T. I. : The Stomach and Upper Alimentary Canal, London, 1925.
5. Harrison, G. A. : Chemical Methods in Clinical Medicine, London, 1930.
6. Bloomfield, A. L., and Keefer, C. S. : Jour. Clin. Invest., 1928, v., 295.
7. Hurst, A. F., and Stewart, M. J. : Gastric and Duodenal Ulcer, London, 1929.
8. Boldyreff, W. N. : Quart. Jour. Exp. Physiol., 1915, viii., 1.
9. Bolton, C., and Goodhart, G. W. : THE LANCET, 1922, i., 420.
10. Maclagan, N. F. : Quart. Jour. Med., 1934, xi., 321.
11. Vanzant, F. R., Alvarez, W. C., Eusterman, G. B., Dunn, H. L., and Berkson, J. : Arch. Internal Med., 1932, xlix., 345.
12. Polland, W. S. : Ibid., 1933, li., 903.
13. Bennett, T. I., and Ryle, J. A. : Guy's Hosp. Rep., 1921, lxxi., 286.
14. Baird, M. McC., Campbell, D. M., and Hern, J. R. B. : Ibid., 1924, lxxiv., 23.
15. Apperley, F. L., and Semmens, K. M. : Med. Jour. Australia, 1928, ii., 226.
16. Stewart, M. J. : THE LANCET, 1931, ii., 617.
17. Sagal, Z., Marks, J. A., and Kantor, J. L. : Ann. Internal Med., 1933, vii., 76.
18. Koyihar, A. J. : Guy's Hosp. Rep., 1926, lxxvi., 65.
19. Lander, F. P. L., and Maclagan, N. F. : THE LANCET (in press).
20. Comfort, M. W., and Osterberg, A. E. : Jour. Amer. Med. Assoc., 1931, xcvii., 1141.
21. Fisher, R. A. : Statistical Methods for Research Workers, London, 1932.
22. Palmer, W. L., and Heinz, T. E. : Arch. Internal Med., 1934, liii., 269.

TETANUS TREATED WITH CURARE

BY LESLIE COLE, M.D. Camb., F.R.C.P. Lond.

PHYSICIAN TO ADDENBROOKE'S HOSPITAL, CAMBRIDGE

CURARE is an arrow poison used by the natives of South America to paralyse their game. They prepare it in the form of a black resinous extract from the bark of plants of the genus strychnos, which they store in gourds, earthenware pots, or bamboo sticks. A number of plants may be used in preparing the extract, and the strength of the crude preparation varies considerably in different samples. Boehm [1] found that different preparations might contain different alkaloids, most of which have a paralysing action and are typified by curarine. Their action is similar to that of the crude drug. One of them, however, curine, is a weaker poison and has an entirely different effect, for it acts upon the heart.

The chief effect of curare is to paralyse voluntary movement by blocking the passage of impulses from the peripheral nerves to the muscles. The point of action is thought to be the end-plates of the motor nerves. The voluntary muscles are first paralysed and later the respiratory muscles, death taking place from asphyxia.

The idea of using curare to control the spasms of tetanus is not new, for it is mentioned in several older medical text-books. Hunter [2] used it in a few desperate cases, but apart from this, accounts of cases in which it has been used are difficult to find.

Hartridge and West [3] have used curare to control tetany in parathyroidectomised dogs. They found considerable variation in strength of different samples and that two specimens out of seven possessed the power of removing tetany in the dog without causing paralysis. West [4] used one of these two samples in the treatment of 17 cases of muscular rigidity, resulting from diseases of the pyramidal and extrapyramidal motor systems. In doses which caused no detectable weakness or loss of power there was considerable reduction of rigidity while under the influence of the drug. He suggests that some samples of curare may contain a second active principle which has a selective action in that it can abolish rigidity in certain rigid states without causing paralysis, and mentions the possibility of using curare in tetanus. These observations show that different samples of curare vary considerably both in strength and action, and the dose is therefore a question of difficulty.

The sample used in the case here described was given me by Dr. J. F. Gaskell [5] and was of the "gourd" variety. It was the most potent of ten samples whose paralysing power had been compared by injection into leeches. Doses up to 32 mg. had been given to a patient with pyramidal rigidity, and this observation formed the basis of dosage in these cases. Prof. Hartridge tested the potency of this sample for frogs and found that 0·005 mg. is the lethal dose for a frog weighing 26 g., and that it paralyses frogs from that amount to 0·0025 mg.

THE FIRST CASE

A labourer, aged 39, in the afternoon of Monday, Jan. 15th, while cutting reeds, cut the tip of the second finger of the left hand on a reed. The wound was a deep one. He treated it by soaking it daily in hot water. On Monday, Jan. 22nd, he found difficulty in opening his mouth, and his throat felt stiff on swallowing. On the 23rd the stiffness of the jaw and the difficulty with swallowing were much worse and he had spasms of pain in the neck and back. On the 24th all these symptoms were worse, and he was admitted to Addenbrooke's Hospital at 1 P.M.

State on admission.—Severe spasm of masseters. Risus sardonicus. Back arched and rigid, abdomen boardlike. No relaxation between spasms. Some stiffness of arms and legs but no local tetanus. Whitlow of tip of second finger of left hand, fluctuant and full of pus. Scar of wound on lateral aspect of finger. No œdema of hand or lymphangitis. No teeth present in upper jaw.

Treatment on admission.—200,000 units of antitoxin were given intravenously and 2000 subcutaneously on either side of the infected finger. Half an hour later the whitlow was incised and washed out with hydrogen peroxide. No further antitoxin was given.

Progress.—Spasms began shortly after admission and increased rapidly in severity. By the evening the patient was having severe spasms which were brought on by the slightest sound or movement, and these occurred every minute or so. Opisthotonos occurred during the spasms, the back was rigid and arched between spasms, and the abdomen boardlike.

The sedatives used during the course of the illness were avertin and paraldehyde given rectally and occasional small doses of morphia. 7·3 c.cm. of avertin (full dose for basal anæsthesia) was given every night for eight nights. From three to five drachms of paraldehyde were given rectally dissolved in normal saline every day for ten days. Food in the form of glucose lemonade, milk, and egg and milk were given hourly when the patient was awake. The fact there were no teeth in the upper jaw made feeding a good deal easier.

By Jan. 26th, however, the spasms were getting more frequent and severe, and the patient was showing signs of exhaustion. Treatment with curare was therefore begun. Four doses of 32 mg. were given subcutaneously at six-hourly intervals beginning at midday on the 26th.

Within two hours of starting this treatment the spasms were less severe, the rigidity of the arms and abdomen was less, and the spasm of the masseters was less, so that feeding was made a good deal easier. The patient had less pain and was more comfortable. He complained of no abnormal sensations after injection and there was no evidence at any time of difficulty in breathing. The pulse-rate however continued to rise. Observations on the blood pressure and reflexes could not be made. This improvement continued for 48 hours, but on the 29th spasms and rigidity began to get worse again. He was therefore given three more injections of 32 mg. of curare at six-hourly intervals. Following this the same effects were observed and the same improvement occurred, but the pulse-rate still remained rapid. On Feb. 1st spasms and rigidity again began to get worse, and so one more injection of 32 mg. was given. Following this there was steady improvement and the spasms gradually became less and ceased on Feb. 6th. The rigidity of the abdomen and back and the opisthotonos gradually passed off and had disappeared by Feb. 17th. No abnormal symptoms were observed during convalescence, but the wasting and weakness of the forearms and legs were very marked. Before discharge on Feb. 28th the patient could walk about the ward and the central nervous system showed no abnormality. One month later he was perfectly well but for some weakness of the arms and legs.

THE SECOND CASE

The patient, a boy aged 7, on July 12th fell off his bicycle and grazed his left elbow, knees, and right heel on the road. The wounds were slight and superficial, except that on the heel which was rather deep. No treatment was given. On the morning of the 14th he seemed out of sorts and complained of stiffness of the jaw on trying to eat, and pain in the neck, shoulders, and left side of the chest. These symptoms grew steadily worse and he was admitted to hospital on the 15th.

State on admission.—Continuous rigidity of the abdomen and back with stiffness of the jaw and risus sardonicus. The stiffness was made worse by noise or manipulation, and occasional slight spasms with opisthotonos occurred. The wounds had scabbed over.

Treatment and progress.—100,000 units of antitoxin were given intravenously and the wounds were cleaned. Rigidity and spasms became more severe and frequent. At 10.30 P.M. the jaw was continuously clenched, the back arched and rigid, the abdomen boardlike, and the limbs stiff. Spasms of the most intense severity occurred every 30 seconds and were caused by the slightest sound or touch. The attempt to give water with a spoon brought on severe spasms, swallowing was impossible, and attempts to suck fluid through a tube had the same effect. Perspiration was profuse, temperature 104° F., and pulse-rate 140–50.

At 11.30 P.M. 7·5 mg. of curare were given subcutaneously. Five minutes later the spasms were less severe, the reflex excitability was less, and the limbs were less rigid. At 11.40 7·5 mg. were given; at 11.50 15 mg.; and at 12.10, 15 mg., with progressive improvement. After the last injection of curare the rigidity of the abdomen had disappeared between spasms, the limbs were relaxed, the mouth could be opened, and fluid could be sucked and swallowed without bringing on spasms. Reflex excitability had almost disappeared, and the arms and legs could be manipulated freely. Only occasional slight spasms occurred throughout the night. At 1 A.M. there was some respiratory difficulty, but this improved. The pulse, however, grew weaker and more rapid, and the temperature rose steadily to 108° F. at 5.30 A.M. The respiration then began to fail and the child died at 6.20 A.M.

DISCUSSION

These cases of tetanus are 2 of a series of 19 cases I have treated during the last six years. Of the 19 patients 11 recovered. All of them, including the two which received curare, were treated on the same general lines, each being given a large dose of antitoxin by the intravenous route as early as possible and before the wound had been touched. The first case treated with curare and described above was certainly the most severe of those which recovered.

In both cases here described, curare seemed to reduce the continuous rigidity of the limbs, abdomen, and jaw muscles, to lessen reflex excitability, and to lessen the frequency and duration of the spasms. In Case 2 the severe spasms, induced by attempting to suck fluid and even by the sight of fluid, were stopped and swallowing was made possible. In Case 1, in which the dose was relatively small, the action of the drug was first apparent about two hours after the first injection. The effects appeared to last about forty-eight hours. In Case 2 the effects first appeared five minutes after the injection.

It is possible that in Case 1 the action was sufficient to tide the patient over the critical period of the illness by preventing exhaustion and by allowing more food to be given. No unpleasant symptoms were observed while the drug was being given and respiration did not appear to be effected in any way. No serious after-effects were noted, though it is possible that the rather prolonged weakness and wasting of the muscles of the arms and legs may have been due to the curare.

The second case was of such rapid onset (incubation period 48 hours) and intense severity that there was no chance of recovery. Treatment might have been more effective in prolonging life if it had begun a few hours earlier. Given however when rigidity was continuous, and reflex spasms of the most intense severity were occurring every thirty seconds, curare checked the spasms, stopped the reflex excitability, and made the rigidity very much less. Respiratory failure only occurred seven hours later when the heart had begun to fail.

Observations on these two cases are encouraging and confirm the suggestion that curare or its alkaloids will be useful in the treatment of tetanus. Dosage however is at present a difficult problem, and will remain so until standardised preparations are available and more is known of the particular actions of its various alkaloids.

I am indebted to Dr. Gaskell for the curare used in these cases, and for allowing me to treat Case 2, and to Prof. Hartridge for testing the potency of this sample on frogs.

REFERENCES

1. Boehm, R.: Arch. f. exp. Path. u. Pharm., 1895, xxxv., 16 ; 1908, lviii., 265 ; 1910, lxiii., 177.
2. Hunter, H.: British Guiana at the Paris Exhibition, London, 1878, Preface, p. 80.
3. Hartridge, H., and West, R.: Brain, 1931, liv., 312, 508.
4. West, R.: Proc. Roy. Soc. Med., 1932, xxv., 39.
5. Gaskell, J. F.: Philosoph. Trans. Roy. Soc., B., 1914, ccv., 191.

SPINAL MANIPULATION

WITH SPECIAL REFERENCE TO LUMBOSACRAL STRAIN AND BRACHIAL NEURITIS

By THOMAS MARLIN, M.D. Glasg., D.P.H., D.M.R.E.

MEDICAL OFFICER IN CHARGE OF THE MASSAGE, LIGHT, AND ELECTROTHERAPEUTIC DEPARTMENTS OF UNIVERSITY COLLEGE HOSPITAL

IN a study of the methods commonly used for manipulating the spine, whether it be by the "osteopath's twist" or by the forcible movements under an anæsthetic as practised by orthopædic surgeons, one cannot help feeling that generally an unnecessary amount of force is used. This does not mean necessarily that the operator uses too much force to gain his end by his particular technique, or that no benefit accrues from such manipulation. But it seemed that it would be a great advantage if a method could be devised, which, while still effective in producing the movement, would be more pleasant to the patient and produce less reaction in the surrounding tissues. This is important, for a patient who has once been hurt naturally resists if the manipulation be attempted on a subsequent occasion. Hence we desire a movement which can be done with the minimum amount of force. Then certain parts of the spine are difficult to manipulate. Different workers, using different techniques, and many of them displaying much ingenuity, have managed to produce a movement at practically every intervertebral joint, but two regions for various reasons have always presented difficulties. These two regions are the lumbosacral junction and the first dorsal segment including the first rib. Accordingly it would be an advantage in devising any new method if such technique could embody a principle which would make it effective for those two regions.

Working in collaboration with H. Goehring of Pennsylvania I have developed a method which apparently meets the case. It is not unpleasant to the patient, does not cause much discomfort or reaction afterwards, and can be used effectively for the whole spine except the cervical region, where several other methods are in vogue. We early came to the conclusion that of all forms of forcible movements, traction or extension was the least disagreeable to the patient. In our own fingers, for example, we could produce a separation of the joint surfaces of the inter-phalangeal or metacarpo-phalangeal articulations by flexing those joints and then forcibly pushing them a little further into flexion. Such a proceeding caused considerable discomfort, whereas the same result could generally be attained by pulling on the digits, and this was not in the least degree painful.

Now most spinal manipulations rely for success on such movements as flexion or extension, rotation or twisting, or on thrusts of various kinds, and it occurred to us that, taking a lesson from what we had found in our fingers, we might try to exploit the principle of traction ; but the difficulty was to be able to fix the spine at any given level.

For instance, with a patient on his back, if we took hold on of his head, one hand beneath the occiput and the other under his chin, and made traction, it was possible by giving little tugs on the head to produce movement at various levels of the cervical spine. With this procedure, however, we were not able to control the exact level at which movement took place.

A similar problem arose with respect to the rest of the spine. If the patient were on his back and we tugged on the feet, sometimes movement might take place at the ankle or the knee, very often it occurred at the sacro-iliac joints, and sometimes at the lumbars or lower dorsals. The site at which movement took place probably varied with the point of friction between the patient and the couch, and the height at which the feet and legs were held when the tug was administered, but certainly was not within the control of the operator.

Various methods and devices were tried with a view to fixing the spine at different levels while the pull was being administered. The body was put into different positions, the trunk held at varying angles to the horizontal, and straps applied in a number of ways, but nothing appeared to fulfil the purpose till the idea suggested itself that the end might be achieved if two operators took part in the manipulation. Each operator must be capable of doing either part of the manipulation, and each should know exactly what the other is expecting to do or feel. Once this absolute understanding has been established between them the method is simplicity itself.

A strong couch is required, suitably padded, and with detachable pillow, so that the patient can lie quite flat. It is essential to have the covering of the

680   THE LANCET]   [SEPT. 21, 1935

SPECIAL ARTICLES

PLASTER TECHNIQUE IN THE MODERN TREATMENT OF FRACTURES

BY K. H. PRIDIE, M.B. Lond., F.R.C.S. Eng.

SURGICAL REGISTRAR TO THE FRACTURE CLINIC AND ORTHOPÆDIC DEPARTMENT OF THE BRISTOL ROYAL INFIRMARY

THE great advance in traumatic surgery during the last few years has resulted from the adoption of the principles and methods of Dr. Lorenz Böhler, director of the Hospital for Accidents in Vienna. In his book on the treatment of fractures, which is available in translation to English readers,* he emphasises the vital importance to the community of the organised treatment of fractures, which should no longer be left to junior house surgeons to treat. There is probably no branch of surgery where the difference between efficient and inefficient treatment is so marked ; for instance, a man with a simple fracture of the leg, instead of being back at work in three months, may be crippled for life with an ununited fracture or a painful leg. The saving of compensation and of lost wages repays the cost of the clinics many times over.

It is the organisation of these special clinics that is so important ; first, because it is not economic to apply the method to individual and isolated cases, and secondly, because a great factor in the success of the method is psychological. To see other patients with leg injuries similar to his own walking without pain after a few days has such a good effect on the new patient that he is no longer a mental invalid, and very rarely is the compensation neurotic encountered. Many cases of Pott's fracture and fracture of the tibia can walk home the same day as their injury, and need not stay in bed one day. Many of them are able to carry on their work and women patients are able to look after their housework. But no amount of physiotherapy, electrical treatment, or massage will restore full function to a

---

* The Treatment of Fractures, by Dr. Lorenz Böhler. Fourth English edition. Translated from the German by E. W. Hey Groves, emeritus professor of surgery, University of Bristol. Bristol and London. 1935. (Reviewed in THE LANCET, 1935, i., 992.)

patient whose fracture has been incompletely reduced. It is waste of time and money for a patient with an unreduced Colles's fracture to receive massage and physiotherapy, for the end-result will only bring discredit to the masseuse.

A childish superstition of reverence surrounds a padded piece of wood. Often a patient is sent up to hospital in a splint whose weight is causing painful displacement of the bone-ends, for example, a back-splint and foot-piece used for a below-knee fracture. In the case of a Pott's fracture, a firm bandage over wool gives far more support than a back-splint and foot-piece where the foot is anchored to the splint and the tibia is free to rotate and cause displacement and pain. Patients in these splints dread being touched, and frequently remove them when the doctor has gone. Böhler has introduced the unpadded cast as a method of fixation after reduction. Plaster-of-Paris is unequalled for the fixation of fractures, but the method of application has to be learnt, and unless the surgeon knows how to apply these casts the results will be poor. After the application of unpadded casts the patients feel comfortable, they sleep at night, and no longer dread being touched.

The removal of splints for massage is wrong ; there is risk of displacement of the fractured bone-ends. The only massage the patients need is the massage of function. Massage should not be allowed till the bones are firmly united ; then, if the reduction has been satisfactory, and the patient has been using the limb, there will be full range of movement two weeks after removal of the plaster.

It is so essential for the teaching of students to secure a plaster of standard weight, strength, and application, that a bandage of constant composition must be used. Hospital-made bandages vary in different institutions, and even in different wards of the same institution. For these reasons I have adapted my technique to the three-yard Cellona bandage.† Cost and comfort have been the main factors in the evolution of this technique. The cost of the entire treatment is greatly diminished for these reasons :

1. The surgeon's time is only spent on reduction and fixation of the fracture.

2. Using these methods the majority of fractures can be treated as out-patients, hospitalisation being avoided.

3. Patients' visits and travelling expenses are reduced to a minimum.

4. Physiotherapy (a costly form of treatment) is only required in about 5 per cent. of cases, as compared with 100 per cent. using the old methods. The patient by his activity performs his own physiotherapy.

5. The majority of patients are able to follow their own occupation, without consequent loss of wages, and in any case disabilities and invalidism are avoided. Women can perform their household duties without outside help, and children can continue to attend school.

Besides this it is possible with the technique to produce casts of a

---

† The Cellona bandage, which is made by the manufacturers of Elastoplast (T. J. Smith and Nephew Ltd., Neptune-street, Hull), contains 90 per cent. by weight of plaster ; the setting time may be regulated as desired ; and although exceptionally strong, it is the lightest plaster bandage yet produced.

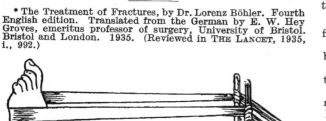

FIG. 1.—Böhler extension apparatus : position for application of standard below-knee cast, in cases not needing skeletal traction for reduction.

cough-reflex abolished by hypnosis : by then all is ready for an impending low-grade pneumonia which will carry him off. When surgery is finally demanded as " un dernier ressort," is it little wonder that fatality ensues ?

Increasing experience confirms the cherished conviction that the continuous blood-drip, aided by appropriate and timely surgery, is solving the ulcer-hæmorrhage problem and rationalising the treatment of these anxious cases, which have hitherto so frequently dismally disappointed the all-too-sanguine expectations of a futile and complacent inactivity ; to this inert policy I was myself for a time idly, hopefully, disastrously partisan. Finsterer's " first forty-eight hours " is still the optimum period for surgical attack in hæmatemesis, and the golden age of gastric surgery will have been attained only when all cases of hæmorrhage from chronic ulcer come to operation within that space of time.

Let there be no procrastination, for delay is fraught with peril ; early enterprise is the prelude to success.

REFERENCES

1. Pauchet, V.: Clinique, Paris, 1927, xxii., 363.
2. Gutman and Demole : Bull. et mém. Soc. méd. hôp. de Paris, 1930, xlviii., 576.
3. Delore, X.: Lyon Chir., 1933, xxx., 480.
4. Finsterer, H.: Jour. de Chir., 1933, xlii., 673.
5. Marriott, H. L., and Kekwick, A.: THE LANCET, 1935, i., 977.
6. Hurst, A. F., and Stewart, M. J.: Gastric and Duodenal Ulcer, London, 1929, p. 253.
7. Quoted by Hurst and Stewart (ref. 6).
8. Bulmer, Ernest : THE LANCET, 1927, ii., 168 ; Brit. Med. Jour., 1933, i., 848.
9. Middlesex Hospital Series, quoted by Gordon-Taylor, Proc. Roy. Soc. Med., 1934, xxvii., 1524.
10. Cooke, A. M.: Proc. Roy. Soc. Med., 1934, xxvii., 238.
11. Aitken, R. S.: THE LANCET, 1934, i., 839.
12. Hellier, F. F.: Ibid., 1934, ii., 1271.
13. Wilkie, D. P. D.: Brit. Med. Jour., 1933, i., 771.
14. Bolton, C.: Proc. Roy. Soc. Med., 1934, xxvii., 225.
15. Behrend, M.: Jour. Amer. Med. Assoc., 1930, xcv., 1889.
16. Alessandri, R.: Personal communication.

AN OUTBREAK OF
SCABIES IN A MENTAL HOSPITAL

BY FRANK E. KINGSTON, M.B. Lond., D.P.M.

ASSISTANT MEDICAL OFFICER, WEST RIDING MENTAL HOSPITAL, WAKEFIELD

THE problem of scabies in an institution has certain distinctive features. On the one hand, disinfection of all individual bedding and clothing is readily accomplished ; the patients, moreover, are under constant observation and one can readily satisfy oneself that any treatment prescribed is carried out in detail. On the other hand, there is the wide range of dissemination from the undetected scabetic through accidental interchange of clothing and bedding, and the impracticability of treating all such possible contacts—as one can in the small family—as if they were actually infected.

In the mental hospital there are two further difficulties. The patients rarely complain of any discomfort and thus do not come forward for treatment ; and, secondly, with a few exceptions, they do not coöperate. Not a few patients are actively hostile and resistive to any sort of attention ; and the difficulty of applying any treatment which depends upon the opening-up of all burrows need not be stressed. Below is given briefly an account of an outbreak of scabies in the chronic female block of Wakefield Mental Hospital, comprising 12 wards and containing some 650 patients.

It may be mentioned here that the particular technique of sulphur ointment treatment followed was that recommended by Sequeira [1] of three rubbings with soft soap, three baths with thorough scrubbing, and three liberal applications of unguentum sulphuris B.P. at intervals of 24 hours. The only detail omitted was the use of gloves and stockings after the application of the ointment. Clothing and bedding were autoclaved.

HISTORY OF THE OUTBREAK

The position at the end of April, 1934 (when I took over the charge of the block), was that of the dozen or so cases of scabies which had appeared in four separate wards since the beginning of the year, all had been energetically treated with sulphur-potash baths and sulphur ointment for periods of a week or more and were regarded as cured.

Early in May a patient was reported to have a rash, and examination showed well-advanced generalised scabies. Microscopical examination of a scraping revealed the sarcoptes. The patient was isolated in bed and the routine sulphur ointment treatment given. The following day the limbs of all the other patients in the ward were systematically examined. Two clinically certain and four doubtful cases were found. All six were isolated and treated. During the next few days all previously suspected or treated cases were thoroughly examined, and wherever a suspicious case was found the limbs of all other patients in the ward were examined without delay. All cases, whether certain scabies or only doubtful, were submitted to the routine treatment.

In this way some 30 cases were netted and isolated. Treatment was repeated at fortnightly intervals in all cases which appeared clinically to be still active and which showed, in addition, the sarcoptes or unhatched eggs in scrapings from the burrows. Isolation in bed was maintained for a week after all suspicious lesions had disappeared.

After about a month had elapsed it became apparent that while nearly all of the " doubtful " cases had cleared up hardly any of the clinically " certain " cases had done so, and not one of the cases in which microscopical evidence of the parasite had been found showed any permanent improvement ; nor did stricter supervision of the treatment and the opening-up of all visible burrows with the scalpel give results commensurate with the time and energy expended.

The position in July can be summed up as follows : of ten cases in which the diagnosis had been confirmed microscopically not one had been cured by two courses of treatment. Five had been cured after 3, 3, 3, 4, and 5 courses respectively, while five remained active after 2, 2, 3, 3, and 5 courses respectively.

Treatment was now tried, tentatively at first, using a combination of sulphur and turpentine. The latter was chosen for the reason that it is capable of holding sulphur in solution and that it penetrates the skin.[2] It had the further recommendation that it is itself used as a parasiticide (for ringworm).[2] The application finally used (referred to as S.T.P.) was prepared as follows :

Thirty grains of sublimed sulphur were melted in a wide test-tube. To this, small quantities of oil of turpentine B.P. were added, well boiled, cooled by the addition of more turpentine, and decanted. This process was repeated until all the sulphur was dissolved, 6 fluid ounces of turpentine being used, and the volume made up to 8 fluid ounces with liquid paraffin B.P. The resultant preparation of sulphur, turpentine, and paraffin is a clear deep amber fluid with a pungent odour. The percentage of sulphur dissolved in the turpentine is about 1 per cent. If more is dissolved it crystallises out on cooling.

The three-day scheme of treatment, using S.T.P. in place of sulphur ointment, was adhered to, commenc-

816   THE LANCET]   DR. F. E. KINGSTON : SCABIES IN A MENTAL HOSPITAL   [OCT. 12, 1935

ing with a single bath and scrubbing. Later this was found to be unnecessary and no attempt was made to open up burrows beyond that required for diagnostic purposes. In view of the observation made that vesicles will continue to form—apparently as irritative phenomena from fragments of sarcoptes left in the skin—the treatment, whenever possible, was completed with one or more baths and scrubbings to get rid of the dead parasites.

It soon became evident that S.T.P. was a more effective medicament than sulphur ointment, and had the initial netting of infected patients been complete the outbreak would rapidly have ended. As it was, in addition to one or two cases drafted from another block, fresh cases appeared both in the wards previously infected and in others. (This last fact is not surprising in view of the severe overcrowding, and the fact that structural defects of the block necessitate the constant intermingling of one ward with another.) The chief problem was no longer the treatment of the individual but the netting of the cases as yet undetectable. To do this, whenever scabies appeared the " hands and feet " examination of the ward was repeated at fortnightly intervals until two consecutive examinations were negative. Treated patients were re-examined more thoroughly and over a longer period. In this manner, after several phases of premature optimism, the outbreak was gradually quashed, the last four cases appearing in the early months of 1935. Doubtful cases should, of course, have been treated ; but in view of the experimental nature of the treatment this was withheld until the disease was confirmed microscopically.

Many of the cases netted by systematic examination were very early ones. On the other hand, cases appearing in a ward not yet " scabies-minded " were often remarkably extensive, and this was particularly so in the wildly excited and resistive cases. Of 23 patients treated, 9 were cured after one course of treatment, 10 were cured after two courses. Of the remaining 4, 3 were cured on the third course and the other was treated and cured with Mitigal after the second failure of S.T.P. One other case was cured with mitigal after failure with sulphur ointment, the choice of treatment being determined by the presence of a severe eczema of the legs.

Unpleasant results appear to have been confined to the appearance in two of the earlier cases of a crop

It is worth noting that of the total 29 patients, 13 exhibited scabetic lesions of the palm or sole. Of further interest is the fact that only one patient complained of itching, although several admitted this when questioned. One patient, an intelligent but depressed post-encephalitic, complained not of itching but of general ill-health. She was examined and found to have generalised scabies.

Table showing Survival Times of Adult Female Parasites in Different Media

Medium.	Number of experiments.	Viability.				
Soft paraffin B.P.	1	44 hours. (46)				
Sulphur ointment.. B.P.	4	5 (18½)	11 (20½)	18 (18)	26½ hours. (28)	
Mitigal	4	4 (6)	6½ (17½)	18 (19)	18½ hours. (21)	
2 per cent. K₂S(fresh)	2	10 (13)	12½ min. (15)			
2 per cent. K₂S(stale)	1	70 min. (Sarcoptes lost.)				
S.T.	3	5 (5)	5½ (5½)	7½ min. (7½)		
S.T.P. (1 : 1)	5	4 (5)	5 (6)	9 (11)	12½ (17)	30 min. (33)
S.T.P. (1 : 4)	3	2½ (3½)	20½ (21½)	27 hours. (29½)		

2 per cent. K₂S = 2 per cent. solution of sulphurated potash in water.
S.T. = 1 per cent. solution of sulphur in oil of turpentine B.P.
S.T.P. (1 : 1) = equal parts of S.T. and liquid paraffin B.P.
S.T.P. (1 : 4) = one part of S.T. to four parts liquid paraffin B.P.

EXPERIMENTAL OBSERVATIONS

The examination of the effect of various substances on the isolated living sarcoptes was suggested by the chance finding, in a scraping from a patient already under sulphur ointment treatment, of a vigorously active parasite completely embedded in sulphur ointment when the scraping was examined an hour or so after it had been obtained. From this time on, whenever a favourable case presented itself, examinations were made at the bedside on the living sarcoptes immediately after its capture from the patient. The parasite was at once mounted on a slide in the medium chosen, without any coverglass, and examined under a low-power microscope. All but those which showed active movement at room temperature or on slight warming were discarded, and except for an occasional careful warming in the prolonged experiments (to supply evidence of continued life) all the experiments were carried out at a constant room temperature of between 60° and 70° F.

Considerable variation in vitality in a given medium was found, depending possibly upon the age of the parasite, but in spite of this a significant difference in viability in various media was found. The accompanying Table gives the observed viability of adult female parasites. For each medium the upper row of figures gives the time to the last observed sign of life, while the lower row gives the time to the observation of death. Any muscular movement, whether of

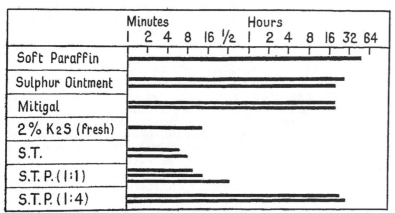

Survival times of sarcoptes in various media (logarithmic scale).

of indolent boils. This was attributed to vigorous rubbing, which was subsequently avoided. Wherever possible the patient's urine was tested both before and after treatment, which was not intended for any case with kidney disease ; but no such case was discovered, nor did any patient show albuminuria subsequently.

limb, jaw, or internal muscles, was regarded as a sign of life. Where observation was continuous the last observed movement was taken as the time of death.

If the survival times of the most viable examples in each medium are represented (roughly) on a logarithmic scale, giving the times between 1 minute and 64 hours, the results shown in the Figure are obtained.

No comparative experiments on the viability of the eggs were carried out. The following observations, however, are worth recording.

Eight eggs were captured and embedded in a film of sulphur ointment. They were left for four days at a temperature of about 60° F., at the end of which time four of the eggs were found to have hatched out, the larvæ having escaped.

Two eggs showing little differentiation of their contents were embedded in sulphur ointment. Each day they were put in an incubator at 100° F. for five minutes. One egg showed no further change. The other, on the fourth day, showed the distinct outline of the developing embryo. On the fifth day development appeared complete and slight warming resulted in repeated movements of the jaw. Hatching did not occur and on the following day there were no signs of life.

COMMENTARY

The object of this paper is to stress the inadequacy of sulphur ointment in the treatment of scabies rather than to advocate a new treatment which is far from ideal. It is not suggested that the experimental results with isolated parasites are strictly parallel with the activity of the medicaments concerned when applied to the skin; and in this connexion it should be mentioned that mitigal, which figures badly in the experiments, has been in the few cases in which I have tried it and in the experience of my colleagues an efficient preparation in the curing of scabies. In view, however, of the dogmatic optimism to be found in text-books of dermatology with regard to the treatment of scabies by sulphur ointment, the following of the recorded observations may well be emphasised:

Out of ten certain cases of scabies in mental patients not one was cured by two courses of sulphur ointment treatment.

A total of 33 courses of treatment resulted in five cures and five failures.

At room temperature an adult female sarcoptes will survive complete embedding in sulphur ointment for 24 hours.

At room temperature the eggs will survive and continue to develop for four days in sulphur ointment, and it does not prevent the larvæ hatching out. On the other hand, sulphur ointment is more lethal for the sarcoptes than Vaseline, killing the parasite in half the time.

Two per cent. sulphurated potash in water is markedly toxic for the parasite, but loses its potency if allowed to become neutralised by the carbon dioxide of the atmosphere. This fact prevented any satisfactory experiment with the reagent at the strength of the sulphurated potash bath as usually prescribed (i.e., about 1 in 1500).

Clinically S.T.P. (sulphur, turpentine, and paraffin) has been disappointing. Apparently potent when applied directly to the parasite at a concentration which caused little or no irritation to the skin, it frequently failed to cure the patient even when given as quite liberal applications on three successive days. On the other hand, for a certain type of patient it is undoubtedly superior to sulphur ointment. The treatment may be repeated the following week without ill-effect, and this course is probably advisable in any well-established case. The preparation is simple and cheap, and the opening-up of burrows, although doubtless of benefit, is not an essential factor in the treatment.

I wish to thank the medical superintendent, Dr. C. J. Thomas, for his permission to publish these results, and my colleagues for their interest and help. I should also like to compliment the nursing staff on its coöperation in somewhat trying circumstances.

REFERENCES
1. Sequeira, J. H.: Diseases of the Skin, London, 1927.
2. Hale-White, W.: Materia Medica, London, 17th ed., p. 525.

ANÆSTHESIA BY CLOSED METHOD

By T. A. B. HARRIS, M.B. Melb.

ANÆSTHETIST TO GUY'S HOSPITAL AND ST. PETER'S HOSPITAL
FOR STONE; ASSISTANT ANÆSTHETIST TO THE
WEST LONDON HOSPITAL

DISREPUTE has been brought upon the closed method of anæsthesia by excessive emphasis on its economy. It is certainly economical, but its importance lies in the exact and rational use that can be made of that hormone of the respiratory system, carbon dioxide.

USE OF THE SODA-LIME CANISTER

Failure to realise that economy is not the whole story has led to the adaptation of a soda-lime canister, often of faulty design, to a machine which has been designed for open anæsthesia. The result of this can only be a makeshift, often physiologically incorrect and therefore unsatisfactory. Closed anæsthesia is, as a result, condemned, although the real fault lies in an incorrect physiological design which renders a sound principle ineffective.

In order to apply the chemical principle of the absorption of carbon dioxide by soda-lime, a closed system of respiration is essential, and in such a system two factors must be fulfilled: (1) the carbon dioxide of each expiration must be completely absorbed; (2) the volume of oxygen used at each inspiration must be replaced by the introduction of a corresponding volume of oxygen.

One may employ a single-phase or a two-phase circuit of breathing. In the single-phase circuit, which is in effect an ebb-and-flow arrangement, the soda-lime canister is set between the mask and the bag. Breathing is from mask to bag and from bag to mask. One breathing tube is used and the direction of the air stream changes with inspiration and expiration. Both the inspired and the expired air are subjected to the resistance and chemical action of the soda-lime. In the two-phase circuit the expiratory and inspiratory phases run in the same direction. An expiratory and inspiratory one-way valve directs expiration from the mask through the soda-lime to the bag, whereas the inspiratory phase runs direct from the bag to the mask. Either circuit can be designed according to correct physiological principles, but the two-phase circuit makes it easier to combine correct physiological with convenient mechanical principles, and a more flexible unit is possible.

Volatile anæsthetic agents are excreted by the lungs almost completely, and in exactly the same form as that in which they were absorbed. In a closed system, therefore, the same amount of anæsthetic may be cleansed and used again and again. In designing such a system five factors are of importance: (1) the system must be airtight; (2) resistance to breathing must be reduced to the smallest possible proportions; (3) the absorptive properties of the soda-lime must always be active; (4) artificial dead

THE LANCET]   [NOV. 16, 1935   1151

NOTES, COMMENTS, AND ABSTRACTS

KWASHIORKOR

A NUTRITIONAL DISEASE OF CHILDREN ASSOCIATED
WITH A MAIZE DIET

BY CICELY D. WILLIAMS, B.M. Oxon., M.R.C.P.,
D.T.M. & H. Lond.

THE name "kwashiorkor" indicates the disease the deposed baby gets when the next one is born, and is the local name in the Gold Coast for a nutritional disease of children, associated with a maize diet, which was first described in December, 1933.[1] An attempt is here made to compare the disease with other conditions, and to indicate the differential diagnosis.

Kwashiorkor is usually observed between the ages of six months and four years, the youngest case noted being nine weeks and the eldest five years old. Some sixty cases have been observed in three years among patients at the Children's Hospital, Accra, the mortality being about 90 per cent. The history always includes defective feeding. The mother is sick, old, and malnourished, or has become pregnant again while the patient is still very young; or the mother may have died, breast-feeding being supplied by an unsuitable foster-mother, very often a senile grandmother; for among these African women some mammary secretion may be present in a woman who has not had a child for 20 years. Supplementary feeds consist mainly of a gruel made from partially fermented white maize, called arkasa, or, for older children, a thick dough of the same called kenki or kon. The child at first appears to progress normally. After a variable interval it ceases to gain weight and becomes irritable. Some swelling of the hands and feet and face appears. This always passes off, both in the event of improvement and in the terminal stages of fatal cases. There may be attacks of diarrhœa; there may be photophobia; and there was sloughing of the cornea in two cases. The most obvious feature is the skin condition. Small, black, thickened, crumpled patches appear first about the knees and elbows, afterwards along the extensor surfaces and the buttocks. These are areas exposed to irritation and pressure. They have no relation to exposure to light, in contrast to the lesions of pellagra. The skin is soft and pliant, but tends to peel off, leaving a moist, raw surface. There is no "branny desquamation." Small sores at the corners of the eyes and mouth and about the vulva are usual. There may be a trace of albumin in the urine. Malaria, bronchitis, and worms are frequent complications; in uncomplicated cases there may be a slight irregular pyrexia. The blood count is little affected; there is no great anæmia and no leucocytosis. The W.R. is negative. Post mortem the only constant

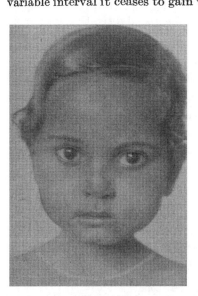

FIG. 1.—A half-caste child, aged 5, suffering from kwashiorkor, with sores at the corners of the mouth.

finding is an extreme fatty infiltration of the liver.

Cases seen very early react well and promptly to an improved diet, rich in accessory substances. Nestlé's sweetened condensed milk with cod-liver oil and malt seemed to be the most successful line of treatment. Unfortunately the condition is an insidious one, and once the dermatitis has set in there is not much hope of recovery. Butter, eggs, tomato, orange, liver, Marmite, yeast, Bemax, iron, and arsenic have also been tried in the treatment.

Figs. 1 and 2 show the condition in a half-caste child of five who died two months later. It is just possible to see the sores at the corners of the mouth. The dark thickened patches of skin are seen on the legs and buttocks. There are none in the areas typical of pellagra. The microphotographs are of the liver (Fig. 3) and of a section of skin (Fig. 4) from the same case. Some points in the differential diagnosis between kwashiorkor and pink disease, vitamin-A deficiency, pellagra, and vitamin-C deficiency are set out below.

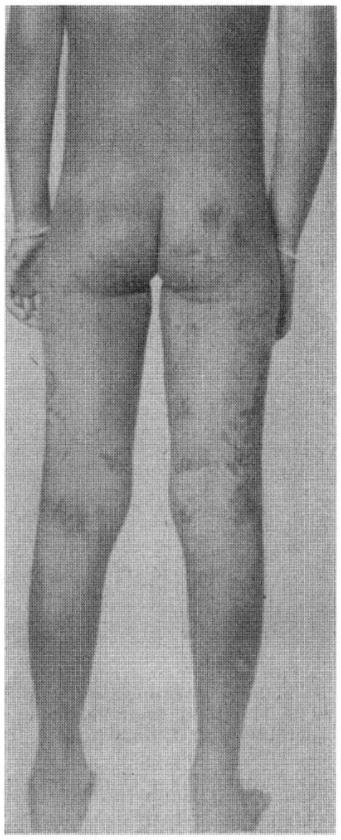

DIFFERENTIAL DIAGNOSIS

Pink disease.—Characteristics common to pink disease and kwashiorkor, both of which occur in young children, are irritability, irregular pyrexia, and skin lesions. The latter reacts well to *early* treatment, whereas the former runs a prolonged course, unaffected by treatment. In kwashiorkor photophobia is seen only occasionally, skin lesions are distinct and typical, and desquamation is extensive, deep, and severe; whereas in pink disease photophobia is pronounced, skin lesions are different, and desquamation is slight.[2]

Vitamin-A deficiency.—Characteristics common to both kwashiorkor and vitamin-A deficiency are the lack of animal fats in the diet, the occurrence of skin lesions, attacks of enteritis, and improvement under cod-liver oil. Phrynoderma, Bitot's spots, night-blindness, and xerophthalmia, often described in connexion with vitamin-A deficiency, occur in other members of the same population, but have not been observed in kwashiorkor, nor does the liability to skin infections appear to be increased.[3-10]

Vitamin-A and -B deficiency of Sierra Leone has in common with kwashiorkor stomatitis, conjunctivitis, and skin lesions, but it occurs in adults; many cases show eversion of the eyelids, and the desquamation is relatively slight.[11] [12]

Vitamin-B deficiencies.—The differential diagnosis from beri-beri, which also causes œdema and affects children and infants, is that beri-beri, unlike kwashiorkor, may lead to sudden death in infants; may be very acute in onset; causes polyneuritis; and produces no skin lesions.[13] Moreover beri-beri responds to treatment in hours instead of in weeks.

Vitamin-B_2 deficiency differs from kwashiorkor in that the diet leading to the condition contains

FIG. 2. — Dark thickened patches of skin on the legs and buttocks of the same child.

no milk or yeast, whereas the diet of the children described above usually includes milk, though its quality is probably defective; and arkasa and kenki do contain yeasts, which have not, however, yet been cultured or tested for biological value.[14][15]

Other deficiencies.—Kwashiorkor cannot be due to deficiency of vitamin C or vitamin D, because the victims show no evidence of either scurvy or rickets. No tests for mineral or protein deficiencies have yet been made.

Pellagra has in common with kwashiorkor the occurrence of œdema, sores at corners of mouth and

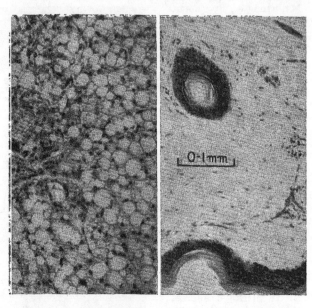

FIG. 3.—Photomicrograph of the liver showing extreme fatty infiltration.

FIG. 4.—Photomicrograph of the skin.

eyes, skin lesions, irritability, and an association with maize diet and with diet poor in protein. The differences are set out below in tabular form.

Differences between Kwashiorkor and Pellagra

KWASHIORKOR	PELLAGRA [16][28]
Affected skin black, rugose, and soft.	Affected skin rough, dry, and branny.
Extensor surfaces and points of irritation and pressure affected.	Face, necklace area, and dorsum of hands and feet affected.
Skin not photosensitive.	Skin photosensitive.
Occurs in children under five years.	Rare in children.
Usual under two years.	Almost unknown under two years.
Reflexes unchanged.	Peripheral neuritis common.
Dementia not observed.	Dementia common.
Patients may be largely on a breast milk diet.	Very rare with milk diet.
Arkasa (preparation of maize) in diet contains yeasts.	Yeasts said to be curative.
Fatty infiltration of liver severe and constant.	Fatty infiltration of liver may be present, but is generally mild.
Never seen in adults.	Common in adults.
Common condition in the Gold Coast.	Never yet described in the Gold Coast.

It has been suggested that kwashiorkor is in fact pellagra,[30] but the points of difference appear to be more numerous and more striking than the points of similarity. The series of cases seen in East Africa by Dr. R. U. Gillan present apparently many points of resemblance to those described above[31] and a perfectly typical case of kwashiorkor has been described by Dr. Dyce Sharp in Cape Coast.[32]

I am indebted to the director of medical and sanitary services for permission to publish this article.

REFERENCES

1. Williams, C. D.: Arch. Dis. Child., 1933, viii., 423.
2. Thursfield, H., and Paterson, D.: Diseases of Children, London, 1934.

(Continued at foot of next column)

SKELETAL REMAINS OF BISHOP JAMES KENNEDY

STRUCTURAL alterations at the University of St. Andrews in 1930 provided an opportunity for an almost complete anthropometric examination of the remains of Bishop James Kennedy, " the most eminent man in Scotland " in the first half of the fifteenth century. Kennedy was of royal descent, his mother being James I. of Scotland's elder sister, whose second husband was Sir James Kennedy. He took an active part in the development of St. Andrews University founded in A.D. 1411 under a Papal Bull, and was appointed one of the regents of the kingdom during the minority of James III. He was a great churchman and statesman, and was thought to have been the means of preserving the Stuart dynasty on the throne. In 1465 he was buried in St. Salvator's Chapel and when the tomb was opened in 1930 a massive casket of dark oak, engraved " Jacobi Kennedy " fell apart owing to dry rot, and the skeleton lay exposed. Prof. David Waterston was invited to examine the bones during the restoration of the tomb and describes his findings (Trans. Roy. Soc. Edin., 1935, lviii., 75).

No evidence of senile changes were seen in the skull or jaws. The limb bones indicate a man 5 ft. 8 in. in height, whose shoulders had been broad with powerfully developed muscles. The areas of attachment of the pronator quadratus on the left ulna was better developed than on the left, the difference being due to a special movement such as fencing. That he was probably a horseman is indicated by an excessive bone formation on the medial surface of the femora. An old oblique fracture is apparent in the right clavicle caused by indirect violence and sustained within the last few years of his life; there is an excess of callus but the fragments are in a position creditable to the surgeon of the day. For some years before his death he had suffered from chronic ill-health; the thoracic vertebræ are the seat of ossifying spondylitis, the sixth to the twelfth being fused together owing probably to some chronic pulmonary affection; there are also signs of a slight arthritis of the hip-joints.

The endocranial cast shows exceptional development of the areas of Broca and Wernicke, which are

REFERENCES (*continued from previous column*)

3. Wilson, J. R., and Dubois, R. O.: Amer. Jour. Dis. Child., 1923, xxvi., 431.
4. Frazier, C. N., and Hu, C. K.: Arch. Int. Med., 1931, lviii., 507.
5. Andrews, G. C.: Diseases of the Skin, London, 1930, p. 861.
6. Pillat, Arnold: Chin. Med. Jour., 1929, xliii., 907.
7. Wright, R. E.: Brit. Jour. Ophth., 1932, vi., 164.
8. Hsu, K. L.: Chin. Med. Jour., 1927, xli., 825.
9. Mackay, H. M. M.: Arch. Dis. Child., 1934, ix., 65.
10. Goodwin, G. P.: Brit. Med. Jour., 1934, ii., 113.
11. Wright, E. J.: West African Med. Jour., 1928, ii., 127.
12.   ,,   ,,   : A and B Avitaminosis Disease of Sierra Leone, London, 1930.
13. Bray, G. W.: Trans. Roy. Soc. Trop. Med., 1928–29, xxii., 13.
14. Goldberger, J.: Pub. Health Reports, 1927, xlii., 2193.
15. Kagan, S. R.: Med. Life, 1933, xl., 434.
16. Mellanby, E.: Nutrition and Disease, London, 1934.
17. Niles, G. M.: Pellagra, London, 1916.
18. Goldberger, Wheeler, and Sydenstricker: Pub. Health Reports, 1920, xxxv., 648, 1650, 2673.
19. Sandwith, F. M.: Trans. Roy. Soc. Trop. Med., 1911–12, v., 120.
20. Arkroyd, W. R.: Nutrition Abstracts and Reviews, 1933–34, iii., 337.
21. Wilson, H.: Jour. Egypt. Med. Assoc., 1932, xv., 405.
22.   ,,   ,,   : Ibid., 1932, xv., 490.
23. Wheeler, S. A.: South Med. Jour., 1933, xxvi., 648.
24. Stannus, H. S.: Trans. Roy. Soc. Trop. Med., 1913–14, vii., 32.
25. Monauni, J.: Wien. klin. Woch., 1933, xlvi., 1413.
26. Spies, T. D., and De Wolf, H. F.: Amer. Jour. Med. Sci., 1933, clxxxvi., 521.
27. Fakhry, Assad: Jour. Egypt. Med. Assoc., 1932, xv., 53, 427.
28. Ruffin, J. M., and Smith, D. T.: Amer. Jour. Med. Sci., 1934, clxxxvi., 512.
29. Chick, H.: THE LANCET, 1933, ii., 341.
30. Stannus, H. S.: Arch. of Dis. Child., 1934, ix., 115.
31. Gillan, R. U.: East Africa Med. Jour., 1934, xi., 88.
32. Dyce Sharp, N. A.: Trans. Roy. Soc. Trop. Med., 1934, xxviii., 411.

THE LANCET]   [JUNE 6, 1936

ADDRESSES AND ORIGINAL ARTICLES

TREATMENT OF HUMAN PUERPERAL INFECTIONS, AND OF EXPERIMENTAL INFECTIONS IN MICE, WITH PRONTOSIL*

By Leonard Colebrook, M.B., B.S. Lond.

MEMBER OF THE SCIENTIFIC STAFF, MEDICAL RESEARCH COUNCIL

Méave Kenny, M.R.C.S. Eng., M.C.O.G.

RESIDENT MEDICAL OFFICER, ISOLATION BLOCK, QUEEN CHARLOTTE'S HOSPITAL, LONDON

AND THE MEMBERS OF THE

HONORARY STAFF OF QUEEN CHARLOTTE'S HOSPITAL

EARLY in 1935 a startling chemotherapeutic success was announced by Domagk [1] in Germany. Hæmolytic streptococci of human origin were injected into the peritoneum of 26 mice. An hour and a half later 12 of them received by stomach-tube a single dose of a dark red dye, the hydrochloride of 4′-sulphamido-2 : 4-diaminoazobenzol—which had been synthesised by Mietzsch and Klarer (see Hörlein [2]), and all survived, at any rate for seven days. (Their ultimate fate is not stated.) Of the remaining 14 animals which served as untreated controls 13 were dead of their streptococcal infection within three days, and the last 1 on the fourth day. It is of interest to note that some of the treated animals received only 0·02 mg. of the drug—i.e., at least 100 times less than the maximum tolerated dose. So far as we are aware this is the only animal experiment which has been reported from Germany. Domagk described the substance—which was named Prontosil—as showing an " elektive Wirkung " upon streptococcal sepsis but as having some action also on staphylococcal infections in the rabbit.

In France, Levaditi and Vaisman,[3] using a similar compound synthesised by Girard and working with a streptococcus " M " of human origin, obtained curative results in mice which were somewhat similar to those of Domagk but less completely successful. The treated animals did not as a rule survive indefinitely after a single dose of the drug but lived a few days longer than the controls. A little later Nitti and Bovet [4] showed that with hæmolytic streptococci of comparatively low mouse-virulence, freshly isolated from human infections, very little or no curative effect was obtained in mice, while with a strain of high mouse-virulence definite prolongation of life was obtained as in Levaditi and Vaisman's experiments. In their most recent paper Levaditi and Vaisman [5] have claimed that by the subcutaneous administration of a large dose (50 mg.) of prontosil in suspension, mice are frequently protected against a fatal dose of streptococcal culture injected 5–10 days later.

In addition to the reports of animal experiments, there have appeared about a dozen papers in Germany referring to the use of the drug in human infections—e.g., erysipelas, puerperal fever, and so forth (Schreus,[6] Anselm,[7] Schranz,[8] Scherber,[9] Fuge,[10] Kramer,[11] and others). These clinical reports are unanimously favourable, but their evidential value must be regarded as small since, in most cases, the recovery of patients is unhesitatingly ascribed to the treatment, and too

little allowance is made for the tendency to spontaneous cure of these infections. The bacteriological and clinical data supplied are nearly always very scanty—e.g., we are not told whether the cases were all infected by hæmolytic streptococci, whether those organisms were present in the blood before the treatment was commenced, nor in how many of the cases there was present any clinical condition, such as generalised peritonitis, which habitually connotes a very high mortality. The papers do serve, however, to indicate that the drug is well tolerated by the human subject and what dosage has given apparently good results.

Laboratory Experiments

The following laboratory experiments and clinical trials have been carried out at Queen Charlotte's Hospital.

CURATIVE EXPERIMENTS ON MICE

Trials were first made with strains of streptococci freshly isolated from human puerperal infections—i.e., after only two or three passages upon artificial nutrient media.

Mice were inoculated into the peritoneum with an amount of culture which preliminary experiments had shown to contain approximately 10–100 minimum lethal doses. A single dose of prontosil or the more soluble related compound (issued for a time under the name of Streptozon S) was given 1½ or 2 hours after, either by stomach-tube or by subcutaneous injection. In later experiments a series of doses was given—e.g., 1½, 5, 24, 48, 72 hours, and so forth after the injection of culture.

Results.—Although occasionally the treated animals survived a little longer than the untreated controls, there were practically no survivals, and the experiments were regarded as negative, failing to confirm Domagk's claim. Six different strains were employed in such tests.

It is important to note that Domagk's original paper refers to two quite distinct substances, both of which gave curative effects in infected mice. The one, prontosil, has the structural formula shown below (I.) and is only slightly soluble in water (to 0·25 per cent.) ; the other, issued for a time under the name Streptozon S, but now as prontosil solubile, is the disodium salt of 4′-sulphamido-phenyl-2-azo-7-acetylamino-1-hydroxynaphthalene 3 : 6-disulphonic acid and is represented by the formula II. below. This is soluble up to 4 per cent.

Formula I

$$SO_2NH_2 \diagdown\diagup N=N \diagdown\diagup NH_2.HCl$$
$$NH_2$$

Formula II

$$OH$$
$$SO_2NH_2 \diagdown\diagup N=N \diagdown\diagup NH.COCH_3$$
$$NaO_3S \qquad SO_4.Na$$

In our animal experiments we have used only prontosil solubile obtained from Germany, and *the French equivalent of prontosil* prepared by Girard. It is possible that the latter substance differed slightly from that used by Domagk in his published experiment. For the *clinical* trials reported in this paper both substances have been administered to every patient—prontosil by the mouth and prontosil solubile by injection—and both had been prepared in Germany.

* A preliminary report to the Therapeutic Trials Committee of the Medical Research Council.

Z

TABLE I.—*Curative Effect of Prontosil Solubile*

	Deaths in each 24-hour period.									
—	1	2	3	4	5	6	7	8	9	—
4 mice were infected with 4000 streptococci (" Richards ") intra-peritoneally : and 1¼ hours later received 7·5 mg. of prontosil solubile subcutaneously. Further doses were given after 1¼ hours, 5 hours, and 1, 2, 3, 4, 6 days.	0	0	0	1	0	0	0	0	0	3 remained well and were killed on 60th day.
4 mice were infected as above : and received prontosil solubile (15 mg.) by stomach-tube 1¼ hours later—and also the following day.	1	0	2	1	..	..	..	..	..	—
7 control mice (no prontosil). { 4 infected with 4000 streptococci (approx.)	1	3	..	..	..	..	..	..	..	—
{ 3 infected with 400 streptococci	0	2	0	0	0	0	0	0	0	1 survived.

At this point we were informed by the courtesy of Dr. Buttle, of the Wellcome Physiological Research Laboratories, that he had obtained more success with a streptococcal strain " Williams " which we had formerly isolated from a puerperal fever case and sent to him. This strain differed from those we had previously employed in that it had been transmitted through a series of 23 mice and had acquired a very much higher virulence for those animals. Our next experiments were therefore carried out with a similar highly virulent passage strain " Richards " (a different serological type from " Williams "). With this strain we began at once to get striking curative results in mice, although the animals only survived indefinitely if a series of 6 or 7 doses was given over a period of several days. Typical results are given in Tables I. and II.

Comment.—The results shown in these tables—and others like them, not set out here—seem to indicate quite clearly that the administration of the drug does exert some curative effect upon infections by these hæmolytic streptococci in the mouse, which normally terminate in peritonitis and septicæmia. They can be checked in the majority of the animals if treatment is commenced within three hours of the injection of culture. If delayed much beyond that time the death of the animals may be postponed for a day or two but it is not usually avoided. It is of interest to note that one mouse survived after treatment although hæmolytic streptococci were already present in the circulating blood in considerable numbers (a small drop of blood from the tail gave colonies equivalent to 400 per c.cm.) *before the drug was administered.*

PROPHYLACTIC EXPERIMENTS ON MICE

Mice were injected subcutaneously with 50 mg. of prontosil (kindly supplied by Dr. Girard) in aqueous suspension (10 per cent.)—and four days later were given a dose of streptococcal culture into the peritoneum. The mice showed no toxic effect of the drug at any time. The results are shown in Table III. It will be seen that whereas 9 out of 12 of the animals which did not receive the drug were dead within three days, only 2 of the 12 treated mice succumbed to streptococcal infection within that period. (Two died somewhat later.)

When the surviving animals were subsequently killed there was a large deposit of undissolved prontosil at the site of injection, and it seems probable that the prophylactic effect shown in the table was due to slow absorption from this depôt. The urine had an orange colour during the whole 26 days after the mice received the drug.

ANIMAL EXPERIMENTS WITH p-AMINOBENZENE-SULPHONAMIDE

In view of the discovery by Trefouel and his collaborators [12] (since confirmed by Goissedet and others [13]) that the diazo linkage in prontosil was not essential for its therapeutic efficacy in animals and that the parent sulphonamide (a colourless compound) was equally effective, we have carried out a few experiments with this latter compound kindly prepared for us by Dr. Harold King, F.R.S., of the National Institute for Medical Research.

The curative effect upon infections by the " Richards " strain is clearly shown in Table IV. No prophylactic effect was obtained when 40 to 50 mg. of the drug was given in aqueous suspension subcutaneously four days before the injection of culture. Probably this was due to absorption of the drug from the subcutaneous depôt more rapidly than in the case of prontosil.

TABLE II.—*Curative Effect of Prontosil Solubile*

	Deaths in each 24-hour period.										
—	1	2	3	4	5	6	7	8	9	10	—
8 mice were infected intraperitoneally with approx. 2160 streptococci (" Richards ") and 1½ hours later received 7·5 mg. of prontosil solubile subcutaneously. Further doses were given after 5 hours, 20 hours, and 2, 3, 4, 6 days.	0	0	0	0	1	2	0	0	0	0	5 remained well and were killed on 42nd day.
6 mice were infected with streptococci as above ; and received the first dose (7·5 mg.) of prontosil solubile 3 hours later. Further doses were given after 7½ hours, 24 hours, and 2, 3, 4, 6 days.	0	0	0	0	0	0	0	0	0	2	4 remained well and were killed on 42nd day.
6 control mice (no prontosil). { 4 infected with 2160 streptococci (approx.)	2	0	1	0	0	0	0	0	0	0	1 survived.
{ 2 infected with 216 streptococci (approx.)	0	2	0	0	0	0	0	0	0	0	—

1282 THE LANCET] DR. L. COLEBROOK & OTHERS: PRONTOSIL IN PUERPERAL INFECTIONS [JUNE 6, 1936

TABLE V.—*Summary of 38 Cases Treated with Prontosil and Prontosil Solubile*

No.	Age.	Pathological condition.	Blood culture.	Day of puerperium.	Prontosil, grammes.			Days of administration.	Result.	Remarks.
					By injection.	Orally.	Total.			
1	28	Local uterine infection with threatened spread to general peritoneum.	−	4th	6	20·4	26·4	12	R	Very ill, S.R.; T. 104°–106°, P. 140–150 for 24 hours; T. normal without further rise after 0·5 g. i.v. (8 c.cm. antitoxic serum also given).
2	29	,, ,,	−	6th	2	17·2	19·2	4	R	Very ill, S.R.; T. 104°–105°, P. 140–150 for 24 hours. T. normal without further rise on 4th day of treatment.
3	33	Septicæmia with threatened general peritonitis.	+ (a)	5th	3·75	18	21·75	10	R	Very ill, debilitated and anæmic; T. 103°–104° for 5 days. T. and P. normal without further rise, and blood culture negative after 4 days' treatment.
4	30	Local uterine infection.	−	3rd	5·25	25·2	30·45	14	R	Very ill, several rigors, delirium; T. 104°. T. and P. persistently normal after 24 hours.
5	35	,, ,,	−	4th	4	23·4	27·4	13	R	Very ill, debilitated and anæmic after severe p.p.h.; P. 130–140 for 24 hours, T. over 104°. T. persistently normal after 3 days' treatment.
6	36	Septic endometritis, pelvic cellulitis, and tonsillitis.	−	8th	2·5	17·4	19·9	10	R	Very ill, debilitated, delirious. After admission condition grew worse for 3 days before prontosil. Spectacular improvement, cellulitic mass resolved rapidly.
7	40	Septic endometritis with extensive infected lacerations.*	−	6th	2·5	7·2	9·7	4	R	Condition fair on admission, became steadily worse; T. over 104°. After 1st dose prontosil T. fell rapidly and general condition remarkably improved.
8	40	Septicæmia with pulmonary emboli and multiple metastases.	+	11th	6·25	24·6	30·85	11	R	Very ill. General condition improved steadily; blood cultures negative on 3rd day of treatment. Metastatic abscesses resolved rapidly.
9	30	Pelvic peritonitis threatening to generalise.	−	6th	4·25	18	22·25	10	R	Very ill; T. 103°–104°, P. 120–130 for 48 hours. T. persistently normal after 24 hours' treatment. Threat of general peritonitis rapidly abated.
10	34	General peritonitis.	−	7th	21	23·4	44·4	13	R	Desperately ill. After massive doses of prontosil signs of peritonitis rapidly abated. A very striking result.
11	24	Acute septic endometritis with extensive infected lacerations.	−	4th	5·5	21·6	27·1	12	R	Severe case, drowsy and toxic, S.R. T. and P. fell in 24 hours, but general improvement flagged.
12	29	Pelvic cellulitis, threatened general peritonitis.	−	11th	3·25	27	30·25	16	R	Very ill, S.R. Remarkable improvement in general condition after 24 hours' treatment; signs of peritonitis rapidly disappeared. Treatment suspended too early, cellulitic mass resolved slowly.
13	29	Early generalising peritonitis.	−	7th	1	1·8	2·8	1	R	Very ill. Signs of peritonitis abated within 24 hours. Treatment stopped on account of albuminuria which was present before 1st dose.
14	32	Early generalising peritonitis with septicæmia.	+ (b)	4th	5·5	18	23·5	10	R	Very ill on admission; T. 104°, P. 140, rising; diarrhœa. Spectacular remission of symptoms and signs within 24 hours. Steady improvement followed.
15	28	Local uterine infection.	−	11th	2·5	11·4	13·9	7	R	Very ill on admission; T. 104°, P. 130–140 for 48 hours. Several rigors. T. persistently normal after 2 days' treatment. General improvement striking.
16	31	Acute generalising peritonitis.	−	5th	8	18·0	26	10	R	Ill-nourished woman, very ill. Spectacular and rapid abatement of signs of peritonitis.
17	38	Local uterine infection.	−	11th	3	21·6	24·6	12	R	Moderately severe case; T. 103°–104° for 4 days. T. and P. settled rapidly. No spread of infection.
18	28	Septic endometritis with infected lacerations.	−	4th	2·25	12·6	14·8	7	R	Mild case; T. 102°–103°, P. 110–120 for 5 days. T. and P. settled without further rise 48 hours after administration of prontosil.
19	28	Local uterine infection.	−	5th	2·75	18·0	20·75	10	R	Moderately severe case. T. and P. subsided without further rise on 3rd day of treatment. General condition improved rapidly.
20	21	Local uterine infection and tonsillitis.	−	6th	4·25	18	22·25	10	R	Moderately severe case; T. 102°–103°, P. 120. T. and P. persistently normal in 48 hours.
21	26	Local uterine infection.	−	4th	1·75	13·8	15·55	8	R	Mild case. T. and P. persistently normal after 24 hours' treatment. Rapid general improvement in debilitated patient.

* Group B, hæmolytic streptococci.

of death had no connexion with hæmorrhage or the operation the mortality is still 20 per cent. In 6 cases anæmia was the sole cause of death, and in all of these there was erosion of a large artery at the base of a penetrating ulcer ; 5 cases were operated on before 1924 when blood transfusion was first introduced. It is questionable whether the serious damage to the parenchymatous organs caused by anæmia could have been repaired by blood transfusion ; for in the sixth case, operated on a year ago, three blood transfusions were unavailing. In spite of the bad results of late operation I have never refused to operate in a single instance, where medical treatment failed, no matter how bad the condition of the patient. In such cases the general condition may be improved sufficiently to render operation possible by previous blood transfusion or by continuous drip infusion of citrated blood.

It is necessary to discriminate between acute profuse gastric hæmorrhage and those cases of recurrent slight hæmorrhage causing severe secondary anæmia. The absolute indication for operation in such cases has been generally accepted since the time of Krönlein and Mikulicz. These cases of severe anæmia are much rarer to-day because patients are operated on earlier. I have had 51 such cases in which bleeding had lasted for weeks with a hæmoglobin percentage of 20 to 30 and 1·5 to 2·5 million erythrocytes. Before the war in these cases I performed gastro-enterostomy. Of 5 cases one was a woman aged 43, operated on in 1911 who died eight days later of severe hæmorrhage. Autopsy revealed erosion of the splenic artery at the bottom of an ulcer penetrating the pancreas. In 44 cases of resection there were 2 deaths—mortality of 4·5 per cent. In 2 cases of unresectable duodenal ulcers with severe anæmia, resection for exclusion was performed and a permanent cure resulted. Operation for secondary anæmia in elderly patients also gives good results provided general anæsthesia is not used. I have brought about a cure by operation in 10 cases between 60 and 74 years of age, using gastro-enterostomy twice and a typical gastric resection in the other 8.

I believe these remarkably good results of operation for acute hæmorrhage were only obtained because local anæsthesia was invariably used. For anyone who is unfamiliar with the enormous advantages of local anæsthesia these results must seem almost impossible, and this may explain the doubt as to the correctness of my figures. It can be readily seen from my report that I have never attempted to embellish my statistics by omitting the fatal cases which may possibly have no direct connexion with the hæmorrhage. I have reported all cases in which death occurred (in both early and late operations), stating the cause, in order that physicians who are the first to see patients with gastric hæmorrhage may be convinced that, in acute hæmorrhage from a chronic ulcer, immediate operation can prevent death from hæmorrhage or perforation and, given proper technique, is more likely than medical treatment to lead to recovery.

DUDLEY GUEST HOSPITAL.—The building extensions at this hospital are making good progress. The adolescent ward, modern theatre suite, and new X ray and massage departments are nearly finished. A further ward unit is in course of erection, and it is hoped to begin shortly on the administration block. Workpeople's contributions for 1935 were £8435, an increase of £772 over the previous year.

THE LOCATION OF CEREBRAL TUMOURS BY ELECTRO-ENCEPHALOGRAPHY

By W. GREY WALTER, M.A. Camb.

ROCKEFELLER FELLOW AT THE CENTRAL PATHOLOGICAL LABORATORY OF THE LONDON COUNTY MENTAL HOSPITALS

(*From the Central Pathological Laboratory and the Hospital for Epilepsy and Paralysis, Maida Vale*)

Berger in 1929 was the first to show that the electrical activity of the human brain could be detected from the outside of the skull.[1] He called the record of this activity—obtained with a galvanometer or amplifier and oscillograph—the Elektrenkephalogram, abbreviated as " EEG " by analogy with the electrocardiogram—ECG. In English-speaking countries the term has come to be " electro-encephalogram." Berger [2] has renounced and condemned the name " Berger rhythm " which is still sometimes used for the phenomenon.

The most prominent feature of the normal human EEG is what Berger called " α waves." These have an amplitude of from 10 to 100 microvolts and a frequency of about 10 Herz (10 cycles per sec.). Their exact frequency varies in different individuals, but is remarkably constant in any given individual. They are nearly sinusoidal and usually come and go at irregular intervals (Fig. 1). Berger regards them as being in some complex way connected with the activity of the whole cortex. Adrian and Yamagiwa,[3] however, have presented very good evidence that the α waves normally originate only in the occipital lobes near the Area 19 of Vogt, and that they are inhibited by visual or intense mental activity. They are really most likely, therefore, to be indicative of a state of physiological rest in an area of the cortex associated with one function.

Berger also described faster " β waves." These are not seen as regularly as the α waves and their origin and significance are doubtful. They appear to arise somewhere in the frontal lobes of some subjects (see Fig. 4 a).

As regards pathological conditions, Berger himself has made several interesting observations on epilepsy [4] and anæsthesia.[5] Gibbs, Davis, and Lennox [6] have also shown how the EEG may be profoundly affected by anæsthesia and by some types of epileptic attack. It is not proposed to go into the contents of these and the other similar publications which have appeared from time to time, since their clinical importance cannot yet be assessed. It is satisfactory, nevertheless, to note that, at least, an abnormal state of the brain is associated with abnormal EEG's.

THE PRESENT INVESTIGATION

In the course of work at the Central Pathological Laboratory on other aspects of electro-encephalography, Dr. F. L. Golla, the director, suggested that records be taken from a case of suspected cerebral tumour. These records were so far from normal (Fig. 2) that it was decided to continue on this line of study. Through the courtesy of the staff of the Hospital for Epilepsy and Paralysis, Maida Vale, it has been possible to take EEG's from seven cases of intracranial tumour.

Three independent amplifiers were used with a triple cathode-ray tube unit ; the amplifiers were home-made but the tube-unit and its power equipment were specially designed and built by Standard Telephones and Cables. The input stages are modified push-pull units similar to the type described by Matthews.[7] This arrangement not only eliminates intercoupling between the amplifiers, but greatly reduces electrical interference, so that satisfactory records may be obtained from a patient

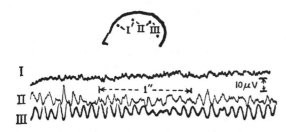

FIG. 1.—An example of a left EEG from a normal subject. Lead I. shows traces of β waves, leads II. and III. α waves moving over the parieto-occipital region. The subject's eyes were closed.

on the operating table without any screening. The amplifiers are resistance-capacity-coupled and battery-driven, but the power for the oscillographs and their associated circuits is obtained from the mains. The oscillograph screens may be observed and photographed at the same time. The maximum overall potential

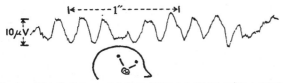

FIG. 2.—The first record taken from a patient with a cerebral tumour. Note the slow waves from an area which normally shows only the fast β waves.

amplification is of the order of 5×10^7, and the maximum overall time constant is 2 sec. Silver-silver chloride pad electrodes were used for the skull leads, held on by a Butywave cap and moistened with saline. For leading off from the exposed brain during operations, sterilised silver-silver chloride wick electrodes were used, filled with sterile normal saline, and supported by an adapted Bestlite reading lamp.

The following results have been obtained :—

1. Records have been taken (a) leading from the skull just before operations, and (b) leading from the exposed brain beneath the same point during operations (Fig. 3). This has been done in both general and local anæsthetic cases. In all cases we have found that records obtained from the skull leads closely resemble those obtained directly from the underlying brain, except in regard to the size of the potential changes, which are attenuated by the skull. The potential changes recorded with the direct leads are of the order of 1 to 10 millivolts, those with the skull leads, 10 to 100 microvolts. It may be said, therefore, that records obtained from the skull are fairly faithful miniature copies of the electrical events in the brain below, except that, as Tönnies[8] has pointed out, the "spread" of the potentials is increased by the complex resistance network of the dura, skull, and scalp.

2. Under a local anæsthetic the potential changes from all but the occipital lobes are mostly irregular, but occasional rhythms can be detected (Fig. 3 i). In one case it was possible to lead directly from a subcortical glioma. As Foerster and Altenburger[9] found, the tumour is much less active electrically than the comparatively normal tissue around it. Probably many of the irregular " base line fluctuations " in skull leads are really due to electrical changes in the brain.

3. Under a general anæsthetic, particularly with ether, rather less with nitrous oxide, very large, often rhythmic potential changes are found (Fig. 3 ii). These involve the whole cortex and may appear at any point on the surface, travel a short distance and subside, to be succeeded by fresh disturbances. When regular, these waves have a frequency of from 3 to 4 per sec. and as lead from the skull an amplitude of up to 100 μV.

4. Similar large quasi-regular disturbances involving the whole cranium are found in cases of raised intra-cranial pressure (see Fig. 7). When the pressure is relieved by intravenous hypertonic solutions or other osmotic means, these disturbances subside. These " pressure waves " are distinguishable from the " anæsthetic waves " though they are very similar. It is probable that they are the result not merely or only of the raised pressure, but of the secondary changes which accompany it.

5. In cases of intracranial tumour in which the cerebral cortex was affected by invasion or by proximity, and where the pressure was still moderate or had been reduced, slow potential waves (of the order of 10 to 20 microvolts in size and occurring at the rate of 2 to 3 per sec.) have been led off from the skull immediately over the place where the tumour was subsequently found at operation or autopsy. Since this finding may turn out to be of clinical interest, the relevant cases will be summarised.

SUMMARY OF CASES

CASE 1. (Examined with single recorder only.)— A man, aged 48, under the care of Dr. Russell Brain. Left EEG : normal in all areas (Fig. 4 a). Right EEG : frontal, normal but for few slow waves posteriorly ; parietal, few slow waves anteriorly ; temporal, slow waves anteriorly (Fig. 4 b) ; occipital, normal. By moving the electrodes about over the temporal region it was possible by " presence or absence " observation to delimit the area over which the slow waves could be found. This was a point

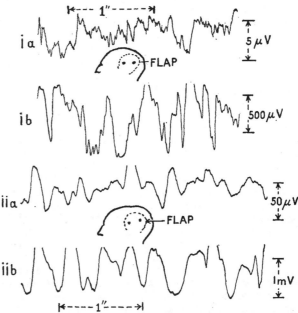

FIG. 3.—(i) Patient A. Man aged 48. (a) From the skull with high amplification. (b) During operation. From the corresponding area on the cortex with much lower amplication. There was only a local anæsthetic and morphine, and the eyes were closed in both records.
(ii) Patient B. Man aged 55. (a) From the skull. (b) From the underlying brain at operation, both when the patient was under nitrous oxide and ether.

PRINCIPLES OF MEDICAL STATISTICS

I.—THE AIM OF THE STATISTICAL METHOD

"Is the application of the numerical method to the subject matter of medicine a trivial and time-wasting ingenuity as some hold, or is it an important stage in the development of our art, as others proclaim ? "

WHATEVER may be our reactions to that question, propounded by Prof. Major Greenwood in these columns [1] fifteen years ago, it must be admitted that in the years intervening between 1921 and to-day there has been a substantial increase in the number of papers contributed to medical journals of which the essence is largely statistical. Not only does there appear to be an enhanced knowledge of and respect for the national registers of life and death which the Registrar-Generals of the United Kingdom annually publish and analyse, but there is an increasing number of workers who endeavour to apply numerical methods of analysis to their records obtained in clinical medicine. The great majority of such workers, however, have had, naturally enough, little or no training in statistical method and many of them would find the more mathematical methods of the professional statistician, as has been said, "obscure and even repellent." Often enough, indeed, the argument is put forward that the use of such mathematical methods is quite unjustifiable, that the accuracy of the original material is not sufficient to bear the weight of the treatment meted out to it. This assertion is not strictly logical. If a collection of figures is worth a statistical analysis at all, it is, obviously, worth the best form of statistical analysis—i.e., the form which allows the maximum amount of information to be derived from the data.

Whether mathematical statistical methods *are* the best form in particular cases or may be regarded as an unnecessary elaboration must turn rather upon this question : Can we in any of the problems of medical statistics reach satisfactory results by means of relatively simple numerical methods only ? Or upon this question : Can we satisfactorily test hypotheses and draw deductions from data that have been analysed by means of such simple methods ? Personally I believe the answer to these questions is an unqualified yes, that many of the figures included in medical papers can by relatively simple statistical methods be made to yield information of value, that where the yield is less than that which might be obtained by more erudite methods which are not at the worker's command the best should not be made the enemy of the good, and that even the simplest statistical analysis carried out logically and carefully is an aid to clear thinking with regard to the meaning and limitations of the original records. If these conclusions are accepted, the question immediately at issue becomes this : Are simple methods of the interpretation of figures only a synonym for common sense or do they involve an art or knowledge which can be imparted ? Familiarity with medical statistics leads inevitably to the conclusion that common sense is *not* enough. Mistakes which when pointed out look extremely foolish are quite frequently made by intelligent persons, and the same mistakes, or types of mistakes, crop up again and again. There is often lacking what has been called a " statistical tact, which is rather more than simple good sense." That tact the majority of persons must acquire (with

a minority it is undoubtedly innate) by a study of the basic principles of statistical method.

It is my object in these articles to discuss these basic principles in an elementary way and to point out by representative examples taken from medical literature how these principles are frequently forgotten or ignored. I very much fear that the discussion will often appear too simple and that some of the mistakes to which space is given will be thought too futile to need attention. I am only persuaded that such is not the case by the recurrence of these mistakes and the neglect of these elementary principles, a feature with which every professional statistician is familiar in the papers submitted to him by their authors for " counsel's opinion."

Definition of Statistics

Whereas the laboratory worker can frequently exclude variables in which he is not interested and confine his attention to one or more controlled factors at a time, the clinician and social worker have to use records which they know may be influenced by factors which they cannot control but have essentially to be taken into account. The essence of the statistical method lies in the elucidation of the effects of these multiple causes. By statistics, therefore, we mean " quantitative data affected to a marked extent by a multiplicity of causes," and by statistical method " methods specially adapted to the elucidation of quantitative data affected by a multiplicity of causes " (G. U. Yule : An Introduction to the Theory of Statistics, 1927). For example, suppose we have a number of children all of whom have been in contact with measles and to a proportion of them is given an injection of convalescent serum. We wish to know whether the treatment prevents the development of a clinical attack. It is possible that the risk of developing an attack is influenced by age, by sex, by social class and all that that denotes, by duration and intimacy of contact, by general state of health. A statistical analysis necessitates attention to *all* these possible influences. We must endeavour to equalise the groups we compare in every possibly influential respect except in the one factor at issue— namely, serum treatment. If we have been unable to equalise the groups ab initio we must equalise them to the utmost extent by the mode of analysis. As far as possible it is clear, however, that we should endeavour to eliminate, or allow for, these extraneous or disturbing causes when the experiment is planned ; in a carefully planned experiment we may determine not only whether serum is of value but whether it is more efficacious at one age than another, &c. It is a serious mistake to rely upon the statistical method to eliminate disturbing factors at the completion of the work. *No* statistical method can compensate for a badly planned experiment.

Planning and Interpretation of Experiments

It follows that the statistician may be able to advise upon the statistical lines an experiment such as that referred to above should follow. Elaborate experiments can be planned in which quite a number of factors can be taken into account statistically at the same time (R. A. Fisher : The Design of Experiments, 1935). It is not possible to discuss such methods here and attention is confined to the type of simple experimental lay out with which medical workers are familiar. Limitation of the discussion to that type must not be taken to mean

---

[1] Medical Statistics (1921) *Lancet*, 1, 985.

that it is the best form of experiment in a particular case.

The essence of the problem in a simple experiment is, as emphasised above, to ensure beforehand that, as far as is possible, the control and treated groups are the same in all *relevant* respects. The word *relevant* needs emphasis for two reasons. First, it is obvious that no statistician can be aware of all the factors that are, or may be, relevant in particular medical problems. From general experience he may be able to suggest certain broad disturbing causes which should be considered in planning the experiment (such as age and sex in the example above) but with factors which are narrowly specific to a particular problem he cannot be expected to be familiar. The onus of knowing what is likely to be relevant in a specific problem must rest upon the experimenter who is, presumably, familiar with that narrow field. Thus, when the statistician's help is required it is his task to suggest means of allowing for the disturbing causes, either in planning the experiment or in analysing the results, and not, as a rule, to determine what *are* the relevant disturbing causes.

The second point that must be observed as regards the equality of groups in all relevant respects is the caution that must attend the interpretation of statistical results. If we find that Group A differs from Group B in some characteristic, say, its mortality-rate, can we be certain that that difference is due to the fact that Group A was inoculated (for example) and Group B was uninoculated ? Are we certain that Group A does not differ from Group B in some other character relevant to the issues as well as in the presence or absence of inoculation ? For instance, in a particular case, inoculated persons might, on the average, belong to a higher social class than the uninoculated and therefore live in surroundings in which the risk of infection was less. We can never be *certain* that we have not overlooked some relevant factor or that some factor is not present which could not be foreseen or identified. It is because he knows a complex chain of causation is so often involved that the statistician is, as it appears to many persons, an unduly cautious and sceptical individual.

The reason why in experiments in the treatment of disease the allocation of alternate cases to the treated and untreated groups is often satisfactory, is because no conscious or unconscious bias can enter in, as it may in any selection of cases, and because *in the long run* we can fairly rely upon this random allotment of the patients to equalise in the two groups the distribution of other characteristics that may be important. Between the individuals within each group there will often be wide differences in characteristics, for instance in body-weight and state of health, but with *large* numbers we can be reasonably sure that the numbers of each type will be equally, or nearly equally, represented in both groups. If it be known that certain characteristics will have an influence upon the results of treatment and on account of relatively small numbers the distribution of these characteristics may not be equalised in the final groups, it is advisable to extend this method of allocation. For instance, alternate persons will not be treated but a division will be made by sex, so that the first male is treated and the second male untreated, the first female is treated and the second female untreated. Similarly age may be equalised by treating alternate males and alternate females at each age, or in each broad age-group if individuals whose ages are within a few years of one another may in the particular case be regarded as equivalent.

AN EXAMPLE

Even if in planning the experiment factors such as age and sex have thus been equalised in the two groups, the analysis of the results should never be directed only to the effects of treatment upon the totals. It is possible that treatment may be more effective at one age than at another and this difference will be lost sight of if the groups as a whole are alone compared. As far as the number of observations allow, comparison should be made between sub-groups differentiated by any factors that may be of importance. As an example of this experimental method and analysis may be cited the report of the Therapeutic Trials Committee of the Medical Research Council on the serum treatment of lobar pneumonia (*Brit. med. J.* 1934, **1**, 241). In each of three centres, London, Edinburgh, and Aberdeen, it was arranged that alternate cases taken in order of their admission to hospital should be treated with serum, both treated and untreated being so far as possible in the same wards and under the care of the same physicians. " It was thought better not to attempt a deliberate sorting of cases in respect of mildness or severity, but to trust that the distortion of chance scatter would become almost negligible in a fairly large number of cases." Age, it will be observed, was not equalised in the allotment of cases, and as fatality from lobar pneumonia certainly varies with age the analysis must first show whether the serum and control groups are equivalent in that respect. The random allocation of patients has, in fact, not quite equalised the groups in that factor. Taking the figures for London and Aberdeen (in Edinburgh the method was not fully carried out) and combining Types I and II, the numbers in two broad age-groups were :—

Age.	Number of patients.		Percentage in each age-group.	
	Controls.	Serum treated.	Controls.	Serum treated.
20–40 ..	104	123	65	75
40–60 ..	55	40	35	25
Total ..	159	163	100	100

Roughly 35 per cent. of the control cases were of ages 40–60 and only 25 per cent. of the serum-treated. It follows that the comparison of results must essentially be made within, at least, these two age-groups. If a lower fatality-rate is found in the serum-treated when the total groups are compared, this result may merely be a reflection of the fact that 10 per cent. less of these patients belonged to the ages at which fatality is normally higher and, correspondingly, 10 per cent. more belonged to the ages at which fatality is normally lower. In other words, as the method of allotment has not equalised the groups in an important respect with regard to fatality, the method of analysis must do so.

It is impossible to ignore the fact that in the random allocation of patients to the treated and untreated categories a difficult moral issue is often raised. The treatment is usually based on a priori evidence which suggests that it should have some curative effect. Can it, then, be justifiably withheld from any patient ? And if it is withheld how extensive a trial is justifiable ? There are no easy answers to these questions. There can be no doubt that any new therapeutic measure *should* be given a period of trial before coming into general use. If the results of such a measure are dramatic in the light of all past experience, then clearly the trial period will not need to be prolonged. But one must be careful of the interpretation of "dramatic"; it must imply something strikingly different from all previous experience, not merely a run of a few successes where some failures might well have been expected. Such dramatic events are unfortunately the exception. More usually the effect of the new measure will be relatively small, though none the less important, and therefore its presence (or absence) be difficult to detect in small-scale tests. Such tests may well give contradictory and confusing answers. They may enable a useless measure to hold for years a position it does not merit (sometimes, perhaps, to the exclusion of more worthy measures); they may even prevent a really valuable form of treatment obtaining the general recognition it deserves. A well-planned and extensive trial (such as has been carried out with measles serum) would obviate such undesirable results, and thereby possibly save more suffering in the long run than is incurred in the trial itself, and more speedily than the indeterminate results given by inadequate tests would allow.

Summary

The statistical method is required in the interpretation of figures which are at the mercy of numerous influences, and its object is to determine whether individual influences can be isolated and their effects measured. The essence of the method lies in the determination that we are really comparing like with like, and that we have not overlooked a relevant factor which is present in Group A and absent from Group B. In experiments involving the treatment of a number of patients who are to be compared with controls not given the specific treatment, any deliberate choice of individuals to be treated may lead, unconsciously, to the treated group differing from the untreated group in some characteristic which, known or unknown, has an influence upon the results. If the series of cases is large, a random allocation of individuals—e.g., by cases being alternately placed in the treated and untreated groups— may reasonably be relied upon to equalise the two groups in all characteristics except the one under examination. Such a method of allocation does not obviate the necessity of testing in the statistical analysis of the results whether in fact the groups are equal in all characteristics which are believed to be relevant.

A. BRADFORD HILL.

SPECIAL ARTICLES

INCIDENCE OF ANÆMIA IN PREGNANCY

INFLUENCE OF SOCIAL CIRCUMSTANCES AND OTHER FACTORS

BY W. J. S. REID, B.Sc., M.D. Aberd., M.R.C.P. Lond.

HON. PHYSICIAN TO ANCOATS HOSPITAL, MANCHESTER; AND

JEAN M. MACKINTOSH, M.D. Glasg., D.P.H.

ASSISTANT MEDICAL OFFICER FOR MATERNITY AND CHILD WELFARE, COUNTY BOROUGH OF STOCKPORT

A SERIES of 1108 pregnant women was examined. There was no selection of cases either as to social circumstances or as to parity, the patients being those who attended the Stockport corporation antenatal clinics. The Haldane hæmoglobinometer was used, and the hæmoglobin estimations were all made by one of us (J. M. M.). The examinations extended over about two years, and were more or less evenly distributed throughout the seasons. About half the women were examined in the forenoon and the rest in the afternoon. Some 72 per cent. of the examinations were made between the twenty-sixth and the thirty-second week of pregnancy, and only 7 per cent. after the thirty-sixth week. The age and parity distribution of the women is shown in Table I.

Incidence of Hyperchromic Anæmia.—In all cases showing a reading of 70 per cent. of hæmoglobin and under, blood films were prepared and examined by one of us (W. J. S. R.). No case of pernicious anæmia was found. It may be recalled that Evans, who examined 4083 patients, "found no case of severe anæmia."

Incidence of Hypochromic Anæmia.—Amongst our cases we found that 45·9 per cent. gave a hæmoglobin reading of 86 per cent. and over, 43·9 per cent. showed a reading between 70 and 84 per cent., and 10·2 per cent. gave a reading below 70 per cent. Davidson and his colleagues in Aberdeen (1935) in an examination of 819 pregnant women, found 17·5 per

cent. with a hæmoglobin reading below 70 per cent. Helen Mackay (1935) in London examined 109 pregnant women and found 4·6 per cent. with a hæmoglobin reading below 70. Boycott (1936), also working in London, in a series of 222 cases found 11 per cent. of his cases gave a reading below 70. All these workers used the Haldane method. American investigators, Moore (1929), Lyon (1929), Galloway (1929), Adair,

TABLE I

Age-group.	Parity.													Total
	1	2	3	4	5	6	7	8	9	10	11	12	13	
20 and under.	75	14	2	—	—	—	—	—	—	—	—	—	—	91
21–25	205	92	27	12	2	1	—	—	—	—	—	—	—	339
26–30	117	99	79	25	18	11	—	—	—	—	—	—	—	349
31–35	31	40	29	36	28	10	12	7	4	1	1	—	—	199
36–40	8	19	6	14	11	11	8	3	6	3	3	4	—	96
41 and over.	4	1	5	2	6	4	3	2	1	3	2	—	1	34
Total	440	265	148	89	65	37	23	12	11	7	6	4	1	1108

Bland, Goldstein, First (1930), with various methods of estimation, examined groups of cases ranging from 100 to 1176 in number, and found a much greater incidence of anæmia in pregnancy. They give figures ranging from 19 to 81 per cent. of patients with less than 70 per cent. hæmoglobin.

Effect of Social Circumstances.—In order to determine whether economic circumstances had any effect, we divided our patients into two groups, according to the average income per head of the family per week after deduction of rent. Group I. comprised those women whose family income amounted to an average of 12s. per head per week or less; Group II. those with an average over 12s. per head. It was possible to assess the income in each case with a considerable degree of accuracy from office

THE LANCET]   DRS. PETERS AND HAVARD : PROSEPTASINE IN STREPTOCOCCAL INFECTIONS   [MAY 29, 1937   1273

CHEMOTHERAPY OF STREPTOCOCCAL INFECTIONS WITH p-BENZYLAMINO-BENZENE-SULPHONAMIDE

BY B. A. PETERS, M.D. Camb., D.P.H.

MEDICAL SUPERINTENDENT TO THE HAM GREEN HOSPITAL AND SANATORIUM, BRISTOL ; AND

R. V. HAVARD, M.R.C.S. Eng.

ASSISTANT RESIDENT MEDICAL OFFICER, HAM GREEN HOSPITAL AND SANATORIUM, BRISTOL

DURING the past winter 150 cases of scarlet fever, 47 cases of erysipelas, and 18 cases with other types of streptococcal infection were treated with Proseptasine (p-benzylamino-benzene-sulphonamide), an ample supply of which was placed at our disposal by the makers, Messrs. May and Baker.

SCARLET FEVER

In the scarlet fever test group no antitoxic serum was given. As controls, 150 alternate cases were treated with serum when considered necessary (56 cases) and the remainder expectantly. The dose given was 0·75 to 6 g. per day according to age by mouth in tablet form, divided into four-hourly doses. The full dose was given for two days, and half the quantity for another two to four days according to the course of the illness. The maximum quantity given in all to any one patient was 22·5 g. The results are shown in the Table.

It will be observed that in the test series, 53 (35 per cent.) developed one or more of the complications tabulated, whilst 84 (56 per cent.) of the control cases showed some complications. This difference is statistically significant. The sum of the individual complications is almost identical, but the complications in the test series occurred in fewer patients. The mean duration of the primary fever from onset to termination was twelve hours longer in the test series. Since antitoxin was administered to a third of the control series, this might be expected, for antitoxic serum undoubtedly reduces pyrexia. Our results would suggest, therefore, that the drug has some effect on the invasive side of this streptococcal infection and the results might be better if the drug could be given earlier. If spaces such as nasal sinuses, the middle ear, or bone are infected, the organism is probably less accessible to the drug. Possibly a combination of drug and serum would be more effective, and this is now being investigated.

ERYSIPELAS

The results here were very striking. A series of 47 cases of erysipelas of varying severity, from mild to very severe, was treated with similar doses of the drug. The youngest patient was four months ; three were 70, 81, and 87 respectively. In 31 cases the temperature was normal within twenty-four hours, in 12 within forty-eight hours, in 3 within seventy-two hours, and in 1 only did pyrexia continue until the fifth day. The spread of the disease was arrested within twenty-four hours in every case. Two developed relapses ten days after the primary attack, which responded at once to further doses of the drug. All the cases made satisfactory recoveries, even the aged ones.

OTHER STREPTOCOCCAL INFECTIONS

In 15 severe cases of *tonsillitis*, notified as diphtheria, there was recovery within forty-eight hours of treatment with the drug.

In one case of *puerperal sepsis*, showing signs of early involvement of the broad ligament, which gave a pure growth of hæmolytic streptococcus from the cervix, the temperature settled within eighteen hours and the patient made an uninterrupted convalescence with rapid resolution of the infiltrated broad ligament.

One very ill patient with *cellulitis* involving the fauces arising from an impacted wisdom tooth lost his fever within seventy-two hours and recovered.

In one case of influenzal pneumonia with a turbid *pleural effusion*, from which a pure growth of hæmolytic streptococci was cultured, the effusion dried up after two aspirations following the administration of the drug and the patient recovered. In our former experience, such effusions invariably became purulent and necessitated operation for cure.

TEST SERIES OF SCARLET FEVER CASES TREATED WITH PROSEPTASINE

Cases showing complications

CONTROL SERIES (56 CASES RECEIVED ANTITOXIC SERUM)

Cases showing complications

AGES	0–5	5–10	10–15	15–20	Over 20	All ages.	0–5	5–10	10–15	15–20	Over 20	All ages.
Cases	27	72	24	9	18	150	28	67	33	9	13	150
Cases with complications ..	12	25	8	2	6	53	14	44	16	4	6	84
Mean day of disease on admission	2·1	2·4	2·2	1·6	2·3	2·3	1·7	2·9	3·3	1·4	2·5	2·6
Mean duration of pyrexia after admission	3·2	3·6	2·8	3·1	3·2	3·3	3·0	2·2	2·2	3·4	3·3	2·5
Adenitis	9	17	2	1	—	29	10	8	6	2	1	27
Otitis	5	5	—	—	1	11	2	4	4	—	—	10
Secondary tonsillitis	2	2	1	1	3	9	1	—	2	2	3	8
Endocarditis	1	2	—	—	—	3	3	4	—	1	1	9
Rheumatism	—	—	1	—	2	3	—	2	4	2	2	10
Albuminuria	1	8	3	—	—	12	5	4	5	2	3	19
Nephritis *	—	3	2	1	—	6	—	4	1	—	—	5
Mastoiditis	—	1	—	—	—	1	—	1	—	—	—	1
Died	—	—	—	—	—	—	1†	1‡	—	—	—	2

* 1 case of nephritis developed uræmia.

† Abdominal case died after exploration.
‡ Died following nephritis.

Y 2

TOXIC EFFECTS

One child with erysipelas developed a macular rash ; two very fat women complained of nausea and vomited once ; no case showed any cyanosis or clinical signs suggesting sulphæmoglobinæmia. It seems, therefore, that the drug produces few toxic symptoms in the doses we gave and is well borne at all ages.

SUMMARY

The administration of proseptasine to scarlet fever patients reduced the number of patients having complications from 56 per cent. in the control series to 35 per cent. The drug seems to affect chiefly the invasive stage and results might be better if it could be given earlier.

In erysipelas the spread of the disease was arrested in 24 hours in all of 47 cases. In 31 cases the temperature was normal within 24 hours and in a further 12 within 48 hours. A similar result was seen in other types of streptococcal infection.

SOME OBSERVATIONS ON A CASE OF PULMONARY ŒDEMA

BY GEORGE GRAHAM, M.D. Camb., F.R.C.P. Lond.
PHYSICIAN, ST. BARTHOLOMEW'S HOSPITAL ; AND

RONALD BURN, M.R.C.S. Eng.

WE have made two observations on a patient with pulmonary œdema which seem so important that we are recording them now, as it may be long before we have the opportunity of making detailed investigations on another patient with this condition.

The patient, a woman aged 64, has been seen at intervals by one of us (G. G.) since 1925. In that year she developed the symptoms of a mild toxic goitre, and was treated by Sir Thomas Dunhill with rest and iodine. Glycosuria and hyperglycæmia were also present at that time, and were treated with dietetic restrictions and insulin. The symptoms abated, and after two to three years did not cause any further trouble. The diabetic condition improved greatly with insulin, and she was able to take 180 g. of carbohydrate without insulin in 1928. Since then the diabetic condition has become worse and in January, 1936, she needed 18+16 units for a diet containing 130 g. of carbohydrate. At that time she was complaining of lassitude and had a slight degree of pyrexia. No cause for this fever was discovered and the temperature gradually decreased and the symptoms abated. In March she was again feeling unwell with slight pyrexia, and then had an acute attack of B. coli pyelitis, which lasted for five weeks. An intravenous pyelogram showed that she had a large cyst of the kidney, which was thought to be congenital. The B. coli infection was at first treated with alkalis and later with mandelic acid ; the symptoms were quickly relieved with mandelic acid but it was not until August that the urine was rendered sterile.

Her general health had greatly improved, but she was still easily tired, and was only up for about five hours in the day. She had occasionally noticed a little wheezing and tightness of the chest when falling asleep.

On Dec. 1st, 1936, she had a slight coryza, and on Dec. 4th at midnight a feeling of tightness of the chest. This was followed at once by an acute attack of pulmonary œdema. She became ashy grey in colour. P. 140, R. 36, B.P. 180/100. Many r, and atropine gr. 1/150. The acute attack lasted about two hours and she gradually recovered. She was seen two days later by Sir Maurice Cassidy, who agreed that the attack was one of acute pulmonary œdema. The electrocardiogram was quite

normal. She was kept in bed for 4 weeks but was then allowed to resume her ordinary convalescent life. She still had a slight pyrexia (99–99·5° F.). Blood pressure was 160 to 180/80 ; hæmoglobin, 82 per cent. ; colour-index, 0·7 ; red cells, 5,600,000 ; and white cells, 23,000.

On Feb. 6th, 1937, she had another acute attack which started suddenly at midnight. The respiration was 40, pulse 144. Many r, coramine 2 c.cm., atropine gr. 1/150. The attack passed off in about 2 hours. She was very unwell the next day, vomiting several times and passing a great deal of sugar in the urine, and was seen by G. G. on this account. The following were the results of examinations made of the blood : sugar, 230 mg. per 100 c.cm. ; urea, 52 mg. per 100 c.cm. ; alkali reserve, 63·5 vols. (Dr. H. E. Archer).

The blood-urea had been estimated several times during the previous illness and was usually between 32 and 36 mg. per 100 c.cm. The rise to 52 mg. suggested that the kidney might have failed because of the acidæmia which was probably present during the acute attack of dyspnœa. As both the attacks started so suddenly the possibility of her being sensitive to some substance was considered. Her rooms were always full of flowers, but no unusual flower had been brought into the rooms in the last few days.

A week later the general condition was better. The blood-urea was 32 mg. per 100 c.cm. and the diabetic condition was under much better control with 22+23 units of insulin. The blood pressure was 170/80. The patient was allowed to get up after tea on this day, and while walking in her room complained of a tight sensation in her chest. She was put to bed at once and given, at 5.50 P.M., morphine gr. ¼, atropine gr. 1/50, adrenaline 0·5 c.cm. In spite of this treatment the symptoms developed rapidly, and when she was seen by R. B. at 6.5 P.M. was in great distress. She was given, at 6.5, coramine 1·7 c.cm. ; at 6.20, morphine gr. 1/6, atropine gr. 1/100 ; at 7.10, atropine gr. 1/100. The blood pressure was 200/80, a rise of 30 mm. from the morning. The pulse-rate was 140 and feeble, and the respiration 46. Moist rs were heard all over both lungs. During the next one and a half hours she vomited two or three times, bringing up a good deal of fluid. Two hours after the onset she was seen by G. G. The attack was then passing off, although she was still very ill. The respiration was 40 and the pulse 140 ; moist rs were heard all over the lungs. Ten c.cm. of blood was collected at this stage for analysis. An injection of adrenaline 0·5 c.cm. was then given subcutaneously, after ascertaining that the point of the needle was not in a vein by first withdrawing the plunger of the syringe. Ten minutes later the breathing was quieter and she said she felt better. The blood pressure at this stage was 170/100, pulse-rate 144. Half an hour later another 0·5 c.cm. of adrenaline was injected, using the same precautions, and the condition continued to improve. An hour later she was well enough to be left although the pulse was still 120 and the blood pressure 170/80.

When the estimation of the blood-sugar was made that night it was noticed that the blood flowed up the pipette with difficulty. This condition had been observed before in a case of diabetic coma (Graham, Spooner, and Smith 1926) and a week previously in a case of severe vomiting after influenza (G. G.). The hæmoglobin was estimated at over 130 per cent. on a Sahli apparatus, and the next day by Dr. H. F. Brewer, using a standard Haldane apparatus, at 135 per cent. When the blood had stood for a while the amount of plasma was very small compared with the number of red cells, but a hæmatocrit estimation was not made. The alkali reserve was 49 vols. ; blood-urea was 36 mg. per 100 c.cm., and blood-sugar 260 mg. per 100 c.cm. The hæmoglobin had been 82 per cent. in January and two days after the attack was 80 per cent.

DISCUSSION

The two observations to which we wish to draw attention are the rise in the blood pressure and the increase in the hæmoglobin percentage, as we believe they may throw light on the cause of the condition.

THE LANCET]   [MARCH 26, 1938 749

CORRESPONDENCE

OUR COLLEAGUES IN AUSTRIA

To the Editor of THE LANCET

SIR,—In view of recent events, we the under-signed members of the medical profession desire to express our alarm at the possible fate of our colleagues in Austria. There are in that country many revered physicians and surgeons who are likely to fall into disfavour with the National Socialist Government either on account of their medical or social views or on account of their belonging to the Jewish race. Judging from what has happened in Germany in the past, we are afraid that serious discrimination will be exercised against them and that even the chance to leave a country which is no longer hospitable to them may be refused.

We beg our colleagues in all countries to watch the progress of events with the closest attention and to do all in their power, whether by public protest or by public or private assistance, to stand by any member of our profession who may suffer hardship under the new régime.

We are, Sir, yours faithfully,

(Signed) W. RUSSELL BRAIN,   HORDER,
     W. McADAM ECCLES,   ALAN MONCRIEFF,
     ARTHUR ELLIS,   J. P. MONKHOUSE,
     RICHARD W. B. ELLIS,   E. P. POULTON,
     DAVID FORSYTH,   H. E. ROAF,
     R. D. GILLESPIE,   JOHN A. RYLE,
     DONALD HUNTER,   ADRIAN STEPHEN,
     ARTHUR HURST,   C. P. WILSON,
     ROBERT HUTCHISON,   W. H. WYNN.

March 21st.

THROMBOSIS AND HEPARIN

To the Editor of THE LANCET

SIR,—I was most interested to read the two articles in your issue of March 19th on the treatment of thrombosis by heparin. Drs. Holmin and Ploman in reviewing a case of thrombosis of the central retinal vein state :

"It is hardly necessary to discuss the diagnosis, thrombus in the main trunk of the central vein of the retina. The sudden decrease in vision indicates a circulatory disturbance and the ophthalmoscopic finding is characteristic."

Surely it is just this question of diagnosis which requires the fullest discussion. If actual thrombosis of the central retinal vein had occurred it is difficult to believe that any amount of heparin would have been capable of restoring circulation in the manner which they describe. Repeated observation compels the conclusion that in those cases where vision returns either spontaneously or as a result of treatment no actual thrombosis can have occurred, and that the observable circulatory disturbance in its early stages, and in probably the majority of cases, must rather be attributed to obliteration of the lumen of the vessel either by local vaso-spasm or by œdema of surround-ing tissues. The same argument must be true of so-called thrombosis in other vessels, as for example the cerebral or coronary arteries. In the presence of arterial disease subsequent thrombosis may occur extremely quickly, but it is often astonishing how long it may be delayed.

I well remember being called to see a lady of 72 with a very high blood pressure who for five days had been deeply unconscious with a left hemiplegia. I read the death sentence to a large gathering of relatives before administering my routine treatment of intensive amyl nitrite. Much to my astonishment and confusion the patient became semi-conscious in 10 minutes, was talking in half an hour, and was as well as ever in three days.

While subscribing to the value of heparin in the treatment of these conditions I submit that its principal value lies rather in the prevention of clot formation in a stagnant circulation and only to a very much less extent in the inhibition of increment to a clot which has already formed (as in Dr. Magnusson's case). In other words I regard it as an auxiliary to, but by no means a substitute for, existing lines of treatment which must still be directed at the urgent relief of the underlying vaso-spasm. That the latter measures by themselves were adequate, provided that the patient was seen in good time, is evident from my own small group of cases of "thrombosis" of the central retinal vein. Far from being " unique to witness the disappearance of hæmorrhages and the increase of vision to its normal value in so short a time as five to six weeks " I am led to believe that such a result should be anticipated with reasonable confidence in patients who report as early as the hospital nurse under review.

Finally I cannot refrain from hazarding the guess that the underlying vasomotor instability of both subjects is of climacteric origin. The nasal catarrh and unilateral grinding headache in the nurse aged 52 and the recent onset of mild diabetes in the neurological case aged 48 would strengthen this assumption. If this be so then further vascular crises can be predicted with reasonable certainty unless this tendency can be adequately controlled by the correct employment of œstrogenic substances.

I am, Sir, yours faithfully,

Manchester, March 21st.   H. R. DONALD.

PURPURA FOLLOWING SEDORMID

To the Editor of THE LANCET

SIR,—I have seen, within the last few weeks, two cases of severe thrombocytopenic purpura following the use of Sedormid for insomnia. Both patients were middle aged ; both had been taking sedormid each night unknown to their medical attendants, one for three months, the other for three weeks ; both showed a profuse purpuric rash which involved the skin as well as the mucous membrane of the mouth ; and both had severe bleeding from the kidneys. Both recovered quickly when the sedormid was withheld ; no other treatment was used except a high calcium diet. Only in the first case were blood counts taken ; these showed a progressive anæmia to 50 per cent. of normal and a drop in the platelet count to 80 per c.mm. Loewy described three such cases in your columns (*Lancet*, 1934, **1**, 845) ; but, as far as I can find, this is the only English reference to this condition, though Lieberherr (*Med. Klin.* 1937, **33**, 475) gives seven references to this allergo-toxic reaction. As sedormid, allyl-isopropyl-acetyl-carbamide, is usually considered to be non-toxic I think it is, perhaps, worth while reminding your readers that its use is not unattended by the danger of severe purpura developing in those who are susceptible to its action.   I am, Sir, yours faithfully,

Wimpole-street, W., March 19th.   JAMES TORRENS.

FAMILY ALLOWANCES

THE enormous strain placed on the resources of a family of small means by three or more children was the theme of an address given last week by Sir ROBERT KINDERSLEY, president of the National Savings Committee. With wages based on the type of employment and the grade of the worker within his occupation, every additional child means a lowering of the standard of living, in a material sense, for the family as compared with others similarly earning. Consequently the children in such households suffer most from poverty and malnutrition ; they pay the penalty of their parents' procreativity. The time is past when procreation at any level of society can be condemned as improvidence, unless we are content to see the race move at an accelerated pace to extinction. Sir ROBERT commended the example of a firm in St. Helens, Lancs, which pays allowances for children in addition to the ordinary wage. In a pamphlet [1] published by the Family Endowment Society, Miss GREEN gives a concise account of the general measures of this kind already adopted in France, Belgium, and Italy, in New South Wales and New Zealand, and also of a few occupational schemes in England. She mentions, further, that family allowances are paid in some occupations in Germany, Holland, Luxembourg, Poland, Switzerland, Hungary, Czechoslovakia, and Jugoslavia. It appears that none of the workers' organisations in countries which have experience of the scheme believes that the total income going to their members has been reduced. At any one time only a small percentage (actually about 5) of the workers in this country have dependent children, and it is suggested that an allowance for each of them would not be an impossible burden for either industry or the State. Miss GREEN'S argument is that the future adults are the human capital of industry, and industry or the State should husband it not only by social services but also by a redistribution of wages as family allowances in proportion to the number of persons they have to maintain.

The proposal seems more practicable, and more in conformity with the modern attempt to correlate income with needs, than the idea underlying Mr. J. KUCZYNSKI's calculations [2] that every man over 21 years of age should have an income big enough to support a wife and three children whether he has them or not. Clearly, however, the estimate of needs would have to be less exiguous, in times of peace, than that provisionally made by Mr. SEEBOHM ROWNTREE last year [3] in support of his argument not for family allowances but for a minimum wage. The lack of any agreement on what is meant by a standard of living and on the means of measuring it is discussed in a recent report from the International Labour Office.[4] The report points out that while subjective satisfactions have an important bearing on the adequacy of living conditions, they are not readily measurable. Comparisons have, therefore, to be confined to items of an objective character—viz., (1) the level of consumption, or the composite of goods and services of a specific quantity and quality consumed by an individual family or group within a given period ; (2) social services and free services, particularly those which relate to health, education, and recreation ; and (3) working conditions which affect not only the worker's health and earning capacity but also the size and regularity of his income. On such items a large amount of information exists, but it is heterogeneous and considerable gaps remain to be filled in all countries before an adequate picture can be drawn. At present there is danger in making comparisons as between different times or different national groups or different countries. As a practical scheme it seems logical for the purposes of social policy to establish " norms of consumption "—i.e., for nutrition, housing, clothing, &c.—on the basis of expert opinion, and apply them to the preparation of standard budgets, so setting up national minima at different levels—comfort, decency, and subsistence

ANNOTATIONS

LEGAL REPRESENTATION OF MEDICAL MEN AT INQUESTS

THERE is a class of inquest which is held because allegations of carelessness in treatment or error in diagnosis are, through misunderstandings on the part of the household or gossip on the part of the neighbours, made against the medical attendant of the deceased. The coroner is obliged to intervene and investigate. Occasionally substance is found in the complaints ; but far more often, after hearing the evidence and particularly the disinterested testimony of the pathologist's report, the members of the dead man's family express themselves as entirely satisfied that nobody was to blame. Thus the public is reassured, though at the cost of grave anxiety to the medical practitioner, whose professional reputation was placed in issue. When he received a summons to attend the court, he would be aware that he was likely to be cross-examined in unfamiliar and possibly unfriendly surroundings by somebody who is doing his best to find material for charges of negligence. It would not be surprising if, with this prospect in view, the practitioner sought in his helplessness to enlist the help of a legal representative at the inquest.

It is an old saying in the legal world that a man who is his own lawyer has a fool for a client. Experts nevertheless advise that, in the case of a medical man whose professional work is likely to be challenged in a coroner's court, he does better to stand upon his own feet than to lean for support upon a legal representative whose opportunities of advocacy will be severely restricted by the procedural traditions of an inquest. The report presented on Tuesday to the

---

[1] Family Allowances. By Marjorie E. Green. The Family Endowment Society, 72, Horseferry-road, London, S.W.1. 1938. 6d.

[2] Hunger and Work. By Jürgen Kuczynski. London: Lawrence and Wishart. 1938. Pp. 132. 3s. 6d.
[3] See Lancet, 1937, 1, 1411.
[4] The Worker's Standard of Living. Studies and Reports, Series B (Economic Conditions) No. 30. The International Labour Office, Geneva. London: P. S. King and Son. 1938. 2s.

information. This can be applied to any organism which, when grown in blood, alters it so that the colonies are recognisable in slide-cells. Most of the pyogenic cocci, hæmolytic *B. coli*, diphtheria bacilli and others can be tested in this way.

We suggest that when time does not press it would be good practice to test the sensitivity of the infecting organism to M. & B. 693 or sulphanilamide by the method we have described, either in normal human defibrinated blood or in the patient's own blood. If the organism is very sensitive the chemical could be administered with the expectation of a good result. If the organism is only moderately sensitive then it is likely that, to obtain a good result, serum or vaccine treatment would have to be combined with chemotherapy, while if the infecting organism is quite insensitive there would be little hope of benefit accruing from the administration of the drug, and the patient might be spared its possible toxic manifestations.

Summary

A method is described by which the sensitivity of a microbe to M. & B. 693 can be tested in vitro. By this method pneumococci have been found to vary enormously in their sensitivity to the drug and this variation is not associated with the *type* of pneumococcus but with the individual *strain*. Experiments in mice confirm the results obtained in vitro.

It is suggested that wherever possible such a test should be carried out and according to the result obtained forecasts can be made as to the result likely to be obtained with 693 treatment. If the infecting organism is very sensitive simple treatment with the drug will probably be effective ; if it is only moderately sensitive it is very likely that some increase in immunity will be necessary in addition to 693 treatment ; but if the organism is insensitive to 693 in concentrations which can be attained in the human body there is no justification for embarking on a course of 693 treatment, which cannot do good and may have serious toxic effects.

In the second part of the paper it is shown that a single dose of pneumococcus vaccine given to mice or rabbits profoundly affects the course of an experimental infection in these animals when treated with M. & B. 693, and a strong case is made out for the combined use of vaccines and M. & B. 693 in all cases of pneumonia in man.

In the concluding part experiments are cited which prove that pneumococci can, in an infected animal treated with 693, readily establish a tolerance or fastness to the drug. This makes it essential that the initial doses should be large, and also—as M. & B. 693 merely interferes with the growth of the bacteria and the body has to do the actual killing—it is essential that the immunity should be raised to as high a degree as possible by any means, active or passive, specific or non-specific, so that the destruction of the bacteria may be complete before they have established tolerance to the drug.

REFERENCES

Barach, A. L. (1931) *J. exp. Med.* **53**, 567.
Cokkinis, A. J., and McElligott, G. L. M. (1938) *Lancet*, **2**, 355.
De, S. P., and Basu, V. P. (1938) *Brit. med. J.* **2**, 564.
Fleming, A. (1938a) *Lancet*, **2**, 74.
— (1938b) *Ibid*, p. 564.
Loewenthal, H. (1939) *Ibid*, Jan. 28, p. 197.
de Smidt, F. P. G. (1938) *Brit. med. J.* **2**, 1140.
Whitby, L. E. H. (1938a) *Lancet*, **1**, 1210.
— (1938b) *Ibid*, **2**, 1095.
Willcox, W. H., and Morgan, W. P. (1909) *Ibid*, **2**, 471.
Wynn, W. H. (1936) *Brit. med. J.* **1**, 45.

A NEW TILTABLE BED :
ITS MEDICAL USES

BY F. C. EVE, M.D. Camb., F.R.C.P.

SENIOR CONSULTING PHYSICIAN TO THE ROYAL INFIRMARY, AND
SENIOR PHYSICIAN TO THE VICTORIA HOSPITAL FOR
CHILDREN, HULL

WE call ourselves clinicians—from the Greek κλίνη, a bed—but do we not forget that the bed is our chief clinical implement ? It has remained unaltered during the twenty-five centuries since Tutankhamen ; hence we are apt to take the all-important bed for granted and to leave it too much to the nurses. True, we now have the excellent cardiac beds which lift the knees and back ; but these are costly, complicated, and liable to rust, and wrongly assume a constant length of thigh. Moreover they do not provide the invaluable head-down tilt. Bed-blocks give the very ineffective tilt of 1 in 6 (10 degrees). Hence I have designed a cheap and simple tiltable bed, now manufactured to clinical requirements by Messrs. Siddall and Hilton, of Sowerby Bridge, Yorkshire. The figure shows how it can be tilted and clamped at any desired angle, head-up or feet-up. A check-cord is an additional, if redundant, precaution.

I found that such a bed was useless without an efficient and adaptable bed-donkey, which did not exist. This was contrived (see figure) from an inverted hammock of webbing, supported between two arched iron rods. In the foot-down tilt the patient reclines on the bed and sits on the donkey, which also supports his legs. If his thighs are short, two lateral straps are slackened and the whole hammock lowers to fit him. His heels touch neither bed nor donkey, thus avoiding heel-pain or bedsores. If his legs are extra long, a pillow under his buttocks makes him fit the donkey. The Fowler or cardiac posture is thus attained (see figure) with much of his weight transferred from his buttocks to his thighs. This avoids bedsores and the wearisome pains in the bent lower back. On an ordinary bed the Fowler position usually entails a bent spine and hence a bulging abdomen, conducive to flatus and stretched stitches. Moreover a helpless patient slips and needs that exhausting and repeated hoisting which is such a reproach to the clinician. This is prevented absolutely by two cords or straps that secure the donkey to the bed-frame. The hot bottle (coverless) is housed under the arch of the donkey, where it cannot touch the patient's skin, but the warmth rises. An arched rod takes off the weight of the bedclothes.

Foot-drop is prevented by a pillow or board (15 × 11 in.) tied to the arches of the donkey by four strings. In swollen legs or phlebitis the donkey is reversed to provide an effective slope, quickly emptying a " white leg." In the tropics this donkey would be much cooler for the legs than is the usual " Dutch wife " bolster. In the afternoon rest of tired ladies the donkey, on bed or couch, produces a restful relaxation of every muscle. This I confirmed by finding that the stimulus needed to produce a knee-jerk is, in anxious patients, a half or a third of that needed in the crossed-knee sitting posture. This perfect relaxation should help patients during psycho-analysis or for hypnosis.

SOME MEDICAL USES

The *feet-down tilt* secures without slipping the cardiac posture needed in bad hearts, asthma, and pneumonia. In a case of renal anasarca with ascites, under Dr. D. C. Muir, multiple punctures in the legs—with a mackintosh leading to a bucket at the bed-foot—yielded 10, 8, and 6 pints of fluid on the first, second, and third days respectively. The tilt also caused the ascites to empty. Sir Arthur Hurst tells me that he has never seen sepsis occur in these incisions; neither have I. For bed-weary patients, perhaps with backache or congested lungs, the mere change of tilt is useful; all the pressure-points and directions of pull and sag are altered. I have observed distended patients belching abundantly when shifted from the horizontal to the Fowler posture.

In the *head-down position* the tilting bed opens up new possibilities. In abscess of the lung, bronchiectasis, or difficult expectoration postural drainage is secured. After certain poison gases the excessive and suffocating bronchial secretion should drain mouthwards. In diphtheria with pharyngeal paralysis a head-down tilt may save life by draining away mucus. Bed-blocks are often inadequate.

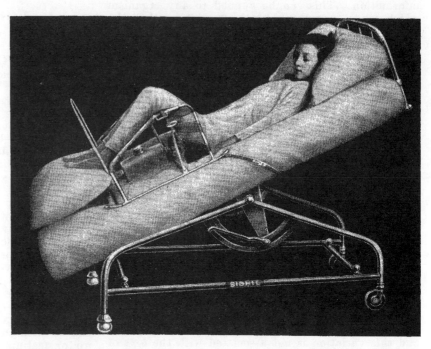

Composite photograph of Fowler position. Patient reclines on bed with straight spine and flat abdomen without fear of slipping. General muscular relaxation saves energy and encourages sleep which does not alter posture.

The "death rattle" is produced by thin mucus surging up and down the trachea, which the patient is powerless to expel. This need not be assumed to be fatal, for a head-down tilt soon stops the horrible noise, and complete recovery may follow—as I have seen in diphtheritic paralysis of the diaphragm and in severe meningitis. Deglutition pneumonia may be avoided by a steep head-down tilt (blocks being useless) because I have found that the patient can easily swallow uphill, but the fluid food cannot flow into the trachea uphill. A desperate meningitis case, needing 15 cisternal punctures in the first month, was saved by this uphill feeding (Eve 1937).

Artificial respiration can be performed with the tiltable bed by my rocking method (Killick and Eve 1933). The bed is merely rocked about 30 degrees up and down a dozen times a minute by relations or other volunteers. The weight of the abdominal contents pushes and pulls at the inert diaphragm, securing a pulmonary ventilation equal to or exceeding Schaefer's method. After a few days of this, recovery is quite likely to occur—in two days after my first diphtheritic diaphragm case (Eve 1932) and after eight days' rocking in Dr. Kerr's recent severe poliomyelitis case at Grimsby (Kerr 1939).

Thus a tilting bed can meet these tragic emergencies with the necessary promptitude, and the rare long cases can later be put into an "iron lung" if preferred. But this demands so much storage and such very expert nursing (Gauvain 1938) that I believe a rocking bed will prove the cheapest and simplest solution of this problem. The bed fits any patient and allows access to any nurse anywhere. Enterprising Grimsby has already authorised one driven by a small electric motor.

The rocking method of artificial respiration has been criticised as likely to produce sea-sickness. I have not seen it occur, and Mr. W. Riley tells me that in his extensive experience of the rocking stretcher with trainees and resuscitations at the Wakefield Central Rescue Station he has met with only one case —that of carbon-monoxide poisoning in a youth who recently had a heavy meal (treatment successful). I can only surmise that this curious immunity may be due to hyperventilation—similar to the 75 per cent. cure of sea-sickness by oxygen inhalation recently reported by Boothby (1938) of the Mayo Clinic. Hence, if sea-sickness did occur with rocking, the addition of oxygen by mask or nasal catheter should alleviate.

To sum up, the tiltable bed and donkey have been designed to convert gravity—that ancient enemy of the nurse and of her helpless patient in bed—into a friend. Clinicians can conduct their postural therapy in three dimensions rather than in two. A new field, which might be called gravitational nursing, needs developing.

I wish I could here thank individually all those doctors and nurses at the Hull Royal Infirmary and at our Isolation and Children's Hospitals who have helped so much—besides the manufacturers—to worry out these mechanical, medical, and nursing problems.

REFERENCES

Eve, F. C. (1932) *Lancet*, **2**, 995.
—— (1937) *Clin. J.* **66**, 426.
Gauvain, H. (1938) *Lancet*, **2**, 1327.
Kerr, J. A. (1939) *Ibid*, Jan. 7, p. 24.
Killick, E. M., and Eve, F. C. (1933) *Ibid*, **2**, 740.

THE Rockefeller Foundation have announced that during the next seven years they will grant a sum not exceeding £12,000 to the Imperial College of Science and Technology, South Kensington, for research on vitamins, sterols, and related compounds. The work will be carried out under the direction of the professor of organic chemistry, Prof. I. M. Heilbron, F.R.S.

CONTROL OF *STAPHYLOCOCCUS AUREUS* IN AN OPERATING-THEATRE

By E. A. DEVENISH, M.S. Lond., F.R.C.S.
FIRST ASSISTANT TO THE SURGICAL UNIT, UNIVERSITY
COLLEGE HOSPITAL, LONDON ; AND

A. A. MILES, F.R.C.P.
PROFESSOR OF BACTERIOLOGY, UNIVERSITY COLLEGE
HOSPITAL MEDICAL SCHOOL

THE investigation described in this paper was prompted by the occurrence of suppuration in a large proportion of patients after " clean " operations by the surgical unit of University College Hospital. In most wounds the suppuration was obvious on the fourth to the fifth day after operation, though in some it appeared later. It was relatively superficial in some—e.g., in the rectus sheath in most of the laparotomies—though in one case staphylococcal peritonitis developed. The infection was usually deep in suppurating thyroidectomy and thoracoplasty wounds. With the exception of one *Streptococcus pyogenes* infection, suppuration was due to *Staphylococcus aureus*. We have recorded the results of the investigation because our conclusions differ from those of recent American investigators who indict the air as the main source of staphylococcal infection in operation wounds.

Sources of *Staph. aureus*

The routine sterilisation of instruments, ligatures, lotions, dressings, gowns, masks, and gloves was reviewed and found satisfactory. Broth cultures from ligatures, instruments, and instrument-rinsing saline were made at the end of a number of operations and found free of *aureus*. There remained for consideration the air of the theatre, the skin of the patient, and the skins and upper respiratory tracts of the theatre staff.

Methods of sampling and identification of cultures.—Direct plating on 5 per cent. horse-blood agar was employed whenever possible. Broth cultures were not more sensitive in revealing small numbers of organisms and gave no idea of the number of organisms originally present. The skin was sampled with a broth-moistened swab rubbed with a circular motion twenty times over an area 4 cm. in diameter. The swab was plated as soon as possible after taking. The nose was sampled with one swab through both nostrils.

All plates were incubated for a day at 37° C. and for two days at 18° C. in a north light to facilitate the production of pigment. All golden and white colonies consisting of typically arranged monomorphic cocci 1μ in diameter were tested in mannitol ; and all strains that fermented mannitol within three days were tested for the production of coagulase. We have called *Staph. aureus* only those organisms which produced coagulase. A few coagulase-positive white strains have been included in the *aureus* group. In effect, this is the practice of Cowan (1938a), who found that the correlation between the production of coagulase and that of hæmolysin was complete, and who grouped the hæmolysin-producing staphylococci, irrespective of the production of pigment, into one species, *Staph. pyogenes*. Since most of our coagulase-positive strains yielded golden colonies, we have for the present retained the more familiar label of *Staph. aureus*.

The production of coagulase is not a constant feature of those cocci that on all other counts should be classified as pathogenic *Staph. aureus*, but in most recent surveys of staphylococci (Cowan 1938a, Chapman et al. 1938) the proportion of coagulase-negative strains has been small. Moreover, since all those strains from the suppurating wounds that we tested were coagulase-positive, the disposition of coagulase-positive staphylococci in the operating-theatre seemed likely to reflect the disposition of all pathogenic *Staph. aureus* adequately enough for the solution of our problem.

AIR

Plates were exposed near the instrument table during operations ; twenty-five for an hour, forty-nine for half an hour, and thirteen for 35–120 minutes. Half-hour plates, being least crowded with colonies, are best for investigation. The plates were counted after incubation for a day at 37° C. and three days at 18° C.

A total of 4894 colonies, mostly of air saprophytes, grew on plates exposed for a total of 63·6 hours, an average of 77 per hour. Eleven plates showed *Staph. aureus* : 4 colonies twice, 2 colonies twice, and 1 colony seven times ; a total of 19 in 63·6 hours, or 0·3 *aureus* colonies per hour on a plate 12 sq. in. in area.

This is the best available estimate of the continuous risk of infection by *aureus* from the air, though it must vary with the state and staff of the theatre. The area of an operation exposure is also usually about 12 sq. in. and the direct settlement on it of one *aureus*-bearing particle every three hours is not an obvious danger.

But air-borne *aureus* settling on instruments, on swabs, and on the gloves and sleeves of the surgeon may also be carried into the wound. Meleney (1935) assumed that patient, surgeon, assistants, tables, and instruments constituted the area at risk, which he estimated at 4000 sq. in.—i.e., 333 times the plate area. On this basis $0·3 \times 333 = 100$ *aureus* menaced the wound in an hour.

But in fact only a few of the objects in this area are introduced into the wound. It is unlikely that the total area of wound and objects introduced into it will be more than say, that of a 24×18 in. instrument table—i.e., 432 sq. in., which is 36 times the plate area. On this basis $0·3 \times 36 = 11$ *aureus* menace the wound every hour.

PATIENT'S SKIN

Twenty-four to forty-eight hours before operation the skin was shaved, washed with ether soap and water, ether and alcohol, and finally a 1 in 1000 solution of flavine in spirit. The area was sterilised a second time with the flavine paint when the patient was on the table. Swabs were taken immediately before the second application of antiseptic, and *aureus* was found in 4 of 50 skin-plates (9, 2, 1, and 1 colony). Swabs taken after the second application were heavily charged with flavine and usually sterile. It may be assumed that the antiseptic preparation is reasonably effective in killing *aureus* on the superficial layers of the skin.

Staph. aureus may survive in crypts of the skin, to be released during operation by sweating or by section of a crypt during incision. The low incidence of *aureus* in the partly sterilised skin does not account satisfactorily for a high incidence of *aureus* suppuration.

NOSE AND SKIN OF THEATRE STAFF

At the time of maximal incidence of sepsis skin samples from the back of the right wrists and nasal swabs were taken from forty persons, including senior operating staff, theatre and ward nurses, dressers, and a few adult patients in the male ward. Eighteen of these were more or less pronounced nasal carriers, and two of these were skin-positive ; one nose-negative person was skin-positive.

With these tests an estimate was made of the incidence of staphylococci infesting various situations. The infestation was high in the nasal cavities, and the carrier-rate agrees with that found in larger surveys of *aureus* carriers (see McFarlan 1938) ; it was low on the skins tested and in the air. It was impossible to discover whether the particles in the air giving rise to *aureus* colonies contained more than one coccus. But the slow development of, and the uniform size attained by, the *aureus* colonies, compared with the growth-rates of colonies from experimentally seeded single cocci, exclude the possibility that

initially there were very large numbers of cocci in each colony-producing particle. We have already assumed that the *Staph. aureus* air menace was, on the average, eleven particles an hour. Even if each consisted of twenty cocci, they would be unlikely to settle in one part of the wound, and the odds against an inoculum of twenty cocci getting a foothold in relatively healthy tissue must be high. The rarity with which very small doses of known pathogens can be made to infect susceptible animals, even after passage, makes it unlikely on a priori grounds that *aureus* infection would occur readily in such circumstances. We have, however, no direct evidence on the point. Aside from these speculations we have evidence that the air was not responsible ; for, whereas its average *aureus*-content remained constant, the suppuration disappeared, although no attempt was made to prevent the access of air bacteria to the operation wounds. In any event the constancy of infection at the outset of this investigation suggested a source of *aureus* more constant than the air proved to be. On the other hand, the danger from a pronounced nasal or skin carrier in the operating staff should be minimised by the use of masks, gloves, and gowns. The implication of any one source, in the absence of more extensive data, would have been a matter of conjecture had not the incidence of infection proved to be closely associated with one surgeon. Most of the operations were performed by surgeon A or surgeon B, and in table I the association of sepsis with A is clearly seen (see also fig. 1A). Of 54 " clean " operations performed by A in a five months' period, 14 were infected by *Staph. aureus*, and only 1 of 41 operations by B in the same period.

Table V shows that, during the year under consideration, the operations performed by A and B were comparable ; hence the suppuration in A's case was not due to a difference in the operative material of the two surgeons. Both A and B used the same staff and theatre, and often both operated in the same session. The infection apparently depended on the intimate contact of operator with patient, for at many of the operations B assisted A and A assisted B. The difference in the incidence of infection in A's and B's cases is such that the odds against it arising by chance are over 200 to 1. The cause of the infection was therefore to

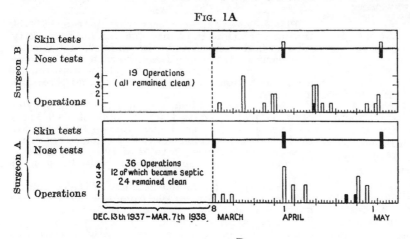

FIG. 1A

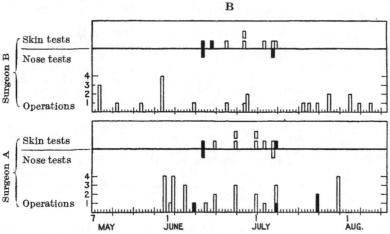

B

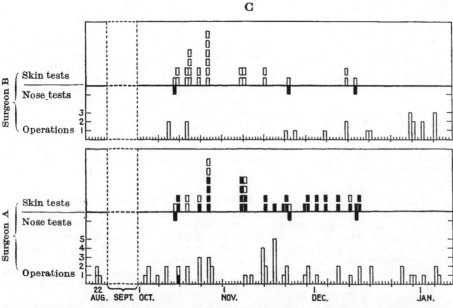

C

FIG. 1—Chart of operations and nose and skin tests for the presence of *Staphylococcus aureus*. White columns indicate (1) negative results of tests, and (2) operations not followed by suppuration. Black columns indicate (1) positive results of tests, and (2) operations followed by suppuration due to *Staph. aureus*. A, Preliminary period under ordinary conditions ; B, period during which operators wore battiste oversleeves and cellophane in masks ; C, period in which additional manipulative care was taken.

1090 THE LANCET]   MR. DEVENISH & PROF. MILES : *STAPH. AUREUS* AND THE OPERATING-THEATRE   [MAY 13, 1939

be looked for in some essential difference between A and B ; it was unlikely that *aureus* in the air, on instruments, or on the skin of the patient was responsible.

Both A and B were persistent nasal carriers of *Staph. aureus*, and platings of their nasal swabs

TABLE I—INCIDENCE OF *Staph. aureus* SUPPURATION IN CLEAN CASES (DECEMBER, 1937, TO MAY, 1938)

Surgeon	*Aureus* cases	Non-infected cases	Totals	Sepsis (per cent.)
A ..	14	40	54	25·9
B ..	1	40	41	2·4
Totals ..	15	80	95	15·3

$n = 1$, $\chi^2 = 8·00$, and $P = 0·0047$ (see Hill 1937).

showed several hundred *aureus* colonies. B's nose was the more infested of the two, the swabs often yielding an apparently pure culture. The results of swabbing A and B and the incidence of *aureus* infections in their patients are shown in fig. 1, which records the *aureus* history of the two surgeons from Dec. 13, 1937, to Jan. 11, 1939, omitting the month of September, 1938.

Staph. aureus might fall from the nose or mouth on to the wound in heavy droplets spat through the mask or pass from the skin through holes in rubber gloves or through the sleeves of an operating-gown. These possibilities were investigated as follows.

Masks specially designed to prevent the discharge of infected droplets are usually tested by placing culture plates in the line of possible discharge and instructing the wearer to cough (for references to recent work on mask tests see Arnold 1938). We adopted a more stringent test of permeability. After use the mask was laid nasal side upwards over a blood-agar plate and its outer surface lightly and evenly pressed on to the agar by a sterile 3½ in. rubber bung. By this means all the *aureus* capable of being brushed off the outside of the mask were sampled, and any mask that was *aureus*-free on its outer surface after operation might be safely assumed to be impermeable to the coccus. Nineteen tests were made on 4 carriers wearing masks without efficient cellophane. On the average the masks were worn for 100 min. *Staph. aureus* was found on six occasions ; the colonies totalled 126. Of sixteen tests on 2 carriers with efficient cellophane in the masks, fifteen were negative. The masks were worn for 110 min. on the average, and in the single positive test only one *Staph. aureus* colony was found.

The ordinary theatre masks, made of two layers of butter muslin, let *aureus* through. A loose sheet of cellophane introduced between the folds of the muslin just before operation was ineffective, for it crumpled and slipped during the operation, and the mask was still permeable to *aureus*. A 6¾ by 8¾ in. sheet of cellophane (No. 600 P.T. Messrs. Pakcel Ltd.) was sewn into a 7 by 9 in. pocket made in the middle of the upper border of a mask of double-folded muslin, 36 by 15 in. and sterilised in situ. The resulting mask was impermeable to *aureus*.

In the sixteen tests of A and B in these masks only one *aureus* colony was found on the outside ; other colonies consisted of typical air saprophytes. Press-plates of the inside of these masks showed nasal and mouth flora, with *aureus* present in all those tested that had been worn by carriers.

The air discharged laterally from the edges of the mask might carry very fine droplets containing *aureus*. Blatt and Dale (1933) find this lateral discharge to be " practically sterile," but even if *aureus* escaped from the carriers in this way it would contribute merely to the already determined air-infesta-

tion, for droplets small enough to be carried out on this lateral discharge would have insufficient weight to fall directly on to the wound.

In the small number of mask tests there was no obvious difference between A and B.

Gown sleeves.—The gowns were of coarse linen, 48 meshes to the inch. The irregularity of the threads and the large size of the holes in this cloth are illustrated in the photomicrograph (fig. 2).

Press-plates of the outside of gown sleeves alone and of stockinette oversleeves worn over gown sleeves showed *aureus* at the end of the operation, but the introduction of battiste (British Pharmaceutical Codex 1934, p. 1136) oversleeves to cover the gown sleeves reduced the incidence of *aureus* on press-plates to one colony in forty-one tests on A and B.

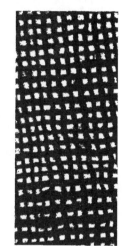

FIG. 2—Photomicrograph of linen sleeve of operating-gown. (× 5.)

The difference between A and B (table II) is obvious. There was a similar difference in the skin swabs of A and B, 6 of 8 skin swabs of A, but only 2 of 10 swabs of B, being positive in a period of seven months. Moreover, on five occasions scalpel-scrapings of B's skin were *aureus*-free.

These results suggest that the relevant difference between A and B was that, though both were nasal carriers, the skin of A was the more constantly infested with *aureus*, and that *aureus* was sweated through the gown sleeve of A during operation. This belief was strengthened by the results of testing the hands of A and B.

Operating-gloves.—*Staph. aureus* that survived scrubbing-up and disinfection of the surgeon's hands could get into a wound only through a puncture in the glove. Glove puncture is a relatively common accident. The leaks are more certainly discovered if an under-water test is made. In table III the puncture-rate in 6965 gloves is recorded.

The first series contains those worn in the main hospital theatres over a period of four months and includes both patched and unpatched gloves, 6585

TABLE II—GROWTH ON PRESS-PLATES FROM THE OUTSIDE OF LINEN AND STOCKINETTE SLEEVES AND OF BATISTE ARMLETS

Surgeon	Sleeve material	Tests	Average time worn (min.)	*Staph. aureus* Times found	*Staph. aureus* Total colonies
B	Linen, &c.	16	64	2	2
	Battiste	13	62	0	0
A	Linen, &c.	31	71	8	50
	Battiste	28	60	1	1
5 others	—	11	45	0	0

in number ; in these the incidence of puncture was 24 per cent. The second and third series comprise tests on unpatched gloves worn by A and by B, chief assistants, and instrument nurse in sixty-nine operations ; 14·5 per cent. were punctured. In the last two series 48 of the 55 punctures were in the thumb, index, and middle fingers : 22 on the right hands, 26 on the left.

There is thus the opportunity for the leakage of *aureus* from the skin of the hand. It remains to be shown that (1) *aureus* was present on the hands of A but not of B, and (2) it could leak through punctures.

(1) The infestation of sterilised hands by *Staph. aureus* was tested by making 121 press-plates of the inside of A's and B's gloves immediately they were

TABLE III—INCIDENCE OF PUNCTURES IN OPERATING-GLOVES

Wearers	Gloves tested	Punctures and per cent.	Consecutive operations
Hospital staff in main theatres	6585	1593 (24·2)	—
Surgeon A	81	11 (13·6)	42
Surgeon B, chief assistants, and instrument nurses	299	44 (14·7)	69

peeled off at the end of an operation. The number of colonies developing depended more on the amount of sweat in the glove than on the length of time the glove had been worn. A glove that was dry after two hours' wear might yield 20 colonies, whereas a sweating glove worn for only 30 minutes might yield 500–1000. Moderately wet gloves often yielded colonies grouped in clusters, which were composed of only one or two types of colony. Clustering appeared in 60 per cent. of moderately crowded plates and gave the impression that each cluster had arisen from a circumscribed area on the skin, such as a pocket or crypt filled with one or two kinds of micro-organisms. Table IV records the tests on the right- and left-hand gloves of A and B after operations lasting 20–180 minutes. A's hands " excreted " *aureus* 30 times in 42 tests, the number of colonies varying from 5 to 5000. The total number of colonies was about 1·5 to 5 times the number of *aureus* colonies, the commonest non-*aureus* organism being a non-mannitol-fermenting coagulase-negative strain of *Staph. albus*. B excreted far fewer colonies, counts of more than 100 being rare ; and *Staph. aureus* was never found. His common organisms were *Staph. albus*, pleomorphic gram-positive cocci, and diphtheroids, in that order of frequency. As

TABLE IV—GROWTH ON PRESS-PLATES FROM THE INSIDE OF GLOVES AFTER OPERATION

Surgeon	Tests	Aver. time worn (min.)	Distribution of plates according to approximate number of colonies thereon						Times *Staph. aureus* found
			Colonies ..	0	1–50	51–500	501–5000	5001 +	
A	42	80	*Aureus* cols.	12	4	16	7	3	30
			All cols. ..	1	7	15	16	3	—
B	29	77	*Aureus* cols.	29	0	0	0	0	0
			All cols. ..	4	20	5	0	0	—

soon as the danger from A was realised, additional care was taken to avoid glove-puncture during operation : fingers were introduced into wounds as little as possible and instruments used for manipulation wherever possible (fig. 1c). The capacity of *aureus* for leaking through holes in the gloves was estimated by experimental puncture.

(2) During a period when the infestation of A's hands by *Staph. aureus* was pronounced experimental punctures were tested as follows. At the finish of an operation the gloves were washed before removal, rinsed with alcohol, and dried on a sterile towel.

The finger-tips and knuckles were lightly pressed on to a blood-agar plate as a control culture and then punctured and pressed on to a second plate. After puncture press-plates were made of the inside of the glove, as described above. Twelve tests were made. Test 1 is illustrated in fig. 3. Large holes were made by a needle, and several hundred *aureus* came through. Smaller needle pricks were ineffective in two tests. In surgical practice a very small hole might be temporarily enlarged when the rubber immediately surrounding it is stretched during operative manipulation. Accordingly, in four tests a sterile 2 in. glass disk was manipulated after the puncture in such a way as to stretch the rubber at the finger-tips, and its surface was rubbed over blood agar ; in two tests *aureus* leaked through. In five further tests the puncture was made with a No. 25 × 1 in. hypodermic needle, and 0·2 c.cm. of sterile saline was introduced. The fingers were lightly massaged together and then stroked on to a plate. *Aureus* leaked through in all five tests. In all, leakage occurred in eight of twelve tests.

The leakage of *aureus* apparently depends on a sufficiency of organisms and fluid— i.e., sweat in the natural condition —inside the glove

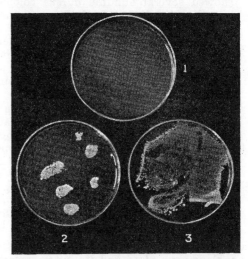

FIG. 3—Photographs of press-plates. (1) Culture from outside of glove before pricking ; (2) culture from outside of glove after pricking ; (3) culture from inside of glove. About half the colonies are of *Staph. aureus*.

and on the coincidence of the puncture with an *aureus*-producing area of the hand. With excessive sweating the *aureus* is disseminated throughout the space between rubber and skin, and any prick may be the site of an *aureus* leak. The average number of cocci escaping through leaks in A's gloves was very much greater than that likely to fall on to one spot in a wound from the air, or to be introduced on air-infected instruments, or on sleeves through which *aureus* has been sweated. Both the *aureus* infestation and the opportunity for implantation in the wound were greater in the hand than in all other sources tested. In the light of the available evidence it is the *Staph. aureus* on A's hands that must be considered to be the chief source of the suppuration.

Effect of Precautionary Measures

Except emergency operations and those in which there was a possibility of wound infection from conditions found at operation, all " clean " operations performed by the staff of the surgical unit from Dec. 13, 1937, to Jan. 11, 1939 (September, 1938, excluded), have been watched, and the subsequent progress of the wound followed, by one observer. Of 262 operations performed by four surgeons, 22 suppurated frankly and small pustules round the stitches developed in 7. Disregarding these 7 cases, since necrosis from excessive tension on the stitch probably contributed to the lesion, 8·4 per cent. of the cases suppurated. This figure is about the same as that reported by other observers for the general incidence of suppuration in clean operation wounds (Ives and Hirshfeld 1938, Meleney 1935). The record for each of the four surgeons is as follows:—

Surgeon A .. Total 141 .. Suppurated 20
  ,,   B .. ,,   84 ..   ,,   1
  ,,   C .. ,,   22 ..   ,,   0
  ,,   D .. ,,   14 ..   ,,   1

Fig. 1 and table V record the operations of A and B. It will be noted that 4 wounds in A's series suppurated after the introduction of cellophane masks and batiste sleeves (fig. 1B) and 1, a thyroidectomy wound made on Oct. 14, 1938, after the modification of the operative technique (fig. 1C) described in the text. After this operation the left index finger of the glove was found punctured, and a press-plate of the inside of the gloves yielded a heavy growth of *Staph. aureus*. Between Oct. 14, 1938, and Jan. 11, 1939, A performed 45* clean operations without suppuration, even though during this period *Staph. aureus* was repeatedly grown from the inside of his gloves and his gloves were occasionally punctured. This observation confirms the conclusion reached by the tests—namely, that the leakage of an infective dose of cocci from a skin carrier is determined by more than mere puncture of the glove.

Discussion

Staph. aureus was found in various parts of the operating-theatre and its staff. A precise definition of the infection risk from the different sources of *Staph. aureus* is impossible, for the discovery of a likely source was necessarily followed by immediate attempts to stop it. Nevertheless, the staphylococcal history of surgeons A and B in the operating-theatre strongly suggests that the main danger lay in the *aureus* infestation of A's skin. Wells and Wells (1936, 1938) have in the past few years emphasised the importance of the air as a vehicle of pathogenic bacteria, and Hart (1937) has advocated the sterilisation of the air in operating-theatres by ultraviolet light. Without minimising the importance of the Wells's observations or denying the efficacy of Hart's methods of sterilisation it is questionable whether postoperative *Staph. aureus* suppuration is necessarily due to air-borne cocci. Our experience is limited to one surgical unit, but the striking decline of the sepsis-rate, in the face of a continued *aureus* menace in the theatre, suggests that in other cases the improvement due to a greater nicety of operative technique may have been wrongly attributed to the elimination of air-borne pathogens. Indeed Hart, in his latest report (1938b), attributes his avoidance of sepsis to "meticulous operating room asepsis, development of a delicate atraumatic technique, and the use of the least irritating suture material" besides "the elimination of air-borne contamination." It is obvious that surveys of a number of operating units should be made (cf. Hart 1938a) to decide on the incidence and importance of air-borne *aureus*. For this purpose it is important to fix a standard method of measuring the number of air organisms present and criteria for the recognition of pathogenic strains. The air centrifuge of Wells and Wells is at present

too expensive for general adoption as a means of sampling the air.

We suggest that the best readily available measure of the infestation-rate by *aureus* is the average number of colony-forming particles falling into a 4 in. petri dish per hour, calculated from colony counts of blood-agar plates exposed for 30 min. each. A limited number of experiments we have made indicates that four such plates grouped round the patient, at operation-table level, provides a representative sample of the air organisms. The proportion of plates contaminated with a given pathogen has been used as a measure of infestation of the air, but this figure gives a false impression of the risk. For example, from our data, 17 per cent. of 63 one-hour plates would have shown *Staph. aureus* in the 63 hours tested, a misleadingly impressive figure compared with an average rate of 0·3 *aureus* per hour. The definition of potentially pathogenic *Staph. aureus* must, in the present state of classification of the staphylococci, be more or less arbitrary. A study of over 800 plates seeded with material from air, dust, skins, and nasal cavities has convinced us that neither *Staph. aureus* nor *Staph. albus* can be safely identified by the appearance of the colony and the stained smear (criteria apparently adopted by many observers). The most useful single criterion is provided by the coagulase test. This may be combined, if desired, with the test for production of α-hæmolysin (McFarlan 1938), and all golden, yellow-gold, and white colonies, made up of mono-morphic cocci that ferment mannitol, should be so tested. There is the same need for agreement about the criteria for recognising other air-borne pathogens. It is obvious from recent work that hæmolytic strepto-cocci cannot be regarded as potentially pathogenic unless they belong to the A, B, C, or G groups of Lancefield and Hare (Topley and Wilson 1936). If a relatively high degree of *aureus* infestation were demonstrated in the air of any theatre, a high risk of wound infection would not necessarily be implied. A properly controlled test of the infectivity of small doses of *aureus* in human tissue is impossible. We must rely on circumstantial evidence, and from the result of our own experience we suggest that, before the air is indicted as a source of danger, the sources we have demonstrated in our own theatre should be tested and stopped.

The evidence pointing to the skin infestation of surgeon A, as the feature distinguishing him from the non-infective surgeon B, not only rules out air-borne cocci and those on the patient's skin but also those in the noses of both A and B as causes of the suppuration. But in other circumstances the patient's own cocci and the surgeon's nasal cocci might well be dangerous, though risk of direct infection from the nose can be removed by the use of an efficient mask. The mask we devised is both efficient and comfortable. The skin carrier presents a greater problem. *Staph. aureus* can be sweated through a gown sleeve, and the conditions inside a surgical rubber glove promote the "excretion" of *Staph. aureus* from a previously well sterilised skin.

Apart from the solution of our immediate problem, the general applicability of our conclusions depends on the prevalence of *aureus* skin infestation among practitioners of surgery. Surgeon A is not an isolated example of *aureus* skin infestation. About the middle of 1938 surgeon D was nose- and skin-negative. Shortly before an attack of *Staph. aureus* boils he operated on one patient whose wound subsequently suppurated. After the attack he was found to be a nasal carrier and subsequently sweated *Staph.*

* From Jan. 11 to April 17, 1939, surgeon A performed 35 consecutive "clean" operations. His skin was still infected with *Staph. aureus*; no suppuration developed in any of the wounds.

aureus into his gloves at operation. The discovery of surgeon A's nose and skin infestation followed an attack of boils some months previously. It may be that heavy infestation of the skin is the result of recent manifest infection.

A's nasal and skin strains behaved identically in all the tests applied. They were coagulase-positive ; both produced α-hæmolysin and leucocidin to the same high titre in parallel tests ; and both were type IIIa by Cowan's (1939) slide agglutination-test. It is of interest that the nasal strains of A and D, who were skin carriers, produced high-titre leucocidin of the Panton-Valentine type. B was a heavily infected nasal carrier. He rarely had *aureus* on the skin, and his nasal strain was leucocidin-negative. It is tempting to relate the dependence of skin infestation in nasal carriers to the pathogenicity of the nasal strain, as indicated by the production of leucocidin (Valentine 1936) ; but B's carrier state followed an acute staphylococcal sinusitis complicated by orbital cellulitis and osteomyelitis of the frontal bone, and, if the carrier strain is the

TABLE V—CLASSIFIED OPERATIONS PERFORMED BY A AND B FROM DEC. 13, 1937, TO JAN. 11, 1939 (SEPTEMBER, 1938, EXCLUDED)

Type of operation	Surgeon A		Surgeon B	
	Healed	Sup-purated	Healed	Sup-purated
Herniotomy, inguinal and femoral	15	1	12	0
Herniotomy, scar	2	1	1	0
Excision of plantaris tendon	13	2	5	0
Partial thyroidectomy ..	9	4	8	1
Phrenic avulsion	2	0	3	0
Other operations on neck ..	1	3	4	0
Thoracoplasty	8	3	3	0
Extrapleural artificial pneumothorax	12	0	2	0
Other chest operations ..	5	0	0	0
Radical mastectomy ..	3	0	2	0
Other operations on breast..	3	0	3	0
Laminectomy	4	0	0	0
"Cold" appendicectomy ..	3	0	3	0
Laparotomy and intra-abdominal operations ..	15	6*	4	0
Operations on limbs and limb-joints	20	0	27	0
Other operations	6	0	7	0
Totals	121	20	84	1

* In one case of these six the infection was due to *Strep. pyogenes* ; the remainder listed in the table were *Staph. aureus* infections.

same as the original infecting strain, its lack of leucocidin here at any rate does not indicate lack of pathogenicity. The relationship between nasal and skin infestation, and between recent skin infection and the skin carrier state, cannot be discussed profitably on such scanty data ; these problems are being investigated. The evidence so far obtained indicates that there is an appreciable skin carrier-rate in the hospital community, though it does not approach the rate of 30–40 per cent. found in the nasal cavities.

Turning to the surgical aspect of the problem, it will be seen from table V that thyroidectomy, thoracoplasty, and laparotomy wounds suppurated most

often. It is perhaps significant that in these operations the amount of stitching necessary, and therefore the risk of glove puncture, is relatively great, though of course stitching is not the only procedure during which gloves may be damaged. The possibility of infecting a wound by a leak of bacteria through a glove puncture has long been recognised. When in 1895 Lane (1909) introduced his method of plating simple fractures he was well aware of this danger and in the description of his technique emphasised that the fingers should never be introduced into the wound and that "the instruments should be long . . . in order to avoid any contact with the wound by the portion of the instrument grasped by the hand since . . . the gloves are liable to be damaged." This accident is more frequent than is generally supposed ; thus 24 per cent. of the gloves used in the theatres of the main hospital were punctured. It may be objected that this figure includes gloves worn by students and nurses, and that the surgeon would be less likely to puncture his glove ; yet of the surgeon's gloves alone 14 per cent. were punctured at a time when special care was being taken to avoid damage. In a few instances the puncture was discovered immediately it was made, but most of the holes were found on testing the gloves at the end of the operation, by which time there had been maximum opportunity for leakage. Leakage is a danger only in skin carriers of pathogenic organisms like *aureus*. Our results show that the carrier state may be more certainly demonstrated if press-plate cultures of the inside of rubber gloves into which the subject has sweated are substituted for the usual procedure of skin swabbing.

There remain for consideration a few other measures that have been advocated for the reduction of sepsis. If the air can be shown to be the source of infection (Cowan 1938b) its sterilisation by such agents as ultra-violet light (U.V.L.) or aerosols (Pulvertaft et al. 1939) is of obvious importance. It is possible that the success of Hart's U.V.L. is due less to air sterilisation than to the sterilisation of bacteria that have reached the wound from all sources, though the relatively poor penetrative powers of U.V.L. make it unlikely that heavy inocula will be destroyed. Hart (1938b) records that in one of the thoracoplasty wounds which suppurated badly in spite of U.V.L. irradiation, it was known that the wound was contaminated with sweat escaping from a torn glove. Meleney (1935) stated that the substitution of silk for catgut as ligature material reduced the incidence of wound infection. We have no evidence that the ligature material has any influence on the incidence of wound infection, which depends on the introduction into the wound of an infective dose of bacteria. In the light of our experience we would attribute the success of Meleney's technique to the greater nicety of operative procedure that he found necessary with silk. Hart (1938a) has suggested that so far as possible nasal carriers of *Staph. aureus* should be excluded from the theatre. The risk from this source is not necessarily great, and in view of the high *Staph. aureus* carrier-rates recorded in hospital communities such exclusion may be impracticable. For example, in one week during the period recorded we should on this account have excluded the two senior surgeons, one house-surgeon, one theatre sister, two nurses, and one dresser out of a staff of fourteen.

The removal of *Staph. aureus* from the skin of a carrier presents a problem yet to be solved. A course of U.V.L. had no effect on the coccal infestation of Surgeon A's skin. There remains the possibility of applying antiseptics, such as Dettol cream, to the hands before operation, as recommended by Colebrook and Maxted (1933); but in view of the marked infestation of A's hands with *Staph. aureus* we were unwilling to risk any damage to the skin tissues that might have an infective sequel. The problem was less urgent than it might have been, for other prophylactic methods were completely successful. However, so long as the skins of A and D remain infested, we cannot expect a continued freedom from wound suppuration. The problem of carrier cure is still under investigation.

Summary

(1) A high incidence of suppuration due to *Staph. aureus* in "clean" operation wounds was found to be due to the leakage of *Staph. aureus* through glove punctures from the skin of one surgeon who proved to be a skin carrier.

(2) The *Staph. aureus* present in the air of the theatre and on the skin of the patients operated upon apparently played no part in the incidence of suppuration.

(3) Nasal carriers of *Staph. aureus* among the theatre staff do not constitute a danger, provided that masks are made impermeable to direct droplet discharge from the nose and mouth.

(4) All the strains of *Staph. aureus* recorded fermented mannitol and produced a coagulase for human plasma.

(5) Skin carriers, negative by the ordinary swabbing tests, may sometimes be detected by cultivating the sweat from the inside of rubber gloves at the end of operation. This method has the advantage of excluding positive results due to temporary superficial contamination of the skin.

(6) The frequency of glove puncture during operation was found to be as high as 24 per cent.; this was reduced to 14 per cent. by precautions to avoid puncture.

(7) The following measures were followed by disappearance of the sepsis: (*a*) the introduction of cellophane sheets into butter-muslin masks; (*b*) the wearing of batiste (B.P.C.) sleeves over linen gowns to prevent the escape of skin cocci in sweat; (*c*) the avoidance of glove puncture during operation by special attention to operative technique; and (*d*) the avoidance, so far as possible of direct handling of the tissues.

We are indebted to Dr. S. T. Cowan and Dr. F. C. O. Valentine for serological and leucocidin-production tests on some of our *aureus* strains; and to Dr. O. Khairat for fig. 3.

REFERENCES

Arnold, L. (1938) *Arch. Surg.*, Chicago, **37**, 1008.
Blatt, M. L., and Dale, M. L. (1933) *Surg. Gynec. Obstet.* **57**, 363.
Chapman, G. H., Berens, C., Nilson, E. L., and Curcio, L. G. (1938) *J. Bact.* **35**, 311.
Colebrook, L., and Maxted, W. R. (1933) *J. Obstet. Gynæc.* **40**, 966.
Cowan, S. T. (1938a) *J. Path. Bact.* **46**, 31.
— (1938b) *Lancet*, **2**, 1052.
— (1939) *J. Path. Bact.* **48**, 169.
Hart, D. (1937) *Arch. Surg.*, Chicago, **34**, 874.
— (1938a) *Ibid*, **37**, 521.
— (1938b) *Ibid*, p. 956.
Hill, A. B. (1937) *Principles of Medical Statistics*, London, p. 93.
Ives, H. R., jun., and Hirshfeld, J. W. (1938) *Ann. Surg.* **107**, 607.
Lane, W. A. (1909) *Ibid*, **50**, 1106.
McFarlan, A. M. (1938) *Brit. med. J.* **2**, 939.
Meleney, F. L. (1935) *Surg. Gynec. Obstet.* **60**, 264.
Pulvertaft, R. J. V., Lemon, G. C., and Walker, J. W. (1939) *Lancet*, Feb. 25, p. 443.
Topley, W. W. C., and Wilson, G. S. (1936) *The Principles of Bacteriology and Immunity*, London.
Valentine, F. C. O. (1936) *Lancet*, **1**, 526.
Wells, W. F., and Wells, M. W. (1936) *J. Amer. med. Ass.* **107**, 1698.
— — (1938) *Amer. J. publ. Hlth* **28**, 343.

ABDOMINAL RESECTION FOR RECTAL CANCER *

BY E. G. MUIR, M.S. Lond., F.R.C.S.
ASSISTANT SURGEON TO KING'S COLLEGE HOSPITAL, LONDON
SURGEON TO THE BOLINGBROKE HOSPITAL

THE operation of abdominal resection for a high rectal growth has had more advocates on the Continent than in this country. Sometimes known as Hartmann's operation (Hartmann 1923), or anterior resection, it has been ignored by many of our text-books, though descriptions of it have been given at various times by Rankin (1929), Gordon-Taylor (1929–30), and Gabriel (1937). This operation has certain advantages and my object is to suggest that it should be adopted more often in the treatment of rectal cancer.

It is common practice to speak of cancer of the terminal sigmoid as a pelvi-rectal growth, and it is not possible to make a sharp distinction between some high growths of the rectum and those of the terminal sigmoid. In order to avoid confusion the term rectal cancer is used here to mean that the actual surface of the growth can be touched with the finger on rectal examination. I propose to limit my remarks to such cases, though it is obvious that a growth half an inch higher may require the same treatment.

No operation for cancer can be regarded as efficient if it does not aim at removing not only the growth but also the potentially involved lymphatics and glands. Of late years increasing attention has been paid to the lymphatic drainage of the rectum and its involvement by growth. It will be germane to consider some of the findings.

According to Miles the lymphatic drainage of the rectum takes place mainly in an upward direction along the superior hæmorrhoidal artery, but also laterally along the levatores ani muscles and downwards in the region of the ischio-rectal fossæ. In 1925, as the result of injections of the rectal lymphatics, Villemin, Huard and Montagné suggested that the rectum should be regarded as two parts, each having a different lymphatic drainage. The lower part, the ampullary portion and the ano-rectal region, drains upwards but also laterally and downwards, while the upper, that part of the rectum above the lowest valve of Houston, drains only in an upward direction along the superior hæmorrhoidal artery. From the dissection of specimens removed by perineo-abdominal resection, Gabriel, Dukes and Bussey (1935) considered that the spread of rectal cancer took place first into the regional lymph-nodes in the close vicinity of the growth and then in an upward direction along the superior hæmorrhoidal artery, lateral and downward spread only taking place when the lymphatics above were blocked by growth.

Recently the same view has been taken by Gilchrist and David (1938). Out of 47 specimens removed by abdomino-perineal resection they found 2 in which, as the result of metastases above the growth, a retrograde spread to lymphatic glands below the growth had occurred. They found evidence, however, to suggest that a lateral spread in the region of the levator ani muscle was more frequent when the growth was at that level. Present belief seems to be that the main lymphatic spread of any rectal growth

* Communicated to the Royal Society of Medicine, section of proctology, on May 10.

so distinct that we hoped to demonstrate such a difference by relatively crude methods of inquiry ; but, beyond showing a 50 per cent. higher habitual consumption of " fresh " milk (practically all the milk used by both these groups was pasteurised) in the caries-free group, our results by such methods were inconclusive. Indeed it appears practically impossible to obtain by any method short of direct observation even a moderately accurate qualitative and quantitative dietary history in a human being beyond the age of infancy.

In view of the often repeated assertion of a relationship between irregular dentition and caries, the mouths were charted and the following results obtained :—

	A	D
Regular dentition	9 ..	9
Very irregular dentition	4 ..	6
Others (not perfectly regular)	12 ..	10

Similarly unconvincing were the findings with regard to oral hygiene : 16 of the 25 children with perfect teeth had never used a toothbrush regularly, and 12 not at all.

Perhaps the most interesting findings are yielded by inquiry into the histories of past history of common illnesses :—

	A	D*			A	D*
Measles	22 ..	25		" Pneumonia " ..	2 ..	7
Measles complicated				Diphtheria	1 ..	0
by bronchopneu-				Scarlet fever ..	2 ..	1
monia	0 ..	3		Chronic cough ..	3 ..	8
Pertussis	8 ..	13		Rickets	0 ..	7

The average age-incidence of measles was 4·5 years and of pertussis 5·5 years in group A, and 3·2 and 3·4 years respectively in group D*, and cases of measles in children under 4 years numbered 8 in group A and 14 in group D*. The incidence of other past illnesses in the two groups is also very illuminating :—

	A	D*		D*
Acute appendicitis ..	1..		" Anæmia "	4
" Tonsils and adenoids "	1..	4	Chronic abscesses.. ..	1
Diabetic (12 months' his-			Meningitis..	1
tory, on 150 g. of carbo-			Bronchiectasis †	1
hydrate and insulin) ..	1..		Empyema..	1
Mastoid		2	Cœliac disease †	1
Tuberculous glands ..	..	1		

† Confirmed by hospital investigations.

These figures reveal a spectacular amount of past illnesses among the 25 D* " normal " children picked out from their 1842 fellows for examination solely on account of their dental condition. Although in some cases the onset of noticeable caries seemed to be directly traceable to some severe illness, no causal relationship can be defined on the basis of this data. Nevertheless, reviewing the whole series of cases and the ages at which the illnesses occurred, it is difficult not to conclude that this high incidence of illness was probably a causal factor in the development of caries. Even the maternal health during pregnancy is shown to be different in the two groups :—

	A	D*
Toxæmia of pregnancy	1 ..	5
" Unwell " during pregnancy, ranging from " anæmia " and " malnutrition " to " tuberculosis "	0 ..	6

SUMMARY

Examination of two groups of 25 children between the ages of ten and fourteen, one group with complete freedom from dental caries and the other group suffering from gross caries, demonstrates certain factors which were apparently associated with freedom from dental caries : (1) good family dental history (not apparently of such significance as good general hygiene and diet) ; (2) careful infant feeding, especially breast-feeding ; and, probably above all, (3) absence of severe illness and an early incidence of infectious fever. No difference of present economic status was demonstrable between the two groups, but a point of importance appeared to be that children with bad teeth were often the younger members of a family, whereas those with good teeth were frequently first children. In this series of cases irregular dentition and inadequate oral hygiene did not appear to exercise any unfavourable effect on the degree of freedom from caries.

We wish to thank Dr. G. C. M. M'Gonigle and Dr. J. C. Spence for helpful criticism and advice, and the Newcastle-upon-Tyne education committee for the facilities afforded to us.

REFERENCES

Miller, H. G. (1938) Brit. med. J. **2**, 718.
Read, T. T., and Knowles, E. M. (1938) Brit. dent. J. **64**, 185.

MEDICAL SOCIETIES

ROYAL SOCIETY OF MEDICINE

SECTION OF SURGERY

AT a meeting of this section held on July 6, Mr. CLAUDE FRANKAU being in the chair, Dr. GORDON MURRAY, of Toronto, read a paper on

Heparin in the Prevention of Thrombosis

The properties of heparin as an anticoagulant had, he said, been discovered in 1916 ; he had become interested in it because of the help it afforded in experimental work on blood-vessel anastomosis. One of the most important steps had been the obtaining of heparin in a pure state whereby its toxicity had been eliminated. The crystalline barium salt which had been produced had a constant potency. Opinions differed as to whether heparin was an antithrombin or an antiprothrombin. It might be injected subcutaneously, applied to surfaces, or injected into vessels. In vessels its action might be restricted to a length of vessel, or, by injection into the general circulation, it might act by altering the clotting-time of the blood. This general effect had been found the most useful. Veins and arteries could be divided and sutured under the influence of heparin ; Dr. Murray gave illustrations of perfect healing with complete patency and no evidence of clotting. Without the use of heparin, such results were rare ; with heparin they occurred in over 90 per cent. of cases. In grafting experiments—e.g., of a length of jugular vein into a gap in the carotid artery—without heparin thrombosis occurred every time within three hours ; with previous administration of heparin for 7–9 days by constant intravenous drip—admittedly a difficult procedure to carry out successfully in animals—complete patency of the grafted vessel was assured. Dr. Murray had followed the histological changes in these grafts up to one year after the operation and was able to demonstrate how the grafted vein gradually assumed the characters of the artery. A thrombus produced experimentally by insertion of a foreign body at the bifurcation of a peripheral artery, such as the femoral, could be successfully removed in the heparinised animal even after it had remained in situ for twenty-four hours and had become attached to the intima. Experiments on the splenic vein suggested that heparin had a similar anticoagulant effect in the portal system; in the transplantation of organs also heparinisation ensured success. One valve of a heart had been removed and a new valve substituted and the animal continued to live without thrombus formation in the heart.

Clinically, heparin had been given by continuous intravenous drip to more than 400 patients without toxic effects; superficial veins near the wrist were used, and no vein had thrombosed up to two weeks. Without heparin it was usual for the veins to thrombose at the end of 26–48 hours. As a preventive of postoperative thrombosis and pulmonary embolism he thought heparin was of value. It had been found that the incidence of pulmonary embolism in 600 major operations was 2 per cent.; in 400 cases in which patients received intravenous heparin after operation no case of pulmonary embolism occurred. Embolectomy was a field of surgery where the use of heparin had been most helpful; 60 per cent. of these operations were successful in heparinised patients. The heparin was administered twenty-four hours after the operation, so as to guard against undue bleeding at operation. The clotting-time returned to normal in one and a half hours, and there was no negative phase later on.

In 72 cases of thrombophlebitis in which heparin had been administered the results had been impressive. Pain, temperature and œdema had rapidly subsided. The clot was not absorbed. In pulmonary embolism Dr. Murray claimed no operative success, but in some cases of repeated embolism he believed that heparin had proved of value in preventing further attacks. In mesenteric thrombosis, necessitating large bowel resection, success was rare; he had seen only one case recover. But four consecutive cases were alive and well in which the resection had been done and heparin administered. Two subsequent cases died, one after nine days, from peritonitis. In splenectomy and in blood-transfusion heparin had proved its value, and there might be a field for its use in coronary thrombosis. The rationale of its use in coronary disease was not clear, but if it were true that occlusion at the commencement was incomplete then heparin might prevent complete occlusion. In cases in which heparin had been used, all they could say was that the clinical course and the electrocardiograms had been unusual. He described a case in which he had excised a popliteal aneurysm and grafted a length of the jugular vein to re-establish the continuity of the artery. The patient subsequently developed an aneurysm in the lower end of the venous graft. This was sutured and the man returned to the Bush with a perfectly normal leg.

Summing up, Dr. Gordon Murray said it was proved that heparin was non-toxic, both in animals and human beings; that it prevented thrombosis; that it was valuable in determining success in operations on blood-vessels, and in cases in which thrombosis was a feature.

DISCUSSION

The CHAIRMAN confirmed the value of heparin in the operation of embolectomy. He congratulated Dr. Murray on the brilliance of his work, which he said was well recognised in Toronto.

Mr. G. GORDON-TAYLOR said he did not feel so despondent as Dr. Murray about mesenteric thrombosis: almost half his cases had recovered.

Sir JAMES WALTON said he knew of no piece of experimental work in surgery which had been so rapidly and successfully carried through or so rapidly applied to clinical use as had Dr. Murray's.

In reply to various speakers, Dr. MURRAY said that there was still great difficulty in assessing accurately the heparin content of blood; possibly however in cases with thrombosis the heparin content might not be a significant factor. In Toronto they had found it best to determine the individual clotting-time for a patient and aim at doubling or trebling that, rather than at producing a standard clotting-time. The simplest possible method of estimating clotting-time had proved the most satisfactory; they had given up complicated machines. The average case required 750–1000 units of heparin per hour intravenously. The price of heparin was as real a difficulty in Toronto as here; he was afraid it would not be appreciably lower till a synthetic preparation came on the market. There had been successes in septicæmic cases—as, for example, in septicæmia following carbuncles; and physicians were hoping that heparin given in vegetative endocarditis might prevent the thrombus forming on the valve and thus destroy the nidus for the growth of organisms.

OXFORD OPHTHALMOLOGICAL CONGRESS

As is now customary, this congress gathered at Keble College, Oxford, where on July 5 the members met informally and dined in hall. The discussions and demonstrations took place at the School of Anatomy, beginning next day with the installation of Mr. PERCIVAL HAY (Sheffield) as master, in succession to Dr. C. G. RUSS WOOD, who died shortly after last year's meeting.

Chiasmal Lesions

The Doyne lecture was delivered this year by Mr. F. A. WILLIAMSON-NOBLE (London), who took as his subject the Ocular Consequences of Certain Chiasmal Lesions. The characteristics of the chiasmal syndrome, he said, include defective central vision, optic atrophy (with or without papillœdema), and very numerous and varied defects of the visual field. The common causes are :—

(a) *Meningiomas* which grow from the dura covering the circle of sinuses surrounding the pituitary diaphragm. As they enlarge, these raise the chiasma and stretch both it and the optic nerves. Irregularity of pressure accounts for corresponding asymmetry of the field defects.

(b) *Suprasellar pituitary adenomata* occur either as outgrowths from the stalk of the gland, or from its upper part. In either case there may be a strange absence of signs at first, the most likely evidence being field changes. Small test objects and the use of the two-metre screen are valuable in this connexion.

(c) *Craniobuccal pouch cysts*, enlarging from remnants of the hypoglossal duct, form a third group. They are commonest in childhood, and tend to calcify.

(d) *Arachnoiditis* of the chiasmal region may arise from many causes. The clinical features appear as the result of adhesions or cyst formations. General neurological findings may be absent.

(e) *Aneurysms of the circle of Willis* arise and yield signs after the age of 30 as a rule. Suddenness of onset and pain are the chief features. Radiography may reveal calcification in the aneurysmal wall.

(f) *Chiasmal glioma* is rare. The age-period is youth and there is a tendency towards enlargement of the optic foramina.

FIBRIN SUTURE OF PERIPHERAL NERVES

MEASUREMENT OF THE RATE OF REGENERATION *

By J. Z. Young, M.A. Oxfd ; and

P. B. Medawar, M.A. Oxfd

(*From the Department of Zoology and Comparative Anatomy in the University of Oxford*)

To reduce the difficulties of nerve suture and to minimise the disorganisation of the fibres which is apt to be produced by stitches, even if restricted as far as possible to the epineurium, a method has been devised by which stumps can be held together with concentrated coagulated blood plasma. The method consists simply in holding the cut stumps together and pouring round them plasma which has just been mixed with a little strong tissue-extract. In about ½–2 min., according to the age of the plasma and the strength of the extract, the plasma clots to a firm jelly, which sticks to the nerves and holds the stumps together. The plasma is freely permeable and during the subsequent days is dissolved away, although remaining long enough to allow a firm union to be established between the divided ends.

METHOD

The gel formed by ordinary plasma is not sufficiently strong to maintain union under tension, but it can be fortified by dissolving in it sufficient fibrinogen to increase its normal concentration by anything up to ten times. In the experiments so far undertaken cockerel plasma has proved to be more satisfactory than that of mammals. Blood is withdrawn from the carotid artery through oiled cannulæ into large centrifuge tubes. These are packed in ice for 10 min. and then spun. The supernatant plasma, which separates easily, is stored in waxed test-tubes on ice and keeps for at least six weeks. The animal should be starved for thirty-six hours before operation. A normal yield under ether anæsthesia is 100–150 c.cm. of whole blood. No heparin need be used.

The concentration is effected by the precipitation of fibrinogen (with prothrombin) from part of the plasma and by its re-solution in a smaller volume. The concentration thus concerns the protein constituents only. The method of salting out by half-saturation with sodium chloride is unsatisfactory, because the excess of salt, which cannot be easily removed, interferes with clotting. Accordingly Mellanby's (1917) method is used, 1 volume of plasma being mixed with 9 volumes of redistilled water and then, slowly, with 0·10–0·15 volume of a solution of acetic acid in redistilled water containing 1% by volume. The fibrinogen forms a flocculate, which is centrifuged out very firmly after standing for 5 min. The supernatant fluid is discarded and replaced with water, which is then also taken off with a fine pipette. The fibrinogen may now be either used directly or stored under distilled water at 4° C. It keeps for at least ten days in this condition without changing its properties, except that it becomes progressively more difficult to redissolve.

---

* This work was assisted by a grant from the Rockefeller Foundation.

REFERENCES : *continued from previous page*

Lewis, D. (1920) *J. Amer. med. Ass.* **75**, 73.
Marie, P. and Foix, C. (1916) *Rev. neurol.* **29**, 159.
Medical Research Council Committee on Injuries of the Nervous System (1920), *Spec. Rep. Ser. med. Res. Coun., Lond.*, No. 54.
Platt, H. (1921) The Surgery of Peripheral Nerve Injuries of Warfare, Bristol.
—— and Bristow, W. R. (1923) VIᵉ Congrès de la Société Internationale de Chirurgie, **3**, 184.
Rosenstein, A. (1935), Bumke and Foerster's Handbuch der Neurologie, Berlin, vol. i, p. 261.
Sherren, J. (1906) *Edinb. med. J.* **20**, 297.
Spielmeyer, W. (1918) *Münch. med. Wschr.* **65**, 1039.
Stookey, B. (1922) Surgical and Mechanical Treatment of Peripheral Nerves, Philadelphia.
Stopford, J. S. B. (1920a) *Brain*, **43**, 1.
—— (1920b) *Lancet*, **2**, 1296.
—— (1930) Sensation and the Sensory Pathway, London.
Tinker, M. B. and Tinker, M. B. jr. (1937) *Ann. Surg.* **106**, 943.

Before use, the fibrinogen is dissolved in the appropriate volume of plasma—not in saline, because in the presence of serum the fibrin clot is stronger and much more stable. For use with rabbit nerves a $6 \times N$ concentration has proved satisfactory—i.e., one produced by dissolving in 1 volume of plasma the fibrinogen precipitated from 5 volumes. During the first stage of solution the precipitate becomes hydrated and swells ; to prevent it from forming a tough gelated mass, it should be broken up with the tip of a pipette and sucked in and out as rapidly as possible. The entire set of operations, which are rapid and simple, should be performed aseptically and the reagents subjected to routine bacteriological tests for sterility.

The quick and even coagulation of the plasma is ensured by mixing it thoroughly just before application with not more than a tenth of its volume of a concentrated tissue-extract, although such a procedure is not absolutely necessary. Chicken-embryo extract in saline (2 c.cm. per 10-day embryo) is very satisfactory, because it is a powerful clotting agent which is sterile in the first instance. The extract retains almost full potency for a week if it is stored just above 0° C. and the saline is buffered. The slight precipitate which invariably forms after the first day of storage may be disregarded.

RESULTS

The plasma method has been found to give very satisfactory junction of the cut sciatic nerve of the rabbit, even under conditions in which the stumps retract 1 cm. or more from each other. The stumps are held together with fine forceps, and the plasma, after mixing with the embryo extract, is dropped in from a sterile pipette in such a way that it remains as a small pool round the ends. It is desirable to dry the site of application as far as possible with gauze. The forceps are carefully withdrawn through the coagulum which forms ; sharp watchmaker's forceps are useful, because they come out easily. Plasma 0·5 c.cm. is a full allowance for the union of the sciatic nerve of the rabbit. Very good apposition of the cut ends can be obtained in this way. To ensure that the ends are held properly in place, the epineurium of both stumps can be gripped with one pair of forceps, which is then fixed with a clip while the epineurium is seized again on the opposite side of the nerve trunk, held together, and clipped. If the junction is for any reason unsatisfactory, it can be broken and remade without any damage to the nerve.

Little or no plasma penetrates between the cut stumps, and no barrier to regeneration is presented. The plasma is usually wholly dissolved away ; hence in rabbits opened two or three weeks after operation no trace of it is seen. Small whitish masses sometimes remain after this period, but they do not appear to set up any reaction. To test the possibility of a general reaction to cockerel plasma, 2 rabbits were each injected intravenously with 1 c.cm. of heparinised cockerel plasma a week for six weeks. No detectable response corresponding to sensitisation was seen, and the rabbits remained apparently completely normal.

Experiments on joining the sciatic nerve of the dog have proved a severe test of the plasma method, not so much because of the size of the nerve and the tension between the cut ends as because of the activity of the animal in the days after the operation. These experiments show that it would probably be necessary to restrict movement in the limb for a few days, though no special precautions of this sort have to be taken with the rabbit.

Histological study (figs. 1 and 2) shows that the junctions made by the plasma method are readily crossed by nerve-fibres. It is impossible in any nerve junction to ensure that all the fibres pass straight from the central to the peripheral stump, but in the fibrin junction there is a near approach to this condition, with none of the whorls and deviation of large bundles of fibres which are unavoidable with stitching unless the epineurium alone is sutured—a difficult achievement with small nerves.

RATE OF REGENERATION

To judge the effectiveness of regeneration after different procedures—such as suture and the fibrin method just described—we have measured how far from the point of junction a reflex response can be elicited.

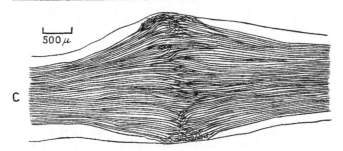

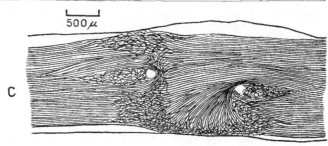

FIG. 1.—Right sciatic nerve of a rabbit. Junction made with plasma twenty-five days previously. The fibres have grown forwards with little deviation except at the edges. C, central stump. This and fig. 2 are tracings from photographs of sections stained by Bodian's method for showing axons.

FIG. 2.—Left sciatic nerve of same rabbit as in fig. 1. Junction made with fine silk stitches. The stitches interrupt the outgrowth and the pressing together of the ends produces whorls and deviation of bundles.

C, central stump.

This is most easily done by exposing the nerve under light anæsthesia and by pinching it with fine forceps, first far peripherally and then nearer and nearer to the junction, until the reflex response is obtained. The first response is usually a contraction of the flexors of the same side or a turning of the head. The method thus presumably shows the distance to which pain fibres have regenerated. Stimulation by electrical methods gave results similar to those of pinching, but with the disadvantage that either very strong faradic shocks or long and strong condenser discharges must be used, because the young fibres, being small and unmedullated, are difficult to excite electrically. Because of the spread of the current it is therefore difficult to determine in this way the exact point from which a response can first be elicited ; but it can be established that responses cannot be obtained to electrical stimulation from a point peripheral to that at which pinching is effective. In fact the reverse is usually the case.

Study of sections of the pinched region by Bodian's method has shown that the region giving a response when pinched usually contains very few nerve-fibres,

and that few or no fibres are found beyond this point. The pinching test therefore gives a sensitive indication of the distance to which the fibres have reached.

With this method it has been found that there is no significant difference between the rates of regeneration of the fibres of the tibial and the peroneal nerves in the rabbit. Moreover the rate of regeneration is very similar between different individuals. The rabbits were usually operated on both sides, the tibial portion of the sciatic being cut in the middle of the thigh and the stumps joined on one side with plasma and on the other with stitches—usually two of fine white silk. Examination was made at various later dates, usually at the fifteenth and twenty-fifth days. Fig. 3 shows that after a latent period the fibres grow out regularly through the peripheral stump. Since the growing region is of constant cross-sectional area, it is reasonable to assume that the growth-rate is constant, and it may therefore be calculated by determining the regression coefficient of distance of outgrowth on age. This has been done separately for the nerves joined by stick and stitch sutures and has given rates of 3·86 and 3·89 mm. a day respectively. The difference between the rates is not significant, and indeed we should not expect that the type of junction would influence the rate of growth in the peripheral stump. It is also possible to calculate the time at which the new fibres first appear in the peripheral stump ; this is 8·1 and 9·6 days for the plasma junctions and the sutures respectively. The data so far collected are not sufficient to establish the statistical significance of this difference, but they certainly suggest that the latent period is shorter with the plasma method—i.e., with it the fibres cross the scar more readily than they do after stitching.

The histological studies of Cajal (1928) showed a rate of growth of fibres through the scar of the order of 0·2 mm. a day, which agrees with our estimate of the latent period. Previous estimates of the rate of growth within the peripheral stump have mostly been based on the time of recovery of function—i.e., they do not take separate notice of the delay in the scar or at the end-organ. The figures reported are of the same order as those here found ; for instance, Dustin (1917) gives 2–4·5 mm. daily for the ulnaris and 4–5 mm. for the musculospiral in man. One can therefore calculate the time of expected recovery on a basis of ten days or more (according to complications) for crossing the scar and a rate of 4 mm. a day in the peripheral stump. The delay at the end-organ is not definitely known but is perhaps not great.

The rate of growth of the new fibres is not the only criterion of successful regeneration, and the method we have used gives no test of exactness of apposition of funiculi or other factors conducive to successful functional recovery. However, the results of histological examination give assurance that the fibrin method provides junctions even better than those obtainable with stitches, and it may be concluded that the method outlined is effective for the rabbit and dog, besides having the great advantage of rapidity and ease of execution. There appears to be no reason why it should not be used for larger nerves, especially if the stumps can be brought together without undue tension and the limb kept still for a few days after operation. We have found the method very convenient when making nerve grafts in which the ends can be approximated without tension ; and it is especially

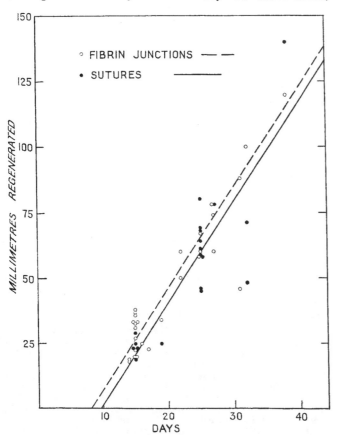

FIG. 3.—Graph showing distances reached by new fibres at various times after stitching the nerves or sticking the ends together with plasma. The lines shown are the regression lines arithmetically calculated. Regeneration begins in the fibrin junctions about a day earlier than in the stitched junctions, and thereafter the rates of growth through the peripheral stump are similar.

spaces full. Impaired resonance R. axilla and R. base. X ray : no abnormality.

CASE 27.—Blast. Fracture R. hip. No chest symptoms. Fullness of lower chest. Diminished air-entry both bases. X ray : no abnormality.

DISCUSSION

Symptoms relating to the chest.—Cough and expectoration were noticed by 6 patients, and in 1 of these there was shortness of breath and general restlessness. The symptoms appeared between the second and fifth days. In no instance were they noticed on the day of the bombing. No-one complained of pain in the chest or of spitting bloodstained sputum.

Physical signs.—In 16 cases there were abnormal physical signs of a recognised character. In only 3 of these were the signs marked. In 15 cases the chest seemed fuller than normal, especially in the lower parts (fig. 1). In 1 case the intercostal spaces seemed to share this fullness. Diminished diaphragmatic movement was present in 10 cases, in 2 affecting the right side, in 4 the left side, and in 4 both sides. There was no tenderness to suggest fracture of the ribs and no evidence of this was found in the radiograms ; there was no surgical emphysema. There was generalised hyper-resonance in 1 case. In 3 cases there was impaired resonance either at one or both bases. Loud harsh breath-sounds were present in 1 case. In 7 patients the breath-sounds were faint and almost inaudible. Added sounds were heard in 6 patients—i.e., coarse or fine crepitations at one or both bases and in 2 cases diffusely scattered rhonchi. In no case was a pleural friction sound heard.

One patient (case 23) was clearly the subject of old chest trouble as confirmed by X-ray examination, and the findings were discounted. Case 18 had patchy areas of dullness at both bases, especially the right, with fine crepitations and diminished air-entry resembling a bronchopneumonia. This was confirmed on X-ray examination. Another (13) had signs of collapse in the left lower lobe also confirmed by X ray.

Radiological findings.—X-ray examination presented difficulties, for the patients had to be examined in bed, on account of their injuries, and they could not have their position in bed adjusted as required. Standardisation of position, therefore, could not be attained and allowance had to be made for this in scrutinising the radiograms. Abnormal radiological appearances were found in 14 out of the 27 cases. Of these, 2 showed obvious changes ; 1 case (13) had a fairly dense area in the lower left lung field due to consolidation of part of the lung, probably the lower lobe (fig. 2), while case 18 showed the congestive changes of a bronchopneumonia (fig. 3). The remainder showed changes similar to an early pleurisy—a diminution of rib-expansion on the affected side, together with a slight loss of translucency (figs. 4 and 5). In nearly all the cases this appearance was on the left side.

SUMMARY AND CONCLUSIONS

1. A series of 27 patients who were under treatment for burns or other injuries resulting from the bursting of high-explosive bombs at close quarters are reviewed with special regard to the state of their chests. In only 2 patients was the question of exposure to blast doubtful, in the remainder severe blast had been experienced.

2. Only 6 patients complained of symptoms related to the chest ; 16 showed some abnormal physical signs and 14 showed abnormal radiological appearances.

3. Evidence of serious or gross pathological changes in the chest was absent in all but 2 cases ; 1 of these had the signs of collapse of a lobe of the lung, the other had the signs of a patchy consolidation of the bronchopneumonic type.

4. The relative importance of the three factors to which the patients were exposed—blast, burns, and immersion—in relation to the chest conditions is impossible to assess. It will be difficult to find cases in which there are no external injuries. Immersion may have played an important part in case 18, for example, but only 3 suffered this experience and the other 2 showed neither symptoms nor signs of chest involvement. Burns were extensive though superficial,

but in case 17 with burns which involved almost the whole skin of the chest, there was no X-ray evidence of chest involvement. Physical examination was impossible in this case.

5. Attention is specially drawn to :

(*a*) The relative disproportion in frequency between the symptoms and physical signs in the cases studied. This may be due to the fact that all were the subject of serious injuries which would tend to direct their attention away from the chest. Moreover, they were all confined to bed. Chest complications may arise after explosion blast without definite warning symptoms and this should encourage the performance of routine examinations even in those who are apparently unaffected by the blast.

(*b*) The physical signs, judging from what we have seen, that may be expected are : diminished movement of the diaphragm ; fullness of the chest giving it an emphysematous appearance ; and impairment of resonance at one or both bases, with or without crepitations.

(*c*) The frequency of a " blown-up " or ballooned appearance of the chest, especially at the lower costal margins after such injuries. This may be related to the posture the patients adopted in bed, or to the presence of an already existing emphysema, though this seems unlikely since they were all young men and in good health before being injured. This appearance was often associated with diminished movement of the diaphragm. It may be that some true traumatic emphysema results in these cases.

(*d*) The radiological appearances of a diminution of rib-expansion, together with slight loss of translucency, particularly on the left side. This is an appearance that theoretically should be produced by a pleura slightly thickened by bruising and " bruised pleura " may be the pathological condition present. The explanation of the frequency of this appearance on the left side may be that this was the side exposed to the blast, but we have been unable to confirm this point.

PENICILLIN AS A CHEMOTHERAPEUTIC AGENT

BY

E. CHAIN, PH.D. CAMB.   M. A. JENNINGS, B.M. OXFD,

H. W. FLOREY, M.B. ADELAIDE,

A. D. GARDNER, D.M. OXFD, F.R.C.S.   J. ORR-EWING, B.M. OXFD,

N. G. HEATLEY, PH.D. CAMB.   A. G. SANDERS, M.B. LOND.

(*From the Sir William Dunn School of Pathology, Oxford*)

IN recent years interest in chemotherapeutic effects has been almost exclusively focused on the sulphonamides and their derivatives. There are, however, other possibilities, notably those connected with naturally occurring substances. It has been known for a long time that a number of bacteria and moulds inhibit the growth of pathogenic micro-organisms. Little, however, has been done to purify or to determine the properties of any of these substances. The antibacterial substances produced by *Pseudomonas pyocyanea* have been investigated in some detail, but without the isolation of any purified product of therapeutic value.

Recently, Dubos and collaborators (1939, 1940) have published interesting studies on the acquired bacterial antagonism of a soil bacterium which have led to the isolation from its culture medium of bactericidal substances active against a number of gram-positive micro-organisms.[1] Pneumococcal infections in mice were successfully treated with one of these substances, which, however, proved to be highly toxic to mice (Hotchkiss and Dubos 1940) and dogs (McLeod et al. 1940).

Following the work on lysozyme in this laboratory it occurred to two of us (E. C. and H. W. F.) that it would be profitable to conduct a systematic investigation of the chemical and biological properties of the antibacterial

---

1. See *Lancet*, 1940, **1**, 1172.

RESULTS OF THERAPEUTIC TESTS ON MICE INFECTED WITH *Strep. pyogenes, Staph. aureus* AND *Cl. septique*

Expt.	—	Dose of infecting culture (c.cm.)	Interval before starting treatment (hrs.)	Duration of treatment	Single dose (mg.)	Total dose (mg.)	No. of mice	Survivors at end of— hours			days								
								6	12	24	2	3	4	5	6	7	8	9	10
Strep. pyogenes—Lancefield, Gp. A.																			
1	Controls	0·5	..	..	..	..	25	..	15	9	8	6	..	5	..	4	..	..	4[1]
	Treated	0·5	1	12 hrs.	2	10·0	50	..	..	..	49	42	..	34	30	28	..	26	25
2	Controls	0·5[2]	..	..	..	..	25	24	3	0[3]	..	..	..	..	..	..	..	..	0
	Treated	0·5	2	45 hrs.	0·5	7·5	25	24	24	..	..	..	..	..	..	..	..	..	24
Staph. aureus [4]																			
1	Controls	1·0	..	..	..	..	24	21	1	0[3]	..	..	..	..	..	..	..	..	0
	Treated	1·0	1	55 hrs.	0·5	9·0	25	25	25	12	..	11	..	10	..	..	..	..	8
2	Controls	0·2[2]	..	..	..	..	24	23	15	5	0	..	..	..	..	..	..	..	0
	Treated	0·2	1	4 days	0·5	11·5	24	24	..	23	22	..	..	21	..	..	..	..	21
Cl. septique																			
1	Controls	see text	..	..	..	..	25	..	21	0[5]	..	..	..	..	..	..	..	..	0
	Treated	..	1	10 days	0·5	19	25	..	..	24	21	..	18	..	..	..	..	..	18
		..	1	10 ,,	1·0	38	25	..	..	..	..	..	24	..	..	..	..	..	24

1. A control mouse which was killed by mistake at 24 hrs. is counted as a survivor. Heart-blood culture strongly positive.
2. Between experiments 1 and 2 the virulence of the organism was raised by passage.
3. Controls all dead within 16 hrs.
4. A bovine strain exceptionally virulent to mice kindly supplied by Dr. H. J. Parish of the Wellcome Laboratories.
5. Controls all dead within 17 hrs.

substances produced by bacteria and moulds. This investigation was begun with a study of a substance with promising antibacterial properties, produced by a mould and described by Fleming (1929). The present preliminary report is the result of a coöperative investigation on the chemical, pharmacological and chemotherapeutic properties of this substance.

Fleming noted that a mould produced a substance which inhibited the growth, in particular, of staphylococci, streptococci, gonococci, meningococci and *Corynebacterium diphtheriæ*, but not of *Bacillus coli, Hæmophilus influenzæ, Salmonella typhi, P. pyocyanea, Bacillus proteus* or *Vibrio choleræ*. He suggested its use as an inhibitor in the isolation of certain types of bacteria, especially *H. influenzæ*. He also noted that the injection into animals of broth containing the substance, which he called " penicillin," was no more toxic than plain broth, and he suggested that the substance might be a useful antiseptic for application to infected wounds. The mould is believed to be closely related to *Penicillium notatum*. Clutterbuck, Lovell and Raistrick (1932) grew the mould in a medium containing inorganic salts only and isolated a pigment—chrysogenin—which had no antibacterial action. Their culture media contained penicillin but this was not isolated. Reid (1935) reported work on the inhibitory substance produced by Fleming's mould. He did not isolate it but noted some of its properties.

During the last year methods have been devised here for obtaining a considerable yield of penicillin, and for rapid assay of its inhibitory power. From the culture medium a brown powder has been obtained which is freely soluble in water. It and its solution are stable for a considerable time and though it is not a pure substance, its anti-bacterial activity is very great. Full details will, it is hoped, be published later.

EFFECTS ON NORMAL ANIMALS

Various tests were done on mice, rats and cats. There is some œdema at the site of subcutaneous injection of strong solutions (e.g. 10 mg. in 0·3 c.cm.). This may well be due to the hypertonicity of the solution. No sloughing of skin or suggestion of serious damage has ever been encountered even with the strongest solutions or after repeated injections into the same area.

Intravenous injections showed that the penicillin preparation was only slightly, if at all, toxic for mice. An intravenous injection of as much as 10 mg. (dissolved in 0·3 c.cm. distilled water) of the preparation we have used for the curative experiments did not produce any observable toxic reactions in a 23 g. mouse. It was subsequently found that 10 mg. of a preparation having twice the penicillin content of the above was apparently innocuous to a 20 g. mouse.

Subcutaneous injections of 10 mg. into two rats at 3-hourly intervals for 56 hours did not cause any obvious change in their behaviour. They were perhaps slightly less lively than normal rats but they continued to eat their food. Their blood showed a fall of total leucocytes after 24 hours, but after 48 hours the count had risen again to about the original total. There was, however, a relative decrease in the number of polymorphs, but the normal number was restored 24 hours after stopping the administration of the substance. One of these two rats was killed for histological examination ; there was some evidence that the tubule cells of the kidney were damaged. The other has remained perfectly well, and its weight increased from 76 to 110 g. in 23 days. It is to be noted that these rats received, weight for weight, about five times the dose of penicillin used in the curative experiments in mice. No evidence of toxic effects was obtained from the treated mice, which received penicillin for many days.

Other pharmacological effects.—On the blood-pressure, heart-beat and respiration of cats no effects have been observed after intravenous injection of 40 mg.—enough to bring up the concentration in the blood just after injection to 1/5000. *Perfusion* of the isolated cat's heart, with Ringer-Locke solution containing 1/5000 penicillin produced progressive slowing during 15 minutes and at the end of that time the heart looked as though it would stop beating ; however, it was quickly revived by perfusing with Ringer-Locke solution alone. The same depressant action was seen at 1/10,000 dilution but the effect was less than at 1/5000. Solutions are absorbed from the intestine in the rat without causing any observable damage to the mucosa. They are also readily absorbed after subcutaneous injection and the substance can be detected in the blood. It is excreted by the kidneys, the urine becoming bright yellow. At least 40–50 % appears in the urine in a still active form. *Human leucocytes* remain active in a 1/1000 solution for at least 3 hours.

It must be emphasised that the results of these preliminary tests have been obtained with an impure substance and such slight toxic effects as have been noted may possibly be due, in part at least, to these impurities.

EFFECTS ON BACTERIA IN VITRO

In view of this slight evidence of tissue toxicity it is all the more striking that the substance in a dilution of one in several hundred thousand inhibits in vitro the growth of many micro-organisms, including anaerobes. Of those so far tested in this laboratory the following are sensitive to the inhibiting action of our preparation : *Clostridium welchii* (2 strains) ; *Cl. septique* (1 strain, Nat. coll. type-cultures No. 458) ; *Cl. œdematiens* (1 strain, N.C.T.C. No. 277) ; *C. diphtheriæ* (1 strain, mitis type) ; *Streptococcus pyogenes* (Lancefield group A) ; *Str. viridans* (1 strain from tooth) ; *Str. pneumoniæ* (type 8) ; staphylococci (3 strains). Penicillin is not immediately bactericidal but seems to interfere with multiplication.

THERAPEUTIC EFFECTS

From all the above tests it was clear that this substance possessed qualities which made it suitable for trial as a chemotherapeutic agent. Therapeutic tests were therefore done on mice infected with streptococci, staphylococci and *Cl. septique* ; the results are summarised in the accompanying table, the preliminary trials on small numbers of mice being omitted.

Bacteriological methods : streptococcus and staphylococcus.— The staphylococcus was kept in culture in meat extract broth and the streptococcus in the same with serum. Both organisms were repeatedly passed through mice and were used for experiment 2–4 days after the last passage. The experimental infection was induced with 20–24 hour broth cultures injected intraperitoneally. According to opacity measurements with Brown's tubes, doses of 450 and 350 million cocci, living and dead, were given respectively in the two streptococcal experiments, and doses of 760 and 200 million in the staphylococcal experiments.

Pathogenic anaerobes.—The therapeutic effects were tried in mice infected with spores of *Cl. septique* in the manner described by Henderson and Gorer (1940). Attempts to carry out similar tests with *Cl. welchii* were temporarily abandoned owing to the difficulty of establishing in mice a type of infection which is both certainly fatal and allows adequate time before death for treatment to take effect. A spore suspension of *Cl. septique* was made by anaerobic growth at 37° C. for 48 hours on Dorset's egg slopes, suspension of the growth of each slope (surface about 15 sq. cm.) in about 1 c.cm. of sterile distilled water, centrifugalisation, once washing with distilled water, recentrifugalisation and resuspension in the original volume of distilled water. The suspension was then heated to 75° C. for one hour. The virulence of the suspension, when injected with an equal volume of 5% calcium chloride was roughly titrated by injection into the thigh muscle of mice, and a dose was chosen for the therapeutic experiment such as would kill for certain without being unnecessarily severe, viz., 0·05 c.cm. of the suspension diluted one in three, mixed with 0·05 c.cm. of the calcium chloride solution. This was injected into the thigh muscles of the 75 mice whose subsequent fate is recorded in the table.

Treatment.—The general principle has been to keep up an inhibitory concentration of the substance in the tissues of the body throughout the period of treatment by repeated subcutaneous injections. No extended tests have been made to determine the minimum effective quantities or the longest intervals possible between injections. The doses employed have been effective and not toxic ; they may have been excessive. The solution contained 10 mg. per c.cm. of substance.

In the first streptococcal experiment the treatment was continued for 12 hours only. That this was inadequate was shown by deaths occurring during the arbitrarily chosen 10-day period. In the second experiment the time of treatment was lengthened, with improved results. In this and the two staphylococcal experiments injections were given 3-hourly for the first 32–37 hours, then at longer intervals.

In preliminary experiments with *Cl. septique* it was found that the infection could be satisfactorily held in check so long as penicillin was being given (i.e., for 2 days) but when the administration was stopped the infection developed. In the experiment quoted, therefore, the injections were given for 10 days, 3-hourly for

41 hours, then at longer intervals, and twice daily for the last 2 days of the period. No deaths have subsequently occurred (22 days after beginning of experiment).

The behaviour of the mice infected with streptococci and staphylococci was interesting. For some hours after the start of treatment they looked sick—some even appeared to be dying—but as the experiment went on they progressively improved till at the end of 24 hours in the case of the streptococci and about 36 to 48 hours with the staphylococci it was difficult or impossible to distinguish them from normal mice. The survivors of the *Cl. septique* infection on the other hand remained well throughout, except for a few in which leg lesions appeared near the site of injection and cleared up in a few hours.

Summarising the data given in the table we see that in the final streptococcus experiment (no. 2) whereas 25/25 controls died, 24/25 treated animals survived. With *Staphylococcus aureus* the final experiment (no. 2) shows 24/24 deaths of the controls and 21/24 survivals among the treated. Lastly, with *Cl. septique* when the larger doses of penicillin were given (bottom line) the figures are 25/25 control deaths and 24/25 treatment survivals.

CONCLUSIONS

The results are clear cut, and show that penicillin is active in vivo against at least three of the organisms inhibited in vitro. It would seem a reasonable hope that all organisms inhibited in high dilution in vitro will be found to be dealt with in vivo. Penicillin does not appear to be related to any chemotherapeutic substance at present in use and is particularly remarkable for its activity against the anaerobic organisms associated with gas gangrene.

In addition to the facilities provided by the university we have had financial assistance from the Rockefeller Foundation, the Medical Research Council and the Nuffield Trust. N. G. Heatley has held a Rockefeller fellowship. To all of these we wish to express our thanks. We also wish to acknowledge the technical assistance of D. S. Callow, G. Glister, S. A. Creswell, J. A. Kent, and E. Vincent.

REFERENCES

Clutterbuck, P. W., Lovell, R. and Raistrick, H. (1932) *Biochem. J.* **26**, 1907.
Dubos, R. J. and Cattaneo, C. J. (1939) *J. exp. Med.* **70**, 249.
Fleming, A. (1929) *Brit. J. exp. Path.* **10**, 226.
Henderson, D. W. and Gorer, P. A. (1940) *J. Hyg., Camb.* **40**, 345.
Hotchkiss, R. D. and Dubos, R. J. (1940) *J. Biol. Chem.* **132**, 791, 793.
McLeod, C. M., Mirick, G. S. and Curnen, E. I. (1940) *Proc. Soc. exp. Biol.* **43**, 461.
Reid, R. D. (1935) *J. Bact.* **29**, 215.

MENINGOCOCCAL MENINGITIS STARTING AS DIABETIC COMA

BY CECIL W. WARD, M.B. Leeds

AND

ALBERT A. DRIVER, M.B. Leeds, D.P.H.

ASSISTANT MEDICAL OFFICERS AT SEACROFT HOSPITAL, LEEDS

THE following unusual case of meningococcal meningitis presented a difficult problem in diagnosis.

A well-developed athletic man, aged 19, was apparently in perfect health on the morning of Feb. 26. He had little appetite for his midday meal and in the afternoon complained of a slight headache and drowsiness. During the evening this drowsiness became more pronounced, and when first seen by the doctor at 10.30 P.M. he was comatose and could only be roused with great difficulty.

The patient was admitted to Seacroft Hospital about midnight. He did not respond to any stimulation. Pupils half dilated and did not react to light. Swallowing reflex present ; knee, ankle, and abdominal reflexes present but sluggish ; plantar responses not obtained. Uniform flaccidity of all four limbs, with no perceptible difference between the two sides. No rigidity of neck. Breathing deep and regular ; smell of acetone in breath and dryness of tongue led to immediate catheterisation. Sugar 3% and acetone bodies found in urine. Temperature 99·8° F., pulse-rate 84, respiration-rate 32.

Diabetic coma having been diagnosed with some hesitation, the patient was given saline containing 25 g. of glucose to the pint by the intravenous drip method and 25 units of insulin

subject, therefore, has 50 × 63·5, or 3175 c.cm., of plasma, containing about 222 g. of proteins. The percentage increase in the plasma proteins after the transfusion of one bottle of fluid is shown above.

Obviously it is the use of serum which calls for most care. Once introduced, plasma protein cannot readily leave the circulation, and by virtue of its osmotic pressure retains the water injected with it ; this means extra work for the heart. The lungs act as the immediate safety valve, and if the volume of plasma protein solution in circulation exceeds a certain level fluid rapidly passes into the pulmonary alveoli, causing œdema of the lungs. We cannot say what percentage increase of protein in the plasma will cause a dangerous degree of pulmonary œdema, but probably even one bottle of serum may be deleterious. There can be little doubt that in severe secondary shock one bottle in excess of the amount required to replace lost plasma may endanger life. In patients suffering from " primary " shock only, where there is no evidence of loss of cells or plasma from the circulation either by internal hæmorrhage or œdema, it cannot be too strongly emphasised that there is no rational basis for treatment by transfusion.

CONTROL OF DOSAGE

Ideally, dosage would be regulated by repeated determinations of plasma-volume or blood-volume, but unfortunately really simple methods for estimating these do not exist. The urgent need for transfusion often precludes the use even of such methods as are available. Of these, one of the best is that of Hill [1] for determining the blood-volume during transfusions of whole blood ; as Hill suggests, the same principle might be used in assessing the plasma-volume during serum transfusions. In the absence of such precise information, other and less reliable indications have to be considered. No single test is a sure guide : pulse-rate, hæmoglobin percentage, red-cell count and hæmatocrit determinations are of value, but their interpretation is at times very difficult. A mental estimate of the amount of plasma and red cells which may have left the circulation is useful, but may be difficult to make. Even the immediate response of the blood-pressure to transfusion affords no certain indication either that enough fluid has been or that more should be administered. Early in " primary " shock the blood-pressure may be subnormal—a factor making differentiation from circulatory shock difficult. If no time is allowed for observation of such a patient, and a transfusion is given at once, the subsequent rise in blood-pressure may wrongly be ascribed to satisfactory treatment of circulatory shock. Conversely, even if the blood-pressure fails to respond favourably, transfusion should be discontinued once the volume permissible on the grounds discussed here has been administered.

While it is difficult, then, to assess dosage on the basis of any or all of these various signs, we shall probably avoid transfusing an excessive amount if we administer, of any medium, only sufficient to make good the maximum probable protein loss from the circulation.

SUMMARY

In cases of hæmorrhage or circulatory shock, the lasting restoration of the blood-volume to its normal value by transfusion depends on the replacement of dissolved protein lost from the circulation as a result of injury.

Since equal volumes of serum, citrated plasma, citrated whole blood and defibrinated whole blood contain different amounts of dissolved protein, the volume to be transfused in any given case will depend on the medium chosen.

Bearing in mind the blood-volume of the patient in health, and the maximum probable loss of fluid from the circulation at the time of transfusion, it is possible to state how much of any one of these media can be administered with safety. These maximum volumes are : serum 3·4, citrated plasma 5·1, citrated whole blood 8 and defibrinated whole blood 6·6 bottles.

This estimate may serve as a check against the transfusion of excessive amounts when the interpretation of the clinical indications for dosage is difficult and the case-history unknown.

1. Hill, D. K. *Lancet*, 1941, **1**, 177.

CIVILIAN PSYCHIATRIC AIR-RAID CASUALTIES

By FELIX BROWN, D.M. Oxfd, M.R.C.P.
REGISTRAR IN PSYCHOLOGICAL MEDICINE AT GUY'S HOSPITAL;
PSYCHIATRIST UNDER E.M.S.

THE psychological reaction of civilians to air-raids has been observed in the south-eastern sector, and it is now possible to classify the types of casualties occurring and make some suggestions for their treatment. The swarms of hysterics which were by some expected to follow bombing have not appeared, but nevertheless there are certain psychiatric disorders attributable to air-raids.

ACUTE EMOTIONAL SHOCK

The symptoms in mild cases of shock are tremor, sometimes violent, dilated pupils, and tachycardia, with an emotional state of fear, perhaps mixed with anxiety about relatives and property. There is usually extreme sensitivity to noise and considerable restlessness. This reaction may occur in anyone who has been in a bombed building, especially if he is anxious about an injured wife or husband.

CASE 1.—A man, aged 35, of previously normal personality was bombed while in a public-house. His wife had a flesh wound in the back. He was extremely tremulous and anxious, chiefly about his wife. Reassurance, a night in hospital and a strong sedative (Nembutal gr. 6) enabled him to recover and return to his normal life next day.

In this fear reaction there is no hysterical amnesia for the events.

ACUTE TRANSIENT HYSTERICAL REACTIONS

Some cases seen shortly after a bombardment are in a limp semistuporose state, usually with a tremor. These patients are acutely scared and seem to be groping for hysterical symptoms to give them peace of mind and forgetfulness of the incident.

CASE 2.—A married woman, aged 40, was seen half an hour after a raid. She complained of trembling of her hands, which she said were going stiff. She had dilated pupils and looked terrified. She held her fingers stiffly extended. She said " I was writing. I heard the bomb coming down, the crash came. Then all the windows came in on me. I ran for the door and the blast came in from outside. I went into my neighbour's flat, but she seemed to have a fit. I seemed to go all dizzy and collapsed. I thought I had a stroke." Her mother had died of a stroke ; two of her sisters had had St. Vitus's dance. For the past 10 years she had complained of headaches and depression ; she did not get on well with her husband, and resented sexual intercourse. Her symptoms had been better recently until this incident, as she had been able to mix with others in the public shelters.

No attempt was made to get rid of her hysterical symptoms at once, but she was reassured and given gr. 30 each of chloral hydrate and potassium bromide. It was not possible to admit her to hospital, but she was allowed to sleep for 3 hours in the outpatient department. On waking up and having a cup of tea she had lost her symptoms and was able to discuss her experience without terror ; she had recovered enough to go to a friend's house. This patient had a previous history of psychoneurotic traits, and developed her shock in circumstances by no means exceptionally disturbing. The hysterical symptoms, however, were only of short duration.

CASE 3.—A hospital porter, aged 19, was seen about five minutes after being bombed. He was pale, looked shocked, his pupils were dilated and his pulse was of good volume, rate 70 per min. There was a slight superficial scratch on his forearm but no other physical abnormality. At first he was mute, gazing with a vacant stare at the ceiling. With some persuasion he was able to give his name and address slowly and with a severe stammer. After about ten minutes he was persuaded to give his history, still with a bad stammer. He had been within a few yards of one of a salvo of bombs which had hit a hospital building. He went among the wreckage, and was trying to rescue a woman trapped under a sink when another bomb exploded and blew him out of the window. He picked himself up, unhurt but dazed. After sitting down in an office he collapsed and was unconscious for a few minutes. When this history was being obtained he at first said " I don't

consumption of green vegetables. The amounts of phosphorus in the diets were almost identical in the two surveys. Both total and inorganic iron were higher in the war-time dietaries. The iron acquired from the increased bread and vegetables more than made up for the iron sacrificed by the shortage of meat.

VITAMIN C

The question has often arisen as to whether the war-time dietary is deficient in vitamin C. To obtain some information on this point the vitamin C intakes of the individual women have been calculated as accurately as possible from the 1935 and 1941 records. The most reliable figures which are available for the vitamin C in raw and cooked fruit and vegetables were kindly supplied by Miss M. Olliver. A sliding scale was adopted for potatoes, since it has been shown that the vitamin C in this vegetable varies greatly from one time of year to another. Table VI shows the results. The amount of the vitamin C derived from various sources on the two occasions is also shown. It will be seen at once that the average intake in 1941 was only half what it had been in 1935.

In 1935 fruit supplied ten times as much vitamin C as it did in 1941, and the women in the first survey got

TABLE VI—AVERAGE VITAMIN-C INTAKES (MG. PER DAY)

Source						Women 1935		Women 1941
Fruit	..	..	..	..	..	37·5	..	2·8
Vegetables	..	..	..	..	..	15·6	..	19·4
Jam and marmalade	..	..	..	..	1·5	..	1·5
Milk	..	..	..	..	.:	2·4	..	3·2
Total from all sources	..	..	..	57	..	26·9
Maximum..	..	..	..	..	..	140	..	85·2
Minimum ..	..	..	..	..	..	10·2	..	7·7
Standard deviation	..	..	..	..	31	..	9·4

more from this source alone than those in the second obtained from the whole of their diet. The amounts provided by vegetables and milk were a little higher in 1941, due to an increased consumption of these foods. Jam provided the same amount on the two occasions in spite of the increased consumption of this food. This was because the vitamin C in jam varies widely according to the fruit from which it is made. In 1935 more black-currant jam, rich in C, was eaten.

Fig. 4 shows the frequency distribution of the vitamin C intakes. It will be seen that in 1935 9 women were having less than 25 mg. a day, 39 between 25 and 75 mg., and 15 more than 75 mg. In 1941 26 out of 57 women had less than 25 mg., and only one had more than 75 mg. ; this was the woman who ate 300 oz. of potato during the week, and she derived 43 mg. of ascorbic acid a day from this source alone.

The Technical Commission (1938) suggested that the vitamin C requirement of adults was covered by 30 mg. of ascorbic acid daily. The present results suggest that this is true, but that very much smaller amounts will suffice, for in the 1941 survey 41 women were having less than 30 mg. a day, and had probably been having so for 3–6 months. There were, moreover, no manifest signs of scurvy among them, nor indeed have there been any reports of scurvy, even among sections of the community less privileged than the women here investigated. Fox (1940) also came to the conclusion that the vitamin C requirement was much less than others (Harris 1939, Bacharach 1940) have supposed.

The vitamin C intake in war-time must be expected to vary from one season to another, as it has ceased to do in peace-time. This survey was carried out in the lean season. There was no fresh fruit, or raw vegetable salads, and even potatoes were at their lowest ebb. No doubt the intakes would have been much higher in the summer and autumn.

SUMMARY

The records of a dietary survey carried out in 1935 on 63 men and 63 women of the English middle class have been re-analysed. At that time the men were eating an average of twice as much sugar and bacon, three times as much meat, butter and jam, and five times as much cheese, as the rations allowed them in spring 1941. The women were eating less of these foods, but the quantities of all of them except sugar exceeded their rations in spring 1941.

An individual dietary survey was carried out in spring 1941 on 57 women of a similar social class. They were found to be eating much less raw fruit, and less un-rationed meat, fish and sweets and chocolates than the women surveyed in 1935. Milk, bread and other cereal foods, potatoes and other vegetables were being consumed in larger amounts in the 1941 survey.

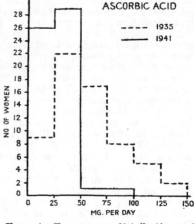

FIG. 4—Frequency distribution of vitamin-C intakes.

The women in the 1941 survey had maintained their calories at their prewar level by substituting unrationed carbohydrate for rationed fat. Their protein and phosphorus intakes were unchanged, their calcium and iron intakes were higher than they had been in 1935. The amount of animal protein was less in the war-time dietary.

The average vitamin-C intake in 1935 was 57 mg. a day, and 27 mg. in 1941. This decrease was due entirely to the disappearance of raw fruit from the market. Three-quarters of the women in the 1941 survey were having less than 30 mg. a day.

We are grateful to all those who have participated in this investigation by weighing their food. We wish to thank Dr. R. A. McCance for his advice and assistance in the preparation of the results for publication. We are indebted to the Medical Research Council for grants and expenses.

REFERENCES

Bacharach, A. L. (1940) *Food*, 9, 110.
Fox, F. W. and Dangerfield, L. F. (1940) *Proc. Transv. Mine med. Offrs' Ass.* 19, 1.
Harris, L. J. (1939) British Encyclopædia of Medical Practice, vol. XII, 570.
McCance, R. A. and Widdowson, E. M. (1940) *Spec. Rep. Ser. Med. Res. Coun. Lond.* No. 235.
— —. (1941) *Ibid.* In press.
Technical Commission on Nutrition (1938) *Bull. Hlth Org. L.o.N.* 7, 461.
Widdowson, E. M. (1936) *J. Hyg. Camb.* 36, 269.
— and McCance, R.A. (1936) *Ibid*, 36, 293.

SNEEZING AND THE SPREAD OF INFECTION

R. B. BOURDILLON,   O. M. LIDWELL,
D.M. OXFD   PH.D. OXFD

(From the National Institute for Medical Research)

RECENT developments in flash photography [1] have increased our knowledge of the particles projected in human sneezing to a point which justifies some practical conclusions as to the best methods of preventing infection from sneezes. American workers [2] have shown that in an ordinary sneeze many thousands of droplets are projected at an initial velocity which may occasionally be as high as 150 ft. per sec., and that most of these droplets come from the mouth. Our own studies have given similar results in many instances, and have shown further points as follows.

Sources of spray.—While in most photographs the

1. Edgerton, H. E., Germeshausen, K. J. and Grier, H. E. *J. appl. Physics*, 1937, 8, 2.
2. Jennison, M. W. *Sci. Mon. N.Y.* 1941, 52, 24.

366   THE LANCET]   DRS. BOURDILLON AND LIDWELL : SNEEZING AND THE SPREAD OF INFECTION   [SEPT. 27, 1941

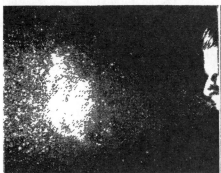
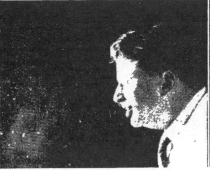
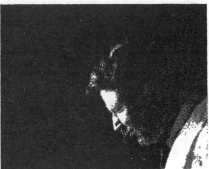

FIG. 1—Discharge chiefly from mouth.   FIG. 2—Discharge from both mouth and nose.   FIG. 3—Discharge from nose only.

majority of the droplets come from the mouth as in fig. 1, in some cases a purely nasal discharge is seen as in fig. 3, and in others a mixed oral and nasal discharge is seen as in fig. 2. In this photograph it is evident that the nasal discharge is being blown forward by the air stream from the mouth, and so goes forwards rather than downwards. It is evidently not justifiable to conclude, as has been suggested, that nasal discharges are unimportant in ordinary sneezes.

Size of droplets varies greatly in different sneezes. Tightly closed teeth or lips and high expiratory pressure

good health and free from cold (in August), but the serum-agar plate after 14 hours incubation showed over 19,000 colonies. These colonies came from at least 19,000 separate droplets, and no attempt was made to estimate the number of bacteria per droplet. While in this case the bacteria are mostly harmless ones from the front of the mouth, it is clear that very many of the droplets in a sneeze do contain living bacteria. It seems reasonable to infer that in acute infections of the upper respiratory tract droplets from sneezes are highly infective.

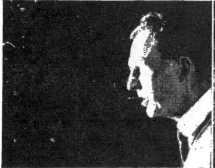
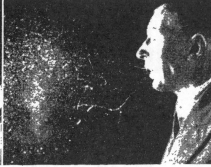
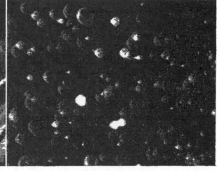

FIG. 4—Teeth open, pressure low. Large drops with few small ones.   FIG. 5—Strings of mucus are common.   FIG. 6—Part of fig. 2 enlarged to two-thirds life size.

give a fine spray as in fig. 1. Open jaws and lips and moderated expiration give relatively few large drops as in fig. 4. Thus a sneeze with open mouth is probably less dangerous to other people, owing to the rapid fall to the ground of large drops, as well as being safer for the subject, owing to the reduced pressure in nose and throat. Strings of mucus are common, as seen in fig. 5. Fig. 6* shows the remarkable appearance of the droplets when photographed while in motion. The pointed outline of the faster moving droplets is possibly an artefact.

Distance projected.—In a vigorous sneeze very large numbers of droplets will hit a vertical plate 3 ft. distant from, and a few inches lower than, the subject's mouth. A small number of large droplets reach a plate 5 ft. distant and 1–1½ ft. below the subject's mouth. The range of danger from direct projectile infection is not less than 4 ft. but will rarely exceed 6 ft. for a person at the same height as the sneeze.

Infectivity of spray.—Fig. 7 shows a culture plate of 9 in. diameter which was placed vertically in the path of the sneeze shown in fig. 1, at a distance of 3 ft. from the subject's nose. The subject was in

Presence of droplet nuclei.—Tests have been made with a subject sneezing in a small closed room of 800 cu. ft. capacity, with floor and table oiled as a precaution against dust. Culture plates of 9 in. diameter were exposed on a table 5 ft. from a subject who sneezed twice. On one plate uncovered only for the 20 min. period from 10 to 30 min. after the sneezes no less than 493 colonies grew. A similar plate exposed for 15 min. in a control test without the sneezes showed only 5 colonies. A series of tests of this type have shown conclusively that a large number of the bacteria-carrying particles from a sneeze are small enough to remain suspended for

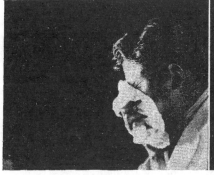
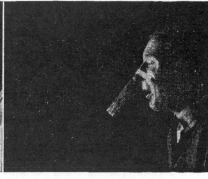

* The enlargement is such that the subject's head if included would be two-thirds life size, but the true size of the droplets may be less than their apparent size, if they are appreciably out of the focal plane.

FIG. 8—A sneeze well covered with an ordinary handkerchief.   FIG. 10—A sneeze into a cheap mask. Note three droplets only escaping downwards.

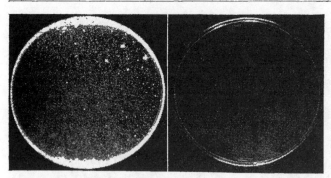

FIG. 7—19,000 colonies of bacteria on a culture plate exposed to the sneeze shown in fig. 1.

FIG. 9—One colony only, on a culture plate exposed to a sneeze as in fig. 8.

over 15 min. before falling on the culture plates. Such particles come within the category defined by Wells[3] as " droplet nuclei," and are certainly capable of conveying infection under suitable conditions.

HYGIENIC MEASURES

To prevent the spread of infection when sneezing indoors one or more of the following measures is usually adopted. We have placed them in order of estimated efficiency.

Sneezing directly into a coal or gas fire (from a short distance) does, in our opinion, ensure sterilisation of nearly all the droplets, since, owing to the chimney draught, few droplets will escape being carried into the fire or up the chimney.

The careful use of a large handkerchief.—Figs. 8 and 9 show that this method can be very efficient. In fig. 8 the subject is sneezing vigorously at the moment of exposure, but no droplets can be seen escaping. Fig. 9 shows a culture plate similar to that shown in fig. 7 but exposed in front of a sneeze trapped by a handkerchief as shown in fig. 8. This plate contained one colony only.

A transparent mask.—Fig. 10 shows a vigorous sneeze covered by a cheap mask of cellulose acetate $5\frac{1}{2}$ in. $\times$ $5\frac{1}{2}$ in., such as has been provided in reserve for London shelter populations. The droplets from the sneeze can be seen collected inside the mask except for three which are seen below the mask in line with its surface. The high apparent efficiency of this type of mask is rather surprising, and it is possible that some very fine droplets are escaping sideways without being visible in the photograph.

A gauze mask of good quality can be fairly efficient for a single sneeze, but becomes messy and unpleasant after multiple sneezes, since, unlike a transparent plastic, gauze cannot be wiped clean and dry.

The hand.—Figs. 11 and 12 show how very inefficient the hand is as a sneeze guard. With the closed hand in fig. 11 inefficiency would be expected, but with the open hand placed in position well before the sneeze occurred, as in fig. 12, more protection might be expected. Its failure is due to the upward deflection of the air stream, which can be seen in this photograph, and has been confirmed in another instance.

TECHNIQUE

Few people can sneeze regularly in front of a camera, owing to the ease with which the sneezing reflex is inhibited. We found a number of subjects who could do it occasionally after taking snuff, and two who could sneeze regularly, one after taking snuff, and one after inhaling minute quantities of ω-bromaceto-6-methoxyquinoline hydrobromide.

A stroboscope lamp was used with mercury kathode and a special igniting electrode, supplied by British Thomson-Houston Ltd. The flash was made by discharging through this a battery of 100 $\times$ 1 μf dry condensers charged to 2100 volts from a series of dry batteries and accumulators. A

3. Wells, W. F. *Amer. J. Hyg.* 1934, **20**, 611.

cylindrical parabolic reflector of duralumin was placed behind the lamp with small electric heaters at the sides to keep the lamp gently warmed. The flash was timed with a hand-controlled switch by an observer who watched the onset of each sneeze. The camera C, lamp L, and subject S were placed at the corners of a triangle of dimensions approximately as follows : LC 55 in., LS 36 in., CS 41 in. The subject sneezed on a line passing close to the lamp, but between it and the camera. The lamp reflector was just to the left of the portions of the photographs reproduced here. This system gives maximum illumination as the droplets approach the lamp—i.e., at the farthest distance included in the photograph. It is in contrast to the system used by most American workers, who place the lamp very close to the subject's head. Owing to the very brief duration of the flash the subject is not dazzled, even if his eyes are open.

SUMMARY

The droplets from a sneeze contain many fine bacteria-laden particles which remain suspended in the air for more than ten minutes. A large handkerchief carefully used prevents the scattering of these droplets, and a simple impermeable mask collects the vast majority of

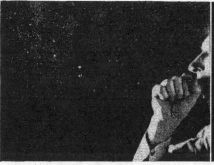 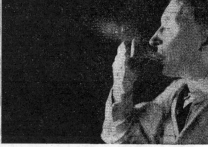

FIG. 11—The closed hand is very inefficient.

FIG. 12—The open hand may only stop a fraction of the particles, and deflect the rest upwards.

them. The use of the hand for checking such scattering is very inefficient.

We wish to thank the research staff of British Thomson-Houston Ltd. for advice on the use of this lamp, and the various subjects who have patiently sneezed for this study. We are also indebted to Mr. S. F. Wilkinson for suggesting the taking of some of these photographs.

CORROSIVE STRICTURE OF THE STOMACH

WITHOUT INVOLVEMENT OF THE ŒSOPHAGUS

C. A. R. SCHULENBURG, M.B. Cape Town, F.R.C.S.
LATELY SURGEON IN AN E.M.S. HOSPITAL

CICATRICIAL stricture of the œsophagus following ingestion of corrosive acids or alkalis is well known, and lesions of the stomach in association with an œsophageal stricture have been reported (Sager and Jenkins 1935, Vinson and Hartmann 1928), but stricture of the stomach with an unharmed œsophagus seems to be very rare, at any rate in England, though the condition is fully dealt with in a number of foreign papers.

The only recorded case in the English language is described by Vinson and Harrington (1929). A man of 59 accidentally swallowed formaldehyde, subsequently developing signs of obstruction in the stomach ; barium meal 4 weeks after the episode showed a double stricture of the stomach, which was confirmed at operation ; there had been no permanent damage to the œsophagus. There is also a case in the autopsy records at Guy's Hospital (Bishop, P. M. F., personal communication) of a woman of 61 who swallowed hydrochloric acid and developed signs of pyloric obstruction ; she died 4 weeks after admission from bronchopneumonia. At autopsy the œsophagus was found to be free from any lesion, while the stomach showed a tight, fibrous, annular stricture for 3 cm. above the pylorus. Prof. Grey Turner, who has had extensive experience of strictures of the œsophagus and other lesions following the ingestion of corrosives, tells me that he knows of only one case where pyloric stenosis

THE LANCET]   FIRST-AID TREATMENT OF BURNS   [SEPT. 27, 1941 377

Special Articles

FIRST-AID TREATMENT OF BURNS

A. H. McINDOE,

M.B. N.Z., M.S., M.SC. MINNESOTA, F.R.C.S., F.A.C.S.

CIVILIAN CONSULTANT PLASTIC SURGEON TO THE R.A.F.;
SURGEON IN CHARGE, MAXILLO-FACIAL UNIT,
EAST GRINSTEAD

DURING the past year much thought has been given to the treatment of burns. This has culminated in recommendations made by the War Wounds Committee of the Medical Research Council after a prolonged survey of the results produced by various methods, under both civilian and Service conditions. It is not surprising that, considering the special causes and unusual types of burns encountered, these recommendations have modified established procedure, though not as extensively as many seem to believe. Careful perusal of the E.M.S. pamphlet (343)[1] will show that coagulation therapy, far from being condemned, remains an important method of treatment, particularly in the extensive burns of the 1st and 2nd degree on the trunk and extremities common in civilian life, where shock and toxæmia are liable to follow. Exception was, however, taken to its use in encircling burns of the hands and feet and in other areas of functional importance, such as the face, flexures, perineum and genitalia, where experience showed that undesirable complications might follow. It was not suggested that burns of all degrees in these special areas showed equally bad results when coagulated, for many have not done so, but certainly some of the more severe burns in which function has been endangered have been further compromised by coagulants.

Most competent observers will agree that it is relatively easy to distinguish between a 1st and 3rd degree burn, but often extremely difficult, even under the best conditions, to decide between those of the 2nd and 3rd degrees. If the surface is contaminated with dirt and oil it may be impossible to make an accurate diagnosis of any degree. This problem is much more acute at first-aid posts and advanced dressing stations, where cleansing facilities are often inadequate, light is poor, and examination is perforce superficial. When the patient is admitted to hospital the degree of involvement must be determined and the appropriate treatment decided on. It is thus vitally important that first-aid treatment should not compromise hospital treatment.

Experience shows that tannic acid is not a panacea for war burns, whatever its results in civil practice. It certainly takes its place, however, in the pattern of treatment which is being slowly evolved. This pattern has not yet reached finality. Alternative methods are still under investigation and it is not intended here to express dogmatic opinions as to their relative value. The wholesale distribution of tannic-acid preparations and vital dye coagulants to homes, first-aid posts and dispensaries has, however, created considerable confusion in the minds of many as to whether coagulants should be applied as a first-aid measure or whether other dressings should be substituted. The desire to make some sort of immediate local application to the burned area is strong, and admittedly the patient may be greatly relieved thereby. The ideal local application would be a quick-drying, flexible and elastic seal, incorporating bacteriostatic and anæsthetic agents. It should be painless to apply, and should resist, when dry, ordinary handling for two to three days without renewal and during that period prevent loss of tissue fluids and the entrance of organisms into the burned area. Especially, it should be water or oil soluble so that it can be easily removed at the hospital where adequate treatment of the burn is undertaken. Whether coagulation should be an essential part of its action is open to question.

None of the variety of suggested preparations exactly fulfils these requirements, and until the ideal substance is produced, obviously the simplest form of easily removable dressing is to be preferred. One can therefore agree with almost any coagulative or non-coagulative treatment which personal preference might dictate in the case of minor burns not requiring admission to hospital, but the first-aid application of any local treatment other than easily removable dressings to those major burns requiring hospital treatment should be discouraged. This is particularly true of those more positive coagulative agents applied hurriedly and inadequately over unclean surfaces in such a way as to be detrimental to the success of subsequent treatment in hospital. While there may be some disagreement between those who believe in universal coagulation and those who do not, they are united in the opinion that first-aid tanning of serious burns is a handicap to the definitive hospital treatment, because once they are applied the crust is difficult to remove.

The function of the first-aider is therefore, first, to distinguish between minor burns which do not require hospital treatment and to treat them efficiently; secondly, to transfer major burns to the nearest hospital or burn unit as soon as possible, limiting treatment to measures of a general nature and to simple local applications, avoiding anything which may be difficult to remove.

The problem is not altogether simple, for while the majority of badly burned patients can be transported to hospital within a short time, it may be days before others can reach suitable hospital facilities. Thus first-aid may be required for burns at sea or in the desert under such difficult conditions that treatment considered inadvisable where quick transport is available might be desirable where there is great delay. An attempt is being made to suggest a reasonable first-aid programme adequate for burns of various types occurring under varying circumstances.

MINOR BURNS

A minor burn is defined as one of the 1st or 2nd degree, covering an area not greater than 1% of the total body surface—i.e., an area corresponding in the adult to one side of the hand or about 28 square inches. It should not involve any of the special areas already mentioned : the hands, face, feet, flexures, perineum and genitalia. Shock is not in evidence and sepsis is uncommon. Pain is usually severe. Healing is rapid by regeneration from the undamaged portion of the skin whatever local application is used.

General treatment.—If pain is not controlled by aspirin or Veganin, then morphine gr. $\frac{1}{6}$–$\frac{1}{3}$ should be given (for an adult).

Local treatment where cleansing facilities are available.—Since these burns are not sent on to hospital, first-aid treatment is as a rule definitive. Whatever is applied should be regarded as the final dressing. Some form of coagulant is therefore safe, simple and satisfactory. Coagulation seals the surface, abolishes pain, prevents secondary infection, and enables the patient to carry on with his work within a short time.

If the burned area is likely to be contaminated, it should be carefully and gently washed, together with the surrounding skin, with soap and water. An application is then made of one of the coagulants in tube form, usually available at most first-aid posts, such as Tannafax, Amertan, gentian-violet jelly, or triple-dye jelly. It is either smeared directly on the burn or applied on a single layer of lint or gauze. Alternatively, the surface may be daubed with 10% tannic acid, 5% silver nitrate, or both, or painted with gentian violet 2% or triple dye (gentian violet 1/400, brilliant green 1/400, neutral acriflavine 1/1000). If tannic acid or silver nitrate is used no dressing should be applied over the burned area.

Non-coagulant dressings may also be used, such as Vaseline gauze, tulle gras, Ambrine, or soft paraffin, but care must be taken to ensure the sterility of the dressings. If sulphanilamide powder is liberally sprinkled over the burn before their application the risk of sepsis will be negligible, and possibly the rate of epithelialisation greater than with coagulant dressings. It is certainly true of the sulphanilamide, tulle gras, saline sequence now in wide use. Nevertheless, the coagulants have a decided advantage over non-coagulant dressings as a first-aid dressing for minor burns, in that once applied they do not require renewal or much aftercare and are not so liable to contamination from outside sources.

The newer preparations, such as Euglamide, a paste incorporating Albucid and a local anæsthetic, and the

---

1. See *Lancet*, 1941, 1, 425.

water-soluble jellies containing sulphanilamide alone or in combination with an antiseptic, have given good results but are not altogether suitable for first-aid purposes, because of their messiness and inability to remain in situ for long.

Local treatment where cleansing facilities are not available. —Not infrequently, burns of this type are badly contaminated with oil or dirt, under such difficult conditions that adequate cleansing facilities are not at hand—for instance, at a thoroughly disorganised first-aid post, where the water has failed, in the desert, or at sea in an open boat. If any form of cleansing is impossible, it is foolish to coagulate a heavily contaminated burn of any type, and thereby seal up organisms on the damaged surface. In any case, the presence of oil will prevent coagulation. It might be pointed out that in the desert where mechanical transport is usually near, benzene or petrol are excellent cleansing agents, and are also practically painless when applied to injured surfaces. Under such circumstances, one of the non-coagulant dressings should be used, and if flies constitute a menace the whole area can be sealed off with a piece of oiled silk, or, if it is available, enclosed in a Bunyan-Stannard envelope. At sea, failing all else, a compress of sea water would be excellent provided it was kept wet.

CLASSIFICATION OF MAJOR BURNS

Burns of any greater extent or depth than minor burns or any burns of the hands, face, flexures, genitalia or perineum should be regarded as of major importance and dispatched to the nearest hospital or burn unit as soon as possible. As opposed to minor burns, the first-aid problem centres round the patient's general condition and the question of how soon he can be transferred. Local treatment is of secondary consideration except under unusual circumstances, and should be concerned only with the protection of the burns from further trauma and secondary infection. Major burns may be classified as follows :—

(*a*) Major burns without serious shock where transport is available. These form the majority of war burns and are easily dealt with.

(*b*) Major burns with serious shock rendering transport dangerous. There are very few cases of this type. They become noticeably fewer the greater the experience of the observer and the more prompt the transport arrangements.

(*c*) Major burns with or without shock, occurring in situations where transport is delayed or is not available. With severe shock every moment which passes before the administration of plasma or serum increases the risk to life. Hence it is better to undertake a difficult journey than to allow blood-volume to fall and hæmoconcentration to rise. Naturally these are difficult problems and much depends on local facilities, mode of transport and distance to the nearest hospital.

SHOCK

Although shock has been divided into primary and secondary forms the former is not commonly seen ; if it does occur it resembles a fainting attack due to neurogenic and traumatic factors. It usually passes off quickly under the influence of rest, heat and morphine. True wound shock (called secondary shock) has all the characteristic signs of ordinary wound shock—rising pulse-rate and respiration-rate, pallor, thirst, anxious restlessness, falling blood-pressure, and so on. It must always be regarded as serious, for it is responsible for 60% of all deaths from burns. It may appear within an hour of injury but does not usually show itself for 6 hours or more. During this time the patient feels and looks well and may even have walked several miles to a dressing station with burns of the most extensive type. This is common in Service casualties. The detection of incipient shock in such cases is difficult without hæmoglobin estimations but the possibility of its clinical development, either slowly or suddenly, must always be borne in mind. Shock results from failure of the circulation in the face of hæmoconcentration and falling blood-volume. The "trigger" which usually induces it is rapid loss of body heat from exposure to cold or further trauma to the already injured skin surface. Undressing the patient to examine the burns in first-aid posts, or any rough handling of burnt areas, should therefore be sedulously avoided. As a rule there is a

relatively safe period in the first 6 hours in which the patient, though severely burned, can stand a reasonably long journey (20–30 miles) by road ambulance. There are few cases to which this does not apply. The patient may suddenly become shocked during transfer, but this is not necessarily the result of the journey. It would probably have happened anyhow. The likelihood of shock supervening rapidly may be judged from the extent and situation of the burns, but as it is dangerous to undress a burned patient, only a very rough estimate of this can be made. In general, shock is liable to be serious if more than 25% of the body surface is involved. In estimating this percentage the following table may be useful :—

	Per cent.		Per cent.
Head	6	Entire front of trunk	19
Both hands	6	Entire back of trunk	19
Both arms	18	Thighs	19
Lower legs	18	Feet	6

Burns of the face, precordial area and abdomen are more dangerous than those of the arms, legs or back. The depth of the burn is not so important as its extent.

If for any reason there is delay at the first-aid post and shock is feared, the pulse and respiration should be noted every half hour, and the B.P. taken as often as possible. With burns of the hands and arms this may be impossible.

GENERAL TREATMENT OF MAJOR BURNS

Pain.—All patients with major burns should receive a full dose of morphine immediately ($\frac{1}{3}$–$\frac{1}{2}$ gr. for an adult). Anything less is futile and the dose can be repeated. Many patients with severe burns are not conscious of pain until the shock phase is over but moderate burns without shock are usually extremely painful.

Shock.—If this is likely to occur while waiting for transport to arrive the patient should lie down on a stretcher or cot and be covered with blankets, with hot-water bottles to keep him warm. Unless the clothing is soaked in water or other fluids it should not be removed, and then only if something warmer can be substituted. Hot sweetened drinks such as tea or coffee should be given freely. Plasma or serum injection is rarely possible or advisable in first-aid posts, and if required should be obtained by means of a mobile unit from the nearest hospital. Rapid transfer of the patient to the hospital is certainly the better plan. In the Services, all station sick quarters, many advanced dressing stations and some ships are suitably equipped for intravenous therapy in the places where delay in transport is likely. Plasma should be used wherever it is indicated. The usual preliminary dose is two bottles of dried plasma or liquid human serum given according to M.R.C. Memorandum No. 1. This may in serious cases be increased to ten or twelve bottles.

LOCAL TREATMENT OF MAJOR BURNS

Major burns should not be coagulated as a first-aid measure. The local conditions are almost always totally unsuitable for this procedure and in the majority of cases more harm than good will be done. Burns on exposed parts dispatched forthwith to hospital should be powdered with sulphanilamide and covered with a sterile towel or wet compress of sodium bicarbonate or saline. Since contact with air is painful the burn surface may be more efficiently protected with simple vaseline gauze strips or tulle gras over the layer of powder. The Bunyan-Stannard oilsilk envelope is a useful added protection during transport, and indeed may be used alone for this purpose.

The problem of the burned patient when transfer to hospital will be delayed for days—e.g., at sea, in the desert or in isolated spots—is difficult, and will depend on the facilities at hand and the severity of the burn. For the patient's comfort it may be necessary to coagulate the whole area, in which case the vital dyes or silver nitrate 10%, which are themselves antiseptic, are most suitable. It will be best to avoid an anæsthetic if possible, for this will undoubtedly increase the risk of shock. Flies will usually constitute a major danger, hence the oilsilk envelope will have considerable value. First-aid treatment in these circumstances will constitute an unhappy compromise between what is possible and what should be done.

the war are analysed. They represented 8·5% of all admissions. The monthly average throughout the period was 52 and was more or less constant.

Of these, 397 (42·5%) were considered to be cases of peptic ulcer. This percentage fell in the successive six-monthly periods, being 46%, 44% and 33%. After the first two months of the war only 7% of these cases were sent back to duty ; the rest were discharged from the Army.

Of the total ulcer cases 13·3% had gastric, 15·3% pyloric and 71·4% duodenal ulcers ; most of these gave a history of many years' duration.

A group of 534 (57·5% of the total dyspeptics) were considered to have no peptic ulceration ; 90% of these were returned to duty, mostly without any lowering of category, the rest being discharged from the Army.

Every case of dyspepsia of more than a month's standing should be examined clinically and radiologically. If possible a fractional gastric analysis should be carried out.

Of all men discharged from the Army through a particular command medical board during a particular period, 14·2% were suffering from peptic ulcer ; 54% of these were discharged after less than 12 months' service.

There is no evidence of an increase in peptic ulceration as a result of the war, but the war has revealed the unsuspected commonness of peptic ulcer and gastritis in the civilian population before the war began. It is vitally necessary that the cause of the great increase in peptic ulceration since the last war should be determined.

I wish to thank Major Hugh Morris, Major W. F. Mair, and Major R. W. Fairbrother for their help.

REFERENCES

Allison, R. S. and Thomas, A. R. (1941) Lancet, i. 565.
Graham, J. G. and Kerr, J. D. O. (1941) Brit. med. J. i, 473.
Maingot, R. (1941) Ibid. i, 533.
Morris, H. (1940) Ibid, ii, 235.
Payne, R. T. and Newman, C. (1940) Ibid, ii, 819.
Spillane, J. D. (1941) Ibid, i, 333.
Turner, H. M. S. (1941) Ibid, i, 605.
Willcox, P. H. (1940) Ibid, i, 1008.

DISTURBANCES OF THE BODY SCHEME
ANOSOGNOSIA AND FINGER AGNOSIA

JOHN D. SPILLANE, M.D. WALES, M.R C.P.
MAJOR, R.A.M.C.

THE term " body scheme " was introduced by Head and Holmes (1911) to signify the concept which a person develops of his own body. The body " scheme," " image " or " pattern " means the picture of the body which is formed in the mind. It became evident to these observers while studying the sensory activity of the human cortex that " one of the faculties which we owe to cortical activity is the power of relating one sensation to another, whether they arise simultaneously or consecutively." The sensory cortex becomes a storehouse of sensory experience ; it receives impressions, stores them and judges new ones in the light of its experience. A standard is formed against which incoming impressions are modified and subsequent conduct determined. In the formation and maintenance of this plastic body image the importance of optical and postural impressions is therefore to be expected. An obvious corollary is that distortion of our own postural model may be associated with loss of orientation in regard to the bodies of other people. Finally, lesions of the sensory cortex may be expected to result occasionally in disorders of the body scheme.

ANOSOGNOSIA

The term " anosognosia " was first used by Babinski (1914) and means unawareness of disease. He reported the cases of 2 hemiplegics who were unaware of their paralyses. Unawareness of blindness had been described by C. von Monakow (1885) in a patient with bilateral disease of the occipital lobes, and unawareness of deafness by Anton (1899) ; the latter also described lack of recognition of hemiplegia following Pick's original observation in 1898. It has been pointed out (Nielson 1938) that anosognosia is a general term, applied to disease as a whole, but that Babinski used it in a specific sense. By anosognosia Babinski meant unawareness

of hemiplegia and as such the term has remained. Cases have since been reported, however, in which, as Meige suggested in the discussion following Babinski's paper, the limbs and not the paralyses have passed out of consciousness. In its mildest form the disorder may merely be a periodic " forgetting " of a limb (Alajouanine et al. 1934, von Stockert 1934, Ives and Nielsen 1936), a delusion that can be corrected by persuasion and argument. In such cases the limb disappears from the attention rather than from consciousness. In other cases one whole side of the body may disappear from consciousness (Barkman 1925)—a negative condition (Koch and von Stockert 1935) to be distinguished from a positive feeling or delusion of absence of the side, such as was observed in 2 cases by Ives and Nielsen (1937). In most reported cases a period of disturbance of consciousness preceded the development of the anosognosia, but there are exceptions (Babinski 1918, and von Hagen and Ives 1937).

Where there existed true imperception of hemiplegia the paralysis was always on the left side, together with homonymous hemianopia. In the only 4 cases in which autopsy reports are available a lesion of the right optic thalamus was observed. Pick's case had chronic diffuse meningitis with softening in the right thalamus and first and second right temporal convolutions. Pötzl's (1924) second case revealed superficial softenings in the right parietal and occipital lobes with a large area of vascular necrosis in the right thalamus. In his first case there were left hemianæsthesia and in the second homonymous hemianopia. The case described by von Hagen and Ives showed left homonymous hemianopia, left hemiplegia and hemianæsthesia, unawareness of hemiplegia. At autopsy there were several metastatic cerebral abscesses, one involving the right thalamus, caudate nucleus, globus pallidus, internal capsule and adjacent structures. Thus, in genuine anosognosia (imperception of hemiplegia) the constant finding of a lesion in the right optic thalamus suggests that the trouble lies in the failure of sensory impulses from the paralysed side to reach consciousness.

In the second type of case—that in which there need be no hemiplegia and no unawareness of disease but in which there is periodic " forgetting " or absence from consciousness of a limb or of one side of the body—the lesion does not so constantly affect the thalamus. It is usually more superficially situated in the parietal cortex so that the disturbance is not merely one of non-perception of impulses. There is then a true distortion of the body scheme resulting from a lesion at a higher level. In the first of the 2 cases reported by Ives and Nielsen (1937) the causative lesion was an area of vascular softening in the right retrolenticular portion of the internal capsule partly involving the thalamus. The patient was aware of his paralysis (left hemiplegia) but denied that the paralysed limbs belonged to him ; he thought they belonged to the doctor. In their second case the patient similarly refused to acknowledge that his paretic left arm was really his own : " Someone is substituting this arm for my left arm," he repeatedly stated. At autopsy there was diffuse vascular softening of the right cerebral hemisphere. It involved the lenticular nucleus but not the thalamus.

CASE 1

An officer-cadet was admitted to a military hospital in May, 1940, complaining of severe occipital headache of sudden onset a few hours previously. Temperature 99° F., pulse-rate 90 per min. He showed neck rigidity, spinal tenderness, brisk knee- and ankle-jerks and a positive Kernig sign ; plantar responses were normal. Lumbar puncture produced a sterile blood-stained fluid. He remained fairly well for a week and further puncture indicated that there had been no fresh bleeding. Then signs of severe meningeal irritation developed, with bilateral extensor responses, extreme spinal rigidity and much headache. It was found necessary to tap him daily, for papilloedema rapidly developed with retinal hæmorrhages, recurrent coma and general deterioration. He lost flesh alarmingly and was gravely ill for several months. Unconscious periods occurred frequently and on a few occasions he ceased breathing. Artificial respiration was repeatedly employed and frequent lumbar puncture released deeply stained fluid under high pressure (360 mm.) of water. There was every indication of a constant seeping of blood from an intracranial aneurysm over a period of two months. Root

been good with high dosage. Finally, we grew yeast on a basis of soya-bean mash and fed it to these patients along with the medium on which it was grown. Even this had to be limited as to dosage, but good results were achieved in almost every case ; only in one or two were the results not as good as could have been wished.

Curiously enough, these patients showed few or no stigmata of dietary deficiency otherwise, again offering a contrast to Dr. Wilkinson's cases.

We learned, when in Stanley Camp, by devious ways, that many cases of serious nutritional eye defect had also occurred among the military internees on the Island. It seems likely that these would be of a similar type. One cannot help speculating on the ultimate outcome of these cases if left untreated or inadequately treated.

When they are ultimately released from internment Dr. Hargreaves and Dr. Yaroogsky-Erooga will undoubtedly publish their findings and I am sure the details will be of great interest, especially when compared with those of Dr. Wilkinson and Dr. Au King.

Hospital for Sick Children,   A. V. GREAVES.
    Toronto, Canada.

TRANSMISSION OF INFECTIVE HEPATITIS TO HUMAN VOLUNTEERS

EFFECT ON RHEUMATOID ARTHRITIS

SIR,—G. F. Still in 1897 and Wishart in 1903 remarked upon the relief of pain in patients with rheumatoid arthritis who developed spontaneous jaundice. Hench in America has more recently made the same observations in a large group of cases of rheumatism, and attempted to reproduce the effect by inducing artificial hyperbilirubinæmia by intravenous injection of bile-salts and bilirubin. Only slight transitory relief, which was not comparable with that produced by the spontaneous jaundice, resulted. Thompson and Wyatt, who originated the method used by Hench, obtained slightly more satisfactory results. Hanssen, who induced jaundice with 'Lactophenin,' also claimed transitory relief. There was however no reliable or reasonably safe method of inducing jaundice.

Though there have been reports from Germany of transmission of infective hepatitis to canaries and white mice, workers in other countries have failed to confirm these experiments, and because of the lack of a susceptible animal, human volunteers have been used in an attempt to obtain more information regarding causes and natural modes of transmission of communicable jaundice. Cameron (1943) has injected blood, and Voegt (1942) blood, urine and duodenal juice from infective hepatitis. Similar studies on the so-called homologous serum jaundice have been made by Findlay and Martin (1943) who inoculated nasal washings by the nasal route, and Oliphant, Gilliam and Larson (1943) and MacCallum and Bauer (1944) who inoculated icterogenic serum and tissue cultures of such serum subcutaneously and intranasally.

In the latter series (MacCallum and Bauer 1944) some volunteers who were suffering from rheumatoid arthritis were deliberately included. Pooled dried transfusion serum known to be icterogenic produced jaundice according to expectation and with beneficial effect on the arthritis. Patients with rheumatoid arthritis have been included in further investigations using materials from cases of infective hepatitis. The results obtained with these materials are tabulated below. Groups I to V have been under observation for 3–4 months, group VI for 7 weeks and group VII for 12 weeks.

The materials were collected from several individuals in the preicteric stage of infective hepatitis or within 24 hours of the appearance of jaundice ; they were stored at –20° C. for 7–10 days and pooled before use except in group VII where specimen (a) was kept 48 hours only at –20° C. and specimen (b) 24 hours at 0° C. before use. The material in the different groups was not from the same patients. The material used in groups V and VI was an ether-treated 20% saline suspension flavoured with vanillin.

Although frank jaundice resulted only when fæces or serum were used, the two subicteric cases which followed spraying of nose and throat with nasopharyngeal washings suggest that this material was also infectious. Further

Group	Infective hepatitis — Stage collected	Material	Route and dose (c.cm.)	Volunteers inoculated	Induced hepatitis — Positive	Induced hepatitis — Jaundice	Induced hepatitis — Incubation period (days)
I	1st day	Saline naso-pharyngeal washings	N.2·0 P 2·0	7	+2	0	24 & 28
II	" "	"	N.2·0 P 2·0	9	0	0	..
III	" "	Urine	N.2·0 P.2·0 O.5·0	19	0	0	..
IV	" "	(a) Serum pool from 2 individuals	S.1·25	4	0	3	64,75,92
		(b) " "	S.1·5	2	0	0	
V	24–72 hours after jaundice	(a) Pooled fæces from 2 individuals	N.2·0 P.2·0	6	0	0	..
		(b) "	N.2·0 P.2·0	6	0	0	..
		(c) Pool of (a) & (b)	N.2·0	2	0	2	27 & 31
VI	(a) Pre-icteric	Pooled fæces from 3 individuals	N.2·0 P.2·0	7	0	1	28 (approx.)
	(b) "	Pooled fæces from 2 individuals	N.2·0 P.2·0	5	0	0	..
VII	(a) Pre-icteric (b) 1st day jaundice	Nasopharyngeal washings	N.2·0				
		"	P.5·0	6	0	0	..

Route—N. and P. =sprayed into nose and pharynx respectively. O. =oral administration.   S. =Subcutaneous inoculation.
+ Positive =symptoms and/or rise in serum bilirubin but no jaundice.
Incubation is the number of days from inoculation to onset of symptoms or rise in serum bilirubin.

experiments are being carried out with nasopharyngeal washings, urine, fæces and blood collected earlier in the preicteric stage.

The arthritis of the 6 patients who developed jaundice was considerably improved. Jaundice was mild in all 6 cases, and the amelioration of arthritis was not directly proportionate to the rise in serum bilirubin.

This note is a preliminary announcement of work in its very early stages which was done under the auspices of the Medical Research Council's jaundice committee. We are greatly indebted to the volunteers and the numerous colleagues who have collaborated.

MRC Jaundice Committee,   F. O. MacCallum.
    Cambridge.   W. H. Bradley.

REFERENCES

Cameron, J. D. S. (1943) Quart. J. Med. 12, 139.
Findlay, G. M. and Martin, N. H. (1943) Lancet, i, 678.
Hanssen, P. (1942) Acta med. scand. 109, 493.
Hench, P. (1938) Brit. med. J. ii, 394 ; (1940) Med. clin. N. Amer. 24, 1209.
MacCallum, F. O. and Bauer, D. J. (1944) Lancet, i, 622.
Oliphant, J. W., Gilliam, A. G. and Larson, C. L. (1943) Publ. Hlth Rep., Wash. 53, 1233.
Still, G. F. (1897) Trans. R. med. chir. Soc. 80, 47.
Thompson, H. E. and Wyatt, B. L. (1937) J. Amer. med. Ass. 109, 1482.
Voegt, H. (1942) Münch. med. Wschr. 89, 76.

PHYSIOTHERAPISTS AND "RUBBERS"

SIR,—This letter is dictated by a debt which I have owed for over twenty years to an élite of physiotherapists. Misapprehension of the part these persons play, though natural to laymen in and out of Parliament, is less amusing or excusable when it affects ourselves. Yet I have found that quick informed appreciation of their many-sided work is limited—like speed in streams— to relatively narrow channels. Only a fractional percentage of surgeons and physicians could fail, we might suppose, to be apprised ; but everywhere one seems to meet this fractional per cent.

I thus was fortunate of late in finding someone with a view on this as welcome as the sight of an oasis. Sir Thomas Carey Evans, by his keen support, concurred in making possible that every patient in my wards should have the earliest chance of duly graded exercise : exercise in breathing before and after operation, exercise

THE LANCET]   PARA-AMINOSALICYLIC ACID IN THE TREATMENT OF TUBERCULOSIS   [JAN. 5, 1946 15

EFFECT OF 1·6 MG. SODIUM SALICYLATE ON THE OXYGEN
UPTAKE OF DIFFERENT PATHOGENIC AND NONPATHOGENIC
HUMAN AND BOVINE STRAINS OF THE TUBERCLE BACILLUS

Strain	Patho-genicity	Bovine or human strain	Culture medium	Age of culture (weeks)	Salicylate effect. Increase in $O_2\%$
H.W.	Path.	Human	Glyc. broth	5–6	72–157
H.W.	Path.	Human	Souton	3	82
H₃	Path.	Human	Souton	12	90
K₂	Path.	Bovine	Glyc. broth	12	38
R	Nonpath.	Human	Souton	12	0*
R	Nonpath.	Human	Glyc. broth	16	0
102	Nonpath.	Human	Glyc. broth	2–7	0
B.C.G.	Nonpath.	Bovine	Glyc. broth	2–3	0
B.C.G.	Nonpath.	Bovine	Souton	2–6	0

* Within the limits of about ± 5%.

It cannot as yet be decided whether benzoates and salicylates act as catalysers or as metabolites. If the latter
is the case it must be assumed that the pathogenic strains
can open the benzene ring in these compounds.

The differences found seem to open up new pathways
for studying the biochemistry of the pathogenicity of the
tubercle bacillus.

On the basis of the stimulative effect of benzoates
and salicylates more than 50 derivatives of these substances were investigated for their inhibitory effect on
the growth of tubercle bacilli (competitive enzyme
inhibition). Preliminary results of these experiments—
bacteriological as well as clinical—are presented in an
accompanying paper (Lehmann 1946) with special regard
to p-aminosalicylic acid as the most effective inhibitor.

REFERENCES

Bernheim, F. (1941) J. Bact. 41, 387.
Dieckmann, H., Mohr, H. (1933), Zbl. Bakt. 129, 185.
Lehmann, J. (1946) Lancet, i, 15.
Loebel, R. O., Shorr, E., Richardson, H. B. (1933) J. Bact. 26, 167.
Nakamura, T. (1938) Tohuku J. exp. Med. 34, 231.

Preliminary Communication

PARA-AMINOSALICYLIC ACID IN THE TREATMENT OF TUBERCULOSIS

IN 1940 Bernheim [1] showed that salicylic (2-hydroxy-
benzoic) acid and benzoic acid increase the oxygen
consumption and carbon-dioxide production of the
tubercle bacillus, whereas the homologues 3- and 4-
hydroxybenzoic acid were inactive. It was concluded
that salicylic and benzoic acids were oxidised as metabolites and that similar chemical configurations possibly
play a part in the metabolism of the bacillus.

On the basis of these experiments I have investigated
more than 50 derivatives of benzoic acid with the purpose
of finding a substance possessing bacteriostatic properties
against the tubercle bacillus. The substances were
synthesised by K. G. Rosdahl, of Ferrosan Co., Malmö.
An attenuated bovine strain (B.C.G.) grown on Souton's
medium was used for the experiments. The substances
investigated were added to the medium in concentrations from 10^{-2} to 10^{-6} mol. The area, or the dry weight,
of the bacilli was determined when the surface of the
control flasks (100 ml. medium in 250 ml. flasks) was
covered with a somewhat packed film of the bacilli—
i.e., after 12–20 days.

The most active substance found was 4-aminosalicylic
acid (p-aminosalicylic acid) producing an inhibition of
50–75% in a concentration of 10^{-5} mol. (1 in 650,000 or
0·15 mg. per 100 c.cm.). The bacteriostatic effect was
completely abolished if the amino group was placed in
position 3 or 5, or if its place was taken by NO_2. Substitutions in the 4-amino group (by CH_3 or stearic acid)
reduced the bacteriostatic effect only slightly or not
at all. If the hydroxy group in the 2- position was
replaced by CH_3 activity was retained, but not if it was
replaced by NH_2 or Cl. Substitutions in the hydroxy

1. Bernheim, F. Science, 1940, 92, 204.

group decreased the activity considerably. If the
hydroxy group was placed in position 3 instead of 2
the effect was diminished. If the carboxy group was
replaced by a sulphonic acid group the activity was
abolished. Substitutions in the carboxy group (methyl,
ethyl, and furfuranylanhydride) changed the activity
only slightly. Double molecules of 4-aminosalicylic
acid linked together at position 3 were as effective as
4-aminosalicylic acid but highly toxic to animals.

Animal experiments showed that 4-aminosalicylic acid
was not toxic to rats when given for 1–2 months in a
concentration of 5% in a synthetic food. A blood
concentration of 3–7 mg. of free aminosalicylic acid
per 100 c.cm. was found when analysed by Ehrlich's
dimethylaminobenzaldehyde reagent. Guineapigs were
more sensitive as they showed a decrease in appetite
and in growth. No changes in the blood-cells or hæmoglobin were observed either in the rats or in the guinea-
pigs. The substance could be administered by mouth,

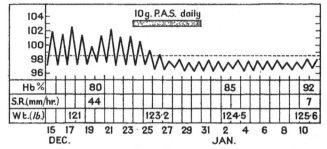

Fig. 1—Chart in case 1, showing effect of third course of para-
aminosalicylic acid.

subcutaneously, intramuscularly, or intravenously. The
treatment of experimental tuberculosis in guineapigs
and rats is in progress.

Clinical trial.—The treatment of tuberculosis in man
was started parallel with the animal experiments.
Tuberculous abscesses after thoracoplasty up to 50–60 ml.
in volume have been treated daily with a neutral 10%
solution of p-aminosalicylic acid and showed healing
after some months even when they had remained
unchanged for 3–6 months before treatment. It has been
given by mouth to 20 patients since March, 1944, at the
Renstroemska Sanatorium in Gothenburg (Superintendent Dr. G. Vallentin). A blood concentration of
2–7 mg. per 100 c.cm. was achieved by giving 10–15 g. a
day. Periods of 8 days' treatment were followed by
free intervals of 8 days. It is too early to follow up
the results. In many cases, however, a prompt fall in
temperature—temporary or permanent—coincided with
the periods of treatment and was accompanied by

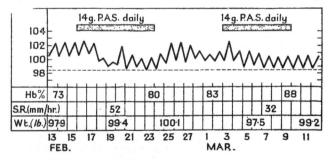

Fig. 2—Chart in case 2.

improvement in the patient's general condition as indicated
by a gain in appetite and weight, an increase in the red
cells and hæmoglobin and a decrease in the erythrocyte
sedimentation-rate.

Two illustrative cases follow.

CASE 1.—A woman, aged 24. Onset of tuberculosis in
May–June, 1944. X-ray examination on July 3, 1944, showed
an acute general dissemination of cloudy processes in both
lungs. Remittent fever 97·5°–101·5° F from July 3 to
Nov. 26, when treatment with p-aminosalicylic acid (P.A.S.)
was given in three periods with concomitant falls in temperature; the last period is illustrated in fig. 1. Normal
temperature has been maintained up to the present since this

treatment. Artificial pneumothorax instituted on March 7, 1945, on the right side for an apical cavity ½–1 in. in diameter.

CASE 2.—A man, aged 35. Bilateral pleural effusion; onset June, 1944. Guineapig test positive on the exudate from both sides. No manifest tuberculosis in the lungs. P.A.S. treatment started Feb. 16, 1945, followed by general improvement (fig. 2). Gain in weight 15½ lb. in two months.

None of the usual effects of salicylates (sweats, ear symptoms) were observed even with a high dosage of *p*-aminosalicylic acid (15 g. daily). The fall in temperature was therefore thought not to be due to a salicylate effect.

The work here recorded was done at the Sahlgrenska Hospital, at the Research Laboratories of the Ferrosan Co. at Malmö, and at the Renstroemska Sanatorium, Gothenburg.

JÖRGEN LEHMANN,
Sahlgrenska Hospital, Gothenburg, Sweden.

Medical Societies

ROYAL SOCIETY OF TROPICAL MEDICINE AND HYGIENE

AT a meeting of the society on Dec. 13 with Dr. C. M. WENYON, F.R.S., the president, in the chair, a discussion on the

Teaching of Tropical Medicine

was opened by Dr. L. E. NAPIER, who said that in the United States of America a serious attempt is being made both to improve the teaching of the subject to the undergraduate and also to develop its postgraduate teaching. In Great Britain, however, tropical medicine appears to have been relegated to the place of a specialty about which the general practitioner need know nothing and with which the ordinary student need not be burdened. These shortcomings require remedying urgently. To avoid overloading the undergraduate curriculum the student should be introduced in his premedical years to selected parasites of man, and the essential clinical diagnostic methods used in tropical medicine should be included in the teaching of clinical pathology. This would leave the pathology, symptomatology, and therapeutics of important tropical diseases to be taught in the systematic lectures on medicine and in the clinical departments as the occasion arose. At this stage it seems entirely wrong to segregate tropical medicine as it has been segregated in the past and to teach the student virtually nothing of the pathology, symptomatology, and therapeutics of tropical diseases. Tropical diseases furthermore could provide excellent examples for teaching the general principles of preventive medicine. Scarcity of clinical material must not be used as an excuse for avoiding clinical teaching ; the student of general medicine fails to see examples of many diseases which he will be expected to diagnose and treat later in his practice. Much can be done by the use of lantern slides and cinema films. The future will also bring an increasing number of tropical diseases among those whom the war has taken to the tropics, while rapid air transport may allow cases of tropical disease to enter the country unsuspected during the incubation period. Interest in tropical medicine must be fostered by all means. Short-term exchanges of personnel, research-workers, and teachers between this country and the tropics should be encouraged. As an artificial way of maintaining interest in tropical diseases examining bodies should demand a sound knowledge of the commoner tropical diseases. Turning to postgraduate teaching Dr. Napier said there are few if any places in the world where one can see a better selection of tropical diseases than in London, but owing to the war there is at present no suitable hospital where the available clinical material can be collected ; a crying need today is for a " tropical medical centre." Special provision should be made for those who are proposing to specialise in tropical hygiene. Dr. Napier ended by emphasising the necessity for making the undergraduate and his teachers conscious of the existence of tropical diseases, and for the early establishment of a hospital in London that would act as a centre for teaching and research in tropical medicine ; meanwhile the society should prepare a memorandum on the teaching of tropical medicine and try to obtain representation on all committees considering the matter.

Sir PHILIP MANSON-BAHR thought that the medical student's burdens should be not increased. but agreed that more emphasis should be laid in the premedical studies on the parasites associated with disease in man. He disagreed with the statement that tropical medicine is entirely neglected in the present undergraduate curriculum, pointing out that in practically every medical school in London lectures on tropical diseases are already given to the undergraduate, and that in the examinations of the last few years questions on the more important diseases have always been included. In the postgraduate courses it is also necessary to avoid overloading the curriculum. The best days of teaching tropical medicine were those when the tropical school was a compact self-contained unit, with the laboratory and clinical work closely linked ; a plethora of visiting lecturers, however specialised their knowledge, leads to overlapping and overloading of the curriculum. In teaching tropical medicine differential diagnosis is most important, and the practical value of microscopy cannot be overstressed. Any difficulty of obtaining clinical material would largely be overcome if the general hospitals were more willing to transfer tropical cases to a tropical hospital for teaching purposes.

Prof. R. M. GORDON also agreed that the course in zoology should include the simpler parasitology of man, and that the teaching of tropical medicine should be extended, especially in the undergraduate's final year. The graduate student would then require an amplification of his general knowledge, and such teaching would be well covered by the present D.T.M. & H. course, which does not make a specialist but only a good practitioner for the tropics. He did not believe that the situation in which tropical medicine finds itself in London now that the war is over necessarily means that the subject is in danger throughout the country ; the Liverpool School flourished during the war and is confident of its own future. The dearth of living material in this country for the teaching of parasitology and entomology necessitates the artificial maintenance of strains. This involves much labour, and loss of a strain is a disaster unless it is maintained in more than one place ; some institution, such as the Wellcome Laboratories of Tropical Medicine, should interest itself in this matter. The Colonial Office and all firms operating in the tropics should insist on a diploma in tropical medicine for their medical officers.

Dr. G. MACDONALD supported broadening the undergraduate curriculum to include more instruction in tropical medicine. He did not admit that the teaching of tropical medicine in London is in a parlous state, but he urged the restoration of facilities lost directly owing to the war and deplored that, outside the special group of those intimately concerned with tropical medicine, interest in the subject has been lost, even the writers of the Goodenough report failing to consider the matter seriously. There must be a centre of clinical research in London to replace that lost in the war, but on a better and more fully equipped scale, and it should coöperate with the existing School of Tropical Medicine as now constituted. Postgraduate teaching in tropical medicine should round off a general medical education and fit the student to practise medicine in the tropics, rather than create a specialist ; the specialist requires, in addition to special knowledge of tropical diseases, a high qualification in general clinical medicine. Similarly those specialising in tropical hygiene should hold a D.P.H. as a basis, supplemented by a D.T.M. & H. and experience overseas before taking up independent work in tropical hygiene. The society should form a policy committee to examine and foster the development, teaching, and standards required in tropical medicine and hygiene.

Lieut.-Colonel VERE HODGE, while agreeing that the establishment of an Imperial centre for tropical medicine should be the ultimate object, thought that immediate steps are required to deal with the large numbers of repatriates who may be returning with latent tropical infections ; after a long absence from home these persons will not want to be sequestrated in special centres, and this will necessitate a number of tropical units throughout the country. The limitations of teaching tropical medicine in this country will make it necessary to have subsidiary centres abroad, but even short courses in this country would give practitioners going abroad an advantage. Three types of teaching in tropical medicine are

THROMBOSIS
EARLY DIAGNOSIS AND ABORTIVE TREATMENT WITH HEPARIN

GUNNAR BAUER
M.D.

From the Mariestad Hospital, Mariestad, Sweden

BY earlier diagnosis and the use of anticoagulants it should be possible to reduce the mortality from thrombosis of deep veins and consequent pulmonary embolism, which has been stationary for many decades.

It was long believed that thrombosis usually originates in the large pelvic veins or in the upper part of the femoral veins. Of late years, however, it has been shown by many workers that it often starts in the veins of the lower leg. My own investigations have led me to conclude that it almost always arises in the deep veins of the lower leg, and only in about 3% of cases in the thigh or pelvis.

In these studies (Bauer 1940, 1942) I used phlebography. The normal anatomy of the venous channels of the leg was first investigated in over 100 subjects, and fig. 1 is a schematic drawing from the X-ray pictures obtained. Anatomical studies showed that the double fibular vein is by far the most important blood channel from the muscles of the lower leg. In normal phlebograms this vein is seen to be well filled with contrast medium ; but when a thrombus is developing in the lower leg the blood containing contrast fluid is unable to flow through the vein, which is no longer visible on radiography (figs. 2 and 5). This opens up the prospect of being able to detect an incipient deep thrombosis at a very early stage.

From combined phlebographic and clinical examination of 150 patients with fresh thrombosis I have reached the following conclusions, since confirmed by Hellsten (1942).

The process begins with formation of a thrombus, for some unknown reason, in a muscle vein. This thrombus projects into the lumen of one of the large venous trunks of the lower leg, and extends through it in the direction of the blood-stream. Even this first, embryonic, stage can be demonstrated in a phlebogram, though it will probably evade diagnosis by other methods.

During the next stage the large veins of the lower leg are progressively filled ; the thrombus gradually occludes the entire lumen and becomes attached to the vessel wall. Concurrently there is longitudinal growth up the femoral vein, which will sooner or later contain, freely waving in the blood-stream, an eel-like formation 40–50 cm. long, dark red in colour, and with a slippery surface. The thrombus forms, as it were, a cast of the lumen of the large vein, though it does not completely occlude it ; the wall of the vein is as yet not involved in any way, and the thrombus is only anchored at its lowermost end, far down in the lower leg. This condition, which entails great risk of embolism, appears to be commoner than was formerly supposed, and cannot be diagnosed by the ordinary clinical methods ; but phlebography helps to detect it.

The waving thrombus, by breaking off at some point or other and floating up towards the heart, may give rise to an embolus. Much more often, however, it grows in thickness, blocks the femoral vein, begins to involve the endothelium, and becomes firmly attached to the vessel wall along its whole length. A typical phlegmasia alba dolens then arises. Phlebography now gives the kind of picture represented in figs. 3 and 6.

Often the thrombosing process extends still further, and invades the pelvic veins ; but there may be no prominent clinical evidence of its extension unless this goes so far as to occlude veins essential to life such as the renal and hepatic veins. Not infrequently, too, the process becomes bilateral ; but phlebographic evidence suggests that in these cases thrombosis in the second leg always begins in its lower part.

The various stages after the thrombosis has become manifest clinically are well known. The temperature usually falls after a few weeks, and it has been customary to let patients get up when they have been fever-free for about a fortnight. For those who survive, the illness lasts on an average 6–7 weeks. After a further period of convalescence, patients have been allowed to leave hospital, with one or both legs still swollen ; and most of them are eventually able to resume their work.

It is now known, however, that even then the disease is not overcome. On the contrary, it passes into a *chronic* stage, and most of those who have suffered from thrombosis have to look forward to serious after-effects. Of these sequelæ our knowledge is regrettably deficient ; but Homans (1939) suggested that chronic ulcers on the lower leg are sometimes the result of deep thrombosis earlier, and Birger (1941) thought that at least a third of such ulcers are caused by a pre-existent thrombotic condition.

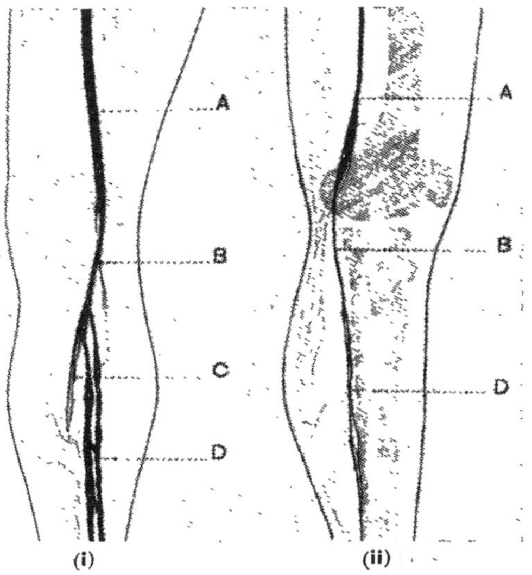

My phlebographic studies (Bauer 1942) show that once the deep veins of the leg have been destroyed by thrombosis, recanalisation hardly ever occurs. For the

Fig. 1—Normal phlebogram. (i) Postero-anterior view. (ii) Lateral view. A, femoral vein ; B, popliteal vein ; C, posterior tibial vein ; D, fibular vein.

rest of the patient's life the venous blood from the lower leg is drained through an accessory system of subcutaneous veins, usually with the great saphenous vein acting as the chief channel of return (fig. 3). So long as these superficial veins are intact they can transport the blood satisfactorily. But a mild state of venous stasis is always present, causing chronic œdema in the lower leg. Through constant overloading, the superficial veins become distended and tortuous, and the valves defective (fig. 4). Drainage deteriorates, venous stasis is accentuated, and œdema of the lower leg steadily increases, with eventual appearance of leathery indurative lesions.

In the centre of the induration, tissue disintegration usually takes place after two or three years, and a leg ulcer is formed. These ulcers, which have hitherto been attributed to varices, are the result, I believe, in 80–90% of cases, of an earlier deep thrombosis. The term "varicose ulcer" should be changed to "post-thrombotic ulcer."

Of 100 patients showing late thrombosis, all, from the beginning, had swelling of the leg, which if anything increased as the years passed. Five years after the acute stage of the disease 45 had indurative lesions on the lower leg ; after ten years 72 showed these changes ; and later the number rose to 91. Leg ulcers broke out in 20 patients during the first five years, and in 52 within ten years, and finally 79 had open sores.

they are not encapsuled—the cells infiltrating slightly at the sites from which they arise. They are therefore not true neoplasms, and not analogous to uterine fibromyomas; and it seems questionable, at least, whether they have any right to retain their provisional title of tumours, even if that title is ascribed to them only by implication. This does not of course exclude the possibility that human fibromyomas may yet be found to be due to a hormonal derangement; but in that case the uterine fibroids would also lose their status in pathology as tumours and would become hormone-conditioned hyperplasias like the experimental hyperplasias of the pituitary which were once thought to be adenomas.

The discovery of these curious focal fibrous proliferations in guineapigs has been valuable in several ways. It suggested a possible cause of uterine fibroids that had not been thought of; it can be used in demonstrating what is and what is not a true tumour; and it provides in the guineapig a kind of indicator of hormone action and antagonisms. As regards these various uses, it must be admitted that we do not yet know what is the cause of uterine fibroids; and, while it is known that hyperplasias may become converted into true neoplastic tissue, there is no evidence of this happening in the guineapig lesion. As an indicator of action and reaction of the sex hormones of the guineapig these fibrous proliferations enable ingenious experiments to be done, and Professor LIPSCHUTZ in his lectures related a remarkable series. It is of course too early to predict what further knowledge this technique may reveal.

Annotations

A MORAL PROBLEM

NUREMBERG is to be followed by further trials, and among the first to answer charges of atrocious conduct will be some doctors who are said to have misused human beings in scientific experiments. The sort of crimes of which they are accused are described in a collection of narratives by medical survivors from internment camps in Czechoslovakia [1]; and the stories there told suggest a degree of degeneration which few would have thought possible in Europe. Having accepted the Nazi view that extermination of Jews and other enemies was necessary and legitimate, a number of doctors in concentration camps assisted in destroying these lives. From this it was but a step to persuade themselves that the men and women doomed to death should previously be employed as experimental material: if they were killed under controlled conditions—for example, by measured exposure to cold—data could be obtained which might later save the life of a good German soldier. Why should not science, and German arms, make use of this unusual opportunity?

From time to time during the past year or two we have been invited to publish or summarise, for the use of investigators, detailed reports of lethal experiments performed by Germans. None of these has seemed to us, on its merits, worth publicity; for the tests were generally ill conceived and ill conducted and the results no more informative than those already secured by other means. But supposing facts of real value to medicine were still to emerge from the records of the experiments —should they be published or not?

Opinion on this difficult ethical question is divided. Those who favour publication say that the crime has been committed, and that our duty both to the victims and to their surviving friends is to see that all possible advantage is gained from their sufferings, so that they shall not have suffered wholly in vain. If some good can come out of this horror, let it come. Those who would refuse publication argue, on the other hand, that the crime has been committed and that we should make ourselves accessories if we were to profit by it in any way. To do so, they believe, would make it slightly easier for someone in the future to justify another crime of the same kind; and the value of medical progress is as nothing weighed against the harm done to human values by promoting tolerance to systematic murder.

The problem was presented in simple form by a member of our profession in a novel published before the war.[2] Here a hospital doctor kills a patient so as to get information required in his researches—information which proves in fact to be of no small interest and value. After his suicide the hospital's medical committee faces the question whether this information is to be used. "May I remind you," says the chairman, "that our duty to our neighbour, our fellow man, comes before even our interest in science?"; and the papers are solemnly burnt. Now that the same problem may arise in real life, ought we to burn the papers? Or is this a case in which we should take the moral risk eternally involved in trying to extract good from evil?

POTASSIUM AND PARALYSIS

THE association of low serum-potassium with attacks of familial periodic paralysis has been recognised for some years, but there has been a conspicuous absence of authentic reports of paralysis associated with low serum-potassium in other conditions. An example has now been reported by Holler [1] in a diabetic girl of 18 years, admitted to hospital in coma. After the administration of 800 units of insulin in twenty-one hours ketosis was overcome, but respiratory paralysis supervened, so severe that the patient had to be put into a Drinker apparatus. Blood for serum-potassium was taken, but without waiting for the result 1.5 g. of potassium chloride was given intravenously, with great clinical improvement, the diaphragm now moving freely. The serum-potassium report was 2.5 m.Eq. per litre (9.75 mg. per 100 ml.) instead of the normal value of 5 m.Eq. After her removal from the Drinker apparatus the girl's respiratory difficulty recurred and was again relieved by potassium. On her complete recovery from all symptoms five days later her serum-potassium was found to be 5.07 m.Eq. per litre.

Two years ago Brown and colleagues [2] recorded 3 cases of chronic nephritis in which attacks of paralysis occurred spontaneously and were relieved by potassium administration, but the analytical data were somewhat scanty. Though at the time the condition did not seem so well substantiated as in the report of Holler it seems probable that a similar syndrome was involved. On the other hand, as Allott and McArdle [3] pointed out, alkalosis from pyloric stenosis is often accompanied by extremely low serum-potassium levels, without any evidence of paralysis. The syndrome of low serum-potassium with alkalosis has been reported in Cushing's syndrome by Willson and colleagues,[4] and very low serum-potassium levels are observed after testosterone treatment; in both these conditions there is no paralysis.

1. Medical Science Abused: German Medical Science as Practised in Concentration Camps and in the so-called Protectorate. Reported by Czechoslovak Doctors. Prague: Orbis. 1946. Pp. 92.

2. Murder in Hospital. By "Josephine Bell." Penguin Books. 1941.

1. Holler, J. W. J. Amer. med. Ass. 1946, 131, 1186.
2. Brown, M. R., Currens, J. H., Marchand, J. F. Ibid, 1944, 124, 515.
3. Allott, E. N., McArdle, B. Clin. Sci. 1938, 3, 229.
4. Willson, D. M., Power, M. H., Kepler, E. J. J. clin. Invest. 1940, 19, 701.

THE LANCET]

ORIGINAL ARTICLES

[MARCH 8, 1947

SPONTANEOUS COMPRESSION OF BOTH MEDIAN NERVES IN THE CARPAL TUNNEL

SIX CASES TREATED SURGICALLY

W. Russell Brain
D.M. Oxfd, F.R.C.P.
PHYSICIAN TO THE LONDON
HOSPITAL AND THE MAIDA
VALE HOSPITAL

A. Dickson Wright
M.S. Lond., F.R.C.S.
SURGEON TO ST. MARY'S
HOSPITAL AND THE MAIDA
VALE HOSPITAL

Marcia Wilkinson
B.M. Oxfd, M.R.C.P.
MEDICAL REGISTRAR AT THE MAIDA VALE HOSPITAL FOR
NERVOUS DISEASES

In this paper we describe 6 patients, all middle-aged or elderly women, who suffered from bilateral median neuritis due to compression of the nerves under the transverse carpal ligament at the wrist. They were treated by surgical division of the ligament. This operation appears to have been performed on only three occasions previously (Woltman 1941, Zachary 1945), and in those three patients the compression of the nerves was due to fracture or arthritis. In our 6 patients the compression arose spontaneously, but unaccustomed manual work may have helped to cause it. We have seen 8 other patients in whom the lesion has not yet been verified. Most of these add no fresh features, but allusion will be made to one, in whom the compression was secondary to fracture of the scaphoids and osteo-arthritis. The syndrome presents several points of interest in relation, particularly, to its pathogenesis, to the symptoms of slow compression of a mixed peripheral nerve, and to the diagnosis of partial thenar atrophy.

PREVIOUS OBSERVATIONS

Ramsay Hunt (1909, 1911, 1914) drew attention to syndromes which he described as "the thenar and hypothenar types of neural atrophy of the hand." The hypothenar type, which he ascribed to compression of the deep branch of the ulnar nerve, does not concern us further. He reported (1911) three examples of the thenar type. In two the wasting was bilateral, in the third unilateral. The limitation of the wasting to the abductor pollicis brevis, the opponens pollicis, and the outer head of the flexor brevis pollicis, together with the absence of sensory loss, led Hunt to place the lesion, hypothetically, in the thenar branch of the median nerve, which he supposed to be compressed where it passed over the palmar border of the transverse carpal ligament. Later (1914), however, he attributed the paralysis to a lesion of the thenar branch beneath the ligament. Marie and Foix (1912) reported ten examples of "isolated non-progressive atrophy of the small muscles of the hand," with four necropsies ; but in only two of their patients was the wasting limited to the thenar eminence, and these were not among those on whom a pathological examination was made. Marie and Foix concluded that the lesion was in the spinal cord and was a localised destruction of anterior-horn cells, mainly of the 8th cervical segment.

A year later, however, Marie and Foix (1913) reported a case in which the lesion was in the median nerve.

Their patient was a woman, aged 80, admitted to hospital with a cerebral vascular lesion and found to have also bilateral wasting of the thenar eminences. Unfortunately, sensory testing was impossible.

Outside the central nervous system there was no lesion except in the median nerves, which showed, immediately above the transverse carpal ligament, a thick and firm nodular swelling or neuroma, while beneath the ligament there was a narrowing due to a "strangulation" which contrasted with the swelling above.

Microscopically the swelling was characterised by great overgrowth of interfascicular and intrafascicular fibrous tissue, with destruction of myelin sheaths. At the level of the ligament there was still much intrafascicular fibrosis, but it was less marked than above. Weigert-Pal stain showed that the myelin sheaths diminished progressively from the upper limit of the neuroma and disappeared at the level of the ligament.

It was clear that the thenar atrophy in this case was due to an interstitial neuritis at the level of the ligament, causing a strangulation of the nerve beneath the ligament and a neuroma above it.

Brouwer (1920) reported 14 cases. His first 4 patients were tailors ; 2 of his female patients did much washing, and 3 had arthritis. Brouwer emphasised the importance of occupation, and considered that the thenar muscles, being of recent phylogenetic development, were especially liable to undergo degeneration as a result of trauma.

Harris (1926) described wasting of the thenar muscles due to neuritis of the median nerve caused by intermittent pressure on the ball of the thumb by an instrument such as a trowel-handle or a scrubbing brush. He also mentioned wasting of the abductor and opponens pollicis as a result of motor neuritis secondary to arthritis of the trapezio-metacarpal joint at the root of the thumb.

Lhermitte and de Massary (1930) reported a case of senile non-progressive thenar atrophy, without sensory loss, associated with an atrophy of the posterolateral group of cells in the anterior horn of the 6th cervical segment of the spinal cord on the affected side.

Dorndorf (1931) reported 16 cases of isolated paralysis of the ball of the thumb. All his patients were women at or near the menopause. He was inclined to attribute the disorder to ischæmia, without reaching a conclusion about the site of the lesion. If it were in the median nerve, he thought the absence of sensory loss must be attributed to a higher resistance of sensory fibres or to a selective damage to the motor fibres.

Wartenberg (1939) reported 7 cases of "partial thenar atrophy." His paper included an anatomical report on the muscular branch of the median nerve to the thenar eminence by Saunders, who has found that this branch arises independently from the volar aspect of the median nerve beneath the middle of the transverse carpal ligament. It then proceeds distally beneath the ligament to its distal border, to pass through a definite canal in the lateral attachment of the ligament to the trapezium. After this it is reflected to pursue a recurrent course to its division to supply the individual muscles. In this part of its course the position of the nerve is variable in its relation to the flexor brevis muscle. Winckler (1930) has reported a case in which the thenar branch actually pierced the anterior carpal ligament. Wartenberg observes that these facts show that the thenar branches of the median nerve may be so unfavourably placed in a normal person as to be subject to trauma by the ordinary use of the hand. Nevertheless he concludes that the evidence that such is the cause of the thenar atrophy is unconvincing. The occurrence in some patients of paræsthesiæ not necessarily confined to the distribution of the median nerve suggests the presence of some unknown nocuous factor to which Wartenberg supposes the thenar muscles to be specially susceptible owing to their late development in the evolution of man.

Moersch (1938), who reported another case, accepted Hunt's view that the motor branch was injured as it passed over the distal edge of the anterior carpal ligament.

Woltman (1941) reported 2 cases of median neuritis with both motor and sensory symptoms. The first patient had acromegaly, and her hands eventually improved after X-ray treatment of the pituitary. The second patient had unilateral median neuritis, secondary to arthritis of the wrist, with motor, sensory, and trophic symptoms which disappeared after section of the transverse carpal ligament.

Zachary (1945) reported 2 cases similar to the last. His first patient had bilateral motor and sensory symp-

H

TWO ESSAYS ON
THE PRACTICE OF MEDICINE

ROBERT PLATT

M.D. Sheff., F.R.C.P.

PROFESSOR OF MEDICINE, MANCHESTER UNIVERSITY

IT has seemed to me for a long time that good doctors differ from bad ones in two major respects. The time they devote to history-taking and their ability to interpret a history correctly is the first. The second is their ability to formulate a plan of treatment. I have written down my thoughts on these two subjects in the form of two short essays.

On History-taking

I know that I am not alone in thinking that history-taking is the greatest art in medicine. Generations of clinical teachers have acknowledged its importance and have tried to pass on the art to their pupils. Yet there are teachers, doctors, and students who still fail to appreciate its major place in diagnosis.

Many physicians select for their ward teaching cases with good physical signs and reject or pass over the cases with a good history and no signs at all. In the outpatient department they allot cases to their clinical clerks so that in effect the clerks are doing the same in that department as they do in the wards. In this way it is possible for a medical student to go through his whole course without ever hearing a patient interrogated *ab initio* by an expert clinician.

My students have to understand that they come to the outpatient department to learn the art of consultation, and above all to hear me taking case-histories. After the history has been taken, we discuss the provisional or possible diagnosis *before* examining the patient.

There are some who may regard this procedure with astonishment if not with horror, but it is really only an illustration of the process whereby all good doctors arrive at a diagnosis. It is quite impossible for an intelligent physician to take a history without diagnostic possibilities being presented to his mind. Far more mistakes are made by putting too much significance upon doubtful physical signs and neglecting the clear indications of the history than by the opposite process. After the examination we reconsider the diagnosis in the light of our further findings.

There is a special reason why the value of history taking needs to be emphasised today. We are embarking upon a National Health Service in which laboratory facilities will be freely available for the first time to ordinary patients in general practice. The practitioner is sometimes under the illusion that the consultant's work is relatively easy—he has the resources of the laboratory and the X-ray department at his disposal and has only to set the machine in operation for the correct diagnosis to be produced for him. The consultant of experience knows full well that it is not so. He knows how wasteful and misleading the ancillary services may prove if due care has not been given to the initial examination of the patient and above all to the history. If laboratory and X-ray services are to be intelligently used, history-taking must become more, not less, important and it is a task which in difficult cases can never be delegated.

AN INQUIRY

In order to emphasise the importance of history-taking, I have recently in my outpatient department noted the provisional diagnosis after taking the history ; the diagnosis after examination ; and the final diagnosis after all investigations were carried out, the patient being admitted to hospital if necessary. These diagnoses I have recorded in 100 consecutive cases, but I have of course only used cases presenting a diagnostic problem.

Cases sent solely for treatment, where a full diagnosis had already been made, were not included, neither were those in which the doctor's letter supplied foreknowledge of a physical sign of major importance, such as significant hypertension.

Most doctors send patients to the outpatient department with only a brief outline of the main complaint, and all such cases were suitable for the inquiry. The results are as follows :

The diagnosis reached after history-taking alone was unchanged by examination or investigation in 68 cases out of 100. For example :

Diagnosis after history : bronchiectasis.
Examination : basal râles.
X ray (bronchogram) : bronchiectasis.

In addition to these 68 cases, the diagnosis after history-taking was *substantially* correct in another 6. For example :

Provisional diagnosis : rheumatic heart disease with early failure.
After examination : mitral stenosis with early failure.

In a further 8 cases, the provisional diagnosis was correct, but examination and investigation contributed important findings to the final diagnosis, unsuspected during the history-taking. For example :

Provisional diagnosis : osteo-arthritis of spine.
After examination : the same plus glycosuria.
After investigation : osteo-arthritis of the spine plus diabetes.

In 1 case the provisional diagnosis was correct, but examination was misleading, and a change of diagnosis was made which turned out to be wrong, the sequence being duodenal ulcer ; gallstones ; and (after two X rays) duodenal ulcer.

In 12 cases no provisional diagnosis could be arrived at after taking the history—only a number of vague possibilities presented themselves. Examination provided the clue in 5, investigation in another 5, and the remaining 2 were still vague at the end of the diagnostic process.

In 5 the provisional diagnosis was frankly wrong and had to be amended—in 2 cases by the examination and in 3 after further investigation. For example :

Provisional diagnosis : cervical root pain.
After examination : the same.
After X ray : pulmonary tuberculosis. (Re-examination failed to show physical signs but the possibility should have been considered before it was revealed by X ray.)

COMMENT

Before attempting to assess the significance of these results, we must bear several things in mind.

The first is that history-taking comes first in the diagnostic sequence. There is no intention of belittling the importance of examination. If examination came *before* history-taking, the results might be equally striking, but no sane physician works in that order.

Secondly, what we call history-taking really takes into account much more than the statements of the patient. We do not take histories with our eyes shut. We know how old the patient is; how he walks into the room, whether he is pale or flushed, thin or fat, healthy looking or cachectic, and in some cases we may know a great deal more, that he has a facial paralysis for instance or a tremor of the hands. All this is observed before the provisional diagnosis is made.

Thirdly, it must be emphasised that the diagnosis made after history-taking is in any case only provisional, and requires confirmation before any competent physician would act upon it. One would not give insulin on a history of thirst and polyuria, nor liver extract upon breathlessness, pallor, and paræsthesia. Again let it be emphasised that no case is being made out for neglect of diagnostic care and precision. On the contrary, the claim is put forward that because history-taking will lead to the right diagnosis in so many cases, it is an art to be acquired, taught, and constantly exercised, and never on any account to be neglected whatever may be the facilities available for investigation.

Finally, let it be remembered that these cases were all diagnostic problems sent for solution, and seen by me for the first time, and that the histories were taken not in the leisured atmosphere of the consulting-room but in a busy outpatient department in the presence of numerous students. With some help in routine examinations (blood-pressures, reflexes, &c.) the average time spent on each patient is unfortunately less than twenty minutes and this includes teaching and the dictation of brief notes.

On Therapeutics

How many doctors today think that they have the modern outlook in therapeutics because they treat sore throats with penicillin lozenges and prescribe stilbœstrol for menopausal flushing ? And how many show their complete misunderstanding of all that modern therapy implies by prescribing vitamin B₁ for sciatica, by giving digitalis in inadequate doses to the wrong patients, and by retaining a belief in expectorant mixtures, not pausing to consider whether their results are due to the treatment prescribed, to its psychological effect, or to spontaneous recovery ?

The new therapy, instead of being hailed as a welcome revolution in medicine, has simply been looked upon as an addition to knowledge, in no way modifying the use of the older remedies. In this year of 1947, I read in the examination paper of a final-year student the words " diuretics such as pot. cit. or mersalyl," as if these were equivalent. It is like saying : " The journey can be made by stage-coach or by aeroplane." And from two current textbooks I cull the following information :

(In angina pectoris) " the daily bath should be advised to keep the skin active " (no comment).
(In acute nephritis) " diuretics should not be used *at least until diuresis is established* " (italics mine).

In other words, if you use a drug be sure to use it at such a time and in such a way that you will be quite ignorant of its value and almost certain to deceive yourself as to its efficacy. So long as that is the teaching in therapeutics from the writers of textbooks, we cannot expect rational therapy from the majority of the profession.

We, the teachers of medicine, are often criticised, and often deservedly, for not applying ourselves sufficiently to the problems which the student will later meet in general practice. It is a fact that some teachers are too prone to discuss Cushing's syndrome when they should be teaching the causes and treatment of headache, but if the critics infer that we ought to be teaching how to write a prescription for a diaphoretic in bad Latin, I for one refuse to waste my time on such anachronisms. Yet we cannot hope to get rid of the bottle-of-medicine tradition without facing the problem and giving the prospective practitioner something to put in its place. It is not sufficient for us to teach the use of parenteral penicillin and blood-transfusion, leaving the student quite ignorant of how we, his teachers and exemplars, would tackle the problem of treatment in general practice ourselves.

CHANGES IN OUTLOOK

The therapeutic revolution to which I have referred has necessitated certain fundamental changes in outlook.

Firstly, diagnosis is far more important nowadays than ever before. For instance, before penicillin, a missed diagnosis of bacterial endocarditis was unimportant ; today it may amount to malpraxis. In the old days the immediate diagnosis of pneumonia or meningitis was not essential ; today it may be life-saving. With more potent and specific remedies the need for accurate diagnosis and control should require no emphasis.

Secondly, these remedies must be properly used. With *mist. expect.* it matters little whether ¹/₂ oz. or 1 oz. is given, and whether every four hours or three times a day. With sulphonamides, with insulin, with iron, with digitalis, with thiouracil, the dosage, frequency, and mode of administration are all-important.

Thirdly, in the old days when we had no real remedies for anything, we had to treat everything. Today when we can efficiently treat so many illnesses we can usually afford to admit honestly when we are beaten. There is less excuse than ever for the diaphoretic mixture, the febrifuge, and the aperient.

Fourthly, there is a healthy tendency nowadays to admit the importance of psychological factors in the cure of disease instead of ascribing the cure to something else. We should therefore try to realise when we are employing psychotherapy so that we may use it rationally.

We who have the privilege—the very great privilege—of working in a well-equipped hospital with every diagnostic and therapeutic aid, with a team of young men to help in treatment and investigation, and above all with the advantage of being able to discuss our problems with junior and senior colleagues, have a duty to those who are in the more isolated practice of medicine, to pass on to them if not our facilities, at least the trend of our thought, and to apply ourselves to their problems as well as our own, so as not to disapprove without at least attempting to show the way.

POSSIBLE REFORMS

What reforms then might be made in the teaching and practice of therapeutics ?

First, I would divide the pharmacology textbooks and the *British Pharmacopœia* into two parts : the first dealing with remedies in current use, the second with remedies which are no longer used in modern practice. In the second category, I would put drugs like strychnine, calomel, hexamine, and strophanthus whose action it may be as well that pharmacologists should not forget, though I would not have them teach it to medical students. This would give the necessary authority for the omission of obsolete information from the curriculum, thereby defeating even the retarding effects of external examiners.

Secondly, I would inculcate the principle that therapy should always be approached as a scientific experiment. Often enough the result of the experiment will be known in advance, but at least it should be planned so that the answer will be as clear as possible at the end. With this aim in view, it stands to reason that major remedies should ordinarily be given one at a time unless their various actions are clearly distinguishable. In planning a therapeutic experiment, the following considerations seem to me to be universally applicable :

1. (*a*) *Is there a specific remedy for this complaint ?*—Under the heading of specific remedies would come hormone therapy in clearly defined syndromes (insulin in diabetes, thyroid in myxœdema) ; vitamins in deficiency states such as rickets, pellagra, scurvy ; penicillin and sulphonamides in the appropriate infections; antisyphilitic treatment ; quinine and mepacrine ; iron and liver used specifically each for its corresponding anæmia. Some operations come into this group.

(*b*) *Is there a specific remedy known to do good in the majority of cases, though not necessarily curative ?*—For instance, gold in rheumatoid arthritis, or barbiturates in epilepsy, &c.

2. (*a*) *Although there may not be a specific treatment, is there some major corrective to the disordered physiology of the disease ?*—Here we have digitalis (properly used) in heart failure ; mercurial diuretics in œdema ; salines in dehydration ; adrenaline in asthma ; blood-transfusion in anæmia and hæmorrhage ; plaster and physiotherapy in arthritis ; and some minor or major operations.

(*b*) *In this connexion, is there a way of life which I should advise the patient to adopt or to avoid ?*—For instance rest in bed, exercise, diet, weight reduction, change of environment, or occupation.

3. *Symptomatic treatment.*—In the absence of treatment which is known to modify the course of the disease, or while waiting for a diagnosis to be made or for cure to take place, what can be done to relieve the symptoms ? Here we have analgesics from aspirin to morphine, hypnotics, aperients occasionally, a linctus or inhalation, and many simple nursing and dietary measures.

4. *What psychological treatment is necessary ?*—This applies both to organic and to psychogenic disease. It can be divided into : (*a*) psychotherapy, which may be anything from simple explanation and reassurance to treatment in a mental hospital, and (*b*) therapy by placebos. The latter has to be distinguished from symptomatic treatment.

The frequency with which placebos are used varies inversely with the combined intelligence of the doctor and his patient. The more intelligent the doctor, the more will he make use of explanation, reassurance, and, when necessary, an honest statement as to why medicine will do no good. The more intelligent the patient, the more will he heed the doctor's statement and advice. In this connexion, intelligence and social status do not always go together. The point is that the prescription of a placebo should be a deliberate act and not a conditioned reflex, and it should be an invariable rule that it must be something which can *do no good*. The greatest obstacle to the intelligent practice of medicine is the habit of giving something which *might* do good. Then if the patient improves, the reason remains obscure (but see under 5 below).

It must be clearly understood that a placebo is given for the mental comfort of the patient, not of the doctor, and that whereas it may occasionally be expedient to deceive the patient it should never be done at the risk of deceiving oneself. Placebos should therefore consist of the simplest possible ingredients such as infusion of gentian.

The above principles are primarily designed for the case in which a diagnosis has been made. In other cases a plan of therapy is just as necessary. The first question often is : how can an accurate diagnosis be established ? And the second : am I justified in withholding therapy until it has been made ? The answer is often unequivocal. In suspected pernicious anæmia or carcinoma of the stomach, it is always mischievous, sometimes criminal, to treat before investigating. In other cases the decision is not so easy, for instance in a case of high fever. Here the decision will depend upon the degree of likelihood that the provisional diagnosis is correct, the availability of diagnostic aids, the danger of non-intervention, and the danger of wrong-intervention. In a remote country district or on active service, I would give sulphaguanidine for an acute febrile diarrhœa. In an urban practice I would at least send a stool for bacteriological examination before doing so, even if, in a severe case, I decided to start treatment while awaiting the result. Finally in such cases treatment may often be designed to give diagnostic information, which comes under the important heading of :

5. *The therapeutic test.*—This is usually wrongly carried out. The tendency is for therapeutic timidity to accompany diagnostic doubt—" I gave a small dose of sulphathiazole in case it turned out to be pneumonia " is atrocious therapy.

The right approach to the therapeutic test is this : " I am not certain. Therefore I will give remedy X in *full doses* for *x* days " (the usual period in which a response is likely to occur). " If it is disease X, then he will respond and I will know the diagnosis and continue treatment. If there is no response I will try remedy Y in the same way—or I will make further investigations into the cause."

I make no apology for this elementary explanation because I know how rarely a therapeutic test is properly applied. The point is that, used intelligently, every treatment becomes a therapeutic test, thus aiding stage by stage in the diagnosis. For instance, it may be suspected that a headache is psychogenic. If the placebo contains aspirin, no useful information is obtained ; the diagnosis is merely obscured. If it is dispensed on correct placebo principles (paragraph 4(*b*)) and the headache is regularly relieved, the diagnosis of psychoneurosis can be made with some confidence.

Finally, there is :

6. *Experimental therapy designed for the purposes of research.*

It is beyond the scope of this essay, but if such trials were properly planned with the necessary controls an enormous amount of valuable information could come from careful experiments in general practice, particularly as to the value of many accepted or advertised remedies in minor ailments.

I can think of no disorder in general practice that cannot be dealt with according to the scheme which has been described. Set out at length, it may appear extravagant of time ; but actually it is merely a mental habit once the principles are grasped, and it is quite unnecessary to *think* in terms of 1, 2, 3, and 4. Nevertheless, lack of time is usually made the excuse for bad work. It is quicker to prescribe a bottle of medicine than to examine the patient properly and explain the nature of the illness. This is equivalent to an admission of failure, and let it be noted that the patient for whom the bottle of medicine has been prescribed will probably return for another and another, and what is more serious, an anxiety state may be induced, whereas explanation and reassurance might have finished the treatment in one consultation, thus saving time in the long run. Perhaps we must admit that many of us still have one more category which is :

7. *Treatment hastily prescribed without regard to principle or consequence.*

None of us is perfect. Let us realise that no. 7 exists, but is something to be ashamed of. I suspect that in not a few practices it is the category which most nearly corresponds with normal therapeutic procedure.

No-one's considered opinions are entirely original ; they evolve gradually and are much influenced by discussion. Prof. J. C. Spence first used the words " teaching the art of consultation " to me, though I have practised the method for years. Dr. G. W. Rippon, of Sheffield, himself a general practitioner, first gave me the phrase " therapy designed not to deceive oneself."

SOCIAL MEDICAL TEACHING

W. MELVILLE ARNOTT
B.Sc., M.D. Edin.,
F.R.C.P.E., M.R.C.P.
PROFESSOR OF
MEDICINE

THOMAS McKEOWN
M.D. Birm., D.Phil. Oxfd,
Ph.D. McGill
PROFESSOR OF SOCIAL
MEDICINE

F. A. R. STAMMERS
C.B.E., B.Sc., Ch.M. Birm., F.R.C.S.
PROFESSOR OF SURGERY

From the University of Birmingham

BOTH the Goodenough Committee and the General Medical Council have emphasised that the scope and method of undergraduate teaching in social medicine " are matters in which there is much room for experiment." In addition to a fuller discussion of the preventive services, they anticipated that instruction should be extended to include the more ambitious aim of influencing the clinical teaching so that due emphasis is given to the relation of the social environment to individual cases. In our view this aim can be realised only if accepted as the responsibility of all clinical departments. We here describe briefly the experience of a first year of joint social and medical teaching in the departments of medicine, social medicine, and surgery at the University of Birmingham.

We state first on what grounds we value this teaching Since it has been supported by considerations in which

toxins per se. Some other factor appears to precipitate the paralysis. That this factor may be fatigue is suggested by the transfer of paresis seen in crossing over. Also, in considering the anatomical elements involved in deglutitional complications, the groups affected suggest a continuity of weakness along one physiological system independently of the nerve-supply to its various components—e.g., palate to pharynx, pharynx to elevators of the hyoid. The view that fatigue is a prominent factor in promoting paralysis is also supported by the common observation that allowing patients to read too early promotes paralysis of accommodation.

Since my return to England my attention has been directed to an observation by Scholes (1927), whose series of diphtheria cases number 33,477. He was also impressed with the importance of usage as an ætiological factor—" continued functioning of the muscles after the damage has been done."

SUMMARY

Palatal paresis in diphtheria mainly consists of two types : defective elevation of the palate and deviation of the uvula.

Reversal of uvular deflection has been noted in 5 cases during the course of palatal paresis. It is suggested that its ætiology lies in fatigue.

Nasal regurgitation in deviation cases can be prevented by simple postural treatment.

Movements of the thyroid cartilage have been observed in diphtheria, and deflection of the cartilage is sometimes observed in severe paralysis.

The effects of diphtheria toxin generally on the musculature are discussed, and it is suggested that the effect of fatigue on affected end-plates is a prominent factor in paralysis.

REFERENCES

Cameron, J. D. S., Muir, E. G. (1942) *Lancet,* ii, 720.
Oldfield, M. C. (1941) *Brit. J. Surg.* 29, 197.
Ronaldson, G. W. (1925) *Rep. metrop. Asylums Bd.*
— Kelleher, W. H. (1935) *Brit. med. J.* i, 1019.
Scholes, F. V. G. (1927) Diphtheria, Measles, Scarlatina. Melbourne, p. 26.
Walshe, F. M. R. (1918) *Quart. J. Med.* 11, 191.

CLINICAL EXTRACORPOREAL DIALYSIS OF BLOOD WITH ARTIFICIAL KIDNEY

NILS ALWALL
M.D.

With the collaboration of

LEMBIT NORVIIT   ADOLFS MARTIN STEINS

From the Medical Clinic of the University of Lund, Sweden

SEVERAL workers have tried to construct an efficient apparatus for the dialysis of a patient's blood outside the body. Abel (1913) seems to have been the first to call such a device an artificial kidney ; and Kolff invented one capable of being used clinically (Kolff and Berk 1944, Kolff 1946).

Various ill effects, such as hæmolysis, lowered blood-pressure, shock, and pulmonary œdema, were reported by Kolff to follow dialysis with his apparatus. These drawbacks are minimised by the method of construction of Alwall's dialyser, which we have used, with modifications, since 1945 (Alwall 1947, Alwall and Norviit 1947).

The first apparatus was built as follows :

The 'Cellophane' tube through which the blood flowed was wound round a cylinder of wire netting immersed in a glass container filled with saline solution kept constantly moving by a motor-driven propeller. A mantle of wire netting held the cellophane tube compressed so that the layer of blood was very thin, independently of the pressure in the tube. In this way the conditions for a quick dialysis were very good. The cylinder was fixed in a box with a close-fitting lid which prevented evaporation and allowed saturation of the saline solution with oxygen and carbon dioxide.

The necessary fluid balance between the blood in the cellophane tube and the saline solution could be obtained by adjusting the dialyser at the required level below that of the patient.

For use with human patients the apparatus measured 42 cm. (about 16½ in.) high and 20 cm. (about 8 in.) in diameter. The container held about 600 ml. of blood, and about 25 litres of salt solution. Dialysis area about 6500 sq. cm.

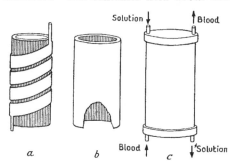

Fig. 1—Diagrams showing construction and assembly of Alwall's dialyser: (*a*) inner cylinder with cellophane tube wrapped round it ; (*b*) outer cylinder, grooved on inner aspect ; (*c*) cylinders assembled with top and bottom.

All the results reported here refer to the apparatus described above. The apparatus was later simplified and improved as follows :

The cellophane tube, through which the blood is to flow, is wound round a vulcanite or metal cylinder bearing on its outer surface longitudinal grooves, and is placed inside a second cylinder similarly grooved on its inner surface. The two cylinders are held firmly in position by tightly fitting top and bottom (fig. 1).

The space between the two rigid cylinders is so calculated that the cellophane tube can contain only a thin layer of blood of predetermined thickness which cannot be altered.

During dialysis, while the blood flows through the cellophane tube, a thin stream of saline solution flows in the opposite direction along the grooves on the cylinders.

With this construction fluid balance between the blood in the cellophane tube and the saline solution in the grooves on the cylinders is obtained in the manner described above ; the osmotic water attraction of the blood is compensated by a corresponding hydrostatic pressure.

In the latter construction it is possible to combine the positive pressure of the blood in the cellophane tube with the negative pressure of the saline solution outside the cellophane tube. A screw clip on the rubber supply tube controls the speed with which the saline solution flows to the apparatus. The saline solution flows off through a long rubber tube which discharges at a lower level than that of the apparatus (the tube, for instance, is lowered into a discharge-pipe). The length of this rubber tube thus determines the negative pressure of the saline solution on the cellophane tube.

Before dialysis is started the patient is heparinised to prevent coagulation of the blood in the dialyser.

Before the apparatus is connected with the patient or the animal the cellophane tube as a rule is filled with blood. The arterial pressure drives the blood from the radial artery through the apparatus back to the median cubital vein. When dialysis is interrupted a short-circuit is opened between the glass cannulæ in the blood-vessels.

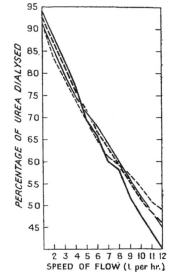

Fig. 2—Dialysis of urea solutions of 125, 250, 500, and 750 mg. per 100 ml. at different speeds of flow.

The operation for exposing the blood-vessels is done the day before dialysis if possible, to prevent excessive bleeding after the heparinisation.

By adding citrate to the saline solution it may be possible to reduce the risk of coagulation in the apparatus and do away with the need of heparin and, consequently, the danger of bleeding in uræmic colitis and so on.

ADVANTAGES

This apparatus is relatively small and easy to handle and has a great dialytic capacity. The blood is continuously distributed throughout the whole cellophane tube in an unvarying thin layer. The whole of the cellophane tube is in continuous contact with the salt solution. Since the saline solution is in uninterrupted motion and is changed at suitable intervals, it should be possible to make use of the maximal capacity of the cellophane tube.

The blood does not have to pass any rotating cylinder, rotating couplings, or rotating Beck-pump as it has to in Kolff's apparatus. The arterial pressure drives the blood through the apparatus back to the vein; thus there is no hæmolysis. There is less risk of coagulation. The heparin dosage can be considerably reduced in comparison with that used by Kolff; thus there is less risk of bleeding.

The cellophane tube can be exposed to arterial pressure direct without any increase in its content, which is controlled and constant. Thus the blood-pressure does not fall during the treatment, there are no such dangerous shock complications as Kolff reports " when too much blood is allowed to run from the patient into the kidney."

The apparatus offers the essentially new and practically important possibility of maintaining, by means of adjusted hydrostatic pressure, a fluid balance between the blood in the cellophane tube and the surrounding saline solution.

The apparatus is furnished with a tightly fitting lid which prevents evaporation and allows saturation of the saline solution with a suitable mixture of oxygen and carbon dioxide for regulation of the pH through CO_2—bicarbonate. Kolff's cylinder rotates in an open tank.

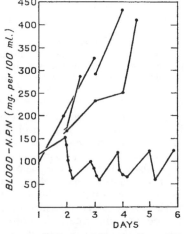

Fig. 3—Dialysis of blood of a rabbit with both ureters ligated (lowest curve), compared with four controls in which dialysis was not used.

TESTS WITH UREA SOLUTION

Fig. 2 gives the results of the tests with solutions of urea in water in concentrations of 125, 250, 500, and 750 mg. per 100 ml., and at speeds of flow from 1 to 13 litres an hour. The urea solution was dialysed against water at 40°C. At low speeds of flow 90% or perhaps somewhat more of the urea was removed by dialysis; at a speed of flow of 5 litres an hour about 70%; at 10 litres an hour about 50%; and so on.

The speed of flow from the radial artery through the apparatus in clinical dialysis is about 8–10 litres.

The percentages of urea eliminated decreased with increasing speed of flow, but the dialytic action, expressed as the absolute quantity of eliminated urea, increased with the speed of flow within the limits investigated.

TESTS ON ANIMALS

Ligation of Ureters.—One rabbit was treated with dialysis of the blood for 4–6 hours daily for 4 successive days. There were four untreated controls. The treated rabbit died after 138 hours from hæmorrhage in the abdominal cavity; the heparinisation contributed towards the bleeding. The results are shown in fig. 3.

Acute Mercurial Poisoning.—One rabbit was treated with dialysis of the blood for 6 successive days. There

were seven untreated controls. The results are shown in fig. 4.

CLINICAL USE OF DIALYSIS IN URÆMIA

Case 1.—A man, aged 49, moribund with chronic nephritis and uræmia, diffuse silicosis of the lungs, chronic bronchitis, and bronchopneumonia. During 6 hours' dialysis about 45 g. of non-protein nitrogen (N.P.N.) was

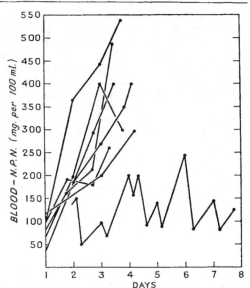

Fig. 4—Dialysis of blood of a rabbit with acute mercurial poisoning (lowest curve), compared with seven controls in which dialysis was not used.

eliminated, and the content in the blood decreased by 98 mg. per 100 ml. to 320 mg. per 100 ml. The œdema round the eyelids practically disappeared during the treatment. The general condition obviously improved. Patient died next day of uræmia and bronchopneumonia.

Case 2.—A woman, aged 54, with hypertonia and probably chronic nephritis and acute nephritis, with pneumonia, who was passing only small amounts of urine and had a rising blood-N.P.N. level, increasing œdema of her face, and her general condition deteriorating, was comatose when dialysis was applied. Owing to a technical mishap only about 60% of the cellophane tubing in the dialyser could be used.

During 8 hours of dialysis 18 g. of N.P.N. was eliminated, and the blood-N.P.N. level sank from 235 to 182 mg. per 100 ml. The daily output of N.P.N. in the urine before treatment was only 2–3 g.

Her general condition improved considerably, and the œdema decreased. After a later temporary deterioration patient regained her health, with a normal blood-N.P.N. level but reduced renal function, as shown by tests.

In cases 1 and 2 the speed of flow of the blood through the dialyser was low.

Case 3.—A woman, aged 44, with two years' history of symptoms of cancer uteri, a history of nephrectomy, and a month's history of decreasing amounts of urine owing to compression of the remaining ureter.

Her blood-N.P.N. level was gradually increasing. Progressive deterioration of general condition during the last few weeks with constant nausea and vomiting.

On examination patient was comatose. Blood-N.P.N. levels: 131 mg. per 100 ml. on Jan. 14; 240 mg. per 100 ml.

TABLE I—DETAILS OF CASE 3

Blood levels	First dialysis treatment (5 hours on Feb. 8)		Second dialysis treatment (8 hours on Feb. 9)	
	Before	After	Before	After
Non-protein nitrogen (mg. per 100 ml.)	346	182	200	77
Xanthoprotein (units)	140	80	120	70
Indican	+ +	+	+ +	+
Uric acid (mg. per 100 ml.)	13·3	7·3	9·3	4·6
Bicarbonate (m. mol.)	12·1	19·1	15·7	20·3
Total base (m. mol.)	157	157	161	158
Chloride (mg. per 100 ml.)	369	369	387	404
Sugar (mg. per 100 ml.)	240	300	290	290

on Jan. 22 ; 225 mg. per 100 ml. on Jan. 31 ; 346 mg. per 100 ml. on Feb. 5 and Feb. 7.

Treatment.—Dialysis (flow speed about 6 litres of blood an hour) for 5 hours on Feb. 8 eliminated 34 g. of N.P.N., and for 8 hours on Feb. 9 eliminated 28 g. of N.P.N. During treatment the general condition improved in a striking manner, the patient becoming bright and lively. For details see table I.

During the week which followed the dialysis the patient said she had " not felt so well for a long time " and could eat " better than she had done for the last month." Improvement in general condition continued, and patient was satisfied with the result. During the last two days of her life she had a change for the worse, and she died suddenly on Feb. 18.

Case 4.—A woman, aged 57, with congenital polycystic disease of the kidneys which had progressed to the stage of advanced renal insufficiency, had had severe progressive symptoms of uræmia for at least two weeks. She was comatose when dialysis was applied.

During 20 hours' continuous dialysis, with a speed of flow of the blood about 8–10 litres an hour, about 70 g. of N.P.N. was eliminated, and the blood-N.P.N. level decreased from 222 to 57 mg. per 100 ml. Her general condition improved considerably, and after some days patient could leave her bed for several hours every day.

The improvement in her general condition continued, and she felt quite well during the following month in spite of a

TABLE II—RESULTS OF DIALYSIS

Case no.	Diagnosis	Blood-N.P.N. level (mg. per 100 ml.)		Dialysis	
		Before treatment	After treatment	N.P.N. eliminated (g.)	Length of treatment (hours)
1	Chronic nephritis	418	320	45	6
2	Chronic and acute nephritis ..	235	182	18	8
3	Cancer uteri and anuria—				
	Feb. 8 ..	346	180	34	5
	Feb. 9 ..	200	70	28	8
4	Polycystic disease of kidneys	222	57	70	20
5	Chronic nephritis	234	71	80	20
6	Acute and subacute nephritis	364	100	70	17
		292	118	64	10
7	Nephrosclerosis	125	83	13	4
8	Renal hypoplasia and chronic nephritis	230	133	55	18*

* For 14 hours only 60% of the cellophane tubing could be used.

blood-N.P.N. level of about 100–125 mg. per 100 ml. During the last two weeks of her life her condition gradually deteriorated and her blood-N.P.N. level rose. She died of uræmia and bronchopneumonia.

Case 5.—A man, aged 59, with a long history of chronic nephritis and uræmia. During 20 hours' dialysis about 80 g. of N.P.N. was eliminated and the blood-N.P.N. level fell from 234 to 71 mg. per 100 ml. His general condition improved considerably.

The results obtained in these and three further cases are shown in table II.

SUMMARY

Alwall's dialyser or artificial kidney is described.

After successful preliminary tests with a solution of urea, followed by dialysis of blood in tests on animals, the dialyser was used to treat eight patients with uræmia.

REFERENCES

Abel, J. J. (1913) *J. Pharmacol.* **5**, 625.
Alwall, N. (1947) *Acta med. scand.* **128**, 317.
— Norviit, L. (1947) *Ibid,* suppl. 196, p. 250.
Kolff, W. J. (1946) The Artificial Kidney, Kampen.
— Berk, H. T. J. (1944) *Acta med. scand.* **117**, 121.

SENSITISATION OF PENICILLIN-RESISTANT BACTERIA

A. VOUREKA
M.D. Athens
BRITISH COUNCIL RESEARCH SCHOLAR
From the Laboratories of the Wright-Fleming Institute for Microbiology, St. Mary's Hospital, London

MANY observers have made organisms insensitive to penicillin in vitro, but no methods have yet been published of rendering penicillin-insensitive bacteria sensitive, except by repeated culture. I report here experiments showing that penicillin-sensitivity can be restored to some insensitive bacteria by association with other bacteria or their products.

The original idea was that penicillin-sensitivity might depend on the presence of a chemical or physical factor. If this were correct, it might be possible, in certain circumstances, for bacteria short of or devoid of this chemical factor to borrow it from other bacteria possessing it, or it might be that growth in association with a sensitive microbe would alter, in some way, the physical structure.

In choosing the bacteria it seemed wise to start with resistant strains of an organism of which most strains are known to be penicillin-sensitive.

On the assumption that during growth of a penicillin-sensitive organism a chemical substance is produced which might be transferred to, or act on, the resistant strain, the general procedure adopted was to grow the resistant and the sensitive organisms together in mixed culture and then isolate the resistant one and test its sensitivity. The control was provided by subculturing the resistant bacterium in a similar manner and growing it on the same medium but without the sensitive strain.

FINDINGS

1. *Change in a Resistant Streptococcus Grown with a Staphylococcus.*—In the first experiment a resistant strain of hæmolytic streptococcus was used. This was grown for 24 hours with a sensitive staphylococcus (standard Oxford strain) in broth and then subcultured on half a blood-agar plate, while on the other half the resistant streptococcus was grown alone. Single streptococcus colonies were then selected from each side, planted one on each half of another blood-agar plate, and a penicillin solution containing 10 units per ml. was poured on half the plate (so as to cover half of either section) to test the sensitivity of the bacteria.

After 24 hours' incubation there was growth throughout the whole length of the control culture, while the strepto-

INCREASE IN SENSITIVITY OF FOUR PENICILLIN-RESISTANT STRAINS OF STAPHYLOCOCCI GROWN WITH A HÆMOLYTIC STREPTOCOCCUS (MILNE)

Resistant strains of staphylococci		Growth in broth containing different concentrations of penicillin (units per ml.)							
		500	100	20	4	0·8	0·16	0·03	Control
6652	Control ..	−	+ +	+ +	+ +	+ +	+ +	+ +	+ +
	Treated*	−	−	−	−	−	−	+	+ +
7007	Control ..	−	+ +	+ +	+ +	+ +	+ +	+ +	+ +
	Treated*	−	−	−	−	−	−	+	+ +
6821	Control ..	−	−	+ +	+ +	+ +	+ +	+ +	+ +
	Treated*	−	−	−	−	−	−	+	+ +
44	Control ..	−	+ +	+ +	+ +	+ +	+ +	+ +	+ +
	Treated*	−	−	−	−	−	−	+	+ +
Standard Oxford strain		−	−	−	−	−	−	+	+ +

* Grown in mixed cultures with hæmolytic streptococcus.

THE LANCET]   SALICYLIC ACID FOR CORONARY THROMBOSIS?   [JUNE 19, 1948   965

THE SITUATION

SIR,—It might be useful to inquire as to the actual position of the profession today as the result of the recent action taken by the representative body of the British Medical Association.

We had two alternatives before us early this year —and this whether we consider the progress of medicine, the best service for the public, or our own freedoms— either to get the present Act so amended that these things would be safe for a considerable period or to give the Minister a blank cheque and be in perpetual doubt as to whether we could honour it, in other words, watch every regulation with critical eyes for an indefinite time. In February we had no doubt that the first alternative was the proper one, and we said so. In April the hurried plebiscite, with its implication that the position had changed materially, and the volte-face of the council, which the chairman was powerless to oppose, broke the all too tenuous thread which held us united, and in May, through the representative body, we chose the second alternative.

How, now, are we to clarify the position and regain our self-respect and the respect of the public? There is a large section of the profession which feels that these things should not be left in the hands of men who, despite all their arduous deliberations, did " take the wrong turning." Confidence in them has been badly shaken. There are many doctors asking for guidance, both for themselves and for their sons and daughters, thinking of medicine as a vocation. To these are to be added many members of the public. There will shortly be a third group—men who will leave the service they have too hastily joined out of fear and not conviction.

What is the best way of dealing with the situation? Will you allow me, Sir, to say through the medium of your columns that I shall welcome the views of any of your readers sent to me privately. Such a step as this seems to me desirable before any action is taken in which I am concerned.

32, Devonshire Place, W.1.   HORDER.

SALICYLIC ACID FOR CORONARY THROMBOSIS?

SIR,—It appears that two processes are involved in the pathology of coronary thrombosis—atheromatous arterial degeneration and blood coagulation. We seem unable to control the former, but recently we have learnt something about the control of the latter. Much remains obscure about coagulation, but it is reasonable to suppose that the coagulability of the blood is controlled by the liver, the factory of prothrombin and presumably, too, of heparin.

Clinical experience suggests that coagulability varies in degree from time to time; for the occurrence of thrombotic states, characterised by multiple thromboses, is fully recognised. In 1933 Strickland Goodall[1] suggested that such a blood change may be a primary cause of coronary thrombosis. This seems reasonable; for though it is easy to imagine the gradual occlusion of a diseased artery by the accretion of platelets, it is difficult to understand the sudden development of local fibrinous thromboses except as the result of increased coagulability of the blood as a whole. In the treatment of coronary thrombosis dicoumarol is steadily gaining favour, but its dangers are not yet fully understood or controllable. It is thought to act by preventing the conversion of vitamin K into prothrombin by the liver. It seems that salicylic acid has a similar action,[2] and it is known that these two products are structurally related. It has even been suggested that dicoumarol effects its specific action by being degraded to salicylic acid in the liver. However that may be, clinicians know that salicylates given in full dosage sometimes induce an obvious hæmorrhagic state. With these facts in mind, I would suggest that at least until we know more about dicoumarol we might use salicylic acid for the treatment of coronary thrombosis: it could do no harm and might well do good. We might even go further than this; for if Goodall was right in supposing that a thrombotic state precedes the occurrence of coronary thrombosis, and if in fact the liver

does control the coagulability of the blood, it follows that in the prevention and treatment of this condition we should direct our attention to the liver. It may be of more than passing interest that salicylates not only induce hypoprothrombinæmia but are also reputed to have a cholagogue action.

It is probable that this idea of substituting salicylic acid for dicoumarol in the treatment of coronary thrombosis has occurred to others; and so I venture to cast my bread upon your waters in the hope that I may see it again after many days.

Torquay.   PAUL GIBSON.

TOXIC EFFECTS OF MYANESIN

SIR,—The principal toxic effect of ' Myanesin ' is described as hæmolysis with hæmoglobinuria. Pugh and Enderby[1] point out that the high threshold value for the excretion of hæmoglobin by the kidney prevents its appearance in the urine unless considerable lysis has taken place.

I have been investigating the effect of myanesin on hysterical motor paralysis, to see if the alleged muscle-relaxing power of that drug[2] would facilitate return of movement at the fixed joints.

The patient selected was a man, aged 35, with motor hysteria. He had a pseudo-poker-back from spasm of the nuchal and paravertebral muscles. There was no evidence of organic disease. Pulse-rate 68 per min., regular. At the start of the trial the urine was found to contain neither albumin nor blood; thereafter every specimen was tested.

May 1.—6 ml. of 10% solution of myanesin, injected intravenously, produced no effect on the patient's voluntarily abducted arm. A slight improvement was noted in rotation of the cervical spine, but not appreciably more than had been observed previously with thiopentone-induced hypnosis. Five min. later 8 ml. of the same solution produced a similar effect.

May 3.—10 ml. of the solution produced no relaxation of the patient's abducted arm. There was freer and a more extensive range of head-turning movement, but no change in the spastic antagonistic muscle-groups whose simultaneous contractions soon brought any rotation of the cervical spine to an abrupt halt.

May 4.—At 11 A.M. 17 ml. of same solution gave an effect no different from that of the previous day. At 12.30 P.M. the patient passed wine-red urine. Tests for blood pigment were strongly positive; microscopical examination of a centrifuged specimen showed only one or two red blood-cells per field. No spectroscope was available, but one could assume that hæmolysis had taken place, with overflow of some blood pigment into the urine. Red blood-cells 4,496,000 per c.mm.; Hb 80%; colour-index 0·9. General condition satisfactory. Pulse-rate 52 per min., irregular, showing 3 : 1 alternating with 4 : 1 partial heart-block. Copious fluids and large doses of alkalis were administered.

At 1.15 P.M. the urine was still wine-red and was neutral to litmus. Pulse-rate 52 per min., regular. At 2.15 P.M. the urine was straw-coloured and alkaline, containing no red cells or blood pigment. Pulse-rate 56 per min., regular. At 4 P.M. the urine was as at 2.15 P.M. Pulse-rate 58 per min., regular. Red blood-cells 4,432,000 per c.mm.; Hb 81%; colour-index 0·9.

May 5.—General condition satisfactory. Urine as at 4 P.M. on the previous day. Pulse-rate 68 per min., regular.

Though the results of this trial do not shed any further light on the problems of hysteria, nor on the site of action of myanesin, they do include two items which are, I believe, of interest. (1) It seemed that, as Pugh and Enderby suggest, the amount of blood lysed, and therefore hæmoglobinuria, is directly proportional to the dose of myanesin injected. (2) I had not previously come across partial heart-block shortly after the intravenous administration of myanesin. Hunter and Waterfall[3] state that myanesin has produced bradycardia, but make no mention of alteration in cardiac rhythm. I do not know whether a degree of hæmolysis *per se*

1. Goodall, J. S. *Brit. med. J.* 1933, ii, 892.
2. Fawns, H. T. *London Hosp. Gaz.* 1948, **51**, 37.

1. Pugh, J. I., Enderby, G. E. H. *Lancet*, 1947, ii, 387.
2. Berger, F. M., Bradley, W. *Ibid*, 1947, i, 97. Leading article, *Ibid*, March 27, p. 487.
3. Hunter, A. R., Waterfall, J. M. *Ibid*, March 6, p. 366.

THE LANCET

LONDON : SATURDAY, JULY 3, 1948

Our Service

IN shelters, fo'c'sles, barrack-rooms, and other places of common resort, the talk often turned to the shortcomings of society. " But it will be different after the war," we used to say. And in the anxious winter of 1942 BEVERIDGE showed how it might be made different—how the nation could ensure that all its members, whether old or young, ill or unfortunate, should have a basic minimum of food and care. Being older and wiser, we now know that in times like these even social security is insecure ; its money benefits would quickly be made worthless by inflation or external bankruptcy, and its stabilising influence in time of trial has to be weighed against its possible effect in discouraging effort when effort is so badly wanted. Moreover, in seeking Freedom from Want one may lose other freedoms, and Britain's recent advances towards Equality and Fraternity have been made at some cost to Liberty. The balance proper to our day and generation is hard to strike, and it may be long before we reach equilibrium. Yet with all these reservations it is certainly a source of strength to a country for its people to feel that, in peace as in war, the necessities of life will be shared according to need ; and we can all be proud at least of the impulse behind the legislation that comes into force next Monday.

The new arrangements confer a great benefit on medicine by lessening the commercial element in its practice. Now that everyone is entitled to full medical care, the doctor can provide that care without thinking of his own profit or his patient's loss, and can allocate his efforts more according to medical priority. The money barrier has of course protected him against people who do not really require help, but it has also separated him from people who really do : and only time can show the relative proportions of the two classes. But though, as we hope, removal of this barrier will help to bring medicine to those who need it most, a truly satisfactory application of medical knowledge and resources demands much reorganisation and development both in general and hospital practice. Given time, the rationalisation of hospital services under State ownership should mean real progress in applied medicine, and anyone who has studied the membership of the boards and committees charged with their management must agree that our profession has been given a full opportunity for leadership. If we continue to think of the National Health Service as a State service it will fail ; but if we recognise it as our own service we can make it a great and increasing success. For this we shall require all the sense of duty that training and tradition can inspire, and the result will ultimately depend on the standards of the teaching schools. But our tradition is strong because it is a good tradition ; and it will prevail.

History at Geneva

CLINICIANS generally think of medicine as a personal art : " take care of the patients," they say, " and the populations will take care of themselves." For clinicians this may be right and proper and wise ; but it is only penny wisdom if it blinds them to the benefits of the communal approach to health. Similarly a national outlook is .pound-foolish if it discourages an international approach that would be for the general good ; and only the most perversely insular will deny the immense potential significance of the World Health Assembly which opened in Geneva last week. The constitution of the World Health Organisation was signed two years ago by 61 nations—probably the greatest number that have ever agreed on any set of principles—and the new body is unique among United Nations special agencies in containing representatives of the Soviet republics. To everyone it appeals as a constructive effort ; and it is a good basis for working together, because, as the Chinese delegate said, " no nation by gaining health takes it from another."

In our own country the public-health movement arose early last century from recognition that disease in the poorer sections of the community was a peril to all. In the same way the international movement is based first on the fact that " unequal development in different countries in the promotion of health and control of disease, especially communicable disease, is a common danger." Today, in a world growing rapidly smaller with the development of transport, there is increasing need of centralised epidemiological information and a central body able to take the kind of action required by last year's cholera epidemic in Egypt. As a defensive organisation W.H.O. assumes functions previously carried out by several others, including the Office International d'Hygiène Publique and the Health Organisation of the League of Nations, and it will also be continuing previous work when it provides us with international standards for drugs and biological products, an international pharmacopœia, and an international classification for diseases and causes of death. But although there are obvious advantages in having all these necessary tasks undertaken by a single organisation, there is admittedly nothing very new or exciting about them. What is really novel about W.H.O. is the size of its ultimate objective—" the attainment by all people of the highest possible levels of health." Nowadays not only do we know how to prevent the spread of infections, at relatively low cost, but also we know that scientific medicine, wherever it is applied, is capable of greatly increasing the health and strength, and therefore the prosperity, of mankind. The duty laid by its founders on W.H.O. is to spread more widely the advantages now enjoyed by relatively few. The old negative conception is thus supplemented by a new positive one, and the World Health Assembly will have to decide exactly where, in this present year of grace, the emphasis should be placed.

Two widely different lines of policy might be followed. Some of the participating countries—including some with long experience of international endeavour—believe that W.H.O. would do well to concentrate at first on the tasks which cannot possibly be undertaken by nations individually—epidemiological information, sanitary conventions, standardisation, and the like. The right course, as they see it, is to proceed quietly with this unspectacular work which may not interest the public but is unquestionably essential and is also inexpensive. At the other end of the scale are countries which see in W.H.O. a means of bringing the resources of science to vast populations now living in medical darkness. From the statement that W.H.O. makes no distinctions of race, political belief, or social condition they deduce that it should direct its gaze towards the East rather than the West, forming regional branches which could undertake big schemes for eradicating tropical diseases, training medical workers, and perhaps even subsidising hospital care. Between these extremes is the compromise policy placed before the assembly by the W.H.O. interim commission which has gone on with the work during the two years that have preceded ratification of the constitution.

Under the able chairmanship of Dr. ANDRIJA STAMPAR, of Yugoslavia, who was last week unanimously elected president of the World Health Assembly, this commission has not only carried on defensive epidemiological services but has maintained technical missions in many countries and has initiated a very successful scheme of fellowships by which already 250 doctors and other health workers have gone abroad to gain experience or information. The fellowships and missions, which have hitherto been financed from the residual funds of UNRRA, must undoubtedly be continued, and the missions ought to be extended to other than UNRRA countries. In addition, however, the interim commission suggests that in the immediate future W.H.O. should tackle four major problems—malaria, tuberculosis, venereal disease, and the health of mothers and children. In so doing it would follow the example of the Rockefeller Foundation ; rather than embark on large schemes of its own it would help countries to help themselves, and use its experts and its funds as catalysts. To fulfil this compromise programme the interim commission proposes a budget of some 6,500,000 dollars in 1949—a small enough sum when one considers the cost of national medical services or of other agencies of the United Nations. But even this modest demand now seems unlikely to be granted ; for in the United States the World Health Organisation has unfortunately come under suspicion as a potential exponent of " socialised medicine," and in ratifying its constitution the Congress has made regrettable reservations, one of which is that the American contribution shall be limited to 1,920,000 dollars per annum while another is that the United States reserves the right to withdraw on a year's notice. If the United States contribution is scaled down, others are likely to be reduced in proportion.

Ratification with reservations is not exactly ratification ; and though the U.S. delegation was last week provisionally admitted to full membership of the World Health Assembly its members find themselves in a slightly equivocal position. The U.S.A. has nevertheless set a valuable example by sending to Geneva an exceptionally large number of delegates, including representatives of unofficial bodies such as the American Medical Association. The assembly will have to decide whether in future years non-governmental medical agencies should be entitled to attend as observers—and if so which of them should be invited. Though this may seem a small matter, it is closely related to the question whether W.H.O. is going to remain a smallish official organisation with strictly limited functions, or is going to develop rapidly with the stimulating support from public opinion which it could easily enlist. In such a project, at such a time as this, it is very necessary to keep both feet on the financial ground ; yet those responsible for the new venture must be well aware that money usually comes in the end to those who can prove that they would use it profitably. Nowhere more than in international effort is there need of faith, and Dr. STAMPAR was right in saying that if the World Health Organisation adopts a negative attitude, and does not treat health problems as of global importance, " it is bound to experience setbacks right from the beginning, and we shall gradually lose the faith in it which all of us express at present." In mutual aid between nations, as between individuals, lies our only real hope for the future, and the World Health Organisation has it in its power to play a notable part in the process of civilisation. In President TRUMAN's words, we look to it " with hope and expectation."

Surgical Physiology of the Stomach

THE flow of gastric juice is under dual control. There is a psychic flow, produced by the taste, sight, and even thought of food ; and a chemical flow, provoked by the arrival of certain foods, particularly meat extracts, in the stomach. The psychic flow results from the passage of nerve impulses down the vagi, and can be imitated by stimulating the vagi electrically or abolished by cutting them. EDKINS showed in 1906 that the chemical flow is due to gastrin, a hormone which is formed by pyloric mucosa in contact with appropriate foods and enters the blood-stream to reach the glands of the gastric fundus. The existence of gastrin, for long in doubt, has been confirmed by cross-circulation experiments and by the preparation of the hormone in a considerable degree of purity and free from histamine. It is a protein and is water-soluble. Experimentally it works only on intravenous injection and it stimulates the parietal cells only, the juice produced by its injection being poor in enzyme content. Gastrin is also responsible, as a humoral intermediary, for the psychic flow. Vagal stimulation induces a flow of gastric juice by causing the prepyloric antrum to elaborate gastrin. Thus excision or cocainisation of the prepyloric antrum almost abolishes the nervous flow from the fundus ; whereas, if the antrum is isolated with its blood and nerve-supply intact, stimulation of the vagi produces an ample flow from the fundus. Cross-circulation experiments show that stimulation of the vagi of the donor animal will produce a flow of gastric juice in the recipient animal. Such experiments, repeated with a variety of modifications, have yielded the results, negative or positive, which the underlying theory would lead one to expect. Gastrin extracted from the human pylorus and duodenum, when injected into animals, will excite a flow of gastric juice which ceases thirty minutes after the injection. Though injection of purified gastrin will provoke only the parietal cells to activity, vagal stimulation yields gastric juice of

specimens in the later stages of the investigation. Messrs. Glaxo Laboratories Ltd. supplied the penicillin.

REFERENCES

Bigger, J. W. (1944) *Lancet*, ii, 497.
— (1946) *Ibid*, i, 81.
McSweeney, C. J. (1946) *Ibid*, ii, 114.
Rammelkamp, C. H., Helm, J. D. jun. (1943) *Proc. Soc. exp. Biol., N.Y.* **54**, 31.
Thomas, J. C., Hayes, W. (1947) *J. Hyg., Camb.* **45**, 313.
Zaslow, J., Counseller, V. S., Heilman, F. R. (1947) *Surg. Gynec. Obst.* **84**, 140.

MATERNAL RUBELLA AND CONGENITAL DEFECTS

DATA FROM NATIONAL HEALTH INSURANCE RECORDS

A. BRADFORD HILL   T. McL. GALLOWAY*
D.Sc., Ph.D. Lond.   M.B. Edin., M.R.C.P.E., D.P.H.

From the Department of Medical Statistics, London School of Hygiene and Tropical Medicine

SINCE the original observations of the Australian workers on the association between rubella in the pregnant woman and the occurrence of congenital defects in the child, many similar, but rather haphazardly observed, cases have been reported from the U.S.A., Great Britain, and elsewhere. That evidence, which we need not review here, seems to us sufficiently strong to substantiate the association—i.e., that rubella early in pregnancy can cause defects in the fœtus. What we regard as still undetermined with any accuracy is the frequency with which the disease will lead to abnormalities.

From the evidence then available Swan et al.[1] concluded that rubella contracted within the first two months of pregnancy would almost invariably lead to a defective child, whereas in the third month the chance might be about 50%. Many of these, and other, important original observations were, however, made retrospectively—by noting the congenital deformity in the new-born child and then obtaining the history of the mother during pregnancy. By such a method it is clearly impossible to obtain the required probabilities of a defect arising. To take a simple example, 20 women might have rubella in the first two months of pregnancy and 10 give birth to defective children. The true, required, probability is 50%. On the other hand, if we work retrospectively solely from the 10 defective children we should automatically reach a 100% association—all their mothers had rubella. In other words, a fundamental requirement for the measurement of the risks involved is a forward mode of inquiry. The attack of rubella must first be observed in the pregnant woman ; the condition of the child born to her must subsequently be noted.

Such an inquiry is extremely difficult to carry out, for very large numbers of women must be observed, and it is specially important that the occurrence of the disease in them be recorded at a time when they may not even know that they are pregnant. These difficulties are clearly apparent in an investigation made this way by Fox and Bortin[2] in Michigan, where out of some 22,200 notified cases of rubella in 1942–44 these workers could finally detect and trace only 11 women who were pregnant at the time of their illness.

A similar inquiry by Ober et al.[3] gave results on a larger scale. Starting from some 35,000 notified cases of rubella in Massachusetts in 1943, they identified from the notification returns 3068 women aged 17–49.

* Holding a Rockefeller Foundation fellowship in preventive medicine.
1. Swan, C., Tostevin, A. L., Moore, B., Mayo, H., Black, G. H. B. *Med. J. Aust.* 1943, ii, 201.
2. Fox, M. J., Bortin, M. M. *J. Amer. med. Ass.* 1946, **130**, 568.
3. Ober, R. E., Horton, R. J. M., Feemster, R. F. *Amer. J. publ. Hlth*, 1947, **37**, 1328.

Approaching these women by mail they collected 49 instances of rubella during pregnancy, and to these they added another 5 discovered by other methods. Less than half the women approached, however, chose to reply to the letter. Hence it is not known whether the cases finally discovered are a representative group of all such cases. The probabilities might well be affected in this way ; but, the sample being accepted as it stands, the results show that of 5 women who had rubella during the first month of pregnancy 2 aborted, 2 had defective infants, and only 1 had a normal infant. In the second-month attacks 2 infants were stillborn, 2 were defective, and 4 were normal. In the third-month attacks 2 mothers aborted, 1 child was defective, and 6 children were normal. In the later attacks, from the fourth to the ninth month, there were 25 normal infants, only 2 doubtful defects, and 3 losses by abortion or stillbirth.

Clearly one of the main difficulties is to secure sufficient cases for investigation without a prohibitive amount of work. An additional difficulty in this country is that rubella is not notifiable (Manchester, we believe, is the only exception to this rule). It is therefore impossible to follow the examples cited above from the U.S.A. and to collect cases from notifications of infectious disease. The method of observing carefully all women attending prenatal clinics is not likely to be of much help, since the women do not attend the clinics often enough for this purpose during the early weeks of pregnancy. Some other method of case-finding must therefore be found.

PRESENT METHOD OF INQUIRY

It occurred to us that one way of securing records of rubella in pregnancy and the birth of a child was to use the data collected by the approved societies operating under the National Health Insurance Acts before July 5, 1948. If an employed and insured married woman drew benefit for a sickness which caused her to be absent from work she had to present a sickness certificate giving the precise dates of her illness and the general practitioner's diagnosis. If she subsequently gave birth to a child she would be entitled to draw maternity benefit, and the date of the birth would also be recorded. Thus whether she was in the first month of pregnancy and unaware of it, or in the ninth and under no illusions, the occurrence and the dates of the two events would be recorded.

The drawbacks were that : (1) we were necessarily limited to employed insured women and might therefore not get enough cases ; (2) we should observe only cases of rubella severe enough to cause absence from work ; and (3) we should have to rely on the general practitioner's diagnosis. Perhaps (2) and (3) to some extent cancel one another, leaving us with only the more clear-cut cases to work on and freeing us from dealing with fleeting and doubtful rashes.

We concluded that this method of approach was at least worth a trial, for it was simple to operate and would lend itself to the observation also of other diseases than rubella during pregnancy. That is clearly an important point, since the evidence concerning the possible effects on the fœtus of other infectious diseases in pregnancy—e.g., measles and mumps—is at present both scanty and unconvincing. We therefore asked some large approved societies to take special note of all cases of rubella and measles in married women, and to observe whether any of these women gave birth to a child within 12 months of the end date of the recorded illness. For these " double-event " cases they filled in a " notification " form and returned it to us. We made the post-illness interval 12 months for ease of operation and because we thought that some of the immediate preconception illnesses might be of interest. No controls were needed, because our sole interest lay in the relative

THE LANCET]   PUBLIC HEALTH   [DEC. 31, 1949   1237

sympathising to some extent with this objection, the committee points out that " the National Insurance (Medical Certification) Regulations, 1948 (S.I. 1948, no. 1175), provide, in paragraph 3 of the Schedule, that if, in the practitioner's opinion, a disclosure to the claimant of the precise cause of incapacity would be prejudicial to his well-being, the certificate may contain a less precise statement."

PARA-AMINOSALICYLIC ACID AND STREPTOMYCIN IN PULMONARY TUBERCULOSIS

A CLINICAL trial of p-aminosalicylic acid (P.A.S.) and streptomycin in pulmonary tuberculosis was undertaken in 1948 by the Medical Research Council, with the coöperation of the British Tuberculosis Association. The trial is not yet completed but some of the results already obtained are so important that the joint committee responsible for guiding the trial has decided to issue the following preliminary statement.

A major disadvantage of streptomycin is that the period of effective therapy is limited in many patients by the emergence of streptomycin-resistant strains of tubercle bacilli after five or more weeks of treatment. Many workers have suggested that the addition of another tuberculostatic agent might suppress the resistant strains, which in the initial phases are present in very small numbers ; published reports on a few cases treated with P.A.S. and streptomycin have been encouraging. The present investigation was planned to examine, by the method of controlled trial, the possibility that P.A.S. has this property, and at the same time to assess the clinical effect of this drug alone and in combination with streptomycin.

PLAN OF TRIAL

Three treatment groups of over 50 cases each were observed : (a) P.A.S. alone (20 g. of the sodium salt daily) ; (b) streptomycin alone (1 g. daily) ; and (c) both drugs together (20 g. of the sodium salt of P.A.S. and 1 g. of streptomycin daily). The methods were similar to those employed in the first M.R.C. clinical trial of streptomycin in pulmonary tuberculosis,[1] and the type of case was again defined as follows : acute rapidly progressive bilateral pulmonary tuberculosis, of recent development, unsuitable for collapse therapy, in young adults aged 15–30. After acceptance for the trial by a panel, patients were allocated to one or other of the three treatment groups by a method of random selection. The prescribed treatment was given for three months in each group. Clinicians and pathologists at eleven hospital centres have coöperated in this investigation, keeping uniform records, using standard clinical and bacteriological procedures, and reporting results at regular intervals to the council's Tuberculosis Research Unit, where the grouped results have been analysed.

PRELIMINARY RESULTS

For this well-defined type of case of pulmonary tuberculosis, the trial has demonstrated unequivocally that the combination of P.A.S. with streptomycin considerably reduces the risk of development of streptomycin-resistant strains of tubercle bacilli during the six months following the start of treatment. This conclusion is applicable so far only to the acute form of disease treated, and it remains to be seen whether the same results are obtainable in other forms of tuberculosis amenable to streptomycin therapy. Furthermore, the conclusion is applicable only to the large dose of P.A.S. used ; this dosage causes discomfort in some

1. Brit. med. J. 1948, ii, 769.

patients and it has been agreed to find out, by further trials, whether smaller doses would achieve a same result. It must be stressed also that streptomycin is effective only in certain forms of tuberculosis, and the finding reported here must not be interpreted as indicating that a combination with another drug will be effective in those forms for which little result would be expected from streptomycin alone.

THE NEW ZEALAND ELECTION

FROM OUR NEW ZEALAND CORRESPONDENT

AT this general election on Nov. 30, the National Party was returned with the substantial majority of 46 seats to Labour's 34, the latter figure including all the 4 Maori seats. The Labour government's fourteen years of office thus came to an end, and Mr. S. G. Holland has assumed office as prime minister. The new minister of social security and health is Mr. J. T. Watts, of Christchurch, a barrister and solicitor about 40 years of age with a distinguished academic record, who entered parliament six years ago.

The National Party's election policy emphasised prevention and research, and promised a complete reorganisation of the hospital system on a basis of regional control and decentralisation. It supported recent Acts for the more economical management of medical and pharmaceutical benefits, and promised help for the elderly, for the Post Graduate Women's Teaching Hospital in Auckland, and for a number of other projects. With recent and forthcoming appointments inside the health department—notably that of the new director-general, Dr. J. Cairney—the field is open for much-needed progressive development.

The Labour Party's fourteen years saw the introduction, in spite of war-time difficulties, of an almost complete series of medical and allied benefits under social security, specialist services being the only major gap. The fee-for-service principle in maternity and medical benefits was dominant. Little change in hospital organisation and planning was undertaken, though during this era the government came to be much more responsible for finance than formerly.

Public Health

Typhoid on a Liner

WHEN the liner s.s Mooltan arrived in the Port of London on Dec. 16, three sick members of the crew were removed to hospital for observation. On subsequent days further members of the crew were admitted to hospital, and a diagnosis of typhoid fever has now been confirmed in some of them. On Dec. 22 a total of eleven confirmed cases were under treatment, and five further members of the crew were under observation in hospital. The organism is Vi-phage type A. Retrospective inquiries suggest that the dates of onset of illness were during the last ten days of the voyage. One passenger has been admitted to hospital as a suspected case of enteric fever. The names and addresses of passengers and members of the crew who left the vessel have been notified to medical officers of health of the destinations to which they were proceeding.

Poliomyelitis

In the week ended Dec. 10 notifications in England and Wales numbered : poliomyelitis 124 (141), polio-encephalitis 10 (15). Figures for the previous week are shown in parentheses. The total of 134 notifications of poliomyelitis and polioencephalitis together may be compared with figures of 76 in the corresponding week of 1947 and 36 in 1948. In 1926 the corresponding

THE LANCET]   THE CARNAGE ON THE ROADS   [FEB. 25, 1950 367

Points of View

THE CARNAGE ON THE ROADS

C. G. LEAROYD
M.R.C.S.

CHILDREN in this country are robbed of some fifty thousand years of life each year by motor traffic. Motor-cycles kill 500–1000 young men a year—twice the number of car drivers killed, though there are over four times as many cars licensed. Pedestrians, cyclists, and passengers make up well over three-quarters of the carnage. The driver of the goods vehicle has the highest average killing capacity ; the private car driver comes second. The motor-bike is the most lethal form of transport ; a bus can go fifteen times further before killing anybody. The ratio of killed to injured is about 1 to 30 ; but one or two of the 30 are economically dead.

Statistics may be convincing, but they are not so compelling as remembered scenes. We doctors in general practice collect in our memories quite a number of tragic roadside groups, snaps of crippled servitude, and cameos of homes in tears. There is always a contrasting element in them—the live animal and the pulped thing ; the triviality of the error and the heavy sentence ; the trip for pleasure and this. Three recent ones in my mind are : (1) a lovely English lane and a young man sprawled over a twisted motor-bike, the grey of his brain showing ; (2) a nursery head and body with crushed thighs on a slab midst disinfectant smells ; and (3) a dazed cluster in a cottage on the night before the inquest. We go on collecting them all our lives and can fling them in the faces of those who say : " This is an engineering or educational or legislative problem and does not particularly concern you."

Parrots say " This is a blot on our civilisation," but I am not sure that it is not part of an industrial civilisation ; something of the impersonality of the machine and the ruthlessness of huge production affects its concentrated populations. The more machine-minded a nation is, the more careless of life, in that respect, it becomes ; in the U.S.A. 40 million vehicles killed 32,300 people and wounded 1,150,000 in 1947.

People, however, react as strongly as ever to the isolated personal tragedy. Queen Victoria was most indignant and said that mountaineering ought to be stopped by law when Whymper left some dead friends on the Alps, but there was not any general indignation at the myriad lives halved by lead poisoning in the potteries ; thousands burn with resentment at the injustice done to a Winslow boy but are left comparatively cold by " Pedestrians (under 7), 609 killed on the roads in 1948, 60·4% by goods vehicles." Most people are only capable of compassion within their own group—except in war, when the group is enlarged into the nation. This is probably defensive, for a man with a universal compassion would hardly have enough energy left to paddle out of his tears. Most doctors in their first few weeks of a job in a mental hospital feel like this.

When death, in the form of an industrial disease or a habit like gin-drinking or this road-killing, keeps stealing victims from among a moderately indifferent community, certain people with a surplus of compassion, often relatives of the victims, band themselves together and become nuclei of societies, which stimulate the Government to its duty. Eventually the Government takes on the whole job. We have not reached that stage with road casualties yet and probably will not do so for another ten years. Meanwhile the Royal Society for the Prevention of Accidents and other agencies are doing splendid work in helping to reduce the deaths, which fell from 6500 in 1938 to 4500 in 1948, though how many of the lives were saved by lack of petrol cannot be known. The individual also has his part to play, especially we doctors with our compelling pictures.

WHAT CAN BE DONE ?

The problem of accident-prevention is being tackled in this country under three main headings : engineering, education, and enforcement.

Under engineering come the road schemes, the erection of a thousand signs, the robot schoolmasters of our erring feet and wheels.

" Under education, which is considered to be the main weapon in the present economic condition, a comprehensive organisation has been set up throughout the country for conducting the road-safety campaign, which was launched in 1945. Most local authorities now have their road-safety committees ; the police and school-teachers play a large part in their work of educating both children and adults in correct road behaviour." [1]

Our job here is to make instructed asides, and there is one small psychological point, probably dating back to the time when man was nomadic, which is the basis of a big proportion of road accidents—the feeling and display of superiority in those with the swifter forms of transport. You see it in the small boy with his scooter, and in primal form in the proud mien of the rider to hounds ; you may remember it as an ecstasy of movement when you first took to cycling, skating, or driving a car. In others it incites envy, hatred, and admiration.

There is a simple bit of child psychology which could be turned to good account in accident-prevention education. Children and young people have a natural taste for horror stories. This is not primarily ghoulish or morbid, it is their way of learning from the experience of others. If they had to learn from their own experience there would be a terrible casualty list, and few of us would be here. The almost pleasurable apprehension of the story is kept up until it is satisfactorily topped off with an explanation or a moral, which cannot be forgotten. I remember over fifty years ago being told a satisfying story of a boy who was drowned because he ate three pounds of cherries with the stones before swimming. The modern version is : " . . . so he stepped into the road, but he was walking with the stream of the traffic and not against it, and he did not look behind him, so the Big Blue Bus . . ." Most of the children killed on the road are under seven. Cannot some genius provide them with a new set of nursery stories—*Red Riding and the Wicked Rolls* ; or *Goody Twoshoes and the Bad Goods Vehicle* ?

ENFORCEMENT

Excellent as all this education of children and parents is, it must cause sardonic laughter in Heaven that we train the children from earliest years and then let off the person who does the killing with half an hour's test, generally under non-testing conditions.

All that is being done for road safety now may slowly lessen the casualty list or keep it more or less stationary while the number of cars increases, but attention to the strict training of drivers would halve it in a year.

Turning a person loose with a car after the present elementary tests is like licensing a surgeon as soon as he knows the Red Cross book and how to hold a knife. Even these tests were opposed by the A.A. and the R.A.C. " They argued that tests would be of very doubtful practical utility and a source of considerable expense. They declared that the chief requisite of safe driving is ' road sense, which can only be acquired on the road

---

1. Part of a letter from the secretary of the Royal Society for the Prevention of Accidents, to whom I am also indebted for many of the statistics quoted.

itself ' " [2]—i.e., by practice on the public. Yet between Nov. 1, 1946, when tests were resumed, and Nov. 26, 1949, the examiners made 976,220 tests and failed 38% of the candidates.

Tests of Fitness and Accident-proneness

The questions on the present application forms for a driving licence—Can you read so-and-so ? Do you suffer from epilepsy ?—are silly. The driver fills in and signs his own certificate of fitness to drive, and the person with a prohibitive but not too obvious defect has merely to lie. The only object of these questions is to cover the officials, so when the epileptic driver kills a pedestrian they can say : " We are not to blame. He signed this." It is their job to find out these things themselves—to insist on a proper medical examination, including visual and auditory tests, and an examination of past history with a right to see the panel card, besides an ordinary physical examination as for life insurance.

What a medical examination will not discover is accident-proneness. In an investigation in the U.S.A. it was found that 50% of the accidents were caused by 7% of the drivers. And the Industrial Health Research Board,[3] reporting on accident-proneness, says that if a large number of people are exposed to the same risks something like 10% of them will have 75% of the accidents. Accident-proneness, the board's report continues, is a relatively stable quality ; those who have an undue number of accidents in one period of exposure will tend to do so in other periods. Further, those who have an undue number of minor accidents also tend to have an undue number of major ones.

The National Institute of Industrial Psychology devised a series of tests which can pick out the accident-prone driver. These tests are truly psychosomatic. One of them tests the time from ocular stimulus to muscular action ; the lag is never less than $^3/_5$ second and the average is $1^1/_5$ seconds. Thus, with a car going at 30 m.p.h., if the driver sees a child run out in front of him, the car will move forward 26 feet before the brakes start to act with a quick-reacting driver, 53 feet with an average driver, and 80 feet with a slow-reacting driver. Other tests are for visual acuity and for judgment of spatial relationships, relative size, and speed. There is a series of tests in a dummy car with a moving picture of a road in front. The track followed by the driver and the speed attained are automatically recorded. Sir Ernest Graham-Little proposed in Parliament some sixteeen years ago that certain of these tests should be made compulsory for all applicants for driving licences, and if his advice had been taken there would be a good many more people alive today. The tests pick out the potential homicide and show others in what way they are inclined to be homicidal. There is abundant foreign experience to justify their imposition.

Lectures

Then there should be a series of lectures on Roadery and Road-craft with a written examination and a viva at the end. One lecture might well be on " Alcohol and the Driver," and, if there is merit in having insight into one's own condition, another on " The Bad Driver." I can imagine a page from the notes of a putative candidate on this :

Over 90% of fatal accidents would not have happened if the Highway Code had been obeyed.

Six types of bad driver :

(1) The Thruster. Generally male. Example of male aggressiveness. Hurts his pride to be overtaken.

(2) The Hurrier. Usually with nothing to hurry for. Associated with restlessness and acquisitiveness. (Shown

aerial film of London-Brighton road on a Sunday, 50 miles of continuous traffic in which one " hurrier " overtook eight times to gain half a mile in the queue.)

(3) The Downtrodden at Home who is a hell of a fellow behind ten horse-power.

(4) The Dreamer. You cannot see mental pictures and real ones clearly at the same time. Malcolm Campbell's definition of a good driver : " Concentration and again more concentration. Your mind must not wander for a second."

(5) The Speed Merchant who enjoys speed for its own sake. Generally immature. Speed is the biggest single factor in fatal accidents.

(6) The Exhibitionist. The man or youth who wants others to think he is a dare-devil.

Anyone who thinks that road-craft consists in sitting behind a wheel and steering is on a par with those who think all a judge has to do is to dress up and look wise. Road-craft requires the skill of a cricketer, the intuitions and knowledge of conventions of the bridge player, and the imperturbable patience of a dry-fly man.

The tests of accident-proneness and lectures on road-craft should be given also to the children of 14–15 at school, where Roadery and Road-craft should rank with the three Rs. Boys have a natural aptitude for these subjects, and embryo drivers would thus start their training early. In any case, safety on the road affects them vitally : " It is estimated that at the present rate every fourth or fifth child born in Great Britain is destined to be killed or injured in a road accident."[4] The Highway Code might be learnt by heart, as the Catechism used to be, or set to music.

Then to the actual driving test on the road should be added a dusk and night test ; dusk is a peak hour for killing and it is absurd to let a driver loose until he has been tested in it.

There is also much to be said for laying out special tracks for testing drivers. London omnibus drivers have or had one and part of it was greased, so that they could practise rectifying skids. With india-rubber children and dogs scudding about, operated from a central control tower, and with other delights, it could be made a real test for a driver's reaction to emergency conditions.

Some years ago I admitted to a mental hospital a young woman with acute hysteria, who had just killed a bread-winner cycling home in the dusk. Whatever the merits of the accident—and there were no witnesses—I am absolutely certain she should not have been a driver. In the proposed course she would have failed on past history, in the medical examination, in the body-mind tests, probably in the written examination and viva, and certainly over the emergency track. She had passed the usual test.

A word must be said about the motor-bikes, which are the most lethal instruments on the road. Unless the tester rides pillion it is impossible to make the driving test for motor-cyclists a real one, and therefore it is all the more necessary to make the rider's factual knowledge as complete as possible. It is just murder allowing these boys of 16 to go on the road without letting them know what they are in for. They are, however, at an age when, though the sense of adventure is at its strongest, a wise nature has also quickened their sense of self-preservation, which expresses itself as a love and memory for horrors, warnings from vicarious experience. The lectures to them would be on these lines :

" You may get a grand thrill going round a bend at 60 m.p.h. and banking at 60°, but just remember what you may be running into—the greasy patch and the skid, sheep, the car on the wrong side, playing children."

Then follow a dozen short films of real motor-bike smashes —the roadside confusion, the twisted metal shorn of glory, close-up of the stertorous head, the ambulance, a glimpse

2. Vernon, H. M. Accidents and Their Prevention. London, 1936 ; p. 154.

3. The Personal Factor in Accidents. Industr. Hlth Res. Bd emerg. Rep. no. 3, 1942.

4. Vernon, H. M. Accidents and Their Prevention. London, 1936 ; p. 101.

through a door at a sheeted figure, the glimpse that does not disclose finally but suggests endlessly.

" If you want to be bold and bad, go and do it in the boxing ring or on the football field or on a horse. Only 23 people were killed in these ways last year, whereas on motor-bikes there were . . ."

At the end of the courses for drivers and riders, when they were handed their licences, they would be given a little slip telling them—quite cheerfully—that the most dangerous time for them would be not when they first went on the road but shortly afterwards, when the caution of the novice had worn off.

The whole course would take about ten days, and a driver's licence would be on a par with a pilot's certificate, and as worth guarding as a minor professional qualification.

Any motoring offence, especially exceeding the limit on restricted roads, where two-thirds of the deaths occurred last year, should automatically involve a testing or re-testing. This would make the old driver who was uncertain of passing the test extraordinarily careful. It would also threaten the livelihood of the careless goods-vehicle driver, who is the biggest killer of children. This should be made mandatory on our amateur justices, the bulk of whom are drivers themselves and can be lenient to the point of flabbiness.

CONCLUSION

The whole question is this : Having regard to the facts that 4500–5000 people are killed and some 150,000 wounded on the roads each year and that 90% of these accidents are preventable, is driving a sufficiently lethal occupation to demand skilled drivers who are adequately tested ?

Whether the Minister of Transport and a Parliament of drivers are brave and selfless enough to do anything about it is another matter.

Meanwhile twelve people going about their tasks today are destined to be killed on the roads tomorrow.

Public Health

Supplies of B.C.G. Vaccine

ACCORDING to an announcement by the Department of Health for Scotland, " reports and letters appearing in the press indicate that there is a belief that the temporary stoppage of supplies of B.C.G. vaccine is due to financial reasons.

" This belief," says the announcement, " has no foundation. As has been previously stated, the stoppage is entirely due to production difficulties of a technical nature. Everything possible is being done to overcome these difficulties, and the Department of Health hope that as a result further supplies of B.C.G. will be available in the near future."

Scottish Report on Poliomyelitis

In a report on the 1947 epidemic of poliomyelitis, the Department of Health for Scotland notes that the disease seemed to attack small, rather than large, family groups : and " it was obvious that poliomyelitis was a disease especially of persons living in four apartment houses, particularly those with less than six occupants." Compared with previous years, there was a significant increase in the percentage of cases among people over 15 years of age. In the 1947 epidemic, 6·5% of cases were among children under 1 year of age, 35·8% among those aged 1–4 years, 34·6% among those aged 5–14 years, and 23·1% among people aged 15 years or more. Paralytic poliomyelitis was a disease principally of the cities. The focal attack of the outbreak in cities was in children under 5 years of age, whereas in rural areas it was in older patients.

Estimate of Births

The Registrar-General's return for the week ended Feb. 4 gives the following estimates for live births in England and Wales : final estimate for the quarter ending March 31, 186,000 ; provisional estimate for the quarter ending June 30, 183,000.

In England Now

A Running Commentary by Peripatetic Correspondents

I HAVE been following the activities of my colleagues, and others who are offering themselves at the hustings, with purely academic interest, because, like everyone else, I made up my mind which way to vote before the campaign had even started and quite irrespective of the candidates' oratorical powers. I have been sadly disappointed at the low standard of repartee in dealing with hecklers, which is perhaps attributable to the modern habit of politicians of haranguing defenceless audiences over the wireless. Such retorts as " Shut up ! ", " Oh *do* shut up ! ", and " You silly woman " represent a stage in the development of repartee that most of us left behind at our prep-school and are asking for the radio rejoinder : " You clot ! "

There seems to be a lack of subtlety and originality in the posters, too. When Lord Addison was standing in the 1910 election his opponent put up a poster saying : " Dr. Addison asks for support on the ground that he is used to cutting up bodies. Will you let him cut up the Empire ? Don't vote for Addison who Cuts Up the Stomach, but vote for Hay who will See it is FILLED." People (including the Editor of *The Lancet*) wrote to the *Daily Chronicle* about it. You can read the angry headlines in the faded cuttings in that fascinating store of medical miscellanea, the scrap-books in the Royal College of Surgeons library in London. I fancy that one of the attractions of electioneering is that sticking up posters for passers-by to see gives vent to a primitive urge. There is surely the same underlying motive in sticking slogans on outdoor walls at election times and in scribbling other things on other walls at other times.

* * *

My wife has undertaken to distribute milk to the more needy coloured infants at what may be called a welfare clinic in the grounds of our excellent maternity unit. The maximum age is about three years. Since she started this I have often been surprised to hear smatterings of pidgin-Arabic floating round the house, to the amusement of the servants, because with commendable enterprise my wife took on the job not knowing much more than *imshi* and the more useful *fissa*.

In my own ignorance I had carefully explained to her that a certain amount of organisation was needed if she was to make up, distribute, and annotate the issue of milk to upwards of fifty screaming infants whose escorts had never learnt the art of queueing. The maths involved in mixing dried milk with water, being psychic as to the number who would turn up, and opening sufficient tins in advance occupied more than one whole evening.

We need not have worried. All our planning went by the board. The children appeared with escort— usually some relative about a year older than the eldest child taking part in this new whim of the mad British. Sometimes the escorts would appear without infants but with filthy bottles in lieu, so the order went out : " No chicos, no milk." On the next few mornings the provision of " chicos " was accomplished with such speed that the only honest explanation could have been that all the " patients " lived just outside the hospital compound.

The proceedings are enlivened by the occasional appearance of the clinic doctor—a very hard-worked lady—whose method of communication can at least be said to quell the riot for a few seconds. She resorts to a flow of language, pitched in a voice even higher than that of the indigenous population, which leaves all mute and gaping with awe. The method adopted by one of the interpreters, who gave a helping hand the first few mornings, is equally effective ; this consists in beating a rapid tattoo with both hands on the heads of all children in reach. The milk is distributed in emptied butter tins, and woe betide the doler-out-of-milk if, in a fit of temporary aberration, she hands out an Australian butter tin when a South African one was handed in. The very small infants are given bottles— with careful instructions as to which is the teat and which the valve. The finest sight of all is the row of babies

THE LANCET] GENERAL PRACTICE IN ENGLAND TODAY [MARCH 25, 1950 555

GENERAL PRACTICE IN ENGLAND TODAY
A RECONNAISSANCE

JOSEPH S. COLLINGS *

M.B., B.Sc. (Agr) Sydney

GENERAL medical practice is a unique social phenomenon. The general practitioner enjoys more prestige and wields more power than any other citizen, unless it be the judge on his bench. In a world of ever-increasing management, the powers of even the senior managers are petty compared with the powers of the doctor to influence the physical, psychological, and economic destiny of other people.

But unlike the manager, who exercises his controls over whole groups of society, the doctor exercises his in a microcosm and in relation to individuals ; and for this and other reasons he is largely free from the limitations which democratic principles set on the acquisition of power.

General practice is unique in other ways also. For example, it is accepted as being something specific, without anyone knowing what it really is. Neither the teacher responsible for instructing future general practitioners, nor the specialist who supposedly works in continuous association with the G.P., nor for that matter the G.P. himself, can give an adequate definition of general practice. Though generally identified with the last-century concept of " family doctoring," usually it has long ceased to be this. Nevertheless its stability and its reputation rest largely on this identification.

While other branches of medicine have progressed and developed, general practice, instead of developing concurrently, has adapted itself to the changing patterns ; and sometimes this adaptation has in fact been regression.

There are no real standards for general practice. What the doctor does, and how he does it, depends almost wholly on his own conscience.

The conduct of general practice and of the individual practitioner is inextricably interwoven with commercial and emotional considerations, which too often negate the code of medical ethics by which the public are supposedly safeguarded and from which the high reputation of medicine stems. Hence material and moral issues have become inseparable, and it is impossible to discuss general practice without discussing morals, and therefore without moralising. In this report the issues are kept separate as far as possible, but this is not very far.

Section I describes how the observations were made ; section II is an account of general practice as I found it ; and section III deals with the National Health Service in relation to general practice as I found it. I contrast this with the usual endeavour made to interpret the Act in terms of what general practice is supposed to be or what we might like to think it is.

I know well that many of my deductions rest on subjective impressions rather than objective fact, though I have tried to keep the two apart. Very little statistical evidence is used—principally because little valuable evidence of this kind is available, and secondarily because the major problems of general practice are not soluble in terms of statistics.

My observations have led me to write what is indeed a condemnation of general practice in its present form ; but they have also led me to recognise the importance of general practice and the dangers of continuing to pretend that it is something which it is not. Instead of continuing a policy of compensating for its deficiencies, we should admit them honestly and try to correct them at their source. If I do no more than convey this, I shall be satisfied.

I. SCOPE AND METHOD OF STUDY

At the outset I was advised that no accurate picture could be obtained by detailed inquiries in the London area, with its aggregation of teaching hospitals and many other complicating factors peculiar to a city of this size. I therefore decided to work outside London, in regions selected so that a mosaic might be constructed which would present the general picture. Having no knowledge of British geography or economy, I was guided by various advisers who knew the country, and eventually decided on three regions—in the north, the north-west, and the south. For purposes of comparison I also spent some time in Scotland.

Thanks to the willing coöperation of all the doctors approached, I have been able to see their work, both in their surgeries and in the homes of their patients, to become conversant with their difficulties, professional and personal, and to learn a great deal about their individual and collective attitudes to the new service.

Though others were visited, I have studied in some detail the work of 55 English practices, operated by 104 doctors. These 55 may be classified as :

Industrial	..	..	..	16
Urban-residential	..	..		17
Rural	..	..	..	..	22

The 16 industrial practices can be further divided into complete industrial 9 and " mixed " (industrial better-class residential) 7. The 22 rural practices can be divided into rural-town 8 and isolated rural 14. Some 30 of the practices were run by individual practitioners ; the rest were partnerships or partner-assistantships with 2–6 doctors working together.

The 55 practices visited varied greatly in size (both number of patients and area) and in history and development.

Of the one-man practices some had full lists (4000) while others ranged down through 3000 and 2000 to less than 1000. Examples of different sizes were seen in all areas, though in the industrial areas only two practices were seen where the doctor's list was less than 2000, and in the rural areas only three where the lists approximated to or exceeded 3500. The partnerships and partner-assistantships studied covered much the same wide range of patient numbers, though very few had less than 2000 per partner.

In terms of area covered by a practice and accessibility of patients, conditions ranged from the most compact type of practice, in densely populated urban areas, to remote rural practices with less than 1000 patients living miles apart.

The history and development of the practices showed a similar wide range of variation. Some were over a century old ; others had been established before the war but had since been entirely re-established. Many of the industrial practices had had large " panel " and " club " lists since the early days of the old National Health Insurance scheme, and had depended on these for the greater part of the income ; but there were various gradations of the panel-private ratio through to completely private practice.

---

* At present research fellow, Harvard School of Public Health, Boston, Mass.

THE LANCET]   MUNCHAUSEN'S SYNDROME   [FEB. 10, 1951   339

Special Articles

MUNCHAUSEN'S SYNDROME

Richard Asher
M.D. Lond., M.R.C.P.

HERE is described a common syndrome which most doctors have seen, but about which little has been written. Like the famous Baron von Munchausen, the persons affected have always travelled widely ; and their stories, like those attributed to him,[1] are both dramatic and untruthful. Accordingly the syndrome is respectfully dedicated to the baron, and named after him.

The patient showing the syndrome is admitted to hospital with apparent acute illness supported by a plausible and dramatic history. Usually his story is largely made up of falsehoods ; he is found to have attended, and deceived, an astounding number of other hospitals ; and he nearly always discharges himself against advice, after quarrelling violently with both doctors and nurses. A large number of abdominal scars is particularly characteristic of this condition.

That is a general outline ; and few doctors can boast that they have never been hoodwinked by the condition. Often the diagnosis is made by a passing doctor or sister, who, recognising the patient and his performance, exclaims : " I know that man. We had him in St. Quinidine's two years ago and thought he had a perforated ulcer. He's the man who always collapses on buses and tells a story about being an ex-submarine commander who was tortured by the Gestapo." Equally often, the trickster is first revealed in the hospital dining-room, when, with a burst of laughter, one of the older residents exclaims : " Good heavens, you haven't got Luella Priskins in again, surely ? Why she's been in here three times before and in Barts, Mary's, and Guy's as well. She sometimes comes in with a different name, but always says she's coughed up pints of blood and tells a story about being an ex-opera-singer and helping in the French resistance movement."

DIAGNOSIS

It is almost impossible to be certain of the diagnosis at first, and it requires a bold casualty officer to refuse admission. Usually the patient seems seriously ill and is admitted unless someone who has seen him before is there to expose his past. Experienced front-gate porters are often invaluable at doing this.

The following are useful pointers :

1. (Already mentioned) a multiplicity of scars, often abdominal.
2. A mixture of truculence and evasiveness in manner.
3. An immediate history which is always acute and harrowing yet not entirely convincing—overwhelmingly severe abdominal pain of uncertain type, cataclysmal blood-loss unsupported by corresponding pallor, dramatic loss of consciousness, and so forth.
4. A wallet or handbag stuffed with hospital attendance cards, insurance claim forms, and litigious correspondence.

If the patient is not recognised by an old acquaintance, the diagnosis is only gradually revealed by inquiries at other hospitals. Some have given so much trouble elsewhere they have been placed on hospital black-lists. Often the police are found to know the patient and can give many helpful details. Gradually the true history is pieced together and the patient's own story is seen to be a matrix of fantasy and falsehood, in which fragments of complete truth are surprisingly imbedded. Just as the patient's story is not wholly false, so neither are all the symptoms ; and it must be recognised that

these patients are often quite ill, although their illness is shrouded by duplicity and distortion. When the whole truth is known, past history sometimes reveals drug-addiction, mental-hospital treatment, or prison sentences, but these factors are not constant, and the past may consist solely in innumerable admissions to hospitals and evidence of pathological lying. Often a real organic lesion from the past has left some genuine physical signs which the patient uses (to quote Pooh Bah) " to give artistic verisimilitude to an otherwise bald and unconvincing narrative."

SOME CHARACTERISTIC FEATURES

Most cases resemble organic emergencies. Well-known varieties are :

1. The acute abdominal type (laparotomophilia migrans), which is the most common. Some of these patients have been operated on so often that the development of genuine intestinal obstruction from adhesions may confuse the picture.
2. The hæmorrhagic type, who specialise in bleeding from lungs or stomach, or other blood-loss. They are colloquially known as " hæmoptysis merchants " and " hæmatemesis merchants."
3. The neurological type, presenting with paroxysmal headache, loss of consciousness, or peculiar fits.

The most remarkable feature of the syndrome is the apparent senselessness of it. Unlike the malingerer, who may gain a definite end, these patients often seem to gain nothing except the discomfiture of unnecessary investigations or operations. Their initial tolerance to the more brutish hospital measures is remarkable, yet they commonly discharge themselves after a few days with operation wounds scarcely healed, or intravenous drips still running.

Another feature is their intense desire to deceive everybody as much as possible. Many of their falsehoods seem to have little point. They lie for the sake of lying They give false addresses, false names, and false occupations merely from a love of falsehood. Their effrontery is sometimes formidable, and they may appear many times at the same hospital, hoping to meet a new doctor upon whom to practise their deception.

POSSIBLE MOTIVES

Sometimes the motive is never clearly ascertained, but there are indications that one of the following mechanisms may be involved :

1. A desire to be the centre of interest and attention. They may be suffering in fact from the Walter Mitty syndrome,[2] but instead of playing the dramatic part of the surgeon, they submit to the equally dramatic rôle of the patient.
2. A grudge against doctors and hospitals, which is satisfied by frustrating or deceiving them.
3. A desire for drugs.
4. A desire to escape from the police. (These patients often swallow foreign bodies, interfere with their wounds, or manipulate their thermometers.)
5. A desire to get free board and lodgings for the night, despite the risk of investigations and treatment.

Supplementing these scanty motives, there probably exists some strange twist of personality. Perhaps most cases are hysterics, schizophrenics, masochists, or psychopaths of some kind ; but as a group they show such a constant pattern of behaviour that it is worth considering them together.

ILLUSTRATIVE CASE-RECORDS

Three cases of the abdominal type of Munchausen's syndrome are described below ; for they show clearly the typical features of the advanced form of the disease. Many other milder forms have been encountered, but it would be tedious if more were described. All the

1. Raspe, R. E., et al. (1785) Singular Travels, Campaigns and Adventures of Baron Munchausen. London : Cresset Press. 1948.

2. Thurber, J. The Secret Life of Walter Mitty. My World and Welcome to It. London, 1942.

names used in these case-histories have been altered, though most of the names were false to start with ; but doctors who have met any of the patients may find that the changed name gives a clue to the original one.

I

A man of 47, giving the name Thomas Beeches, was transferred to the Central Middlesex Mental Observation Ward on May 16 from Harrow Hospital. He had been admitted there on May 13 with suspected intestinal obstruction; laparotomy had shown nothing abnormal. After the operation he had accused the ward sister of tampering with his wallet while he was under the anæsthetic, he had become truculent and demanded his discharge, and because of his violence, and his foolhardiness in wanting to walk out with a day-old laparotomy, he was sent for mental observation.

On examination he was rational and convincing. His abdomen was a mass of scars of various vintage. He explained that while in the Merchant Navy in 1942 he had been torpedoed, suffering multiple abdominal injuries. He was then taken prisoner by the Japanese and kept in Singapore till 1945. Throughout this time he had multiple discharging fæcal fistulæ. In 1945, after the liberation of Singapore, he had been taken to Freemantle where he had eleven operations in 7 months (to close the multiple fistulæ), since when he had been continuously at sea till 4 days previously.

The characteristic Munchausen flavour of this history led to further inquiries which revealed that only 8 days previously, while supposed to be at sea, he had been in St. James' Hospital, Balham, complaining of acute abdominal pain ; and that a year before that he had been in the same hospital and again behaved in the same way. It was further found that in 1943, when he should have been in Singapore, he had been admitted to the Central Middlesex Hospital complaining of "bursting open of an old torpedo wound" with a discharging sinus in the right iliac fossa. He had then told such a bewildering series of different stories that he had been transferred to Shenley Hospital as a chronic delinquency psychopath, where he was observed for 2 months and then discharged. At Shenley it was discovered that he had a long history of delinquency and had three past convictions for crime, as well as having been twice in West Park Mental Hospital. (He had escaped both times.) On this present occasion no certifiable abnormality could be found and he was discharged on May 19, 3 days after admission. No doubt he is still going from one hospital to another.

A fortnight later, a surgical registrar, knowing my interest in Munchausen's syndrome, produced the notes of a case he had encountered at the Norfolk and Norwich Hospital. It was interesting but not surprising to find that it was the same patient. The notes showed that a Thomas Beeches had been admitted on June 23, 1949, as a case of acute intestinal obstruction. He told a story of having been 33 years in the R.A.F. and of having been shot down over Mannheim in 1942, after which he needed "eight abdominal operations and three short-circuits." After treatment with morphine, intravenous drip, and gastric suction, he refused a laparatomy and discharged himself against advice on June 26.

II

A woman of 29, giving the name of Margaret Coke, was admitted on June 13, 1948, complaining of 3 days' severe abdominal pain and vomiting. Her abdomen was a mass of scars. Though admitted from an Edgware address, she gave a home address in Houston, Texas, and said that all her previous operations had been done there, some of them by a "horse doctor." Clinically, she appeared to have subacute intestinal obstruction and was treated with morphine and a Miller-Abbot tube ; but she discharged herself on June 19 at her own request.

Three weeks later, on July 3, a woman calling herself Elsie Silverborough was admitted to another ward at the Central Middlesex Hospital, having been found collapsed in the street by the police. She gave a home address in Lancashire. It was found she had discharged herself that day from Wembley Hospital, where she had been admitted on the previous day for suspected acute

intestinal obstruction. As before, she had been found by the police collapsed in the street. Elsie Silverborough told a story of having had all her previous operations at the Manchester Royal Infirmary, but a surgical registrar recognised her as the Margaret Coke who had been operated on by the Texas horse doctor, and they were proved to be one and the same person.

Inquiries at Manchester Royal Infirmary revealed no trace of either Margaret Coke or Elsie Silverborough having been there, but the day after the identities of these two persons had been merged, a surgical houseman recognised the patient as a certain Elsie Packoma whom he had encountered twice at the Royal Northern Hospital on Oct. 27, 1947, and Nov. 13, 1947. On both occasions she arrived in casualty smelling of drink and complaining of retention of urine. On the first occasion she was catheterised and then refused all treatment, refused to sign the book or to be admitted, and said she was going to a hotel to call in her private doctor. On the second occasion, she was recognised by the casualty officer and made off before a doctor had seen her. Further inquiries at the Manchester Royal Infirmary revealed that an Elsie Packoma, with a scarred abdomen and a Manchester address, had been admitted as a case of intestinal obstruction on Nov. 15, 1947—two days after discharging herself from the Royal Northern Hospital. No operation had been performed. She had been treated with morphine, Ryle's tube, and enemata, and discharged herself against advice 2 days after admission.

The triad of Margaret Coke, Elsie Silverborough, and Elsie Packoma was discharged from the Central Middlesex Hospital on July 6, 1948, and nothing further has been heard of it. She told us before she went that she had lived in Piccadilly nearly all her life, working as a prostitute.

III

A woman of 41, giving the name Elsie De Coverley, was admitted to the Central Middlesex Hospital on Feb. 7, 1950, having collapsed on a bus. She gave a history of 2 days' melæna and 1 day's severe abdominal pain with vomiting of dark blood. On examination she was apparently in severe pain. Her abdomen was a mass of scars and her veins showed marks of many "cutting down" operations. Her heart showed a mitral presystolic murmur. She told us that in the last 5 years she had had two operations for perforation, one for gastro-enterostomy and one for intestinal obstruction, all done at the Royal Devon and Exeter Hospital, where she said she was due to return for a partial gastrectomy.

At first she was diagnosed as a case of a bleeding ulcer with probably a small perforation, but despite her severe pain there was no abdominal rigidity and radiography showed no gas under the diaphragm. Her hæmoglobin was 96 % and her stools gave only a weakly positive benzidine test. A telephone message to the Royal Devon and Exeter Hospital revealed that she had only once been there in 1944 and had never had an abdominal operation there, but that many other hospitals had made inquiries about her. The patient continued to complain of severe abdominal pain, and a barium meal and gastroscopy had been arranged when she discharged herself against advice on Feb. 15, saying that nobody really thought she had pain.

Since that time an attempt has been made to find out about her past, and here the Royal Devon and Exeter Hospital have been most helpful, because they have been able to trace much of her progress round the country by noting the hospitals that asked after her. More inquiries at these hospitals have each disclosed more admissions at other hospitals, and the complexity of the patient's wanderings grew in the manner of a snowball. I had not the time or the patience to pursue the meanderings completely and the fact that she was found to use nine different names made the project more formidable. The following list of some of her activities is probably incomplete :

In February, 1944, she was admitted to the Royal Devon and Exeter Hospital as Elsie De Coverley from Exeter Prison, with epistaxis.

On April 9, 1947, she was admitted to the Croydon General Hospital as Miss Joan Morris, a shorthand typist, giving a long history of dyspepsia and hæmatemesis. While being treated with rest and diet she discharged herself 2 days later.

From Oct. 31 till Nov. 16, 1947, she was in the Royal Sussex Hospital, giving the name Joan Summer, and suspected of having a bleeding leaking ulcer ; but at operation the findings were subacute obstruction from adhesions and scarred duodenal ulcer. Gastrojejunostomy was performed. She discharged herself on Nov. 16 against advice, still complaining of severe abdominal pain.

On Dec. 10, 1947, she was admitted to the Croydon General Hospital with acute abdominal pain, " doubled up in agony," as Mrs. Elsie Layton, a district nurse. She said she was awaiting a partial gastrectomy in Birmingham Hospital. Efforts made to contact her relatives showed that the names and addresses were all false and the patient discharged herself on Dec. 12. She was admitted to Redhill County Hospital a few days after leaving Croydon. She again gave a similar story and discharged herself within a few days.

From Jan. 29 to March 29, 1948, she was in Paddington Hospital, again as Joan Summer, and a laparotomy for bleeding duodenal ulcer was performed ; later she complained of severe anginal pain and discharged herself after giving much trouble in the ward.

In March, 1948, she was in the West London Hospital as Joan Lark with alleged pain and bleeding, and discharged herself.

From April 6 to 9, 1948, she was in Fulham Hospital as Joan Summer giving a history of having all her previous operations in York (inquiries at York failed to trace her), and again presenting with alleged abdominal pain and hæmatemesis. On April 9 she was recognised by a surgeon as Joan Lark of the West London and discharged herself that day.

On July 10, 1948, she was admitted to Guy's Hospital as Joan Malkin, but later said this was an assumed name and gave the name Joan De Coverley, and said all her previous operations had been done at Edinburgh (Edinburgh denied knowing her). At Guy's she was suspected of having a perforated ulcer, but a laparotomy on July 10 showed nothing abnormal except a mass of adhesions, and she discharged herself on July 13, only 3 days after the operation, and never returned to have her stitches out.

On Jan. 6, 1950, she was admitted to the Royal Free Hospital as Elsie De Coverley, with the usual story. She complained of continuous pain and discharged herself on Jan. 11, saying her sister had just died. (At many hospitals she has given a story of a dying sister.)

On Jan. 18 she was admitted to St. Mary Abbots Hospital still as Elsie De Coverley, having collapsed in Kensington High Street with alleged pain and vomiting of blood. On Jan. 20, when told she was not going to have an operation, she pulled out her stomach tube and demanded her immediate discharge.

Later the same day, she was admitted to University College Hospital, and she had a laparotomy on Jan. 25 for suspected perforation. Nothing was found except adhesions. The usual self-discharge followed on Jan. 30.

The same day she was admitted to St. Bartholomew's Hospital and discharged herself on Feb. 2.

From Feb. 7 till 15 . she was in the Central Middlesex Hospital—see the description at the beginning of this story.

Since leaving us she has remained active, because on March 7 she arrived at the Elizabeth Garrett Anderson Hospital as Jean Hops and was transferred via the Emergency Bed Service to the Royal Free Hospital. The transfer was unfortunate for her because she was recognised by the ward sister and registrar at the Royal Free, where she had been under another name in January this year, and she discharged herself immediately.

On March 27 she was admitted to Middlesex Hospital as Elsie De Coverley, with the usual story of pain and hæmatemesis, where she remained for three days. She discharged herself when she learnt that inquiries were being made about her at the Royal Devon and Exeter Hospital.

On April 12 she was admitted to the Croydon General, saying she was awaiting a partial gastrectomy at the Royal Devon and Exeter Hospital, and giving a history of severe abdominal pain and bleeding. The Croydon General rang the Royal Devon and Exeter Hospital and while the telephone conversation was being conducted she got out of bed, dressed, and made off.

On April 17 she turned up in Hackney Hospital as Elsie Shackleton, and that is the last that has been heard of her.

Probably she is now careful to avoid mentioning the Royal Devon and Exeter Hospital, who have repeatedly exposed her in the past, and, with new names and a slightly different story, is continuing to deceive the few remaining hospitals which she has not yet visited.

It seemed worth publishing this rather tedious itinerary in full to show the lengths to which a case of Munchausen's syndrome can develop, and also because it may be a help to surgeons and physicians who are confronted by her case in the future.

CONCLUSION

The syndrome of Baron von Munchausen has been described and three typical cases reported.

These patients waste an enormous amount of time and trouble in hospitals. If any correspondence follows this account, exposing other cases, perhaps some good will have been done. It would be even better if an explanation for the condition could be found, which might lead to a cure of the psychological kink which produces the disease.

I wish to thank the many doctors and records officers who supplied information about these cases, particularly Mr. K. P. S. Caldwell who traced most of the migrations of case 3.

COST OF HOSPITALS

Some Facts from Scotland

THE Department of Health in Edinburgh has been working away industriously at hospital " cost " statistics. The obligation to make good use of the material now coming to hand in respect of the six Scottish regions for 1949–50 is clearly felt strongly. The department deserves a good mark—not yet earned by the Ministry of Health in London, or by any of the regions in England and Wales—for coming forward and offering its efforts for publication and criticism.

Much of this material is of considerable interest. It is based on the first full year's figures available— i.e., 1949–50, when the total bill for Scotland, including specialist services, was £21,933,000. A total showing the relative importance of the several elements in the hospital cost proper, which amounted to £17,691,000, shows the following picture :

		% of total	
Patients' food	..	9·8	
Patients' clothing and laundry	..	3·1	
Drugs, dressings, surgical appliances, &c.	..	6·1	
		—	
1. COSTS ATTRIBUTABLE TO PATIENTS	..		19·0
Maintenance of buildings and grounds	..	2·7	
Domestic repairs and replacements	..	6·0	
Fuel, light, and power	..	8·2	
		—	
2. COSTS ATTRIBUTABLE TO BUILDINGS	..		16·9
3. MISCELLANEOUS—administration, transport, travelling, amenities, trading services, rent, and rates, &c.	..		4·9
Staff food, laundry, and uniforms	..	4·5	
Salaries and wages—junior medical staff	..	2·3	
—nursing staff	..	28·8	
—administrative staff	..	4·3	
—other staff	..	19·3	
		—	
4. COSTS ATTRIBUTABLE TO STAFF	..		59·2
		—	
Total	..		100·0

Commenting on these figures the Secretary of State has pointed out that it is thus clear that most of the money is going on staff salaries and upkeep and that control over staff establishment is therefore of decisive importance as a means of ensuring economy. Expenditure, however, on the salaries of those who are solely concerned with administrative and clerical work of the hospitals represents only some $2\frac{1}{2}\%$. " In the light of these figures," he said, " it does seem to me to be sheer nonsense to talk wildly of saving millions on the Health Services by slashing administrative waste in the hospitals."

THE LANCET]   SPECIAL ARTICLES   [MAY 5, 1951 1007

Special Articles

OBSERVERS' ERRORS IN TAKING MEDICAL HISTORIES

A. L. COCHRANE   P. J. CHAPMAN
M.B. Camb.   M.B. Brist.

P. D. OLDHAM
M.A. Oxfd

From the Pneumoconiosis Research Unit of the Medical Research
Council.

ALTHOUGH medical disagreement has long been recognised as common and was publicised by Alexander Pope (1732), there appears to be some general reluctance to recognise it as due to the subjectivity of medical judgment and even more reluctance to investigate it quantitatively. Certain recent tendencies have, however, made the recognition and measurement of medical error desirable.

In the work of our unit, for instance, it is necessary to correlate medical observations on workmen with the physical characteristics and quantity of the dust they have breathed. In doing this, just as the imprecision of the physical measurements must be allowed for, so, similarly, it is necessary to estimate how much one medical observer varies when he repeats his observations on the same material (intra-observer error) and how much his observations differ from those of another (inter-observer error); for in large-scale surveys several observers must coöperate and their results must be comparable.

Although relatively few studies have been published on the subject of medical error, several different approaches can be distinguished. In some cases—e.g., in the study of cyanosis (Comroe and Botelho 1947)—it has been possible to compare a clinical estimate with some objective accurate measurement of the same characteristic. Similar but less-accurate measurements have been used by Birkelo and Rague (1948) and Cochrane et al. (1949) to estimate the accuracy of radiological prognoses by following up minimal tuberculous lesions. Cochrane et al. introduce a slight refinement in technique in that an estimate was made of the number of prognoses that would have been made accurately by chance, the results being expressed as the percentage of the errors expected of a "blind" radiologist which were avoided by the reader. Such a refinement is obviously necessary when there are relatively few possible choices.

In other studies no objective standard was possible and attention was focused chiefly on the inter-observer error. These studies were mainly confined to estimates of human nutrition (Bean 1948, Derryberry 1938, Jones 1938), although Britten and Thompson (1926) and Sydenstricker and Britten (1930) have suggested that a similar error is attached to routine clinical examinations.

Recently there have been several detailed studies of the intra-observer and inter-observer errors in the diagnosis of pulmonary tuberculosis (Birkelo et al. 1947), pneumoconiosis (Fletcher and Oldham 1949), and pulmonary fibrosis (Hebert 1939). In all these cases the simple repeat technique was applicable, for the subjects of the examinations were not altered by the first investigation. Difficulties arise when the first examination is likely to affect the results of the second, as is clearly the case in taking a medical history. The general problem is discussed at some length by Kinsey et al. (1948), who emphasise that the second interview is influenced by the first, and require a minimum of eight months between interviews.

In large-scale surveys of coalminers carried out by this unit we wished to know the proportions of men complaining of various symptoms and showing various degrees of radiographic abnormality at a particular time, and a method such as Kinsey's would be impossible.

We have therefore approached the problem from a rather different point of view. If a population is divided into groups by some purely random method, the proportion giving a positive answer to questions asked by the same observer should be very similar in each separate group. The limits outside which the proportions have a small probability (say 5%) of falling by chance can be calculated. If then the population is divided into groups at random and each group is seen by a different observer, proportions of positive answers differing by more than the amount expected will be assumed to show that observers are either obtaining different answers from patients in the same clinical state or are interpreting the patients' answers differently.

MATERIAL AND TECHNIQUE

During a survey of an English coalmine 993 underground workers were interviewed. Observers A, B, and C did the bulk of the interviewing. Three other observers, who saw somewhat fewer miners, are called "observer D." The numbers of miners seen by each observer were as follows:

Observer		No. interviewed
A	..	261 (26·3%)
B	..	250 (25·2%)
C	..	300 (30·2%)
D	..	182 (18·3%)
Total		993

All the interviews took place in the same room under apparently identical conditions. Usually a queue formed, and the men took the places in order as they fell vacant. At slack periods it was rather difficult to tell whether the men chose the observer or the observer the man. There was probably a little of both. Three observers were usually present in the room at the same time and could easily overhear each other's questions, and every effort was made to standardise technique. The men were asked, in such a way that simple positive or negative replies could be made, whether they had cough, sputum, pain in the chest, tightness of the chest, or shortness of breath, and whether they had a history of bronchitis, pneumonia, pleurisy, or dyspepsia. The interviewing had to be done very quickly, since miners were usually seen at the end of a shift, when they were anxious to get home. The average time taken was about 5 minutes per man.

TABLE I—AGE-DISTRIBUTION OF MEN IN EACH GROUP

Age (yr.)	No. of men seen by observer				
	A	B	C	D	Total
14–19	21 (8·0%)	18 (7·2%)	14 (4·7%)	5 (2·7%)	58 (5·8%)
20–24	19 (7·3%)	20 (8·0%)	22 (7·3%)	23 (12·6%)	84 (8·5%)
25–29	29 (11·1%)	31 (12·4%)	49 (16·3%)	33 (18·1%)	142 (14·3%)
30–34	26 (10·0%)	23 (9·2%)	34 (11·3%)	23 (12·6%)	106 (10·7%)
35–39	40 (15·3%)	44 (17·6%)	48 (16·0%)	29 (15·9%)	161 (16·2%)
40–44	35 (13·4%)	38 (15·2%)	42 (14·0%)	27 (14·8%)	142 (14·3%)
45–49	36 (13·8%)	41 (16·4%)	39 (13·0%)	19 (10·4%)	135 (13·6%)
50–54	20 (7·7%)	12 (4·8%)	24 (8·0%)	10 (5·5%)	66 (6·6%)
55–59	16 (6·1%)	12 (4·8%)	12 (4·0%)	7 (3·8%)	47 (4·7%)
60–64	11 (4·2%)	7 (2·8%)	12 (4·0%)	4 (2·2%)	34 (3·4%)
65–69	8 (3·1%)	3 (1·2%)	4 (1·3%)	2 (1·1%)	17 (1·7%)
70 or more	— —	1 (0·4%)	— —	— —	1 (0·1%)
Total	261	250	300	182	993

TABLE II—NUMBER AND PROPORTION OF MEN IN EACH GROUP WHO COMPLAINED OF CERTAIN SYMPTOMS

Symptom	No. of men seen by observer				Probability (%)
	A	B	C	D	
Cough ..	61(23·4%)	70(28·0%)	121(40·3%)	60(32·9%)	<0·1†
Sputum ..	34(13·0%)	50(20·0%)	108(36·0%)	76(41·9%)	<0·1†
Tightness of chest	39(14·9%)	42(16·8%)	69(23·0%)	40(21·9%)	5·4
Pain ..	18 (6·9%)	16 (6·4%)	28 (9·3%)	30(16·5%)	0·1—. 1·0†
Dyspnœa*	40(15·5%)	45(18·0%)	42(14·0%)	18 (9·9%)	10—20

* Excluding three cases with no record of dyspnœa.
† Significantly small.

RESULTS

To discover whether observers A, B, C, and D had been interviewing similar samples of the total population, the age-distribution of those seen by each observer was determined (see table I). Although the men seen by observer B had a slightly higher mean age than the others, the difference is not statistically significant, for it might occur once in eight times by chance alone. Years underground and the prevalence of pneumoconiosis have found to be closely related to age, and it seemed reasonable to proceed on the assumption that the necessary random clinical composition of the groups seen by each observer had been attained.

Fig. 1 and table II show the percentages of men in each observer's group who gave a positive answer when asked whether they had cough, sputum, pain in the chest, tightness of the chest, or shortness of breath on exertion.

Fig. 2 and table III show the percentages of men in each group who gave a past history of bronchitis, pleurisy, pneumonia, and dyspepsia. The probability that these differences were due to chance is given in the last column of each table. Accepting as the level of significance that the difference would not have occurred more often than once in twenty times by chance, we find that there was a significant difference in the observers' recordings

of the frequency of cough, sputum, pain in the chest, and dyspepsia.

DISCUSSION

Our results suggest that the recording of patients' answers to simple questions may, in some cases, give results that are unaffected by the observer. In the case of a past history of bronchitis, pleurisy, or pneumonia the question " Have you ever had. . . . ? " is straight-forward, and the answer in most cases will be " Yes " or " No," which will be thus recorded.

The consistency between the observers' recordings, however, does not mean that the answers are necessarily correct. Their accuracy must have depended on the memory and coöperation of the men who were asked the question, but men with good and bad memories or high and low levels of coöperation were presumably randomly distributed throughout the group. In the other questions, however, the observer had to interpret the man's answer before recording it. For instance, to the question " Have you a cough ? " or " Do you spit ? ", the man might reply " Only an ordinary cough " or " Only after work " (for miners commonly cough up a little black phlegm after the shift). The observer would then have to ask supplementary questions to decide whether or not the severity of the cough constituted a symptom

TABLE III—NUMBER AND PROPORTION OF MEN IN EACH GROUP WHO GAVE A HISTORY OF HAVING HAD CERTAIN DISEASES

Disease	No. of men seen by observer				Probability (%)
	A	B	C	D	
Bronchitis	32 (12·2%)	26 (10·4%)	31 (10·3%)	21 (11·5%)	80—90
Pleurisy	24 (9·2%)	21 (8·4%)	31 (10·3%)	23 (12·6%)	50
Pneumonia	30 (11·5%)	36 (14·4%)	45 (15·0%)	24 (13·2%)	50—70
Dyspepsia	26 (9·9%)	40 (16·0%)	70 (23·3%)	49 (26·9%)	<0·1*

* Significantly small.

of chest disease, and his ultimate recorded answer would depend as much on his judgment as on the man's answer. This is presumably why, in these cases, we find very different frequencies recorded by different observers.

In the case of shortness of breath on exertion, which is normal to some extent in health, the observers had agreed before the survey on a careful grading. The miners were asked if they could keep up with their fellow workers of their own age while walking. Our results seem to show that such a system helps to reduce observer error if it is properly used. Errors due to faulty answers will remain.

In the case of dyspepsia there is once more an infinite gradation from healthy men who feel bloated after Christmas dinner to the true case of peptic ulcer ; hence the observer's judgment once more enters into his recorded answer. Presumably the error that we have shown could have been lessened by more careful definition, as in the case of dyspnœa.

We believe that our results demonstrate that, at least in this particular survey, the recorded answers to several questions commonly asked in taking clinical histories were not reproducible from one observer to another, so they could not be considered objective scientific observations. Possibly if the observers had been more experienced clinicians, or if they had worked more slowly, their results would have been better. Observer A was an experienced clinician of consultant-physician status, and observers B and C could fairly claim to be well trained in academic scientific medicine, which might be considered at least as important as clinical experience for the accurate and consistent recording of men's answers. The composite observer D would be expected to be exceptionally accurate, for the

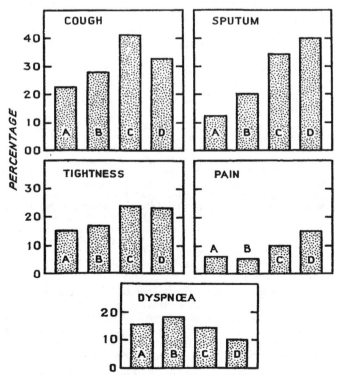

Fig. 1—Symptoms found by each observer.

THE LANCET]   SPECIAL ARTICLES   [MAY 5, 1951   1009

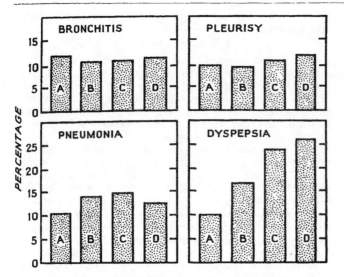

Fig. 2—Past medical history found by each observer.

proportions found by D are a kind of average of those found by the three observers included in D, the inter-observer error of the three being thus partially averaged out. For this reason the discrepancies found are likely to be underestimated. In view of the slightly higher mean age of the men seen by observer B it is interesting to observe that his results are in only one case more extreme than those of observers A, C, and D.

The work was certainly done quickly, but little faster than some of the work done in hospital outpatient departments or in the consulting-rooms of general practitioners. Possibly miners are a particularly difficult group, because so many of them have the slight degree of cough and expectoration after work to which we have already referred.

In spite of these reservations we believe that our findings have some general application; they are certainly important in clinical field surveys. Unless different observers can obtain consistent answers to questions from comparable groups of witnesses, their findings are of little scientific value. If this were generally recognised, a great deal of misplaced research endeavour would be saved, and many publications would gain in validity what they lose in length. We suggest that the technique we have adopted is suitable for investigating the reproducibility of clinical findings.

The application of our results to history-taking in general is less certain, but many doctors must remember certain curious discrepancies between the histories taken by them as students and those elicited later from the same patients by the house-physician or the registrar. This inter-observer error of hospital history-taking would merit investigation particularly if there were any possibility of the histories being used for research purposes later.

A further possibility is in the field of medical education. A great deal is taught about the art of history-taking; its science is badly neglected. It should not be difficult to arrange demonstrations for students to show the dangers of leading questions and the invalid deductions that can be made owing to the lack of reproducibility of clinical findings.

SUMMARY

A clinical survey of a large number of coalminers was made by several medical observers who interviewed different groups of men. The age-distributions of the groups were similar. The observers all asked the miners in their groups the same questions.

The answers to some of these questions showed that the observer's bias was influencing the frequency with which a positive answer was recorded. Other questions were more consistently answered in the different groups.

These results are discussed, and it is suggested that more attention should be paid to possible lack of reproducibility in the answers that patients give to questions commonly asked in clinical practice, and that, for research purposes, answers which are not reproducible are worthless.

In such large-scale coöperative work it is difficult to apportion credit fairly. We should, however, like to mention Dr. C. M. Fletcher, Dr. J. C. Gilson, and Dr. K. J. Mann, of this unit, and the 993 miners who answered our questions so patiently and so surprisingly.

REFERENCES

Bean, W. B. (1948) *J. appl. Physiol.* **1**, 458.
Birkelo, C. C., Chamberlain, W. E., Phelps, P. S., Schools, P. E., Zachs, D., Yevushalmy, J. (1947) *J. Amer. med. Ass.* **133**, 359.
— Rague, P. O. (1948) *Amer. J. Roentgenol.* **60**, 303.
Britten, R. H., Thompson, L. R. (1926) *Publ. Hlth Bull., Wash.* no. 162.
Cochrane, A. L., Campbell, H. W., Stein, S. C. (1949) *Amer. J. Roentgenol.* **61**, 153.
Comroe, J. H. jun., Botelho, S. (1947) *J. Amer. med. Sci.* **214**, 1.
Derryberry, M. (1938) *Publ. Hlth Rep., Wash.* **53**, 263.
Fletcher, C. M., Oldham, P. D. (1949) *Brit. J. industr. Med.* **6**, 168.
Hebert, G. T. (1939) *Tubercle,* **20**, 145.
Jones, R. H. (1938) *J. roy. Statist. Soc.* **101**, 1.
Kinsey, A. C., Pomeroy, W. B., Martin, C. E. (1948). Sexual Behavior in the Human Male. Philadelphia and London.
Pope, A. (1732) Epistle 3 to Lord Bathurst. London.
Sydenstricker, E., Britten, R. H. (1930) *Amer. J. Hyg.* **11**, 73.

IMPERIAL CANCER RESEARCH FUND

IN his summary of the work done during the past year in the laboratories of the Imperial Cancer Research Fund,[1] Dr. James Craigie, F.R.S., the director, reports investigations on tumour transplantation, tumour induction and progression under hormonal influences, and chemical carcinogenesis in the liver.

Dr. A. M. Begg, Miss P. E. Lind, and Miss Margaret Hayward, PH.D., have collaborated with Dr. Craigie in exploring the possibility of developing quantitative methods for the study of transplantable tumours. For this purpose a better knowledge of conditions governing cell survival in vitro is essential. It was found that tumours could be preserved as cell suspensions in the frozen state provided that dextrose solution was used. It was noted that cell suspensions contained a small number of highly refractile bodies similar in size and contour to tumour cells. Retention of viability in vitro depended on maintenance of this refractility as seen by phase-microscopy. Refractile cells were resistant to dextrose solution and to freezing and drying in dextrose—manipulations which kill normal tumour cells.

The discovery of a resistant state raises many questions.

Doubtless before doing any further work along these lines, the facts have been taken into consideration that normal cells—liver, for example—as well as tumour cells of all kinds actually develop this curious refractile change with obscured nuclear detail in dextrose, sucrose, and glycerin solutions; that the appearance is completely reversible by washing out the sugars or glycerin; that it is not to be confused with a similar but irreversible appearance natural to dead pyknotic cells; that no normal liver cells, whether highly refractile or not, are resistant to immersion in dextrose solutions, and to freezing and partial drying as measured by growth after animal grafting. And therefore high refractility is not likely to underlie any property peculiar to tumour cells.

Dr. Leslie Foulds has extended his studies on the progression of tumours towards malignancy and on their responsiveness to various physiological conditions. Observations extended over long periods of intermissions of breeding have confirmed the previous findings that some mammary tumours that regressed after parturition

1. Imperial Cancer Research Fund : 48th Annual Report, 1950–51. Issued by the Fund. Royal College of Surgeons, Lincoln's Inn Fields, London, W.C.2.

THE LANCET]   ORIGINAL ARTICLES   [JULY 28, 1951   151

thetic agents were required to keep the patients in the desired plane of anæsthesia, and this probably explains why there was no delay in their recovery from anæsthesia.

The longest operation, a difficult extrapleural pneumonectomy, lasted three and a half hours. Although the optimal low blood-pressure was maintained throughout, the period of recovery did not differ from cases which had taken a much shorter time ; hence it seems that protracted hypotension has no deleterious effect.

The patients were aged 18–40, and in this age-group any difference in response to the hypotensive drug was not related to age. Dosage was often related to the patient's weight but depended much more on his sensitivity to the drug, and this sensitivity varied greatly in different cases. For this reason it is important to give a test dose of only 20 mg., as emphasised above. In one case this test dose alone proved adequate to bring the systolic pressure to the optimal 60 mm. Hg. In the present series the largest total amount of hypotensive drug given to a single patient during an operation was 300 mg. of pentamethonium bromide. In 6 cases the response to the hypotensive drug was unsatisfactory, the systolic pressure falling only to about 90–95 mm. Hg, and further doses produced no response. It can therefore be assumed that, if no satisfactory response is obtained after 150 mg. has been given, the patient is not sufficiently sensitive to the drugs at present available and should not be subjected to further doses.

A blood drip is instituted in each case because in the hypotensive state the loss of even a small quantity of blood may be dangerous, and by the use of a blood drip any blood-loss can be immediately replaced. The rate of the drip is kept as low as blood-loss necessitates ; otherwise the added blood would tend to neutralise the effect of the hypotensive drug.

The postoperative rise of the blood-pressure is very gradual and takes 3–8 hours to reach its preoperative level. This slow rise allows adequate time for the sealing of the minute blood-vessels, and this prevents reactionary hæmorrhage and excessive postoperative oozing.

CONCLUSIONS

The use of hypotensive drugs to produce an optimal low blood-pressure not only minimises blood-loss, thus diminishing the necessity for extensive blood-transfusion, but also should shorten the operation by providing a clearer field and reducing time taken in obtaining hæmostasis. In a case of pneumonectomy the clamp was inadvertently taken off the inferior pulmonary vein before ligation, but no difficulty was encountered in controlling the hæmorrhage, there being no sudden gush of blood from the venous stump.

In the past, one of the fundamental concepts of surgery, especially of thoracic surgery, has been the importance of maintaining the blood-pressure, but this does not seem to hold with the use of the technique described here. Shock seemed to be much less, compared with similar cases where the hypotensive technique was not used, possibly owing to the minimising of loss of blood and tissue fluid.

It is problematical why a smaller amount of anæsthetic agent is required ; it may be due to lowered cellular metabolism or to a diminution in nervous reflex irritability.

This form of control of the circulation seems to be particularly suitable in thoracic surgery, because the diminution of respiratory movements reduces the venous return to the heart and aids the maintenance of hypotension. Further, the position of the patient that gives the best hypotensive effect is only a modification of the position in common use in thoracic surgery.

My thanks are due to Mr. J. Howell Hughes, surgeon to the thoracic unit, and Dr. J. H. Hawkins, physician-superintendent, of the North Wales Sanatorium, Denbigh, for their coöperation and helpful suggestions.

REFERENCES

Arnold, P., Rosenheim, M. L. (1949) *Lancet,* ii, 321.
Burt, C. C., Graham, A. J. P. (1950) *Brit. med. J.* i, 455.
Enderby, G. E. H. (1950) *Lancet,* i, 1145.

THE MULTIPLE-PUNCTURE TUBERCULIN TEST

FREDERICK HEAF
M.A., M.D. Camb., F.R.C.P.
DAVID DAVIES PROFESSOR OF TUBERCULOSIS, UNIVERSITY OF WALES

ONE of the disadvantages common to most methods of determining if a person is a non-reactor to tuberculin is the number of tuberculin tests that have to be made. These have been reduced to two, but even so it is necessary to make three visits to the clinic. If these tests are followed by B.C.G. vaccination, many more visits are necessary ; in fact, the full programme for B.C.G. vaccination, as outlined in the *Ministry of Health Memorandum 322/B.C.G./revised*, requires seven visits to the clinic. Most people find such a schedule very trying, and it is not improbable that some will refuse to comply with it. If it is possible to determine tuberculin sensitivity by one test, considerable simplification of the routine can be effected. The multiple-puncture tuberculin test has been devised with this object. So far the results have been encouraging, and the simplicity of the technique should make it useful in mass surveys.

APPARATUS REQUIRED

The equipment required for the test is as follows : 1 platinum loop of 2 mm. diameter, 1 spirit lamp, 1 multiple-puncture apparatus, some spirit, cotton-wool, and 1 ml. of adrenalised pure Old Tuberculin. It is an advantage, but not a necessity, to have a small petri dish to obtain a shallow reservoir of spirit about 5 mm. deep for sterilising the needles of the multiple-puncture apparatus. The petri dish assures that the needles are not immersed too deeply in spirit and thereby collect too great a quantity of the fluid, which when ignited heats the whole of the end apparatus and makes it too hot to use. This is avoided if the needles are dipped only to a depth of 5 mm. and then flamed.

The *multiple-puncture apparatus* * provides an automatic punch mechanism whereby six needles are released to puncture the skin evenly to a depth of 1 or 2 mm. as desired. The needles are arranged in a circle of 6 mm. diameter. One set of needles remains sharp for about 2500 punctures. The battery of needles is easily exchanged for a reserve set while the first set is sharpened. The apparatus is simply constructed and easy to use.

---

* The apparatus may be obtained from Messrs. Allen & Hanburys, Wigmore Street, London, W.1.

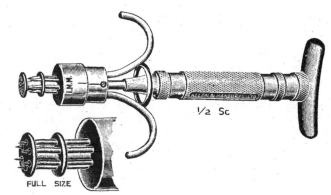

1/2 Sc

FULL SIZE

Multiple-puncture apparatus.

D 3

apparently not available, but it seems probable that patients with intractable ulceration are liable to develop similar ulceration again, even if the trouble has been temporarily healed by the drip. Perhaps, therefore in practice the greatest value of the drip is in treating those victims of severe ulceration who refuse operation or have other ailments making operation inadvisable. The drip may also possibly be of help as a preliminary to operation, by making this less difficult technically.

Much conflicting advice has been variously given as to the indications for gastrectomy. And no doubt many factors should be taken into account, such as the patient's age, build, temperament, and occupation, and the presence or absence of chronic bronchitis or other significant second condition. Nevertheless, unless one of these factors provides a strong argument against gastrectomy, the reasonable criterion for this operation seems to be that the patient *cannot be made well and kept well by frequent doses of alkali while living his normal life.* There are, of course, weighty arguments for operation which are generally accepted—typically recurrent hæma temeses and pyloric stenosis—but since those so affected do not remain well while living their normal lives, the criterion suggested covers these eventualities.

THE ONUS OF PROOF

The " orthodox " medical management of peptic ulcer involves long, and often repeated, periods of rest in bed and longer spells of absence from work, an artificial and more or less unpleasant diet, often to be continued indefinitely, and the avoidance or restriction of tobacco and alcohol—all of which tend to give the patient the impression that he is an invalid. Quite apart from the arguments advanced against this management in the present paper, it must be asked on whom must the onus of proof lie when the value of remedies are in doubt— on those who advocate them or on those opposed to them ?

Elsewhere (Todd 1951) I have pointed out that, whereas in respect of new drugs it is universally agreed that the onus of proof should rest on their advocates, the attitude widely adopted towards old and traditional remedies, and in particular régimes and diets, is to accept them as valuable until evidence is advanced that they are not. I concluded that this difference of approach is unsound, and that the advocates of all remedies should produce evidence of their claims. If such evidence is lacking, remedies should be abandoned, no matter how widely they are used, and no matter what pronounce- ments as to their value appear in textbooks. (Admittedly in practice the doctor, especially if he is young and lacks prestige, can hardly be blamed for treading carefully the paths of unorthodoxy ; but there is no reason why he should think on orthodox lines, even if discretion makes him act on them.)

If these arguments are sound, the advocates of bed rest, staying away from work, dropping commitments, changing the habits of life, eradicating septic foci, omitting tobacco and alcohol, and eating artificial diets should be required to provide proof of their views, and until such proof is advanced it is sound practice not to prescribe these remedies for peptic ulcer. Moreover, the treatment recommended in this paper—that large doses of alkali should be taken throughout the day— is so much simpler and pleasanter for the patient than taking frequent meals that the onus of proof should surely lie on the advocates of frequent meals, not on the advocates of frequent alkali.

Probably only a minority of patients are advised to undergo the full rigours of orthodoxy, especially in the matter of staying in bed and being away from work. (Those treated by general practitioners are, one may suppose, more fortunate in this respect than those treated by some of the specialists in gastro-enterology whose advice appears in textbooks and journals.) No doubt, too,

a high proportion of patients who are ordered the whole orthodox ritual ignore much of what they are told. It seems, indeed, that the ordinary instincts of the patient may sometimes give better results than the considered opinions of his medical advisers and that the practical understanding which the general practitioner has of his patients' problems may make his treatment better than that derived from the more theoretical calculations of the specialist.

Summary and Conclusions

Of the various methods of treating peptic ulcer only three are of proven value—diminishing the gastric acidity, gastrectomy, and psychotherapy (which has only a very limited application).

As a routine for the medical management of peptic ulcer, it is suggested that the patient, while carrying on with his work, should take alkaline tablets at hourly intervals throughout his waking hours (except at the usual meal-times, when he has his ordinary food instead). He should continue to do this until his ulcer is thought to be healed, and thereafter he should be told that the more closely he adheres to this régime, the less will be the chances of relapse.

The view is advanced that the onus of proving the value of rest in bed, absence from work, an artificial and monotonous diet, phenobarbitone, the eradication of septic foci, the avoidance of tobacco and alcohol, and the other orthodox remedies, should rest on their advocates, not on those who are opposed to them.

This paper is an elaboration of ideas which I have previously expressed elsewhere (Todd 1949). I wish to thank Dr. James Dow for his advice and criticism, and my father for his valuable help in revision.

REFERENCES

Bentley, F. H. (1950) *Practitioner,* **165,** 624.
Blackford, J. M., Bowers, J. M. (1929) *Amer. J. med. Sci.* **177,** 51.
Davies, D. T. (1936) *Lancet,* i, 521.
— Wilson, A. T. M. (1937) *Ibid,* ii, 1353.
Douthwaite, A. H. (1947) *Brit. med. J.* ii, 43.
Ferriman, D. (1940) *Ibid,* i, 210.
Gill, A. M. (1947) *Lancet,* i, 291.
Ivy, A. C., Grossman, M. I., Bachrach, W. H. (1950) Peptic Ulcer. London.
Jones, F. A. (1949) *Brit. med. J.* ii, 1463.
Nicol, B. M. (1939) *Lancet,* ii, 881.
Palmer, W. L., Kirsner, J. B., Levin, E. (1951) *J. Amer. med. Ass.* **145,** 1041.
Stolte, J. B. (1950) *Lancet,* ii, 58.
Todd, J. W. (1949) Rational Medicine. Bristol.
— (1951) *Lancet,* ii, 438.
Winklestein, A., Cornell, A., Hollander, F. (1942) *J. Amer. med. Ass.* **120,** 743.

INTRA-OCULAR ACRYLIC LENSES AFTER CATARACT EXTRACTION *

HAROLD RIDLEY
M.D. Camb., F.R.C.S.
OPHTHALMIC SURGEON, ST. THOMAS'S HOSPITAL, LONDON ;
SURGEON, MOORFIELDS, WESTMINSTER AND CENTRAL EYE
HOSPITAL, LONDON

No surgical operation surpasses modern cataract extraction in doing what it is designed to do, for the defective part is removed under local anæsthesia in a single stage through an incision which heals with an invisible scar. But the lens, an important part of a highly specialised organ, is lost and cure is complete only when another lens is substituted. Extraction alone is but half the cure for cataract.

CATARACT OPERATIONS

Operations for cataract have been practised for 3000 years. " Couching," or surgical dislocation of the opaque lens into the vitreous chamber, was in early times the only possible measure, but the proportion of successful results must have been small. Even in the present century this operation, or modifications of it, was used in India and

---

* A fuller account of this work will appear in the *British Journal of Ophthalmology.*

other countries where the people are backward and surgeons few and where only surgery which is quick is relatively safe from sepsis, and does not necessitate postoperative convalescence, is practicable.

In 1748 Daviel described the first cataract extraction ; but, as is often the case, his operation, though an evident improvement, was not at first well received, and couching continued to be the method of choice. Apart from the risk of sepsis the absence of anæsthesia must have made Daviel's operation difficult and dangerous, and one cannot but admire his courage in performing it. Little improvement took place until the last quarter of the 19th century, when cocaine was introduced as a local anæsthetic, rendering the operation not only painless but also less hazardous. Since then the results of cataract surgery have become increasingly successful.

Extracapsular Extraction

At first extracapsular extraction seemed the only possible method, and with its many modifications and improvements it is still widely used today. After a corneoscleral section the anterior capsule is incised and the opaque lens expressed through the pupil and out of the eye. For many years surgeons would not operate until the cataract was mature, when the entire cortex could be extracted in one piece. This, however, entailed the patient waiting perhaps years in almost complete blindness ; for, if the operation were performed too soon, only the nucleus would be expressed. The remaining cortex might block the pupil, set up anaphylactic iridocyclitis, and possibly prevent proper healing of the wound, leading to further complications, including even sympathetic ophthalmia.

Two major improvements have since been made : better asepsis has rendered possible the removal of residual cortex with a jet of sterile saline solution, and removal of a large central area of the anterior capsule with toothed capsule-forceps has made a clear pupil probable. It is found that, if only the thin posterior lens capsule is left, needling of " after cataract " is seldom required. In suitable cases the modern extracapsular extraction gives excellent results, and the posterior capsule remains as a useful bulkhead in the eye, keeping the vitreous in place and reducing the risk of aphakic glaucoma and retinal detachment.

Intracapsular Extraction

Early in the 20th century intracapsular extraction was introduced. In this operation the intact anterior capsule is grasped with non-toothed forceps, and by a combination of traction from in front with pressure from behind the entire lens enclosed in its membrane is removed. This improvement, which permits extraction of quite immature cataracts as soon as the patient can no longer read, was at first considered unjustifiably dangerous and has only in recent years become more popular than the well-tried and generally successful extracapsular extraction. There is no doubt that in the hands of inexperienced operators the risk is considerably greater, but with perfected technique the acme of cataract extraction has been attained.

Now since 1949, 200 years after Daviel's first extraction, it has proved possible successfully to substitute for the missing lens an artificial intra-ocular lenticulus.

APHAKIA

An eye which has undergone cataract extraction suffers many disadvantages. Accommodation is inevitably lost, but this is of small practical importance since the loss is physiological in most persons of cataract age. The eye is completely out of focus without a spectacle lens of about +11 D and, when washing or bathing, the patient is almost blind. Cataract glasses are cumbersome, disfiguring, and heavy, and, what is more important, function only at their best when the view is through the optical centre. Oblique views produce aberration and apparent displacement of objects which make patients feel uncertain of the position of steps and other obstacles and give rise to lack of confidence in traffic. For these reasons, though 6/6 vision is often attained, the sight is not so good as this high acuity suggests. If the other eye is normal or has even moderate vision, the two eyes when focused are incompatible, for in addition to producing aberrations the aphakic spectacle lens magnifies the retinal image by a third. A contact lens would considerably reduce these disabilities, but the image of the aphakic eye would still be magnified by a sixth. Moreover most cataract patients cannot insert contact lenses or do not persevere with them, because of the irritation they cause. Surgeons are often loth to remove even a mature cataract if the other eye has moderate sight, for patients often prefer to continue using the eye which has not undergone operation and has an acuity as low as 6/24 rather than the aphakic eye which can read perhaps 6/6. The new technique of inserting an artificial intra-ocular lens is particularly indicated in monocular cataract or when the other eye still has fair sight, for patients generally have no difficulty in coördinating the two eyes and appreciate binocular vision from the start.

ARTIFICIAL LENTICULI

All the disadvantages of aphakia, except lack of accommodation, can be overcome by the use of an intra-ocular lens. Human lens grafts are impracticable, certainly at present, and an artificial prosthesis is the only solution. The problem to be solved is threefold : (1) to select a suitable transparent material which will not produce a tissue reaction in the eye ; (2) to determine the size and refractive power of the lens ; and (3) to devise a method of inserting it and retaining it steadily in position within the eye.

The only materials available at present which are suitable for such a lens are glass and " plastic " polymethyl methacrylate compounds, generally known as ' Perspex ' or ' Plexiglass." Both are inert in the body. Fragments of glass have remained in eyes for years, often overlooked even with careful examination, and cause no trouble unless a sharp edge lies against a sensitive and mobile portion such as the iris. Rather less is known about methacrylate, but some knowledge has been gained from eye injuries caused by aircraft accidents. Methacrylate spheres can be used to fill up Tenon's capsule after enucleation of an eye and have been extensively used in orthopædic surgery not only for filling gaps in flat bones but also to take the place of the head of the femur. In joint cavities movement and the presence of synovial fluid provide some resemblance to conditions within the eye.

Physically glass and perspex are similar in their almost perfect transparency and in their constant optical properties and ease of working. Perspex is the softer and therefore more easily scratched ; but it has the overwhelming advantage of light weight, its specific gravity being 1·19, only half that of glass and little exceeding that of the aqueous. For this reason methacrylate was preferred.

On inquiry, the manufacturers of perspex (Imperial Chemical Industries) advised their product ' Transpex I ' as the variety of polymethyl methacrylate best suited to the purpose, because its composition and optical properties are constant, and, being unpolymerised, it avoids the risk of gradual liberation of free polymeriser which might cause chemical irritation. The refractive index is 1·49 and the specific gravity 1·19. It cannot be boiled without risk of distortion, and it is affected by certain organic solvents, including alcohols. For cleansing and sterilisation it is recommended that 1% cetrimide be used for at least half an hour. Other sterilising fluids are under experiment, but clinically cetrimide has proved satisfactory.

120   THE LANCET]   ORIGINAL ARTICLES   [JAN. 19, 1952

The design of the artificial lens to replace the natural is not the simple problem it might appear. The human lens is a complex structure composed of differing layers of anterior and posterior capsule, cortex, and nucleus, and therefore has no constant refractive index. It is thought that, when the lens is in the eye and unaccommodated, its diameter is about 9·4 mm., its thickness 4 mm., the radius of the anterior curve 10 mm., and the radius of the posterior curve 6 mm. The refractive index is approximately 1·42, and the refractive power is variously estimated between 16·01 D and 19·11 D in the aqueous fluid.

In designing the intra-ocular lenticuli it was decided to make them about 1 mm. less in diameter than the natural, for ease of insertion and to obviate pressure on the ciliary region and filtration angle, which might tend to produce cyclitis and glaucoma. The earliest lenses were made 8·35 mm. in diameter and with curvatures of the radii attributed to the natural lens. But in the human eye it was found, as it could be in no other way, that such a lens was too strong. Calculating from the refraction resulting from this prototype within an otherwise normal eye the present lens specification was evolved :

Material	Transpex I
Diameter	8·35 mm.
Thickness	2·40 mm.
Radius of anterior curve..	17·8 mm.
Radius of posterior curve	10·7 mm.
Refractive power in aqueous (1·33 refractive index) ..	24·0 D

A peripheral groove is cut in both sides of the lens before polishing so that it may be grasped in forceps. The lenses are individually worked from solid transpex I and finished to fine limits of accuracy by Messrs. Rayner, London.

It is evident that this lenticulus is not a copy of the human lens and that its refractive surfaces cannot occupy the same positions. The compound system produced by this and the ocular media, however, closely and consistently reproduces the normal, judged by the refraction of the other eye. Up to now the object has always been to render the two eyes refractively similar and capable of working together again ; in future, if the pre-cataract refraction is accurately known and it is intended to insert acrylic lenses in both eyes, it may be desirable to produce lenses to individual specification to attain postoperative emmetropia.

OPERATION

The acrylic lenticulus may be inserted immediately after extraction of the cataract or at a second operation some time later. The two-stage operation is recommended only when the cataract has been caused by a perforating wound, or when it has proved impossible at the extraction to remove all lens matter and time has to be allowed for absorption of cortical remnants. In two-stage operations difficulty may be experienced in freeing the iris from the lens capsule, for synechiæ may be found not only at the pupillary margin of the iris. Before operation the acrylic lens, and a spare, should be placed in a special rack (Rayner) correctly oriented so that it can be readily grasped in forceps with the flatter surface forwards. The difference in the curvatures can be seen fairly easily in profile, but a valuable check is to observe the two reflections of a source of light from the anterior and posterior lens surfaces. When these are markedly dissimilar the flatter anterior surface is in front. If the lens were inserted back to front, the resulting refraction of the eye would be greatly affected. The rack containing the lenses is sterilised in 1% cetrimide, thoroughly rinsed in sterile water, and placed with the cataract instruments, which include in addition special lens-insertion forceps and an iris hook (Messrs. Weiss, London).

Extracapsular extraction is recommended, but the intracapsular has been used on two occasions. The pupil should be dilated to at least 5 mm. in diameter with homatropine. Anæsthesia is provided by 4% cocaine drops, no retrobulbar injection being required. A procaine injection is given over the neck of the mandible to prevent orbicularis spasm, and a simple stitch is inserted through the upper lid so that it can be strapped to the cheek to ensure closure of the eye after operation. Two half-thickness corneoscleral mattress sutures of the finest silk are inserted, and a normal cataract section is cut, including where possible a conjunctival flap. Very complete removal of the anterior lens capsule is effected with toothed capsule forceps, and after expression of the nucleus great care is taken to wash out all cortical remnants so that only the thin posterior capsule remains in the pupil. If these stages have proceeded satisfactorily, the lens may now be inserted : if not, the eye must be closed and the operation completed at a later date. The lens is grasped by its peripheral groove with the insertion forceps, the corneoscleral wound is held open with an iris repositor, and the acrylic lens is gently introduced with a slight side-to-side movement through the pupil so that it rests partly behind the iris below (fig. 1). The grip can now be relaxed ; and, while the lens is steadied with a repositor, the iris above and laterally is manipulated over the lens with the hook (fig. 2). When the pupil has been made circular, a small peripheral iridectomy is done, and, after centring of the lens by external pressure on the cornea and sclera and a final irrigation, the sutures are tied. Penicillin is instilled, but miotics are not generally necessary or desirable. The patient is allowed out of bed on the third or fourth day, and the sutures are removed on the eighth day.

COMPLICATIONS

The operation is clearly more complex than simple extraction. The key to success is to introduce the lens beneath the lower part of the iris before the forceps' grip is relaxed. If, however, the lenticulus is found to be entirely in the anterior chamber, it is advisable to grasp it again by the peripheral groove and to reinsert it, for otherwise it is very difficult to hook the lower edge of the pupil over the lens. The iris hook has a pliable stem so that it may be bent to facilitate this manœuvre if necessary.

With 2 exceptions, all the operations so far performed have proceeded satisfactorily. In the first, in which too large a lens was inserted and no corneoscleral sutures were used, the patient developed an iris prolapse, but the eye by good fortune has healed satisfactorily and is now free from inflammation. In a later case, a rather feeble

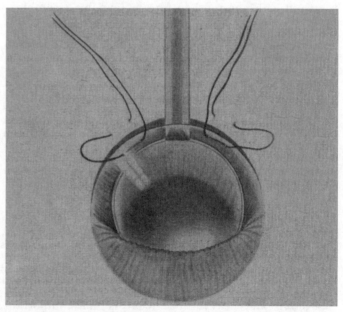

Fig. 1—Insertion of acrylic lens beneath lower part of iris.

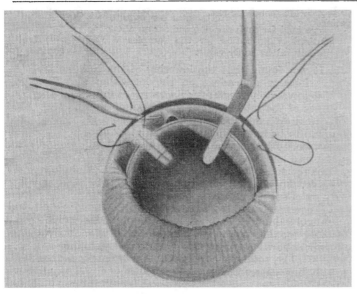

Fig. 2—Upper part of iris hooked in front of acrylic lens, which is steadied by iris repositor.

patient, aged 75, developed glaucoma because the corneoscleral wound did not unite in the usual time, and when the sutures were removed the iris became adherent to the cornea, causing a false filtration angle and glaucoma. Many, but not all, of the others have developed a transitory serous iritis, but in no case has this persisted or recurred. It has, however, led to the deposition of exudate and iris-pigment granules on the anterior surface of the lens, which is sometimes slow to clear. Subconjunctival injections of cortisone 10 mg. are valuable in these cases, which, however, seem to have a strong tendency to clear spontaneously. Adhesions forming between the iris and the lens may assist in keeping the lens in position, though they are not essential.

Thickening of the posterior capsule is an evident possibility. If this is feared, a central capsulotomy could be performed before the lens is inserted, and in one early case it has been necessary later to incise the capsule from behind under direct observation through the pupil. In the other cases this operation, which entails risk of damaging or dislocating the acrylic lens, has not been required. It must be remembered that the posterior lens capsule, unlike the anterior, which has also an inner cellular layer, is a simple hyaline membrane of minute thickness, the central area measuring only 4 μ, and that the presence of the acrylic lens tends to keep it taut and free from wrinkles.

There has been no case of dislocation of the prosthesis. The lenticulus is held steadily in the patellar fossa by even pressure from the muscular iris in front against the natural curve of the posterior lens capsule behind. Since the specific gravity of the lens is only slightly greater than that of the aqueous, there is little tendency for it to sink, and the stability is shown by the constancy of the refraction, for even a slight tilt of a powerful lens would cause marked astigmatism.

The early operations were done only on patients with monocular cataracts, for those whose eye was completely normal had less to lose should complications ensue, whereas success, in addition to other advantages, would restore single binocular vision. The risks were explained beforehand.

RESULTS

Of the 25 eyes which have so far undergone this operation at St. Thomas's Hospital and Moorfields, Westminster and Central Eye Hospital the first 2 are unsatisfactory; for the experimental lenses inserted, which were made with the same curvatures and thickness as the human lens, proved in practice to be too strong, producing postoperative myopia. In conjunction with the other eye the visual result is no better, though little worse, than would have resulted from simple extraction.

Of the remaining 23, only 1 has given serious trouble : as noted above, the patient was an old man whose corneoscleral wound did not heal properly. The other 22 cases are all successful in that binocularly the visual result is better than it would have been with simple extraction alone.

A more stringent criterion, however, is to judge each eye individually and not as one of a pair and to assess the performance of the organ rather than of the patient.

These 22 eyes are surgically satisfactory, having circular or nearly circular pupils, acrylic lenses in good position, normal tension, and no active iridocyclitis. In several there is a deposit of fibrinous exudate coloured by iris pigment on the front of the lens, but even in the worst cases this is gradually dispersing, and there seems good prospect that all will clear in time and that every eye may obtain high acuity. At present two eyes can see 6/36 letters, one 6/24, three 6/18, two 6/12, five 6/9, five 6/6, and two 6/5. One 6/36 eye is technically perfect with an intracapsular extraction but has myopic degeneration. Two recent cases have not yet been tested for acuity. All but three underwent the one-stage operation.

The compound lens system resulting from the conjunction of the acrylic lens described and the ocular media must necessarily differ from the normal, since the lens is certainly not the same as the natural one in shape and thickness and may not occupy precisely the same position in the eye. The effect, however, is most satisfactory, the resulting refraction being generally within 2 dioptres of the pre-cataract refraction, judged by the other eye. Many patients see quite well without spectacles or with those they used before cataract developed. Astigmatism averages about 1 dioptre— rather less than with simple extractions. Binocular vision is usually appreciated as soon as the eye is ready for use, and in some cases accurate sight is regained very early. It is a new experience to hear a cataract patient remark at a postoperative dressing : " I can see the faces of all you gentlemen quite clearly."

DISCUSSION

The introduction of intra-ocular acrylic lenses is capable of producing an improved result in all types of case. In monocular or nearly monocular cataract the advantages are overwhelming, for by no other method is it possible to restore almost perfect binocular vision. Convalescence is not prolonged and the dangers of operation seem comparable to those of simple cataract extraction. Though the technique is still in its early stages, and improvements are being made continually, the experience here recorded shows that a satisfactory lens can be inserted and retained in place without apparent harm to the eye. In 1 case two years have elapsed since the lens was introduced.

SUMMARY

It is now possible to substitute for the opaque crystalline lens an artificial intra-ocular lenticulus capable of producing an excellent visual result.

Such a lens can remain in an eye for at least two years without causing irritation.

My sincere thanks are due to Mr. J. Pike, of Messrs. Rayners, 100, New Bond Street, London, W.1, for constructing and perfecting the intra-ocular lenses and designing the lens rack ; to Messrs. John Weiss & Son, 287, Oxford Street, W.1, for making the special lens forceps and iris hook ; and to Imperial Chemical Industries for supplying suitable acrylic compounds. Miss J. Trotman has kindly drawn the illustrations.

BIBLIOGRAPHY

Ridley, H. (1951) *Trans. ophthal. Soc. U.K.* **71** (in the press).
—— (1951) *St. Thom. Rep., Lond.* **7** (in the press).

THE LANCET]   SPECIAL ARTICLES   [JAN. 3, 1953   37

Special Articles

A PRELIMINARY REPORT ON
THE 1952 EPIDEMIC OF POLIOMYELITIS IN COPENHAGEN
WITH SPECIAL REFERENCE TO THE TREATMENT OF ACUTE RESPIRATORY INSUFFICIENCY

H. C. A. LASSEN
M.D. Copenhagen
PROFESSOR OF EPIDEMIOLOGY IN THE UNIVERSITY OF COPENHAGEN ; CHIEF PHYSICIAN, DEPARTMENT FOR COMMUNICABLE DISEASES, BLEGDAM HOSPITAL, COPENHAGEN

THE 1952 epidemic of poliomyelitis in Greater Copenhagen has been the largest and most severe local epidemic ever recorded in Denmark.

ADMISSIONS

The metropolitan area of Copenhagen has a population of 1,200,000 people served by a single hospital for communicable diseases, the Blegdam Hospital. Between July 24 and Dec. 3 2722 patients with poliomyelitis were admitted to this hospital—866 with paralysis and 1856 without. In 316 of the 866 paralytic cases we had to resort to special measures, such as tracheotomy, artificial respiration, postural drainage, or combinations of these. The enormous load of severely ill patients is well illustrated by the fact that in four months we treated three times as many cases with respiratory insufficiency, paralysis of the ninth, tenth, and twelfth cranial nerves, and involvement of the bulbar respiratory and vasomotor centres as in the preceding ten years. At times we had 70 patients requiring artificial respiration, and we still have from 50 to 60 requiring it. To my knowledge nothing comparable has ever been seen in Europe.

The great number of severely ill patients pouring in made therapeutic improvisations necessary. During these months we have in fact been in a state of war, and at the beginning we were not nearly adequately equipped to meet an emergency of such vast proportions. Fig. 1 shows that the epidemic culminated about Sept. 1. During the week Aug. 28–Sept. 3 our hospital admitted 335 patients or nearly 50 cases daily. The descending branch of the epidemic curve is, as usual, less steep than the ascending branch. At the time of writing, Dec. 7, the epidemic seems to be nearing its

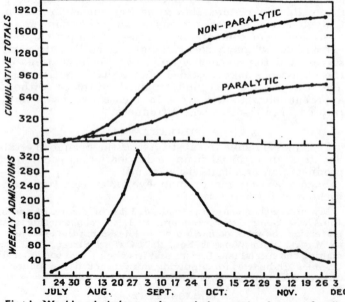

Fig. 1—Weekly admissions and cumulative totals of cases of poliomyelitis in 1952.

end. During the last two months the proportion of paralytic in relation to non-paralytic cases has grown steadily, but as a whole the ratio is 1 : 2. Naturally the number of patients admitted with non-paralytic poliomyelitis does not give an accurate picture of the true incidence of such cases in the epidemic area.

TREATMENT OF RESPIRATORY INSUFFICIENCY AND BULBAR DISEASE

In former years our therapeutic results in cases with respiratory insufficiency and involvement of the lower cranial nerves and the bulbar centres have always been very bad.

During the eleven years 1934–44 respirator treatment was used in 76 cases with a mean mortality-rate of 80%. Only cuirass respirators were used.

It is generally agreed that respiratory insufficiency of spinal origin is far easier to treat than respiratory insufficiency due to the involvement of the lower cranial nerves and the bulbar centres. Table I shows clearly the extremely grave prognosis of the pure bulbar and combined forms of respiratory insufficiency. With very few exceptions all our patients belonging to these groups died.

In 1948 we started using tracheotomy in all cases where it proved impossible to maintain an open airway because of pooling of secretions and aspiration into the lungs. In the U.S.A. this procedure seems to have had

TABLE I—RESULTS OF RESPIRATOR TREATMENT OF POLIOMYELITIS 1934–44

Type of disease	No. of cases	No. of deaths
Respiratory paralysis without bulbar involvement	17	5 (28%)
Respiratory paralysis with bulbar involvement	51	48 (94%)
Respiratory paralysis of undetermined type	8	8 (100%)

a beneficial influence on prognosis. In our hands this has not been so.

Table II shows that all the patients treated by tracheotomy and with respirators died, whereas treatment with respirators alone had a somewhat better prognosis, 1 man and 4 children surviving. Of these 5 patients 4 had respiratory insufficiency of purely spinal origin, and 1 patient had transient slight impairment of swallowing.

Thus the prognosis of poliomyelitis with respiratory insufficiency was rather gloomy at the outbreak of the present epidemic in Copenhagen. At our disposal we had one tank respirator (Emerson) and six cuirass respirators. This equipment proved wholly insufficient when the epidemic developed into a major catastrophe.

Fig. 2 shows the admission dates of the 316 poliomyelitis patients requiring special treatment—i.e., tracheotomy, artificial respiration, postural drainage, and combinations of these forms of treatment. The chart exclusively comprises patients with respiratory insufficiency, paralysis of the lower cranial nerves, the respiratory or vasomotor bulbar centres or combinations of these forms of paralysis. During the epidemic tracheotomy was performed in about 250 cases. The indication for this operation was invariably stagnation of secretions in the upper airway, leading to inadequate ventilation. By far the greater number of the patients had simultaneously paralysis of the respiratory muscles. The 316 cases did not all come from the metropolitan area, because in recent years we have done much to centralise the treatment of such patients. Consequently fig. 2 includes 75 cases brought in from localities outside our usual area. These admissions account for the three peaks of the curve.

Until the last week of August we used the therapeutic methods practised in 1948–50, but during these terrible weeks the situation became increasingly critical. The

Public Health

DECEMBER FOG IN LONDON AND THE EMERGENCY BED SERVICE

G. F. ABERCROMBIE
M.D. Camb.

CHAIRMAN, EMERGENCY BED SERVICE COMMITTEE,
KING EDWARD'S HOSPITAL FUND FOR LONDON

IN the first half of December, 1952, a violent and untimely "epidemic" smote the people of London, and applications to the Emergency Bed Service (E.B.S.) for the admission of general acute cases far exceeded all previous records. In what follows, E.B.S. admissions only are considered; there must have been a great number of direct admissions of which the E.B.S. has no knowledge.

Fig. 1 shows day by day the applications for this month of December (7992 applications, 6852 [85·73%] admitted) compared with those for the previous August (2946 applications, 2815 [95·53%] admitted). Plotted thus, the graphs are too erratic to be of use in predicting how many requests the service is likely to receive in the immediate future; but if, instead, a "moving" weekly total is calculated and charted, the more extreme irregularities

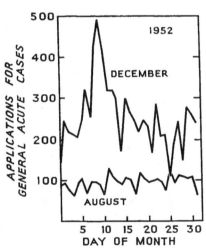

Fig. 1—Totals of daily applications for admission of general acute cases in August, 1952, and in December, 1952.

disappear and the general trend becomes discernible. Fig. 2 shows the moving weekly totals each winter from 1949 to December, 1952. Each point on these tracings shows the total applications received during the previous seven days: for example, the weekly total up to Nov. 30, 1952, was 1313, and next day 243 applications were received; adding these and subtracting the 220 received on Nov. 24, the moving weekly total for Dec. 1 is 1336.

The annual rhythm is now fairly clear. After a quiet summer the line begins to move upwards as winter approaches; there is usually (though not in 1951) a characteristic fall just at Christmas, and then the line rises steeply to its peak in early January, after which it declines more or less steadily to reach the summer levels in April.

WARNING SYSTEM

After January, 1951, when 7064 applications were received and only 65·5% of patients were admitted, the service evolved a warning system which is now on trial. When the percentage of admissions to applications, calculated on the moving weekly totals, falls below 85%, a "white" warning is sent to the appropriate hospital authorities. This is a precautionary signal, saying in effect: "E.B.S. is hard pressed and may be in serious difficulty in the next day or two." If the percentage falls below 80% a "yellow" warning is issued, and if below 75% a "red" warning. These are urgent calls for help and mean: "The situation is serious, the resources of E.B.S. are rapidly being exhausted, and for one patient in five—or four—no bed can be found." On receipt of these warnings, regional-board hospitals take pre-arranged action to provide more accommodation by

slowing down admissions from the waiting-list, by putting up extra beds, and so on. Teaching hospitals are also informed and coöperate as far as possible.

THE FIRST YELLOW WARNING

In 1952, owing to the prevalence of cold weather since early November the work of the service rose steadily throughout that month with the result that on Dec. 1 243 general acute applications were received instead of the normal 130 or so. This rise continued until Dec. 6, when the fog settled on London, and the number of

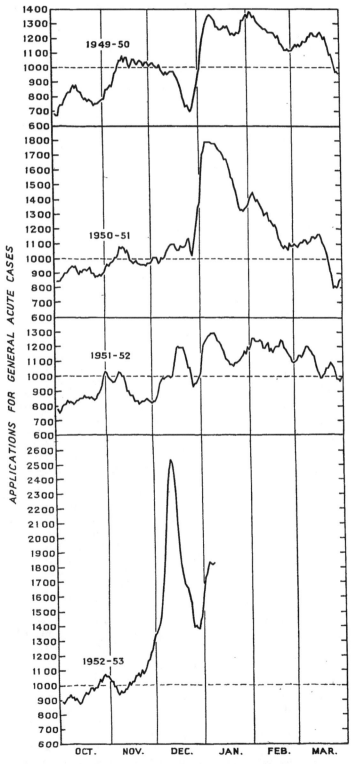

Fig. 2—Moving weekly totals of applications for admission of general acute cases in each of the winters from 1949-50 to 1952.

THE LANCET]   PUBLIC HEALTH   [JAN. 31, 1953   235

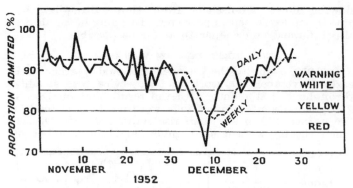

Fig. 3—Percentage of patients admitted to hospital in November and December, 1952, (a) daily and (b) by moving weekly totals.

applications rose very rapidly, reaching an unprecedented peak on Dec. 9, when 492 were received. Applications continued in abnormally high but diminishing numbers until the 13th, after which a fairly stable state was reached (fig. 1).

On Dec. 1 the admission-rate was 88·5%, and in spite of increasing pressure it was kept above 85% until Sunday, the 7th, when it fell to 84·9%; a "white" warning was issued at 11 A.M. next day (fig. 3). On Tuesday, the 9th, the rate was 79·9%, and the "yellow" warning was issued. The response was such that, despite the high total of applications, the admission-rate fell only a further 1·5%. The "yellow" warning was cancelled on the 15th, and the "white" on the 17th.

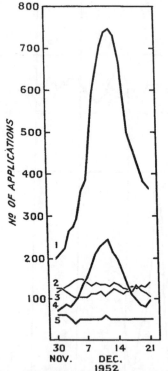

Fig. 4—Weekly totals of applications in December, 1952, by types of disease. (1) Respiratory disorders. (4) Cardiac disorders. (3) Other acute medical disorders. (2) Acute surgical disorders. (5) Cerebral hæmorrhage.

Prior to these warnings the admission-rate had been maintained above 85% by the action of the regional medical admission officers, who freely used the power to refer any given case to the group medical referee for immediate admission. This must have been a very severe burden on the regional-board hospitals.

It is interesting to note that, whereas on Jan. 1, 1951, at the height of the influenza epidemic, 293 applications were received by the E.B.S. and 185 cases were admitted, on Dec. 9, 1952, at the height of the fog "plague," 492 applications were received and 390 cases were admitted. The highest weekly total of admissions previously recorded was 1169 on Jan. 2, 1951; but in the week ended Dec. 13, 1952, 2019 cases were admitted.

TYPE OF ILLNESS

The increase in sickness was due almost entirely to respiratory disease, which was nearly quadrupled (fig. 4). The rise in heart-disease to about three times the normal numbers, though less spectacular, should not be overlooked. As in the winter of 1951–52,[1] the

1. See Abercrombie, G. F. Lancet, 1951, ii, 1175.

increase in sickness was almost exclusively confined to the over-45 and under-5 age-groups.

CONCLUSION

The warning system appears to be satisfactory, and the magnificent response by the hospitals undoubtedly saved the day.

EFFECTS OF A SEVERE FOG ON A GENERAL PRACTICE

JOHN FRY

M.B. Lond., F.R.C.S.

GENERAL PRACTITIONER, BECKENHAM, KENT

THIS is a report on the effects of a severe fog on a general practice of 4500 patients in the south-eastern outskirts of London. The fog reduced visibility at times to nil, and persisted for five days from Dec. 5 to 9, 1952. It was preceded and accompanied by intense cold; illness was widespread, and there was an increase in the number of deaths. In the week ending Dec. 13 there were 4703 deaths in Greater London, compared with 1852 in the corresponding week of 1951; and during the same week the Emergency Bed Service dealt with 2007 hospital admissions, compared with 917 in 1951.

VOLUME OF WORK

There was a remarkable increase in the work of the practice during the period of the fog and the following two weeks. This was largely accounted for by the increased number of visits that were necessary. The normal average number of weekly visits for this time of year is 75; during the week of the fog the number rose to 125. The number of attendances in the surgery did not vary from the anticipated average, which is 250 consultations per week.

TYPE OF WORK

There was a considerable increase in the prevalence of two conditions—namely, the upper respiratory tract affections and the respiratory disorders. The former included all coughs and colds with no abnormal chest signs and with relatively little constitutional upset; "respiratory disorders" means all conditions with symptoms referrable to the lungs and where abnormal signs were detected.

Table I shows clearly this rise during the period of the fog compared with the number of attendances for the preceding three weeks. Of course, these figures give no idea of the total number of people affected by the fog, for very many did not seek medical advice.

Upper Respiratory Tract Affections

Between Dec. 1 and 22 201 people sought medical advice for symptoms referrable to the upper respiratory tract. The chief complaint was a very irritating cough, with little sputum; what sputum there was was black or grey mucoid material. Nasal discharge and sore throat were the other prominent symptoms. All ages were affected, but there was a high proportion of patients in the 40–50 age-group. No abnormal signs were detected in the chests of these patients.

TABLE I—ATTENDANCES FOR UPPER RESPIRATORY TRACT AFFECTIONS AND FOR RESPIRATORY DISORDERS

Week	Nov. 10–16	Nov. 17–23	Nov. 24–30	Dec. 1–7	Dec. 8–14	Dec. 15–21
No. of attendances for upper respiratory tract affections ..	36	48	47	68	94	75
No. of attendances for respiratory disorders	19	29	30	51	93	62

TABLE II—AGE-DISTRIBUTION OF RESPIRATORY DISORDERS

Age	0–4	5–9	10–19	20–29	30–39	40–49	50–59	60–69	70–79	Over 80
No. of patients	—	3	—	1	—	2	8	13	12	4

Digestive Disorders

6 patients were seen during this period with sudden attacks of vomiting. This came on at the peak of the fog, and it was not accompanied by other digestive disturbance, such as abdominal pain or bowel alterations. Presumably the cause was gastric irritation produced by swallowing fog.

Respiratory Disorders

It was here that the fog produced its most serious effects. 43 patients, with varying degrees of illness, were seen with signs of involvement of the lower respiratory tract. They very often gave a history of previous chest trouble : in 37 of these patients there was a history of either recurrent productive winter coughs and dyspnœa— i.e., chronic bronchitis—asthma, bronchiectasis, or one of the forms of pulmonary fibrosis. In this practice there are 105 people with these chest troubles, and 37 of them were affected.

The *age-distribution* is shown in table II, which shows how the elderly suffered most.

The *sex-distribution* showed a 2 : 1 preponderance of men, there being 29 men and 14 women in this group.

The majority of the illnesses had a fairly sudden onset on the third or fourth day of the fog. This latent period has been noted during other fogs ; and it may be due to the fact that by the third or fourth day the concentration of atmospheric contaminants reaches a certain threshold level, or it may simply be that it takes this period for the respiratory defences to be overcome. The symptoms and signs seemed to arise from a combination of :

(1) Mucosal irritation (cough and sputum).
(2) Bronchial obstruction (dyspnœa, cyanosis, and loud rhonchi during both inspiration and expiration).
(3) Infection (fever and general constitutional upset— probably a secondary factor superimposed on the local irritation).
(4) Cardiac failure (evident in many of the more elderly patients).

On clinical assessment, 16 patients were severely ill, with considerable distress, and in some danger ; the other 27 had only a moderate degree of dyspnœa and general disturbance. Quite a number of these were able to remain up and about in their homes, and some even went out to work.

The severe cases were medical emergencies with paroxysmal dyspnœa, accompanied by an irritating and distressing cough and blackish mucopurulent sputum. Cyanosis was obvious in some patients, and in all of them the pulse-rate was around 120, the respirations were between 35 and 40 per minute, and the temperature varied from 100° to 104°F.

There were loud rhonchi all over both sides of the chest in both phases of respiration. Râles were noted in some cases, especially after a few days' illness. In no case were signs of clinical consolidation detected. The picture was therefore one of severe asthma, if asthma is taken to mean a condition of dyspnœa produced by bronchial obstruction ; but these patients did not respond to the usual antispasmodics.

It was impracticable to carry out any radiological or pathological investigations : there was so little time and so much work.

Most patients improved slowly and it took four to nine days for the symptoms and signs to clear up. This course was not influenced in any obvious way by the treatment adopted. This was directed to controlling the infection by using antibiotics—procaine penicillin in the first instance and chloramphenicol if there was no improvement after four days—and to attempting to relieve the bronchial obstruction with antispasmodics such as adrenaline, ephedrine, isoprenaline, and amino-phylline, whose effects were at the most very short-lived. The less severely ill were not treated with antibiotics, but with simple hot saline expectorants, combined with antispasmodics. It was not possible to use oxygen in these cases.

Of this group of 43 patients, 2 died and 1 was admitted to hospital. A man, aged 66, with a past history of pulmonary fibrosis which had caused great disability for some three years, died within four hours of the onset of symptoms. An old lady of 76, who had had a severe pneumonia four years previously, which had left her prone to winter coughs and dyspnœa, died on the eighth day of illness from cardiac failure. The patient admitted to hospital was an elderly man, who was too ill to be nursed at home by his even older wife.

CONCLUSION

These observations agree with the analysis of the effects of the November fog of 1948.[1] The effects of a fog, in association with cold weather, are principally on the respiratory and gastric mucosæ. Irritative symptoms, such as cough, nasal discharge, and vomiting, are the primary results ; but in cardio-respiratory invalids secondary infection and other complications often appear in the lungs and bronchi. The most severe cases are found in the elderly, deaths being rare under the age of 45. It is remarkable that although there are quite a number of asthmatic children in this practice none of them was affected ; in fact, there was less illness than usual in children during this period. The same observation was made during the influenza epidemic of 1950–1951, when there was widespread illness in adults but less than usual in children.

Influenza

Last week reports of widespread influenza on the Continent and in the United States were quickly followed by news of large numbers of cases in this country, especially in the south of England. There is so far no evidence that the disease is taking a severe form, and recovery from the acute symptoms within 48 hours seems usual. In some patients the respiratory symptoms have been followed (not accompanied) by gastro-intestinal disturbance. Early laboratory evidence suggests that an A-prime virus is responsible.

The latest figures from the 160 great towns of England and Wales show 72 deaths from influenza in the week ended Jan. 17, compared with 51 in the preceding week. There were 76 deaths from influenza in the great towns in the corresponding fortnight of 1952. Deaths from pneumonia showed no significant increase up to Jan. 17. Notifications of pneumonia (primary or influenzal) in England and Wales numbered 1204 in the week ended Jan. 17, compared with 1167 in the preceding week and 869 in the corresponding week of 1952.

These figures give no indication of the rapid spread of mild influenza that is taking place. One doctor on the outskirts of London reports that Monday, Jan. 26, was his heaviest day in 15 years of general practice. On Jan. 27 the Emergency Bed Service issued a " red " warning to hospitals. This warning is given when the service finds that London hospitals can take less than 75 % of the cases referred to the service for admission. Regional boards have asked their hospitals to respond to this warning by bringing into action plans for restricting the admission of non-urgent cases and for freeing as many beds as possible.

On the Continent epidemics are reported in France and Germany (where the U.S. zone is particularly affected). An influenza vaccine has been distributed for the inoculation of American troops in Europe.

1. Logan, W. P. D. *Lancet*, 1949, i, 78.

THE LANCET] ANNOTATIONS [FEB. 6, 1954 301

and adjusted to give the cost per inpatient per week, based on the total number of beds with deductions for vacant beds and a notional allowance for outpatient work. If the actual cost for outpatient work is known this figure is used, but the report gives no clue when this has been done. This costing figure may provide some basis for accountancy comparison; but it does not reflect the efficiency of the hospital, which could be better shown by calculating the cost per patient treated. The hospital that appears expensive is often the efficient hospital with a rapid turnover and high bed occupancy; and here the cost per patient treated may, in fact, be under half that of a poorly staffed and ill-equipped, but much cheaper, hospital. The figures published may be of some value in calculating costs for road accidents or pay-beds, but the present overemphasis on cost per bed per week constitutes a real injustice to the efficient hospital. It would be of considerable interest to find hospitals in each of the different categories where both the profession and the Ministry agree that the level of staffing and equipment is optimal for really good work, and to use these costs as a basis for comparison.

One of the principal objects of publishing these statistics is to enable hospital authorities to make broad comparisons in terms of performance, staffing, and so on, between hospitals for which they are responsible and similar hospitals elsewhere, and in this way to consider the possibilities of increased efficiency. For any constructive criticism, however, comparison of two hospitals needs a very intimate knowledge of their particular circumstances. The Ministry is now considering how best to present these statistics for 1953 and future years to enable an accurate comparison to be made. The editions published so far have revealed any gross differences in costs, and for these there have usually been adequate explanations. It is very doubtful whether such a detailed breakdown of figures is necessary at all; it would be valuable to have a much simplified analysis with emphasis on figures which demonstrate volume and efficiency of the hospital service, as shown, for example, by the bed-occupancy rate, bed-turnover rate, and cost per patient treated, giving some comparison with previous years. Such an analysis, together with regional summaries, in one volume, could be both informative and digestible.

There is no limit to the statistical analyses which could be made of public services : it might be interesting, but it would not necessarily be useful, to know the number of letters handled per postman in each postal district or the running-costs of every railway station. Although full of fallacies, the figures for hospitals that have hitherto been issued have served a good purpose by focusing attention on the need for better costing systems and improved turnover; but the time has surely come for complete revision of the method of presentation.

THE ANATOMY OF FACIAL PALSY

THE commonest cause of facial weakness in an otherwise healthy adult is Bell's palsy. This eponym was assigned to the disorder well over a century ago; yet the cause is still obscure. Usually the patient feels a vague ache behind the ear, which is accompanied or followed by a facial weakness that often rapidly becomes more severe; previous exposure to draught is common. If, in addition to the facial palsy, there is some loss of taste on one side of the tongue, the diagnosis is further confirmed. This clinical picture portrays only the site of the lesion—namely, between the geniculate ganglion, through which taste-fibres leave the nerve-trunk, and the origin of the chorda tympani, at which they join it. Taste is not always involved, however, and it seems that in Bell's palsy the nerve may be attacked at different levels, at any rate between the geniculate ganglion and the stylomastoid foramen.

Tschiassny [1] suggests that lesions of the facial nerve can be defined by carefully analysing the type of palsy and its accompanying signs. In addition to the well-known supranuclear lesion, with preservation of emotional and paralysis of voluntary movement and relative escape of the forehead, he lists seven levels at which lesions may be recognised. At the nucleus, though all movement is abolished, reflex "tearing" and taste are unaffected, since fibres for these join the nerve in the midbrain and at the geniculate ganglion respectively. Extracerebrally, but above the geniculate ganglion, tearing is lost but taste preserved. At the ganglion taste is also lost. Below this, tearing is again unaffected since fibres for this pass via the ganglion to the greater superficial petrosal nerve. Further down, the nerve to stapedius leaves the facial trunk, and lesions below this level no longer cause hyperacusis to loud sounds. Next, the chorda tympani segregates taste-fibres and lesions after this no longer cause loss of taste. Finally, just at the stylomastoid foramen a motor branch passes to the digastric muscle, and below this level the slight deviation of the chin caused by paralysis of the digastric is absent.

Application of these signs to cases of Bell's palsy tends to confirm that the site of the lesion varies. In practice, however, the tests described by Tschiassny often give equivocal results. The important distinctions are of upper from lower motor-neurone lesions, and of Bell's palsy from other types of lower motor-neurone lesion. Fortunately, both these distinctions can usually be made on the history and clinical findings.

HUMAN BIOCHEMICAL GENETICS

THE pathologist's long-term aim is to describe all disease in terms of the physics and chemistry of the cell. His first successes are likely to come in disorders due to the primary action or inaction of a genetic factor, rather than in the disorders where some external agent, such as infection, is important. Genetic factors must operate first among the chemical elements in the nucleus; and mutations, changes in genetic factors, must produce some variation from the normal in cell biochemistry. Work on lower organisms, such as the fungus neurospora, suggests that in many instances one genetic factor controls the production or functions of one enzyme. In man it is difficult to study what is going on in the cell, and knowledge of biochemical variation is mostly limited to that which can be studied in blood, saliva, and urine. The first biochemical disorder to be recognised was alkaptonuria, because here the abnormal metabolite not only appears in the urine but turns this black on standing. These abnormalities were first fully discussed by Garrod.[2] Harris has now ably summarised present knowledge in a monograph from the Galton Laboratory.[3]

The genetically determined variations in metabolism can be placed in certain broad groups. One group are those in which the end-product differs from the normal, or, if there is no normal, may be present in several alternative forms. Another group are those in which there is an apparent block at some intermediary stage so that normal metabolites accumulate in abnormal amounts.

A good example of the first group are the variants of hæmoglobin. That found in patients with sickle-cell anæmia and, in smaller amounts, in those with the sickle-cell trait differs from normal adult hæmoglobin in its much slighter solubility in the reduced state and also in the electrophoretic properties of some of its derivatives. This physical difference in solubility is chemically important, but it must depend on only small differences in the chemical composition of the molecules. Chemical analysis of these types of hæmoglobin shows

1. Tschiassny, K. Ann. Otol., &c., St. Louis, 1953, 62, 677.
2. Garrod, A. E. Lancet, 1908, ii, 1, 73, 142, 214.
3. An Introduction to Human Biochemical Genetics, by H. HARRIS, M.A., M.D. Eugenics Laboratory Memoirs, XXXVII. Cambridge University Press. 1953. Pp. 96. 15s.

only differences in the relative proportions of the different amino-acids found, and X-ray analysis of the crystals gives a picture identical in every detail. Different individuals with the sickle-cell trait vary in the proportion of sickle-cell hæmoglobin present. This depends on other genes present, since within families there is less variation in this respect. Two other genetically determined abnormal types of hæmoglobin are known. Another example of genetically determined variation, chemically small but clinically important, is that between the A, B, and O blood-group substances. These substances have been thoroughly analysed, and again the only differences found are in the relative proportions of the different amino-acids present. Yet another example is the congenital methæmoglobinæmia that has been found in four generations of one family where the globin moiety differed from that in normal hæmoglobin. It is noteworthy that the examples in this group, comprising variations in the end-products of metabolism, are mostly due to genetic factors which take appreciable effect in the heterozygous state and in this sense are dominant.

The best examples of the second group come at the moment from the biochemistry of the amino-acid, phenylalanine. Alkaptonuria represents a block at a late stage in the breakdown of phenylalanine. In phenylketonuria, on the other hand, the block appears to be at the first stage of its metabolism—the conversion to tyrosine. Phenylalanine in normal people is an essential constituent of diet, and tyrosine is not ; but in phenylketonuria any phenylalanine fed can be recovered from the urine in the same quantity, as phenylalanine or one of its near derivatives, such as phenylpyruvic acid. In addition to these two well-known conditions one case of tyrosinosis has been described in which tyrosine and p-hydroxyphenylpyruvic acid were present in the urine in amounts which varied according to the amount of tyrosine or phenylalanine fed ; here the block must lie at a stage between that in phenylketonuria and that in alkaptonuria. Fructosuria, pentosuria, and the recessive type of congenital idiopathic methæmoglobinæmia also probably depend on enzyme deficiencies. So presumably do the storage diseases such as glycogen-storage disease, the amaurotic family idiocies, Gaucher's disease, and gargoylism. In this group, comprising blocks in intermediary metabolism probably due to specific enzyme deficiencies, the genetic factors responsible mostly take effect only in the homozygous state, and in this sense are recessive. In some pedigrees, however, alkaptonuria and also Gaucher's disease behave as if due to dominant genetic factors.

Harris includes in his account a third group in which the essential abnormality appears to be failure of renal tubular function. These are errors of metabolism in that the specific dysfunction of the renal tubular cells probably depends on the failure of one or other of the syntheses which normally makes possible the reabsorption of these substances from the glomerular filtrate. The details of these syntheses are not yet known. In this group he places renal glycosuria and also the type of cystinuria in which cystine stones often form and in which greatly increased amounts of the three amino-acids, cystine, lysine, and arginine, are found in the urine, although the plasma levels of these three substances are within normal limits. There is at the moment no obvious reason why these three particular amino-acids should be affected together ; presumably their reabsorption involves the same biochemical synthesis. The inheritance both of renal glycosuria and of the cystine-lysine-arginine type of amino-aciduria is not straightforward.

Advances in histochemistry are certain to lead to rapid advances in biochemical genetics. When these come the geneticist will no longer be limited to the study of conditions in which chemical variations can be detected

in the blood, saliva, and urine. It is reasonable to suppose, for example, that in achondroplasia, due in most instances to a dominant factor, and in Morquio's disease, due in most instances to a recessive factor, specific biochemical abnormalities will be found in the osteoblasts and osteoclasts. In the same way specific abnormalities in the nerve-cells will be found, for example, in Huntington's chorea, which is dominantly inherited, and in Kinnier-Wilson's disease, which is recessively inherited.[4] In Kinnier-Wilson's disease there is in fact already some evidence that there is abnormal deposition of copper in the brain and liver and an abnormally low level of protein-bound copper in the plasma. Bearn suggests that the sequence is a low level of copper in the plasma, increased absorption of copper from the gut, deposition of copper in the tissues with damage to the basal nuclei of the brain and to the liver, and increased excretion of copper in the urine bound to amino-acids. No doubt the time will come when individual differences in resistance to infection—for example, to the tubercle bacillus—can be described in terms of individual variations in biochemistry, but that is looking some way ahead.

"SMOKER'S COUGH"

TOBACCO-SMOKING is a hazardous pastime. While contributing to the yearly £617 million tobacco tax, the smoker may, it seems, raise his blood-pressure, diminish his vital capacity, have anginal pain, and lay the foundations of a bronchial carcinoma. He may also suffer from "smoker's cough," chronic pharyngitis, wheezing, shortness of breath, and a tendency to respiratory infections—a combination that has been termed "smoker's respiratory syndrome." Waldbott[5] has found the pharyngeal and bronchial mucosa in this condition fiery red and streaked with mucopus ; the patients had wheezing, a productive cough in the mornings, "rhythmic darting and angina-like" chest pains, and a sensation of constriction beneath the sternum. When they stopped smoking two-thirds of them improved, and most became completely well. Some who did not improve had advanced emphysema, and Waldbott assumes that this was the end-result of chronic irritation by nicotine, pyridine, collidine, ammonia, and hydrocyanic acid.

"Smoker's cough" is not new. A German who visited London in 1598 noted that the English were constantly seen smoking the "nicotean weed" and puffing out the smoke along with "plenty of phlegm and defluction from the head." Nor are smokers unaccustomed to having their indulgence attacked, though seldom so vehemently as in King James's "Counterblaste to Tobacco." Smoking was very widespread at that time. According to a declaration introducing the tax of 6s. 8d. a pound in 1604, it was "through evil custom and the toleration thereof, excessively taken by a number of riotous and disorderly persons . . . who do spend most of their time in that idle vanity . . . and also do consume [their] wages . . . not caring at what price they buy the drug." It has been suggested that the very excess of smoking by all classes in the 17th century may have led to the growth of the snuff habit, which gradually replaced smoking in the 18th. Snuffing itself also developed to fashionable excess, but yielded to cigarette-smoking in early Victorian times. The immoderate cigarette-smoking of the 20th century may some day become unfashionable and snuff-taking return—but perhaps not on the lavish scale of the past, when Samuel Johnson carried his snuff loose in his waistcoat pockets, Coleridge suggested that snuff might be the final cause of the human nose, and a certain Mrs. Thompson requested that at her funeral her faithful servant should walk before the coffin and distribute every twenty yards a

4. Bearn, A. G. Amer. J. Med. 1953, 15, 442.
5. Waldbott, G. L. Ann. intern. Med. 1953, 39, 1026.

THE LANCET]   ORIGINAL ARTICLES   [JULY 9, 1955 57

extensors of the toe, often producing perceptible small movements up or down, probably in an effort to utilise active joint sense to compensate for the failure to appreciate passive movement.

These observations indicate that impairment of passive joint sense is of little practical importance to the individual. In the course of a neurological lesion it is the loss of active joint sense which results in functional disability. Lesions of the posterior columns of the spinal cord may produce loss of both these modes of sensation, together with blunting of tactile discrimination, and it is the loss of all three (particularly perhaps the last) which causes inability to respond in the ordinary clinical test of passive movement in the great toe.

Conclusions

Clinical testing of appreciation of passive movement of the great toe, when carefully performed, may demonstrate impairment to which no pathological significance can be attached. On the other hand, in patients with known lesions of the central or peripheral nervous system, clinical testing as ordinarily performed may suggest the presence of normal sensation even when this is impaired or absent. It would therefore appear that testing passive joint sense at the metatarsophalangeal joint gives no reliable evidence of neurological changes.

REFERENCES

Boyd, I. A., Roberts, T. D. M. (1953) *J. Physiol.* **122**, 38.
Browne, K., Lee, J., Ring, P. A. (1954) *Ibid*, **126**, 448.
Hutchison, R., Hunter, D. (1949) Clinical Methods. London; p. 346.
Lee, J., Ring, P. A. (1954) *J. Physiol.* **123**, 56P.

SMEARS FROM THE ORAL MUCOSA IN THE DETECTION OF CHROMOSOMAL SEX

KEITH L. MOORE
M.Sc., Ph.D. Western Ontario
RESEARCH FELLOW OF THE NATIONAL CANCER INSTITUTE, DEPARTMENT OF MICROSCOPIC ANATOMY

MURRAY L. BARR
M.Sc., M.D. Western Ontario
PROFESSOR OF MICROSCOPIC ANATOMY

UNIVERSITY OF WESTERN ONTARIO, LONDON, CANADA

THE skin-biopsy test of chromosomal sex is being used with increasing frequency as an aid to differential diagnosis in errors of sex development, such as hermaphroditism and gonadal dysgenesis (Moore et al. 1953, Barr 1954, 1955, Marberger and Nelson 1954, Polani et al. 1954, Wilkins et al. 1954, Bromwich 1955, Ehrengut 1955, Grumbach et al. 1955, Sohval et al. 1955). The epidermal nuclei of females contain a mass of sex chromatin that is inconspicuous in nuclei of males (Moore et al. 1953, Emery and McMillan 1954). The nuclei of epidermis are similar to those of other human tissues in this respect (Moore and Barr 1954). A sex difference in nuclear morphology has been found in several other mammals (Barr et al. 1950, Graham and Barr 1952, Moore and Barr 1953, Prince et al. 1955). The sex chromatin of female cells is thought to be formed by heterochromatic portions of the two X chromosomes adhering to each other in intermitotic nuclei. For reasons that are only partly understood, the XY sex-chromosomes of male nuclei do not form a distinctive mass of chromatin.

In our experience, the skin-biopsy test is reliable if the sections are of good technical quality. Experience has also shown, however, that difficulty is sometimes encountered in obtaining sections that display fine nuclear detail. The use of smears from the oral mucosa has been investigated in the hope of simplifying the cytological detection of chromosomal sex.

Procedure

In 140 subjects (81 males and 59 females) the mucosa of the cheek was rubbed firmly with the edge of a wooden tongue depressor. The material obtained was smeared gently on microscopic slides that had been coated with a thin film of Mayer's egg-albumin. 13 of the smears were from infants aged 2–7 days; the ages of the other subjects ranged from 2 months to 62 years. The Ayre spatula was a useful substitute for a tongue depressor when dealing with infants.

The slides were immersed immediately in Papanicolaou's fixative (equal parts 95% ethyl alcohol and ether). Drying of the smear was avoided. The period of fixation was not critical; times of from two to twenty-four hours were satisfactory. The fixed smears were passed through 70% alcohol, 50% alcohol, and distilled water, five minutes in each, with two changes of distilled water.

The following staining procedure resulted in good nuclear detail:

(1) Staining in a 1% solution of cresyl echt violet (Coleman and Bell) for five minutes.

(2) Differentiation in 95% alcohol (two changes) for about five minutes.

(3) Further differentiation in absolute alcohol, checking at intervals with the microscope until the details of cell structure were sharply defined.

(4) Clearing in xylene (two changes).

(5) Mounting in picolyte or neutral balsam.

Some smears were stained by the Feulgen method for desoxyribose nucleic acid.

If the slides are to be mailed to a laboratory for staining and microscopic study they should be transferred from distilled water to a 15% solution of glycerin in water for about two minutes. The excess solution is drained off. This treatment protects the smears from drying while in transit. The slides should be washed free of glycerin with distilled water before the smears are stained. The procedure of Ayre and Dakin (1946) for cervical smears may be used.

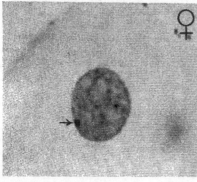 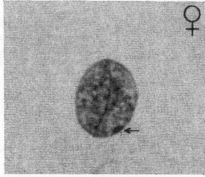 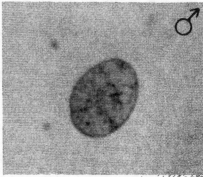

Figs. 1–3—Epithelial cells, stained with cresyl echt violet, in smears from the oral mucous membrane (× 2000). Fig. 1, adult female. Fig. 2, female infant, aged 2 days. Fig. 3, adult male.

58 THE LANCET]   ORIGINAL ARTICLES   [JULY 9, 1955

Observations

Each of us examined independently the series of 140 smears without reference to the sex of the subjects. The sex was correctly diagnosed in 100% of cases by both examiners.

Males

The appearance of the nuclei varied from cell to cell, and to some extent from one smear to another. As expected, some nuclei were shrunken and pyknotic and unsuitable for study. In other nuclei, however, the general chromatin was distributed evenly as small particles throughout the nucleoplasm, with a predilection for the inner surface of the nuclear membrane. One or more irregular clumps of chromatin of larger size were seen in various positions within the nucleus in some cells. Nucleoli were inconspicuous. An epithelial cell characteristic of smears from males is illustrated in fig. 3.

Females

The typical female-sex chromatin was a feature of many nuclei. The intensity of staining and sharpness of outline of the sex chromatin varied from cell to cell. The sex chromatin was located in various positions in relation to the periphery of the nucleus as seen in optical section. It was most definite and easiest to recognise when at the periphery of the nucleus, as illustrated in figs. 1 and 2. The sex chromatin was identified in this location in 40–60% of nuclei that were suitable for the study of morphological detail. A roughly planoconvex shape was most characteristic, the more flattened surface being adherent to the inner surface of the nuclear membrane. In some cells the sex chromatin was very much flattened, appearing as a local thickening of the nuclear membrane. Other shapes were encountered. The sex chromatin was Feulgen-positive. Measurements of a hundred masses of sex chromatin (ten cells in ten smears) with a filar micrometer eyepiece produced a mean value of $0.7 \times 1.2 \mu$. Moore and Barr (1955) found that the average size of the female-sex chromatin was $0.7 \times 1.2 \mu$ in sections of several human tissues.

Discussion

We believe that, with reasonable care, chromosomal sex can be diagnosed from smears of oral mucosa with very little chance of error. The preparation of mucosal smears has the advantage over skin biopsies of simplicity. On the whole, smear preparations are easier than skin biopsies to interpret, and they require less experience in cytology. Further smears can be easily obtained from a patient if the first preparations are technically unsatisfactory, and smears can be prepared in the rare instances where permission for a skin biopsy is refused. The mucosal-smear method of detecting chromosomal sex is suggested, therefore, as an alternative to skin biopsy, over which it has certain distinct advantages. The results obtained from study of a smear from the oral mucosa will no doubt have the same significance, in differential diagnosis, as does the interpretation of a skin biopsy (Barr 1954, 1955).

Summary

Smears were prepared from the oral mucosa of 140 persons (81 males and 59 females) and stained with cresyl echt violet.

The characteristic female-sex chromatin was clearly visible in the epithelial-cell nuclei of females, while a similar chromatin mass was not seen in the cells of males.

This method has the advantage of simplicity. It is suggested as an alternative to skin biopsy for the detection of chromosomal sex in congenital errors of sex development.

We are indebted to Mr. J. E. Walker and Mr. C. E. Jarvis for expert technical assistance. This work was supported by grants from the National Cancer Institute and the National Research Council of Canada.

References at foot of next column

THE ERYTHROCYTE-SEDIMENTATION RATE IN HYPOTHYROIDISM

STUART G. McALPINE
M.B. Glasg., F.R.F.P.S.
REGISTRAR IN MEDICINE, UNIVERSITY DEPARTMENT OF
MEDICINE, THE ROYAL INFIRMARY, GLASGOW

IT is well known that acceleration of the erythrocyte-sedimentation rate (E.S.R.) may occur in a variety of conditions associated with increased tissue destruction or with alterations in the blood chemistry. In endocrine disorders the E.S.R. is variable. In thyrotoxicosis, for example, a number of writers have noted that it is sometimes raised (Whitby and Britton 1950). In hypothyroidism, however, so far as I am aware, the only reference in the literature to elevation of the sedimentation rate is by Gram (1929) who noted increased sedimentation values in 4 of 9 cases with low basal metabolism. Wood (1950), on the other hand, has remarked on the normal E.S.R. in myxœdema. For these reasons it is considered that the experience of this clinic, in which acceleration of the E.S.R. has been noted in a high proportion of cases of hypothyroidism, merits publication.

Methods

The sedimentation rate was performed throughout by a standard Westergren technique.

4 ml. of blood was added to 1 ml. of 3.8% sodium citrate solution, graduated glass tubes, appropriately marked, being used. The citrated blood was drawn into Westergren tubes as soon as practicable after withdrawal, and the reading in mm. recorded after the tube had stood vertically for one hour at room-temperature.

Normal values for this method are 3–5 mm. for males and 4–7 mm. for females, but only values in excess of 10 mm. are generally regarded with significance. For the purpose of this paper therefore 10 mm. has been taken as the upper limit of normal.

The Patients

19 patients with hypothyroidism and 4 patients with pituitary hypofunction, in which hypothyroidism was part of the clinical picture, were included in the inquiry. 22 of these patients were female. Their ages ranged from 13 to 76 years. The diagnosis was made on the clinical picture, and in the majority of cases supported by a low basal metabolic rate (B.M.R.), and in every case confirmed by the response to thyroid extract given orally. The youngest in the series, a girl of 13, had had her ectopic thyroid gland removed surgically in the erroneous belief that it represented a thyroglossal cyst.

Results

The E.S.R. was recorded in all patients before treatment was begun, with the exception of 1 patient who

DR. MOORE, PROF. BARR : REFERENCES

Ayre, J. E., Dakin, E. (1946) *Canad. med. Ass. J.* **54**, 489.
Barr, M. L. (1954) *Surg. Gynec. Obstet.* **99**, 184.
— (1955) *Anat. Rec.* **121**, 387.
— Bertram, L. F., Lindsay, H. A. (1950) *Ibid*, **107**, 283.
Bromwich, A. F. (1955) *Brit. med. J.* i, 395.
Ehrengut, W. (1955) *Münch. med. Wschr.* **97**, 162.
Emery, J. L., McMillan, M. (1954) *J. Path. Bact.* **68**, 17.
Graham, M. A., Barr, M. L. (1952) *Anat. Rec.* **112**, 709.
Grumbach, M. M., Van Wyk, J. J., Wilkins, L. (1955) *J. clin. Endocrin. Metab.* (in the press).
Marberger, E., Nelson, W. O. (1954) *Anat. Rec.* **118**, 399.
Moore, K. L., Barr, M. L. (1953) *J. comp. Neurol.* **98**, 213.
— — (1954) *Acta anat.* **21**, 197.
— — (1955) *Brit. J. Cancer.* (in the press).
— Graham, M. A., Barr, M. L. (1953) *Surg. Gynec. Obstet.* **96**, 641.
Polani, P. E., Hunter, W. F., Lennox, B. (1954) *Lancet*, ii, 120.
Prince, R. H., Graham, M. A., Barr, M. L. (1955) *Anat. Rec.* (in the press).
Sohval, A. R., Gaines, J. A., Gabrilove, J. L. (1955) *Amer. J. Obstet. Gynec.* (in the press).
Wilkins, L., Grumbach, M. M., Van Wyk, J. J. (1954) *J. clin. Endocrin.* **14**, 1270.

THE LANCET]   ORIGINAL ARTICLES   [APRIL 21, 1956   461

and it might properly be called " rational radical mastectomy." The term " extended radical mastectomy " might be reserved for those procedures in which attempts are made to remove more than the primary lymphatic drainage areas—e.g., where a supraclavicular dissection is included.

Rational radical mastectomy is still experimental. Whether it will improve the results of treatment remains to be seen. All that can be claimed at present is that the procedure rests on a sound theoretical basis and can be carried out with no significant addition to the mortality, morbidity, or deformity of the Halsted operation.

Summary

A new technique is described for excision of the internal mammary lymph-nodes in primary operations for carcinoma of the breast.

57 patients have been operated upon without mortality; in 55 the primary tumour was either in the inner hemisphere or in the central area of the breast.

The disability, deformity, and morbidity of the operation are no greater than after the classical radical mastectomy.

Invasion of the internal mammary lymphatic chain was found in 23 cases (40%).

It will not be possible to assess the value of the operation in terms of cure-rate until further time has elapsed.

We are greatly indebted to the Bland-Sutton Institute of Pathology of the Middlesex Hospital Medical School, and in particular to Dr. A. C. Thackray, for the histological work incorporated in this paper ; and to Miss E. Hewland, the hospital medical artist, for the drawings of the operative technique.

REFERENCES

Abrao, A., Gentil, F. (1955) Rev. paulist. Med. 46, 217.
Andreassen, M., Dahl-Inverson, E., Sørensen, B. (1954) Lancet, i, 176.
Brenier, J. L. (1953) Rev. Chir., Paris, March-April, p. 72.
Handley, R. S., Thackray, A. C. (1954) Brit. med. J. i, 61.
McDonald, J. J., Haagensen, C. D., Stout, A. P. (1953) Surgery, 34, 521.
McWhirter, R. (1955) Brit. J. Radiol. 28, 128.
Margottini, M., Bucalossi, P. (1949) Oncologia, Roma 23, 70.
Patey, D. H., Dyson, W. H. (1948) Brit. J. Cancer, 11, 7.
Redon, H., Lacour, J. (1954) Mem. Acad. Chir. 80, 568.
Sugarbaker, E. D. (1953) Cancer, 6, 969.
Urban, J. A. (1951) Ibid, 4, 1263.
Wangensteen, O. H. (1949) Ann. Surg. 130, 315.

" . . . Men meet together for many reasons in the course of business. They need to instruct or persuade each other. They must agree on a course of action. They find thinking in public more productive or less painful than thinking in private. But there are at least as many reasons for meetings to transact no business. Meetings are held because men seek companionship or, at a minimum, wish to escape the tedium of solitary duties. They yearn for the prestige which accrues to the man who presides over meetings, and this leads them to convoke assemblages over which they can preside. Finally, there is the meeting which is called not because there is business to be done, but because it is necessary to create the impression that business is being done. Such meetings are more than a substitute for action. They are widely regarded as action. The fact that no business is transacted at a no-business meeting is normally not a serious cause of embarrassment to those attending. Numerous formulas have been devised to prevent discomfort. Thus scholars, who are great devotees of the no-business meeting, rely heavily on the exchange-of-ideas justification. To them the exchange of ideas is an absolute good. Any meeting at which ideas are exchanged is, therefore, useful. This justification is nearly ironclad. It is very hard to have a meeting of which it can be said that no ideas were exchanged."—J. K. GALBRAITH, The Great Crash, 1929. London, 1955.

A AND B BLOOD-GROUP ANTIGENS ON HUMAN EPIDERMAL CELLS
DEMONSTRATED BY MIXED AGGLUTINATION

R. R. A. COOMBS
Ph.D Camb., M.R.C.V.S.
ASSISTANT DIRECTOR OF RESEARCH

DONALD BEDFORD
RESEARCH ASSISTANT

DEPARTMENT OF PATHOLOGY, UNIVERSITY OF CAMBRIDGE

L. M. ROUILLARD
M.A. Camb., F.R.C.S.E.
CONSULTANT PLASTIC SURGEON, UNITED CAMBRIDGE HOSPITALS

STUDIES of the antigenic structure of body cells other than red cells have awaited the development of new methods. The technique reported here for demonstrating intra-species differences in the antigenic structure of human epidermal cells offers certain possibilities.

Isolated epidermal cells or aggregates of these cells prepared from small sheets of split skin do not give cellular suspensions suitable for agglutination tests. The inhomogeneity of the suspension, the irregular shapes of the cells, and the difficulty in obtaining suspensions in sufficient quantity militate against the use of this reaction. On the other hand, if it were possible to obtain a specific link or attachment between antibodies combining with even a few epidermal cells and different but specially selected indicator cells, the interaction of the individual cells should be easy to observe under the microscope. Such specific mixed agglutination or combination between two cell types should occur if both cell types possess a particular antigen in common. For instance, Wiener and Herman (1939) showed that horse anti-pneumococcus type-14 serum would form mixed agglutinates between type-14 pneumococci and human red cells because both these cells possess a common antigen.

If skin epidermal cells of a person of blood-group A possess the A antigen, then, accepting that ordinary agglutinating antibodies are at least bivalent, we would expect such epidermal cells to be capable of being linked by anti-A to group-A red cells. Thus on theoretical grounds the phenomenon of specific mixed agglutination or combination should provide a means of revealing whether epidermal cells do in fact contain the A and B blood-group antigens on their membranes.

The procedure which we have adopted for testing epidermal cells for the A (and B) antigen is illustrated diagrammatically in fig. 1. A suspension of epidermal cells from a group-A person is exposed to anti-A, and the cells are subsequently washed free from uncombined antibody. Only epidermal cells possessing the A antigen should adsorb anti-A and consequently, after being washed, possess free extending " receptors " with affinity for the A antigen. Group-A red cells added at this stage should combine with extending anti-A receptors on the treated epidermal cells. On the other hand, group-B and group-O red cells should not adhere to the treated epidermal cells.

The results recorded here substantiate this reasoning and appear to offer conclusive evidence for the existence of the A and B antigens on epidermal cells of group-A and group-B persons respectively.

Materials and Methods

Preparation of Isolated Epidermal Cells from Human Skin

The skin available for this study consisted of small fragments of stored thin split skin procured for plastic

996 THE LANCET]   PRELIMINARY COMMUNICATION   [JUNE 23, 1956

Preliminary Communication

DETERMINATION OF FŒTAL BLOOD-GROUP

BY examining the desquamated cells in the amniotic fluid for the specific sex chromatin discovered by Barr and his associates,[1] it has become possible to diagnose the sex of a fœtus. This method has been described by two of us,[2] and independent development of the method simultaneously in various parts of the world has amply confirmed its reliability.[3-6] We have since tried to develop a method for determining the fœtal blood-group, and we report here the preliminary results of antenatal ABO-grouping in the last months of pregnancy from desquamated cells in the amniotic fluid.

If the fœtal blood-group can be determined as early as the sex—i.e., from the fourth month of pregnancy—and amniotic fluid can be withdrawn at this stage without disturbing the pregnancy (which we believe but have not yet proved), then it will be possible to diagnose both sex-linked and blood-group-linked hereditary diseases at a stage when pregnancy can be safely interrupted.[7]

No simple and reliable method for determining the blood-group from tissue cells was available until Coombs and his co-workers recently described a method by which A and B antigens could be demonstrated on human epidermal cells by mixed agglutination.[8] Coombs et al. believed that this method could be applied to most tissue

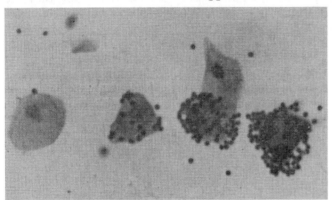

Fig. I—Mixed agglutination of erythrocytes and amniotic-fluid cells. Cells do not all participate in agglutination.

cells and thus afford a useful tool in studies of the antigenic structure of tissue cells. In our hands, this method has made it possible to detect A and B antigens in the cells of amniotic fluid, all of which are of fœtal origin.

Amniotic fluid was obtained by inserting a catheter into the amniotic cavity from below in cases where labour was to be induced, and by transabdominal puncture in a case of hydramnios. 2-5 ml. of each sample was centrifuged for three minutes at 1500 r.p.m. in silicone-coated conical glass tubes. The vernix and the supernatant were removed and the cellular sediment was resuspended in Ringer's solution and centrifuged again. This procedure was repeated once or twice. 10 drops of a suitable cell suspension was then incubated for one hour at 20°C with a similar quantity of anti-A immune serum, and another aliquot with anti-B serum. After this the samples were centrifuged again for three minutes, and the sediments were washed twice with Ringer's solution. Erythrocytes of groups A, B, and O were washed twice, and 1% suspensions with Ringer's solution were made. 4 drops of the cell suspensions was then mixed with similar amounts of the erythrocyte suspensions in silicone-treated test-tubes in the following way :

(1) Amniotic cells incubated with anti-A + A erythrocytes.
(2) Amniotic cells incubated with anti-B + B erythrocytes.
(3) Amniotic cells incubated with anti-A + O erythrocytes.
(4) Amniotic cells incubated with anti-B + O erythrocytes.

The tubes were centrifuged and the sediments were then carefully resuspended in the supernatant by gently shaking the tubes. A drop of each cell-erythrocyte mixture was inspected on a slide under cover with an ordinary light microscope or a phase-contrast microscope.

Where agglutination occurred, appearances very similar to those described by Coombs et al.[8] were seen (figs. 1 and 2). The erythrocytes adhered in large numbers to

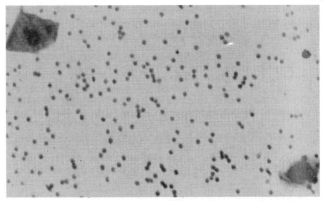

Fig. 2—Cell-erythrocyte mixture showing no agglutination.

the surface of the much larger amniotic-fluid cells, but no agglutination of erythrocytes or of cells alone was seen. When agglutination occurred in mixture no. 1, a fœtal blood-group of A was diagnosed ; agglutination in mixture no. 2 was diagnosed as group B ; agglutination in both as group AB ; and no agglutination as group O. No agglutination occurred in mixtures nos. 3 and 4 in any instance, thus providing a control.

So far we have studied twelve samples of amniotic fluid, six of which were examined by two of us independently of each other. One sample was found at the first centrifugation to contain blood ; contamination with maternal blood was assumed, and this was confirmed by the subsequent examination. In one case very weak agglutination was obtained in mixture no. 1 by both investigators. Postnatal blood-grouping of umbilical-cord blood indicated group A. In all the remaining cases except one the results agreed with the blood-groups determined postnatally on cord blood. Only in one case did one of the examiners fail to obtain agglutination in mixture no. 2, where the blood-group later turned out to be B. In two instances one of us saw slight erythrocyte agglutination in cases of group O, but no mixed cell-erythrocyte agglutination which alone is taken as a positive test.

Although the number of samples is small there is no doubt that the fœtal ABO blood-group can be diagnosed by this method. How early in pregnancy it can be done is not known, nor has any attempt been made to determine the Rh-group as yet. A knowledge of the fœtal Rh-group would be of practical value in cases of Rh-immunisation. At present we induce labour in such cases about two weeks before term if the fœtus is estimated at 2800 g. or more ; but even in cases where the mother has a high titre of antibodies the fœtus may be Rh-negative, and antenatal diagnosis of the Rh-group would make it possible to avoid induction of labour in such cases.

1. Moore, K. L., Graham, M. A., Barr, M. L. Surg. Gynec. Obstet. 1953, 96, 641.
2. Fuchs, F., Riis, P. Nature, Lond. 1956, 177, 330.
3. Shettles, L. B. Amer. J. Obstet. Gynec. 1956, 71, 834.
4. Sachs, L., Serr, D. M., Danon, M. Science, 1956, 123, 548.
5. Makowski, E. L., Prem, K. A., Kaiser, I. H. Ibid, p. 542.
6. Dewhurst, C. J. Lancet, April 21, 1956, p. 471.
7. Edwards, J. H. Ibid, April 28, 1956, p. 579.
8. Coombs, R. R. A., Bedford, D., Rouillard, L. M. Ibid, April 21, 1956, p. 461.

FRITZ FUCHS
M.D. Copenhagen
ERIK FREIESLEBEN
M.D. Copenhagen
ELSE E. KNUDSEN
M.D. Copenhagen
POVL RIIS
M.D. Copenhagen

Department A, Royal Maternity Hospital and Blood Bank, Rigshospitalet, Copenhagen; and Department F, Copenhagen County Hospital, Denmark

THE LANCET]   PRELIMINARY COMMUNICATION   [SEPT. 1, 1956 447

Preliminary Communication

MALIGNANT DISEASE IN CHILDHOOD AND DIAGNOSTIC IRRADIATION IN UTERO

PUBLIC-HEALTH departments all over the country are engaged in an environmental survey which will eventually cover some 1500 children who died of leukæmia or malignant disease before the age of 10 in the years 1953–55. As yet only approximately a third of the case-material has been gathered, but preliminary analysis has yielded a result which should, we feel, be reported without further delay.

The survey covers the whole of England and takes the following form.

The addresses of all children certified as dying from leukæmia or malignant disease during the three years 1953–55 have been collected and the attendant doctors asked for permission to approach the parents. Where the request has been approved, the mother is invited to coöperate by allowing a doctor from the local-authority health department to call and interview her. An interview by the same doctor is also arranged with the mother of a control child of the same age and sex, chosen at random from a list of births in the town or rural district in which the affected child's parents were living when the death occurred.

Of necessity a large number of doctors are conducting these interviews, but they are all following the same conventions and using standard schedules. Provided the parents of the dead child have not moved out of the area, only one doctor interviews each case-control pair. The questionnaires for the children who have died are designed to elicit information about the child's health before the onset of the fatal illness, and the mother's health before and during the relevant pregnancy. All investigations and treatments are recorded, and wherever possible X-ray data are checked with hospital notes. A note is also made of any cases of leukæmia and malignant disease in the family, any degree of consanguinity between parents and grandparents, and certain features of the child's diet and home background. The schedules for the controls ensure that the same facts are obtained up to the age when the corresponding case first showed signs of the fatal illness.

PAST HISTORIES* OF X-RAY EXAMINATIONS AND ANTIBIOTICS IN 547 CHILDREN WITH MALIGNANT DISEASE AND 547 CONTROLS MATCHED FOR AGE, SEX, AND LOCALITY

No. of mothers and children X-rayed		Leukæmia		Other malignant diseases		All malignant diseases	
Period	Type of exposure	269 cases	269 controls	278 cases	278 controls	547 cases	547 controls
Antenatal	Diagnostic— Abdomen	42	24	43	21	85	45
	Other	25	23	33	32	58	55
Before conception of survey child	Therapeutic	..	..	..	1	..	1
	Diagnostic— Abdomen	17	24	28	30	45	54
	Other	103	88	108	119	211	207
Postnatal (children only)	Therapeutic	1	..	1	..	2	..
	Diagnostic	45	49	46	50	91	99
	Shoe-fittings	55	52	40	46	95	98
†Total no. of mothers		140	130	160	154	300	284
Total no. of children		89	91	75	84	164	175
Either mother or child X-rayed		179	172	194	198	373	370
Postnatal medication (children)							
Sulphonamides		51	45	42	42	93	87
Antibiotics		68	52	50	58	118	110

* i.e., before the onset of the fatal illness in the affected child or equivalent period in the control child.
† Since a mother or child may appear in more than one X-ray category, the totals in this category are less than the sum of totals in the three preceding ones.

One reason for attempting a nation-wide survey was the possibility that the peak of leukæmia mortality in early life noted by Hewitt[1] might be explained if weak irradiation could initiate malignant changes in a fœtus or very young child. Hence this preliminary analysis of the completed schedules is focused mainly on the X-ray histories. The accompanying table shows the numbers of cases and controls with a history of irradiation of the mother or child. It also gives the numbers of children who received antibiotics or sulphonamides before the onset of the fatal illness or the equivalent date.

It will be seen that although they are alike in other respects, there is one important difference between the children who died and their controls : the number of mothers who had an X ray of their abdomen during the relevant pregnancy was 85 for the cases and only 45 for the controls. In the group labelled Other Malignant Diseases the corresponding figures for growths in different parts of the body were :

	Cases	Controls
Brain and appendages	11	9
Kidneys	10	2
Suprarenals	9	4
Lymph-nodes	4	2
All other sites	9	4

So large a total difference between the cases and controls can hardly be fortuitous. Nor, in view of the other resemblances, is it likely to be due to faulty choice of controls or to bias in recording. It could, however, be explained if children who are X-rayed before they are born are more prone to develop leukæmia and other malignant diseases than children who have not been X-rayed in utero.

DISCUSSION

The following facts have been known for some time. First, excessive exposure to radioactive materials may cause not only immediate radiation sickness and death but also the subsequent development of leukæmia and cancer. Secondly, the immediate ill-effects of radiation are disproportionately great when the whole body is exposed. Thirdly, therapeutic irradiation of pregnant women is liable to cause microcephaly and other congenital defects in the fœtus.[2]

In the last twelve months two other disturbing facts about X rays have come to light. In the first place it is now known that radiotherapy can cause leukæmia in adults[3] and cancer in children.[4] Secondly, the dose of irradiation received by the fœtal gonads during diagnostic pelvimetry frequently exceeds 2·5r.[5] The present investigation suggests that, besides causing genetic damage, this apparently harmless examination may occasionally cause leukæmia or cancer in the unborn child.

We acknowledge with gratitude all the help we have received from the health departments of counties and county boroughs, from the mothers of the survey children and from the General Register Office. We also thank the Lady Tata Memorial Trust for contributing generously towards the cost of the survey.

One of us (J. W.) receives a grant from the Medical Research Council.

ALICE STEWART
M.D. Camb., F.R.C.P.
JOSEFINE WEBB
M.B. Lond.
DAWN GILES
B.A. Oxfd.
DAVID HEWITT
M.A. Oxfd.

Department of Social Medicine, University of Oxford

1. Hewitt, D. Brit. J. prev. soc. Med., 1955, 9, 81.
2. Murphy, D. P. Congenital Malformations. Philadelphia, 1947.
3. Court Brown, W. M., Doll, R. Medical Research Council Report. Cmd. 9780. H.M. Stationery Office, 1956 ; p. 87.
4. Simpson, C. L., Hempelmann, L. H., Fuller, L. M. Radiology, 1955, 64, 840.
5. Osborn, S. B., Smith, E. E. Lancet, 1956, i, 949.

THE LANCET] ORIGINAL ARTICLES [DEC. 15, 1956

POLIOMYELITIS AND PROPHYLACTIC INOCULATION

AGAINST DIPHTHERIA, WHOOPING-COUGH, AND SMALLPOX

REPORT OF THE MEDICAL RESEARCH COUNCIL COMMITTEE ON INOCULATION PROCEDURES AND NEUROLOGICAL LESIONS *

THE reports of Hill and Knowelden (1950), Anderson and Skaar (1951), Korns, Albrecht, and Locke (1952), and Grant (1953) all supported the evidence brought forward by Martin (1950), Geffen (1950), and McCloskey (1950) that there was occasionally a causal relation between paralytic poliomyelitis and the inoculation of prophylactics against diphtheria and whooping-cough given singly or mixed. These observers were unable to give an accurate assessment of the risk or to be sure whether some prophylactics were more likely to be followed by the occurrence of paralysis than others, because they had no accurate information about the number of inoculations given.

Early in 1951 medical officers of health in England and Wales agreed to collaborate with the Medical Research Council in a study of the problem and to provide information on all notified cases of poliomyelitis. The information requested included details of diphtheria and pertussis prophylactics † and of smallpox vaccine given 84 days (12 weeks) or less before the onset of symptoms.

Medical officers of health, or their health visitors or sanitary inspectors, visit the homes of poliomyelitis patients as a routine soon after cases have been notified, and complete reports. It was therefore easy for them to add to the usual list of questions one about inoculations given before the onset of symptoms. For children inoculated at welfare centres or school clinics, and for most of those inoculated by general practitioners the medical officer of health was able to check the patient's story, or that of his parents or relatives, with the records in the health department. When no record was available in the health department the history was checked with the general practitioner or hospital medical officer concerned. One of the secretaries of the Committee, or Dr. D. Thomson, Ministry of Health, visited the areas in England from which cases were reported, and Dr. I. A. Bolz visited the areas in Wales; in collaboration with the medical officers of health and hospital clinicians or general practitioners they obtained as full a history as possible of the inoculations given and of the clinical and general epidemiological findings.

In addition a special request for information on the number of inoculations given to children was made to the medical officers of health for the county boroughs of England and Wales, for the administrative counties of London and Middlesex, and for the five non-county boroughs with populations of over 100,000—Dagenham,

Ilford, Leyton, Luton, and Walthamstow. Between May, 1951, and December, 1953, these medical officers of health supplied week by week a record of all inoculations given in welfare or school clinics. Records of children inoculated by their own doctors were not asked for, because the long interval which sometimes elapses before general practitioners submit their records of immunisation to the local authority would have made it difficult to relate the returns to the weeks in which the inoculations were given. The records from clinics gave the numbers of inoculations in detailed age-groups, as well as for the separate prophylactics, and indicated whether the inoculations were the first, second, or third of a primary course or were reinforcing. For convenience, the clinics in these different areas will be referred to as "county-borough clinics."

Cases in England and Wales 1951-53

NUMBER OF CASES NOTIFIED AND NUMBER INVESTIGATED

During the study, from April 1, 1951, to Dec. 31, 1953, 7023 paralytic and 3757 non-paralytic cases in patients of all ages were notified (corrected notifications) in England and Wales; the Committee obtained reports on all but 152 paralytic and 101 non-paralytic cases. Those for which reports were not received were usually in rural or small urban districts where often only one or two cases were notified during the inquiry. The prophylactics mentioned are, with the exception of smallpox vaccine, seldom given to persons over 15 years of age; this report is therefore based on children up to 15 years of age reported to us as cases of poliomyelitis and known to have had inoculations of one or more of the stated prophylactics within 12 weeks (84 days) before the onset of symptoms. Of the 478 such cases reported 66 were excluded from the analysis—24 because the diagnosis was changed, 10 because the diagnosis was doubtful, and 32 because they were not reported until more than three months after the onset of symptoms, or because it was impossible to obtain accurate information about them. Altogether 412 cases, of which 354 were paralytic and 58 non-paralytic, were fully investigated and included in the analysis. Table I provides information on the age of the patients at onset of symptoms, the type of illness (paralytic or non-paralytic), and the prophylactics used. From the table it is clear that most of the children investigated were between 6 months and 2 years old or between 4 and 6 years old. These are the ages at which primary courses and reinforcing doses are commonly given.

INTERVAL BETWEEN INOCULATION AND ONSET OF POLIOMYELITIS

The 355 paralytic cases (one child given inoculations of two different prophylactics at the same time has been included as two separate cases) are shown in table II by the interval in days between the date of the last— that is the most recent—inoculation and the date of the onset of symptoms, and by the type of prophylactic inoculated. They have been divided into three further groups: (a) those in children who did not complete the primary course before the illness began; (b) those in children who developed symptoms after the final inoculation of the primary course; and (c) those in children who developed symptoms after a reinforcing dose. The 58 non-paralytic cases are shown in the same table but, as there were not many of them, they were not grouped under the different prophylactics. Without laboratory confirmation it was difficult to be sure that so-called non-paralytic poliomyelitis was due to the poliomyelitis virus, and nothing is to be gained by considering these cases further in this report.

For primary immunisation against diphtheria or whooping-cough two or three inoculations are given,

---

* The members of the committee are: Dr. G. S. WILSON (chairman), Dr. W. H. BRADLEY, Dr. E. A. CARMICHAEL, Dr. E. T. CONYBEARE, Prof. F. GRUNDY, Prof. A. BRADFORD HILL, F.R.S., Dr. F. O. MacCALLUM, Dr. W. RITCHIE RUSSELL, Mr. H. J. SEDDON, Dr. I. N. SUTHERLAND, Dr. IAN TAYLOR, Dr. J. F. WARIN, and Dr. W. C. COCKBURN and Dr. J. KNOWELDEN (joint secretaries). The plans of the studies were prepared by the joint secretaries, who analysed the information and prepared the report.

† Information was asked about alum-precipitated toxoid (A.P.T.), purified diphtheria toxoid aluminium phosphate precipitated (P.T.A.P.), diphtheria toxoid-antitoxin floccules (T.A.F.), formol (diphtheria) toxoid (F.T.); pertussis vaccine, plain suspension; mixed diphtheria-pertussis vaccine with alum, mixed diphtheria-pertussis vaccine without alum.

Conclusion

Such is a very rough-and-ready sketch. I am profoundly aware that already a few courses organised on these lines exist and that much may be learned from them. I am also aware that the best results of such a course could be obtained only if it interlocked with the teaching in the clinical years far more closely than does the present preclinical course. Such interlocking is implicit in the structure of the new course's third year: much of the sociology, for example, would be taught by medical men from the fields of social medicine and of the psychology of industrial and group relations. Doubtless some crusading zeal could be lavished on the last years of our present curriculum too! But I am trying to be very strictly practical; everything I have suggested could actually be put into practice—as an experiment—without too much trouble with regulations, I believe, at any of a number of medical schools in the United Kingdom.

The General Medical Council in its 1957 *Recommendations as to the Medical Curriculum* has removed its previously rather detailed recommendations about the teaching of particular subjects. The present recommendations have been drawn up specifically to foster experimentation with the curriculum: they " refrain from specifying the period of time to be allotted to particular subjects or the sequence in which they should be taught . . . and from specifying subjects in which separate examinations should be held ". The Council make a particular point of asking schools not to regard their activities as " in any way limiting their own right, which may equally be described as a duty, to experiment with different courses and various methods of teaching ".

The present proposals should be viewed in the light of this recommendation. Summing them up one could say they imply a three-year preclinical course covering all the present ground of 1st M.B., 2nd M.B., and general pathology, but reorientated in consecutive courses entitled Cellular Biology, Organisation of Mammals, and Organisation of Man. Biochemical genetics enters the course at the start; ethology is part of it all along. The growth process is used to introduce anatomy and physiology and at the same time behavioural development. The concepts of maturation and learning introduce normal psychology, family studies, sociology, and finally a discussion of the role of the doctor—or various sorts of doctors—in our society.

I am sure much more thought and a great deal of experiment must go towards making a real course in human biology for doctors; but I think we ought to face squarely the implications of the modern nature of medical practice in our society. I believe we should seriously consider giving thought to the reorganisation of the curriculum from the point of view of the human biologist. We might further invite the views upon this of a variety of disciplines outside our own to see what their representatives conceive of as the doctor's role and his training for it. In this way we would gradually work towards the time when we could envisage setting up an experimental training in line with these emerging conceptions, and in which studies of human biology would exert their true usefulness in the training of medical men.

This essay has benefited much from the constructive criticism of a number of persons who have long thought about problems in medical education. In particular I would like to thank Dr. C. F. Harris, Prof. A. A. Moncrieff, Prof. J. Z. Young, Sir Geoffrey Vickers, and Dr. J. S. Weiner. Needless to say, however, the views above are not to be imputed in whole or part to anyone but myself.

INVESTIGATION OF ABDOMINAL MASSES BY PULSED ULTRASOUND

IAN DONALD
M.B.E., B.A. Cape Town, M.D. Lond., F.R.F.P.S., F.R.C.O.G.
REGIUS PROFESSOR OF MIDWIFERY IN THE UNIVERSITY OF GLASGOW

J. MacVICAR
M.B. Glasg., M.R.C.O.G.
GYNAECOLOGICAL REGISTRAR, WESTERN INFIRMARY, GLASGOW

T. G. BROWN
OF MESSRS. KELVIN HUGHES LTD.

VIBRATIONS whose frequency exceeds 20,000 per second are beyond the range of hearing and therefore termed " ultrasonic ". One of the properties of ultrasound is that it can be propagated as a beam. When such a beam crosses an interface between two substances of differing specific acoustic impedance (which is defined as the product of the density of the material and the velocity of the sound wave in it), five things happen:

(1) Some of the energy is reflected at the interface, the amplitude of the reflected waves being proportional to the difference of the two acoustic impedances divided by their sum (Rayleigh's law). Therefore the greater the difference in specific acoustic impedance between two adjacent materials the higher will be the percentage of energy reflected. This fact makes a liquid-gas interface almost impenetrable to ultrasound and is important in relation to gas-filled intestine within the abdominal cavity.

(2) Much of the energy which is not reflected is transmitted into the second medium but is somewhat attenuated.

(3) Some refraction may occur, particularly when the ultrasonic beam is not at right-angles to the plane of the interface.

(4) Some of the energy may be absorbed and produce heat. The ability to absorb ultrasound varies with different tissues —e.g., that of bone is considerable.

(5) Cavitation may be produced if considerable energies are present at the lower ultrasonic frequencies. This phenomenon, whose mechanism is not yet fully understood, can develop when the negative sound pressure exceeds the ambient hydrostatic pressure, giving rise to small temporary voids in the material. Cavitation becomes increasingly difficult to produce as the frequency of the ultrasound is raised, and usually develops only when the ultrasonic energy is applied continuously or in pulses of much greater duration than those we use. Nervous tissue is more susceptible than other tissues to cavitation (Fry et al. 1950).

For diagnostic purposes reflection and transmission are the important phenomena. Transmission is ruled out in our type of investigation because of the multiplicity of interfaces within the abdominal cavity and the impenetrability of tissue-gas boundaries. The recording and mapping of echoes from the reflecting interfaces is therefore the method of choice, which has been extensively used for many years in industry for detecting flaws in homogeneous materials, particularly metals, and the information so obtained may in some instances be superior to radiography, even with 2,000,000-V X-ray machines.

The use of ultrasonic echoes in studying human tissues promises to be much more complicated because of the great variety of tissues concerned and, it is believed, the not very large differences in specific acoustic impedance between them. It is therefore not surprising that results so far do not appear to have matched the technical ingenuity which has been shown in recent years.

A-scope Presentation

To confirm that echoes were obtainable within the body we started modestly with this method of presentation,

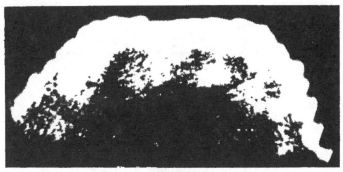

Fig. 11—Gross ascites due to cirrhosis of liver. Ultrasonic beam can penetrate more deeply in random fashion because of fluid between coils of intestine.

By contrast the *healthy abdomen* of one of us (J. M.), scanned at the level of the umbilicus, is shown in fig. 10. We are not yet certain of the identification of the various layers of the abdominal wall shown here, but the noteworthy feature is that deep penetration into the abdomen is prevented by normally situated coils of intestine.

In *ascites*, however, the fluid intervening between the coils of gut allows the ultrasound to penetrate to a much greater depth, yet without producing the clearcut margins of an ovarian cyst. This is shown in fig. 11, taken in a case of portal cirrhosis in which the patient's abdomen was scanned at umbilical level in the presence of gross ascites. This film is almost certainly overexposed and probably exaggerates the picture.

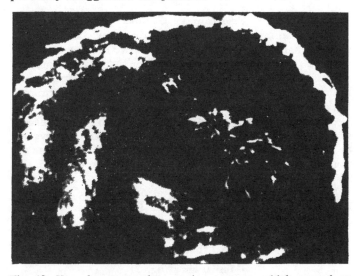

Fig. 12—Very large complex ovarian tumour, which proved at operation to be a multilocular pseudomucinous cystadenoma with almost solid plaques of minute loculi.

A huge and structurally very complicated ovarian tumour is shown in fig. 12. This was a large pseudomucinous cystadenoma of ovary with many areas of very small loculi clustered together so as almost to give the macroscopic impression of areas of solidity. Histology showed the tumour, however, to be benign.

Multiple fibroids are shown in fig. 13. Our findings so far indicate that fibroids tend to absorb and scatter ultrasound, with the result that only faint echoes can be recorded from the posterior surface of the mass (as in this figure) or none at all, in contrast to a fluid-containing cyst, in which the ultrasound is readily transmitted and reflected from its posterior wall. Here the outline of the fibroids can be roughly seen and the thickness of the tumour gauged. Our tentative conclusions at present are

that the ability of fibroids to transmit ultrasound depends on their vascularity.

The *pregnant uterus* offers considerable scope for this kind of work because it is a cystic cavity containing a solid fœtus. In fig. 14 a suprapubic scan is shown of a patient at the 34th week of gestation in whom placenta prævia was suspected; we were trying to see the placenta in the lower segment. We are not yet sure about this, but the outline of the fœtal head shows up very well.

Hydramnios is very vividly shown in fig. 15, in which the transverse section of the baby's body appears within the enormously distended amniotic sac. The period of

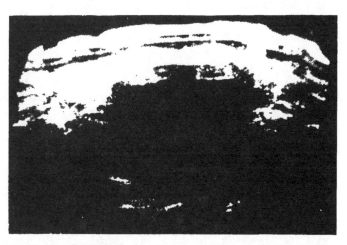

Fig. 13—Multiple fibroids, showing progressive attenuation of ultrasound, with only faint echoes from posterior surface of mass in contrast to ovarian cysts.

gestation in this case was 32 weeks, and the girth of the abdomen 44 inches.

Twins are shown in fig. 16. The scan was taken just above the level of the umbilicus at the 37th week of gestation. Both twins presented by the vertex, and what is visible here is the two breeches at the fundus.

Fig. 17 is very interesting. The patient had had three months' irregular vaginal bleeding and a very hard enlargement of the uterus corresponding in size to about 14 weeks' gestation. A year previously a fibroid had been found within her uterus, and she was now admitted to hospital for myomectomy. A scan taken one inch above the symphysis pubis showed, however, a very different picture: a cystic cavity containing in its left half a mass which is clearly a very early fœtus. The result of the Aschheim-Zondek test ordered was awaited with considerable excitement since clinically the diagnosis was con-

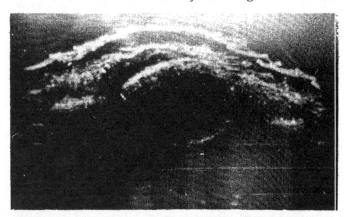

Fig. 14—Outline of fœtal skull in utero at 34 weeks' gestation (suprapubic scan).

TOTAL CARDIOPULMONARY BYPASS IN THE LABORATORY

A PRELIMINARY TO OPEN HEART SURGERY

L. D. ABRAMS
M.B. Birm., F.R.C.S.

F. ASHTON
M.B. Birm., F.R.C.S.

E. J. CHARLES [1]
Ph.D. Birm.

J. FEJFAR

E. J. HAMLEY [2]
Ph.D. Lond.

W. A. HUDSON
M.B. Sheff., M.R.C.P.

R. E. LEE
M.A., B.M. Oxon., F.F.A. R.C.S.

R. LIGHTWOOD

E. T. MATHEWS
M.B. Birm., F.F.A. R.C.S.

A. L. D'ABREU
O.B.E., Ch.M. Birm., F.R.C.S.

*From the Departments of Surgery, Chemical Engineering,
and Physiology, University of Birmingham*

EARLY in 1957 we began work on total cardiopulmonary bypass, hoping that within a year we could employ a heart-lung machine on patients requiring deliberate open cardiac surgery. This limited aim has been achieved, and the techniques learnt in the laboratory have been translated to the operating-theatre. Lillehei et al. (1956) and Kirklin et al. (1956) in the U.S.A. had developed satisfactory bypass techniques well before we started; the most superficial study of their work reveals the stress they placed on painstaking laboratory preparation. We outline here the work done by a team anxious to gain the knowledge necessary to carry out safe total cardiopulmonary bypass.

The Apparatus

We use a Lillehei-deWall pump-oxygenator (deWall et. al. 1957) (fig. 1). The pump, a 'Sigmamotor T-6S',* has identical arterial and venous heads in which a length of latex tube is compressed against a spring-loaded back-plate by each of a series of twelve steel fingers in turn milking the blood along. The speed of action, and thus the delivery-rate of each head is independently variable. Blood passes from the caval cannulæ to the venous pump. (In the last 11 perfusions we have used a gravity drainage venous well [deWall et al. 1958].) From the pump the blood passes up a vertical tube, the oxygenator, into which oxygen is bubbled through a perforated disc at its lower end. During this ascent the blood is oxygenated and then passes down into a wider tube, the debubbler, set at 25° to the horizontal and coated with a silicone antifoam (I.C.I. M430 †) to break the bubbles; it flows from the debubbler into a long spiral tube, the helix, immersed in a thermostatically controlled water bath at a temperature of 41°C. In the helix any remaining bubbles rise, so that blood leaving the base of the helix is bubble-free. The helix also acts as a reservoir in which the volume of blood can be accurately observed. The arterial pump takes blood from the helix and passes it to the arterial cannula through a simple monofilament nylon-mesh filter, which also serves as an additional bubble trap.

Apart from the latex in the pump heads all the tubing is of transparent polyvinyl chloride.‡ The various connections, including the perforated plate for introducing the oxygen, are made of highly polished stainless steel or nylon. All apparatus in contact with blood is sterilised by autoclaving in sealed nylon tubular foil bags.§ Although providing a barrier to bacterial contamination, these bags are permeable to steam during autoclaving and allow subsequent drying.

1. Of the Department of Chemical Engineering.
2. Of the Department of Physiology.
* Sigmamotor Inc., 3, North Main Street, Middleport, N.Y., U.S.A.
† Imperial Chemical Industries Ltd., Nobel Division, 25, Bothwell Street, Glasgow, C.1.
‡ Capon Heaton Ltd., Hazelwill Mills, Stirchley, Birmingham.
§ Portex Plastics Ltd., Bassett House, Hythe, Kent.

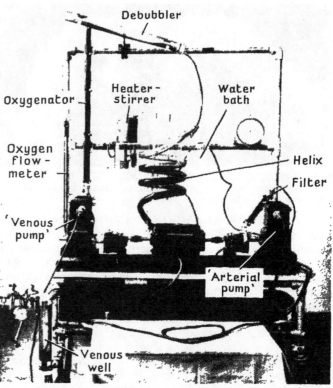

Fig. 1—Lillehei-deWall heart-lung machine, with arterial and venous hoses connected.

Preliminary Studies

Before animal work was started, many hours were spent in handling the machine so that we became familiar with its behaviour. It was found that, with correct adjustment of the back-plates, the pump output was independent of inflow pressures from —50 to +50 mm. Hg and of outflow pressures up to 400 mm. Hg.

Oxygenation was studied using fresh heparinised venous ox-blood. It was found that a ratio of oxygen to blood-flow of 5 : 1 by volume ensured 98% oxygenation at rates of flow between 500 and 800 ml. per min. of 24% oxygenated venous blood.

Mechanical hæmolysis was also studied. Plasma-hæmoglobin levels were less than 150 mg. per 100 ml. after continuous circulation of ox blood, equivalent to perfusion at 900 ml. per min. for one hour. These experiments also showed that debubbling was satisfactory.

Monitoring (fig. 2)

A monitoring technique has been established to give continuous records of the aortic and inferior vena caval pressures, electrocardiogram (E.C.G.), electroencephalogram (E.E.G.), and œsophageal temperature (fig. 2).

The recording apparatus is an Ediswan four-channel pen oscillograph. The manometers used for measuring the pressures are of a valve transducer (R.C.A. 5734) type modified from a design by Arnott et al. (1951). Calibration is effected by connecting each manometer through three-way taps to a system filled with heparinised isotonic dextrose incorporating a pressure bottle and a valve¶ as a precaution against air embolism. This obviates the use of long fluid columns and thus gives a rapid and accurate method of repeated calibration.

The E.C.G. electrodes are safety-pins inserted subcutaneously in each shoulder and the left leg. The E.E.G. electrodes are two tempered-steel pins varnished except for the tips lightly hammered into the frontal and occipital regions of the skull of the

¶ The ' Oxford Safety Dropper ' (Macintosh and Pask 1941), Medical and Industrial Equipment, 10–12, New Cavendish Street, London, W.1.

Special Articles

CYTOLOGICAL SCREENING OF 1000 WOMEN FOR CERVICAL CANCER

A Report by the South-East Scotland Faculty of the College of General Practitioners *

THIS report shows that the cytological detection of early cervical carcinoma can be undertaken in general practice. In this country until now cervical smears have been taken only from groups of hospital patients, from patients attending contraceptive clinics, and from gynæcological outpatients.

Papanicolaou and Traut's 1943 paper on exfoliative cytology demonstrated that cancer cells desquamate from a neoplasm of the cervix. During the past fifteen years or so it has become generally accepted that cervical cancer can be detected as an early preinvasive lesion in the squamous epithelium of the external os. (This pre-

TABLE I—ANALYSIS OF UNSUSPECTED POSITIVES ACCORDING TO THE INDICATION FOR TAKING THE SMEAR

Occasion for taking smear			No. of smears	Unsuspected positives
Postnatal examination	..	..	363	7 (1·93%)
Menopausal complaint	..	..	155	2 (1·29%)
Other reasons	..	..	482	6 (1·24%)
Total	..	..	1000	15 (1·5%)

invasive cancer is also known as intraepithelial cancer or carcinoma-in-situ.) It has been shown by Petersen (1956) that about a third of these lesions can develop into invasive cancers.

The average age in early cases detected by cytological examination is about 38, whilst the average age of presentation for all stages of clinically obvious cervical cancer is 48 years. It seems reasonable to assume that the ten years gained in diagnosis may be of considerable importance.

The Investigation

In 1955 Prof. R. J. Kellar invited the South-East Scotland faculty to take part in a research project on the early detection of cervical cancer. The general practitioners were instructed in the use of a wooden Ayre spatula and the fixing of slides. The slides were sent, with a note of the details of each case, to Professor Kellar's department.

The general practitioners taking part in this investigation took cervical smears during their ordinary consulting hours from three groups of patients:

(1) All women who came for postnatal examination.

(2) As many women as possible who had menopausal problems *without* histories pointing to any disease of the genital organs.

(3) As many women as possible in whom a complete medical examination was indicated for any reason other than gynæcological complaints, or women seeking advice on family planning.

* The following general practitioners took part in this investigation: I. A. D. ANDERSON, A. FRASER DARLING, B. C. HAMILTON, J. GOODBRAND, G. IRVINE, E. V. KUENSSBERG, LOWELL LAMONT, A. H. D. LARGE, A. R. LAURENCE, S. LIPETZ, D. MURRAY, R. MACGREGOR, D. McVIE, D. W. MACLEAN, G. MACNAUGHTAN, M. W. MOSS, C. E. MUNRO, H. NEVE, M. PEARSON, A. D. ROBERTSON, R. SCOTT.

TABLE II—UNSUSPECTED POSITIVES CLASSIFIED BY AGE-GROUPS

Age (yr.)			No. of smears	Unsuspected positives
20 or under	..	..	9	—
21–25	..	..	160	—
26–30	..	..	228	2 (0·88%)
31–35	..	..	180	5 (2·78%)
36–40	..	..	123	4 (3·25%)
41–45	..	..	125	2 (1·64%)
46–50	..	..	98	—
51 or over	..	..	77	2 (2·6%)
Total	..	..	1000	15 (1·5%)

Results

Tables I-III summarise our findings. " Unsuspected positives " were patients who had a healthy cervix clinically (on inspection and palpation) but whose cervical smear was reported as suspicious or frankly malignant. The average age of " unsuspected positive " cases was 35·5 years; of the 7 patients who underwent hysterectomy 37 years; of patients who required amputation of the cervix 36 years; and of those still under surveillance after ring biopsy 32·2 years.

Table III does not show the time interval between the first suspicious smear and the final diagnosis and operation, and it does not give all the grounds on which the final decision to operate rested. In most cases several repeat smears and biopsy specimens were taken. In cases 1–4 the biopsy was in itself sufficient to eradicate the whole suspected area: subsequent cervical smears showed no abnormal cells. Similarly, in cases 5–8. amputation of cervix removed the cancer.

TABLE III—HISTOLOGICAL DIAGNOSIS AND SUBSEQUENT HISTORY OF UNSUSPECTED POSITIVES

Case no.	Age (yr.) of patient	Mode of confirmation of diagnosis	Histological diagnosis	Subsequent history
1	28	Ring biopsy	Preinvasive cancer	Still followed up. Subsequent smears negative
2	30	Ring biopsy	Preinvasive	Still followed up
3	33	Cone biopsy	Preinvasive cancer	Still followed up. Subsequent smears negative
4	38	Ring biopsy	Borderline invasive epithelium	Still followed up. Subsequent smears negative
5	32	Ring biopsy, followed by amputation of cervix	Preinvasive cancer	Still followed up. Subsequent smears negative
6	33	Ring biopsy, followed by amputation of cervix	Preinvasive cancer	Still followed up. Subsequent smears negative
7	38	Ring biopsy, followed by amputation of cervix	Preinvasive cancer	Still followed up. Subsequent smears negative
8	41	Ring biopsy, followed by amputation of cervix	Preinvasive cancer	Still followed up. Subsequent smears negative
9	28	Ring biopsy	Preinvasive cancer	Total hysterectomy
10	29	Ring biopsy	Early invasive cancer	Total hysterectomy
11	32	Ring biopsy	Early invasive cancer	Wertheim hysterectomy
12	36	Cone biopsy	Preinvasive cancer	Total hysterectomy
13	39	Cone biopsy	Preinvasive cancer	Total hysterectomy
14	42	Ring biopsy	Preinvasive cancer	Total hysterectomy
15	53	Ring biopsy	Early invasive cancer	Radium

The following case-history illustrates the routine procedure:

In January, 1956, at a postnatal examination a positive smear was obtained in case 9. This was repeated in hospital and on two subsequent occasions in 1956. However, the patient became pregnant during this period of observation and was allowed to continue with her pregnancy. Postnatal examination yielded a further positive smear and a hysterectomy was finally performed in December, 1957, and the diagnosis of invasive cervical cancer was thus confirmed.

Discussion

Early fears that the Ayre technique would take up too much time, or that it would be resented by the patients, proved groundless. The operation was easily performed after a little practice, and very few slides had to be repeated because they were technically unsatisfactory. The smear was not intended to take the place of gynæcological investigation by a specialist. When the history or physical examination was suspicious, the patient was referred to a gynæcologist even if the cervical smear was negative. Similarly, if the family doctor received a suspicious report on a smear taken from a clinically unsuspected cervix, he referred the patient for further investigation.

Before the general practitioners became accustomed to examining the cervix visually as well as manually they may have had some difficulty in deciding whether or not the cervix looked suspicious. However, in all the 15 cases diagnosed on cytological grounds alone the gynæcologist confirmed that there was nothing clinically abnormal.

Admittedly this series of 1000 cases is still small, but the finding of 15 clinically unsuspected positives and of another 5 atypical cases is worth noting. In British series of hospital or special-clinic patients the incidence has been about half as high (Royal College of Obstetricians and Gynæcologists 1955); and in field-surveys in Georgia, Tennessee, and at the special cancer-prevention clinic in New York the proportion of clinically unsuspected positives was even lower (Erickson et al. 1956, Scapier et el. 1952). An incidence of approximately 2% in women attending for postnatal examination in the present investigation suggests that routine screening of this group is especially desirable.

For several reasons the average age of women who have their babies at home is slightly greater than that of women who are admitted to hospital. This may have given prominence in this series to the age-group 30–40 which included most unsuspected positives; but this underlines rather than detracts from the need for greater vigilance.

It has been said that pregnancy changes in the cervical endothelium are often suspicious but that they regress spontaneously after parturition. All postnatal positive smears in this series were still positive three to six months after delivery. In none of our cases was there spontaneous regression, and treatment was eventually required in all but one. (The exception was case 1, who has now been followed up for two and a half years.)

In the minds of those who have taken part in this investigation there is no doubt whatever about the value of the smear as a routine screening-test: it should be part of every pelvic examination. It was particularly significant to find positive cases in the 30–40 age-group: this suggests a possible lag of ten to twelve years between the first positive smear and the appearance of a clinically detectable cervical carcinoma. Such a latent period has been demonstrated experimentally by Foulds (1951).

Summary

Cervical smears were taken from 1000 women. 15 unsuspected positives for early carcinoma were found—a higher incidence than in previous hospital studies.

To take such smears in general practice is simple and reliable. Cytological reports on such smears should be available to all general practitioners.

We are greatly indebted to Professor Kellar and his staff, in particular Dr. A. F. Anderson who examined the smears, in collaboration with Miss R. MacBryde and Miss K. Cockburn, for their constant advice and encouragement. We are also grateful for the helpful advice of Mr. S. A. Sklaroff, lecturer in the department of public health and social medicine, Edinburgh University. A grant was provided by the Scottish Advisory Committee on Medical Research.

REFERENCES

Erickson, C. C., Everett, B. E., Jr., Graves, L. M., Kaiser, R. F., Malmgren, R. A., Rube, I., Schreier, P. C., Cutler, S. J., Sprunt, D. H. (1956) J. Amer. med. Ass. 162, 167.
Foulds, L. (1951) Ann. R. Coll. Surg. Engl. 9, 93.
Papanicolaou, G. N., Traut, H. F. (1943) Exfoliative Cytology.
Petersen, O. (1956) Amer. J. Obstet. Gynec. 72, 1063.
Royal College of Obstetricians and Gynæcologists (1956) Report of conference. J. Obstet. Gynæc., Brit. Emp. 1956, 53, 3.
Scapier, J., Day, E., Dunfee, C. R. (1952) Cancer, 5, 315.

A HOSPITAL WORKSHOP *

W. V. WADSWORTH
M.B., B.Sc. Manc., M.R.C.P., D.P.M.
MEDICAL SUPERINTENDENT

R. F. SCOTT
B.A. Lond., Dip. Psych.
MANAGER OF REHABILITATION UNIT

W. L. TONGE
M.D. Manc., D.P.M.
DEPUTY MEDICAL SUPERINTENDENT

CHEADLE ROYAL HOSPITAL, CHESHIRE

ALL the different types of sheltered hospital workshops so far established in this country have had to contend with two difficulties: first, they have been completely dependent on a continuous even supply of suitable material from outside industry, and secondly, they have found it hard to provide chronic psychotic patients with simple assembly work in sufficient variety. Our own industrial unit, started two years ago, has on the whole been successful and has raised many interesting points. For instance, though the patients were all doing the same work of assembling umbrellas, or should have been doing the same work (for they were all producing the same end-product), differences in practice crept in, though a standard method was taught originally. Such differences may appear slight and superficial, but when taken with tempo of work, they could easily account for almost all the variation in earnings between patients. On a straight piece-work basis, it is speed, used effectively, that governs the size of the pay-packet. The twin principles of financial payment and speed lift the work done by patients into the same category as work done by outside healthy workers—in distinction from traditional occupational therapy, which, by definition and association, is only done by those ill enough to remain in hospital.

SETTING NORMAL STANDARDS

The problem is, in part, one of communicating to the patients normal outside standards of tempo, which in the leisured setting of occupational therapy have little

* Abridged from paper to the Royal Medico-Psychological Association on April 30, 1958. The Nuffield Provincial Hospitals Trust have given a grant to cover research on this project.

THE CHROMOSOMES IN A PATIENT SHOWING BOTH MONGOLISM AND THE KLINEFELTER SYNDROME

C. E. FORD
Ph.D. Lond.

K. W. JONES
Ph.D. Wales

OF THE MEDICAL RESEARCH COUNCIL RADIOBIOLOGICAL
RESEARCH UNIT, HARWELL

O. J. MILLER
M.D. Yale

URSULA MITTWOCH
Ph.D. Lond.

L. S. PENROSE
M.D. Cantab., F.R.S.

OF THE GALTON LABORATORY, UNIVERSITY COLLEGE, LONDON, W.C.1

M. RIDLER
F.I.M.L.T.

A. SHAPIRO
M.D. Lond., D.P.M.

OF HARPERBURY HOSPITAL, SHENLEY, HERTS

FOR many years the diploid number of chromosomes in normal men and women was believed to be forty-eight. Since the observations of Tjio and Levan (1956) and of Ford and Hamerton (1956), using improved methods, forty-six has been generally accepted as the correct

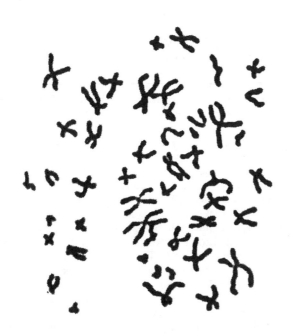

Fig. 1—Mitotic metaphase in a bone-marrow cell.

number, twenty-two pairs of autosomes and one sex chromosome pair. The chromosomes of a case of Klinefelter's syndrome, with skin cells exhibiting the Barr chromatin body as in the female, have been studied by Jacobs and Strong (1959) and found to number forty-seven. This was interpreted as the result of the presence of two X chromosomes as well as one Y. The chromosome complement in mongolism was first investigated by Mittwoch (1952) who reported an approximate diploid number of forty-eight chromosomes in spermatocytes. Techniques at that time were not adequate to give exact results. However, Lejeune, Gautier, and Turpin (1959) reported the finding of a small extra chromosome in tissue cultures from the connective tissue of three cases of mongolism, making a total count of forty-seven.

The patient described here is an imbecile, aged 45, who shows signs typical both of Klinefelter's syndrome and of mongolism. He is fourth in a sibship with three normal sisters. The father was 40 years old and the mother 42 at his birth and they are not consanguineous. The Barr chromatin body is present in cells of the skin and buccal mucosa; leucocytes with drumstick appendages have been identified, as in a normal female. He has small testes, scanty facial, axillary and pubic hair, slight gynæcomastia and feminine distribution of fat. Testicular biopsy revealed advanced atrophy with no spermatogenesis, only ghost tubules and rare interstitial cells. The mongoloid traits are very well marked, including typical palmar patterns, single creases on the minimal digits, fissured tongue, cataract, and slight cyanosis.

Bone-marrow specimens, obtained by sternal puncture, were treated by a modification of the method described by Ford, Jacobs, and Lajtha (1958). Squash preparations were made from the final, Feulgen-stained, cell suspension. These were searched systematically for cells in metaphase of mitosis. More than fifty cells, in which the chromosomes could be counted accurately, were recorded. Each of them contained forty-eight chromosomes. The detailed chromosome morphology was examined carefully in ten cells. Each appeared to contain a normal set of twenty-three pairs, as in a female, with, in addition, a Y chromosome and an extra acrocentric chromosome. There are two very similar pairs of acrocentric chromosomes in the normal complement, one pair probably slightly larger than the other, pairs 22 and 23 of Ford et al. (1958)—alternatively, nos. 21 and 22 of Tjio and Puck (1958). In the present case, these four chromosomes and the additional acrocentric chromosome are almost indistinguishable from one another: it is possible that two are a little longer than the other three. A representative cell is shown in fig. 1. In fig. 2 the chromosomes from this cell are arranged as far as possible in pairs. The five short acrocentric chromosomes are arranged as a pair and a group of three, and the Y chromosome, which, though very similar, is usually distinguishable from them, is shown by itself. Identification of the X chromosome pair is still uncertain: it is believed to be the seventh in order of length and is shown as such in fig. 2.

This appears to be the first time that a human being with two supernumerary chromosomes has been described. He possesses an additional sex chromosome, as found in

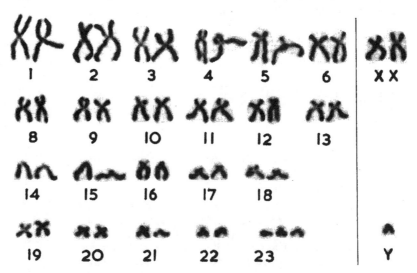

Fig. 2—Chromosomes arranged to size; the X chromosomes are seventh in this order.

Klinefelter's syndrome, and an additional small chromosome which seems likely to be characteristic of mongolism. It is remarkable that the patient's general health should be satisfactory.

The writers wish to thank Mr. B. D. Stutter, Dr. R. F. Welch, and Dr. T. H. Howells for conducting the biopsies at Barnet General Hospital.

REFERENCES

Ford, C. E., Hamerton, J. L. (1956) The chromosomes of man. *Nature, Lond.* **178**, 1020.
— Jacobs, P. A., Lajtha, L. G. (1958) Human somatic chromosomes. *ibid.* **181**, 1565.
Jacobs, P. A., Strong, J. A. (1959) A case of human intersexuality having a possible XXY sex-determining mechanism. *ibid.* **183**, 302.
Lejeune, L., Gautier, M., Turpin, R. (1959) Les chromosomes humains en culture de tissus. *C.R. Acad. Sci., Paris,* **248**, 602.
Mittwoch, U. (1952) The chromosome complement in a mongolian imbecile. *Ann. Eugen., Lond.* **17**, 37.
Tjio, J. H., Levan, A. (1956) The chromosome number of man. *Hereditas,* **42**, 1.
— Puck, T. T. (1958) The somatic chromosomes in man. *Proc. nat. Acad. Sci.* **44**, 1229.

THE SOMATIC CHROMOSOMES IN MONGOLISM

PATRICIA A. JACOBS
B.Sc. St. And.

A. G. BAIKIE
M.B. Glasg., M.R.C.P.E.

W. M. COURT BROWN
M.B., B.Sc. St.And.,
F.F.R.

J. A. STRONG
B.A., M.B. Dubl., F.R.C.P.E.,
M.R.C.P.

From the M.R.C. Group for Research into the General Effects of Radiation, and the Department for Endocrine and Metabolic Diseases, Western General Hospital, Edinburgh, 4, and University of Edinburgh

DURING recent studies of human intersexes it has been found that chromatin-positive cases of Klinefelter's syndrome have a diploid number of 47 and that the additional chromosome is an X chromosome, the chromosome sex in these cases being XXY (Jacobs and Strong 1959, Ford personal communication). These studies were made on marrow cells utilising the technique previously described by Ford, Jacobs, and Lajtha (1958).

Following these studies, and because some cases of Klinefelter's syndrome suffer from mental deficiency (Ferguson-Smith 1958), it was decided to extend such investigations to cases of mongolism. This decision was also conditioned by the reported association between mongolism and leukæmia (Carter 1956, 1958, Krivit and Good 1956, Merrit and Harris 1956, Stewart, Webb, and Hewitt 1958). The presence of an abnormal chromosome number has been reported in one case of acute human leukæmia (Ford, Jacobs, and Lajtha 1958) and further

CHROMOSOME COUNTS IN FOUR MONGOLS

Case no.	Chromosome number and number of cells counted					
	44	45	46	47	48	Polyploids
H 114	1	..	2	41	7	3
H 120	..	1	6	26	2	..
H 122	..	1	2	36	1	4
H 125	..	1	1	34	3	3

examples of such abnormalities have been found in other cases of acute leukæmia (Jacobs unpublished data, Ford personal communication).

The somatic chromosomes have been examined in six typical mongols—three males aged 41, 22, and 20 years, and three females aged 20, 20, and 16. Two of the females had congenital heart lesions. The males were chromatin-negative, and the females chromatin-positive, as determined by an examination of blood and buccal smears.

In all six cases the diploid number was found to be 47: detailed counts for four cases are shown in the accompanying table. Deviations from the diploid number are considered to be due to technical errors (Ford, Jacobs, and Lajtha 1958). Lejeune, Gauthier, and Turpin (1959) have also reported the finding of a diploid number of 47 in three male mongol children. It appears, therefore, that the condition of mongolism is associated with the presence of an extra chromosome.

The additional chromosome, as seen in our material and as reported by Lejeune, Gauthier, and Turpin, is an acrocentric chromosome in the smallest size range, where the Y chromosome is also to be found (Ford, Jacobs, and Lajtha 1958, Tjio and Puck 1958). The remaining 46 chromosomes do not appear different from those in the normal diploid set. It is improbable though not impossible that the additional chromosome in mongolism is a Y chromosome. In the case of females, however, this would result in an XXY female, a sex-chromosome constitution known to be associated with chromatin-positive cases of Klinefelter's syndrome. It is known that the risk of giving birth to a mongol is closely related to increasing maternal age (Penrose 1934) and that the mongol child resembles its mother antigenically more closely than its father (Penrose 1957). Both these facts suggest that the primary disorder may lie in oogenesis. If this is so, the extra chromosome is likely to be an autosome. It may well be that mongols are trisomic for one of the smallest acrocentric autosomes. The trisomic condition is recognised as being due to the failure of both members of a pair of homologous chromosomes to segregate during either meiosis to give a haploid set in each gamete, or in mitosis to give rise to two cells of a chromosome constitution (Swanson 1958). If both chromosomes pass to the same nucleus this may result, in the case of a gamete effecting union with a normal gamete, in an individual with a chromosome number of $2n+1$, the value of n for man being 23. The possibility cannot be entirely excluded at present that the extra chromosome is a supernumerary one. The origin of such chromosomes is unknown: they have been found in a variety of insects and plants, and are said to be of smaller size than other members of the chromosome complement, as well as appearing to be genetically inert (Swanson 1958).

Among the many implications of the reported findings, the association of a predisposition to leukæmia in a group of individuals with an abnormal karyotype is clearly of great interest and potential importance. The significance of this association in relation to possible mechanisms of carcinogenesis—e.g., the two stage mechanism postulated by Armitage and Doll (1957) remains to be elucidated.

We are grateful to Dr. W. M. C. Harrowes for allowing us to study patients under his care, and Dr. N. Maclean for examining the blood and buccal smears. We should also like to thank Miss M. Brunton for technical assistance.

REFERENCES

Armitage, P., Doll, R. (1957) *Brit. J. Cancer,* **11**, 161.
Carter, C. O. (1956) *Brit. med. J.* ii, 993.
— (1958) *J. ment. Defic. Res.* **2**, 64.
Ferguson-Smith, M. A. (1958) *Lancet,* i, 928.
Ford, C. E., Jacobs, P. A., Lajtha, L. G. (1958) *Nature, Lond.* **181**, 1565.
Jacobs, P. A., Strong, J. A. (1959) *ibid.* **183**, 302.
Krivit, W., Good, R. A. (1956) *A.M.A. Amer. J. Dis. Child.* **91**, 218.
Lejeune, J., Gauthier, M., Turpin, R. (1959) *C.R. Acad. Sci., Paris,* **248**, 602.
Merrit, D. H., Harris, J. S. (1956) *A.M.A. Amer. J. Dis. Child.* **92**, 41.
Penrose, L. S. (1934) *Proc. roy. Soc. Lond.* B. **114**, 431.
— (1957) *J. ment. Defic. Res.* **1**, 107.
Stewart, A., Webb, J., Hewitt, D. (1958) *Brit. med. J.* ii, 1495.
Swanson, C. P. (1958) Cytology and Cytogenetics. London.
Tjio, J. H., Puck, T. T. (1958) *J. exp. Med.* **108**, 259.

1960s–2005
From **THALIDOMIDE** to
SARS

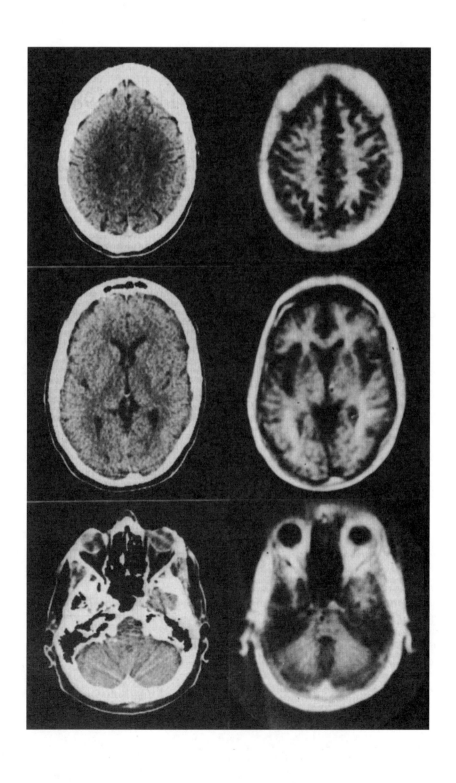

1960s–2005

1970 **Luzzatto, Nwachuku-Jarrett and Reddy: Increased sickling of parasitised erythrocytes as a mechanism of resistance against malaria in the sickle-cell trait.** 379
14.2.1970: 319–322   (Extract: first page only)
Attempt to account for resistance to malaria among people with sickle-cell trait. Patients were children presenting with febrile illness at University College Hospital in central London.

1971 **Tudor Hart: The Inverse Care Law.** 380
27.2.1971: 405–412   (Extract: first page only)
A landmark in awareness of contrasting distributions of healthcare need and healthcare services. Much cited, now invariably without attribution. Sadly, at eight pages, too long to appear here in full.

1972 **Jennett and Plum: Persistent vegetative state after brain damage.** 381
1.4.1972: 734–737
A successful attempt to name a syndrome largely resulting from the human impact of life-support capability. The authors urged study to define predictors for this unhappy condition (PVS).

1972 **Blackwell, Bloomfield and Buncher: Demonstration to medical students of placebo responses and non-drug factors.** 385
10.6.1972: 1279–1282   (Extract: first page only)
Report of an interesting experiment in which medical students were led to expect sedative or stimulant effects from placebo capsules. Thirty percent experienced drug-associated changes. Medical education has always been considered important in *The Lancet*, although clinical and scientific material has somewhat crowded it out in our selection.

1973 **Roberts *et al*.: Simple versus radical mastectomy.** 386
19.5.1973: 1073–1076   (Extract: first page only)
Preliminary results of a two-centre trial comparing two operations: a): the then orthodox radical operation for breast cancer which often caused great discomfort, considerable mutilation, and often, long term problems with the mobility of the arm on the affected side, with b): a less invasive new treatment, designed to conserve tissue, preserve mobility and to result in a less mutilated appearance.
The contest between the proponents of the two operations was ostensibly on grounds of therapeutic value. The importance of this paper was that it showed the tissue-conserving operation had so far proved of equal therapeutic benefit.

1973 **Bierenbaum *et al*.: Ten-year experience of modified-fat diets on younger men with coronary heart-disease.** 387
23.6.1973: 1404–1407   (Extract: first page only)
Key paper on dietary fat, showing the positive impact of lower dietary fat intake.

1973 **Brock, Bolton and Monaghan: Prenatal diagnosis of anencephaly through maternal serum-alphafetoprotein measurement.** 388
27.10.1973: 923–924
Brock had already shown (with Sutcliffe, *Lancet* 29.7.1972: 197–199) that AFP concentrations in the amniotic fluid of foetuses affected by spina bifida and anencephaly differed from unaffected pregnancies. He had drawn attention to the potential value of this finding in early diagnosis and had suggested that a more sensitive test might detect AFP in maternal blood serum, avoiding the risks of amniocentesis. This paper confirmed the hypothesis.

1974 **Teasdale and Jennett: Assessment of coma and impaired consciousness.** 390
13.7.1974: 81–83
This paper presented the 'Glasgow Coma Scale' to assess depth of coma: an important paper which had considerable practical impact, long term, on intensive care for the comatose patient.

1981   **Hymes *et al.*: Kaposi's sarcoma in homosexual men – a report of eight cases.**   406
19.9.1981: 598–600   (Extract: first page only)
A series of sentinel cases, forming a herald epidemic cluster of this (then) uncommon sarcoma, which later turned out to be due to human immunodeficiency virus (HIV).

1981   ***The Lancet*: Editorial – ECT in Britain: a shameful state of affairs.**   407
28.11.1981: 1207–1208
A good example of *The Lancet*'s voice during this era, commenting on a recent audit of electro-convulsive treatment in British mental institutions. The sense of shock and disbelief at such a state of affairs is clear in *The Lancet*'s reaction.

1983   **Warren and Marshall: Unidentified curved bacilli on gastric epithelium in active chronic gastritis.**   409
4.6.1983: 1273–1275
These letters are part of an extraordinary medical story with significant implications for the care of gastric acid reflux and ulcer previously believed to be related to unexplained imbalances in body chemistry. The *bacilli* had been seen before, but thinking them 'curiosities', no-one had perceived their significance. The discovery of a relationship between gastritis and a previously unknown organism – eventually named as *Helicobacter pylori* – led to effective antibiotic treatment.

1984   **Cuckle, Wald and Lindenbaum: Maternal serum alpha-fetoprotein measurement: a screening test for Down syndrome.**   412
28.4.1984: 926–927   (Extract: first page only)
Development of an early pre-natal test for Down syndrome and spina bifida.

1984   **Moser, Fox and Jones: Unemployment and mortality in the OPCS longitudinal study.**   413
8.12.1984: 1324–1329   (Extract: first page only)
This paper demonstrated a connection between the stress of unemployment and raised mortality (including suicide) among unemployed men and their wives. The OPCS was the Office of Population Censuses and Surveys, an office of UK government. A follow-up paper confirmed these findings: see *Lancet* 15.2.1986: 385–386. The paper appeared at a time of high unemployment in the UK.

1985   **Powell-Jackson *et al.*: Creutzfeldt-Jakob disease after administration of human growth hormone.**   414
3.8.1985: 244–246   (Extract: first page only)
Important paper showing transmission to a child of Creutzfeldt-Jakob disease (CJD) from cadaver-derived growth hormone.

1986   **GISSI: Effectiveness of intravenous thrombolytic treatment in acute myocardial infarction.**   415
22.2.1986: 398–402   (Extract: first page only)
Randomised controlled trial of over 11,000 patients showing lower mortality among those given blood-thinning treatment within 12 hours of a heart attack.

1986   **Sommer *et al.*: Impact of vitamin A supplementation on childhood mortality.**   416
24.5.1986: 1169–1173   (Extract: first page only)
This randomised controlled trial revealed childhood mortality in Sumatra could be decreased by as much as 34% by vitamin A supplementation. It was based on earlier findings (*Lancet* 10.9.1983: 585–588). This trial had a significantly greater impact (see *Lancet* 29.2.2005: 649).

1989   **Nelson, Taylor and Weatherall: Sleeping position and infant bedding may predispose to hyperthermia and the sudden infant death syndrome.**   417
28.1.1989: 199–201   (Extract: first page only)
These authors brought together evidence from around the world to support the hypothesis that overheating might be a significant cause of cot death, suggesting that sleeping position might contribute to a baby's inability to control its own temperature, and that overdressing and soft bedding might compound the problem, leading to hyperthermia. These ideas led to the 'Back to Sleep' campaign, whose simple recommendations have saved many lives.

1999

Bang et al.: Effect of home-based neonatal care and management of sepsis on neonatal mortality: field trial in rural India.
4.12.1999: 1955–1961   (Extract: first page only)
By a relatively simple and inexpensive intervention, involving the training of local health workers and traditional birth attendants in neonatal care, and a health education programme, the Bangs and their co-workers were able to cut the number of neonatal deaths in the study region by 50%. The rural Indian population amongst whom this vital work was done is described as malnourished and illiterate. The intervention cost $5.3 per child.

429

2000

Yudkin: Insulin for the world's poorest countries.
11.3.2000: 919–921
A classic paper making the moral argument for cheaper drug availability for the world's poor.

430

2000

Kanitakis et al.: Regeneration of cutaneous innervation in a human hand allograft.
18.11.2000: 1738–1739   (Extract: first page only)
This report demonstrates rapid and functional regeneration of cutaneous innervation in biopsy samples. A telling sign: the patient's recovered sensitivity to pain.

433

2001

Dixon-Woods et al.: Parents' accounts of obtaining a diagnosis of childhood cancer.
3.3.2001: 670–674   (Extract: first page only)
Study illuminating sources of delay in the diagnosis of childhood cancers and how they might be obviated, by interviewing parents of children undergoing cancer treatment. The startling finding emerged that 50% of parents knew something was wrong, but felt their concerns about the seriousness of their child's condition had not been heard by their general practitioner, or taken seriously soon enough. The study has serious implications for consulting methods and standards of diagnosis in general practice.

434

2001

Kuroda et al.: Whole genome sequencing of meticillin-resistant *Staphylococcus aureus*.
21.4.2001: 1225–1240   (Extract: first page and page 1238 only)
A large team of Japanese researchers, led by Kuroda of Tokyo, produced this remarkable genomic analysis of the pathogen MRSA, finding that it has an effective defensive cell wall and an extraordinarily versatile and complex genetic structure, incorporating resistance and virulence genes from other organisms, and capable of producing a considerable array of diverse super-antigens. This analysis revealed a glimpse not only as to why MRSA is such a highly resistant and ubiquitous infectious agent, but also how little we yet understand it.
The Lancet pushed the boat out for the publication of this paper, with several pages of colour printing for the technical details. A colour-adapted version forms the endpapers to this volume.

435

2002

Magpie Trial Collaborative Group: Do women with pre-eclampsia, and their babies, benefit from magnesium sulphate? The Magpie Trial: a randomised placebo-controlled trial.
1.6.2002: 1877–1890   (Extract: first page only)
Impressive trial showing that the risk of pre-eclampsia can be halved without short-term harm.

437

2002

Heart Protection Study Collaborative Group: MRC/BHF Heart Protection Study of antioxidant vitamin supplementation in 20,536 high-risk individuals: a randomised placebo-controlled trial.
6.7.2002: 23–33   (Extract: first page only)
A large study of antioxidants which demonstrated no benefit to patients measured by cancer, heart problems or mortality.

438

2003

Peiris et al.: Coronavirus as a possible cause of severe acute respiratory syndrome.
19.4.2003: 1319–1325   (Extract: first page only)
New virus isolated from severe acute respiratory syndrome (SARS) patients in Hong Kong.

439

2004   **Alonso *et al.*: Efficacy of the RTS,S/AS02A vaccine against *Plasmodium falciparum* infection and disease in young African children: randomised controlled trial.**   455
16.10.2004: 1411–1420   (Extract: first page only)
Reports the first successful vaccine against malaria: safe, well tolerated and immunogenic. Promises great benefit, especially as further funding has been pledged by the Gates foundation.

2005   **Lawn *et al.*: 4 million neonatal deaths: When? Where? Why?**   456
5.3.2005: 891–900   (Extract: first page only)
Across the world, 450 babies die every hour, mostly from preventable causes: every year, 500,000 mothers die from pregnancy-related causes. The authors declare mortality of such extent unconscionable in the 21st century. The Bangs' paper (see *1999*) shows that were funding available, dramatic inroads might swiftly be made into such ghastly losses.

Special Articles

HUMAN RELATIONS IN OBSTETRIC PRACTICE *

NORMAN MORRIS

M.D. Lond., F.R.C.O.G.

PROFESSOR OF OBSTETRICS AND GYNÆCOLOGY IN THE UNIVERSITY OF
LONDON AT CHARING CROSS HOSPITAL MEDICAL SCHOOL, W.C.2

DURING the past twenty-five years changes in obstetric practice have reduced the physical hazard of childbirth dramatically. This achievement has tended to make us a little complacent. Indeed some people even suggest that there are few problems in obstetrics left for us to solve. But are we to measure success simply in terms of life and death? Though the physical care of the patient has advanced, I believe that many serious gaps remain, particularly in our knowledge and understanding of the patient's emotional condition in pregnancy, labour, and the puerperium.

For most women childbirth is their moment of greatest achievement and sometimes of greatest happiness. It is an immensely important emotional as well as physical event. It is a period of great intensity of feeling and reaction. The influences that a woman meets during this time may have a tremendous psychological and social significance, and in my view our present hospital system often fails miserably in its care of the patients' emotions. The joys, hopes, and wonder that the arrival of new life should bring are spoiled, and splintered into loneliness, indignity, and despair. The feeling of personal achievement is lost, drowned in a sea of inhumanity.

My own opinions and observations have lately been reinforced by a collection of extracts from several hundreds of letters sent to a weekly women's journal,† which I have been allowed to study.

ANTENATAL CARE

Antenatal Clinics

Women attend these clinics regularly, often as many as fourteen times. The clinic is usually drab and colourless, painted in bottle green, brown, or dirty cream. There are rows of uncomfortable benches. There is an atmosphere of coldness, unfriendliness, and severity more in keeping with the spirit of an income-tax office. The clinic is often very overcrowded, and at best a crude appointment system is in operation. Despite this, women often wait 1-3 hours. The interview itself is usually extremely brief, and under such conditions there is little encouragement for the patient to ask questions or relieve herself of any nagging fears or doubts. Therefore she often remains in gross ignorance of what is happening to her. The doctors and nurses also remain virtual strangers since she rarely sees the same one at each visit.

The following extracts from the letters describe experiences in antenatal clinics:

" As you entered the doctor was already reading your case-sheet, and we were on and off the examination table in two shakes . . . barely two minutes, when we had waited perhaps

---

* Based on a lecture given at the opening of the new obstetric unit at Charing Cross Hospital on Feb. 23; see *Lancet*, March 5, 1960, p. 556.
† The original letters are available in the offices of the journal, but I have been sent only extracts, and I do not know the name and address of any of the patients or their hospitals.

two hours or more. I did meet one mother, who was on her first visit only three weeks before her baby was due. She had other children who she found it difficult to leave for so long a time. There was no system of appointments."

" The nurses and doctors were very friendly at the antenatal clinic and very helpful—but—we were rather like ' sausages in a sausage machine'. I understood that there were far too many pregnant women and far too few doctors. It was rather amusing to hear the remark of a nurse on seeing one mother-to-be making her face up. She was told ' Don't bother with your face, dear, it's the other end he's interested in '."

" The midwives at the hospital all seem to have too much on their plate to bother with the odd person who wants to know ' why, where and what '. Whenever I go for treatment, it always seems as though I were being put on a conveyor belt and passing through all the different stages—water—blood—examination and out. There seems to be nothing human in them at times."

" I am not wanting to be fussed over, but I do think a friendly reception—with a smile would go a long way to make one feel more confident about the birth. . . . One's reception is so cool, and there seems to be little interest shown at hospital, with hardly an exchange of words. In fact these seem to be minimised to ' Go in, undress, lie down ' (from a very tight-lipped nurse) and ' Are you feeling any kicks? ' (from the gynæcologist). More often than not, I feel like giving him a few kicks myself! "

There is a myth that patients will not keep appointments. This is not true. Appointments will be kept by the patient, if the hospital shows definitely that it intends to honour these appointments on time. Doctors interviewing large numbers of women on an endless conveyor-belt system inevitably lose their sensitivity. Not long ago I heard a senior obstetrician admit that even after seeing about eight patients he began to feel dizzy. Such an arrangement is terribly fatiguing, and yet there is little evidence that much is being done to end this archaic system.

Preparatory Classes

Many hospitals encourage some form of classes for special instruction and preparation for labour, but unfortunately there is often poor liaison between the people who run the classes and the staff of the labour ward. Few obstetricians take an active part in organising and running the classes, though physiotherapists and midwives are doing excellent work despite our lack of support.

Virtually no studies have been done on the average patient's emotional response to pregnancy and labour. We know even less about the ultimate effect of experiences in childbirth on the mother's relationship with her child and family. As a result these preparation classes are very much in their infancy. But even in their present form they do enable women to approach labour with confidence and to bring it under their own control. In my view a hospital that fails to provide such classes is as negligent in an emotional sense as it would be in a physical sense if it failed to test the urine regularly during pregnancy.

Some obstetricians and midwives still doubt the value of preparation classes. They point out that preparation has no effect on the length of labour, the forceps-rate, or the cæsarean-section rate. They are obsessed by purely physical standards. How can we produce statistics to show how many women emerge from labour exalted rather than demoralised, confident rather than afraid?

We can measure the length of labour but not the mother's sense of achievement or wellbeing.

MANAGEMENT OF LABOUR

When the patient arrives at the hospital in labour, she usually goes through a ceremonial, known as " being admitted ". Before this ceremonial can begin she often has to supply " some particulars " to the porter or nurse on duty. She is then undressed, shaved, given an enema and a hot bath. Some more active centres also treat their patients to a castor-oil cocktail. These measures can prove a little unnerving, especially if they are unexpected. When this ritual is completed the patient either goes into a first-stage labour-ward or into the general ward.

In the first-stage ward, usually a large room with several beds, there are often many women in different stages of labour. To a woman in early labour it is extremely frightening to be brought into such close contact with women in the later stages of labour and who may appear distressed and upset.

The following extracts show how much sympathetic management can contribute to the patients' morale:

" Then came the hustling process into a bath, then an enema, with my mental condition indescribable! I thought all this might injure my baby and they could not be bothered to offer the one word of comfort or explanation. From 7 A.M. till noon I did not see a soul, and was told before being left on the labour bed ' Don't keep ringing the bell, we have not the time to answer you '. Eventually, my son, an eight pounder, was safely delivered, but I had been robbed of my peace of mind for many months to come. In fact, to be frank, in my youth and ignorance, I could not bear my husband near me for a long time after the baby's birth . . . "

" . . . I am a young girl of twenty-one and I had my first baby a little over two months ago. I was in labour for two days and nights, and was on my own for the whole time, except for occasional heads being popped round the door, and when my husband could come. I had to lie in pain listening to other women groaning and calling out in pain all down the corridor. I was very very scared! During the last few hours, after calling for a nurse for considerable time, she came bustling in and told me to ' shut up ' and what did I expect when I was having a baby—of course I was in pain '. She then plonked the gas and air machine on my nose, told me the baby would not arrive for ages—and left me."

" Later in the night or early morning, another mother was admitted to the same ward and had her baby with just a screen between us. I was sweating with fear for my forthcoming labour, and it was probably far worse just to hear the sounds and not know what was happening. After this experience my own contractions stopped, probably due to fear."

" The first baby was born in hospital, the second at home. And the third will be at home. I found that in hospital they are more concerned with the second stage of labour than the first. The reasons may—in fact most probably are—due to shortage of staff, but to a woman giving birth to a baby—a first one in most cases—it is extremely terrifying to be left alone. I believe the staff in a maternity ward leave the women on their own for the simple reason that they do not know or understand how lonely they are. Shouldn't part of their instructions be the state of mind of a pregnant woman, as well as her body ? "

" Why not make an appeal to women who have had at least three children, to volunteer to sit with mothers in labour wards of the busy maternity hospitals ?"

" I had a midwife my age and two nurses present at my daughter's birth, and they were wonderful. We all worked as a team, and I can't speak too highly of them. My baby cried when her head popped out, and we all laughed, and suddenly the lump that I had in my tummy became a person. She was there and she was mine, and I was full of beans and wanted to rush around to all expectant mums to tell them not to fear, put themselves in the hands of their doctors and nurses, and enjoy the most wonderful experience of their lives."

" It is the adult approach that appealed to me personally. To be told encouragingly ' you are doing fine with your breathing, everything is coming along nicely ' and ' now the second stage is starting, baby will soon be born '. You feel marvellous, as if you are part of the team, and they are rooting for you! "

" Looking back, it does seem to me the worst of childbirth is that the nurses and doctors tend to forget that you are the body through which life is coming into being, and that you want to be kept in the picture."

Some obstetricians and midwives still do not allow husbands to be with their wives during any stage of labour. Here are some more patients' views:

" Every woman realises that her husband is rather apprehensive the first time when he knows that his wife wants him with her, but it means secretly a lot to a woman that he did not choose to shirk what she could not shirk either."

" My husband said, a few hours after our son's birth—I cannot imagine life without him now; he seems to have belonged to us for ever, seeing him born made him belong to me, too, whereas, when you came home from the hospital with Sarah, she was a little stranger, and I found it hard to realise that I too had a place in her life."

" As for having one's husband at the birth, that's nonsense. Most men couldn't stand it, and that's a fact. My husband was visiting me when labour started, and I thought he would never go away and leave me to it. I can't be bothered with anyone during labour. In fact, I usually doze until it's time to start pushing."

If a husband wants to be with his wife in labour, I am certain that we have no right to deny him this experience. I actively encourage husbands to be present providing they know what to expect.

The following extracts describe the mothers' reactions after the baby has been delivered and in the puerperium:

" When at last I got to the ward, I thought I should see my baby, but they just said, ' he's all right, you'll see him in the morning '. Eventually one sympathetic staff nurse carried him round the ward and I saw him in her arms, but I still didn't have him to hold myself until the morning after he was born (he was born at two in the afternoon). All the ten days I was there, I only held him for a short while for feeding and when I eventually got home, it was some while before I felt he was really mine. My husband, too, had only seen him at a distance, he felt stranger than I did! "

" After each feed in hospital we were expected to express any milk remaining in the breasts, and woe betide us if, when the bowls were handed in, we had not contributed something. It was common practice for the midwife to take the mother's nipple between none too gentle fingers and to painfully extract such milk as remained in the breast. I don't condemn this practice, which seemed to help the breasts from becoming too heavy and painful, but I do object to the manner in which it was carried out. The hospital was modern, efficient, bright and cheerful, but we might indeed have been cattle—and rather tiresome cattle at that. I have no doubt that the nurses and midwives were overworked and the hospital understaffed—and perhaps in these conditions it is hard to be patient with mothers, who, after all, are not ill."

" The nurses should remember that although they are used to the sight of the human body, to many young women, childbirth is their first experience of hospital, and they are extremely shy of exposing themselves."

DISCUSSION

These extracts are only a small sample of the many views which were expressed in the different letters. Perhaps I have painted the picture in too harsh colours, but I feel that if we are really honest, we must admit that there are times when the atmosphere in our maternity units is not very pleasant. The recurrent theme of the letters is lack of rapport between the hospital staff and the patient, and we should do well to consider the reasons for this.

Why are some women left alone in labour and often shown very little kindness and sympathy? Why is there so little thought for the mother as an individual? How far is this situation the end-result of poor training and can it be prevented? Is this unsympathetic attitude a form of defence mechanism against the constant load of anxiety inevitable in every maternity unit? Is it also related to the fact that midwives have to work very hard for long periods under stress, and have to spend valuable time on domestic chores rather than on the actual care of the patients? Nurses in training always seem to be walking about and are seldom encouraged to sit down and talk to their patients. Does this also contribute to the later development of an inhuman attitude?

Why do some hospital doctors appear cold and distant? Are they overworked or badly trained? Do obstetricians in training have enough opportunity to learn much about normal labour and do they develop much insight into women as women? Has the physician-accoucheur been replaced by the surgeon-accoucheur with little interest in normal labour? Do our senses become dulled by constant observation of childbirth? Are some people's reactions to childbirth subconsciously different from what they appear to be on the surface? In fact, do some nurses and doctors find childbirth repugnant and not something rather wonderful? Do midwives who are spinsters past the menopause have to contend with specific emotional complications, which in part are exacerbated by their occupation?

How far are any of us fully aware of the impression we make upon the patient?

Major conflicts do often exist between midwives and doctors, midwives and midwives, and finally between trained midwives and pupils. It is useless for us to pretend any longer that these conflicts do not occur. Does the present training as laid down by the Central Midwives Board really encourage the idea that midwives should cooperate fully with doctors in the joint management of normal labour; or do the present regulations tend to encourage the midwife to think that she is entirely responsible for normal labour and need only call in medical aid (doctors) when things are going wrong? What other factors have resulted in doctors not being present during, or in control of normal labour?

Do the present training methods ensure that matrons, superintendent midwives, and sister-tutors have adequate knowledge of psychology and of the enormous influence that they may have for good or ill on young pupil midwives, who are often coping with emotional difficulties and complications of their own? In fact, should there be an " agonising re-appraisal " of all the present methods of training midwives and obstetricians?

Surely it is not necessary to know the answers to all these questions before we make some attempt to put our house in order. First, all hospital staff must appreciate that the mother-to-be is extremely vulnerable. She is at their mercy for good or for ill. Many of our present procedures, which involve dragooning and regimentation, must be revised. The training of nurses, medical students, and midwives must include a careful study of patient-staff relations and also exactly where these are likely to break down. The importance of *words* and their impact on the patient must be repeatedly emphasised—in particular the extraordinary value of kindness.

We must destroy the illusion that the patient is a human being apart, someone quite unlike ourselves. We must get rid of that awful method of dividing patients into " cooperative " or " uncooperative ", into " easy " or " difficult ". This classification is largely based on how much regimentation the patient will stand without complaining.

I have an enormous respect for the great work that midwives are doing, and the huge burden they are carrying, but I am conscious that there are a few midwives, just as there are doctors, who do let the side down badly. All midwives and doctors, particularly those in charge of labour wards, should have a proper insight into the emotional as well as the physical needs of their patients and staff. We must somehow ensure that no patient is ever at the mercy of a midwife's own frustrations and mixed-up emotions. No senior sister must be allowed to exert her authority by means of a reign of terror, to which even the consultant obstetrician himself sometimes submits.

We must replan our maternity units, so that every department reflects joy rather than sorrow, hope rather than gloom, life rather than death. Somehow we must contrive to reproduce in hospital the natural tranquillity that often develops quite spontaneously with home confinements. Architects must combine with us to experiment in new forms of design.

We must also resolve the conflicts which often exist between midwives and doctors. An obstetric unit must operate as a unit and not as a collection of jealous individuals. The division of obstetrics into " normal " and " abnormal " can only do harm, since obstetricians have come to concentrate their attention more and more on the abnormal. As a result so-called " normal " labour is taken for granted and is conducted on a rule-of-thumb conveyor-belt system. Obstetricians should take much more active interest in the direction and coordination of their units, for a maternity unit is a complex organisation, which calls for continuous leadership and example. Each unit must be encouraged to develop its own philosophy and sense of purpose. Obstetricians were not meant to be reluctant foremen of baby factories, but privileged guardians of the next generation.

If we can use pregnancy as a time of preparation, not only for labour but for all that family life means, and if we can make childbirth a more positive experience, then I think the social repercussions will be remarkable. The next century will undoubtedly see a great advance in our understanding of all the complex factors that influence and govern human relationships. The health, happiness, and possibly even the survival of our children will depend on the success of our studies in this field. Midwives and obstetricians have an especial responsibility, for they are there at the beginning, and probably it is the manner of the beginning that matters most of all.

attributed to any extraneous cause. Many of these discharges (but by no means all) were sent by family doctors, and it may well be that patients with these " simple " discharges come to hospitals less often than those with more severe symptoms. It may be, too, that the growing interest in personal health leads women to complain to their doctors of symptoms which in an earlier age were borne in silence.

Summary

Of 561 specimens of vaginal discharge from women of reproductive age, 9 appeared to be due to bacterial infection. 134 were associated with *Trichomonas vaginalis,* and 64 with *Candida albicans.* The remainder were indistinguishable from normal vaginal secretion in any character except quantity.

13/16 vaginal discharges in children and 15/18 in women over 50 appeared to be due to bacterial infection.

A tentative classification of vaginal discharges based upon the reaction of the host and the parasite is suggested.

It is possible that *C. albicans* is parasitic, not on the vaginal wall, but on the secretions of the vagina.

My thanks are due to Mr. P. M. G. Russell for many interesting conversations on this subject and to Dr. Stella Henderson for supplying material from the Family Planning Clinic.

REFERENCES

Adair, F. L., Hesseltine, H. C. (1936) *Amer. J. Obstet. Gynec.* **32,** 1.
Cruickshank, R., Sharman, A. (1934) *J. Obstet. Gynæc. Brit. Emp.* **41,** 190, 369.
Davis, M. E., Pearl, S. A. (1938) *Amer. J. Obstet. Gynec.* **35,** 77.
Feo, L. G., Dellette, B. R. (1953) *ibid.* **65,** 131.
Hesseltine, H. C. (1933) *ibid.* **26,** 46.
Jeffcoate, T. N. A. (1955) *Med. World,* **82,** 136.
Karnaby, K. J. (1954) *Amer. J. Surg.* **87,** 188.
Kessel, J. E., Gafford, J. A. (1940) *Amer. J. Obstet. Gynec.* **39,** 1005.
Liston, W. G., Cruickshank, L. G. (1940) *Edinb. med. J.* **47,** 369.
McCrea, M. R., Osborne, A. D. (1960) *J. comp. Path.* **67,** 342.
Magath, T. B. (1938) *Amer. J. Obstet. Gynec.* **35,** 694.
Rogosa, M., Sharpe, M. E. (1960) *J. gen. Microbiol.* **23,** 197.
Russell, P. M. G. (1960) Personal communication.

ENDOSCOPIC EXAMINATION OF THE STOMACH AND DUODENAL CAP WITH THE FIBERSCOPE

BASIL I. HIRSCHOWITZ
B.Sc., M.D. W'srand, M.R.C.P., M.R.C.P.E.
ASSOCIATE PROFESSOR OF MEDICINE AND DIRECTOR, DIVISION OF GASTROENTEROLOGY, UNIVERSITY OF ALABAMA MEDICAL CENTER, BIRMINGHAM, ALABAMA

With illustrations on plate

SINCE a previous report on the fiberscope (Hirschowitz, Curtiss, and Peters 1958), work has progressed to the point where a clinically useful model of this completely flexible instrument has been made and used in the examination of the upper gastrointestinal tract. The current experimental model has been used successfully to examine the lower œsophagus, stomach, pyloric canal, duodenal bulb, and both afferent and efferent loops of jejunum for a distance of up to 12 in. beyond gastrojejunal anastomoses, all with sufficient resolution to describe fine mucosal detail. Furthermore, both still and movie photographs in colour have been taken through the instrument of the stomach and duodenum without additional illumination. Among the interesting findings are the observations on duodenal ulcer in situ and of a distinct sphincter at the apex of the duodenal bulb.

The Instrument

The fiberscope superficially resembles a conventional gastroscope, comprising a head which contains a lamp bulb, a prism, and a compound lens which focuses the image on to the distal (objective) end of the fibre bundle. The view is at right angles to the instrument. The shaft of the instrument contains the glass fibre bundle which transmits the image to the eyepiece and is *completely flexible throughout its entire length* (fig. 1).

The bundle is protected by a flexible flat bronze spiral which is also used to transmit torque. It is in turn covered by a

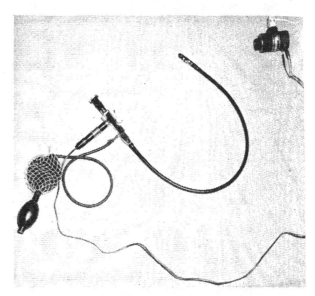

Fig. 1—The fiberscope with air and electrical connections.

smooth plastic sheath. The ocular (proximal) end contains a simple lens for magnifying the image from the proximal end of the fibre bundle, a ratchet for focusing the distal lens, and connections for air and electrical current supplied from a standard 10-volt variable transformer. The overall length is 38 in. (92 cm.) and the diameter just under 0·5 in. (11 mm.)

The image is transmitted through a bundle of glass fibres traversing the length of the instrument and so arranged spatially that the orientation of the fibres is the same at each end, but, being unbound in the middle, the bundle is completely flexible. Each fibre (diameter 0·0006 in. or approximately 14 μ) transmits a spot of light and the image is transmitted as a composite of these spots of light. About 150,000 fibres are used to make one bundle of about 0·25 in. diameter, allowing high optical resolution. Light transmission through the fiberscope is about $2^{1}/_{2}$ times better than through the standard gastroscope, and each fibre is insulated to prevent light scatter from one to another.

The principle of transmission of light through the length of a fibre is that of total internal reflectance which depends on the refraction of light when passing from one optical medium to another of lesser optical density. Light beams are refracted closer to the interface as the angle of incidence becomes smaller. At the critical angle light is refracted along the interface between the two media and at any angle greater than the critical angle, light is reflected back into the medium of origin (in this instance glass). When light enters the end of a rod (or fibre) any light entering at a greater than critical angle (relative to the sides of the fibre) is automatically trapped and perforce has to proceed to the other end of the fibre. Once the light is trapped, curvature or bending of the fibre within wide limits will not cause the light to be lost before it appears at the other end. This briefly is the principle of the instrument used.

Its Clinical Use

Preparation of the Patient

The principal indication for premedication is the prevention of nausea and gagging, rather than analgesia, since the examination is painless. After trying a variety of drugs for premedication, including promazine ('Sparine'), dimenhydrinate ('Dramamine'), barbiturates and pethidine (demerol), either alone or in combination, as well as examining a number of patients without premedication, the following general method has been adopted. When the patient is first seen the activity of the gag reflex is graded 0, +, or ++. For those with little or no gag reflex, preparation is confined to surface anæsthesia of the throat. Those patients with + gag reflex are given 25–50 mg. pethidine and those with ++ gag reflex are given 50–100 mg. pethidine intravenously 5–15 mins. before endoscopy. The throat is then anæsthetised with spray or gargle of the endoscopist's choice (I have no special preference).

Passing the Instrument

A drop of silicone antifoam * is placed on the tip of the instrument to reduce bubbling (Hirschowitz, Bolt, and Pollard 1954). While an assistant holds the headpiece, the lubricated instrument is passed readily into the stomach with the patient sitting on the side of the bed or couch facing the endoscopist (fig. 2). In no instance has there been any difficulty

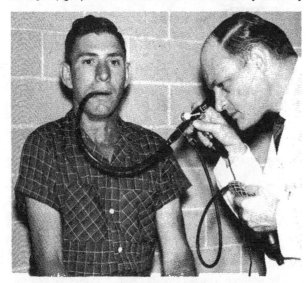

Fig. 2—Stomach of outpatient being examined with the fiberscope.

in entering the stomach, and the blunt end seems preferable to the rubber finger end both for swallowing and for transpyloric passage. Air is pumped into the stomach, as in the standard gastroscopic examination.

Some of the œsophageal mucosa and the whole cardio-œsophageal area can be seen since the focus of the instrument is so arranged to display surfaces in contact with the objective window. By moving the patient into different positions, which can be done without discomfort or danger, a greater area of the stomach can be seen than with the standard gastroscope. The fundus is an area which still cannot be examined, but there are no other "blind" areas. With the patient sitting upright the upper half of the stomach can be seen, but if there is any fluid in the stomach the patient has to lie down on his back or either side for examination of the lower half of the stomach.

Proceeding with the examination, the whole antrum is viewed from a point approximately opposite the angulus on the greater curve. Then, with the patient lying on the right side, the instrument is advanced through the pyloric canal into the duodenal bulb. This has been possible every time it was attempted. The patient is then asked to lie on his back or left side to drain the duodenal bulb.

* Dow Corning.

When there is a gastroenterostomy the instrument can usually, though not always, be passed through the stoma for a distance limited by the respective lengths of the patient and instrument—usually for about 12 in. It is easier to pass the fiberscope into the efferent loop with the patient lying on his back or sitting upright; it is often necessary to advance the instrument into the afferent loop with the patient lying on the right side, and with some help from pressure through the abdominal wall.

Anteroposterior orientation is made relatively easy by observing transillumination through the abdominal wall. Once an organ is distended with air and the light is directed anteriorly, the whole outline of that organ can be readily made out on the abdominal wall. Anatomical sites are readily recognisable when once seen—this applies to the pylorus, duodenal bulb, and the jejunum (see below). Usually the position of the head can be confirmed by observing the outline of the transilluminated organ either jejunum (afferent or efferent loops) or the duodenal cap which is seen to the right of the midline beyond a dark band which represents the pyloric sphincter. The position of the head can also be confirmed by external palpation, and an ulcer can be further identified by finding point tenderness which corresponds to a lesion.

Because of its complete flexibility there is neither discomfort during the procedure nor afterwards. Nearly all the patients examined kept the instrument down for over 20 minutes, some as long as 60 minutes. The patient is not limited to any position, particularly the sword-swallowing one, and spinal deformity or inability to extend the neck no longer preclude examination. The patient can be examined anywhere and our patients have been examined in their beds, in the outpatient clinic, and even sitting in a chair. The instrument is manipulated by pushing and pulling and by rotation of the headpiece from which torque is transmitted to the distal end on a 1:1 ratio by the metal spiral incorporated in its shaft. A certain amount of manipulation can be done through the abdominal wall.

Observations

Œsophagus

Current models of the fiberscope were not designed to provide systematic examination of the œsophagus. Nevertheless, because objects in contact with the objective window can be brought into focus, an adequate view of the cardio-œsophageal area is readily obtained.

Stomach

Body of the stomach (fig. 3).—Resolution of the image is every bit as good as the conventional gastroscope provides, and because of greater light transmission the actual image seen is generally better. Colour reproduction is generally faithful, since transmission of light with wavelength above 5000 Å is close to 100%, being considerably reduced only below 5000 Å. The lesions seen so far include gastric cancer, acute ulcer (fig. 4), chronic ulcer, erosive gastritis, superficial gastritis, gastric mucosal atrophy (in pernicious anæmia), and hypertrophy or mammillation (in duodenal ulcer), and regional enteritis.

Antrum.—The entire pyloric antrum can always be seen and the motility of this area can be studied at leisure since the patient suffers no appreciable discomfort. Close-up views of the sphincter can always be obtained by advancing the instrument into the pyloric canal.

Pyloric canal.—Visible only occasionally with the conventional gastroscope, the pyloric canal can be very readily

MAY 27, 1961   ORIGINAL ARTICLES   THE LANCET   1129

first of all necessitated ureterolithotomy, and later the loss of a kidney. Case 2 was bedridden for a year. In addition to his ruptured urethra and fractured pelvis he had an extraperitoneal rupture of his bladder, fractures of the right femur, right wrist, right fibula, left tibia, and the right fourth and fifth metatarsals. Multiple recumbency calculi developed in his left kidney. Pyelolithotomy was performed nine months after his accident, and he remained well after this with a normally functioning kidney. The pyelitis in case 4 responded to antibiotics and caused no further trouble.

Recumbency calculi are avoidable. They are due to a combination of urinary stasis, a raised level of urinary calcium, and infection. Urinary stasis can be prevented by assuring an adequate intake of fluid, and by the avoidance of a permanent dorsal decubitus position. Decalcification of bone can be prevented by exercise and massage to the uninjured limbs. Urinary acidification will lessen the chances of urinary infection and also will prevent the deposition of soft triple-phosphate calculi (Cordonnier and Talbot 1948).

Impotence

Three out of the twelve cases in this series are completely impotent (one, case 6a, was not available for follow-up, but was still impotent fourteen months after his injury). Case 2 has poor erections, and case 5a is still rather young for certain assessment. Two out of the three patients with impotence can ejaculate. This is of great importance both from a social and from a medicolegal point of view, as these patients might well father a child by A.I.H. In case 3, semen analysis was carried out and the result is shown in the table.

The exact cause of the impotence in these cases remains obscure. Young (1929) considered it due to vascular injury, and Abbott (1921) ascribed it to injury to the greater and lesser cavernous nerves. Because of the lack of evidence of injury to the sympathetic nerve-supply to the prostate, vesicles, and bladder neck in these cases (in spite of complete dislocation of the prostate), vascular damage may well be the likely cause of the impotence.

Summary

The diagnosis and techniques of management of rupture of the posterior urethra are discussed.

The value of urethrography is emphasised, both for diagnosis and later to exclude stricture.

The three principal complications are stricture formation, urinary infection, and impotence.

Urethral dilatation is probably done more often than is necessary, and rupture of the posterior urethra need not be a cause of a " certain stricture ".

Though these patients may be impotent, they may be able to ejaculate.

Twelve cases seen at Preston Royal Infirmary are reviewed, to compare the results of treatment by two different methods: (1) repair of rupture over a urethral catheter as a splint, and (2) repair of the urethra over a Foley catheter which was then put on traction.

All patients had a suprapubic cystostomy. Those treated by method (2) never showed any tendency to stricture formation; whereas four out of six of those treated by method (1) had strictures.

I am indebted to Mr. W. H. Graham for his encouragement in the preparation of this paper, and to Prof. A. M. Boyd for his most helpful criticism. I should also like to thank the department of medical illustration at Manchester Royal Infirmary who prepared the photographs.

References at foot of next column

ARTHROPLASTY OF THE HIP

A New Operation

JOHN CHARNLEY
M.B., B.Sc. Manc., F.R.C.S.

CONSULTANT ORTHOPÆDIC SURGEON TO MANCHESTER ROYAL INFIRMARY, TO PARK HOSPITAL, DAVYHULME, AND TO THE CENTRE FOR HIP SURGERY, WRIGHTINGTON HOSPITAL

IN considering how arthroplasty of the hip can be improved, two facts stand out:

1. After replacement of the head of the femur by a spherical surface of inert material, the failures are essentially *long-term*. At first the patient may notice no difference between the artificial head and the living one which preceded it. Our problem is to make this temporary success permanent.

2. Objectives must be reasonable. Neither surgeons nor engineers will ever make an artificial hip-joint which will last thirty years and at some time in this period enable the patient to play football.

Deductions from Past Experience

The methods from which we have learnt most are those of Smith-Petersen and Judet.

The *Smith-Petersen method* was a refinement of the oldest of all forms of arthroplasty, in which a membrane, or some kind of tissue, is interposed between the head of the femur and its socket. A metal cup, loose-fitting and polished, was placed between the femoral head and the acetabulum, after the femoral head had been reduced in size and the acetabulum had been enlarged by removal of the eburnated lining. The polished hemispherical surfaces of this metal cup induced changes in the fibrous tissue on the exposed surfaces of cancellous bone, which were transformed into a form of articular cartilage.

Smith-Petersen repeatedly emphasised that the moving parts should be made to fit loosely together; in no sense, therefore, could the mechanical arrangement at the finish of this operation be regarded as a mechanically stable ball-and-socket joint. The femoral head inside the cup is capable of slight displacement, and the cup also is capable of displacement inside the socket (fig. 1). In course of time the spaces between the cup and the femoral head and the cup and the acetabulum becomes filled with fibrocartilaginous material and the hip can thus become stable; but unfortunately the periarticular soft tissues often become thick and stiff, and mobility is lost.

In the *Judet operation* the head of the femur is replaced

MR. WILKINSON: REFERENCES

Abbott, A. C. (1929) *Canad. med. Ass. J.* **20**, 634.
Ashurst, A. P. C. (1909) *Ann. Surg.* **49**, 433.
Bailey, H. (1928) *Brit. J. Surg.* **15**, 370.
Berry, N. E. (1930) *Canad. med. Ass. J.* **22**, 475.
Colp, R., Findlay, R. T. (1929) *Surg. Gynec. Obstet.* **49**, 847.
Constantian, H. M., Felton, L. M. (1952) *J. Urol.* **68**, 823.
Cordonnier, J. J., Talbot, B. S. (1948) *ibid.* **60**, 316.
Gilmour, W. R. (1932) *Ann. Surg.* **95**, 161.
Grey Turner, G. (1923) *Lancet*, ii, 82.
Harrison, J. H. (1941) *Surg. Gynec. Obstet.* **72**, 622.
Hartmann, K. (1955) *Arch. klin. Chir.* **282**, 943.
Key, J. A., Conwell, H. E. (1942) The Management of Fractures, Dislocations and Sprains. St. Louis.
McCague, E. J., Semans, J. H. (1944) *J. Urol.* **52**, 36.
MacLean, J. T., Gerrie, J. W. (1946) *ibid.* **56**, 485.
Mason, J. T., Ratliff, R. K. (1949) *Nav. med. Bull., Wash.* **49**, 670.
Noland, L., Conwell, H. E. (1930) *J. Amer. med. Ass.* **94**, 174.
Ormond, J. K., Cothran, R. M. (1934) *ibid.* **102**, 2180.
Peacock, A. H., Hain, R. F. (1926) *J. Urol.* **15**, 563.
Poole-Wilson, D. S. (1952) *Brit. J. Surg.* War suppl. no. 3; pp. 471, 483.
Rexford, W. K. (1939) *Amer. J. Surg.* **46**, 641.
— (1947) *ibid.* **74**, 350.
Rutherford, H. (1904) *Lancet*, ii, 751.
Simpson-Smith, A. (1936) *Brit. J. Surg.* **24**, 309.
Trafford, H. S. (1955) *Brit. J. Urol.* **27**, 165.
Uhle, C. A. W., Erb, H. E. (1944) *J. Urol.* **52**, 42.
Vermooten, V. (1946) *ibid.* **56**, 228.
Wakeley, C. P. G. (1929) *Brit. J. Surg.* **17**, 22.
Wheeler, W. I. de C. (1929) *Brit. J. Urol.* **1**, 126.
Young, H. H. (1929) *J. Urol.* **21**, 417.

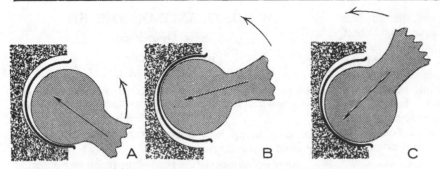

Fig. 1—Defective mechanical design of the Smith-Petersen cup.

When a straight-leg raise is attempted, muscular tone thrusts the femoral head into the socket, and during the initial few degrees of motion the femoral head tends to ride forward in the cup, B. A point is then reached where the femoral head will fall back into position C. This instability will impede the progressive relaxation of the antagonist muscles.

by a prosthesis bearing a polished hemispherical surface. In the original Judet operation the prosthesis was like a gigantic tintack with a hemispherical head (fig. 2) and it was fixed to the femur by driving the spike down the centre of the stump of the femoral neck. The joint formed by this procedure was much more stable than that formed by the Smith-Petersen procedure, because a prosthesis was chosen which was a close fit in the acetabulum. Very soon afterwards many patients could perform circumduction of the hip under full muscle control, against the force of gravity and without pain.

The capacity of the living organism to react favourably to sound mechanical design, and its capacity to reveal incipient mechanical failure by deterioration of function, even before the appearance of frank pain, is a fundamental guide in developing any arthroplasty.

Joint Lubrication

The starting-point of the present research was the well-known observation that after the Judet operation the hip sometimes squeaks. This does not last more than a few weeks and the final result is neither better nor worse than in cases without a squeak. In our experience the squeaks have occurred in the hips of osteoarthritics, but never when the acetabulum was lined with normal articular cartilage as in the treatment of subcapital fractures of the neck of the femur.

A squeak indicates that frictional resistance to sliding is so high that the surfaces are seizing together. Hence it seemed likely that the plastic of the original Judet prosthesis had adverse frictional properties when sliding against the bare bone encountered in an osteoarthritic acetabulum. It seemed possible, too, that the cessation of squeaking might be a sign not of improved lubrication but of loosening of the attachment of the prosthesis to the neck of the femur. In these circumstances the head of the prosthesis would be stationary in the acetabulum and all movement would be taking place between the femoral

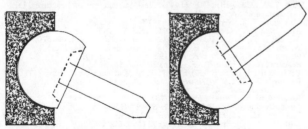

Fig. 2—Judet appliance, showing the improved mechanical design which offers a stationary centre of motion for the femoral head in the acetabulum. This enables the antagonist muscles to relax smoothly and progressively.

neck and the stem or spike by which it was originally attached to the bone. Clearly, the mechanical bond between the prosthesis and the neck of the femur could be broken by a twisting strain, or torque, resulting from high frictional resistance to the turning of the prosthesis in the acetabulum. If there were no such frictional resistance, the mechanical attachment to the femoral neck would be spared any such strains.

Laboratory Experiments

I could find only two references to measurements of the coefficient of friction of normal animal joints (Jones 1934, 1936), and my own experiments closely confirmed the figure of $\mu = 0.02$ reported by Jones, with the possibility that in certain conditions μ might be much less than this. For a skate sliding on ice, μ has been estimated at 0.03, which indicates that an animal joint is rather more slippery than ice. Engineering science knows no way of approaching such low figures for μ in a " plain " bearing when the application concerns reciprocating motion, at slow speeds, and under heavy loads. Nature has solved completely the most difficult set of lubricating conditions which ever face the engineer.

These investigations on lubrication (Charnley 1959) suggested that synovial fluid is not an essential lubricant but rather a product of the activity of joints—a view taken for granted by Sir Arthur Keith in 1919. Emphasis was transferred from the synovial fluid to the properties of articular cartilage, and attention was drawn to the engineering concept of " boundary lubrication " between dry solid surfaces, or between solid surfaces separated by a film of fluid too thin to behave as a fluid. A boundary lubricant reduces friction by entering into physicochemical combination with the surfaces, and diminishes

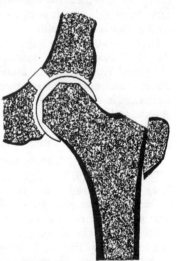

Fig. 3—Original design of polytetrafluorethylene arthroplasty.

Acetabulum lined with thin shell of polytetrafluorethylene and femoral head covered with hollow sphere of the same material. Biological concept of " synthetic " articular cartilage.

the free molecular attraction which may seize the surfaces together. Hence there must be a physicochemical affinity between the lubricant and the solid material of the rubbing surfaces; the lubricant is effective only with certain combinations of solids. Even if synovial fluid is a lubricant in an animal joint, it will not necessarily lubricate a prosthesis.

This was confirmed by experiment on the effect of ox synovial fluid on the frictional resistance between steel and bone and between ' Perspex ' and bone. The coefficient of friction for plastic and steel against bone, moistened with ox synovial fluid, was high ($\mu = 0.4$). On the other hand, when the plastic or steel was tested against

MAY 27, 1961   ORIGINAL ARTICLES   THE LANCET   1131

normal articular cartilage, the frictional resistance was almost as low as in a normal joint ($\mu = 0.02$).

Prosthesis and Socket

These investigations indicated that to give an artificial hip-joint the same kind of slipperiness as a natural joint, we should need a substance with a low coefficient of friction which at the same time could be tolerated in body tissues. For this purpose I chose polytetrafluorethylene—a plastic which

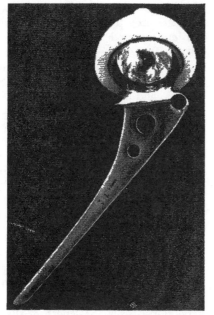

Fig. 4—Penultimate pattern of low-friction arthroplasty. Large metallic femoral-head prosthesis; relatively thin polytetrafluorethylene socket.

looks not unlike articular cartilage (being white and semitranslucent, and capable of being cut with a knife) and is chemically the most inert plastic so far discovered.

The first idea was to use this low-friction material as "synthetic articular cartilage". I lined the eburnated acetabulum of the arthritic hip-joint with a thin shell of polytetrafluorethylene and covered the reshaped head of the femur with a hollow cup of the same material firmly pressed into position (fig. 3). The absolute relief of pain, and the range of active movement under muscular control, were impressive in the first three months; but the most conservative feature of this design was its undoing. Adhering to the conservative principle which Smith-Petersen called "conservation of stock" I had retained the femoral head and refashioned it as a spigot on

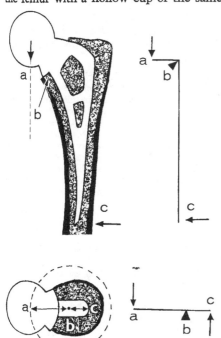

Fig. 5—Forces acting on a femoral-head prosthesis of Austin Moore or Thompson type.

In the frontal plane long levers resist the weight of the body. In the horizontal plane the levers on which the weight of the body act are short, and favour loosening of the prosthetic stem by rotation.

which to press the inner plastic sphere; but this resulted in ischæmic necrosis of the bone inside the inner sphere. As soon as the early good function started to fail, radiological examination always indicated that the head of the femur was necrotic and was becoming loose inside the inner sphere. The poor results of this kind of prosthesis thus resembled the poor results of the Smith-Petersen cup.

Cementing the Prosthesis to the Femur

My next step was to replace the head of the femur with a metallic prosthesis in combination with a low-friction plastic socket (fig. 4). I had for some time been interested in improving the mechanical bond between prosthesis and bone, by using a cement to transfer the weight of the body from the metallic stem of the prosthesis uniformly to the cancellous bone of the interior of the neck and upper end of the femur (Charnley 1960). My object was to get over the defect of the Moore and Thompson types of prosthesis, which is that they have no resistance against stresses tending to twist them in the medullary cavity on its long axis (fig. 5). (Twisting forces of this kind will in particular be experienced when a patient is rising from a sitting position with the femoral shafts horizontal.)

In 3 patients in whom the arthroplasty was re-explored, because of mechanical defects in the socket, I found that the cemented prosthesis had remained absolutely rigid in the femur after taking the full weight of the body during ten or eleven months. Furthermore, experience of over two years, with more than 100 patients, lead me to believe that, as regards infection, this technique is safer than the original one. Infection of an arthroplasty will probably start with multiplication of bacteria in blood-clot within the cavity of the joint. If the prosthesis is

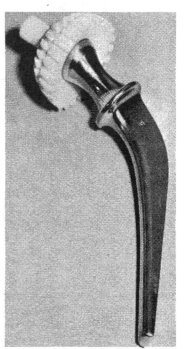

Fig. 6—Final pattern of low-friction arthroplasty. Note thick socket with deep external serrations and small femoral-head prosthesis.

loose in the medulla, the infection will be pumped into the medullary canal at every muscular movement. But where the prosthesis is cemented in position I imagine that the joint might contain pus, and the stump of the femoral neck might be bathed in pus, without any spread of infection to the medullary canal.

Design of the Socket

Though the results of using the arrangement illustrated in fig. 5 were gratifying, it was pointed out to me that the best engineering practice would be to use the smallest diameter of ball which would cope with the expected load. Up to then I had used a standard Moore prosthesis with a ball $1\frac{5}{8}$ in. in diameter, believing that polytetrafluorethylene, being a relatively soft material, would wear longer if the load per unit area of bearing surface were

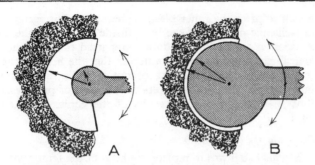

Fig. 7—Illustrating how rotation of the socket against the bone is less likely with a small head and thick socket than with a large head and thin socket as a result of differences in the moment of the frictional force as a result of differences in radii of the parts.

the smallest possible. The recommendation of my engineering colleagues enabled me to make a big improvement in the anchorage of the plastic socket in the bony acetabulum (fig. 6). Resistance to movement of the head in the socket is greatly reduced by reducing the radius of the ball and therefore reducing the " moment " of the frictional force. If at the same time the radius of the exterior of the polytetrafluorethylene socket is made as large as possible, the " moment " of the frictional force between socket and bone will be increased, and this will lessen any tendency for the socket to rotate against the bone (fig. 7). The small remaining shearing force can be resisted easily by the fibrous tissue occupying the deep irregularities on the outer surface of the socket.

Present Operation

The operation is performed through a lateral exposure by elevating the great trochanter. At the end of the operation the trochanter is reattached to the outer surface of the femur in order to enhance the leverage of the abductor muscles. Though this delays rehabilitation, it is of paramount importance in preventing adduction, external rotation, and dislocation.

When the head of the femur has been resected, the acetabulum is deepened and then reamed with special tools to an exact diameter for receiving the polytetra-fluorethylene socket. To enhance the precision of the reaming, the sequence of tools all operate on a $^1/_8$ in. pilot hole which is made in the centre of the floor of the acetabulum, the exact centre being found by a self-centring device. The polytetrafluorethylene socket carries a spigot $^1/_8$ in. in diameter which engages with the pilot hole and ensures correct orientation. The socket is hammered into the acetabulum with a punch, its external surface being deeply serrated to receive the ingrowth of fibrous tissue or bone.

The prosthesis carries a head which at present is no more than $^7/_8$ in. in diameter. Several lengths of neck are available, so that during the operation the one which best suits the depth of the socket can be chosen.

After a trial reduction has shown that everything is satisfactory, the prosthesis is cemented in position and the great trochanter is reattached with wire. The patient is splinted with the leg in abduction for three weeks, and is allowed to take full weight on the hip five weeks after the operation. Recent experiences suggest that plaster is not essential.

Results So Far

Though my experience of using polytetrafluorethylene for arthroplasty of the hip extends over three years, the technique in its present form has been in use only since January, 1960. Since then 97 hips have been operated on.

There have been no deaths, except a coronary occlusion six weeks after operation, and the only serious complication encountered has been deep venous thrombosis.

While the long-term results are still awaited, the method has been restricted to cases of gross disablement by (1) rheumatoid arthritis, (2) severe osteoarthritis in patients over 65, and occasionally (3) bilateral arthritis in middle age. The only disappointing results have been in very difficult " salvage " cases where the absence of normal structures made it impossible to carry out a technically sound procedure. With 1 exception, the only cases of infection have been those in which there have been previous attempts at arthroplasty by other methods.

On removal of the splints, after three weeks, most patients can execute a " straight-leg raise " and have no pain or spasm on passive movement. After a week out of plaster, they have recovered the preoperative range of movement. If the hip has previously been very stiff the final range may be no greater than 30°, but it will be painless and under muscular control. The average stay in hospital is eight weeks, and before they go home most patients can walk the length of the ward without sticks and with only a slight limp.

As regards wear and tear of the socket, working against the metal head of the prosthesis, close scrutiny of the radiographs of patients who have been transmitting the full weight of the body through this implant for ten months has shown negligible wear. The stresses imposed on the hip-joints of patients disabled by arthritis are only a fraction of those borne by the hip-joints of normal subjects or athletes; but even if the method should prove unsuitable for robust patients in middle life, it may have a permanent place in the treatment of the rheumatoid and the elderly, for whom it is particularly suitable, because it requires almost no rehabilitation. Even in the early stages there is no pain on movement, and the procedure is therefore appropriate for subjects with the poor muscles and relatively feeble morale which so often accompany long-continued ill-health or old age.

I am indebted to the Manchester Regional Hospital Board, which has established at Wrightington the centre for the surgery of the hip-joint at which the clinical work described in this paper has been done. In the general ideas behind this project I have been supported by interest shown by Sir Harry Platt, Prof. J. H. Kellgren, and Prof. J. Diamond. The research committee of the Manchester Regional Hospital Board has built and equipped a research workshop in the hospital and has provided the salary for a fitter and turner who will make the surgical implants. With advice from the university department of engineering, we hope to build test " rigs " and other devices for submitting different types of implant to trials of wear.

REFERENCES

Charnley, J. (1959) Institution of Mechanical Engineers: Symposium on
    Biomechanics, April, 17, p. 12.
—   (1960) J. Bone Jt Surg. 42B, 28.
Keith, A. (1919) The Engines of the Human Body. London. 1919.
Jones, E. S. (1934) Lancet, i, 1426.
—   (1936) ibid. i, 1043.
Judet, J., Judet, R. (1950) J. Bone Jt Surg. 32B, 166.
Smith-Petersen, M. N. (1948) ibid. 30B, 59.

" . . . . A new set of problems is confronting the country and medical services through the ' younging ' as distinguished from the ' aging ' of the population . . . By 1970 those of 65 years of age and older (roughly 21,000,000) and those below 20 years of age (roughly 90,000,000) will represent over 50 per cent of the entire population . . . . Contrary to common belief the life expectancy of persons over 50 years of age is now rising very little. In fact, it went down slightly in 1957 . . . . the average remaining lifetime at the age of 65 will be extended only about two years between 1960 and 1970 and only by four years between 1960 and 2000."—*Five-year Review of Activities of Josiah Macy, Jr, Foundation*: New York, 1960.

It is of course possible that some small chromosomal aberration is present, but this reservation is no more than must be made about nearly all current reports of normal human karyotypes. It is of interest that the tumour nuclei in vitro exhibit a relatively high incidence of Barr (sex-chromatin) bodies. In addition the nuclei are fairly uniform, as is so common in thyroid carcinoma. Indeed, the deceptively benign appearance of the nuclei in many thyroid carcinomas is often a diagnostic stumbling block, and to find in them morphologically unremarkable chromosomes will perhaps come as little surprise to the pathologist.

This investigation was supported by a United States P.H.S. research grant C4866, National Cancer Institute and by an institutional grant from the American Cancer Society.

Department of Pathology,
Stanford University School
of Medicine,
Palo Alto, California.   CHARLES P. MILES
ROBERT E. GALLAGHER.

DOWN'S SYNDROME (MONGOLISM)

SIR,—Landon Down's original description of mongolism appeared in a paper entitled "Observations on an ethnic classification of idiots". The features of various groups of "idiots and imbeciles" were compared to the facial appearance of the inhabitants of quite a number of countries other than Mongolia. Thus, Ethiopians, Malayans, and the original races of North America are all mentioned in this connection.

This classification has, of course, little merit and should be abandoned along with the term mongolism. Down undoubtedly made a shrewd and important observation, however, in noting the "mongolian type of idiot", and it is right that his name should be honoured eponymously. Our Russian colleagues have in fact used the term Down's syndrome, or disease, for many years and I suggest we follow their lead.

London, W.5.   A. HOLLMAN.

GLUCOSE-6-PHOSPHATE-DEHYDROGENASE DEFICIENCY

SIR,—Using Motulsky's screening technique on capillary blood samples, Dr. Engleson and Dr. Kjellman (Oct. 21) find that glucose-6-phosphate dehydrogenase (G.-6-P.D.) activity in infants' red cells is slightly less than that in adult life. While these findings are of great interest, it should be pointed out that the Motulsky method, though of great value in the detection of subjects with very low or absent enzyme activity, has not proved to be so reliable in the detection of intermediate ranges of activity. Furthermore, the great variation in hæmatocrit values of capillary blood samples in infancy might be reflected in some slight variation in enzyme activity when assayed by this method. More sensitive spectrophotometric assay methods[1] do give consistently high values for G.-6-P.D. activity in infancy and it would be of great interest to know the results of such assays on the infants studied by Dr. Engleson and Dr. Kjellman.

It is not surprising that G.-6-P.D. deficiency has not been found in association with unexplained neonatal icterus in Sweden since this genetically controlled enzyme deficiency is probably very uncommon in North Europe. Reports from Singapore,[2][3] Greece,[4] Italy[5] and Nigeria,[6] have all pointed to such an association and the recently reported excess of infant over adult deficient subjects in Greece[7] suggests that these infants are at a real disadvantage. It is still not established

1. Zinkham, W. H. Pediatrics, 1958, 22, 453.
2. Smith, G. D., Vella, F. Lancet, 1960, i, 1133.
3. Weatherall, D. J. ibid. 1960, ii, 835.
4. Doxiadis, S. A., Fessas, P., Valaes, T., Mastrokalos, N. ibid. 1961, i, 297.
5. Panizon, F. ibid. 1960, ii, 1903.
6. Gilles, H. M., Taylor, B. G. Ann. trop. med. Parasit. 1961, 55, 64.
7. Zannos-Mariolea, L., Kattamis, C. Blood, 1961, 18, 34.

whether or not hæmolysis can occur in the absence of a sensitising mechanism, but recent studies have shown that the red-cell survival-time in non-sensitised enzyme-deficient Negro adults is definitely shortened.[8] The results of similar studies on enzyme-deficient infant red cells will be of great interest.

Hematology Division,
Johns Hopkins Hospital,
Baltimore.   D. J. WEATHERALL.

THE CATARRHAL CHILD

SIR,—In his interesting book,[9] Dr. Fry drew certain conclusions from his experience which would appear to apply to the whole of this country. In fact the only valid conclusion which can be made applies to the situation in Beckenham, Kent, where this work was done. The problem in other parts of England and in particular in the industrial areas of the North is an entirely different one, and it is most important that this fact should be appreciated.

The College of General Practitioners, through their periodic surveys, are in a unique position to carry out research of this type, and this has already been done in certain parts of Great Britain. It is to be hoped that a complete survey will eventually be made from which it will be possible to draw accurate conclusions.

Doncaster.   PHILIP H. BEALES.

PULMONARY EMBOLISM

SIR,—I was interested in the article of Nov. 4 by Dr. Stevens, in which he discusses the problem of "unheralded pulmonary embolism" in patients who are active and ambulant when chest symptoms begin. Last year I had under my care a patient in whom this dangerous disease had apparently been precipitated by drug treatment.

An unmarried nursing sister enjoyed good general health and was in charge of a busy surgical ward. She was aged forty, and had recurrent endometriosis, for which she had had a laparotomy eight years ago, and subsequent courses of methyltestosterone. During an exacerbation of symptoms treatment was advised with a pseudopregnancy course of 'Enavid' (norethynodrel and ethinylœstradiol 3-methyl ether). Treatment was started with the recommended dose of one tablet (10 mg.) daily for two weeks, followed by two tablets (20 mg.) daily for two weeks. This treatment provoked nausea and vomiting, and she was therefore also given two antiemetic drugs, cyclizine hydrochloride and perphenazine. Despite these measures, a daily dose of 20 mg. caused continued vomiting, and so all treatment was stopped. Vomiting ceased three days later, and for a further week she ate well and led an active country life.

Unfortunately on the tenth day after stopping enavid a severe right-sided pleurisy suddenly developed, and one week later she had a sudden left-sided pleurisy. Treatment with penicillin and tetracycline had little effect, but her condition slowly improved. The diagnosis of bilateral pulmonary embolism with infarction was subsequently confirmed by chest X-ray and electrocardiograph, which showed inversion of T waves in leads 2 and 3 and V_1. Three months later the chest X-ray and E.C.G. had returned to normal. There was no clinical evidence at any time of venous thrombosis in the legs or pelvis, and she had not been confined to bed before the onset of pulmonary embolism. Presumably she had a silent thrombosis secondary to the dehydration and vomiting caused by enavid.

As accompaniments to treatment with norethynodrel, nausea is common, and vomiting not uncommon. The makers suggest ways in which the nausea may be mini-

8. Brewer, G. J., Tarlov, A. R., Kellermeyer, R. W. J. Lab. clin. Med. 1961. 58, 217.
9. See Lancet, Oct. 21, 1961, p. 925.

mised, and Dr. Venning, their medical director, repeated in your columns (Oct. 28) the undesirable consequences of premature interruption of enavid treatment. Because enavid may produce uncontrollable vomiting and provoke pulmonary embolism and infarction, I would counsel caution in the use of this widely advertised drug.

Bungay, Suffolk.   W. M. JORDAN.

SIR,—The letter from Dr. Churcher (Nov. 11) seems to imply that the earliest site of thrombosis is in the upper part of gastrocnemeii. I think many will dispute it. A daily ritual by the residents (on the surgical units at least) of systematically palpating both legs is much more likely to yield fruit by spotting postoperative thrombosis of deep veins.

Incidentally, it is hard to explain why heparin, which is only an anticoagulant, should so dramatically relieve tenderness. After all, four hours is too short a span of time to permit lysis of clot by natural mechanisms.

Gulson Hospital,
Coventry.   J. K. ANAND.

NOMENCLATURE IN GENETICS

SIR,—The nomenclature of specific clinical syndromes due to chromosomal aberrations ought to be uniform, as Dr. Gall [1] maintains. It is my impression that the best way would be to call them by the name of the main authors involved: trisomic 17-18 would be called Edwards' syndrome, trisomic 13-15 Patau's syndrome, and so on. This would avoid some confusion until the autosomes are exactly determined.

Laboratório de Genética Humana,
Universidade do Parana, Brasil.   HOMERO BRAGA.

PREGNANCY AND MALIGNANT MELANOMA

SIR,—Dr. Magnus (Oct. 7) questioned several points in your leading article of Sept. 9 concerning the effect of pregnancy upon melanoma. But he did not refer to two statements in both the papers quoted.

Firstly, in both analyses women were included who became pregnant within one year before diagnosis and five years after diagnosis. A similar period was scanned for pregnancy in the non-pregnancy group. It would therefore seem that similar periods in the history of the disease in the pregnant and non-pregnant groups were covered. Further, in the last paragraph before comment in our paper, we stated that we plotted survival figures for each patient, in both pregnant and non-pregnant groups, to compare length of survival. The same number of women died in the first year after diagnosis in the two groups.

Dr. Magnus's second point, mentioned in our paper, was that those women who were more ill might be less likely to become pregnant is certainly valid, but we do not know of any way this could be controlled. When we compared five-year survivals in pregnant and non-pregnant groups, divided into the stage of the disease, only in those patients with localised disease was there significant five-year survival, and this was slightly better in the pregnant than in the non-pregnant group. It would be difficult to distinguish a doomed patient with localised melanoma from one whose disease has been removed completely, and we cannot, therefore, explain the similarity in survival in the two groups on the basis of one group, being less ill, choosing to become pregnant.

For Dr. Magnus to conclude that the lack of significant difference in five-year survival in the pregnant compared with the non-pregnant patients with melanoma indicated a harmful effect of pregnancy seems totally unwarranted.

Children's Cancer Research
Foundation, Inc.
Boston, Massachusetts.   LAURENS P. WHITE.

1. *Lancet*, 1961, i, 673.

FROM WORDS TO WARDS

SIR,—In *From Words to Wards* of your issue of Oct. 28, the message of words is profound, succinct, and has stirred at least one administrator.

Those of us south of the Border responsible for the programme of hospital building, if we are honest with ourselves, must share the concern that your contributors express. The needs of a human hospital and the ways and means for satisfying them are indeed complex. I would support " the early establishment of a research organisation with adequate resources to initiate experimental inquiry and field studies, and with the freedom of action customarily permitted to research councils ", but my plea is that its members be men and women in touch with the realities of birth, life, and death in the machinery of a hospital.

JAMES FAIRLEY
Senior Administrative Medical Officer,
London, W.2.   South-East Metropolitan Regional Hospital Board.

SELECTIVE VAGOTOMY AND POST-VAGOTOMY DIARRHŒA

SIR,—The findings of Mr. Elliot-Smith and his colleagues (Nov. 4) concerning the incidence and severity of diarrhœa after vagotomy and after gastrectomy differ from those of some other workers. Clark [1] found both greater after vagotomy. So too have we at the West London Hospital. The report of the National Committee on Peptic Ulcer of the American Gastroenterological Association [2] confirms this increased incidence.

Although the contents of the Oxford letter suggest that there is no important difference between the incidence of diarrhœa and pale stools after any of the gastric operations, yet we are told " diarrhœa with frequent loose motions and sometimes extreme urgency and difficulty of control does occur after vagotomy but its incidence is low (2–3%) ". If this is true—and it is—would we not expect a further percentage of less severe yet troublesome cases ?

I support vagotomy in the treatment of chronic duodenal ulceration. I believe that gastric resection has no place in this disease. Yet I would be anxious about the operation if an agreed incidence (2–3%) of very severe diarrhœa and a further perhaps 4–5% of troublesome diarrhœa could not by some means be prevented.

Elliot-Smith et al. are right when they state: " It seems important to define accurately what is meant by diarrhœa. . . ." I think it is because we differ here that we in part disagree. Their definition is " three or more motions daily with loose, watery stools, often urgency or near incontinence . . .". Our experience is that although there is some improvement in these cases over the years, disability persists probably for life. This is indeed a very disturbing state of affairs, and even 2–3% is a serious complication of an operation for simple ulcer.

In all our studies we have found that the usual pattern is one of attacks with 2–4 liquid pale stools daily with urgency. These attacks last for a few days and occur perhaps every few weeks. There is also an early morning pattern with several urgent liquid motions, after which the patient is free from trouble for the day. Some of these patients have great fear of an uncontrolled bowel action before they reach their place of work. The more serious of these cases, added to the 2–3%, bring the incidence of important diarrhœa to a somewhat higher figure.

I do not wish to overemphasise the diarrhœa problem, but we must not shut our eyes to it. I believe that anterior selective vagotomy, bearing in mind the detailed anatomy of the hepatic

1. Clark, C. G. *Brit. med. J.* 1961, ii, 1250.
2. *Gastroenterology*, 1952, **22**, no. 3.

back to form the subject of further discussion. It may not be too much to hope that either the Ministry of Health or the Medical Research Council, or the Ministry through the Medical Research Council, will take the lead.

Department of Surgery,
University of Liverpool.   CHARLES WELLS.

SMOKING BY SCHOOLCHILDREN

SIR,—Your issue of Nov. 25 contains, under Public Health, yet another comment on smoking by schoolchildren. This repeated what has often been said before —namely, that there is an urgent need for increased anti-smoking education of schoolchildren and of the general population if the rising incidence of lung cancer is to be halted and reversed. Such anti-smoking education has been the function of local health authorities for the past three or four years, but there is little evidence that it is having any effect.

In my opinion the principal difficulty is that the power of the local health authority is limited, both in money and manpower, and that opposed to its efforts are those of the cigarette manufacturers who promote cigarette smoking with an energy that the local health authority cannot approach. Your issue of Oct. 28 contains the gist of an exchange in Parliament between Mr. Francis Noel-Baker and Mr. Niall Macpherson, parliamentary secretary to the Board of Trade. The latter was sceptical of the assertion that £20 million was spent on advertising tobacco in 1960 as compared with £1 million in 1953, but he did not deny that £7·7 million was expended on press and television publicity in 1960. The annual report (part I) of the Ministry of Health for 1960 (which, incidentally, devotes just 7 lines to smoking and lung cancer) also shows that local health authorities spent less on providing the midwifery service (£6·5 million) which delivered one-third of the nation's babies than the tobacco manufacturers spent on promoting the consumption of tobacco, and only a little more (£8 million) was spent on home nursing. The local authorities cannot in fact cope with this sort of expenditure devoted to one aspect only of health education, and we are fighting our battle with both hands tied behind our backs. Mr. Macpherson further denied that this advertising had been accompanied by any marked rise in tobacco consumption and gave the figure of 133 million lb. of tobacco smoked in the six months January to June, 1960, compared with 124 million lb. in the corresponding period of 1959. This is, in fact, a rise of 7%, so that the local authorities are making no headway at all!

The complacency of the authorities is difficult to understand. The number of deaths from lung cancer continue to rise from year to year. One can only conclude that even now the connection between smoking and lung cancer is not accepted in high places although, as Sir Derrick Dunlop is reported in *The Guardian* to have said last week (Dec. 1), " To deny that cigarette smoking is an important factor in the ætiology of lung cancer . . . is to carry scepticism to absurd lengths ". The authorities are possibly afraid of losing the revenue from cigarette smoking, but surely it must be appreciated that even with the most energetic efforts the decline in cigarette smoking will be very gradual over the years.

Some help must be given to local health authorities. If, in the interests of liberty (so-called), the advertising industry is to be sacrosanct, then surely an energetic national campaign should be undertaken in the newspapers and on television on the same scale as is put forth by the tobacco manufacturers. Only in this way can we feel locally that our efforts are really worth while.

Public Health Department,   ALFRED YARROW
Hadleigh, Essex.   Medical Officer of Health.

THALIDOMIDE AND CONGENITAL ABNORMALITIES

SIR,—Congenital abnormalities are present in approximately 1·5% of babies. In recent months I have observed that the incidence of multiple severe abnormalities in babies delivered of women who were given the drug thalidomide (' Distaval ') during pregnancy, as an antiemetic or as a sedative, to be almost 20%.

These abnormalities are present in structures developed from mesenchyme—i.e., the bones and musculature of the gut. Bony development seems to be affected in a very striking manner, resulting in polydactyly, syndactyly, and failure of development of long bones (abnormally short femora and radii).

Have any of your readers seen similar abnormalities in babies delivered of women who have taken this drug during pregnancy?

Hurstville, New South Wales.   W. G. McBRIDE.

*** In our issue of Dec. 2 we included a statement from the Distillers Company (Biochemicals) Ltd. referring to " reports from two overseas sources possibly associating thalidomide (' Distaval ') with harmful effects on the fœtus in early pregnancy ". Pending further investigation, the company decided to withdraw from the market all its preparations containing thalidomide.—ED.L.

THE CASUALTY DEPARTMENT

SIR,—Mr. Lamont (Nov. 25) lists a series of likely pitfalls which may befall a doctor but he talks as if these will inevitably beset him. Surely if a registered practitioner (as all casualty officers are) with a whole year of hospital training behind him has no idea how to deal with barbiturate poisoning or of the elementary rules of plastering the fault lies with the present method of medical education, not the method of staffing.

Mr. Lamont actually suggests in his proposed Utopia where all casualty officers will be consultants (able to cock a snook at all and sundry) that their work should be screened by the most junior casualty officer! He is in fact advocating that there should be a casualty department for the casualty department.

The idea that there should be a casualty consultant seems to me absurd. A specialist in not specialising I suppose. What would in fact happen if there were casualty consultants? Would they come to the department at 1 A.M. on a Saturday morning to decide whether or not the drunk has a head injury any more than the present consultants in charge of casualty departments do now? Of course not. Mr. Lamont knows this and so do I. If there is a serious doubt in the casualty officer's mind he will, as now, call in a registrar to help him—be he a medical, surgical, or orthopædic one.

Let me put the other side of the picture. I did casualty work and can honestly say that its very variety is a tonic. Of course one grumbles at the patient who comes to see you late at night complaining of an ache he has had for three days. It so happens that people are like that; and anyone who does not want to treat frail, erratic, stupid, inconsiderate, ungrateful, ill-mannered, but by and large pleasant, people, should take up pathology.

I think the present casualty arrangement is probably one of the most valuable training-grounds there is for any young man. Everyone has got to learn to take responsibility, and once he has registered the sooner the better. What better place than

mend its use as the first choice of procedure in the relief of urinary retention.

Method

The method employs the ' Bardic-Deseret Intracath ', an apparatus designed for venepuncture. It consists of an 8-in. soft, pliant plastic catheter whose end is placed within the lumen of a thin-walled large-bore needle some 2 in. long. Both catheter and needle are protected by plastic guards, and the entire unit is packaged sterile ready for immediate use.

When used in the relief of urinary retention, the introducing needle is inserted directly into the distended bladder through the abdominal wall in the midsuprapubic region. Local anæsthesia may be used to facilitate introduction but is rarely necessary. The catheter is then advanced through the lumen of the needle until several inches lie freely within the bladder cavity. The needle is then withdrawn and passed along the catheter to engage the expanded adaptor at its other end. This adaptor is connected by Luer fitting to a closed system of urine collection. The puncture wound is sealed with ' Nobecutane ' covered by a sterile dressing, and the excess of catheter firmly taped to the abdominal wall to prevent its accidental dislodgement.

Results

This method has been employed as the initial treatment of urinary retention in this hospital for several months and seems to have distinct advantages over urethral catheterisation:

Freedom from infection.—The introduction of infection into the urinary tract is virtually eliminated by adequate preparation of the suprapubic skin and continued sterile protection of the puncture site. Furthermore, bladder drainage may be maintained for long periods without catheter-induced urethritis.

Freedom from pain.—Suprapubic needle-puncture causes much less discomfort than urethral instrumentation, and discomfort can be eliminated completely by local anæsthesia. Moreover, prolonged bladder drainage is infinitely less uncomfortable by this method than by an indwelling urethral catheter.

Freedom from bladder damage.—The soft pliant plastic catheter is non-irritating and cannot damage the bladder wall, while its length prevents its accidental withdrawal into the prevesical space as the bladder contracts.

Freedom from interference with normal micturition.—While urinary retention usually occurs only in patients with mechanical bladder-neck obstruction, its onset is in most cases precipitated by some secondary incident such as alcoholic indulgence, diuresis, constipation, or confinement to bed with some other illness. A common precipitating factor nowadays is the combination of the newer powerful diuretic drugs and bed rest in the treatment of congestive cardiac failure. All surgeons are familiar with the problem of the poor-risk patient who develops urinary retention as a complication of some other grave illness and who has to be submitted to a hazardous prostatectomy after repeated catheterisation has failed to restore normal micturition.

Experience with this method has shown that, if the episode of retention can be relieved without interfering with the normal channels of micturition, the ability to void will return spontaneously in a surprisingly high proportion of patients. The surgical treatment of the underlying obstruction can then be planned at leisure and undertaken at the most favourable time.

Slight modification of the ' Bardic-Deseret Intracath ' would increase its usefulness for suprapubic bladder drainage.

The standard plastic catheter is relatively fine with a single terminal opening, and in some cases it has become blocked by hæmaturia or by the turbid deposit of grossly infected urine. The standard introducing needle being only 2 in. long, difficulty is occasionally encountered in entering the bladder in a particularly obese patient. I have suggested to the manufacturers that a modified version consisting of a longer and larger-bore catheter with lateral openings in its terminal inch, fitted to an introducing needle 3½ in. long, would overcome these disadvantages. This ' Supracath ' modification is undergoing clinical trial at present and is proving very satisfactory.

The ' Bardic-Deseret Intracath ' and its ' Supracath ' modification are manufactured by C. R. Bard, Inc., Murray Hill, New Jersey, U.S.A., and distributed in the United Kingdom by Chas. F. Thackray, Ltd., of Leeds.

FARMER'S LUNG

THERMOPHILIC ACTINOMYCETES AS A SOURCE OF "FARMER'S LUNG HAY" ANTIGEN

J. PEPYS
M.B. W'srand, M.R.C.P., M.R.C.P.E.

P. A. JENKINS
B.Sc. Wales

OF THE MEDICAL RESEARCH COUNCIL RESEARCH GROUP IN CLINICAL IMMUNOLOGY, DEPARTMENT OF MEDICINE, INSTITUTE OF DISEASES OF THE CHEST, BROMPTON, LONDON, S.W.3

G. N. FESTENSTEIN   P. H. GREGORY
M.Sc. S. Afr., Ph.D. Lpool.   D.Sc. Lond., F.R.S.

MAUREEN E. LACEY   F. A. SKINNER
                                     M.A. Cantab., Ph.D. Lond.

OF ROTHAMSTED EXPERIMENTAL STATION, HARPENDEN, HERTS

FARMER's lung results from the inhalation of dust from mouldy hay by persons who have become hypersensitive to antigens in the dust. The hypersensitivity increases with repeated exposure, and in many cases even very limited exposure may provoke severe pulmonary symptoms. Gregory and Lacey (1962, 1963a and b) showed that hay which had caused farmer's lung had evidently become heated spontaneously during maturation, that it had a higher pH than good hay, and that its dust contained more thermophilic moulds and actinomycete spores but not appreciably more herbage fragments. Pepys et al. (1962) found that precipitins against extracts of mouldy hay (known to have produced symptoms of disease) and against extracts of some microorganisms isolated from mouldy hay are present in the sera of patients with farmer's lung. But the antigens held to be important in farmer's lung, because they reacted with about 80% of the sera of affected persons, were not found in extracts of the microorganisms tested. Williams (1963) showed that inhalation by affected persons of mouldy hay extracts containing these additional antigens provoked pulmonary and systemic manifestations akin to those of farmer's lung, but inhalation of extracts of any of the isolated microorganisms which were tested did not. Similar results were reported in experiments with animals exposed to mouldy litter (Parish 1963).

To determine the source of the various antigens in mouldy hay, experimental batches of hay were tested at Rothamsted for their microbial and biochemical changes, and at the Institute of Diseases of the Chest for the development and kind of antigen. The additional antigens in mouldy hay which seem relevant to farmer's lung are here provisionally termed " farmer's lung hay " (F.L.H.) antigen.

In field experiments (to be reported elsewhere) F.L.H. antigen was found to develop in hay that had become heated spontaneously to at least 50°C. The development of F.L.H. antigen was positively correlated with increase of pH from about 6·0 to 7·0 or above, with soluble and volatile nitrogen, and with the numbers of actinomycetes, bacteria, and fungi. Some of these elements were therefore examined for their part in the development of the F.L.H. antigen in mouldy hays produced in the laboratory.

prevent torsion at fixed points, and may also help to keep the functioning coil in a favourable position for drainage.

Water balance in the system is controlled by the glucose in the solution, but the lowest concentration available (1·5 g. per 100 ml.) provides an excessive osmolarity and an undesirable negative balance.

An apparently mild cumulative effect of heparin upon the blood-thrombin time is an incidental point of interest which is receiving further study.

Prolonged peritoneal dialysis is not recommended as a permanent kidney substitute but should be effective in preserving candidates for renal transplant, and as a temporary alternative to intermittent hæmodialysis.

Our thanks are due to Dr. F. W. B. Hurlburt, chief of the department of medicine, and Dr. John Sturdy, director of the department of pathology, for encouragement and support in the project; to Dr. J. E. Newell, clinical biochemist of the hospital, for generous cooperation; and Mrs. D. Scroggs, R.N., and her staff, for management of the exchanges, and for meticulous nursing care. We are grateful to Dr. C. E. Reeve for valuable help; to Dr. Stanford N. Stordy, Dr. E. K. Pinkerton, and Dr. J. P. Piderman for referring cases; and to Mr. Dean Rachel, the hospital photographer.

The tube is manufactured by the W. E. Quinton Instrument Co., 3051, 44th Avenue, Seattle, Washington, U.S.A.

ADDENDUM

Two further communications on peritoneal dialysis in chronic renal failure have appeared. In one case treatment was maintained for 232 days by means of inlying polyvinyl catheters which were changed when necessary; the procedure was ultimately terminated by peritoneal bleeding (C. F. Gutch, S. C. Stevens, F. L. Watkins, *Ann. intern. Med.* 1964, **60**, 289). In another case the patient is being maintained after sixteen months by means of the peritoneal access cannula of Boen et al. (R. R. Schumacher, A. S. Ridolpho, B. L. Martz. *ibid.* p. 296).

RUSSELL A. PALMER
M.D. Vancouver

WAYNE E. QUINTON
B.SC. Seattle

Clinical Investigation Unit,
St. Paul's Hospital, Vancouver,
British Columbia

JOHN E. GRAY
M.D. Vancouver

VIRUS PARTICLES IN CULTURED LYMPHOBLASTS FROM BURKITT'S LYMPHOMA

INTEREST in Burkitt's malignant lymphoma [1] has centred largely on the climatic and geographical factors which determine its distribution,[2][3] since these can be taken to suggest that a transmissible vector-borne agent may be involved in causation.[4][5] As part of an investigation

into this possibility a line of lymphoblasts from a Burkitt tumour has been established in tissue culture [6] for various types of study; this communication gives a preliminary account of virus particles in cells of this line from the first two cultures examined by electron microscopy.

METHODS

Collection of cells.—The cells were taken from two separate stationary cultures after 75 and 82 days in vitro respectively; they were collected in suspension by drawing the culture fluid, in which they grow as free-floating individuals,[6] into a syringe pre-warmed to 37°C.

Preparation for electron microscopy.—The cells were fixed by

1. Burkitt, D. *Brit. J. Surg.* 1958, **46**, 218.
2. Burkitt, D. *Brit. med. J.* 1962, ii, 1019.
3. Burkitt, D. *Nature, Lond.* 1962, **194**, 232.
4. Burkitt, D. *Postgrad. med. J.* 1962, **38**, 71.
5. Burkitt, D. in International Review of Experimental Pathology (edited by G. W. Richter and M. A. Epstein); vol. 2, p. 67. New York and London, 1963.

6. Epstein, M. A., Barr, Y. M. *Lancet*, 1964, i, 252.

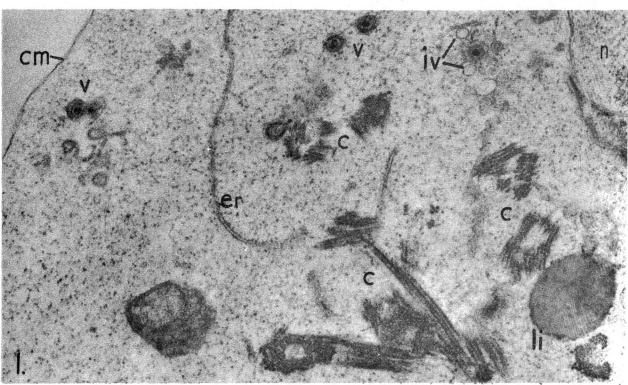

Fig. 1—Part of a cultured lymphoblast derived from a Burkitt lymphoma. The cell membrane (cm) crosses the top left corner and the nucleus (n), bounded by its double membrane, lies in the upper right portion of the field. The intervening cytoplasm contains several mature virus particles (v) within spaces enclosed by fine membranes, some immature particles (iv), and crystals (c) cut in various planes; a large lipid body (li) and endoplasmic reticulum (er) can also be seen. In addition profuse free ribosomes lie scattered throughout the cytoplasmic matrix. Electronmicrograph × 42,500.

in the efferent lymph. However, except for a transient disturbance immediately after irradiation, there was little change in the morphology of the cells of the efferent lymph.

Five preparations were stimulated antigenically 6–140 hours after the lymph-nodes had received 2000r. The resulting increases in antibody titre and the characteristic changes in the cellular composition of the lymph showed that the immunological responsiveness of the nodes had not been altered significantly by irradiation.

These results suggest that the functional capacity of the lymphoid component of a lymph-node depends substantially on the entry of recirculating lymphocytes derived from the pool of lymphocytes in the body rather than on the primary production of lymphocytes within the node.

We are indebted to Dr. R. D. Brock, of the Division of Plant Industry, Commonwealth Scientific and Industrial Research Organisation, for making X-ray facilities available to us, and for his help and advice during the irradiation procedures.

Department of Experimental
Pathology, John Curtin School
of Medical Research,
Australian National University,
Canberra, Australia

J. G. HALL
M.B. Lond.

BEDE MORRIS
B.V.SC. Sydney, D.PHIL. Oxon.

A NEW ADRENERGIC BETA-RECEPTOR ANTAGONIST

PRONETHALOL was shown by Black and Stephenson [1] to be a specific adrenergic β-receptor antagonist which was relatively free from sympathomimetic activity on the cardiovascular system. Clinically, pronethalol has been shown to be of potential value in the treatment of various cardiac disorders.[2-7] The clinical investigation of pronethalol has, however, been limited, partly by the presence of undesirable side-effects in man, and partly because of a particular toxic effect in mice. The side-effects in man include lightheadedness and slight incoordination followed by nausea and vomiting. These side-effects may be due to a non-specific action of pronethalol on the central nervous system, since in animals acute toxicity of central nervous origin occurs with both the $(+)-$ active and the $(-)-$ inactive isomers. Toxicity studies in animals showed that pronethalol was free from chronic toxicity in rats and dogs, but that mice developed lymphosarcomas and reticulum-cell sarcomas, which were first seen in the thymus.[8] A large number of compounds have now been made and tested in an effort to find one with a wider therapeutic ratio than pronethalol and with no carcinogenic potential. Compound I.C.I. 45,520 ('Inderal') has been found to satisfy these criteria.

I.C.I. 45,520 is 1-isopropylamino-3-(1-naphthyloxy)-2-propanol hydrochloride:

$$O \cdot CH_2 \cdot CH(OH) \cdot CH_2 \cdot NH \cdot CH(CH_3)_2 \cdot HCl$$

I.C.I. 45,520.

1. Black, J. W., Stephenson, J. S. Lancet, 1962, ii, 311.
2. Stock, J. P. P., Dale, N. Brit. med. J. 1963, ii, 1230.
3. Dornhorst, A. C., Laurence, D. R. ibid. p. 1250.
4. Alleyne, G. A. O., Dickinson, C. J., Dornhorst, A. C., Fulton, R. M., Green, K. G., Hill, I. D., Hurst, P., Laurence, D. R., Pilkington, T., Prichard, B. N. S., Robinson, B., Rosenheim, M. L. ibid. p. 1266.
5. Payne, J. P., Senfield, R. M. ibid. 1964, i, 603.
6. Honey, M., Chamberlain, D. A., Howard, J. Circulation Res. (in the press).
7. Johnstone, M. G. Brit. J. Anæsth. (in the press).
8. Paget, G. E. Brit. med. J. 1963, ii, 1266.

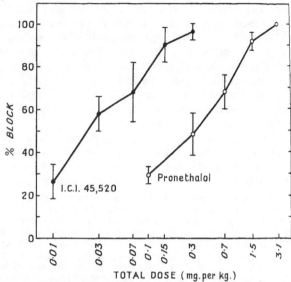

Effect of I.C.I. 45,520 and pronethalol on increments in myocardial tension produced by isoprenaline (results expressed as percentage block of control responses).

This new compound has essentially the same pharmacological properties as pronethalol. The β-adrenergic blocking activity of the two compounds has been compared in anæsthetised dogs and on the isolated sino-atrial-node preparation of the guineapig. Dogs were anæsthetised with intravenous pentobarbitone; and increments in isometric tension, produced by intravenous isoprenaline, were recorded from a strain-gauge arch sutured to the left ventricle. The accompanying figure shows the effects of increasing doses of pronethalol and of I.C.I. 45,520 on the responses to isoprenaline. These findings show that I.C.I. 45,520 is about ten times as active in blocking the inotropic action of isoprenaline. The effect of I.C.I. 45,520 and pronethalol on the chronotropic effect of adrenaline was investigated on an isolated guineapig sinoatrial node preparation. The amounts of pronethalol and I.C.I. 45,520 required to produce 50% antagonism of a maximum increase in rate produced by adrenaline (E.D.$_{50}$) were as follows:

				E.D.$_{50}$ (μg. per ml. bath fluid)
Pronethalol	..	..	..	$0 \cdot 172 \pm 0 \cdot 04$
I.C.I. 45,520	..	..	..	$0 \cdot 015 \pm 0 \cdot 003$

These results confirm that I.C.I. 45,520 is about ten times more active than pronethalol.

Estimates of acute lethal toxicity were made in mice. The L.D.$_{50}$ was 30–40 mg. per kg. body-weight for male mice and 40–50 mg. per kg. for female mice when the drug was given intravenously. Under the same conditions, the L.D.$_{50}$ for pronethalol was 45–50 mg. per kg. body-weight for male and female mice.

I.C.I. 45,520, 200 mg. per kg., was administered orally to thirty male and thirty female mice for sixty-six weeks. No tumours were found in the mice. In a comparable series of experiments with pronethalol, thymic tumours began to appear after ten weeks' treatment.

Experience with this drug in man confirms that effective β-blockade is achieved at about a tenth of the dose needed for pronethalol, and at the effective blocking dose there is no production of lightheadedness or incoordination.

In conclusion, I.C.I. 45,520 is an adrenergic β-receptor antagonist which has a therapeutic ratio about ten times greater than that of pronethalol. It has not caused thymic tumours in mice, and in man does not produce the side-

MAY 16, 1964   NEW INVENTIONS   THE LANCET   1081

effects associated with pronethalol. The evidence suggests that I.C.I. 45,520 should have extended clinical evaluation.

J. W. BLACK
M.B. St. And.

A. F. CROWTHER
M.A., PH.D. Cantab.

R. G. SHANKS
B.SC., M.D. Belf.

L. H. SMITH

A. C. DORNHORST
M.D. Lond., F.R.C.P.

Imperial Chemical Industries, Ltd.,
Pharmaceuticals Division, Research
Department, Alderley Park, Cheshire

Medical Unit, St. George's Hospital,
London, S.W.1

New Inventions

IMPROVED ALARM DEVICE FOR KOLFF TWIN-COIL KIDNEY

DURING dialysis the hydrostatic pressure in the circuit of the Kolff twin-coil artificial kidney must be watched continuously. In particular, if the pressure, which may fluctuate unexpectedly, rises above 300 mm. Hg, the coil may burst. Recently, an alarm device to warn against excessive coil pressures was described by Bienenstock and Shaldon[1]: the electrical circuit was completed when a mercury column rose above a pre-set level; an alarm bell rang and a relay switch cut out the pump motor. Two $4\frac{1}{2}$ V batteries were used to supply the circuit.

Bienenstock and Shaldon's device is simple but has disadvantages. First, after the pump motor has been cut out, the coil pressure falls and the electrical circuit is interrupted: the pump motor re-starts and the pressure rises, whereupon the pump is again cut out. Thus, the motor stops and starts repeatedly until measures are taken to reduce the coil pressure. Secondly, should a fault develop in the electrical circuit of the alarm during dialysis, the pump continues to operate and high pressures may be generated while the attendant medical staff, unaware of the fault, are relying on the alarm.

We have devised compact equipment which overcomes these drawbacks, and which incorporates a mercury manometer to show the coil pressure whether or not the alarm is in use (fig. 1). Circuit details are shown in fig. 2. The relay and bell are supplied with 4 V d.c. from the a.c. mains through a transformer and rectifier, thus dispensing with batteries. One

1. Bienenstock, J., Shaldon, S. *Lancet*, 1963, ii, 815.

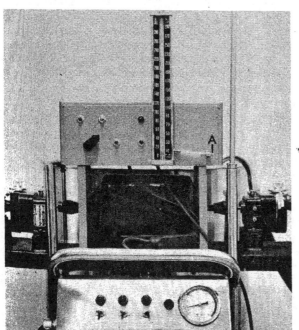

Fig. 1—Alarm equipment incorporating a mercury manometer.

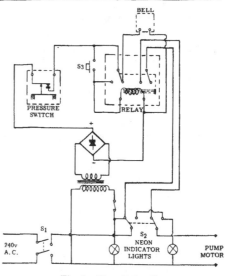

Fig. 2—Circuit details.

set of relay contacts controls the bell and energising coil of the relay itself; the other (heavy-duty contacts) controls the pump motor. A diaphragm-type pressure switch has "normally closed" contacts in series with the relay coil. S_1 is the main switch, and a changeover switch S_2 enables the pump motor to be switched directly on to the mains supply; pilot lights indicate whether the motor is operating directly or through the alarm circuit.

Before the start of dialysis the pressure lead from the bubble-traps is connected with tubing (disposable recipient set extension tubing* is suitable) to the Luer mount at A in fig. 1. When S_1 is closed the bell rings, thus testing the alarm system. Then the push switch S_3 is pressed: the relay is energised and the contacts change over, starting the pump motor and stopping the bell. If the pressure in the system rises high enough (250 mm. Hg in this case) to separate the pressure switch contacts, the relay opens, the bell rings, and the motor stops. The motor cannot re-start until the pressure is lowered and the push switch S_3 is again pressed. The mode of operation ensures that failure in the alarm-circuit supply or discontinuity in the relay-energising circuit immediately shuts off the pump. The device thus "fails safe". In the event of such a failure, however, dialysis may be continued by switching the pump motor directly on to the mains supply through S_2, in the full knowledge that the alarm is not in the circuit.

The alarm is particularly useful when high coil pressures are deliberately used to augment ultrafiltration.

A. J. LOW

N. A. MATHESON
M.B. Aberd., F.R.C.S., F.R.C.S.E.

Departments of Surgery
and Medical Physics,
University of Aberdeen

INSTRUMENT FOR EMERGENCY LARYNGOTOMY

EMERGENCY tracheostomy for the relief of obstructive laryngeal dyspnœa may be needed urgently to save life and can be very difficult. Yet any doctor may, at a moment's notice, be called on to undertake such an operation.

The easiest way of getting air into the lungs in a hurry is to make a small cut in the skin over the larynx in the midline,

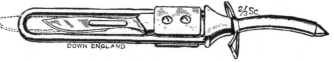

and then open the membrane between the cricoid and thyroid cartilages and slip in a small cannula. This can be left in for a few hours until the patient can be taken to hospital, and, if the obstruction is still present, a leisurely tracheostomy *below* the first ring of the trachea can be carried out in an operating-theatre and then the laryngotomy cannula can be removed.

The small combined instrument shown in the accompanying figure comprises a knife and a laryngotomy cannula and can be carried easily in the pocket or a bag, and in the casualty department and certain wards of hospitals. Though not often needed, it may enable a life to be saved by any doctor at any

* Capon Heaton & Co. Ltd., Stirchley, Birmingham, 30.

1254   JUNE 12, 1965   PRELIMINARY COMMUNICATIONS   THE LANCET

phylactic penicillin and those not so treated. Since other workers have demonstrated the harmful effects of antibiotic prophylaxis, we consider that the use of penicillin prophylactically should be abandoned in the "clean" unconscious poisoned patient.

SUMMARY

In order to determine the incidence of respiratory infection in unconscious poisoned patients, and the value of prophylactic penicillin in the prevention of these infections, 177 consecutive cases were considered.

144 patients were admitted to the trial. Of 71 not given penicillin, 5 became infected; and, of 73 receiving prophylactic penicillin, 3 became infected. In most instances the infection was not severe.

33 patients were excluded from the trial. 18 developed infection, which was often serious.

Unconscious poisoned patients, on admission, can readily be designated "clean" or "unclean"—i.e., already infected or, because of aspiration, likely to be so. Prophylactic penicillin should not be given to the former, but most "unclean" patients develop serious respiratory infections which require energetic treatment.

Preliminary Communications

FOLIC ACID METABOLISM AND HUMAN EMBRYOPATHY

THE effect of folate deficiency on the development of rat embryos has been shown by Nelson.[1] Those embryos which were not resorbed were almost all malformed. Fœtal malformations have also been reported after giving a folic acid antagonist, aminopterin, to pregnant women.[2][3] The malformations were varied, but were all severe.

A study in Liverpool suggested a possible relationship between fœtal malformation and defective folate metabolism in the mother,[4] and we have investigated this possibility in greater detail.

MATERIAL AND METHODS

In 1964, 98 women (in the five main maternity units in Liverpool) gave birth to infants with severe malformations, principally of the central nervous system.

A formiminoglutamic acid (FIGLU) excretion test was done as soon as the malformation was diagnosed prenatally, or within 2 to 3 days of delivery for all 98 mothers. The assay technique, using high-voltage electrophoresis, was that described by Hibbard.[5]

We tried to match each mother with one delivered of a normal infant in the same hospital. These controls were selected with respect to the following criteria: age (± 2 years), parity ($\pm$ one pregnancy, except primiparæ who were matched with primiparæ), and the time of conception and gestation (± 2 weeks).

Of 98 mothers of malformed infants, 54 were matched satisfactorily with controls.

Assays of FIGLU excretion were completed prior to collation with clinical data.

RESULTS

The results of FIGLU excretion tests in these patients are shown in the accompanying table.

DISCUSSION

There seems to be a significant relationship between malformation of the fœtus and defective folate metabolism

RESULTS OF FIGLU EXCRETION TESTS IN 98 MOTHERS OF MALFORMED INFANTS

Mothers	FIGLU excretion test		Total	% FIGLU-positive
	Positive	Negative		
Of all malformed infants ..	61	37	98	62
Of all infants with C.N.S. malformations	48	25	73	66
Matched pairs:				
Mothers of malformed infants	35	19	54	65
Mothers of normal infants	8	46	54	17
Mothers of infants with C.N.S. malformation	24	11	35	69
Mothers of normal infants	6	29	35	17

in the mother. 11·4% of 167 women attending one of the hospitals in this study had positive FIGLU tests.[4] The women delivered of malformed infants show an incidence which is approximately 5 times this normal.

The results are based on the investigation of a metabolic defect present in late pregnancy or immediately after delivery and do not necessarily indicate that such a defect was present at the time of embryogenesis. Furthermore, a positive FIGLU test may indicate defective absorption or metabolism rather than deficient intake of folate. The familial occurrence of serious nervous system malformations might be mediated, in some instances, through a genetically determined defect of folate metabolism.

This investigation could not have been completed without the cooperation of the medical and nursing staff of the obstetric units of Mill Road Maternity Hospital, Liverpool Maternity Hospital, Broadgreen Hospital, Sefton General Hospital, and Walton Hospital. We also thank Miss E. R. Chinn who supervised the collection of specimens and data. We are indebted for financial assistance to the United Liverpool Hospitals Research Committee.

ELIZABETH D. HIBBARD
M.D. Aberd., D.OBST.

Department of Obstetrics
and Gynæcology,
University of Liverpool, and
Alder Hey Children's Hospital,
Liverpool

R. W. SMITHELLS
M.B. Lond., M.R.C.P.,
M.R.C.P.E., D.C.H.

KETOSIS-RESISTANT YOUNG DIABETICS

DIABETICS below the age of 40 ("growth-onset" diabetics), who do not develop ketoacidosis even in the absence of insulin therapy, have recently attracted much attention. In tropical countries some characterisation of such cases is being attempted as regards body-build, insulin-dosage, or response to oral sulphonylureas, although no distinct biochemical or metabolic variation has yet been ascribed to this group.

Stephen and Kinsell[6] have suggested that there is a significant islet-cell reserve in cases which respond satisfactorily to a very low carbohydrate diet and treatment with sulphonylureas.

In this Institute 27% of cases with "growth-onset" diabetes did not develop ketoacidosis when no insulin was given to them for periods of up to 30 days.[7] Plasma-insulin-like activity and response to oral sulphonylureas have been studied in 15 cases of ketoacidosis-resistant "growth-onset" diabetes. This group comprised 8 males and 7 females, with ages ranging from 12 to 32 years (mean 23 years). The duration of the disease in these cases was 2 weeks to 5 years (mean 13·55 months); in 8·cases the duration of the disease was less than 1 year.

The plasma-insulin-activity values, done by the rat-

1. Nelson, M. M. *Ciba Fdn Symp.* 1960. Congenital Malformations. London.
2. Goetsch, C. *Am. J. Obstet. Gynec.* 1962, **83**, 1474.
3. Thiersch, J. B. *Ciba Fdn Symp.* 1960. Congenital Malformations. London.
4. Hibbard, B. M. *J. Obstet. Gynæc. Br. Commonw.* 1964, **71**, 529.
5. Hibbard, E. D. *Lancet*, 1964, ii, 1146.
6. Stephen, C., Kinsell, L. W. *Lancet*, 1963, ii, 764.
7. Ahuja, M. M. S., Varma, V. M., Kumar, A. *Congr. int. Diabetes Fed.* Toronto, 1964.

The Lancet · Saturday 19 February 1966

CHROMOSOME ANALYSIS OF HUMAN AMNIOTIC-FLUID CELLS

MARK W. STEELE
M.D. New York
RESEARCH ASSOCIATE IN CYTOGENETICS,
SOUTHBURY TRAINING SCHOOL, SOUTHBURY, CONNECTICUT

W. ROY BREG, Jr.
M.D. Yale
ASSISTANT CLINICAL PROFESSOR OF PEDIATRICS,
YALE UNIVERSITY SCHOOL OF MEDICINE

WHEN Fuchs and Riis (Fuchs and Riis 1956, Fuchs 1960, Riis and Fuchs 1960) reported on the practicality of six-chromatin determinations on human amniotic-fluid cells obtained by amniocentesis, the cytogenetic study of the human fœtus in utero by culturing these cells became theoretically possible (Austin 1962). In the study reported here we tried to find out: (1) whether human amniotic fluid contained viable cells; (2) if so, whether these could be grown in tissue culture and in quantity for karyotype analysis; (3) whether the cells were fœtal in origin; and (4) whether the technique for determining the sex-chromatin of these cells could be made more reliable.

Methods

Samples of amniotic fluid were obtained by serial abdominal amniocentesis from patients with a suspected erythroblastotic fœtus, starting at 20–37 weeks' gestation. The samples were stored in vacuum containers at 2·5°C for 1 to 3 days, and care was taken to maintain sterility and avoid contamination with maternal cells. So far, 52 specimens have been collected from 35 subjects.

Viability Staining

The amniotic-fluid cell suspension was stained for viability by the trypan-blue method described by Merchant et al. (1960). To 0·1 ml. of amniotic-fluid cell suspension was added 0·02 ml. of 0·4% trypan-blue. After incubating for 5 minutes at 37°C, the stained and unstained cells were counted in all 18 squares of a standard hæmocytometer. Counts were repeated on the 3rd day after amniocentesis. (The cell count × 667 = cells per ml. of amniotic fluid.)

Sex-chromatin Determination

The rest of the amniotic-fluid specimen was centrifuged at 800 r.p.m. for 6 minutes, and the supernatant amniotic fluid was discarded. The residual cell button was resuspended in 2–3 ml. of one of several growth media (see below). Half of this cell suspension was centrifuged at 800 r.p.m. for 6 minutes, and the supernatant growth medium was discarded. The cell button was suspended in 3 ml. of fixative (95% of 95% ethanol and 5% of glacial acetic acid) for 30 minutes. The fixed mixture was again centrifuged, and all but $^1/_4$–$^1/_2$ ml. of fixative was removed. Two drops of the cell suspension on a clean dry glass slide were quickly dried in air, hydrolysed in 5 N hydrochloric acid at room temperature for 20 minutes, stained with thionin for 8 minutes, and mounted. Only well-spread, oval-to-round, lightly stained nuclei were selected for counting. 50 to 100 cells were counted in each case. Fœtal sex was taken to be male if sex chromatin was less than 3%, and female if 12% or more.

7434

Cell Culture

The other half of the cell suspension in growth medium was placed either in a standard ' Pyrex' Leighton tube or in a standard pyrex 199 ml. milk dilution bottle (either empty or containing a layer of irradiated feeder fibroblast cells) for culture. Growth medium at pH 7·2 was added, some of the cultures were gassed with 5% CO_2 in air, and all were incubated at 37°C (see accompanying table).

The following growth media were used:

I. Medium 199 plus the aminoacids, vitamin, and L-glutamine components of an equal quantity of Eagle's basal medium, plus 12% fœtal-calf serum, 12% human serum, and 50 units per ml. of penicillin-streptomycin.

II. A similar medium, but with calf serum instead of fœtal-calf serum.

III. A similar medium, but with 30% calf serum and no human serum.

IV. McCoy's modified medium A, containing L-glutamine and 30% fœtal-calf serum.

V. Diploid Growth Media (GIBCO).

Used media nos. 2 and 4 were also prepared by incubation at 37°C for 24 hours with a human fibroblast culture layer, followed by filtration through a 0·20 μ millipore filter.

Karyotyping

If growth was sufficient for karyotyping the monolayer was removed from the culture container with trypsin, the cells were incubated with 1% sodium citrate for 30 minutes at 37°C, fixed in glacial acetic acid and methanol (1/3) overnight (changing the fixative 2 to 3 times), fixed for another 30 minutes in 45% acetic acid, and resuspended in acetic acid/methanol fixative (1/3). 2 drops of the fixed-cell suspension on a clean glass slide were dried in air or a flame and stained in aceto-orcein for 30 minutes.

Results

Sex-chromatin

Of the 21 babies in our series born so far, our prediction of the fœtal sex has been accurate in all cases. In the 14 boys the fœtal sex-chromatin ranged from 0 to 2%. In the 7 girls it was between 12% and 34%. 1 case showed an intermediate value (6%), but the neonatal sex of the baby, which was stillborn, is not known.

Trypan-blue Viability Staining (fig. 1)

In 9 cases the mean number of unstained cells fell from 20,000 per ml. (range 4300–39,000) 24 hours after

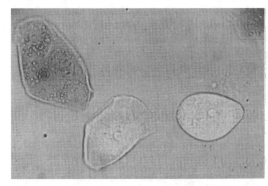

Fig. 1—Amniotic-fluid cells.

One non-viable cell has taken up trypan-blue stain; two viable cells remain unstained.

H

EFFECTS OF SALICYLATES ON HUMAN PLATELETS

J. R. O'BRIEN

M.A., D.M. Oxon., F.C.Path.

CONSULTANT HÆMATOLOGIST,

PORTSMOUTH AND ISLE OF WIGHT AREA PATHOLOGICAL SERVICE, MILTON ROAD, PORTSMOUTH

Summary   Platelet-rich plasma (P.R.P.) normally responds to a variety of agents by aggregation. P.R.P. prepared from the plasma of volunteers who had ingested aspirin responded abnormally to five of these agents (adrenaline, tendon extract, A.D.P., triethyl tin, and centrifugation); the normal response to all these agents is thought to involve release of intrinsic A.D.P. A number of other tests (immediate responses to A.D.P., serotonin, and adrenaline, and the addition of glass beads) were unchanged. Thus it seems that in most, but not all, circumstances A.D.P. is not released by platelets exposed to aspirin; electron-microscopical appearances are compatible with this failure. Sodium salicylate was much less effective than aspirin, so it seems that the short-lived intact aspirin molecule is responsible. Abnormalities, which could be elucidated after ingestion of subclinical (150 mg.) doses of aspirin, were corrected by 10% v/v of normal P.R.P. and, spontaneously, in about the time it would take for new platelets to be formed. These findings suggest that aspirin produces a specific and permanent damage to some enzyme pathway in the platelet or perhaps, at its membrane. Megakaryocyte precursors may also be affected.

Introduction

THE release of adenosine diphosphate (A.D.P.) from stimulated platelets may contribute to the adhesion of more platelets to those already stuck to a site of injury. Such a release mechanism (Grette 1962) clearly could be of great physiological importance. Two waves of aggregation, with independent kinetics, ensue when adrenaline is added to stirred platelet-rich plasma (P.R.P.). O'Brien (1963a) suggested that intrinsic A.D.P. was released from the platelets and caused the second wave. Hovig (1963) and Spaet and Zucker (1964) showed that platelets released A.D.P. when mixed with tendon extract containing collagen. The second wave of aggregation that sometimes happens when a critical concentration of A.D.P. is added to P.R.P. may also be due to the release of intrinsic A.D.P. (MacMillan 1966). The release of A.D.P. and, probably, the degranulation of platelets may, at least in part, be due to the close apposition of platelet to platelet or to some other surface (O'Brien 1968a, Zucker and Peterson 1968); for example, added adrenaline only causes degranulation and release of intrinsic A.D.P. if the P.R.P. is stirred and aggregates form; in unstirred P.R.P. there is no aggregation and no degranulation, and A.D.P. is not released.

Aspirin interferes with this release reaction. (1) Normally when A.D.P. is added to P.R.P., serotonin (5-H.T.) is released from the platelets and factor 3 becomes available; these responses and platelet aggregation induced by connective tissue are inhibited if the donor has previously taken aspirin (Zucker and Peterson 1968). (2) Weiss and Aledort (1967) reported that aspirin ingestion prolongs bleeding-time, confirming the work of Gast (1964), decreases the platelet aggregation caused by adding connective-tissue fragments (collagen), and lowers the release of intrinsic A.D.P., but primary aggregation induced by adding extrinsic A.D.P. is unaffected. (3) Evans et al. (1967) showed that aspirin added in vitro has similar specific inhibitory effects.

These findings, which suggest that aspirin alters platelet metabolism in a specific way, similar perhaps to that produced by chlorpromazine (Mills and Roberts 1967), are not only of great academic interest; they could be of therapeutic value since aspirin medication might alter the course of thrombosis.

The effect of aspirin has been explored further, and enlarges on work briefly mentioned elsewhere (O'Brien 1968b).

Methods

The methods were essentially those of O'Brien et al. (1966) and O'Brien and Heywood (1967). Citrated (final concentration 0·32%) P.R.P. is stirred at 37°C, and the degree of dispersion of the platelets is sensitively and continuously monitored by recording the light transmission with a pen recorder coupled to the photocell. Various aspects of the resulting tracings (fig. 1) can be measured.

The *reaction-time* in seconds is taken from the moment an aggregating agent is added until the first immediate wave of aggregation ceases, when either disaggregation begins or the tracing becomes horizontal. The *slope* is a measure of the rate of aggregation, a high figure indicating rapid aggregation. With adrenaline there is often a *delay* after the first wave of aggregation before a second wave starts. The *slope* of the second wave is also measured. After the addition of a tendon suspension—called " collagen " for short—there is normally a *delay*, measured in seconds, before aggregation begins. This aggregation (with a measured slope) and that of the second wave of aggregation following the addition of adrenaline, normally always proceed to completion with the formation of coarse aggregates when very few free platelets remain.

Aggregation following the addition of 0·46 g. of glass beads requires heparinised blood at 24°C. The tracing obtained is similar to that of collagen with a *delay* and then a wave of aggregation with a measuring *slope*.

The following is a method to show that centrifugation, in the absence of any added aggregating agent, will normally cause the release from platelets of an aggregating agent, presumably intrinsic A.D.P. 1·0 ml. of normal citrated P.R.P. is centrifuged at 3000 r.p.m. for 4 minutes and the tube is then incubated at 37°C for 5 minutes. 0·9 ml. of the supernatant platelet-poor-plasma (P.P.P.) is transferred to 2 ml. of substrate P.R.P. stirred at 37°C. This addition normally causes the substrate P.R.P. to aggregate showing that an aggregating agent has been transferred. If P.P.P. 1-hour old is centrifuged or if the centrifugation of the P.R.P. is omitted then, when samples are transferred to the substrate plasma, no aggregation develops.

Electron Microscopy

P.R.P. after suitable treatment was fixed by rapidly transferring an equal volume of P.R.P. into buffered 2% osmium tetraoxide at 37°C. The platelets were then centrifuged into a button, dehydrated, and embedded in ' Epikote 812 '; the sections were stained with uranyl acetate and then lead citrate.

Serum-salicylate Levels

These were estimated by the method of Trinder (1954).

DR. WALSHE: REFERENCES—*continued*

Uzman, L. L. (1953) Am. J. med. Sci. 226, 645.
— (1957) Archs Path. 64, 464.
— Denny Brown, D. (1948) Am. J. med. 215, 599.
— Hood, B. (1952) ibid. 223, 392.
Varley, H. (1962) Practical Clinical Biochemistry. New York.
Walshe, J. M. (1956) Am. J. Med. 21, 487.
— (1960) Lancet, i, 188.
— (1963) Clin. Sci. 25, 405.
— (1967) Brain, 90, 149.
— (1968a) in International Symposium on Wilson's disease, Tokyo, 1966. New York (in the press).
— (1968b) in Liver Disease (edited by Leon Schiff). Philadelphia and Montreal (in the press).
— Clarke (1965) Archs Dis. Childh. 40, 651.

1174   JUNE 1, 1968   PRELIMINARY COMMUNICATIONS   THE LANCET

injected intravenously was similar in the two groups of animals. Excretion began 1 minute after the injection, reached a peak at the 10th minute, and then decreased rapidly. Again the biliary pigment was made up of 20% unconjugated and 80% conjugated bilirubin. As expected, the pigment concentration in plasma decreased rapidly in both groups of animals.

The unconjugated pigment which appears in the bile of Gunn rats cannot be the fraction injected intravenously

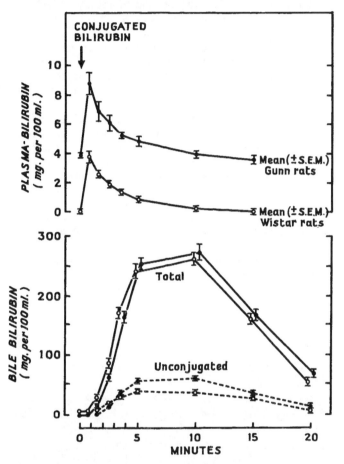

Fig. 2—Mean changes of plasma and bile bilirubin concentrations after intravenous injection of conjugated bilirubin.

with the bile because we had demonstrated in our first experiment that Gunn rats do not eliminate unconjugated bilirubin. Therefore the unconjugated pigment excreted in the bile must have entered the liver as conjugated and must have been deconjugated by passing through.

The presence of a high concentration of β-glucuronidase in the liver is well known. This enzyme may contribute to the intrahepatic hydrolysis of bilirubin glucuronide.

This work was supported by grant no. 4782.3 from the Swiss National Foundation for Scientific Research. We thank Mrs. S. Madarasz-Stucki and Miss M.-M. Bertholet for technical assistance, Prof. E. Fiaschi of the Department of Medicine, the University of Padua, Dr. D. Gardiol, of the Institute of Anatomical Pathology, Mr. A. Gautier, of the Centre for Electron Microscopy, and Dr. D. Regoli, of the Institute of Pharmacology, University of Lausanne, for helpful advice, and Mr. R. L. Pierson, of the National Institutes of Health, Bethesda, U.S.A., for supplying the Gunn rats.

Requests for reprints should be addressed to P.M., Hôpital Nestlé, 1005 Lausanne, Switzerland.

REFERENCES

Acocella, G., Tenconi, L. T., Armas-Merino, R., Raia, S., Billing, B. H. (1968) Lancet, i, 68.
Arias, I. M., Johnson, L., Wolfson, S. (1961) Am. J. Physiol. 200, 1091.
Michaelsson, M. (1961) Scand. J. clin. Invest. 13, 1.
Ostrow, J. D. (1967) J. clin. Invest. 46, 2035.
Schmid, R., Axelrod, J., Hammaker, L., Swarm, R. L. (1958) ibid. 37, 1123.

Preliminary Communications

SURVIVAL OF SKIN HETEROGRAFTS UNDER TREATMENT WITH ANTILYMPHOCYTIC SERUM

Summary   Mice under chronic treatment with anti-lymphocytic serum (A.L.S.) will accept skin grafts from donors of very distant genetical relationships—e.g., from guineapigs, rabbits, or human beings. It is inferred that in this experimental situation, though not necessarily in others, the opposition to heterografts is wholly or predominantly immunological in nature. If this interpretation is valid, it should be possible to induce some degree of immunological tolerance of heterografts in adult animals, so that the grafts remain alive after the administration of A.L.S. has ceased.

INTRODUCTION

IT is now confidently assumed that the factors which normally prohibit the transplantation of homografts are immunological in nature. No such assumption can be made of grafts that transcend a species boundary— "heterografts." It is easy to imagine other than purely immunological reasons why a human skin-graft should be unable to survive transplantation to a mouse—e.g., a heightened form of "allogeneic inhibition",[1] an infection of the graft by viruses carried by but innocuous to mice, the toxicity of metabolites, or a failure of the mouse to supply factors essential for the growth or survival of human tissue. Immunological factors must nevertheless be of real importance, for the survival in mice of rat[2] or human[3] skin or of certain human tumours[4] can be significantly prolonged by the administration of anti-lymphocytic serum (A.L.S.). Our present evidence makes a case for thinking that, in some experimental situations, immunological factors are not merely important but all-important: we find that, under chronic treatment with A.L.S., mice can accept skin-grafts from human beings or guineapigs without immunological opposition.

METHODS

Antiserum against mouse thymocytes was raised in New Zealand White rabbits by the simple method advocated by Levey and Medawar.[3][5] The serum was decomplemented, absorbed with mouse red cells, and sterilised by filtration. All recipients of grafts were adult male CBA mice maintained on 0·25 ml. A.L.S. given subcutaneously twice a week during the period of the experiment, usually after a priming dose of 1·0 ml. spread over the week before grafting. Human skin was in the form of thin split-thickness grafts about 1 sq. cm. in area. (These were kindly supplied by Prof. R. Y. Calne and Mr. J. M. Boak from material left over in skin-grafting operations.) Rabbit and guinea-pig skin-grafts were taken from the ear, and rat skin-grafts from the tail. As with homografts of skin in mice, the grafts were protected for from eight to eleven days by a light plaster casing.

RESULTS

The results of these experiments are illustrated in the accompanying photographs.

Fig. 1 shows a guineapig ear skin-graft six and a half weeks after transplantation. The mice carrying these

1. See Möller, G., Möller, E. Ann. N.Y. Acad. Sci. 1966, 129, 735.
2. Monaco, A. P., Wood, M. L., Gray, J. G., Russell, P. S. J. Immun. 1966, 96, 229.
3. Levey, R. H., Medawar, P. B. Proc. natn. Acad. Sci. 1966, 56, 1130.
4. Phillips, B., Gazet, J-C. Nature, Lond. 1967, 215, 548.
5. Levey, R. H., Medawar, P. B. Ann. N.Y. Acad. Sci. 1966, 129, 164.

grafts had already received and had very slowly rejected guineapig ear skin-grafts over a period of fifty days before the definitive grafts were transplanted, so that the graft illustrated ranks as a " second set " heterograft. The right of the photograph shows the medullated pigmented hairs characteristic of the trunk skin of CBA mice. The guinea-pig graft is distinguished by slender, unpigmented, and non-medullated hairs. Sebaceous glands have differentiated, and new hair-follicles are in process of formation. There is a mild mononuclear reaction in the

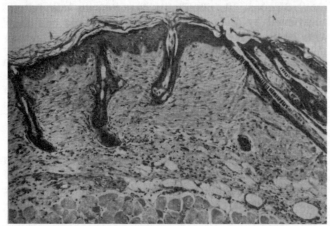

Fig. 1—Guineapig ear skin-graft six and a half weeks after transplantation to a mouse.
Reduced by half from × 140.

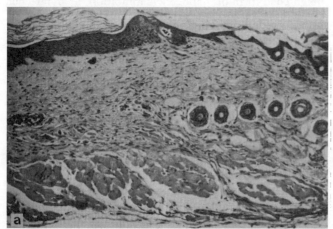

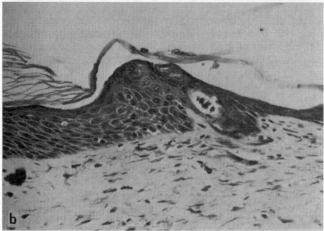

Fig. 2—Human split-thickness skin-graft three weeks after transplantation to a mouse.
(a) Mouse skin on the right. (Reduced by half from × 140.)
(b) Showing two clearly distinguished kinds of epidermal epithelium. (Reduced by half from × 350).

deeper layers of the dermis, which is abnormally thickened. These grafts underwent slow contraction, as if the collagenous matter were being removed by a process perhaps akin to that which causes the slow disappearance of the collagenous remnants of homografts.[6]

Fig. 2 illustrates the condition of human split-thickness skin-grafts three weeks after transplantation. Mouse skin occupies the right side of fig. 2a, and fig. 2b shows that the two kinds of epidermal epithelium can be distinguished down to an intercellular boundary. The human dermal collagen is well preserved and the dermis is unswollen, though it is more cellular than normal skin.

Fig. 3 illustrates the condition of such grafts at two months—i.e., five weeks later. Signs of a cellular reaction in the dermis have now disappeared, but the human epidermis is persistently hyperplastic. Blood and lymphatic capillaries are patent.

Mice such as these, in which graft rejection processes. have been abrogated by chronic treatment with A.L.S., do not discriminate between degrees of " foreignness " in skin-grafts. Distinctions became apparent when inactivation was partial or recovery was allowed to occur. Four sets of mice received 2·0 ml. A.L.S. spread over ten days and were given grafts of A-strain mouse-tail skin, C57Bl6 mouse-tail skin, August rat-tail skin, and rabbit-ear skin, respectively, one day after the first injection of A.L.S. The survival-times of the grafts fell into the order A > C57 > rat > rabbit, the median values ranging from over 50 to under 15 days at the two extremes. It is

6. Medawar, P. B. *J. Anat., Lond.* 1945, **79**, 157.

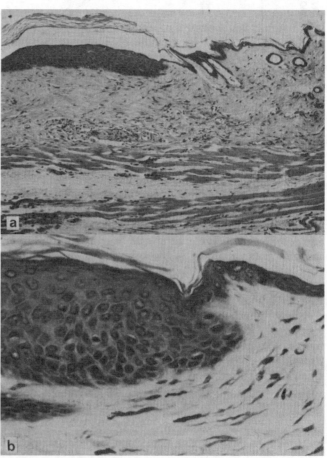

Fig. 3—Condition of graft two months after transplantation.
(a) Reduced by half from × 140. (b) Reduced by half from × 560.

1176   JUNE 1, 1968   PRELIMINARY **COMMUNICATIONS**   THE LANCET

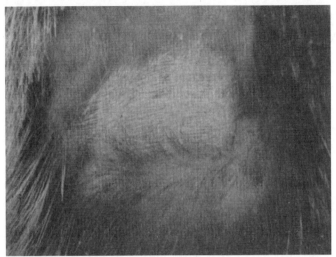

Fig. 4—August rat skin-graft on adult CBA mouse one month after the last injection of A.L.S.

noteworthy that the rabbit grafts enjoyed no special privilege as a consequence of the fact that the A.L.S. injected into their recipients was prepared in rabbits.

Duration of A.L.S. Treatment

Mice cannot be exposed indefinitely to crude unpurified A.L.S. such as we used in these experiments. After about three months pathological changes occur which can be regarded as secondary consequences of the antigenicity of A.L.S. (*quâ* foreign protein) itself.[7] It is now known [8] that these effects can be circumvented by (*a*) using the IgG fraction of A.L.S., in which its immunosuppressive properties reside,[9] and (*b*) inducing tolerance of IgG as such by the prior administration of IgG extracted from *normal* rabbit serum.[10] With these safeguards we believe, but have not yet shown, that immunological factors alone would not set a limit to the life of heterografts. Other factors may do so: it should be borne in mind that the long-term consequences of bringing together tissues of very distant genetic relationship are not known and cannot be foreseen.

Tolerance of Heterografts

The survival of heterografts during the administration of A.L.S. leaves open the question of whether they can be induced to survive after A.L.S. injections have stopped. The conditions under which the administration of A.L.S. alone can abet the induction of immunological tolerance of homografts (i.e., of an antigenically specific non-reactivity which persists after active immunosuppression has ceased) have been studied in some detail.[11] It is known to require the virtually complete inactivation of the central lymphoid organs by a more prolonged administration of A.L.S. than is necessary to exercise a merely peripheral inhibition.[12] In general, the induction of tolerance with the help of A.L.S. obeys the well-established rule that it is difficult in proportion to the antigenic disparity between donor and recipient. To induce tolerance of heterografts is therefore an intrinsically much more difficult enterprise than to induce tolerance of homografts. We have been able to secure a technically significant prolongation of the life of August rat skin-

homografts on adult CBA mice by reinforcing the antigenic dosage with intravenous injections of 100×10^6 August rat thymocytes five to seven days after the cessation of treatment with A.L.S., but the degree of prolongation fell short of anything that might be clinically useful, the longest survival time so far achieved being only about forty days after the last injection of A.L.S. Fig. 4 illustrates such a graft a month after the last injection of A.L.S.: notice the coarse hairs in the distribution characteristic of rat-tail skin. The induction of tolerance by the injection of donor lymphoid cells raises the danger of lethal graft-versus-host reactions. In homograft systems this can be circumvented by the treatment of the lymphoid cell *donor* with antilymphocytic serum, and preliminary results show that this procedure may also be effective when rat lymphoid cells are injected into mice.

COMMENTS

The experiments described here show that the opposition of mice to the grafting of rat, guineapig, or human skin is mainly or wholly immunological in nature and, as such, can be overcome. Heterografts of other, more complex organs, particularly those with secretory products, are certain to raise special difficulties which cannot be expected to yield to so simple a solution: heterografts differ from their recipients by a multitude of strongly antigenic substances, many of which will excite the formation of humoral antibodies and give rise to hypersensitivity reactions of the " immediate " type. (The role of humoral antibodies in the rejection of heterografts is not yet known, but the use of A.L.S. will help to clarify it.) The combination of A.L.S. with conventional immunosuppressive agents may go some way towards meeting these difficulties, which may not be insuperable when (as with grafts of rat tissues into mice, or chimpanzee grafts into human beings) donor and recipient are genetically not too far apart. The work of Reemtsma [13] and of Professor R. Y. Calne and his colleagues [14] raises a reasonable hope that heterografts may one day find use in clinical practice. Our own results, so far as they go, open up a new experimental procedure which is likely to be of some value in developmental biology and in human pathology generally.

E. M. LANCE
M.D.

P. B. MEDAWAR
D.SC.

National Institute for Medical Research,
London N.W.7

PIG-TO-BABOON LIVER XENOGRAFTS

Summary   Seven pig-to-baboon orthotopic liver xenografts are reported. All animals recovered consciousness after operation. Four baboons died from uncontrollable hæmorrhage after 6–30 hours. The remaining three animals, which were given human fibrinogen, did not bleed. Six xenografted livers had centrilobular liver necrosis at postmortem examination; the seventh animal died after $3^1/_2$ days from bronchopneumonia with well-preserved liver parenchyma and round-cell infiltration of the portal tracts.

INTRODUCTION

HEPATIC function has been demonstrated in porcine livers perfused in vitro with human blood from up to 30 hours.[15] Pig livers connected to the arterial and venous

7. Lance, E. M. *Adv. Transplantation*, 1968, p. 107.
8. Taub, R. N., Lance, E. M. Unpublished.
9. James, K., Medawar, P. B. *Nature, Lond.* 1967, **214**, 1052. Lance, E. M. *in* Cell-bound Immunity; p. 103. Liège, 1967.
10. Lance, E. M., Dresser, D. W. *Nature, Lond.* 1967, **215**, 488.
11. Lance, E. M., Medawar, P. B. Unpublished.
12. Levey, R. H., Medawar, P. B. *Proc. natn. Acad. Sci.* 1967, **58**, 470. Brent, L., Courtenay, T. H., Gowland, G. *Nature, Lond.* 1967, **215**, 1461.

13. Reemtsma, K. *Science, N.Y.* 1964, **143**, 700.
14. Calne R. Y., White, H. J. O., Herbertson, B. M., Millard, P. R., Davis D. R., Salaman, J. R., Samuel, J. R. *Lancet.* 1968, i, 1176.
15. Liem, D. S., Waltuch, T. L., Eiseman, B. *Surg. Forum*, 1964, **15**, 90.

AUGUST 24, 1968   OCCASIONAL SURVEY   THE LANCET   449

Occasional Survey

KURU AND CANNIBALISM

JOHN D. MATHEWS

M.B., B.Sc. Melb.

OF THE KURU RESEARCH OFFICE,
PUBLIC HEALTH DEPARTMENT, OKAPA, VIA GOROKA, NEW GUINEA*

ROBERT GLASSE

Ph.D. Australian National

OF THE DEPARTMENT OF ANTHROPOLOGY,
QUEEN'S COLLEGE, CITY UNIVERSITY OF NEW YORK

SHIRLEY LINDENBAUM

Summary   Evaluation of the available evidence supports the hypothesis that cannibalism of kuru victims was responsible for the epidemic spread of kuru through the Fore and their immediate neighbours with whom they intermarry. Clinical disease ensues 4–20 years after ingestion of poorly cooked tissues containing the transmissible agent. The rarity of kuru in men suggests that horizontal transmission of the agent other than by cannibalism is rare, or that it causes kuru of a much longer incubation period. New data suggest that genetic factors are not of major importance in the determination of host susceptibility. Since other cannibal peoples in New Guinea do not suffer from kuru, the kurugenic agent itself may be the unique factor in the ætiology of the disease. Unless vertical transmission to give kuru from mother to offspring or horizontal transmission of an extended incubation period can continue in the absence of cannibalism, kuru should disappear within the next few decades, by which time most people still carrying the agent will have died from kuru.

INTRODUCTION

KURU is a neurological disorder found among the Fore and adjacent peoples with whom they intermarry in the Eastern Highlands of New Guinea; it has been seen in adult women and in young people of either sex.[1-3] To account for the rarity of kuru in adult males, Bennett et al.[2] postulated that kuru was determined genetically as a dominant trait in females but as a recessive trait in males. In the light of evidence for the recent epidemic spread of kuru,[4-7] and for the transmission and passage of kuru to chimpanzees by inoculation of kuru-tissue suspensions,[8 9] purely genetic theories of kuru ætiology [2] have had to be abandoned.[5 10] However, one must still account for the fact that adult males rarely get kuru. One of us (J. D. M.) has suggested that there are two mechanisms of transmission of the kurugenic agent viz., horizontal transmission causing kuru in adult women only, and vertical transmission from mother to offspring, causing kuru in children or young adults.[11] This interpretation is compatible with recent epidemiological data.[12]

EVIDENCE

The possible importance of cannibalism in ætiology of kuru has been the subject of speculation for some time.[13 14] Cannibalism may have had a fundamental role in spreading the virus-like kurugenic agent through the community. Before the suppression of cannibalism in the 1950s people in the Fore region (fig. 1) ate their own dead

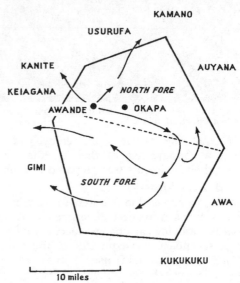

Fig. 1—Schematic map showing Fore and neighbouring linguistic regions.

Arrows indicate the main paths of kuru spread [14 15] from Awande. The Kukukuku have no tradition of intermarriage with the Fore, no tradition of cannibalism and no kuru. Kuru occurs among the Fore, Gimi, Keiagana, Kanite, Usurufa, and Kamano peoples who have a tradition of cannibalism and intermarriage, but the incidence of kuru decreases with the distance from the focus in the South Fore.

kinsfolk for gastronomic reasons, and also to show respect for the dead. It was customary for women and young children to be the main cannibals. Older boys and men rarely took part in these meals, particularly if the victim had been a woman and had died from kuru. Horizontal transmission of kuru could have depended directly on the eating of incompletely cooked human kuru tissue by women,[15] and vertical transmission, in part at least, could have been due to the consumption of kuru material by young children sharing human flesh with their mothers. Experiments to determine the tissue distribution and heat stability of the kuru agent are in progress.[9] By analogy with the properties of the scrapie agent,[16] one might expect the kuru agent to withstand usual Fore cooking procedures [14] without complete inactivation, especially since water boils at less than 95°C in much of the Fore area due to the altitude. Most of the circumstantial evidence of links between the ethnography of cannibalism and the epidemiology of kuru is summarised in the table.

There are, in addition, consistent ethnological accounts of the first kuru cases in certain villages. Consumption of

* Present address: Clinical Research Unit, Walter and Eliza Hall Institute of Medical Research, Post Office, Royal Melbourne Hospital, Victoria. Australia.

1. Gajdusek, D. C., Zigas, V. New Engl. J. Med. 1957, **257**, 974.
2. Bennett, J. H., Rhodes, F. A., Robson, H. N. Am. J. hum. Genet. 1959, **11**, 169.
3. Berndt, R. M. Sociologus, 1958, **8**, 4.
4. Glasse, R. M. The Spread of Kuru Among the Fore: a preliminary report. Department of Public Health, Territory of Papua and New Guinea, 1962.
5. Mathews, J. D. Lancet, 1965, i, 1138.
6. Alpers, M., Gajdusek, D. C. Am. J. trop. Med. Hyg. 1965, **14**, 852.
7. Bennett, J. H., Gabb, B. W., Oertel, C. R. Med. J. Aust. 1966, i, 379.
8. Gajdusek, D. C., Gibbs, C. J., Alpers, M. Nature, Lond. 1966, **209**, 794.
9. Gajdusek, D. C., Gibbs, C. J., Alpers, M. Science, N.Y. 1967, **155**, 212.
10. Fischer, A., Fischer, J. L., Kurland, L. T. J. genet. hum. 1964, **13**, 11.

11. Mathews, J. D. Lancet, 1967, i, 821.
12. Mathews, J. D. Papua New Guinea med. J. 1967, **10**, 76.
13. Gajdusek, D. C. Trans. R. Soc. trop. Med. Hyg. 1963, **57**, 151.
14. Glasse, R. M. Cannibalism in the Kuru Region. Department of Public Health, Territory of Papua and New Guinea, 1963. Glasse, R. M. Trans. N.Y. Acad. Sci. 1967, **29**, 748.
15. Mathews, J. D. To be submitted as an M.D. thesis, University of Melbourne.
16. Hunter, C. D. National Institutes of Neurological Diseases and Blindness Monograph, 1965, no. 2, p. 259.

The Lancet · Saturday 5 October 1968

GROWING CLINICAL SIGNIFICANCE OF METHICILLIN-RESISTANT STAPHYLOCOCCUS AUREUS

E. JACK BENNER
M.D. Oregon, F.A.C.P.

ASSOCIATE PROFESSOR OF MEDICINE AND CONSULTANT IN INFECTIOUS DISEASES, UNIVERSITY OF OREGON MEDICAL SCHOOL, PORTLAND, OREGON*

F. H. KAYSER
M.D. Munich

ASSISTANT MEDICAL DIRECTOR, UNIVERSITY INSTITUTE FOR MEDICAL MICROBIOLOGY, ZÜRICH, SWITZERLAND

Summary   Serious infections caused by methicillin-resistant *Staphylococcus aureus* have been on the increase throughout the Western world. A clinical and bacteriological study of 139 infections in Zürich, Switzerland, documented most as nosocomial problems. Patients in hospital for more than one week with a chronic, debilitating disease were a high risk. Most patients who got pneumonia and/or bacteræmia died, despite intensive therapy with penicillinase-resistant penicillins or cephalosporins. The resistance of the *Staph. aureus* strains was due to a peculiar " tolerance " to β-lactam antibiotics. Most strains had multiple antibiotic resistance and belonged to staphylococcal phage-group III. All 66 strains tested, representing several countries, were inhibited by vancomycin, and only 40% of the strains were inhibited by other commonly used antibiotics.

Introduction

THE extensive use of antimicrobial agents such as benzylpenicillin and erythromycin has often been followed by the appearance of large numbers of *Staphyloccocus aureus* resistant to these agents. If clinical use of the penicillinase-resistant penicillins (methicillin, oxacillin, nafcillin, cloxacillin, dicloxacillin) is often similarly affected, loss of valuable therapeutic agents may be in the making.

In the past, methicillin-resistant *Staph. aureus* strains (which are also resistant to oxacillin, nafcillin, cloxacillin, and dicloxacillin) were thought to be unimportant. However, an increasing frequency of serious clinical infections caused by such staphylococci challenges complacency. Although most strains identified before 1965 were not clearly the cause of clinically significant infections, their presence was established in hospitals (Barber 1964, Courtieu et al. 1964). Moreover, by 1966 such strains were responsible for 10% of the cases of *Staph. aureus* bacteræmia in Denmark (Ericksen 1967). In 1967, there were major infections due to methicillin-resistant *Staph. aureus* in several cities of the United States, and such infections were occurring regularly in England, France, and Switzerland (Benner and Morthland 1967). In

Canton Zürich, Switzerland, methicillin-resistant *Staph. aureus* strains were responsible for 9·7%, 17·3%, and 16·1% of staphylococcal infections during 1965, 1966, and 1967, respectively. Since there is little epidemiological or clinical information available on infections caused by these peculiar strains of staphylococci, 139 cases from Zürich were investigated. In addition, we evaluated certain bacteriological characteristics of the strains from Zürich and additional strains from England, France, and the United States.

Patients and Methods

Although the 139 cases from Zürich were analysed retrospectively, it was possible to define certain clinical and epidemiological features with reasonable certainty, as described in Results.

In-vitro studies were performed on the Swiss cultures (34) by one of us (F. H. K.) in Zürich. The results were confirmed in Portland in a parallel study with reconstituted, lyophilised staphylococci from England (15), France (5), and the United States (12). A standard method (Petersdorf and Sherris 1965) was used for the disc test with the following disc potencies: cephaloridine 30 µg., cephalothin 30 µg., cephalexin (Eli Lilly) 30 µg., chloramphenicol 30 µg., kanamycin 30 µg., vancomycin 30 µg., cloxacillin 2 µg., erythromycin 15 µg., lincomycin 2 µg., methicillin 5 µg., oxacillin 1 µg., and tetracycline 5 µg. Tube-dilution minimal inhibitory concentration tests (M.I.C.s) were done in brain/heart-infusion broth media. The inoculum was 0·5 ml. of a 10^{-2} broth dilution of cells grown at 37°C for 12–18 hours. Replicate plate M.I.C.s were done on Mueller-Hinton agar plates by adding 0·01 ml. of cells grown overnight at 37°C. The basic resistance of each strain was determined by streaking 0·1 ml. of different dilutions of overnight cultures on the surface of agar-plates containing increasing concentrations of oxacillin. The basic resistance was defined as that concentration of oxacillin in µg. per ml. tolerated by 2×10^{7} cells out of 10^{8} cells. Population analysis and minimal bactericidal concentrations (M.B.C.s) were performed as described by Benner and Morthland (1967). The phage-type has been determined according to Blair and Williams (1961).

Results

Kinds of Infections caused by Staphylococci with Methicillin Resistance

139 specimens containing methicillin-resistant strains of *Staph. aureus*, corresponding to individual patients, were received in Zürich during 1965 and 1966. Data adequate for evaluation of the kind of infection were not available in 20 patients. In another 21 patients the abundant yield of methicillin-resistant organisms in the cultured specimen was of uncertain clinical significance. In 98 patients, both the nature of the infection and the ætiological role of the methicillin-resistant isolates of *Staph. aureus* were clearly defined. The kinds of infection in these 98 patients were those to be expected in hospital-acquired problems—that is, there were 38 infections of the respiratory system, 23 surgical-wound infections, 14 bone or joint infections (particularly osteomyelitis or arthritis), 9 infections of skin and muscle, 5 urinary-tract infections,

---

* Present appointment: associate professor of medicine, School of Medicine, University of California at Davis, California.

172   JANUARY 25, 1969   ORIGINAL ARTICLES   THE LANCET

PENETRATION OF
GOWN MATERIAL BY ORGANISMS
FROM THE SURGEON'S BODY

J. CHARNLEY   N. EFTEKHAR

OF THE CENTRE FOR HIP SURGERY,
WRIGHTINGTON HOSPITAL, NEAR WIGAN, LANCASHIRE

Summary   Bacteriological tests show that the fine woven material known as balloon cloth, used extensively in Britain for operating-gowns, can be penetrated by organisms from the surgeon's body. These observations were made possible by the unique circumstances of operating routinely in near-sterile air. It is suggested that the direct transfer of organisms from the surface of a surgeon's gown to the wound can take place even in the presence of sterile air in the operating-room. This route of infection could be avoided by the surgeon wearing a plastic apron beneath his gown or a sterile apron of fine woven cloth over it.

Introduction

IN a prospective study of postoperative wound infection when operating in practically sterile air (Charnley and Eftekhar 1969) it seemed quite clear that a reduction in infection-rates from 9% to 1% could be attributed to clean air. On the other hand, even when the air in the operating-room was to all intents and purposes sterile, there still persisted a postoperative infection-rate of about 1%. It was tempting to assume that this level represented infection originating endogenously in the patient's bloodstream, or exogenously in the patient's skin in the postoperative phase. Before resorting to these explanations we decided to explore the possibility that infection might result from organisms passing through the textile of the surgeon's gown, being then transferred to the wound directly and without being airborne between gown and wound. The operation of total hip replacement involves considerable muscular work; the surgeon pushes his body against a brace-and-bit which is held against the front of his gown and the presence of blood on the gown at this site at the end of the operation confirms this. Inspection of the weave of the fine cotton textile known as " balloon cloth " from which these gowns are made shows apertures up to 50 μ in diameter (see figure).

The feasibility of testing directly this possible route of infection presented itself in the unique circumstances of operating in sterile air. If organisms were recovered from

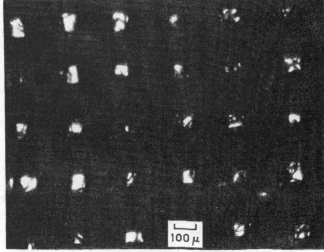

Apertures in weave of the balloon cloth of a surgical gown.

the external surface of the surgeon's gown at the end of an operation performed in sterile air the most likely explanation would be that they had come from inside the gown.

Methods and Results

At the conclusion of an operation the following experiments were done, the surgeon still being inside the sterile air of the operating enclosure while the specimens were being taken.

Experiment 1 (Sampling the External Surface of the Gown by Direct Contact with Nutrient Agar)

The nutrient agar jelly was available as sausages of Oxoid agar base no. 2 according to the technique of Ten Cate (1965) in which the sausage is in a sterile plastic skin so that the cut surface can be applied to a test area and the contaminated surface of the jelly can then be cut off as a slice and deposited for culture in a sterile petri dish. The clean new surface of the sausage can then be used again for further tests in the same experiment. In this experiment the sausage had an average diameter of 4·2 cm. with an average cross-section of 13·8² sq. cm.

Tests were done on an area of the surgeon's gown measuring approximately 30×30 cm. corresponding to the

TABLE I—GROWTH ON SETTLE PLATES USED TO CHECK STERILITY OF OPERATING-ROOM AIR

State of air determined by settle plates	No. of tests	No. of plates	No. of colonies
Both with no growth ..	159	318	0
One with no growth ..	38	38	0
One with growth ..	38	38	47
Both with growth	3	6	9
Total	200	400	56

TABLE II—STATE OF AIR CONTAMINATION WITH POSITIVE AND NEGATIVE GOWN TESTS

State of air determined by settle plates	Gown test	
	Negative	Positive
Both with no growth	91	68
One with growth	18	20
Both with growth	1	2
Total	110	90

anterior chest wall and upper arms. Each newly cut surface of sausage was pressed 15–20 times against the gown surface in different places and three slices of jelly were used in each test. These were then incubated at 37°C for 48 hours, and the colonies were counted.

At the same time a second series of slices was made (but without contact with the gown) and placed in a separate petri dish for control. During every test a pair of blood-agar petri dishes was exposed on the operating-table and left open during the whole of the operation to check the cleanliness of the air during the operation.

Table I shows the cleanliness of the air during the whole of the operation preceding the sampling of the external surface of the surgeon's gown. In two hundred tests (at the conclusion of 200 different operations) 400 settle plates were exposed (2 for each operation) on an average for 60 minutes and 89% of the plates remained sterile with only 11% growing 1–2 colonies per hour. On three occasions only did both settle plates become contaminated. Only once did the number of colonies exceed 2 per plate per hour.

Table II shows the relationship between the contamination of settle-plates and positive and negative tests taken from the surface of the gowns.

should contribute substantially to these changes by ensuring that the population is quantitatively and, above all, qualitatively fit for the tasks of the future.

REFERENCES

Abel-Smith, B. (1967) *Publ. Hlth Pap. W.H.O.* no. 32.
Gabaldon, A. (1955) *Bol. Ofic. sanit. panam.* **38**, 259.
Ohlin, G. (1967) Population Control and Economic Development. O.E.C.D., Paris.
Penchansky, R. (1968) Health Services Administration. Cambridge, Mass.
United Nations (1964) The Economic Development of Latin America in the Post-war Period. New York.

L-DOPA IN POSTENCEPHALITIC PARKINSONISM

D. B. Calne   G. M. Stern

D. R. Laurence

OF THE MEDICAL AND NEUROLOGICAL UNITS, UNIVERSITY COLLEGE HOSPITAL, LONDON W.C.1

J. Sharkey

OF HIGHLANDS GENERAL HOSPITAL, LONDON N.21

P. Armitage

OF THE LONDON SCHOOL OF HYGIENE AND TROPICAL MEDICINE, W.C.1

Summary   Treatment of postencephalitic parkinsonism with oral L-dopa administered over 6 weeks in maximum tolerated doses has been studied in a between-patient double-blind therapeutic trial, involving 40 patients. 7 of the 20 patients receiving L-dopa improved substantially and 3 moderately; 5 showed no useful response, and 5 had to stop L-dopa because of adverse effects. The most notable improvement was in control of movement in walking. Involuntary movements and restlessness were troublesome side-effects. Nausea and orthostatic hypotension were common but transient. It is concluded that L-dopa has a useful role in the management of postencephalitic parkinsonism. Adverse reactions in some patients suggest that treatment should be initiated with caution, if possible in hospital.

Introduction

CONVENTIONAL antiparkinsonian drugs probably act by reducing the synaptic neurotransmitter activity of acetylcholine in the central nervous system (Duvoisin 1967). During the past 10 years accumulating evidence has suggested that dopamine, a catecholamine precursor of adrenaline and noradrenaline present in particularly high concentration in the corpus striatum, is another synaptic neurotransmitter. Acetylcholine exhibits excitatory activity in this region of the brain, and dopamine is predominantly inhibitory (Bloom et al. 1965, McLennan and York 1967).

The amount of dopamine in the basal ganglia of parkinsonian patients is reduced (normal 2·5 µg. per g. wet tissue, 0·01–1·1 µg. per g. in parkinsonism [Hornykiewicz 1966]), and it has been suggested that Parkinson's syndrome might result from an imbalance between cholinergic-excitatory and dopaminergic-inhibitory actions in the direction of cholinergic dominance (McGeer et al. 1961, Barbeau 1962, Arvidsson et al. 1966). This does not necessarily mean that the manifestations of parkinsonism are the result of a primary defect of dopamine metabolism: dopaminergic systems might be particularly vulnerable to damage by viral infections, ischæmia,

trauma, toxin, or idiopathic degeneration. There is evidence that drugs which cause parkinsonism, such as reserpine, tetrabenazine, and phenothiazines, all interfere with the activity of dopamine (Carlsson and Lindqvist 1963, Laverty and Sharman 1965).

On this theoretical basis attempts have been made to treat parkinsonism by raising the level of dopamine in the brain. Oral dopamine does not reach the central nervous system, but L-dihydroxyphenylalanine (L-dopa), its immediate precursor, crosses the blood-brain barrier. Early clinical studies of the therapeutic value of L-dopa produced conflicting results. There are several reports that beneficial effects could be achieved by oral or intravenous dopa (Birkmayer and Hornykiewicz 1961, Barbeau 1962, Gerstenbrand and Pateisky 1962, Friedhoff et al. 1963, Hirschmann and Mayer 1964, Umbach and Baumann 1964), but others have not confirmed this (Greer and Williams 1963, McGeer and Zeldowicz 1964, Fehling 1966, Aebert 1967, Rinne and Sonninen 1968). Most of these studies involved the administration of 50 mg. to 1·0 g. of L-dopa per day over periods of 1 day to 2 weeks. DL-dopa was often used because the racemic mixture is much cheaper than the separated isomers. Monoamine-oxidase inhibitors were sometimes given in an effort to potentiate the dopa.

Cotzias et al. (1967) described their experience with more prolonged treatment using larger doses of dopa. They gave up to 16 g. per day of DL-dopa for several months and reported impressive improvement in 10 out of 16 patients. However, 4 of their patients developed transient granulocytopenia. Recent accounts indicate that up to 8 g. per day of L-dopa, instead of 16 g. per day of the racemic mixture, produce comparable therapeutic effects with less risk of provoking marrow depression (Cotzias et al. 1968, 1969). Duvoisin et al. 1968.

In the present study, maximum tolerated doses of L-dopa were given to a group of patients who were all so disabled by postencephalitic parkinsonism that institutional care had been necessary for many years.

Patients and Methods

40 patients (18 men and 22 women), aged 47–73, took part in the study. They all had a history of illness in the encephalitis pandemic of 1916–26, and they had been in hospital for an average of 29 years. 3 had been admitted in childhood. Half of them were chairbound. None had received stereotaxic surgery. As well as parkinsonism, some patients showed other clinical features: 9 patients had psychiatric disturbances (6 aggressive and uncooperative, 1 obsessional, 1 paranoid, 1 depressive), 4 choreoathetosis, 3 tics, and 6 headache.

Before admission to the trial all patients were screened clinically and biochemically for evidence of cardiovascular, hepatic, and renal disease. Hæmoglobin, total-white-cell counts, and direct Coombs tests were done every 2 weeks.

The trial comprised a double-blind between-patient comparison of L-dopa with placebo. Patients were divided at random into two groups of 20. One group was given L-dopa and the other placebo. Previous antiparkinsonian treatment was not altered; all patients were taking large doses of several synthetic anticholinergic drugs throughout the period of study. L-dopa was administered in 500 or 250 mg. tablets four times a day with meals. Patients who had difficulty in swallowing were given the tablets ground up in food. An initial dose of 1 g. daily was increased every 3rd day until the maximum tolerated dose was attained. Throughout the trial the number of placebo tablets given to the control group of patients was increased in the same way. Nausea and vomiting were treated with cyclizine 50 mg. tablets or 100 mg. suppositories before meals. After an arbitrary period of 47 days all patients were given

every calendar month. For each taker an age-matched, randomly selected control patient is also recruited from the same practice, and both takers and controls must be married or living as married. No other matching is being attempted. Recruitment started on May 1, 1968, and ended on July 31, 1969. Observation on the recruited patients will continue until April, 1973, at the earliest.

All records are forwarded to a coordinating office in Manchester where they are processed for computer input, storage, and analysis. At the time of recruitment each patient is interviewed by her general practitioner who records a number of social and medical factors about her.

RESULT

Besides a number of expected differences between takers and controls in relation to parity and social class, we have encountered a potentially important difference in cigarette consumption at the time of recruitment:

No./day				Takers	Controls
				No. of:	
0	..	..	..	8848 *(52%)*	8742 *(58%)*
1–4	..	..	..	1089 *(6%)*	891 *(6%)*
5–9	..	..	..	1298 *(8%)*	1046 *(7%)*
10–14	..	..	..	2337 *(14%)*	1918 *(13%)*
15–19	..	..	..	1500 *(9%)*	1109 *(7%)*
≥20	..	..	..	2005 *(12%)*	1234 *(8%)*
				17,077 *(100%)*	14,940 *(100%)*

There is a highly significant deficiency of non-smokers and an excess of heavy smokers in the taker group ($\chi^2=189$, $P<0.001$). The mean daily cigarette consumption is 6·18 for takers and 5·09 for controls (ratio 1·21/1). We have examined smoking habits in relation to age, parity, and social class. In every category for each subgroup the mean daily cigarette consumption is significantly higher for takers than for controls, except for social class v where consumption is higher (but not significantly) in the controls.

DISCUSSION

Controls have been recruited later than their corresponding takers, so that until the recruitment phase is completed there will be an unavoidable deficiency of controls (see table). However, in view of the consistent difference in smoking habits between takers and controls throughout the age, parity, and social-class groups, inclusion of the " missing " controls would be unlikely to affect the result materially.

A more serious consideration is that our samples may be unrepresentative. Since there are no suitable published data, either on cigarette smoking or contraceptive usage, we cannot refute this objection, although we are satisfied that our sampling methods are free from obvious sources of error. The participating general practitioners are volunteers who have an interest in research, and their practice populations may in some way reflect this special interest. Nevertheless, the takers and their controls come from the same practices and it is unlikely that these doctors could selectively attract as patients women who both take the pill and have an above-average cigarette consumption, or conversely, women who both smoke little and reject the pill as a method of contraception. It is even less likely that both contingencies could occur simultaneously. We, therefore, believe that the observed relationship between smoking habits and oral contraceptive usage is representative of the population of the United Kingdom at the present time. The same may not be true of other countries and cultures.

We are not here concerned with the sources of the difference in smoking habits: the important factor is the existence of a difference that may influence the morbidity experience of the two groups. We cannot estimate the likely magnitude of this influence since little is known about smoking and morbidity in women of reproductive age. In the United States [1] women aged 17–44 are reported to have a 40% greater number of days of " restricted activity " due to illness than non-smokers, but the nature of the excess morbidity and the number of episodes of illness are not given. The same publication cites evidence that in-vitro thrombus formation and platelet adhesiveness is increased in smokers, but Vessey and Doll,[2] in their extended study, were unable to confirm the suspicion aroused by their earlier observations [3] that oral-contraceptive users were more likely to be smokers than were non-users and that smoking could potentiate the liability of the oral contraceptives to cause venous thromboembolic disease. However, Frederiksen and Ravenholt [4,5] believe that Vessey and Doll's data can be shown to demonstrate such a relationship.

We expect that the effect of smoking on the health of young adult women will be among the results of the present study. In the meantime, it is clear that no observed morbid change can be unreservedly attributed to the use of oral contraceptives if the possible influence of associated smoking habits has not been excluded.

We appreciate the collaboration of the 1400 general practitioners whose observations are providing the data for this study. The study is supported by a grant from the Medical Research Council. The costs of the pilot trials and current supplementary expenditure have been met by the research foundation board of the Royal College of General Practitioners. The board gratefully acknowledges the receipt of funds for research into oral contraception from Organon Laboratories Ltd., G. D. Searle & Co. Ltd., Schering Chemicals Limited, and Syntex Pharmaceuticals Ltd.

Requests for reprints should be addressed to C. R. K., 100 Wilmslow Road, Manchester M14 7DL.

REFERENCES

1. The Health Consequences of Smoking: a Public Health Service Review. Washington, D.C., 1967.
2. Vessey, M. P., Doll, R. *Br. med. J.* 1969, ii, 651.
3. Vessey, M. P., Doll, R. *ibid.* 1968, ii, 199.
4. Frederiksen, H., Ravenholt, R. T. *ibid.* p. 770.
5. Frederiksen, H., Ravenholt, R. T.; Bush, R. D. *ibid.* 1969, iii, 529.

Hypothesis

RELATED DISEASE—RELATED CAUSE?

DENIS P. BURKITT

External Staff, Medical Research Council

Summary   A constant relationship between certain diseases in different geographical areas or in different socio-economic groups suggests some related ætiological factor. Benign and malignant lesions of the large bowel which show such a relationship are examined, and it is suggested that there is epidemiological and other evidence to incriminate low-residue diet as a major ætiological factor.

INTRODUCTION

STUDIES in disease distribution, both geographically in space and chronologically in time, have not been accorded the emphasis they deserve. It is being in-

THE LANCET, DECEMBER 6, 1969

creasingly recognised that most disease is the result of environment rather than genetically determined, and is consequently preventable once the causal factors can be recognised and avoided or eliminated.

The extensive epidemiological studies of Cleave et al.[1] have underlined the important contention that conditions, no matter how apparently divergent, if constantly related geographically or chronologically, are likely to be related to a common ætiological factor. They draw attention to the relationship between such widespread and major diseases of the Western world as cardiac infarction, diabetes, diverticular disease of the colon, and various venous ailments such as hæmorrhoids and varicose veins. In a convincing argument they implicate as a major cause the over-refining of carbohydrate with resultant excessive consumption and removal of the unabsorbable cellulose content.

EPIDEMIOLOGY OF LARGE-BOWEL DISEASE

Epidemiological studies in Africa and elsewhere indicate that many large-bowel diseases which are universally prevalent in the so-called civilised world are almost or totally unknown throughout rural Africa. It is moreover highly significant they all have a similar incidence in the White and Black populations in North America, which inevitably implies dependence on environment.

Joseph Burchenal, in his presidential address to the American Cancer Society in 1966, chose as his title: Geographic Chemotherapy—Burkitt's Tumor as a Stalking Horse for Leukæmia.[2] He suggested that the study of one form of cancer might provide guide-posts to the understanding of another related form.

I should like to extend his concept to the suggestion that the study of certain benign conditions may provide pointers to the cause of related malignant tumours; the former, being considerably more common, render the epidemiological investigation easier. To this end I will endeavour to show a relationship between benign and malignant bowel lesions and suggest common factors which may well be causally related.

Appendicitis, diverticular disease, adenomatous polyps, and bowel carcinoma appear to be directly related to a Western way of life. In highly developed countries appendicitis is one of the commonest surgical emergencies; diverticular disease is said to be present in some 20% of people over the age of forty, adenomatous polyps in the colon are found in over 20% of necropsies, and cancer of the colon and rectum together are, in America and England, second in incidence only to bronchial carcinoma.[3] All these conditions are exceedingly rare throughout rural Africa but have a comparable incidence in the Negro and Caucasian communities in North America. Each will be examined in turn.

Appendicitis

Half a century ago Rendle-Short[4] endeavoured to trace the cause of the rapid rise in incidence of appendicitis in Europe and America in the closing year of the 19th century and the first decade of the 20th. He also made comparisons with the then-known incidence in other countries. With lucid argument and logical exclusion of numerous possible factors he incriminated the lack of cellulose in daily fare which resulted from the growing popularity of refined carbohydrates, and white flour in

particular. Half a century later the urban or educated African is participating in a similar dietary change and is experiencing a similar rise in the incidence of appendicitis. This condition is still almost unknown in rural African communities, and was until recently rare even in larger towns. The incidence, however, is rising rapidly in the larger cities, and Miller[5] reports over 150 cases a year in Nairobi and Bremner[6] an average of 1 a day in Johannesburg.

Diverticular Disease of the Colon

In twenty years' surgical practice in Uganda I never recognised diverticular disease in an African. Of the 52 hospitals in Africa which returned a questionary, 44 had not recorded a single case of diverticular disease. Of the remaining 8, 6 had recorded 1 case only. The remaining 2, where the condition was very rare but not unknown, were large teaching hospitals.

Whereas appendicitis becomes apparent within a few years of Western dietary habits being adopted, diverticular disease probably requires most of a lifetime in a responsible environment since the condition is primarily one of advancing years.

Adenomatous Polyps

Polyps of the colon are exceedingly common in the Western world. In seven large necropsy series the average incidence was over 20%.[7] They are almost unknown in tropical Africa. Keeley[8] found only 1 case of diverticulosis of the colon in 2367 necropsies on Bantu patients in Johannesburg.

Cancer of the Colon and Rectum

In England the incidence of tumours of the colon and rectum in both sexes combined is exceeded only by lung cancer, and such tumours account for over 12% of all malignant neoplasms.[3] Bowel content is the most important environment of intestinal mucosa, and this, being determined by diet, is particularly liable to change when communities migrate from village to city, from lower to higher economic status, or from a less to a more developed country. These tumours are still very rare in Africa and almost unknown in rural communities. Records for four separate rural areas in East Africa showed cancer of the colon and rectum to account for 1·1 to 4·3% of all cancer. It is becoming commoner in large urban communities. Wynder and Shigematsu,[9] in their excellent comprehensive review on the epidemiology of bowel cancer, drew attention to the high incidence of polyps in patients with bowel cancer and vice versa, and asked the pertinent question: Do the factors contributing to the development of cancer of the bowel also contribute to the development of polyps? In Japan colon cancer and polyps are both rare,[10] again suggesting relationship to a common factor. Both conditions are extremely rare in experimental animals,[11] and this is consistent with a related ætiology.

Postulated Common Factor

Stool bulk and content, bacterial flora, total transit-time and intra-lumen pressures can all be profoundly altered by changes in diet, and in particular by the removing of the unabsorable fibre as in much modern food processing.

Increased consumption of refined carbohydrates, and in particular white flour and sugar, are characteristics of so-called civilised communities.

The mechanism responsible for appendicitis is not known; but increased stool consistency, raised bowel pressures, and altered bacterial flora may all play a part. Abnormal pressures within the colon are believed to be the main causal factors in diverticular disease

THE LANCET, DECEMBER 6, 1969

which has been shown to be related to low-residue diet both clinically [12] and experimentally.[13] With regard to bowel tumours, Oettle [14] has pointed out that with Western diet, the greatly delayed transit-time (most of the delay occurring in the distal colon), together with the concentration associated with diminished stool bulk, might enhance the action of any carcinogen by the multiple of these factors. Even if bowel cancer were not related to any ingested carcinogens, these might be metabolised from normal fæcal constituents by the action of bacteria—it is noteworthy that the small bowel with its rapid transit-time and almost abacterial content is a rare site of cancer. Significantly, colon cancer can be induced in rats by administering a carcinogen which is ineffective in germ-free rats.[15] Aries et al.[16] have demonstrated gross differences in the bacterial flora of stools from Uganda woman and Londoners, and postulate that the bacterial flora, in degrading the bile-salts, may convert them into carcinogens.

CONCLUSIONS

There is considerable evidence that diet is related to bowel behaviour and content and that changes in these may in turn be responsible for colon disease. In view of the enormous amount of morbidity and mortality caused by these diseases, it is important to investigate the relationship between diet and bowel disease. To this end studies of bowel behaviour, using the simplest possible methods, are being instigated in many different cultural and ethnic groups throughout Africa and else-where. If a relationship can be established between dietary habits and disease patterns it should not be necessary to await an understanding of the mechanism whereby benign or malignant disease is produced before attempting prevention. The demonstration of a relationship between lung cancer and cigarette smoking has, at least in some quarters, resulted in evasive action, although the mechanism of carcinogenesis is still far from clear.

Requests for reprints should be addressed to D. P. B., Medical Research Council, 172 Tottenham Court Road, London W1P 9LG.

REFERENCES

1. Cleave, T. L., Campbell, G. D., Painter, N. S. Diabetes, Coronary Thrombosis and the Saccharine Disease. Bristol, 1969.
2. Burchenal, J. Cancer Res. 1966, 26, 2393.
3. Doll, R., Payne, P., Waterhouse, J. (editors). Cancer Incidence in Five Continents: U.I.C.C. Report. Heidelburg, 1966.
4. Rendle-Short, A. S. Br. J. Surg. 1920, 8, 171.
5. Miller, J. R. Personal communication.
6. Bremner, C. Personal communication.
7. Bockus, H. L. Gastroenterology; vol. ii. Philadelphia, 1964.
8. Keeley, K. J. Med. Proc. 1958, 4, 281.
9. Wynder, E. L., Shigematsu, T. Cancer, 1967, 20, 1520.
10. Kodaira, T. Cited by Wynder, E. L., Kajitani, T., Ishikawa, S., Dodo, H., Takano, A. ibid. 1969, 23, 1210.
11. Mitra, S. K. Br. J. Cancer, 1966, 20, 399.
12. Painter, N. S. Lancet, 1969, ii, 586.
13. Carlson, A. J., Hoelzel, F. Gastroenterology, 1949, 12, 108.
14. Oettle, A. G. in Symposium on Tumours of the Alimentary Tract in Africans; p. 97. N.C.I. monograph 8, Bethesda, Maryland, 1967.
15. Cole, J. Cited by Wynder et al. (see reference 10).
16. Aries, V., Crowther, J. S., Draser, B. S., Hill, M. J., Williams, R. E. O. Gut, 1969, 10, 334.

Methods and Devices

VARIABLE-HEIGHT EXAMINATION COUCH

JAMES ANDREWS

Geriatric Unit, West Middlesex Hospital, Isleworth

A VARIABLE-HEIGHT examination couch does not seem to be commercially available in Britain; and the second report of the specification working group on Patient Area Furniture (issued by the Department of Health and Social Security), though it states that the most important factor in the design of couches is to safeguard the safety and comfort of patients, makes no mention of height adjustment.

Many patients, and not only those in geriatric departments, have great difficulty in climbing on to a couch of examination-height even with the aid of steps, and so an adjustable couch would be an asset for outpatient departments generally, and for geriatric day wards and outpatients in particular. Not least of its virtues is that it enables one nurse to help a disabled patient on to the couch when, with a fixed height couch, at least two would be needed.

One such couch is shown in the figure. It is made from tubular steel and the dimensions are 198 cm. (6 ft. 6 in.) by 61 cm. (2 ft.) hinged brackrest adjustable to three positions including a 45° position for measuring the jugular venous pressure. The couch is upholstered in green ' Vynide ' (polyvinyl chloride coated fabric) and can have either 2·5 cm. (1 in.) or 5·8 cm. (2 in.) foam padding. The operating handle is at the foot end of the couch. The height, from 56 cm. (22 in.) to 86 cm. (34 in.), is adjusted by a jacking unit fitted at each end of the couch with enclosed winding shaft and gear boxes.

This couch was constructed by Calthena Ltd., Nassau Mills, Patricroft, Eccles, Lancashire.

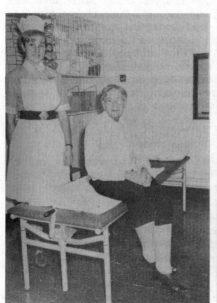
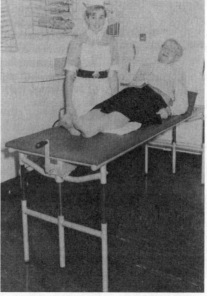

Highest and lowest positions of the couch.
The nurse's height is 163 cm. (5 ft. 4 in.)

The Lancet · Saturday 14 February 1970

INCREASED SICKLING OF PARASITISED ERYTHROCYTES AS MECHANISM OF RESISTANCE AGAINST MALARIA IN THE SICKLE-CELL TRAIT*

LUCIO LUZZATTO   E. S. NWACHUKU-JARRETT

S. REDDY

Subdepartment of Hæmatology, University College Hospital, Ibadan, Nigeria

Summary   Blood-samples from children with the sickle-cell trait (*A/S* heterozygotes) having acute malaria (*Plasmodium falciparum*) were incubated in vitro under anaerobic conditions, such that the number of cells sickled is a linear function of time. The rate of sickling of parasitised cells was found to be 2 to 8 times greater than that of non-parasitised cells within the same blood-sample, indicating that parasitisation of an A/S erythrocyte by *P. falciparum* increases substantially its probability to sickle. It is suggested that parasitised cells, once sickled, will be removed more effectively from the circulation by phagocytosis, and that this is the main mechanism whereby *A/S* heterozygotes are at a selective advantage against subtertian malaria.

Introduction

THE geographical distribution of the gene for sickle-cell hæmoglobin (Hb S) is the expression of the best-documented example of balanced polymorphism in man. The age stratification of the frequency of Hb S, the similarity in the world distribution of the *S* gene and of *Plasmodium falciparum* malaria, and the analyses of parasite-rate, parasite density, and malaria mortality in heterozygous (*A/S*) children all support the concept that these children are protected against death from malignant tertian malaria.[1] Although this concept was suggested by Beet,[2] Raper,[3] and Brain,[4] and fully explored and developed by Allison[5] fifteen years ago, the underlying mechanism is still unknown. Three possibilities have been considered: (*a*) Hb S might be less " palatable " to the parasite than is Hb A[6]; (*b*) there may be a difference in the immune response to malaria between the normal homozygote (*A/A*) and the heterozygote (*A/S*) subjects[7]; and (*c*) parasitisation of *A/S* cells may cause them to sickle and to be removed from the circulation.[8,9]

The third mechanism has the appeal of simplicity, and has been tested previously by counting parasites in

* Preliminary results of this work were presented at the 1st International Conference on Pædiatrics in the Tropics, Ibadan, Nov. 2–5, 1969.

7642

sickled and non-sickled cells after a 24-hour in-vitro incubation[10] and by gametocyte-counts in *A/S* subjects,[9] but with negative results. We have re-examined this model using a different technique, and found that, under defined experimental conditions, parasitised red blood-cells from *A/S* heterozygotes have a higher rate of sickling than do unparasitised cells in the same blood-sample.

Patients and Methods

Patients

Children aged between 1 and 6 years who presented at University College Hospital (general outpatient department) with an acute febrile illness (temperature 38°–40°C) were immediately tested for malaria parasites (at least 4–6 rings of *P. falciparum* per high-power field on a thin blood-film stained by the Leishman method) and for sickling (by the metabisulphite technique[11]). From those children who were positive in both tests venous blood was obtained, and treatment for malaria was started immediately afterwards. A sample of hæmolysed blood was later subjected to electrophoresis,[12] and in all cases an A/S Hb pattern was obtained.

Experimental Conditions

To detect what might prove to be only a small difference in the rate of sickling between parasitised and non-parasitised red blood-cells we had to establish conditions under which sickling would be an orderly, and preferably a linear, process. The following technique proved suitable. 4 ml. of venous blood were collected into 1 ml. of an anticoagulant solution having the following composition: 2·5% trisodium citrate (adjusted to pH 7·4 with 2·5% citric acid), 100 ml.; 10% glucose, 5 ml.; 0·15 M potassium chloride, 4 ml.; 0·15 M magnesium sulphate, 1 ml.; final pH 7·4. 1·75 ml. of the anticoagulated blood was then incubated at 37°C with 0·25 ml. of 8% sodium metabisulphite under a layer of paraffin oil. At the beginning of the incubation, and at six successive 10-minute intervals thereafter, 0·2 ml. samples of the mixture were removed and transferred anaerobically to a tube containing 0·2 ml. of 18% formaldehyde under paraffin oil. After 2 hours' fixation at room temperature, the sedimented cells were washed once with 0·85% sodium chloride, smeared in a very thin film, and stained with Leishman's stain diluted 1/1 with water. In preliminary experiments carried out on non-parasitised blood from a number of A/S heterozygotes, the percentage of cells sickled as a function of time was determined at various concentrations of metabisulphite (fig. 1). Sickling proceeded with an almost linear time-course. The rate of sickling is defined as the slope of the curve at the origin—e.g., in curve C of fig. 1 the rate of sickling is about 1% per minute. The rate of sickling varies in different individuals: however, in two patients tested three times each, it proved self-consistent over a period of 2 weeks. When blood from subjects with sickle-cell disease (*S/S* homozygotes or *S C* heterozygotes) is pro-

G

The Lancet · Saturday 27 February 1971

THE INVERSE CARE LAW

Julian Tudor Hart

Glyncorrwg Health Centre, Port Talbot, Glamorgan, Wales

Summary   The availability of good medical care tends to vary inversely with the need for it in the population served. This inverse care law operates more completely where medical care is most exposed to market forces, and less so where such exposure is reduced. The market distribution of medical care is a primitive and historically outdated social form, and any return to it would further exaggerate the maldistribution of medical resources.

Interpreting the Evidence

THE existence of large social and geographical inequalities in mortality and morbidity in Britain is known, and not all of them are diminishing. Between 1934 and 1968, weighted mean standardised mortality from all causes in the Glamorgan and Monmouthshire valleys rose from 128% of England and Wales rates to 131%. Their weighted mean infant mortality rose from 115% of England and Wales rates to 124% between 1921 and 1968.[1] The Registrar General's last Decennial Supplement on Occupational Mortality for 1949–53 still showed combined social classes I and II (wholly non-manual) with a standardised mortality from all causes 18% below the mean, and combined social classes IV and V (wholly manual) 5% above it. Infant mortality was 37% below the mean for social class I (professional) and 38% above it for social class V (unskilled manual).

A just and rational distribution of the resources of medical care should show parallel social and geographical differences, or at least a uniform distribution. The common experience was described by Titmuss in 1968:

" We have learnt from 15 years' experience of the Health Service that the higher income groups know how to make better use of the service; they tend to receive more specialist attention; occupy more of the beds in better equipped and staffed hospitals; receive more elective surgery; have better maternal care, and are more likely to get psychiatric help and psychotherapy than low-income groups—particularly the unskilled."[2]

These generalisations are not easily proved statistically, because most of the statistics are either not available (for instance, outpatient waiting-lists by area and social class, age and cause specific hospital mortality-rates by area and social class, the relation between ante-mortem and post-mortem diagnosis by area and social class, and hospital staff shortage by area) or else they are essentially use-rates. Use-rates may be interpreted either as evidence of high morbidity among high users, or of disproportionate benefit drawn by them from the National Health Service. By piling up the valid evidence that poor people in Britain have higher consultation and referral rates at all levels of the N.H.S., and by denying that these reflect actual differences in morbidity, Rein [3,4] has tried to show that Titmuss's opinion is incorrect, and that there are no significant gradients in the quality or accessibility of medical care in the N.H.S. between social classes.

Class gradients in mortality are an obvious obstacle to this view. Of these Rein says:

" One conclusion reached . . . is that since the lower classes have higher death rates, then they must be both sicker or less likely to secure treatment than other classes . . . it is useful to examine selected diseases in which there is a clear mortality class gradient and then compare these rates with the proportion of patients in each class that consulted their physician for treatment of these diseases. . . ."

He cites figures to show that high death-rates may be associated with low consultation-rates for some diseases, and with high rates for others, but, since the pattern of each holds good through all social classes, he concludes that

" a reasonable inference to be drawn from these findings is not that class mortality is an index of class morbidity, but that for certain diseases treatment is unrelated to outcome. Thus both high and low consultation rates can yield high mortality rates for specific diseases. These data do not appear to lead to the compelling conclusion that mortality votes can be easily used as an area of class-related morbidity."

This is the only argument mounted by Rein against the evidence of mortality differences, and the reasonable assumption that these probably represent the final outcome of larger differences in morbidity. Assuming that " votes " is a misprint for " rates ", I still find that the more one examines this argument the less it means. To be fair, it is only used to support the central thesis that " the availability of universal free-on-demand, comprehensive services would appear to be a crucial factor in reducing class inequalities in the use of medical care services ". It certainly would, but reduction is not abolition, as Rein would have quickly found if his stay in Britain had included more basic fieldwork in the general practitioner's surgery or the outpatient department.

Non-statistical Evidence

There is massive but mostly non-statistical evidence in favour of Titmuss's generalisations. First of all there is the evidence of social history. James [5] described the origins of the general-practitioner service in indus-

734

THE LANCET, APRIL 1, 1972

Points of View

PERSISTENT VEGETATIVE STATE AFTER BRAIN DAMAGE
A Syndrome in Search of a Name

BRYAN JENNETT

Institute of Neurological Sciences,
Glasgow GS1 4TF

FRED PLUM

New York Hospital—Cornell Medical Center,
New York City, N.Y., U.S.A.

Summary   Patients with severe brain damage due to trauma or ischæmia may now survive indefinitely. Some never regain recognisable mental function, but recover from sleep-like coma in that they have periods of wakefulness when their eyes are open and move; their responsiveness is limited to primitive postural and reflex movements of the limbs, and they never speak. Such patients are best described as in a persistent vegetative state, which should be clearly distinguished from other conditions associated with prolonged unresponsiveness. What is common to these patients is the absence of function in the cerebral cortex as judged behaviourally; the lesion may be in the cortex itself, in subcortical structures of the hemisphere, or in the brain-stem, or in all of these sites. But the exact site and nature of the lesion is unknown to the bedside clinician, and the name for the syndrome should not imply more than is known.

". . . if we have a conception for which no name exists, which we need frequently to speak of, it is not wise, I think, to shrink from an attempt to give it a name."—Sir WILLIAM GOWERS.

NEW methods of treatment may, by prolonging the lives of patients with conditions which were formerly fatal, result in situations never previously encountered. And new situations call for new names if they are to be accurately understood and discussed. Twenty years ago French[1] commented that patients who sustained brain lesions which deprived them of the ability to perform the intuitive and protective functions necessary for survival rarely lived more than a few days or, exceptionally, two or three weeks. He then described five patients who had survived for many months with profoundly altered consciousness, but he did not suggest a name for their clinical condition. With the development of intensive-care units it has now become almost commonplace for patients to survive with devastating brain damage, usually the result of head trauma, a brain-stem stroke, or a cardio-respiratory crisis associated with hypoxia. Clinical and pathological reports about such cases are beginning to accumulate, whilst the ethical, moral, and social issues are provoking comment both in the health professions and in the community at large. Once past the acute stage these patients are neither unconscious nor in coma in the usual sense of these terms, both of which imply a sleep-like insensibility. There is clearly need for an acceptable term to describe their state, in order to facilitate communication, between doctors or with patients' relatives or intelligent laymen, about its implications.

CLINICAL SYNDROME

In the first week or so after injury these patients are in deep coma, never opening their eyes; and when they do react to stimuli they show varying degrees of extensor response in the limbs. However, unless they have bilateral third-nerve paralysis, the survivors begin, within two or three weeks, to open their eyes—at first only in response to pain, then to less arousing stimuli. Soon after this they have periods when, without any provocation, they lie for periods with their eyes open; at other times they seem to sleep. It may be difficult to determine whether their sleep/wake rhythms have a normal diurnal pattern, because such patients are having intensive nursing care; this involves being turned every two or three hours, and the lights in their rooms may never be put out. The eyes are open and may blink to menace, but they are not attentive; although roving movements may briefly seem to follow moving objects, careful observation does not confirm any consistency in this optimistic interpretation. It seems that there is wakefulness without awareness.

The extensor response in the limbs is commonly referred to as decerebrate rigidity, after Sherrington's description of the limb postures of animals after midbrain transection. It can also begin to wear off after two or three weeks, and although for a time some extensor movements may still occur, a noxious stimulus may now provoke a flexor withdrawal, but only after an abnormal delay, and the movement itself is rather slow and dystonic and never takes the form of normal brisk response. A significant grasp reflex often appears, and this may be provoked by chance touch of the bedclothes; to the inexperienced observer or hopeful family the resulting movement may look as though it was initiated by the patient and may even be regarded as purposeful or voluntary. Sometimes fragments of coordinated movements may be seen such as scratching, or even movement of the hands towards a noxious stimulus, and postural alterations in the limbs may be provoked by neck movements. Chewing and teeth grinding are common and may go on for long periods; liquid and food placed in the mouth may be swallowed.

Grunting or groaning may be provoked by noxious stimuli, but most of these patients are silent; they neither speak nor make any meaningful response to the spoken word. Shouting, like a noxious stimulus, may produce a non-specific somatic and vegetative response with eye-opening, grimacing, altered respiratory pattern, and even some stereotyped limb flexion.

Few would dispute that in this condition the cerebral cortex is out of action. Two reported patients with extensive neocortical necrosis had shown this clinical state for several months after cardiac arrest.[2] However, it is also possible for the functions of the cortex to be inactivated without that structure itself being damaged, because, when a critical amount of damage is sustained by the reticular activating system either in the brain-stem or in the basal ganglia or subcortical areas, the cortex thereafter fails to function effectively. Patients with head injury who survive in this state frequently prove to have extensive lesions in the white-matter, with almost complete sparing of the cortex and brain-stem,[3,4] but others have secondary brain-stem compression or extensive ischæmic brain damage in the cortex and subcortical structures.

In the first few weeks after injury the electroencephalo-gram (E.E.G.) may resolve doubts about whether the patient is really attentive; if there is extensive neocortical death the record will initially be flat, as in the two cases of Brierley et al.[2] who had isoelectric records for many weeks. However, this is rare, and there is very little information

THE LANCET, APRIL 1, 1972

about the significance of E.E.G. changes months after the initial incident; there may be high-voltage slow waves or, occasionally, some alpha rhythm, but the activity is unresponsive to visual, auditory, or noxious stimuli. The occurrence of a wakeful E.E.G. record which is unmodified by stimuli, in patients who are unresponsive, has been reported previously with pontine lesions.[5,6]

EXISTING NAMES

A critical review of the terms which are used for this and related disorders gives an opportunity to discuss the differential diagnosis of this condition and to emphasise that none of these terms is quite appropriate. They fall naturally into two categories, the better of which are those that attempt to capture the essence of the syndrome descriptively. Those which imply or impute a particular anatomical or pathological basis, when it is already clear that both the site and the nature of the lesion may vary widely, are obviously less suitable.

Brain Death,[7] Coma Dépasse [8]

This applies to patients in whom structural or anoxic insults have left no evidence of function in the nervous system above the spinal cord: the pupils are fixed, spontaneous respiration has ceased, and the E.E.G. is always isoelectric, but cardiac function may continue for days and there may be stimulus-evoked limb movements due to persisting spinal reflexes. Before concluding that such a state is due to brain death it is essential to be certain that there has been neither excessive dosage with depressant drugs nor hypothermia, because either of these may produce a reversible suspension of brain activity. Brain death is never survived by more than a few days, and then only by reason of respirator support. The syndrome we are discussing may persist for months or even years, provided nutrition is satisfactorily supplied, because respiration is adequate (although some patients have had a short period of assisted ventilation in the acute stage of their illness).

Akinetic Mutism (Coma Vigile)

Coma vigile is an old term, probably first used by the French to describe the state of patients with severe typhus or typhoid fever. Akinetic mutism was coined by Cairns [9] in 1941 to describe an intermittent disturbance of consciousness in an adolescent girl with a craniopharyngioma. She lapsed into this state three times in nine months, and each time she recovered when the cyst was aspirated. Cairns commented on the eyes being open, apparently attentive, and " giving the promise of speech ". Skultety [10] has reviewed the literature which has accumulated since then, and he also reports the attempts which he and others have made to produce this state in laboratory animals. He concludes that the term presents considerable semantic problems and emphasises that akinesia and mutism do not always go together. In particular, the mutism may be only relative—Cairns' patient would answer in whispered monosyllables, whilst some other reported patients would use sign language to communicate. The lesions reported in patients who showed this rather loosely defined and potentially recoverable state range from the brain-stem through the basal ganglia to bilateral cingulate gyrus destruction.

Skultety considered that akinetic mutism was primarily a disorder of responsiveness and that three different types of disorder rather than separate sites of lesions could be recognised. These were loss of critical amounts respectively of the afferent input, of the activating reticular system, or of the efferent mechanisms (but the de-efferented, locked-in syndrome is clinically distinguishable—see below). Attempts to produce the syndrome of akinetic mutism in cats produced a variety of states with akinesia and mutism seemingly independently affected. But animal species at different phylogenetic levels will react differently to having the brain-stem disconnected from the cortex. Furthermore, how closely mutism in a cat (a relatively silent animal) corresponds to speechlessness in man is at best an open question.

Permanent, Irreversible, or Prolonged Coma, Stupor, or Dementia

Certainly we are concerned to identify an irrecoverable state, although the criteria needed to establish that prediction reliably have still to be confirmed. Until then " persistent " is safer than " permanent " or " irreversible "; but prolonged is not strong enough, and unless it is quantified it is meaningless. This state cannot be called " coma ", as ordinarily defined; in particular, it is not a continuation of the coma which characterises the early stages of these particular patients' clinical course. Stupor might be acceptable, but its established use for schizophrenic catatonia might lead to confusion. Dementia by its conventional usage suggests a progressive state of brain dysfunction, and it is in such common use for alert patients who are quite responsive that it seems inappropriate in the present context.

Decerebrate or Decorticate State

These terms are most often applied to different types of motor dysfunction, and, whilst it is usual for the mental state which we are defining to be associated with severe motor disorders, the pattern of this is by no means consistent. Moreover, decerebration was originally used by physiologists to describe the state of animals after brain-stem transection, and if the term were used for the clinical state under discussion it might not only focus attention on the motor dysfunction but it might also misleadingly imply that the lesion was in the brain-stem. The same argument tells against chronic brain-stem syndrome. In any event this is a meaningless tag of jargon, and the same goes for post-traumatic encephalopathy—which might be used for any condition from the postconcussional syndrome to brain death. Both decerebration and decortication might be taken to imply a specific structural lesion: such terms are unsuitable for bedside diagnosis, when the nature of the lesion can seldom be accurately predicted and never be proved.

Apallic Syndrome

This was proposed in 1940 by Kretschmer,[11] a psychiatrist, to describe patients who were open-eyed, uncommunicative, and unresponsive from a variety of lesions, including cerebral arteriosclerosis, lues, and gunshot wounds. His paper was concerned with terms used to describe cortical dysfunction, and he suggested that apallic was in line with the words

736   THE LANCET, APRIL 1, 1972

apraxic and *agnosic,* but that it indicated the simultaneous disturbance of several cortical functions. The full syndrome he considered much less common than partial or incomplete forms, and he implied that recovery was possible because he described the psychiatric features of the recovery period.

The term seems to have been largely neglected until its recent adoption by the Viennese neurologists and neuropathologists to describe survivors of severe head injury,[12,13] anoxic insults, or poisoning. Gerstenbrand [14] also suggests that there are degrees of the syndrome, that considerable amounts of the telencephalon seem still to be functioning in most cases because the E.E.G. is not isoelectric, and that recovery is possible. Ingvar [15] suggests that less severe forms might be termed dyspallic or incomplete apallic, and both he and Gerstenbrand refer to the difficulty of distinguishing this clinical state from the effects of a massive lesion of the dominant cerebral hemisphere, producing global aphasia, apraxia, and agnosia. The characteristics of the complete apallic syndrome, according to Ingvar, are a complete loss of higher (telencephalic) function with an isoelectric E.E.G. and much-reduced cerebral blood-flow and metabolism in supratentorial structures.

Attempts have been made to produce apallic cats by making brain-stem lesions and using intensive-care techniques to ensure prolonged survival.[16] These experiments are most interesting in showing the amount of complex activity which eventually returns after extensive lesions; surgical decerebration of infant monkeys is likewise followed by the return of a considerable repertoire of responsive motor behaviour, and observations on anencephalic humans surviving for some weeks reinforce the view that an appreciable range of activity and responsiveness is possible in the absence of the cortex. However, none of this evidence bears on the problem of mental function in adult man, whilst even at the level of motor behaviour there are difficulties in extrapolating from animal experiments or studies in young infants, because of the varying degrees of dependence of subcortical structures on cortical influence in different species and at different stages of development. Once encephalisation has occurred, phylogenetically or in the individual, it prevents for evermore the return to full function of lower structures that may operate very well in primitive animals. Collicular sight is a good example.

The term *apallic* used in a clinical sense seems to us more to confuse than to clarify the issue under discussion. In the first place, it is an uncommon word even in medicine, and its usage merely adds to the unnecessarily arcane jargon that often makes neurology needlessly difficult for others to understand. In addition, the term is potentially misleading, not only because partial or incomplete syndromes are admitted, but because it assumes an unproved pathology; and there remains ambiguity about whether the structure or the function of the cortex is taken to be absent. As already noted, the clinical syndrome we are describing can be produced by lesions which largely spare the cortex structurally, and the E.E.G. may even show persisting alpha rhythms.

Locked-in Syndrome (De-efferented State)

This term was coined by Plum and Posner in 1965 [17] to describe the tetraplegic, mute but fully alert state which results when the descending motor pathways are interrupted by an infarction of the ventral pons. Such patients are entirely awake, responsive and sentient, although the repertoire of response is limited to blinking, and jaw and eye

movements. One patient [18] still alive after 18 months has full bladder control and signals by Morse code, using blinks and jaw movements, that she appreciates a full range of sensation from skin and joint position. In her, noxious stimuli provoke decerebrate posturing; the E.E.G. is normal, and during 4–6 hours at night shows the usual sleep changes.

PERSISTENT VEGETATIVE STATE

We propose this as the most satisfactory term to describe this syndrome, for several reasons. It describes behaviour, and it is only data about behaviour which will always be available, and in every patient, because such observations are independent of special procedures such as E.E.G. and measurements of cerebral blood-flow or cerebral metabolism. This term presumes neither a particular physio-anatomical abnormality nor a specific pathological lesion, matters which can seldom be settled beyond doubt at the bedside; it therefore invites further clinical and pathological investigation of the condition rather than giving the impression of a problem already completely understood. The word *vegetative* itself is not obscure: *vegetate* is defined in the *Oxford English Dictionary* as " to live a merely physical life, devoid of intellectual activity or social intercourse (1740) " and *vegetative* is used to describe " an organic body capable of growth and development but devoid of sensation and thought (1764) ". It suggests even to the layman a limited and primitive responsiveness to external stimuli; to the doctor it is also a reminder that there is relative preservation of autonomic regulation of the internal milieu. Lastly this term has already occasionally been used to describe patients such as this, although we are unaware of any attempt to define the limits of the syndrome to which it could properly be applied.

Death, recovery, or survival " as a vegetative wreck " were the three outcomes of severe head injury recently recognised by Vapalahti and Troupp [19]; their patients with vegetative survival were described as incapable of communication and without hope of recovery as social human beings. In our view the essential component of this syndrome is the absence of any adaptive response to the external environment, the absence of any evidence of a functioning mind which is either receiving or projecting information, in a patient who has long periods of wakefulness. Akinesia is relative, because postural adjustments and stereotyped primitive withdrawals are usually possible. All the patients are speechless and also fail to signal appropriately by eye movements, although they sometimes follow moving objects in a slow intermittent pattern. Initially the E.E.G. may be isoelectric, but considerable activity and even alpha rhythm may be found once the state has lasted many months. What is common to all patients in this vegetative, mindless state is that, as best can be judged behaviourally, the cerebral cortex is not functioning, whether the lesion be in the cerebral cortex itself, in subcortical structures, the brain-stem, or in all these sites. However, we cannot yet accurately predict the specific pathological substrate or the precise E.E.G. abnormality which will be found in association with the persistent vegetative state.

Exactly how long such a state must persist before it can be confidently declared permanent will have to be determined by careful prospective studies, using the criteria which we have set down here, and we are already undertaking such an investigation. It is already clear that patients destined to make a reasonable recovery (including those who will have considerable permanent disability) do not usually pass through the vegetative state as a phase in their recovery from coma. In these more hopeful cases, once wakefulness returns, there are other signs of returning cortical function, and it is the discrepancy between prolonged periods of wakefulness and the absence of any behavioural or physiological evidence of cortical function or mental activity which characterises the vegetative state. Although we would not deny that a continuum must exist between this vegetative state and some of the others described, it seems wise to make an absolute distinction between patients who do make a consistently understandable response to those around them, whether by word or gesture, and those who never do. It may well become a matter for discussion how worth while life is for patients whose capacity for meaningful response is very limited, but it still seems to us that the immediate issue is to recognise that there is a group of patients who never show evidence of a working mind. This concept may be criticised on the grounds that observation of behaviour is insufficient evidence on which to base a judgment of mental activity: it is our view that there is no reliable alternative available to the doctor at the bedside, which is where decisions have to be made.

It is advantageous to have a term which avoids the mystique of highly specialised medical jargon to describe a condition likely to be discussed widely outside the profession. This is our main objection to *la stupeur hypertonique post-comateuse*, the users of which themselves write: "*Un terme nouveau serait peut-être utile pour nommer ces états*".[20] Certainly the indefinite survival of patients in this state presents a problem with humanitarian and socioeconomic implications which society as a whole will have to consider.[21-23] If it were possible to predict soon after the brain damage had been sustained that, in the event of survival, the outcome would be a vegetative mindless state, then the wisdom of continuing supportive measures could be discussed. Until reliable predictive criteria emerge it is inevitable that the price of reducing mortality from severe brain damage, and enabling many patients to make a reasonable recovery, will be the survival of some patients in a permanent vegetative state.

REFERENCES

1. French, J. D. *Archs Neurol. Psychiat.* 1952, **68**, 727.
2. Brierley, J. B., Adams, J. H., Graham, D. I., Simpson, J. A. *Lancet*, 1971, ii, 560.
3. Strich, S. J. *J. Neurol. Neurosurg. Psychiat.* 1956, **19**, 163.
4. Strich, S. J. *Lancet*, 1961, ii, 443.
5. Chatrian, G. E., White, L. E., Shaw, C.-M. *Electroenceph. clin. Neurophysiol.* 1964, **16**, 285.
6. Kaada, B. R., Harkmark, W., Stokke, O. *ibid.* 1961, **13**, 785.
7. Mohandas, A., Chou, S. N. *J. Neurosurg.* 1971, **35**, 211.
8. Mollaret, P., Goulon, M. *Rev. Neurol.* 1959, **101**, 3.
9. Cairns, H., Oldfield, R. C., Pennybacker, J. B., Whitteridge, D. *Brain*, 1941, **64**, 273.
10. Skultety, M. F. *Archs Neurol.* 1968, **19**, 1.

References continued at foot of next column

Dogma Disputed

THE FOUR QUARTERS OF PREGNANCY

DEREK LLEWELLYN-JONES

*Department of Obstetrics and Gynæcology,
University of Sydney*

IN the days when pregnancy was considered to last nine calendar months, obstetricians found it convenient to divide this period into three trimesters. Even though most obstetric educators now recommend that the duration of pregnancy should be calculated in weeks rather than months, the concept of three trimesters persists, although it is neither chronologically accurate nor particularly valuable as a concept.

For several reasons the time has now come for the division of pregnancy into trimesters to be abandoned, and for medical students to be taught that a pregnancy, which has a mean duration of 40 weeks from the first day of the last menstrual period in a woman whose menstrual cycle is of normal duration, may conveniently be divided into four 10-week periods. We should, in fact, talk about the four quarters of pregnancy.

The reasons for recommending this change can be discussed under several headings.

Abortion.—The World Health Organisation has recommended that "abortions"—referring to the products of conception—should be termed early fetal deaths; and the word abortion should only refer to the process of expulsion. Over 50% of known spontaneous abortions occur before the 10th week of pregnancy, and, where legal abortion is permitted, the morbidity and mortality of the procedure is very much less if the termination is made before the 10th gestational week.[1,2] In fact, many authorities recommend that legal abortion should be induced after the end of the 10th gestational week only if there are strong medical reasons.

Viability.—In Britain the definition of viability requires to be changed. The Registrar-General still accepts that stillbirths are defined as babies born after 28 weeks' gestation who do not show any signs of life after separation from the mother, the presumption being that infants born before this time are not viable. This is not true. Evidence from several nations shows that 7-12% of infants born before the end of the 28th gestational week survive. This fact is recognised by the World Health Organisation, which has recommended that the perinatal mortality shall be calculated by including all infants who weigh 500 g. or

PROF. JENNETT, PROF. PLUM: REFERENCES—*continued*

11. Kretschmer, E. *Zbl. ges. Neurol. Psychiat.* 1940, **169**, 576.
12. Gerstenbrand, F. *in* The Late Effects of Head Injuries (edited by A. E. Walker, W. F. Caveness, and M. Critchley); p. 340. Springfield, Illinois, 1969.
13. Jellinger, K., Seitelberger, F. *ibid.* p. 168.
14. Gerstenbrand, F. Das Traumatische Appallische Syndrom. Vienna, 1967.
15. Ingvar, D. H. *Arch. Psychiat. NervKrankh.* (in the press).
16. Dolce, F., Fromm, H. *Scand. J. Rehab. Med.* (in the press).
17. Plum, F., Posner, J. B. The Diagnosis of Stupor and Coma. Philadelphia, 2nd ed. 1972.
18. Feldman, M. H. *Archs Neurol.* 1971, **25**, 501.
19. Vapalahti, M., Troupp, H. *Br. med. J.* 1971, iii, 404.
20. Fischgold, H., Mathis, P. *Electroenceph. clin. Neurophysiol.* 1959, suppl. 11.
21. *Lancet*, 1971, ii, 590.
22. *ibid.* 1970, ii, 915.
23. Jennett, B. *ibid.* p. 1249.

THE LANCET, JUNE 10, 1972   1279

Only 19 patients (21%) were aborted in National Health Service hospitals; the remainder were terminated privately (64 patients) or abroad (8 patients).

From group A, 8 (9%) had a spontaneous second-trimester abortion and 1 had a clinically incompetent cervix that required a suture. There were no first-trimester abortions. 4 patients went into premature labour, and there was 1 intrauterine death caused by rhesus incompatibility. Clinical details of the abnormal cases are given in table II.

Group B

Of the 91 control patients, 1 had a spontaneous second-trimester abortion and 4 had a first-trimester abortion. 1 patient went into premature labour and there were no stillbirths.

There was a statistically significant increase in the number of second-trimester abortions in group A compared with group B ($\chi^2 = 4.21$ [Yates' correction]. $P < 0.05$).

Group C

Out of the 3223 confinements in this group, there were 32 first-trimester abortions (1%) and 42 second-trimester abortions. After excluding 12 pregnancies ending in the second trimester because of missed abortion, abruptio placentæ, or intrauterine death, there were 30 spontaneous second-trimester abortions—an incidence of 0.9%. 8 of these 30 patients had already had a previous second-trimester abortion; of the remaining 22, 3 had had a vaginal termination of pregnancy, though not immediately before the aborted pregnancy (thus not qualifying for group A).

215 patients (6.7%) went into premature labour and there were 36 stillbirths (1.1%).

DISCUSSION

During 1971 in Queen Charlotte's Hospital there was a tenfold increase in the number of second-trimester abortions in pregnancies which followed a vaginal termination of pregnancy, compared with all patients who delivered in the same year. This increase strongly indicates that temporary or permanent cervical incompetence is induced by the procedure of dilatation of the cervix during termination. This is further suggested by the fact that a control group had significantly fewer second-trimester abortions. The only important difference between the two groups was that the previous-termination patients had had forcible dilatation of the cervix. This result agrees with the finding of Stallworthy et al.[6] that 4.8% of patients had cervical lacerations after vaginal termination of pregnancy. Our abortion-rate of 9% after this procedure is considerably below the 30–40% rate reported by Kotasek,[7] who did not give details of how his figure was determined. The numbers in group A are small because we did not make a retrospective study of this subject. In our experience a significant number of patients do not admit to previous terminations, or refer to them as miscarriages unless specifically questioned about this aspect of their obstetric history. If the 9% incidence of second-trimester abortion in our study is correct, then an additional 10,000 second-trimester abortions may

take place annually in the U.K. over the next few years.

We found no difference between the number of subsequent abortions in patients terminated privately and under the National Health Service. Of the 8 patients in group A who aborted, only 1 had previously been terminated before 10 weeks' menstrual age. Perhaps earlier termination using the Karman catheter will reduce the risk of cervical damage. In our study previous termination was not associated with an increased incidence of premature labour or other complications of pregnancy.

We believe that all patients who have had a vaginal termination of pregnancy should be judged as being at risk of having a second-trimester abortion in their subsequent pregnancy. Digital assessment of the cervix should be performed every two weeks in the subsequent pregnancy for signs of cervical incompetence. This assessment resulted in the early diagnosis and successful treatment of cervical incompetence in case 6 (table II).

Requests for reprints should be addressed to S. C.

REFERENCES

1. Unplanned Pregnancy: report of the working party of the Royal College of Obstetricians and Gynæcologists, 1972.
2. Registrar General's Statistical Review: England and Wales, 1969. Supplement on Abortion. H.M. Stationery Office, 1971.
3. Jurukovski, J., Sukarov, L. *Int. J. Gynæc. Obstet.* 1971, 9, 111.
4. Berić, B. M., Kupresanin, M. *Lancet*, 1971, ii, 619.
5. Sood, S. V. *Br. med. J.* 1971, iv, 270.
6. Stallworthy, J. A., Moolgaoker, A. S., Walsh, J. J. *Lancet*, 1971, ii, 1245.
7. Kotasek, A. *Int. J. Gynæc. Obstet.* 1971, 9, 118.

Medical Education

DEMONSTRATION TO MEDICAL STUDENTS OF PLACEBO RESPONSES AND NON-DRUG FACTORS

BARRY BLACKWELL   SAUL S. BLOOMFIELD
C. RALPH BUNCHER

College of Medicine, University of Cincinnati, Cincinnati, Ohio 45229, U.S.A.

Summary   A class experiment for medical students was devised to demonstrate the influence of the placebo effect and non-drug factors on response to drugs. The subjects were conditioned to expect sedative or stimulant effects, but all received placebo in one or two blue or pink capsules. Predictions about the size and nature of the placebo response and influence of the non-drug factors were made before the experiment and discussed afterwards. Four of six predictions were fully confirmed. Drug-associated changes were reported by 30% of the subjects and were severe in 1 or 2 individuals. Two capsules produced more noticeable changes than one, and blue capsules were associated with more sedative effects than pink capsules. Students rated the experiment highly both as a learning experience and for its relevance to their future practice of medicine.

The Lancet · Saturday 19 May 1973

SIMPLE VERSUS RADICAL MASTECTOMY
Preliminary Report of the Cardiff Breast Trial

M. MAUREEN ROBERTS*   A. P. M. FORREST*

L. H. BLUMGART†   H. CAMPBELL

MARIANNE DAVIES   E. N. GLEAVE‡

J. M. HENK   P. B. KUNKLER§

R. SHIELDS¶

*Department of Surgery, Welsh National School of
Medicine, and Department of Radiotherapy,
Velindre Hospital, Cardiff*

M. HULBERT   C. W. JAMIESON

R. A. SELLWOOD‡

*Departments of Surgery and Radiotherapy,
St. Mary's Hospital, London W2*

Summary   By the end of 1972, 230 patients with breast cancer had been admitted to a clinical trial of simple versus radical mastectomy at centres in Cardiff and London. In both groups adjuvant local radiotherapy was given only if pectoral-node or axillary-node histology indicated metastatic disease. Comment on disease-free survival would be premature. However, there is nothing in the preliminary data to suggest that a conservative surgical approach is inferior to a radical one.

Introduction

IN 1967, a controlled randomised trial was inaugurated to determine if a policy of treatment for primary cancer of the breast, in which a standard operation of simple mastectomy supported by localised adjuvant radiotherapy only if histological examination of the lower axillary nodes indicated metastatic disease, gave results comparable to those of a radical approach.[1] Two centres participated, in each of which a coordinator monitored admission to the trial and supervised its conduct.

Up to Dec. 31, 1972, 230 patients had been admitted to the trial, 187 from Cardiff and 43 from St. Mary's Hospital, London. Although no conclusions regarding disease-free survival-rates can yet be made, preliminary results indicate that the conservative and radical groups are behaving similarly and support our concept that the extent of local treatment can justifiably

be based on the histological findings in the lower axillary (pectoral) nodes.

Patients and Methods

All patients entered into the trial had primary breast cancer of TNM stages I and II (T_1 or T_2, N_0 or N_1), determined by means of a standard form. Each patient was examined twice, and tumour size (measured by callipers), mobility, and skin changes were recorded. The palpability of axillary nodes was recorded and metastatic disease was sought by radiographs of the chest, skull, and pelvis, mammography of both breasts, and liver-function tests. All patients with advanced local disease or metastatic disease were excluded.

Patients were then stratified into twenty-four subgroups according to clinical stage of tumour, clinical palpability of nodes, site of tumour, and menstrual status. Clinical stage of the tumour was defined as T_1 or T_2, palpability of nodes as N_0 or N_1, site of tumour as outer half or others, and menstrual status as premenopausal (periods regular, or up to 2 years since the last menstrual period), menopausal (2–5 years since the last menstrual period), and postmenopausal (over 5 years since the last menstrual period). Patients were randomly selected within these subgroups for one of two policies of treatment.

Conservative Policy

The conservative policy was local mastectomy with selective local radiotherapy. The breast was removed usually from medial to lateral sides through a horizontal incision enclosing the usual ellipse of skin including the nipple. The axillary tail was carefully dissected from between the pectoral and latissimus muscles up to the level of the fascia and was removed with one or two pectoral lymph nodes. These nodes lie on the medial side of the axillary tail at its junction with the axillary fat and just below the outer border of the pectoralis major muscle. They were best defined during the dissection and were sought even if impalpable clinically. In some instances no nodes were identified at this site, yet enlarged palpable nodes were present in the axillary fat. The surgeon was permitted to remove one of these nodes for biopsy, even if this implied breaching the axillary fascia. The nodes were separately placed in formol-saline for histology.

A tissue sample was taken from the edge of the skin ellipse nearest to the tumour and similarly fixed for histological section.

Postoperative radiotherapy was considered when the histology of the nodes and skin were known. If both were negative, no further treatment was given, the patient being treated solely by simple mastectomy. If the axillary nodes were involved radiation was given to the axilla. The protocol of the trial decreed that radiation would be given to the chest wall if the skin were involved; if both axilla and skin were involved, then both axilla and chest wall would be irradiated. In the event, only axillary radiation was given, because all the skin biopsies were negative.

Radiation consisted of 4000 rad from a cobalt source in ten fractions given on alternate days over a 3-week period.

---
* Present address: Department of Clinical Surgery, University of Edinburgh, Royal Infirmary, Edinburgh EH3 9YW.

† Present address: Department of Surgery, University of Glasgow (Royal Infirmary).

‡ Present address: Department of Surgery, University of Manchester (Withington Hospital).

§ Present address: Department of Radiotherapy, University of Leeds (Cookridge Hospital).

¶ Present address: Department of Surgery, University of Liverpool.

1404   THE LANCET, JUNE 23, 1973

Requests for reprints should be addressed to the Boston Collaborative Drug Surveillance Programme, 400 Totten Pond Road, Waltham, Massachusetts 02154, U.S.A.

REFERENCES

1. Vessey, M. P., Doll, R. *Br. med. J.* 1968, ii, 199.
2. Vessey, M. P., Doll, R. *ibid.* 1969, ii, 651.
3. Sartwell, P. E., Masi, A. T., Arthes, F. G., Greene, G. R., Smith, H. E. *Am. J. Epidemiol.* 1969, **90**, 365.
4. Drill, V. A. *J. Am. med. Ass.* 1972, **219**, 583.
5. Preston, S. N. *Am. J. Obstet. Gynec.* 1971, **111**, 994.
6. Friedman, G. D., Kannel, W. B., Dawber, T. R. *J. chron. Dis.* 1966, **19**, 273.
7. Newman, H. F., Northup, J. D. *Int. Abstr. Surg.* 1959, **109**, 1.
8. Kaye, M. D., Kern, F. *Lancet,* 1971, i, 1228.
9. Sampliner, R. E., Bennett, P. H., Comess, L. J., Rose, F. A., Burch, T. A. *New Engl. J. Med.* 1970, **283**, 1358.
10. Robertson, H. E., Dochat, G. R. *Int. Abstr. Surg.* 1944, **78**, 193.
11. Robertson, H. E. *ibid.* 1945, **80**, 1.
12. Hertz, R. *Cancer,* 1969, **24**, 1140.
13. Vessey, M. P., Doll, R., Sutton, P. M. *Br. med. J.* 1972, iii, 719.
14. Arthes, F. G., Sartwell, P. E., Lewison, E. F. *Cancer,* 1971, **28**, 1391.
15. Sartwell, P. E., Arthes, F. G., Tonascia, J. A. *New Engl. J. Med.* 1973, **288**, 551.
16. Mantel, N., Haenszel, W. *J. natn. Cancer Inst.* 1959, **22**, 719.
17. Bottiger, L. E., Westerholm, B. *Acta med. scand.* 1971, **190**, 455.
18. Inman, W. H. W., Vessey, M. P., Westerholm, B., Engelund, A. *Br. med. J.* 1970, ii, 203.
19. Dugdale, M., Masi, A. T. *J. chron. Dis.* 1971, **23**, 775.
20. Aronson, H. B., Magora, F., Schenker, J. G. *Am. J. Obstet. Gynec.* 1971, **110**, 997.
21. Oski, F. A., Lubin, B., Buchert, E. D. *Ann. intern. Med.* 1972, **77**, 419.
22. Zuck, T. F., Bergin, J. J., Raymond, J. T., Dwyre, W. R., Corby, D. G. *Thromb. Diath. hæmorrh.* 1971, **26**, 426.
23. Poller, L., Priest, C. M., Thomson, J. M. *Br. med. J.* 1969, iv, 273.
24. Poller, L., Tabiowo, A., Thomson, J. M. *ibid.* 1968, iii, 218.
25. Poller, L., Thomson, J. M., Tabiowo, A., Priest, C. M. *ibid.* 1969, i, 554.
26. Hedlin, A. M., Monkhouse, F. C. *Obstet. Gynec.* 1971, **37**, 225.
27. Small, D. M., Rapo, S. *New Engl. J. Med.* 1970, **283**, 53.
28. Small, D. M. *Adv. intern. Med.* 1970, **16**, 243.
29. Tritapepe, R., Cesana, A., Gandini, R., Trivellini, G. *Panminerva med.* 1969, **11**, 410.
30. Potter, J. F., Slimbaugh, W. P., Woodward, S. C. *Ann. Surg.* 1968, **167**, 829.
31. Warren, S. *Surgery Gynec. Obstet.* 1940, **71**, 257.
32. MacMahon, B., Cole, P., Lin, T. M., Lowe, C. R., Mirra, A. P., Ravnihar, B., Salber, E. J., Valaoras, V. G., Yuasa, S. *Bull. Wld Hlth Org.* 1970, **43**, 209.
33. Hougie, C. *Am. Heart J.* 1973, **85**, 538.

TEN-YEAR EXPERIENCE OF MODIFIED-FAT DIETS ON YOUNGER MEN WITH CORONARY HEART-DISEASE

MARVIN L. BIERENBAUM   ALAN I. FLEISCHMAN
ROBERT I. RAICHELSON   THOMAS HAYTON
              PORTIA B. WATSON

Atherosclerosis Research Group, Saint Vincent's Hospital, Montclair, New Jersey 07042, U.S.A.

Summary   One hundred men, 30–50 years old, with confirmed coronary-artery disease and past myocardial infarction, were placed on a 28% fat diet after weight reduction. This group was matched with a similar group not under dietary management. Over a period of 10 years there were significant reductions in serum-lipids in the diet-managed group compared with the control group. In this predominantly lipoprotein-phenotype-IV group, using a diet containing less than 9% of calories as saturated fat and less than 400 mg. exogenous cholesterol daily, the degree of unsaturation of the diet did not appear to influence either serum-lipid values or mortality-rates. After 10 years, the diet-managed

group had a 17% greater survival-rate than the control group.

Introduction

EPIDEMIOLOGICAL studies [1-7] have shown a relation between diet, serum-lipids, and the incidence of coronary heart-disease. The ætiology of coronary heart-disease has been shown to be multifactorial, [8-11] and diet is one of the contributing factors. Many of the risk factors have been elucidated by the Framingham study. [12]

Low-fat, relatively unsaturated diets have been successfully used to lower serum-cholesterol in several primary prevention studies. [13-15] In a 12-year secondary prevention study, Morrison [16] reported a significant decrease in the mortality-rate among subjects on a controlled diet who had already had myocardial infarction. Similar results were obtained by Nelson, [17] Lyon et al., [18] and Leren. [19] However, a research committee to the Medical Research Council [20] did not find a significant difference in mortality under similar conditions in a secondary prevention study in London, while Dayton et al., [21] in a primary prevention study, reported a lower incidence of fatal atherosclerotic events but not of total mortality in a group on a diet high in unsaturated fat compared to a control group.

In an earlier 5-year report, Bierenbaum et al. [22] reported a significant lowering in serum cholesterol and triglyceride in a diet-managed group of young men with coronary heart-disease, as compared to a control group, with a concomitant lowering in the reinfarction-rate in the diet-managed group. We report the results of 10 years' experience in a prospective study which compared the effect of two controlled-fat diets, one containing relatively unsaturated fat and the other containing saturated fat, and determined the morbidity and mortality from coronary heart-disease, according to diet group, in young men who had already had at least one confirmed myocardial infarction.

Methods

A study group of a hundred men was assembled in small groups over a period of 18 months. Table I shows the age-distribution of the study and control groups. All individuals had experienced electrocardiographically confirmed myocardial infarctions, with the presence of a Q wave being a prerequisite. They were referred by their own physicians, under whose care they remained throughout the study period.

Dietary pilot studies used a 28% fat diet limited in cholesterol; one diet consisted of relatively unsaturated fat and the other consisted of saturated fat. There was no difference in serum-cholesterol value between the two diet

TABLE I—AGE-DISTRIBUTION OF SUBJECTS UPON ENTRY INTO STUDY

Group	Total	Age-groups (yr.)				
		30–34	35–39	40–44	45–49	50–54
Study	100	1	15 (42*)	26	47 (58†)	11
Control	100	3	15 (49*)	31	46 (51†)	5

* Total in age-groups 30–44.
† Total in age-groups 45–54.

The Lancet · Saturday 27 October 1973

PRENATAL DIAGNOSIS OF ANENCEPHALY THROUGH MATERNAL SERUM-ALPHAFETOPROTEIN MEASUREMENT

D. J. H. Brock

University Department of Human Genetics, Western General Hospital, Edinburgh EH4 2HU

A. E. Bolton

Medical Research Council Radioimmunoassay Team, Edinburgh

J. M. Monaghan

Department of Obstetrics and Gynæcology, Western General Hospital, Edinburgh

Summary   An anencephalic pregnancy was first diagnosed by measurement of α-fetoprotein (A.F.P.) in maternal serum at 16 weeks and then 21 weeks of gestation. After confirmation of the diagnosis by amniotic-fluid A.F.P. measurement and ultrasonic and X-ray scan, the pregnancy was terminated. It is suggested that maternal serum-A.F.P. levels may be useful in the screening of large numbers of pregnancies for possible central-nervous-system malformations.

Introduction

In 1972 Brock and Sutcliffe showed that α-fetoprotein (A.F.P.) concentrations in amniotic fluids of anencephalic fetuses were very much higher than in those from normal fetuses.[1] Most of their samples were obtained between 26 weeks' gestation and term, but one amniotic fluid from a 13-week fetus with spina bifida and one from an 18-week anencephalic fetus[2] suggested that diagnosis based on A.F.P. could be made early enough to allow termination of pregnancy. Subsequently, amniotic-fluid A.F.P. levels have been exploited for the interruption of a number of pregnancies leading both to anencephaly[3,4] and to spina bifida.[5,6]

A.F.P. crosses the placental barrier and can be detected in maternal serum with a sensitive radioimmunoassay.[7] We report an early prenatal diagnosis of anencephaly in which the first indication of abnormality was a raised concentration of maternal serum-A.F.P.

Case-report

The patient's first pregnancy resulted in a normal male, the second in a premature female with congenital heart lesion, and the third in a stillborn anencephalic. During the next pregnancy a sample of blood was taken at 16 weeks' gestation and again at 21 weeks. Serum-A.F.P. was determined by a minor modification of the double-antibody radioimmunoassay described by Ruoslahti and Seppälä,[8] using a purified A.F.P. standard supplied by Dr S. Nishi.

At 16 weeks the patient's serum-A.F.P. was 135 ng. per ml. Mean of thirteen control sera between 14 and 18 weeks' gestation was 38 ng. per ml., with a range of 13–75 ng. per ml. At 21 weeks the patient's serum-A.F.P. was 445 ng. per ml., while a mean of fifteen control sera between 20 and 23 weeks' gestation was 65 ng. per ml., with a range of 14 to 121 ng. per ml. Amniocentesis was performed, and amniotic-fluid A.F.P. was found by immunoelectrophoresis to be 240 μg. per ml. (upper limit of normal at 21 weeks is 18 μg. per ml.).[9] An ultrasonic scan and X-ray examination confirmed anencephaly, while revealing that the mother had spina bifida occulta. The pregnancy was terminated by high-dose oxytocin infusion, and the fetus found to be a male anencephalic without spina bifida.

Discussion

Although anencephaly and spina bifida are relatively common congenital malformations in the U.K., there is no method of identifying most at-risk pregnancies. If the mother has already had an affected child the risk of repetition, calculated empirically, is about 1 in 20. However, more than 90% of infants with anencephaly and spina bifida will be born to mothers with no family history of central-nervous-system malformation. Amniocentesis on all early pregnancies for the purpose of determining amniotic-fluid A.F.P. is out of the question. Although ultrasonic investigation has allowed the diagnosis of anencephaly at 17 weeks' gestation,[10] it is a specialised technique requiring sophisticated interpretation, and is not yet applicable to a large number of patients. The importance of our finding is that it raises the possibility of screening pregnancies through a determination made on a small amount of maternal blood.

The values for the patient's serum-A.F.P., 135 ng. per ml. at 16 weeks and 445 ng. per ml. at 21 weeks, were both substantially above the limited number of controls chosen on the basis that the outcome of pregnancy was known. Ishiguro and Nishimura[11] give an upper limit of normal for 16 weeks of about 50 ng. per ml. and for 21 weeks of about 80 ng. per ml. Garoff and Seppälä[12] report upper limits for these two gestations of 200 ng. per ml. and 300 ng. per ml., respectively. It is probable that as further samples are obtained our normal ranges will be somewhat widened.

It would be unwise to suggest that maternal serum-A.F.P. alone could be used to diagnose anencephaly or spina bifida early in pregnancy. It is not clear whether the raised amniotic-fluid A.F.P. found in these conditions will inevitably be reflected in raised maternal serum levels. Seppälä and Ruoslahti have reported a case of meningomyelocele where amniotic-fluid A.F.P. was considerably increased while the maternal serum level was normal, though this was at 27 weeks of pregnancy.[13] Perhaps more common will be false-positive results, for increased serum-A.F.P. is associated with a number of conditions unrelated to pregnancy—in particular, primary hepatocellular carcinomas,[14] but also other carcinomas,[15-17] and non-malignant diseases of the liver.[18-20] In pregnancy, a raised A.F.P. has been demonstrated to be associated with threatened abortion,[21] non-specific cases of fetal distress, and intrauterine death, and is anticipated where there is fetomaternal transfusion.[13] Most of the false-positives unrelated to pregnancy will be eliminated by amniotic-fluid A.F.P. measurement. Where both maternal serum and amniotic-fluid A.F.P. are raised, the obstetrician is as well to be alerted, whether the outcome of the pregnancy be a spontaneous abortion, an intrauterine death, or an anencephalic infant.

We thank Dr S. Nishi for a gift of highly purified A.F.P., Dr A. F. Anderson for access to his patient, Miss Sandra Brown for technical assistance, and Dr C. Gosden, Mr J. Toop, and Miss M. Watt for their help. The research was supported by grants from the Distillers Company Ltd. and the Association for Spina Bifida and Hydrocephalus.

Requests for reprints should be addressed to D. J. H. B.

REFERENCES

1. Brock, D. J. H., Sutcliffe, R. G. *Lancet*, 1972, ii, 197.
2. Brock, D. J. H., Scrimgeour, J. B. *ibid.* p. 1252.
3. Lorber, J., Stewart, C. R., Milford Ward, A. *ibid.* 1973, i, 1187.
4. Seller, M. J., Campbell, S., Coltart, T. M., Singer, J. D. *ibid.* 1973, ii, 73.
5. Nevin, N. C., Nesbitt, S., Thompson, W. *ibid.* 1973, i, 1383.
6. Allan, L. D., Ferguson-Smith, M. A., Donald, I., Sweet, E., Gibson A. A. M. *ibid.* 1973, ii, 522.
7. Seppälä, M., Ruoslahti, E. *ibid.* 1972, i, 375.
8. Ruoslahti, E., Seppälä, M. *Int. J. Cancer*, 1971, **8**, 374.
9. Brock, D. J. H. Unpublished.
10. Campbell, S., Johnstone, F. D., Holt, E. M., May, P. *Lancet*, 1972, ii, 1226.
11. Ishiguro, T., Nishimura, T. *Am. J. Obstet. Gynec.* 1973, **116**, 27.
12. Garoff, L., Seppälä, M. *J. Obstet. Gynæc. Br. Commonw.* 1973, **80**, 695.
13. Seppälä, M., Ruoslahti, E. *Lancet*, 1973, i, 155.
14. Tatarinov, Y. S. *Fedn Proc.* 1966, **25**, 344.
15. Abelev, G. I. *Cancer Res.* 1968, **28**, 1344.
16. Masopust, J., Kithier, K., Radl, J., Koutecky, J., Kotal, L. *Int. J. Cancer*, 1968, **3**, 364.
17. Bourreille, J., Metayer, P., Sauger, F., Matray, F., Fondimare, A. *Presse méd.* 1970, **78**, 1277.
18. Abelev, G. I. *Adv. Cancer Res.* 1971, **14**, 295.
19. Nayak, N. C., Malaviya, A. N., Chawla, V., Chandra, R. K. *Lancet*, 1972, i, 68.
20. Waldmann, T. A., McIntire, K. R. *ibid.* 1972, ii, 1112.
21. Seppälä, M., Ruoslahti, E. *Br. med. J.* 1972, iv, 769.

CHILDREN OF ADULT SURVIVORS WITH SPINA BIFIDA CYSTICA

C. O. CARTER   KATHLEEN EVANS
Medical Research Council Clinical Genetics Unit, Institute of Child Health, London WC1

Summary A consecutive series of patients with spina bifida cystica, identified from the records of The Hospital for Sick Children and St. Bartholomew's Hospital before 1954, have been studied to estimate the risk of neural-tube malformation in the children of such patients who survive to adult life. The 215 survivors who were traced have had between them 104 children, 2 of whom have a neural-tube malformation. Of 100 male survivors, 14 have between them had 35 children, 1 of whom had spina bifida cystica. Of 115 female patients, 38 have between them had 69 children, of whom 1 had anencephaly. The results of this study combined with two other studies give an estimate for risk to offspring of parents of either sex of about 3%. It appears that the risk to children of male patients is at least as high as that of female patients.

Introduction

SURVIVORS with spina bifida cystica are now asking about the chances of the condition occurring in their children. There is, as yet, little information on which to base an estimate of this risk.

Tünte[1] reported on a series of 32 adults with spina bifida cystica on the genetics register at Münster, Germany, 14 of whom had a total of 24 liveborn and 5 stillborn children. Of the 29 children, 2 had malformations of the central nervous system (C.N.S.), 1 had anencephaly, and 1 had spina bifida cystica (the last 2 cases were both born to the same father). Lorber[2] has briefly reported on 36 adults with spina bifida, ascertained in various ways, who had a total of 86 children. 2 women and 1 man among the 36 patients had had a child with spina bifida.

The present paper describes a study of a series of 202 survivors of spina bifida cystica who had attended The Hospital for Sick Children, Great Ormond Street, between 1940 and 1953, to discover how many of their children had a C.N.S. malformation.

Patients and Methods

We examined all available sources of names of patients with spina bifida attending The Hospital for Sick Children between 1940 and 1953. The 10 who had addresses in South Wales were excluded because they will be included in a survey from Cardiff. A total of 576 (253 boys and 323 girls) was found. Of the 576, 305 were known to be dead and a further 22 were presumed dead because the severity of the malformation made their survival most unlikely and their names do not appear on the National Health Service central register; a further 15 were known to have emigrated; 4 were in the Armed Forces; 5 in institutions for the mentally retarded; 3 refused to give information; 20, who may still be alive, were not traced. This leaves a total of 202 people on whose offspring we can report.

significant correlations between surface area or weight and B.T.T.

Discussion

Japanese migrants to Hawaii—especially their families, the second-generation Nisei—develop disease patterns similar to Caucasians.[6] The Hawaii-Japanese lose the high gastric-cancer risks of Japan and acquire "Western" malignancies such as those of prostate, breast, and colon.[7] The Hawaii-Japanese have more colonic polyps and diverticuloses than Japanese living in Japan.[8]

It would be expected, then, that the more traditional Issei would have a faster B.T.T. than the Nisei and that the Hawaii-Japanese would have transit-times similar to those of Caucasians. We were surprised to find no differences between the Issei and Nisei, and the Hawaii-Japanese had rapid transit-times comparable with those in rural Africans.[2] The B.T.T. differences between the Japanese and Caucasians could not be explained by education, occupation, body-weight, surface area, or the number of bowel movements per day.

With respect to the Hawaii-Japanese experience, B.T.T.s do not seem to be related to the pathogenesis of colonic disease.

We thank Mr Harry Ito of Kuakini Hospital for engineering the stool-collection equipment; and Dr Edgar Childs, Dr Donald Ikeda, and Dr David Sakuda of the Department of Radiology, Kuakini Hospital, for their technical assistance. This work was supported in part by National Institutes of Health contracts E-71-2170 and PH-43-65-1003-C.

Requests for reprints should be addressed to the Japan-Hawaii Cancer Study, Kuakini Hospital, 347 North Kuakini Street, Honolulu, Hawaii 96817, U.S.A.

REFERENCES

1. Burkitt, D. P. Cancer, 1971, 28, 3.
2. Burkitt, D. P., Walker, A. R. P., Painter, N. S. Lancet, 1972, ii, 1408.
3. Worth, R. M., Kagan, A. J. chron. Dis. 1970, 23, 389.
4. Hinton, J. M., Lennard-Jones, J. E., Young, A. C. Gut, 1969, 10, 842.
5. Pryke, E. S., White, H. M. ibid. 1970, 11, 966.
6. Stemmermann, G. N. Archs envir. Hlth, 1970, 20, 266.
7. Doll, R., Muir, C., Waterhouse, J. Cancer in Five Continents; vol. II. Berlin, 1970.
8. Stemmermann, G. N., Yatani, R., Cancer, 1974, 31, 1260.

ASSESSMENT OF COMA AND IMPAIRED CONSCIOUSNESS

A Practical Scale

GRAHAM TEASDALE   BRYAN JENNETT

University Department of Neurosurgery,
Institute of Neurological Sciences,
Glasgow G51 4TF

Summary   A clinical scale has been evolved for assessing the depth and duration of impaired consciousness and coma. Three aspects of behaviour are independently measured—motor responsiveness, verbal performance, and eye opening. These can be evaluated consistently by doctors and nurses and recorded on a simple chart which has proved practical both in a neurosurgical unit and in a general hospital. The scale facilitates consultations between general and special units in cases of recent brain damage, and is useful also in defining the duration of prolonged coma.

Introduction

A WIDE range of conditions may be associated with coma or impaired consciousness. Apart from acute brain damage due to traumatic, vascular, or infective lesions, there are metabolic disorders such as hepatic or renal failure, hypoglycæmia or diabetic ketosis, and also drug overdose. In gauging deterioration or improvement in the acute stage of such conditions, as well as in predicting the ultimate outcome, the degree and duration of altered consciousness usually overshadow all other clinical features in importance. It is therefore vital to be able to assess and to record changing states of altered consciousness reliably.

Need for a Clinical Scale

Impaired consciousness is an expression of dysfunction in the brain as a whole. This may be due to agents acting diffusely, such as drugs or metabolic imbalance; or to the combination of remote and local effects produced by brain damage which was initially focal. Such focal brain damage may affect some of the responses which are used to assess the level of consciousness, and any scale devised for general use must allow for this possibility. A simpler scale might suffice for metabolic or drug coma, when the likelihood of structural brain damage is small, but in an emergency there may be insufficient information to assign patients confidently to a particular diagnostic category. Moreover, coma of mixed origin is not uncommon, as when head injury is suspected of being associated with ingestion of drugs or alcohol, or with a vascular accident. These seem good reasons for devising a generally applicable scheme of assessment.

Existing Systems

The development of equipment for monitoring various functions in critically ill patients has not altered the need for doctors and nurses to assess the level of consciousness. There is an abundance of alternative terms by which levels of coma or impaired consciousness are described and recorded. Systems for describing patients with impaired consciousness are not consistent.[1-14] Indeed, many clinicians retreat from any formal scheme in favour of a general description of the patient's state, without clear guidelines as to what to describe and how to describe it.

In practice, such unstructured observations commonly result in ambiguities and misunderstandings when information about patients is exchanged and when groups of patients treated by alternative methods are compared, or reported from different centres. There is no general agreement about what terms to use, nor are those in common use interpreted similarly by different workers. Almost every report of patients in coma offers yet another classification. Most divide the spectrum of altered consciousness into a series of steps, which in the reports we reviewed ranged from 3 to 17 and were often described in terms which defied clear definition. Many assume the existence of constellations of clinical features which are unique to each "level", whilst

82

others distinguish between coma and consciousness on the basis of only one aspect of behaviour.

The importance of careful and complete neurological examination in determining the nature and site of the lesion causing coma has been described at length by Fisher[5] and Plum and Posner,[13] who emphasised that tests of brainstem function, not usually included in routine examination, can be useful in the diagnosis of stupor or coma. Neither, however, was primarily concerned with repeated bedside assessment of the degree of conscious impairment, which is the subject of our paper.

Glasgow Coma Scale

To be generally accepted, a system must be practical to use in a wide range of hospitals and by staff without special training. But the search for simplicity must not be the excuse for seeking absolute distinctions where none exist: for that reason no attempt is made to define either consciousness or coma in absolute terms. Indeed, it is conceptually unsound to expect a clear watershed in the continuum between these states. What is required instead is an effective method of describing the various states of impaired consciousness encountered in clinical practice. Moreover, this should not depend on only one type of response because this may, for various reasons, be untestable. The three different aspects of behavioural response which we chose to examine were motor response, verbal response, and eye opening, each being evaluated independently of the other. These feature in many previous reports on coma but not in the formal system we propose. This depends on identifying responses which can be clearly defined, and each of which can be accurately graded according to a rank order that indicates the degree of dysfunction.

Motor Responses

The ease with which motor responses can be elicited in the limbs, together with the wide range of different patterns which can occur, makes motor activity a suitable guide to the functioning state of the central nervous system. Indeed, every one of the reported scales which we reviewed included some aspect of motor responsiveness as a criterion.

Obeying commands is the best response possible, but the observer must take care not to interpret a grasp reflex or postural adjustment as a response to command. The terms "purposeful" and "voluntary" are avoided because we believe that they cannot be judged objectively.

If there is no response to command, a painful stimulus is applied. The significance of the response to pain is not always easy to interpret unless stimulation is applied in a standard way and is maintained until a maximum response is obtained. Initially pressure is applied to the fingernail bed with a pencil; this may result in either flexion or extension at the elbow. If flexion is observed stimulation is then applied to the head and neck and to the trunk to test for localisation. In brain death, a spinal reflex may still cause the legs to flex briskly in response to pain applied locally.[15] For this reason, and because the arms show a wider range of responses, it is wise always to test them,

unless local trauma makes this completely impossible.

A localising response indicates that a stimulus at more than one site causes a limb to move so as to attempt to remove it.

A flexor response may vary from rapid withdrawal, associated with abduction of the shoulder, to a slower, stereotyped assumption of the hemiplegic or decorticate posture with adduction of the shoulder. Experienced observers may readily distinguish between normal and abnormal flexion, but for general use in the first few days after brain damage has been sustained it is sufficient to record only that the response is flexor.

Extensor posturing is obviously abnormal and is usually associated with adduction, internal rotation of the shoulder, and pronation of the forearm. The term "decerebrate rigidity" is avoided because it implies a specific physioanatomical correlation.[16]

No response is usually associated with hypotonia and it is important to exclude spinal transection as an explanation for lack of response; and also to be satisfied that an adequate stimulus has been applied.

When recording motor response as an indication of the functional state of the brain as a whole, the best or highest response from any limb is recorded. During a single examination some patients give variable responses, these usually becoming better as the patient becomes more aroused; responses from the right and left limbs may also differ. Any difference between the responsiveness of one limb and another may indicate focal brain damage and for this purpose the worst (most abnormal) response should be noted. But for the purpose of assessing the degree of altered consciousness it is the best response from the best limb that is recorded.

Verbal Responses

Probably the commonest definition of the end of coma, or the recovery of consciousness, is the patient's first understandable utterance; speech figured in nearly all the reported scales which we reviewed. Certainly the return of speech indicates the restoration of a high degree of integration within the nervous system, but continued speechlessness may be due to causes other than depressed consciousness (e.g., tracheostomy or dysphasia).

Orientation implies awareness of the self and the environment. The patient should know who he is, where he is, and why he is there; know the year, the season, and the month. The words "rational" and "sensible" are avoided because they cannot be clearly defined.

Confused conversation is recorded if attention can be held and the patient responds to questions in a conversational manner but the responses indicate varying degrees of disorientation and confusion. It is here that verbatim reporting of the individual patient's responses can be useful.

Inappropriate speech describes intelligible articulation but implies that speech is used only in an exclamatory or random way, usually by shouting and swearing; no sustained conversational exchange is possible.

Incomprehensible speech refers to moaning and groaning but without any recognisable words.

83

Eye Opening

Spontaneous eye opening, with sleep/wake rhythms, is most highly scored on this part of the scale and it indicates that the arousal mechanisms in the brainstem are active. But arousal does not imply awareness, and we believe it is unwise to try to decide whether a patient is attentive on the basis of eye movements. Patients in the persistent vegetative state,[17] who are subsequently shown to be structurally decorticate, have often been believed by relatives, nurses, and even by doctors to be reacting visually to people around them; probably primitive ocular-following reflexes may be executed at subcortical level.

Eye opening in response to speech is a response to any verbal approach, whether spoken or shouted, not necessarily the command to open the eyes.

Eye opening in response to pain should be tested by a stimulus in the limbs, because the grimacing associated with supraorbital or jaw-angle pressure may cause eye closure.

Practical Applications of the Scale

Different observers were able to elicit the responses in this scale with a high degree of consistency, and the likelihood of ambiguous reporting appears to be small. This was demonstrated by having several doctors and nurses examine the same group of patients. Disagreements were rare.[18] This was in pronounced contrast to what happened when the observers were asked instead to judge only whether patients were conscious or unconscious; one in five observers then disagreed with the majority opinion. This 20% disagreement-rate compared with rates of 20–35% which have been reported in various different clinical situations,[19] whilst in one study extensor plantar responses showed only 50% consistency when observations were repeated.[20]

One or other components of this scale may be untestable, and this fact can be recorded. Limbs may be immobilised by splints for fractures, tracheostomy may preclude speech, and eyelid swelling or bilateral third-nerve lesions make eye opening impossible. In the rare "locked-in syndrome," a patient with totally inactive limbs may obey commands to move the eyes and may even be able to signal his needs.[21]

The nurses in our intensive-care unit have willingly adopted this method of formalising observations which they previously used to record as a descriptive comment. They now plot them on a chart (see accompanying figure) somewhat similar in format, but not content, to one proposed by Bouzarth,[1] and which also provides for conventional recording of temperature, pulse and respiration, of the pupil size in mm., and of focal motor signs. This method has already been adopted successfully for making observations on head injuries in a neighbouring general hospital. In such hospitals patients with head injuries form a considerable proportion of acute surgical admissions, and observations there depend on medical and nursing staff who have no special experience of neurology and neurosurgery.

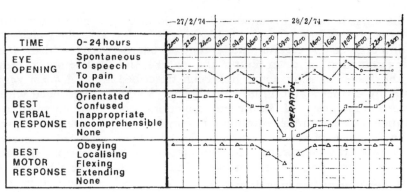

Chart for recording assessment of consciousness.

Discussion

Apart from its practical use in the management of recently brain-damaged patients, this scale allows the duration of coma to be defined more precisely, in terms of how long different levels of responsiveness have persisted. There is evidence that this is a crucial criterion when it comes to predicting the ultimate outcome of coma, particularly after head injury.[22] It would make it possible also to examine critically claims for good recovery after weeks or months "in coma," by enabling the alleged coma to be more accurately assessed. In such cases as we have scrutinised, it has been clear, even retrospectively, that there had been evidence of much earlier recovery, on at least one component of the coma scale, than had been recognised. By resolving the problem of defining "prolonged coma" the scale also makes it possible to distinguish between the various states which this term embraces, such as akinetic mutism and the persistent vegetative state.[17]

Some may have reservations about a system which seems to undervalue the niceties of a full neurological examination. It is no part of our case to deny the value of a detailed appraisal of the patient as a whole, and of neurological function in particular, in reaching a diagnosis about the cause of coma, or in determining the probable site of brain damage. However, repeated observations of conscious level are usually made by relatively inexperienced junior doctors or nurses; these staff are not only few in number but they change frequently even during the course of a day. There are therefore good reasons for restricting routine observations to the minimum, and for choosing those which can be reliably recorded and understood by a range of different staff.

We are grateful to many colleagues for their assistance in developing this scale; particularly Dr Fred Plum of New York, Dr Reinder Braakman of Rotterdam, and Dr David Shaw of Newcastle upon Tyne, in whose units its practical value has also been confirmed. We thank the consultants of the division of neurosurgery, Glasgow, for their cooperation. This scale was devised as part of a study of severe head injuries supported by the National Fund for Research into Crippling Diseases.

Requests for reprints should be addressed to B. J.

REFERENCES

1. Bouzarth, W. F. *J. Trauma*, 1968, **8**, 29.
2. Bozza Marribini, M. L. *Acta neurochir.* 1964, **12**, 352.
3. Bricolo, A. *Minerva neurochir.* 1965, **9**, 150.
4. Fischgold, H., Mathis, P. *Electronecephalogr. clin. Neurophysiol.* 1959, suppl. 11.

References continued overleaf

The distribution of the fatal pulmonary emboli in the controls was pulmonary trunk (5), main pulmonary artery (9), lobar artery (9), and segmental artery (6).

In addition, in 5 patients from the control group and 2 from the heparin group, emboli found at necropsy were considered either contributory to death or an incidental finding, since death in these patients was attributed to other causes. Taking all pulmonary emboli together, 20 in the control group and 2 in the heparin group, the findings are again statistically significant.

Incidence of D.V.T.

D.V.T. was diagnosed clinically by the radioactive-fibrinogen-uptake test and at necropsy. When the 89 patients from the Basle centre, initially included in the M.C.T. analysis, were withdrawn, the significant differences observed between the control and heparin groups remained.

Treatment of D.V.T. and Pulmonary Embolism

Exclusion of the Basle data did not change the highly significant differences which were observed in the number of patients requiring treatment for D.V.T. and/or pulmonary embolism in the two groups.

Operative and Postoperative Bleeding

Exclusion of the Basle data did not influence the previously reported results[1] relating to the incidence of operative and postoperative bleeding.

Conclusion

The evidence that low doses of heparin prevent D.V.T. in most postoperative patients is irrefutable. The main unresolved question was whether this form of prophylaxis also reduces deaths from pulmonary embolism. This question was answered by the M.C.T.[1], and the conclusion of that trial is not affected by our reappraisal of the results: subcutaneous heparin administration before and after surgery significantly reduced the incidence of fatal pulmonary embolism, detected at necropsy. The recent article by Gruber et al.[2] casts doubt on the conclusion of this trial. However, as summarised by Sherry[5] ". . . one is forced to the conclusion that there is a *very high probability* that the differences in the primary end-point (fatal P.E.) between the two groups is real, and that the study should be used to influence the practice habits of the profession for preventing fatal pulmonary embolism following abdominal surgery".

Requests for reprints should be addressed to V.V.K.

REFERENCES

1. International Multicentre Trial *Lancet*, 1975, II, 45
2. Gruber, U. F., Duckert, F., Fridrich, R., Torhorst, J., Rem, J. *ibid.* 1977, I, 207.
3. Rem, J., Duckert, F., Fridrich, R., Gruber, U. F. *Schweiz. med. Wschr.* 1975, **105**, 827.
4. Communication; Rem, J. A. Inaugural dissertation, Faculty of Medicine, University of Basle, 1975, to the Co-ordinating Centre from Basle. Letter received on June 30, 1975, with comments before the publication of the M.C.T. results.
5. Sherry, S. Prophylactic Therapy of Deep Vein Thrombosis and Pulmonary Embolism. D.H.E.W. publications no. (N.I.H.) 76-866, 1975, p. 229.

Preliminary Communications

ISOLATION AND PARTIAL CHARACTERISATION OF A NEW VIRUS CAUSING ACUTE HÆMORRHAGIC FEVER IN ZAIRE

K. M. JOHNSON   P. A. WEBB
J. V. LANGE   F. A. MURPHY

Virology Division, Center for Disease Control, Atlanta, Georgia 30333, U.S.A.

AN outbreak of hæmorrhagic fever with an exceptionally high mortality-rate occurred in southern Sudan and northern Zaire with peak case-rates in September, 1976. A W.H.O. International Commission operated in Sudan and Zaire from October onward.[1][2] Blood and tissue specimens from persons with hæmorrhagic disease were sent to laboratories in Belgium and England, and findings from these laboratories appear in the accompanying reports.[3][4] While these specimens were being studied, Mr E. T. W. Bowen (Microbiological Research Establishment, Porton Down) sent an aliquot of an acute blood specimen from a patient in Zaire (no. 718, patient M.E.) to the Center for Disease Control, Atlanta, for additional study.

This specimen, and all subsequent acute specimens, were inoculated into Vero (African green monkey) cells. Three days later a distinct cytopathic change (focal rounding and refractility) was evident, and an aliquot of supernatant fluid was removed for negative contrast electron microscopy.

ELECTRON MICROSCOPY OF CELL CULTURES

Carbon-coated grids were sequentially floated on droplets of the cell-culture fluid and then on 2% sodium silicotungstate pH 7. Large numbers of filamentous virus particles were seen (fig. 1). They were approximately 100 nm in diameter and varied in length from 300 nm to more than 1500 nm. Many had terminal blebs. Particles had regular surface projections approximately 10 nm long, and when stained they were seen to have internal cross-striations indicative of a helical core structure (fig. 2). In all details, these particles were indistinguishable from Marburg virus particles studied in 1967 (isolates from Germany) and 1975 (isolate from South Africa).[5-7] Two characteristics were more prominent in the 1976 Zaire isolate: there was more branching of the filamentous particles (fig. 1); and more evidence of envelope continuation beyond the ends of the more rigid internal structure (fig. 1, arrow).

Vero cells infected with the same isolate from Zaire were examined also by thin-section electron microscopy. Filamentous virus particles were found budding from the plasma membrane of cells (fig. 3), and many of the cells contained inclusion bodies. These intracytoplasmic inclusions were complex and distinct, and consisted of a finely fibrillar or granular ground substance which condensed into tubular structures. The latter have been considered to be the internal helical structure of mature virus particles. These tubules were sectioned randomly, some in cross-section, some linearly. The virus particles in

TABLE I—COMPARISON OF RECIPROCAL I.F.A. TITRES OF MARBURG ('67, '75) AND MARBURG-LIKE ('76) VIRUS DISEASE SERA

Year of illness	Country	Human sera	Time after onset	Antigen	
				Marburg '67	no. 718 '76
1967	Germany	U	5 mo.	128	<10
		K	5 mo.	64	<8
1975	South Africa	DO	1 mo.	64	<4
		MC	4 mo.	64	<4
1976	Sudan	no. 8	±12 days	<2	16
		no. 9	±12 days	<2	<2
	Zaire	no. 5	1 mo.	4	160

these sections were identical to those observed in the 1967 and 1975 isolates.[6] [8]

POSTMORTEM LIVER SPECIMENS

Evidence of infection was seen by light microscopy in three postmortem human liver specimens from Zaire (received in

formalin). Infection of two of these was confirmed by electron microscopy. Focal eosinophilic hepatocellular necrosis with modest inflammatory infiltration was prominent. Large eosinophilic inclusions were present in many intact hepatocytes, especially near sites of severe necrosis (fig. 4). These rather smooth and refractile inclusions were so characteristic that

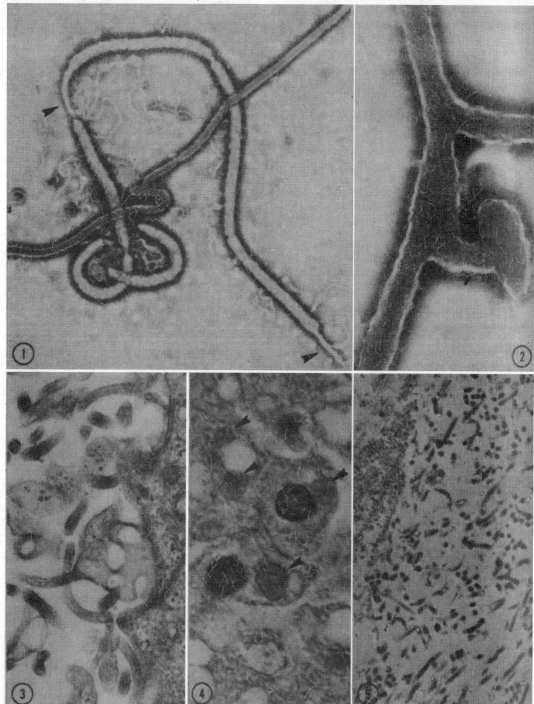

Fig. 1—Ebola virus in first Vero-cell passage after inoculation with patient's blood from Zaire (reduced from × 44 000).

Some filamentous particles in negative contrast preparations were more than 1500 nm long; particles had a uniform diameter of 100 nm and some had ragged ends (arrows).

Fig. 2—Virus particle penetrated by negative contrast medium showing internal cross-striations (reduced from × 115 000).

Fig. 3—Virus particles, in ultrathin section, budding from plasma membrane of Vero cell at 3 days after infection (reduced from × 49 000).

All morphological characteristics were similar to those of Marburg virus as studied in 1967 and 1975.

Fig. 4—Liver from fatal case in Zaire (reduced from × 1100).

Large eosinophilic inclusion bodies (arrows) in many hepatocytes. Focal necrosis and inflammation. Formalin fixation, hæmatoxylin and eosin.

Fig. 5—Virus particles in distended extracellular space in liver from fatal case in Zaire (reduced from × 20 000).

Despite poor tissue preservation, massive numbers of virus particles and characteristic inclusion bodies were identified by electron microscopy of two of three necropsy specimens.

THE LANCET, MARCH 12, 1977

571

TABLE II—COMPARISON OF I.F.A. TITRES OF GUINEAPIGS IMMUNISED (SINGLE INJECTION) AGAINST MARBURG ('67) AND MARBURG-LIKE ('76) VIRUSES

Immunising agent	Guineapig sera	Days after inoculation	I.F.A. titres with antigen of:	
			Marburg '67	no. 718 '76
Marburg '67	G.P. 16	12	>640	5
Marburg-like '76	G.P. 1	10	2	256

they have diagnostic significance. Plastic-embedded formalin-fixed necropsy specimens were examined with the electron microscope. Although preservation of liver tissue was poor, large numbers of filamentous virus particles and inclusion bodies (masses of tubules) were found (fig. 5) which were indistinguishable from those in Marburg virus-infected human and guineapig livers studied in 1967 and 1975.[6-8]

ANTIGENIC COMPARISON WITH MARBURG

An antigenic difference between this isolate and Marburg '67 was demonstrated by indirect immunofluorescence (I.F.A.). An infected Vero-cell suspension was placed in drops on slides, air dried, and then acetone-fixed for 10 min at room temperature. Slides were stored at −70°C until tested. Marburg '67 antigen slides, prepared in like manner, were used for comparison. Reciprocal titres obtained with convalescent human sera drawn during the 1967, 1975, and 1976 outbreaks are listed in table I. With the exception of a weak reaction to Marburg antigen at a 1/4 dilution of the Zaire convalescent serum, the new isolate was distinct from Marburg virus. The homologous Marburg titres of 128 and 64 obtained with '67 and '75 antigens and antisera were comparable to those reported by Wulff and Conrad.[9]

A single-injection immune serum to the new agent was prepared in guineapigs, and reciprocal I.F.A. tests were performed with available similar reagents for Marburg virus. Reciprocal titres (table II) further confirmed the distinctness of the two viruses. Although one of two early convalescent sera from Sudan gave a positive reaction with the Zaire antigen (table I) further work is needed to determine whether the hæmorrhagic-disease agents from the two countries are identical.

EBOLA VIRUS

With the concurrence of Prof. S. R. Pattyn, Institute of Tropical Medicine, Antwerp, and Mr E. T. W. Bowen, Microbiological Research Establishment, Porton Down, the name Ebola virus is proposed for this new agent. Ebola is a small river in Zaire which flows westward, north of Yambuku, the village of origin of the patient from whom the first isolate was obtained. In deference to the countries involved and to the lack of specific knowledge of the original natural source of the virus, it is also suggested that no names of countries or specific towns be used.

REFERENCES

1. Wld Hlth Org. wkly epidem. Rec. 1976, 51, (42), p. 325.
2. Center for Disease Control. Morbidity and Mortality Weekly Report, 1976, vol. 25, p. 378.
3. Pattyn, S. R., Jacob, W., Van der Groen, G., Piot, P., Courteille, Lancet, 1977, i, 573.
4. Bowen, E. T. W., Platt, G. S., Lloyd, G., Baskerville, A., Harris, W. J., Vella, E. E. ibid. p. 571.
5. Kissling, R. E., Robinson, R. Q., Murphy, F. A., Whitfield, S. G. Science, 1968, 160, 888.
6. Center for Disease Control. Morbidity and Mortality Weekly Report, 1975, vol. 24, p. 89.
7. Gear, J. S. S., Cassell, G. A., Gear, A. J., Trappler, B., Clansen, L., Meyers, A. M., Kew, M. C., Bothwell, T. H., Sher, R., Miller, G. B., Schneider, J., Koornhof, H. J., Gomperts, E. D., Isaacson, M., Gear, J. H. S. Br. med. J. 1975, iv, 489.
8. Murphy, F. A., Simpson, D. I. H., Whitfield, S. G., Zlotnik, I., Carter, G. B. Lab. Invest. 1971, 24, 279.
9. Wulff, H., Conrad, L. J. in Comparative Diagnosis of Viral Diseases. New York (in the press).

VIRAL HÆMORRHAGIC FEVER IN SOUTHERN SUDAN AND NORTHERN ZAIRE

Preliminary Studies on the Aetiological Agent

E. T. W. BOWEN   G. S. PLATT
G. LLOYD   A. BASKERVILLE
W. J. HARRIS   E. E. VELLA

Microbiological Research Establishment, Porton, Salisbury, Wiltshire, England

BETWEEN July and September, 1976, sporadic cases of fever with hæmorrhagic manifestations were reported in the areas of Nzara, Maridi, and Lirangu in the southern Sudan. The first cases are believed to have been in agricultural settlements. An outbreak of a similar disease was also reported from the zone of Bumba in northern Zaire.[1] As the epidemic increased in intensity, the disturbingly high percentage of cases reported among hospital personnel suggested direct person-to-person spread of infection. The illness began with an acute fever, malaise, sore throat, muscular pains, vomiting, and diarrhœa. Those severely affected had epistaxis, subconjunctival hæmorrhages, hæmoptysis, hæmatemeses, and melæna. Some patients also had a body rash, tremors, and convulsions.

SOURCES OF SPECIMENS

Specimens from the northern Zaire outbreak were referred to the Microbiological Research Establishment, Porton, by Prof. S. R. Pattyn of the Institute of Tropical Medicine, Antwerp. They were an acute-phase serum (no. 718), cell-culture materials and brains from suckling mice which had already been inoculated with the serum. We later received a specimen of liver from the same patient and also 5 acute-phase blood specimens from Zaire via Professor Pattyn. Specimens from the southern Sudan were mainly collected at Maridi Hospital and sent to us directly by Dr Babiker el Tahir, Dr D. H. Smith, Dr K. Jones, and Dr M. Cornet, who were there to investigate. They consisted of 3 throat swabs, 3 urine specimens, 6 acute-phase blood specimens, and convalescent serum specimens. These specimens were sent on dry ice or in liquid nitrogen. Three laboratories engaged in preliminary studies on the ætiological agent reported the isolation of a virus which was morphologically similar to Marburg virus.[2]

RESULTS OF ATTEMPTS AT VIRUS ISOLATION

Virus isolation from the original human material was attempted in : (1) culture preparations of Vero cells; (2) suckling mice inoculated intraperitoneally (I.P.) and intracerebrally (I.C.); and (3) young guineapigs (200–250 g) inoculated I.P.

Isolation in Guineapigs

So far 5 isolations of the ætiological agent have been obtained in guineapigs: 4 from specimens from northern Zaire and 1 from a specimen from southern Sudan. Guineapigs inoculated with these specimens became febrile 105°F (40.5°C) after an incubation period of 4–7 days. The febrile illness lasted 4–5 days during which the guineapigs failed to thrive and looked ill. 1 of the 12 guineapigs inoculated with original material died on the 12th day after inoculation. The other 11 guineapigs slowly recovered and were subsequently shown to have antibodies detectable by fluorescent antibody tests at titres ranging from 1/64 to 1/128. When whole heparinised blood from febrile guineapigs was inoculated I.P. into other guineapigs it produced a similar febrile illness.

THE LANCET, FEBRUARY 4,   263

Letters to the Editor

TRANSLUMINAL DILATATION OF CORONARY-ARTERY STENOSIS

SIR,—In September, 1977, we introduced a technique for percutaneous transluminal coronary angioplasty (P.T.A.). This technique consists of a catheter system introduced via the femoral artery under local anæsthesia. A preshaped guiding catheter is positioned into the orifice of the coronary artery and through this catheter a dilatation catheter is advanced into the branches of the artery. This dilatation catheter (outer diameter 0·5–1·25 mm) has a sausage-shaped distensible segment (balloon) at the tip.

After traversing the stenotic lesion the distensible segment is inflated with fluid (50% contrast material, 50% saline) to a maximum outer diameter of 3·0–3·8 mm by a pump-controlled pressure of 5 atmospheres (about 500 kPa). This pressure compresses the atherosclerotic material in a direction perpendicular to the wall of the vessel thereby dilating the lumen.

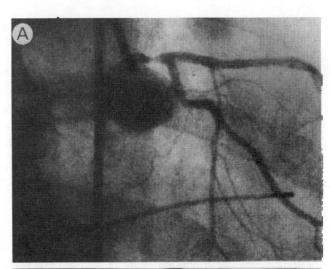

DETAILS OF FIVE CASES TREATED BY P.T.A.

Patient	Age	Sex	Date of dilatation	Stenosis	Primary success
1	38	M	Sept. 16, 1977	L.A.D. 85%	+
2*	44	M	Oct. 18, 1977	L.C.A. 70% (calcified)	—
			Jan. 10, 1978	R.C.A. 80%	+
3	43	M	Nov. 21, 1977	L.A.D. 75%	+
			Nov. 21, 1977	R.C.A. 95%	+
4*	43	M	Nov. 24, 1977	L.C.A. 80%	+
5	61	M	Dec. 20, 1977	L.A.D. 95%	+

L.C.A.=main left coronary artery; L.A.D.=left anterior descending; R.C.A.=right coronary artery.
*Dilatation done at University Hospital, Frankfurt.

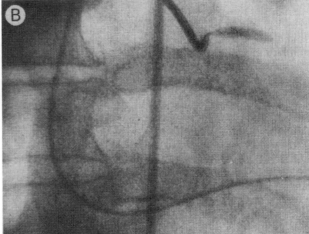

Experience with over 250 peripheral-artery lesions treated by this technique has demonstrated, via morphological studies, that the atheroma can be compressed leaving a smooth luminal surface. The patency-rate, two years after dilatation of iliac and femoropopliteal atherosclerotic lesions, was greater than 70%.[1]

After experimental[2] and intraoperative[3] studies the first percutaneous coronary dilatation was done on Sept. 16, 1977. Five patients with severe stenotic lesions of the coronary arteries associated with refractory angina have so far been treated by coronary P.T.A. (table). Angiograms for one of these patients are shown in the figure. No complications were noted. Follow-up studies by serial stress-testing with myocardial imaging (thallium-201) and angiography suggest that P.T.A. may be an effective treatment in certain patients with severe discrete non-calcified lesions of the coronary arteries.

This technique, if it proves successful in long-term follow-up studies, may widen the indications for coronary angiography and provide another treatment for patients with angina pectoris.

Department of Internal Medicine,
Medical Policlinic,
University Hospital,
8091 Zürich, Switzerland   ANDREAS GRÜNTZIG

1. Grüntzig, A. Die perkutane transluminale Rekanalisation chronischer Arterienverschlüsse mit einer neuen Dilatationstechnik; p. 50. Baden-Baden, 1977.
2. Grüntzig, A., Riedhammer, H. H., Turina, M., Rutishauser, W. Verh. Dt. ges. Kreislaufforschg. 1976, 42, 282.
3. Grüntzig, A., Myler, R., Hanna, E., Turina, M. Circulation, 1977, 56, 84 (abstr.).

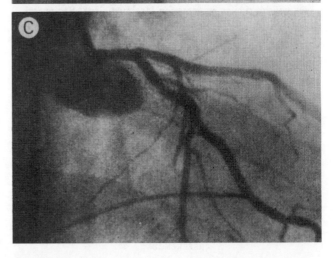

Details of patient 3.

43-year-old man with severe angina pectoris since September, 1977. First angiogram (Nov. 11) revealed severe stenosis of the main L.C.A. and only slight wall abnormalities in some of the branches of L.C.A. After informed consent P.T.A. was done on Nov. 21.

(A) The angiogram before P.T.A. (done under nitroglycerine cover), with the guiding catheter in the orifice showed 80% proximal stenosis of the L.C.A.

(B) After passage of the dilatation catheter the distensible balloon segment was inflated twice to a maximum outer diameter of 3·7 mm. During the dilatation the patient experienced a short period of angina pectoris which quickly disappeared after deflation of the balloon.

(C) The angiogram after the procedure showed a good result without complications. There was no enzyme rise or E.C.G. change after the treatment. A good clinical result has persisted in the following weeks, confirmed by stress tests.

THE LANCET, JULY 15, 1978

119

concentrations of dihomo-γ-linolenic acid (C20:3) as that of E.P.A. were incubated with washed vascular tissue no anti-aggregating material was produced.

Discussion

A.A., the commonest precursor of prostaglandin synthesis, is transformed by the platelets into T.X.A$_2$, a potent pro-aggregating agent,[9] and by the vessel wall to prostacyclin (P.G.I$_2$).[10] The balance between the formation of these two compounds regulates platelet aggregability in vivo and hæmostatic plug formation.[12]

Our present results show that E.P.A. is not pro-aggregating in human P.R.P. even though T.X.A$_3$ is formed,[13] T.X.A$_3$ not being a pro-aggregating agent.[13] However, the vessel wall can utilise E.P.A. to synthesise a potent anti-aggregating agent, probably a Δ^{17}-prostacyclin (P.G.I$_3$).

Clearly, utilisation of E.P.A. rather than A.A. in vivo should displace the balance between pro-aggregating and anti-aggregating forces towards an anti-aggregating condition (fig. 3).

The fatty acid available for prostaglandin biosynthesis in the tissues of Greenland Eskimos (assuming a similar distribution as in plasma fatty acids) is mainly E.P.A. and not A.A., in contrast to that in Caucasians (table). The content of E.P.A. in the blood of Eskimos originates directly from the E.P.A. in the diet, since the dietary content of its possible precursor, linolenic acid (C18:3), is low.[6]

Microthrombus formation on areas of endothelial damage is thought to initiate events which lead to A.M.I.[17] The delayed atherosclerotic process in the vessel wall of Eskimos could be a consequence of several factors, including a favourable lipid profile and low aggregability of the platelets in vivo due to probably the presence of P.G.I$_3$ and to the lack of aggregating activity of T.X.A$_3$. Furthermore, the displacement of the balance of activity towards an anti-aggregating state could account for the hitherto unexplained observations of enhanced bleeding tendency in Eskimos.[7,8]

Dietary manipulation with dihomo-γ-linolenic acid, the precursor of prostaglandins of the "1" series has been suggested[18] as a means of preventing thrombosis since thromboxane A$_1$ (T.X.A$_1$) is not pro-aggregating and P.G.E$_1$ is anti-aggregating. However, this proposition was made before the discovery of prostacyclin and although still maintained by some,[19,20] it is now clear that the P.G.G$_1$ or P.G.H$_1$ are not substrates for the formation of the defensive substance, prostacyclin. E.P.A. has the Δ^5 double bond and can be converted into a potent anti-aggregating substance.

Dietary polyunsaturated fats are generally accepted as being "less harmful" than saturated ones. However, those used in for instance, margarines, are mainly oleic (C18:1) and linoleic acids (C18:2).[21] Linolenic acid (C18:3) is converted to E.P.A. in some species.[22] Thus, E.P.A. and possibly linolenic acid may be more appropriate as beneficial agents than "polyunsaturated fats" in general. Indeed, enrichment of tissue lipids with E.P.A., whether by dietary change or by supplementation may reduce the development of thrombosis and atherosclerosis in the Western World.

We thank Mrs E. A. Higgs for her help.

This study was supported by the Aalborg City Fund for medical research.

REFERENCES

1. Bang, H. O., Dyerberg, J., Nielsen, Aa., B. Lancet, 1971, i, 1143.
2. Bang, H. O., Dyerberg, J. Acta med. scand. 1972, 192, 85.
3. Miller, G. J., Miller, N. E. Lancet, 1975, i, 16.
4. Miller, N. E., Førde, O. H., Thelle, D. S., Mjøs, O. D. ibid, 1977, i, 965.
5. Dyerberg, J., Bang, H. O., Hjørne, N. Am. J. clin. Nutr. 1975, 28, 958.
6. Bang, H. O., Dyerberg, J., Hjørne, N. Acta med. scand. 1976, 200, 69.
7. Berthelsen, A. Meddr. Grønland, 1940, 117, 1.
8. Christensen, P. E., Schmidt, H., Jensen, O., Bang, H. O., Andersen, V., Jordal, B. Acta med. scand. 1953, 144, 429.
9. Hamberg, M., Svensson, J., Samuelsson, B. Proc. natn. Acad. Sci. U.S.A. 1975, 72, 2994.
10. Moncada, S., Gryglewski, R., Bunting, S., Vane, J. R. Nature, 1976, 263, 663.
11. Johnson, R. A., Morton, D. R., Kinner, J. H., et al. Prostaglandins, 1976, 12, 915.
12. Moncada, S., Vane, J. R. Br. med. Bull. 1978, 34, 129.
13. Raz, A., Minkes, M. S., Needleman, P. Biochim. biophys. Acta. 1977, 488, 305.
14. Dyerberg, J., Bang, H. O. Lancet, 1978, i, 152.
15. Vargaftig, B. B., Tranier, Y., Chignard, M. Prostaglandins, 1974, 8, 133.
16. Schrör, K., Moncada, S., Ubatuba, F. B., Vane, J. R. Eur. J. Pharmac. 1978, 47, 103.
17. Ross, R., Glomset, J. A. New Engl. J. Med. 1976, 295, 421.
18. Willis, A. L., Comia, K., Kuhn, D. C., Paulsrud, J. Prostaglandins, 1974, 8, 509.
19. Kernoff, P. B. A., Willis, A. L., Stone, K. J., Davies, J. A., McNicol, G. P. Br. med. J. 1977, ii, 1441.
20. Ibid. p. 1437.
21. Weibranch, J. L., Brignoli, C. A., Reeves, J. B., Iverson, J. L. Food Technol. 1977, Feb., p. 80.
22. Crawford, M. A., Casperd, N. M., Sinclair, A. J. Comp. Biochem. Physiol. 1976, 54B, 395.

β-ENDORPHIN IN HUMAN CEREBROSPINAL FLUID

W. J. JEFFCOATE   LESLEY H. REES
LORRAINE McLOUGHLIN   SALLY J. RATTER
J. HOPE   P. J. LOWRY
G. M. BESSER

Departments of Endocrinology and Chemical Pathology,
St. Bartholomew's Hospital, London EC1A 7BE

Summary   β-endorphin is a brain peptide with potent morphine-like activity structurally related to the anterior pituitary hormone β-lipotrophin (β-L.P.H.). We have developed a radioimmunoassay for human β-endorphin in plasma and cerebrospinal fluid (C.S.F.). Since the antiserum also reacts with β-L.P.H., β-endorphin was distinguished by using a second antiserum which measures β-L.P.H. alone. With these two immunoassay systems and gel chromatography, we found β-endorphin in all 20 C.S.F. samples tested at a concentration always higher than, but with no other relationship to, that in plasma. β-endorphin was found in C.S.F. of patients who had hypopituitarism and undetectable plasma-β-endorphin, suggesting that it is synthesised in the brain rather than in the pituitary.

Introduction

β-ENDORPHIN may be the body's "endogenous opiate". This peptide is structurally related to β-lipotrophin (β-L.P.H.), a larger peptide first isolated in 1965,[1] which is found in the same cells of the anterior pituitary as adrenocorticotropin (A.C.T.H.) and is always secreted in parallel to it.[2-5] β-endorphin binds strongly to opiate receptors in brain and elsewhere[6-8] and has potent morphine-like activity both in vitro and in vivo.[9-11] β-L.P.H. has no defined biological role but it may be the precursor for β-endorphin, the body's natural analgesic.

We have developed a sensitive radioimmunoassay for β-endorphin in human cerebrospinal fluid (C.S.F.) Because the assay measures both β-endorphin and β-L.P.H., the results were compared with the results of a simultaneous N-terminal-β-L.P.H. radioimmunoassay which does not cross-react at all with β-endorphin.

Patients

Samples of C.S.F. from 4 patients who had diagnostic lumbar puncture and 16 who had air encephalography were immediately frozen with dry ice and stored at −20°C. Air encephalography was done under neuroleptanalgesia with diazepam, droperidol, and phenoperidine; lumbar puncture was done while patients were conscious. 3 of the 20 patients had pituitary-dependent Cushing's disease and the remainder had either non-endocrine diseases or endocrine disease not associated with abnormalities of A.C.T.H. secretion.

Blood and C.S.F. were taken synchronously from 2 children with acute leukæmia, 2 adults with hypopituitarism, and 2 women being investigated for hyperprolactinæmia.

Methods

Assay of Immunoreactive β-endorphin

The antiserum to β-endorphin (BNS 4) was raised by immunisation of a rabbit with purified human β-L.P.H. This antiserum shows full molar cross-reaction with human β-L.P.H. and β-endorphin, partial cross-reaction with α-endorphin, and no crossreaction with human γ-L.P.H., methionine enkephalin (Bachem, California), or the A.C.T.H.-related peptides. Human β-endorphin was isolated from a limited tryptic digest of purified human β-L.P.H. and was employed as a standard and as a radioactive tracer. The radioimmunoassay protocol is similar to that for measuring β-L.P.H.[5] Bound and free peptide were separated using dextran-coated charcoal. The assay has a sensitivity of 4 pmol/l (15 ng/l) for a 3 ml sample. At a level of 74 pmol/l the intra-assay and interassay coefficients of variation were 6% and 18%, respectively.

Assay of Immunoreactive β-L.P.H.

The antiserum used to measure β-L.P.H. was raised by immunisation of a rabbit with purified human β-L.P.H. This antiserum shows partial cross-reaction with γ-L.P.H. but none with β-endorphin, methionine enkephalin, or with the A.C.T.H.-related peptides. Human β-L.P.H. was used as a standard and as a tracer.[5]

Chromatography of C.S.F.

Samples of C.S.F. taken at air encephalography from patients being investigated for hyperprolactinæmia were collected into tubes containing 12 mg glycine and 0·56 ml 1 mol/l HCl to prevent proteolysis and immediately chromatographed on 'Sephadex G-75' in 1% formic acid at 4°C. The fractions were assayed for β-endorphin.

Results

β-endorphin and β-L.P.H. in C.S.F.

In the C.S.F. of each of the 17 patients with non-A.C.T.H.-

related diseases the levels of both immunoreactive β-endorphin and immunoreactive β-L.P.H. were higher than in plasma from 16 endocrinologically normal people (range <4–20 pmol/l). In 15 of the 17 patients the apparent β-endorphin concentration exceeded that of β-L.P.H. (fig. 1). In the 3 patients with Cushing's disease the concentration of both peptides in C.S.F. were in the same range as in other patients, even though the plasma β-L.P.H. was abnormally high.

Synchronous Sampling of Plasma and C.S.F.

In all 6 patients C.S.F. concentrations of apparent β-endorphin were higher than those of β-L.P.H. and the concentrations of both peptides exceeded those in

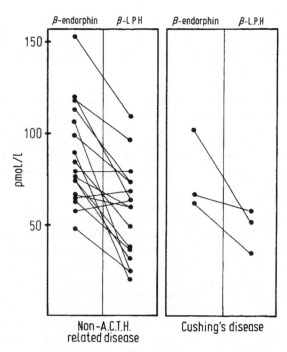

Fig. 1.—Concentrations of immunoreactive β-endorphin and β-L.P.H. in C.S.F.

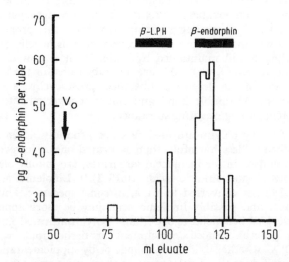

Fig. 2.—Chromatography on 'Sephadex G-75' of material with β-endorphin immunoreactivity in the C.S.F. of a patient with hyperprolactinæmia.

V_0 is void volume.

334

THE LANCET, AUGUST 12, 1978

(5) Non-postphlebitic limbs with normal Doppler ultrasound and abnormal impedance plethysmography need not be investigated by venography and should be treated; if this is done, only 5% will be treated unnecessarily.

(6) A clinical suspicion of D.V.T. superimposed on chronic venous insufficiency is more difficult to manage. When chronic venous insufficiency is detected by Doppler, an abnormal impedance examination is of no value (74% false-positive). Thus, only patients with postphlebitic limbs normal by Doppler and abnormal by impedance testing, and patients with abnormal cardiac hæmodynamics, need proceed to venography for accurate diagnosis of D.V.T.

This plan would allow 3% of limbs with D.V.T. to go untreated and condemn 5% of limbs without D.V.T. to anticoagulant treatment and its inherent risks. Counterbalancing these drawbacks, however, are five advantages of avoiding venography—the significant patient discomfort, radiation exposure, and the possibility of allergic reactions to contrast medium; the risk of inducing phlebitis or worsening existing phlebitis by venography (as high as 20% in one series[12]); non-invasive testing is about one-third the price of venography and does not require a doctor's time other than for interpretation; and contrast venography does not show well the external and common iliac veins in 18% of cases.[8] [11]

In our experience a laboratory approach to guide diagnostic evaluation in patients with clinically suspected acute D.V.T. is possible. In our series, 179 of 207 limbs (86%) could have been spared venography. 2 limbs with D.V.T. requiring treatment would have gone undetected, and 5 normal limbs would have been treated if our selection criteria had been used.

Contrast venography can be deleted from the diagnostic evaluation of D.V.T. only when the alternatives are similar in sensitivity and specificity, cost less, and/or carry fewer risks and complications. For epidemiological or natural-history studies of acute D.V.T., non-invasive testing, which is flow-dependent, will not detect fresh thrombus or thrombi in the soleal sinuses or calf veins, or even major veins if the thrombus is not large enough to impede venous flow. Venography or ^{125}I-fibrinogen remain the best techniques to establish the diagnosis of these conditions.

Supported in part by the Dr Scholl Foundation and the Northwestern University Vascular Research Fund.

Requests for reprints should be addressed to J.S.T.Y., Ward Memorial Building, Medical School, 303 E, Chicago Avenue, Chicago, Illinois 60611, U.S.A.

REFERENCES

1. Alexander, R. H., Nippa, J. H., Folse, R. *Am. Heart J.* 1971, **82**, 86.
2. Wheeler, H. B., Mullick, S. C., Anderson, J. N., Pearson, D. *Surgery*, 1971, **70**, 20.
3. Barnes, R. W., Russell, H. E., Wu, K. K., Hoak, J. D. *Surg. Gynec. Obstet.* 1976, **143**, 425.
4. Yao, J. S. T., Gourmos, C., Hobbs, J. T. *Lancet*, 1972, i, 1.
5. Wheeler, H. B., O'Donnell, J. R., Anderson, F. A. *Prog. cardiovasc. Dis.* 1974, **17**, 199.
6. Cranley, J. J., et al. *Surg. Gynec. Obstet.* 1975, **141**, 331.
7. Barnes, R. W., Hokanson, D. E., Wu, K. K., Hoak, J. D. *Surgery*, 1977, **82**, 219.
8. Hull, R. W., et al. *Circulation*, 1976, **53**, 696.
9. Hull, R., et al. *New Engl. J. Med.* 1977, **296**, 1497.
10. Richards, K. L., et al. *Archs intern. Med.* 1976, **136**, 1091.
11. Benedict, K. T., Wheeler, H. B., Patwardhan, N. A. *Radiology*, 1977, **125**, 696.
12. Albrechtsson, U., Olsson, C. G. *Lancet*, 1976, i, 723.

CONTROLLED CLINICAL TRIAL OF FIVE SHORT-COURSE (4-MONTH) CHEMOTHERAPY REGIMENS IN PULMONARY TUBERCULOSIS

First Report of 4th Study

EAST AFRICAN AND BRITISH MEDICAL RESEARCH COUNCILS

Summary   Five 4-mo regimens of chemotherapy for tuberculosis are compared. The two regimens in which rifampicin was given throughout the 4 mo were associated with bacteriological-relapse rates of 8% in the first 6 mo after stopping chemotherapy, but the three regimens in which rifampicin was given for only the first 2 mo had relapse-rates of 24–32%. There was no evidence that the addition of pyrazinamide in the second 2 mo of chemotherapy reduced the bacteriological-relapse rate. Removal of the streptomycin from the first 2 mo appeared to reduce the bactericidal and sterilising activity of the regimen, although the differences were not statistically significant. The incidence of adverse reactions was very low with all five regimens.

Introduction

THE high level of efficacy of several 6 mo regimens of chemotherapy for pulmonary tuberculosis has been established in studies in East Africa and in many other parts of the world, relapse-rates after the end of chemotherapy being 5% or less.[1-11] It was important, therefore, to investigate regimens of even shorter duration. A pilot study in France[12] of two 3-mo regimens of rifampicin, isoniazid, and streptomycin had had a relatively low overall relapse-rate of 13%. Studies in East Africa[5-7] had also shown that an intensive initial four-drug phase with streptomycin, isoniazid, rifampicin, and pyrazinamide given daily for 2 mo is a very effective component of short-course chemotherapy and that the pyrazinamide plays an important part, as has been confirmed in Hong Kong.[8] The present study was planned to investigate whether adding pyrazinamide to the three drugs studied in France and also increasing the total duration of chemotherapy to 4 mo would improve the results. Even if not uniformly successful, this regimen might still be applicable in developing countries, where standard-duration chemotherapy with regimens known to be 100% effective in antibacterial terms produces relatively low levels of success under programme conditions,[13] default from treatment being a major reason for failure. Thus, a 4 mo regimen that is less than uniformly successful might still constitute a major therapeutic advance. Because daily administration of streptomycin in many developing countries almost invariably requires hospital admission for the duration of treatment, a regimen not including streptomycin was also investigated. This regimen, as well as being applicable to outpatients, provides direct information about the role of streptomycin in the initial intensive phase.

Patients and Methods
PLAN AND CONDUCT OF STUDY

Selection of Patients

Patients selected were Africans aged 15–65, with previously untreated extensive pulmonary tuberculosis believed to be of

366

THE LANCET, AUGUST 12, 1978

Letters to the Editor

BIRTH AFTER THE REIMPLANTATION OF A HUMAN EMBRYO

SIR,—We wish to report that one of our patients, a 30-year-old nulliparous married woman, was safely delivered by cæsarean section on July 25, 1978, of a normal healthy infant girl weighing 2700 g. The patient had been referred to one of us (P.C.S.) in 1976 with a history of 9 years' infertility, tubal occlusions, and unsuccessful salpingostomies done in 1970 with excision of the ampullæ of both oviducts followed by persistent tubal blockages. Laparoscopy in February, 1977, revealed grossly distorted tubal remnants with occlusion and peritubal and ovarian adhesions. Laparotomy in August, 1977, was done with excision of the remains of both tubes, adhesolysis, and suspension of the ovaries in good position for oocyte recovery.

Pregnancy was established after laparoscopic recovery of an oocyte on Nov. 10, 1977, in-vitro fertilisation and normal cleavage in culture media, and the reimplantation of the 8-cell embryo into the uterus $2\frac{1}{2}$ days later. Amniocentesis at 16 weeks' pregnancy revealed normal α-fetoprotein levels, with no chromosome abnormalities in a 46 XX fetus. On the day of delivery the mother was 38 weeks and 5 days by dates from her last menstrual period, and she had pre-eclamptic toxæmia. Blood-pressure was fluctuating around 140/95, œdema involved both legs up to knee level together with the abdomen, back, hands, and face; the blood-uric-acid was 390 μmol/l, and albumin 0·5 g/l of urine. Ultrasonic scanning and radiographic appearances showed that the fetus had grown slowly for several weeks from week 30. Blood-œstriols and human placental lactogen levels also dropped below the normal levels during this period. However, the fetus grew considerably during the last 10 days before delivery while placental function improved greatly. On the day of delivery the biparietal diameter had reached 9·6 cm, and 5 ml of amniotic fluid was removed safely under sonic control. The lecithin: sphingomyelin ratio was 3·9:1, indicative of maturity and a low risk of the respiratory-distress syndrome.

We hope to publish further medical and scientific details in your columns at a later date.

Department of
  Obstetrics and Gynæcology,
General Hospital,
Oldham OL1 2JH   P. C. STEPTOE

University Physiology Laboratory,
Cambridge CB2 3EG   R. G. EDWARDS

SPERM BASIC PROTEINS IN CERVICAL CARCINOGENESIS

SIR,—Dr Reid and his colleagues (July 8, p. 60) have calculated a product-moment correlation coefficient (r) between sperm histone/protamine ratio and socioeconomic class, but this test is not applicable where one of the variables, socioeconomic class, though represented by a number, is really a category, which cannot be used arithmetically. A more appropriate test would be the non-parametric Kruskal-Wallis one-way analysis of variance by ranks, but even this is not applicable when, as here, the relationship between socioeconomic class and two variables (sperm concentrations of histone and protamine) are being examined. Fig. 2 of their paper shows diagrammatically the sperm histone/protamine ratios for the different socioeconomic classes, with what we assume to be the arithmetic means of the ratios; the vertical lines above and below the means, from their symmetry, suggest standard deviations or "normal ranges". We suspect that this ratio fits a skewed, rather than a normal, distribution. In any case the data ought to have been presented in a manner which is clear to readers and permits independent analysis.

The classification of phenomena according to the Registrar General's social classes was a useful procedure when introduced in the 1911 Census and in later medical studies. For instance, it was used to demonstrate neatly and clearly an association between socioeconomic disadvantage and infant ill-health and death. In other words higher rates of infant mortality were associated with evils indicated roughly by the social-class classification which indicated lack of education, poverty, poor housing, hygiene, and nutrition, and so on. This association of low incidence in the professional classes and high incidence in the unskilled was found in many other conditions (e.g., tuberculosis).

Since 1911 jobs have tended to be reclassified because of the illness experienced by those who do them, so statements drawing on the system have tended to become circular. Moreover, socioeconomic changes have rendered the classification less useful. What were often virtually hereditary occupational castes in 1911 (e.g., mining, fishing, and farming) have now so changed that people may be employed in them for only short periods. Mobility, both within and between classes, is common. Income gaps have closed—e.g., in 1948 a consultant in the N.H.S. without a merit award was paid 5 times as much as a coalminer, whereas now, making similar allowances for income tax and other deductions, the differential is $2-2\frac{1}{2}$. Differences in education and skill often remain, especially between social classes IV and V and the rest, and it is often these and the ideologies that accompany them that determine the lifestyle of the different groups.

Some people have suggested that social-class classification asserts differences which have their origins at conception, and we suspect that this is what Reid et al. are on about, though their paper is not clear on this point. This view, once confidently held by the more favoured members of society, can no longer be entertained. A more plausible statement is that social class is a classification of occupations which put their mark on their members in all sorts of obvious and in many subtle ways. For example, there is indeed a social-class association with cervical cancer but it is not as marked as associations between, for instance, the incidence of cervical cancer and early, frequent, and varied experience of sexual intercourse. What a social-class classification can never do is lend itself to precognition. True, medical students will become classified to social class I, provided they pass their exams, but future membership of a profession cannot have any bearing on a protein ratio in sperm. This Aristotelean way of thinking was abandoned by science centuries ago.

How a social-class classification is carried out is important, but Reid et al. give insufficient details of their method. For instance the U.K. subjects are said to have been classified "using the system of the U.K. registrar general", but 100 of them were students who, in the Classification of Occupations 1970,[2] "are coded to the economic position 'Student' and excluded from the classification by occupation". Also in these days of high unemployment it would be astonishing if all the cases could be successfully classified, but all the men studied fit neatly into one or other of the five social classes.

This paper, we feel, fails to match standards we expect from *The Lancet* in respect of its statistics and in its epidemiology.

Department of Community Medicine,
University of Edinburgh,
Usher Institute,   DONALD CAMERON
Edinburgh   IAN G. JONES

ANTURANE REINFARCTION TRIAL

SIR,—Your admirable leader on stroke prevention (July 29, p. 245) concludes with a question which seems to imply tacit acceptance of claims that sulphinpyrazone is of benefit in

1. Reid, B. L., French, P. W., Singer, A., Hagan, B. E., Coppleson, M. *Lancet*, 1978, ii, 60.
2. Office of Population Censuses and Surveys. Classification of Occupations 1970. H.M. Stationery Office, 1970.

The Lancet · Saturday 21 October 1978

HEPATITIS "C" ANTIGEN IN NON-A, NON-B POST-TRANSFUSION HEPATITIS

Ryoichi Shirachi   Hiroyuki Shiraishi
Akira Tateda   Kaneo Kikuchi
Nakao Ishida

Department of Microbiology, Miyagi Prefectural Institute of Public Health, Sendai, Japan; Surgical Clinic of National Sendai Hospital; and Department of Bacteriology, Tohoku University School of Medicine, Sendai

Summary   Evidence for a new hepatitis-specific antigen has been obtained from double immunodiffusion assays between acute and convalescent sera obtained from patients with non-A, non-B post-transfusion hepatitis. The designation hepatitis C (HC) antigen is proposed. HC was found in the acute-phase sera of all 13 non-A, non-B post-transfusion hepatitis patients with longer incubation and duration periods (type 2) tested, but only transiently in 4 out of 10 acute-phase sera obtained from patients with type 1 non-A, non-B hepatitis, with shorter incubation and duration periods. The antigen was also detected in 2 out of 16 single specimens obtained during the acute phase from acute hepatitis patients who had not received a blood-transfusion. This suggests presence of a carrier state. No patients with alcoholic hepatitis and no healthy blood-donor carried HC antigen. The antigen seems distinct from those of hepatitis A and B (surface and core). It migrated in the serum β-globulin region and had a buoyant density of 1·30 and a molecular weight between 100 000 and 300 000. Antibodies against HC antigen were found in only 30% of the type-2 non-A, non-B post-transfusion hepatitis patients and did not persist for long. However, these antibodies were directed specifically against HC antigen and moved in a manner similar to 7S globulin on rate-zonal centrifugation.

Introduction

ONCE the association between hepatitis-B surface antigen (HB_sAg) and type-B hepatitis had been recognised it was expected that screening blood-donors for HB_sAg would eliminate post-transfusion hepatitis. However, even with screening for HB_sAg a 10% frequency of post-transfusion hepatitis has persisted,[1-5] and 90–95% of these cases have been serologically unrelated to hepatitis A or B or cytomegalovirus.[6-8] This suggested the existence of at least one more agent ætiologically responsible for human viral hepatitis. Evidence for a transmissible agent was demonstrated by inoculating blood from patients with non-A, non-B hepatitis patients into chimpanzees.[9][10] However, no serological marker was defined in these studies and no virus particle was observed. Our study was designed to detect a serological marker for this disease.

Material and Methods

Sera

In 1970–77 there were 156 post-transfusion hepatitis patients at the surgical clinic of Sendai National Hospital. 116 were negative for HB_sAg and anti-HB_s antibody (non-B post-transfusion hepatitis), and these could be further divided into two groups, the pattern of serum-glutamic-pyruvic-transaminase (S.G.P.T.) values being monophasic or biphasic[2] (fig. 1). In the monophasic group (type-1 non-B hepatitis) S.G.P.T. values rise rapidly and then fall sharply. The average incubation period was 5·7 weeks and raised S.G.P.T.s persisted for 5·8 weeks.[2] Type-2 non-B hepatitis is characterised by a rapid increase and decrease in S.G.P.T. similar to that of the monopha-

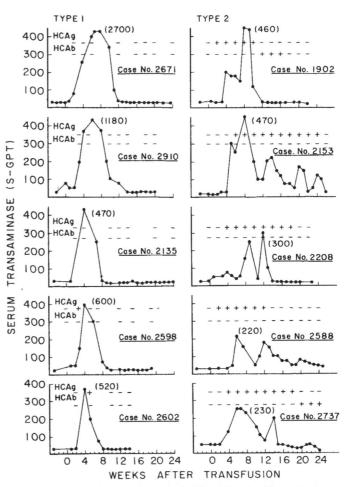

Fig. 1—Clinical courses of type-1 (short incubation and short duration) and type-2 (long incubation and long duration) non-A, non-B hepatitis observed after blood-transfusion.

The Lancet · Saturday 23 & 30 December 1978

CYCLOSPORIN A IN PATIENTS RECEIVING RENAL ALLOGRAFTS FROM CADAVER DONORS

R. Y. Calne   D. J. G. White
S. Thiru   D. B. Evans
P. McMaster   D. C. Dunn
G. N. Craddock   B. D. Pentlow
Keith Rolles

Departments of Surgery and Pathology, University of Cambridge; and Dialysis Unit, Addenbrooke's Hospital, Cambridge

Summary   Seven patients on dialysis with renal failure received transplants from mismatched cadaver donors and were treated with cyclosporin A (CyA), initially as the sole immunosuppressive agent. CyA was effective in inhibiting rejection but there was clear evidence of both nephrotoxicity and hepatotoxicity. A cyclophosphamide analogue was added to the CyA treatment in six of the patients. Five patients are out of hospital with functioning allografts, and two of these have received no steroids. One patient required an allograft nephrectomy because of pyelonephritis in the graft. Another died of systemic aspergillus and candida infection. Further careful study of this potentially valuable drug will be required before it can be recommended in clinical practice.

Introduction

Most transplant clinicians find corticosteroids essential in the prevention of organ-graft rejection, but they have many unwanted effects, and their replacement by safer and more effective chemical immunosuppressants is desirable. A peptide fungal metabolite, cyclosporin A (CyA), has been found to prolong survival of skin grafts in mice,[1] of heterotopic cardiac allografts in rats,[2] of renal allografts in mongrel dogs,[3] and of orthotopic heart grafts in pigs.[4] In dogs given CyA both survival and allograft function were better than in those treated with azathioprine. Rejection and infection were less, and marrow depression was not seen. Since our earlier report,[4] pigs with orthotopic allografts fared well. 3 of 8 have died at days 22, 43, and 72. In the remaining 5 CyA was stopped after 125–197 days, and they remain alive with a median survival in excess of 180 days. In pigs the drug had no obvious side-effects, but 5 (14%) of the 34 dogs with renal allografts became jaundiced.[5] At necropsy 1 proved to have toxoplasmosis in the liver. The other jaundiced animals had areas of focal liver-cell necrosis and cholestasis. 12 (35%) of the dogs died of in-

fection, mostly in the lungs, and 8 (23%) died of rejection, 4 of these being animals in which CyA was stopped 11–14 days after transplantation.

CyA has been studied in two other species with renal allografts—the rhesus monkey (our unpublished observations) and the rabbit.[6][7] In both these species it was powerfully immunosuppressive without obvious side-effects. We felt that the experimental background justified a pilot study of CyA, as the sole immunosuppressant initially, in patients with first cadaveric renal allografts from mismatched donors.

Materials and Methods

CyA was started on the day of grafting, injected intramuscularly dissolved in 'Miglyol' 25 mg/kg for the first 2 to 3 days, until the patients could take the drug orally, dissolved in olive oil, at the same dosage. In two cases the preparation of CyA was changed from olive oil to Sandoz capsules in the third postoperative month. Details of the patients are in table I. The drug dosage in mg/kg was the same as that which achieved good immunosuppressive results with few side-effects in pigs with cardiac allografts and dogs and rabbits with renal allografts. All the kidneys came from donors with complete irreversible cerebral destruction but with intact circulations maintained on mechanical ventilation during nephrectomy. There was therefore no more than a few minutes during which the kidneys were warm and ischæmic. The organs were preserved by flush cooling and ice storage.[8] They were cold and ischæmic for between 1·25 and 16 hours. Liver and renal function were carefully monitored postoperatively and full blood-counts were done daily. In no case could the kidney be regarded as well-matched: all were incompatible for two or more of the four HLA-A, B antigens. The T-cell proliferative responses of peripheral-blood lymphocytes were assessed weekly. Serum samples were studied for their ability to inhibit phytohæmagglutinin (P.H.A.) responses of lymphocytes from normal individuals. Biopsy specimens were taken from six of seven allografts and examined by light microscopy. Two of these had immunofluorescence studies and one was examined by electron microscopy.

Results

None of the biopsy specimens showed severe or extensive mononuclear-cell infiltration of the interstitium, interstitial hæmorrhage, or other histological evidence of severe rejection. When the infiltrating mononuclear cells were sparse and focal a mild cellular rejection reaction was diagnosed. When numbers of cells were increased or the infiltration more diffuse this was regarded as moderate rejection and these cases often had accompanying interstitial œdema (table II). Foci of proximal tubular epithelial degenerations were present in some biopsy

346

represents the best available approach to any prospective research on the physiopathology of cot deaths.

We thank the Foundation for the Study of Infant Deaths and the D.H.S.S. for their financial support. The work reported here depended on the enthusiastic cooperation of the health visitors and the community health staff of Sheffield.

REFERENCES

1. Steinschneider A. A reexamination of "the apnea monitor business". *Pediatrics* 1976; **58**: 1–5.
2. Froggat P. A cardiac cause in cot death: a discarded hypothesis. *J Irish Med Ass* 1977; **70**: 408–14.
3. Carpenter RG, Emery JL. The identification and follow-up of high risk infants. In: Sudden infant death syndrome. Robinson RR, ed. London and Toronto: Foundation for the Study of Infant Death, 1974: 91–96.
4. Carpenter RG, Emery JL. Final results of study of infants at risk of sudden death. *Nature* 1977; **268**: 724–25.
5. Carpenter RG, Gardner A, McWeeny PM, Emery JL. Multistage scoring system for identifying infants at risk of unexpected death. *Arch Dis Child* 1977; **52**: 606–12.
6. Emery JL, Crowley EM. Clinical histories of infants reported to coroner as cases of unexpected death. *Brit Med J* 1956; ii: 1518–21.
7. Carpenter RG, Shaddick CW. Role of infection, suffocation, and bottle feeding in cot death. *Brit J Prev Soc Med* 1965; **19**: 1–7.
8. Froggatt P. Epidemiologic aspects of the Northern Ireland study. In: Sudden Infant Death Syndrome. Bergman AB, Beckwith J, Ray CG, ed. Seattle: University of Washington, 1969: 32–46.
9. Houstek J. Sudden infant death syndrome in Czechoslovakia; epidemiologic aspects. In: Sudden infant death syndrome, pp. 55–63. Berman AB, Beckwith J, Ray CG, eds. Seattle: University of Washington, 1969: 55–63.
10. Carpenter, RG. Sudden death in twins. *M.O.H. Rep Pub Hlth Med Subjcts* 1965; **113**: 51–52.
11. Cameron JM, Watson E. Sudden death in infancy in Inner North London. *J Pathol* 1974; **117**: 55–61.
12. Stanton AN, Downham MAPS, Oakley JR, Emery JL, Knowelden J. Terminal symptoms in children dying unexpectedly at home. *Brit Med J* 1978; ii: 1249–51.
13. McWeeny PM, Emery JL. Unexpected postneonatal deaths (cot deaths) due to recognizable disease. *Arch Dis Child* 1975; **50**: 191–96.
14. Camps, FE. (1972). In: Camps FE, Carpenter RG, eds. Sudden and unexpected death in infancy (cot death). Bristol: Wright, 1972: 2.
15. Carpenter RG, Emery JL. Unpublished.
16. Bergman AB, Rae CG, Pomeroy MA, Wahl PW, Beckwith JB. Studies of the sudden infant death syndrome in King County, Washington. III Epidemiology. *Pediatrics* 1972; **49**: 860–70.
17. Froggatt P, Lynas MA, MacKenzie G. Epidemiology of sudden unexpected death in infants (cot death) in Northern Ireland. *Brit J Prev Soc Med* 1971; **25**: 119–34.
18. W.H.O. Risk Approach for Maternal and Child Health Care. W.H.O. Offset publication No. 39; Geneva, 1978.

Preventive Medicine

HUNTINGTON'S CHOREA

The Basis for Long-Term Prevention

P. S. Harper   D. A. Walker
Audrey Tyler   R. G. Newcombe
Kathleen Davies

Section of Medical Genetics, Department of Medicine, and Department of Medical Statistics, Welsh National School of Medicine, Heath Park, Cardiff

Summary   A long-term programme to reduce the incidence of Huntington's Chorea has been established in South Wales, based on a study of all individuals known to be affected or at high risk in a defined population of 1·7 million people. Systematic but non-directive genetic counselling is being given to all adults at risk, accompanied by regular follow-up to provide both further information and practical support where required. The number of observed and projected new cases of the disorder born between 1900 and 1970 has remained almost constant, despite a progressive reduction in birth-rate in the general population during this period. Prospective monitoring of all births in the high-risk population will allow an estimate to be made of future trends and will show whether preventive measures are having any significant effect on the future incidence of the disorder in the population.

INTRODUCTION

In families afflicted by Huntington's chorea (HC), because of the late onset of the disease and the lack of any established preclinical or predictive test, the number of relatives at high risk is considerably greater than the number who will eventually have or transmit the disorder. Although the mode of inheritance of HC has been known for many years and numerous studies have been undertaken in particular populations, including Wales,[1] there is no evidence that the incidence of the disorder has been or is being reduced as a result of preventive measures. We describe here the basis of a long-term preventive programme in a defined population which may achieve a reduction in future incidence, together with the difficulties and limitations of the programme and the way in which its success can be monitored.

THE STUDY POPULATION

The study population is the residents of Gwent and Glamorgan (now South, Mid, and West Glamorgan)—i.e., almost all of industrial South Wales. It numbered 1 720 901 at the time of estimation of prevalence (1971). Within this area an attempt was made in 1973–78 to obtain complete ascertainment, utilising information from hospital clinicians (principally neurologists, psychiatrists, and medical geneticists), general practitioners, and the records of general and psychiatric hospitals.

We attempted to assess the prevalence of the gene and of the overt disease state in our population at a remote "prevalence date" (April 1971). Among the total of 418 affected individuals identified, who belonged to 10 apparently unrelated kindreds, 130· were alive and had symptoms at that date. The prevalence of HC in the whole study area was estimated at 7·55 per 100 000 and the total heterozygote frequency at 20·2 per 100 000.

THE POPULATION AT RISK

The risks of all family members were computed by a life table method which utilised (a) the prior genetic risk (usually $\frac{1}{2}$ or $\frac{1}{4}$), depending on whether a parent or grandparent had been affected or was known to have carried the gene; (b) the reduction in risk resulting from the age of the individual and (where relevant) the age of an unaffected parent or grandparent.

This life-table (fig. 1) was itself based on the distribution of ages of onset of HC in our study population adjusted to take into account those individuals still at risk of the disease. It does not take into account possible heterogeneity between families for age at onset; this factor may be of importance in genetic counselling of individuals, but is unlikely to affect materially the overall distribution of risks in the population.

1129 living family members had a risk considered high (1 in 8 or greater), of whom 929 lived in Glamorgan and Gwent. 181 individuals living in the area were considered to be at low risk (under 1 in 8). None of the individuals whose nearest affected relative was more remote than parent or grandparent had a life-table risk of over 1 in 10.

for $2\frac{1}{2}$ years after recovery in patient D (fig. 3) agrees with the existence of an asymptomatic carrier state for NANB virus.

Our data support the existence of a virus-specific antigenæmia[5-13] detectable by immunodiffusion in a large proportion of NANB infections. The various NANB viruses may differ in their incubation periods. In the two other studies of the detection of antigenæmia in NANB hepatitis, this incubation period also ranged from 6 to 14 weeks. The timing of antigen and antibody detection was again similar. It seems likely that Shirachi's HC and the NANB Ag/Ab systems are related to the same NANB virus, which is probably the most common one and may be characterised by a long incubation period.*

We thank Dr. L. R. Overby, Dr C. Ling, and Dr R. H. Decker, of Abbott Laboratories, for the anti-HA IgM serological tests and Dr M. C. Van Den Ende for the wedge liver biopsy of chimpanzees and for supervising their plasmapheresis. Linda Richardson and the staff of Vilab II gave expert technical assistance. This study was supported by INSERM, CNRS, UER de Biologie Humaine, The Merieux Foundation, NHLBI, NIH (HE-09011), The New York Blood Center, and Blood Service Inc., Scottsdale, Arizona.

Requests for reprints should be addressed to C. T., Pavilion H, Hôpital Edouard Herriot, 69374-Lyon Cedex 2, France.

*Since this paper was written identity between Shirachi's HC Ag and one of the two antigens of the NANB Ag complex has been demonstrated.

REFERENCES

1. Alter HJ, Purcell RH, Holland PV, Popper H. Transmissible agent in non-A non-B hepatitis. Lancet 1978; i: 459–63.
2. Tabore E, Drucker JA, Hoofnagle JH, April M, Barker LF, Tamondong GT. Transmission of non-A non-B hepatitis from man to chimpanzee. Lancet 1978; i: 463–65.
3. Wike J, Tsiquaye KN, Thornton A, et al. Transmission of non-A non-B hepatitis to chimpanzees by factor IX concentrates after fatal complications in patients with chronic liver disease. Lancet 1979; i: 520–24.
4. Hollinger FB, Gitnick GL, Aach RD, et al. Non-A non-B hepatitis transmission in chimpanzees: a project of the transfusion-transmitted viruses study group. Intervirology 1978; 10: 60–68.
5. Prince AM, Brotman B, Van den Ende MC, Richardson L, Kellner A. Non-A non-B hepatitis: identification of a virus specific antigen and antibody. In: Vyas GN, Cohen SN, Schmidt R, Viral hepatitis. Philadelphia: Franklin Institute Press, 1978: 419–21.
6. Mosley JW, Redecker SM, Feinstone SM, Purcell RH. Multiple hepatitis viruses in multiple attacks of acute viral hepatitis. N Engl J Med 1977; 296: 75–79.
7. Tsiquaye KN, Zuckerman AJ. New Human hepatitis virus. Lancet 1979; i: 1135–36.
8. Feinstone SM, Kapikian AZ, Purcell RH, Alter HJ, Holland PV. Transfusion associated hepatitis not due to hepatitis type A or B. N Engl J Med 1975; 292: 767–70.
9. Knodell RG, Conrad ME, Dienstag JL, Bell CJ. Etiological spectrum of post-transfusion hepatitis. Gastroenterology 1975; 67: 278–85.
10. Hepatitis Laboratories Division, Bureau of Epidemiology Center for Disease Control. Recovery of virus-like particles associated with non A-non B hepatitis. Morbid Mortal Wkly Rep 1978; 27: 199–200.
11. Cossart YE. A new particulate antigen present in serum. International symposium on viral hepatitis, Milan, 1974. Develop Biol Standard 1975; 30: 445–48.
12. Almeida JD, Deinhardt F, Holmes AW. Morphology of the G.B. hepatitis agent. Nature 1976; 261: 608–09.
13. Shirachi R, Tateda A, Shiraishi H, Kikuchi K, Ishida N. Hepatitis "C" antigen in non-A non-B post-transfusion hepatitis. Lancet 1978; ii: 853–56.
14. Wroblewski F, La Due JS. Serum glutamic pyruvic transaminase in cardiac and hepatic diseases. Proc Soc Exp Biol Med 1956; 91: 569–71.
15. Prince AM, Brotman B, Grady GF, et al. Long-incubation post-transfusion hepatitis without serological evidence of exposure to hepatitis-B virus. Lancet 1974; ii: 241–46.
16. Committee on Enzymes of the Scandinavian Society for Clinical Chemistry. Scand J Clin Lab Invest 1974; 33: 291–95.
17. Decker RH, Overby LR, Ling C, Frosner G, Deinhardt F, Boggs J. Serologic studies of transmission of hepatitis A in humans. J Infect Dis 1979; 139: 74–82.
18. Prince AM. An antigen detected in the blood during the incubation period of serum hepatitis. Proc Nat Acad Sci USA 1968; 60: 814–821.

Preliminary Communications

PARENTERAL ACYCLOVIR THERAPY FOR HERPESVIRUS INFECTIONS IN MAN

P. J. SELBY   R. L. POWLES
BERYL JAMESON   H. E. M. KAY
J. G. WATSON   R. THORNTON
G. MORGENSTERN   H. M. CLINK
T. J. McELWAIN

Department of Medicine and Leukæmia Unit, Royal Marsden Hospital, Sutton, Surrey

H. G. PRENTICE   R. CORRINGHAM
M. G. ROSS   A. V. HOFFBRAND

Academic Department of Hæmatology and Microbiology and Department of Medical Oncology, Royal Free Hospital, London NW3

D. BRIGDEN

Wellcome Research Laboratories, Beckenham, Kent

Summary   Acyclovir is a new antiviral agent which is highly active against herpesviruses in vitro and in laboratory animals. Twenty-three cancer patients with cutaneous and/or systemic herpes zoster or herpes simplex infections were treated with parenteral acyclovir. All had received previous specific treatment for their malignant disease and ten had undergone bone-marrow transplantation. The drug seemed to arrest the progress of the infections and was most effective when given early. Although two patients showed transient increases in blood-urea, possibly the result of acyclovir, the drug was remarkably non-toxic in the doses used.

INTRODUCTION

HERPESVIRUS infections cause much morbidity and occasional mortality in immunosuppressed patients.[1] Herpes zoster develops in some 20% of patients with Hodgkin's disease at some stage of their illness and in one-third of these patients the infection becomes disseminated and may lead to life-threatening complications.[2,3] Patients undergoing bone-marrow transplantation are particularly vulnerable to these infections.[4] Topical treatment with idoxuridine may be beneficial for local infections, and adenine arabinoside infusions are probably an effective treatment although they can be difficult to administer and may be toxic.[5] Human leucocyte interferon has been reported to be beneficial but has yet to be evaluated fully.[6]

Acyclovir (9-[2-hydroxyethoxymethyl]guanine), formerly called acycloguanosine, is a guanine derivative with an acyclic side-chain. It is active against herpesviruses in vitro and in laboratory animals.[7,8] Topical application prevented recurrence after wipe debridement of corneal epithelial lesions caused by herpes simplex infections in man.[9] We report our clinical experience of acyclovir treatment of a wide range of herpesvirus infections in immunosuppressed patients.

PATIENTS AND METHODS

Twenty-three patients (aged 7–70 years) were treated with acyclovir (see accompanying table). All had malignant dis-

The Lancet · Saturday 11 July 1981

IMAGING OF THE BRAIN BY NUCLEAR MAGNETIC RESONANCE

F. H. DOYLE   J. C. GORE
J. M. PENNOCK   G. M. BYDDER
J. S. ORR   R. E. STEINER

Departments of Diagnostic Radiology and Medical Physics, Royal Postgraduate Medical School, Hammersmith Hospital, London

I. R. YOUNG   M. BURL
H. CLOW   D. J. GILDERDALE
D. R. BAILES   P. E. WALTERS

Central Research Laboratories, Thorn-EMI Limited, Hayes, Middlesex

Summary   A nuclear magnetic resonance (NMR) machine constructed by Thorn-EMI Ltd was used to produce tomographic images of the brain in eight volunteers and fourteen patients. The use of an inversion recovery technique designed to emphasise variations in the spin-lattice time constant (T_1) resulted in remarkable differentiation between grey and white matter in all subjects examined. White matter was seen both centrally and peripherally to subcortical level and the basal ganglia were clearly demarcated by the surrounding white matter and ventricular system. The posterior fossa was visualised with substantially less artefact than with X-ray computed tomography (CT) and both the brainstem and middle cerebellar peduncle were clearly shown. Pathological appearances in patients with glioblastoma multiforme, cerebral infarction, and cerebral aneurysm were demonstrated and compared with those seen with CT. The technique will require thorough clinical evaluation but appears to have considerable potential in the diagnosis of neurological disease.

Introduction

IMAGING of the brain was transformed by the introduction of the first X-ray computed tomography (CT) head scanner nearly a decade ago. Since that time machine improvements and the use of contrast agents have consolidated the position of CT as the primary diagnostic modality for imaging of the brain. The success of CT has undoubtedly provided a major stimulus for the development of systems which make use of the magnetic properties of the hydrogen nucleus to generate images of sections of the human body. Following research at the Central Research Laboratories of Thorn-EMI Ltd, begun in 1976, brain scans were obtained using a resistive magnet machine and over the past year groups in both Nottingham and Aberdeen have used nuclear magnetic resonance (NMR) techniques to demonstrate intracranial anatomy and pathology.[1-6]

We now report our initial clinical experience with NMR scanning in the demonstration of the anatomical structure of the brain, using a more sophisticated machine based on a cryomagnet, and illustrate some appearances in intracranial disease. The results have been compared with those obtained by CT.

Patients and Methods

After approval by the research ethics committee of the Royal Postgraduate Medical School, eight healthy volunteers and fourteen patients have had NMR brain scans. Informed consent was obtained in all cases and the techniques used followed the guidelines for clinical NMR imaging provided by the National Radiological Protection Board.[7]

CT scans were also performed on two of the volunteers and all of the patients using a Siemens 'Somatom 2' whole body scanner operating in the head mode at 125 kVp and 230 mAs. The scan time for each CT slice was 10 seconds and the slice width 8 mm.

The NMR scanner was developed at the Central Research Laboratories of Thorn-EMI Ltd with the support of the Department of Health and Social Security. The main D.C. or H_0 magnetic field along the long axis of the patient (the Z axis in fig. 1) was provided by a cryogenic magnet built by Oxford Instruments Ltd operating at a field strength of 0·15 tesla (1500 gauss) giving a proton resonant frequency of approximately 6·5 MHz.

The hydrogen nuclei were excited by radiofrequency radiation transmitted by a coil surrounding the head and the signals produced by the excited nuclei were detected as induced electrical currents in a receiver coil lying within the transmitter coil.

In this study, scans were obtained using an inversion recovery technique. This method generates images that are highly dependent on T_1, the spin-lattice relaxation time constant. Protons in the static magnetic field H_0 line up preferentially in the direction of the field, producing a net magnetisation in the $+Z$ direction (fig. 1). A short radiofrequency pulse H_1 (fig. 2) is then applied to rotate the net magnetisation through 180 degrees into the $-Z$ direction. Thereafter the magnetisation returns exponentially to its original state with a time constant T_1, the spin-lattice relaxation time. If, however, a second radiofrequency pulse of half the duration of the first is applied after a short time interval τ (fig. 2), the magnetisation is rotated through 90° into the X-Y plane.

The rotational or precessional motion of the magnetisation in this plane generates a signal which is detected by the receiver coil. The strength of this signal depends both on the number of protons and

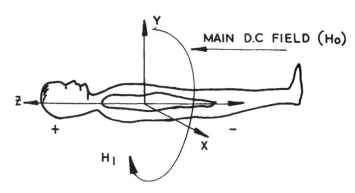

Fig. 1—Body orientation relative to the machine axes.

The main DC field (H_0) is in the longitudinal axis of the body or Z direction. The H_1 field is in the XY plane.

KAPOSI'S SARCOMA IN HOMOSEXUAL MEN—A REPORT OF EIGHT CASES

KENNETH B. HYMES   TONY CHEUNG
JEFFREY B. GREENE   NEIL S. PROSE
AARON MARCUS   HAROLD BALLARD
DANIEL C. WILLIAM   LINDA J. LAUBENSTEIN

Department of Medicine, Divisions of Hematology, Oncology, and Infectious Diseases, New York University Medical Center; Department of Dermatology, Downstate Medical Center, Brooklyn; and Department of Hematology, New York Veterans Administration Medical Center, New York City, New York

Summary   The clinical findings in eight young homosexual men in New York with Kaposi's sarcoma showed some unusual features. Unlike the form usually seen in North America and Europe, it affected younger men (4th decade rather than 7th decade); the skin lesions were generalised rather than being predominantly in the lower limbs, and the disease was more aggressive (survival of less than 20 months rather than 8–13 years). All eight had had a variety of sexually transmitted diseases. All those tested for cytomegalovirus antibodies and hepatitis B surface antigen or anti-hepatitis B antibody gave positive results. This unusual occurrence of Kaposi's sarcoma in a population much exposed to sexually transmissible diseases suggests that such exposure may play a role in its pathogenesis.

Introduction

Kaposi's sarcoma is rare in the United States, where the annual incidence is $0.021-0.061$ per 100 000 population.[1,2] In North America and Europe, this disease commonly presents as tumours of the lower extremities, and the clinical picture is that of a localised disease with an indolent course. Most patients are in their seventh decade. This form of the disease is commonest among Ashkenazi Jews and those of Mediterranean origin, and especially in men.[3,4]

The incidence of Kaposi's sarcoma in African Blacks residing in an endemic region is much higher than among Blacks and Caucasians in North America and Europe. Kaposi's sarcoma makes up 9.1% of all malignancies diagnosed in Uganda.[1] In Africa, about 10% of patients with Kaposi's sarcoma present with the lymphadenopathic form of the disease.[5] They have few skin lesions, which may occur on any part of the body, but extensive lymph node and visceral involvement. Most of the patients are less than 20 years of age, and all reported cases have died within 3 years of presentation.[3,5]

We describe here the features of Kaposi's sarcoma seen in eight young homosexual men in the New York City area.

Methods

Eight patients with Kaposi's sarcoma were seen between March, 1979, and March, 1981, inclusive, at the New York University Medical Center, Brooklyn Veterans Administration Medical Center, and the Mount Sinai Hospital. All were seen and evaluated by at least one of the authors. Routine investigations done in all patients included complete and differential blood counts, serum electrolytes, liver-function tests, and the Venereal Disease Reference Laboratory (VDRL) test. Biopsy specimens and specimens of necropsy tissue were examined by the departments of pathology at the respective institutions. Hepatitis B surface antigen (HBsAg) and anti-hepatitis B surface antibody (anti-HBs) were determined by radioimmunoassay. Cytomegalovirus (CMV) titres

were measured by the complement fixation technique in the New York City Health Department Laboratories.

Clinical Observations

All eight patients with Kaposi's sarcoma reported in this study were homosexual men aged 27–45 years and had multiple sexual partners. All had histories of a variety of sexually transmitted diseases including syphilis, gonorrhoea, viral hepatitis, amoebiasis, *Herpes progenitalis* infection, and condyloma acuminatum. Four of the eight patients were Jewish and one was Italian. The only Black patient in our study was born in America and had never been to Africa. The accompanying table summarises some of the clinical features.

Seven of the eight patients sought medical attention because of skin lesions. The eighth (case 8) presented with *Pneumocystis carinii* pneumonia, and the skin lesions were detected at the first physical examination. In all patients the skin lesions appeared gradually. In six, the skin lesions were numerous when first seen. Case 8 had two discrete lesions on admission but more than twenty new lesions developed during his 3 months in hospital. The skin lesions consisted of nodules and papules in seven patients, and of plaques in case 8. All the skin tumours were non-tender, purplish, and non-ulcerating, and ranged in size from several millimetres to several centimetres in diameter. In several patients the lesions tended to coalesce. Lesions were found in the head and neck in four patients, but no patient showed predominant involvement of the lower extremities.

All eight patients had histologically proven cutaneous and lymph-node involvement. The histological features were typical of Kaposi's sarcoma. Skin lesions showed proliferation of small vessels lined by endothelium and interspersed groups of spindle-shaped pleomorphic cells. There were red blood cells within slit-like spaces not lined by endothelial cells, and haemosiderin-laden macrophages. Lymphnodes showed similar features, with partial to complete effacement of normal nodal architecture and invasion of the capsule. A recent study details the histopathology of this disease.[6]

Seven patients had clinically detectable generalised lymphadenopathy. Six had visceral involvement (spleen, bone, lung, pleura, liver, or gastrointestinal tract) as shown by radionuclide scans, radiographic studies, or histological examination. In case 3 the frontal lobe mass detected by computerised axial tomography (CAT) could represent brain involvement by Kaposi's. Case 8 underwent necropsy.

All the four patients in whom CMV titres were measured had detectable antibody to the virus, but none presented with a mononucleosis-like illness.

Hepatitis B surface antigen was present in one patient and antibody to hepatitis B surface antigen in four.

Four of the eight patients died. Three died from Kaposi's sarcoma despite chemotherapy; the fourth (case 8) died of overwhelming cryptococcosis unresponsive to antifungal therapy before chemotherapy for Kaposi's sarcoma could be started. The average survival of these four patients was 15 months (range 3–20 months).

Four patients are alive 2–30 months after diagnosis. Two patients (cases 1 and 7) are in clinical remission, and one (case 3) has responded partially to chemotherapy. The fourth patient has not yet been treated for his tumour.

The two case-summaries presented below are representative of the clinical spectrum of Kaposi's sarcoma among our patients.

THE LANCET, NOVEMBER 28, 1981

THE LANCET

ECT in Britain: a Shameful State of Affairs

LAST week the Royal College of Psychiatrists published what must be the most complete and thorough medical audit of a particular form of treatment that has ever been undertaken. As an account of the practice of a therapy widely used by British psychiatrists, *Electroconvulsive Treatment in Great Britain, 1980*[1] is deeply disturbing.

The study, conducted by Dr J. PIPPARD and Dr L. ELLAM in 1979 and 1980, had four parts. First, letters were sent to all 3221 members of the Royal College of Psychiatrists, inquiring about their attitudes to and practice of ECT. Second, in a three-month prospective survey, both psychiatrists and hospitals were asked to keep a record of the ECT they actually used. Third, 614 randomly selected general practitioners were questioned about the effect of ECT on recently treated patients. Fourth—and the most revealing part of the study—the investigators visited one hundred ECT clinics and observed the circumstances and manner in which the treatment was given. PIPPARD and ELLAM estimate that in 1979 some 200 000 individual applications of ECT were given in 390 centres, all but 6000 in National Health Service hospitals. Across the country there was a 17-fold difference between the rates of the highest and lowest users of ECT as measured by the number of treatments per annum per 1000 of the population at risk. The Oxfordshire region was consistently the lowest user and North Yorkshire the highest. Nearly all general psychiatrists prescribe ECT and 90–98% expressed generally favourable attitudes to the treatment.

Despite the fact that over twenty studies indicate that unilateral ECT causes less confusion and memory disturbance than bilateral ECT and is no less effective, 80% of ECT clinics rarely or never use it, preferring bilateral electrode placement as a routine. The most disturbing findings come from the series of inspection visits to ECT clinics. 28% of these clinics have an obsolete treatment machine and in 48% the reserve machine is obsolete. (The term obsolete was used of a machine which, though not necessarily unsafe, was no longer manufactured and did not conform to the 1976 safety code for electro-medical apparatus.[2]) 80% of these obsolete machines delivered an untimed stimulus allowing electricity to pass across a patient's head for as long as the operator's finger pressed the treatment button. PIPPARD and ELLAM conclude that many patients were being treated with excessive amounts of electrical energy likely to produce an increase in side-effects such as memory disturbance without increasing therapeutic efficacy. 40% of clinics did not maintain their ECT machine regularly. It was rare to find a consultant psychiatrist involved in the work of an ECT clinic and most treatment was given by untrained or minimally trained junior doctors. 50% of junior staff had no or minimal training and 26% received some tuition but usually not until they had already given ECT several times. Even where a consultant was involved there was little evidence that he was more competent than his juniors.

The report describes clinics of various types and quality and some of the accounts make chilling reading. ECT is given in large open dormitory wards with rows of patients lying on unscreened beds and with the treatment and anaesthetic machines being trundled from bed to bed. Patients waiting before and after treatment can see and hear treatment being given to others. Even in some purpose-built clinics which were fully equipped with modern apparatus, standards were appallingly low. The investigators saw treatment sessions where few patients had a convulsion and where this was not recognised by the medical staff involved—or, if it was, they presumably thought it unimportant. Nursing staff were noted to be bored, apathetic, and hostile to ECT and rarely talked to patients. In an attempt to summarise their findings the investigators made personal ratings on a scale of 0 to 5 on six features of each clinic—premises, equipment, anaesthetist, psychiatrist, nurses, and overall patient care. Only 16% of clinics rated 4 or 5 on all aspects of care, indicating that the investigator was happy, or reasonably so, about the standard of care and safety in the clinic. A further 27% were thought to be generally satisfactory. Less than half the clinics met the minimum criteria specified by the Royal College of Psychiatrists.[3] In 30% standards were unsatisfactory and in 27% there were serious deficiencies such as low standards of nursing care, obsolete apparatus, and unsuitable premises. Of the categories of personnel rated, the psychiatrist came lowest. Only one-third of psychiatrists were thought to be doing their job in a satisfactory way, compared with 64% of nurses and 70% of anaesthetists. The picture painted is one of ECT been given in many clinics in a degrading and frightening way with little consideration for patients' feelings, by bored and uninterested staff, with obsolete machines operated by ignorant or uncaring psychia-

1 Pippard J, Ellam L. Electroconvulsion treatment in Great Britain, 1980. Gaskell (Royal College of Psychiatrists): London, 1981.

2. Hospital technical memorandum no. 8. Safety code for electro-medical apparatus. London: Department of Health and Social Security, 1976.
3. Royal College of Psychiatrists. Memorandum on the use of electroconvulsive therapy. *Br J Psychiatry* 1977; **131**: 261–72

trists. The fact that two recent studies[4,5] have shown that most patients feel they benefit from ECT, do not find it unduly frightening or upsetting, and would be prepared to have the treatment again, should not cause us to doubt the findings of this report. Both were conducted in teaching centres (not in itself a guarantee of good standards of care) with a special interest in ECT research. The views of patients elsewhere may be quite different. As yet they have not been systematically asked for.

The findings of the report were presented to the membership as a special one day meeting of the Royal College on the day of publication. Whether the packed audience was representative of British psychiatry as a whole is doubtful, but there did seem to be genuine concern and a desire to take urgent corrective action. The evidence that ECT works is overwhelming.[6] How it works is less certain. ECT is a complex package consisting of the administration of three drugs, brief unconsciousness, passage of electricity across the brain, and induction of a grand mal seizure, all surrounded by feelings of drama, expectation, and anxiety. The weight of evidence points towards the epileptic seizure being the essential therapeutic ingredient and memory impairment being mainly related to the amount of electrical energy passed through the brain. If this is so, then the aim should be to induce a bilateral epileptic fit lasting for 30–40 s by stimulation of the non-dominant hemisphere with as little electrical energy as possible. (Two other theories were proposed, neither of them new. The first, that therapeutic change is related not to the seizure but to the amount of electrical energy or a combination of the two, has little evidence to support it. The second, that therapeutic change is due to the memory impairment produced, has no evidence to support it.) Despite the evidence, opinion at last week's meeting seemed to be that bilateral ECT with large electrical stimuli is more effective than unilateral ECT with much less electrical energy. If that "clinical opinion" had been based on scrupulous practice in well-run ECT clinics with doctors adequately trained to administer the treatment and observe when a fit had been induced, then it would carry considerable weight. The report makes clear that this is not so. The opinion is based on poor clinical practice and ignorance. There is no doubt that unilateral ECT requires slightly more care and skill to administer and to ensure that a seizure occurs, but it is still a simple, straightforward technique. Scandinavian psychiatrists, many of whom were present at the meeting because of a joint meeting with the Danish Psychiatric Society, use unilateral ECT almost exclusively, and American practice has also slowly shifted to the use of unilateral electrode placement.

Does anyone emerge from this study with credit? Firstly, there are a few clinics where ECT is given with care and consideration by well trained staff. Secondly, the Royal College of Psychiatrists is to be commended for undertaking the study, which was supervised by its research committee, and for making the results freely available. Thirdly, the two investigators must be congratulated. Theirs must have been a difficult task and the fact that such appalling practice was allowed to continue under their eyes says a lot for their investigative skills; nevertheless we must gloomily assume that, since the visits were announced in advance, the true picture is worse than that reported.

What are the implications of this report? The fact that the situation has not been uncovered before must raise doubts about the thoroughness and usefulness of the Health Advisory Service. Why has this body with its regular and expensive visits, not detected such deficiencies; and, if it has and no changes have resulted, what use is it anyway? Clearly, a whole generation of psychiatrists has urgently to be trained in the theory and practice of ECT, but whether their consultants know enough to teach them is doubtful. ECT clinics must be upgraded. The minimum requirements are a safe, regularly serviced up-to-date machine and separate waiting, treatment, and recovery rooms. There can be no excuse for giving ECT in the corner of open wards and behind flimsy screens. If extra money cannot be found then funds should be taken from other treatment facilities which are of less proven value. The report must cast a shadow over many other psychiatric practices. ECT has been the Achilles' heel of psychiatry for many years. One might think that, in view of the publicity and debate that have surrounded its use, psychiatrists would have taken special care to see that their practice of such a controversial treatment was exemplary. Clearly they have not. If this is the casual and offhand way that some British psychiatrists practise a controversial therapy, what must we surmise about their use of treatments which are less in the public eye? Finally, information was gathered for this study on the basis of confidentiality and anonymity, and despite the seriousness of the findings that undertaking must be respected. Dr PIPPARD and Dr ELLAM and the research committee of the College must think very seriously what they are going to do about the malpractice they have uncovered and what action they should take to correct it. Both the Government and the Royal College have set up committees to study the findings but neither of these bodies will have access to details of the clinics themselves where presumably bad practice continues.

Every British psychiatrist should read this report and feel ashamed and worried about the state of British psychiatry. If ECT is ever legislated against or falls into disuse it will not be because it is an ineffective or dangerous treatment; it will be because psychiatrists have failed to supervise and monitor its use adequately. It is not ECT which has brought psychiatry into disrepute. Psychiatry has done just that for ECT.

4. Freeman CPL, Kendell RE. ECT 1. Patients experience and attitudes Br J Psychiatry 1980; 137: 8–16.
5. Hughes J, Barraclough BM, Reeve W. Are patients shocked by ECT? J Roy Soc Med 1981; 74: 283–85.
6. Kendell RE. The present status of electroconvulsive therapy. Br J Psychiatry 1981; 189: 265–83.

THE LANCET, JUNE 4, 1983

UNIDENTIFIED CURVED BACILLI ON GASTRIC EPITHELIUM IN ACTIVE CHRONIC GASTRITIS

SIR,—Gastric microbiology has been sadly neglected. Half the patients coming to gastroscopy and biopsy show bacterial colonisation of their stomachs, a colonisation remarkable for the constancy of both the bacteria involved and the associated histological changes. During the past three years I have observed small curved and S-shaped bacilli in 135 gastric biopsy specimens. The bacteria were closely associated with the surface epithelium, both within and between the gastric pits. Distribution was continuous, patchy, or focal. They were difficult to see with haematoxylin and eosin stain, but stained well by the Warthin-Starry silver method (figure).

I have classified gastric biopsy findings according to the type of inflammation, regardless of other features, as "no inflammation", "chronic gastritis" (CG), or "active chronic gastritis" (ACG). CG shows more small round cells than normal while ACG is characterised by an increase in polymorphonuclear neutrophil leucocytes, besides the features of CG. It was unusual to find no inflammation. CG usually showed superficial oedema of the mucosa. The leucocytes in ACG were usually focal and superficial, in and near the surface epithelium. In many cases they only infiltrated the necks of occasional gastric glands. The superficial epithelium was often irregular, with reduced mucinogenesis and a cobblestone surface.

When there was no inflammation bacteria were rare. Bacteria were often found in CG, but were rarely numerous. The curved bacilli were almost always present in ACG, often in large numbers and often growing between the cells of the surface epithelium (figure). The constant morphology of these bacteria and their intimate relationship with the mucosal architecture contrasted with the heterogeneous bacteria often seen in the surface debris. There was normally a layer of mucous secretion on the surface of the mucosa. When this layer was intact, the debris was spread over it, while the curved bacilli were on the epithelium beneath, closely spread over the surface (figure).

The curved bacilli and the associated histological changes may be present in any part of the stomach, but they were seen most consistently in the gastric antrum. Inflammation, with no bacteria, occurred in mucosa near focal lesions such as carcinoma or peptic ulcer. In such cases, the leucocytes were spread through the full thickness of the nearby mucosa, in contrast to the superficial infiltration associated with the bacteria. Both the bacteria and the typical histological changes were commonly found in mucosa unaffected by the focal lesion.

The extraordinary features of these bacteria are that they are almost unknown to clinicians and pathologists alike, that they are closely associated with granulocyte infiltration, and that they are present in about half of our routine gastric biopsy specimens in numbers large enough to see on routine histology. The only other organism I have found actively growing in the stomach is *Candida*, sometimes seen in the floor of peptic ulcers. These bacteria were not mentioned in two major studies of gastrointestinal microbiology[1,2] possibly because of their unusual atmospheric requirements and slow growth in culture (described by Dr B. Marshall in the accompanying letter). They were mentioned in passing by Fung et al.[3]

How the bacteria survive is uncertain. There is a pH gradient from acid in the gastric lumen to near neutral in the mucosal vessels. The bacteria grow in close contact with the epithelium, presumably near the neutral end of this gradient, and are protected by the overlying mucus.

The identification and clinical significance of this bacterium remain uncertain. By light microscopy it resembles *Campylobacter jejuni* but cannot be classified by reference to *Bergey's Manual of*

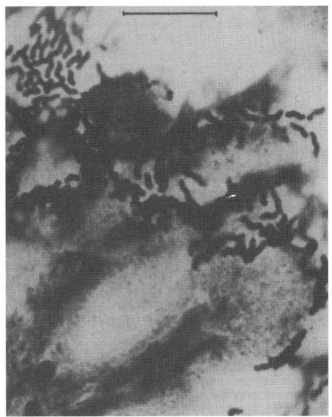

Curved bacilli on gastric epithelium.

Section is cut at acute angle to show bacteria on surface, forming network between epithelial cells. (Warthin-Starry silver stain; bar = 10 μm.)

Determinative Bacteriology. The stomach must not be viewed as a sterile organ with no permanent flora. Bacteria in numbers sufficient to see by light microscopy are closely associated with an active form of gastritis, a cause of considerable morbidity (dyspeptic disease). These organisms should be recognised and their significance investigated.

Department of Pathology,
Royal Perth Hospital,
Perth, Western Australia 6001   J. ROBIN WARREN

SIR,—The above description of S-shaped spiral bacteria in the gastric antrum, by my colleague Dr J. R. Warren, raises the following questions: why have they not been seen before; are they pathogens or merely commensals in a damaged mucosa; and are they campylobacters?

In 1938 Doenges[1] found "spirochaetes" in 43% of 242 stomachs at necropsy but drew no conclusions because autolysis had rendered most of the specimens unsuitable for pathological diagnosis. Freedburg and Barron[2] studied 35 partial gastrectomy specimens and found "spirochaetes" in 37%, after a long search. They concluded that the bacteria colonised the tissue near benign or malignant ulcers as non-pathogenic opportunists. When Palmer[3] examined 1140 gastric suction biopsy specimens he did not use silver stains so, not surprisingly, he found "no structure which could reasonably be considered to be of a spirochaetal nature". He concluded that the gastric "spirochaetes" were oral contaminants which multiplied only in post mortem specimens or close to ulcers. Since that time, the spiral bacteria have rarely been mentioned, except as curiosities,[4] and the subject was not reopened with the

1. Gray JDA, Shiner M Influence of gastric pH on gastric and jejunal flora. *Gut* 1967, **8**: 574–81.

2 Drasar BS, Shiner M, McLeod GM. Studies on the intestinal flora I: The bacterial flora of the gastrointestinal tract in healthy and achlorhydric persons. *Gastroenterology* 1969, **56**: 71–79.

3. Fung WP, Papadimitriou JM, Matz LR. Endoscopic, histological and ultrastructural correlations in chronic gastritis *Am J Gastroenterol* 1979; **71**: 269–79

1. Doenges JL. Spirochaetes in the gastric glands of *Macacus rhesus* and humans without definite history of related disease. *Proc Soc Exp Med Biol* 1938; **38**: 536–38.

2. Freedburg AS, Barron LE. The presence of spirochaetes in human gastric mucosa. *Am J Dig Dis* 1940; **7**: 443–45.

3 Palmer ED. Investigation of the gastric spirochaetes of the human? *Gastroenterology* 1954, **27**: 218–20.

4 Ito S. Anatomic structure of the gastric mucosa. In: Heidel US, Cody CF, eds. Handbook of physiology, section 6: Alimentary canal, vol II· Secretion. Washington, DC: American Physiological Society, 1967: 705–41.

THE LANCET, JUNE 4, 1983

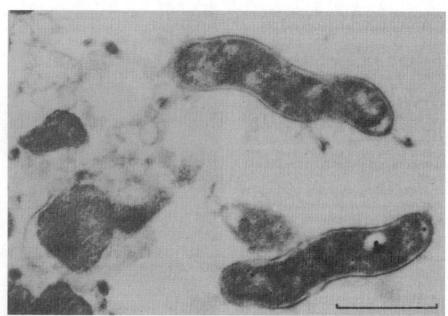

Fig 1—Thin-section micrograph showing spiral bacteria on surface of a mucous cell in gastric biopsy specimen. (Bar = 1 μm.)

advent of gastroscopic biopsy. Silver staining is not routine for mucosal biopsy specimens, and the bacteria have been overlooked.

In other mammals spiral gastric bacteria are well known and are thought to be commensals[5] (eg, Doenges[1] found them in all of forty-three monkeys). They usually have more than two spirals and inhabit the acid-secreting gastric fundus.[5] In cats they even occupy the canaliculi of the oxyntic cells, suggesting tolerance to acid.[6] The animal bacteria do not cause any inflammatory response, and no illness has ever been associated with them.

Investigation of gastric bacteria in man has been hampered by the false assumption that the bacteria were the same as those in animals and would therefore be acid-tolerant inhabitants of the fundus. Warren's bacteria are, however, shorter, with only one or two spirals and resemble campylobacters rather than spirochaetes. They live beneath the mucus of the gastric antrum well away from the

acid-secreting cells.

We have cultured the bacteria from antral biopsy specimens, using *Campylobacter* isolation techniques. They are microaerophilic and grow on moist chocolate agar at 37°C, showing up in 3–4 days as a faint transparent layer. They are about 0·5 μm in diameter and 2·5 μm in length, appearing as short spirals with one or two wavelengths (fig 1). The bacteria have smooth coats with up to five sheathed flagellae arising from one end (fig 2). In some cells, including dividing forms, flagellae may be seen at both ends and in negative stain preparations they have bulbous tips, presumably an artefact.[7]

These bacteria do not fit any known species either morphologically or biochemically. Similar sheathed flagellae have been described in vibrios[7] but micro-aerophilic vibrios have now

5 Lockard VG, Boler RK. Ultrastructure of a spiraled micro-organism in the gastric mucosa of dogs. *Am J Vet Res* 1970; **31:** 1453–62.

6 Vial JD, Orrego H. Electron microscope observations on the fine structure of parietal cells. *J Biophys Biochem Cytol* 1960; **7:** 367–72.

7. Glauert AM, Kerridge D, Horne RW. The fine structure and mode of attachment of the sheathed flagellum of *Vibrio metchnikovii. J Cell Biol* 1963; **18:** 327–36.

8. Shewan JM, Veron M. Genus I vibrio. In: Buchanan RE, Gibbons NE, eds. Bergey's manual of determinative microbiology, 8th ed. Baltimore: Williams & Wilkins, 1974· 341.

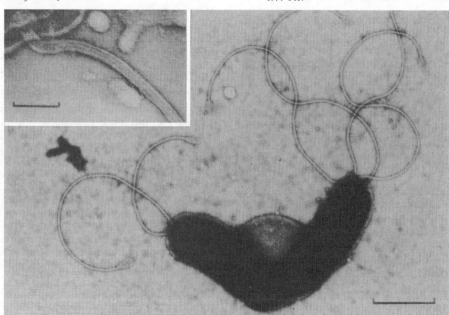

Fig 2—Negative stain micrograph of dividing bacterium from broth culture.

Multiple polar flagellae have terminal bulbs, (2% phosphotungstate, pH 6·8; bar = 1 μm.) Inset: detail showing sheathed flagellum and basal disc associated with plasma membrane. (3% ammonium molybdate, pH 6·5; bar = 100 nm.)

THE LANCET, JUNE 4, 1983   1275

been transferred to the family Spirillaceae genus *Campylobacter*.[8] Campylobacters however, have "a single polar flagellum at one or both ends of the cell" and the campylobacter flagellum is unsheathed.[9] Warren's bacteria may be of the genus *Spirillum*.

The pathogenicity of these bacteria remains unproven but their association with polymorphonuclear infiltration in the human antrum is highly suspicious. If these bacteria are truly associated with antral gastritis, as described by Warren, they may have a part to play in other poorly understood, gastritis associated diseases (ie, peptic ulcer and gastric cancer).

I thank Miss Helen Royce for microbiological assistance, Dr J. A. Armstrong for electronmicroscopy, and Dr Warren for permission to use fig 1.

Department of Gastroenterology,
Royal Perth Hospital,
Perth, Western Australia 6001   BARRY MARSHALL

VASODILATOR PROSTANOIDS AND ACTH-DEPENDENT HYPERTENSION

SIR,—Dr Axelrod (April 23, p 904) proposes that the permissive effect of glucocorticoids on vascular tone is mediated via inhibition of prostacyclin production and that this may contribute to the hypertension of Cushing's syndrome. We became interested in this possibility following the suggestion by Rascher at al[1] that glucocorticoids may produce hypertension as a result of inhibition of phospholipase A_2 and a subsequent reduction in "vasodilator" prostaglandin synthesis. The demonstration by Weeks and Sutter[2] that prostacyclin (epoprostenol) infusion attenuated the development of DOCA (desoxycortone) induced hypertension in the rat was also relevant. We have reviewed the evidence for such a hypothesis in relation to steroid and corticotropin (ACTH) dependent hypertension.[3] Our own studies have been concerned with the mechanism of ACTH induced hypertension in sheep, a form of experimental hypertension and features of glucocorticoid and mineralocorticoid excess but in which these two classes of adrenocortical steroid activity do not appear to account for more than about half of the hypertension.[3] On the basis of detailed experiments in conscious sheep we concluded that although "vasodilator" prostanoids such as prostacyclin appear to modulate the ACTH induced rises in blood pressure they did not play a primary role in the development of the hypertension.

Although in sheep,[4] as in other species, indomethacin enhances vasoconstrictor responses to angiotensin II, ACTH treatment does not alter pressor responsiveness to either angiotensin II, noradrenaline, or arginine-vasopressin.[5-7] Also, indomethacin (3 mg/kg daily for 3 days) had no effect on blood pressure in normotensive sheep.[6] Further, pretreatment of sheep for 24 h with prostacyclin at a dose which lowered total peripheral resistance but not blood pressure did not alter the blood pressure response to

ACTH.[6] This suggests to us that the proposal by Axelrod that ACTH-dependent hypertension is in any way caused by inhibition or prostaglandin synthesis is questionable.

Our evidence that prostaglandins may modulate the severity of ACTH dependent hypertension is based on three series of experiments. The first showed that although indomethacin infusion for 60 min, at a dose which blocks the vasodepressor effect of arachidonic acid, has no effect on blood pressure in normotensive sheep, it produced a further increase in mean arterial pressure of 26 mm Hg in sheep with ACTH-induced hypertension.[6] This rise in blood pressure was entirely due to a rise in total peripheral resistance. In the second series of experiments we showed that in animals pretreated with indomethacin for three days the rise in blood pressure in response to ACTH was significantly greater.[6] Finally we found that although graded doses of prostacyclin, infused for 10 min, produced similar falls in blood pressure in normotensive and ACTH hypertensive sheep, the fall in total peripheral resistance is much greater in the ACTH treated animals.[8] We speculated that plasma levels of vasodilator prostanoids such as prostacyclin may rise in response to ACTH administration. However, measurement of plasma 6-keto-$PGF_{1\alpha}$ (considered by some to reflect prostacyclin production) by Dr Murray Mitchell (Dallas, USA) showed a small but significant decrease with ACTH treatment.[3]

Our studies in sheep suggest a modulating rather than causal role for vasodilator prostanoids in ACTH-dependent hypertension.

Howard Florey Institute of Experimental   B. A. SCOGGINS
  Physiology and Medicine   J. A. WHITWORTH
  and Department of Nephrology,   J. P. COGHLAN
Royal Melbourne Hospital,   D. A. DENTON
Parkville, Victoria 3052, Australia   R. T. MASON

EPOPROSTENOL (PROSTACYCLIN) DECREASES PLATELET DEPOSITION ON VASCULAR PROSTHETIC GRAFTS

SIR,—Prostacyclin (PGI_2) is an important regulator of platelet deposition on vascular surfaces.[9] When a prosthetic vascular graft is inserted, a few weeks are required before the formation of PGI_2 by the pseudovascular wall cells reaches the same level of activity of tissue in the vicinity[10] because of the slow increase in prostacyclin synthetase[11] in the invading cells. Hence platelet deposition on the graft surface may be a significant factor in limiting graft survival[12] and causing early occlusion. PGI_2 can decrease platelet deposition on vascular surfaces,[13] so we wondered if platelet deposition on prosthetic grafts would be affected by a short term infusion of epoprostenol.

We examined nine male and two female patients aged 53–66 years between 48 and 72 h after surgery. Autologous platelet labelling was carried out with 100 µCi ^{111}In-oxine sulphate.[14] Platelet labelling efficiency amounted to 92±2%, and recovery 2 h after re-injection of autologous labelled platelets was 76±4%. 6 h after re-injection of autologous labelled platelets gamma-camera imaging studies were done. Epoprostenol (prostacyclin) 5 ng/kg/min was then infused for 24 h. Gamma-camera imaging was repeated (see figure) during and after prostacyclin infusion. Regions of interest (ROI) were

9 Pead PJ. Electron microscopy of *Campylobacter jejuni*. *J Med Microbiol* 1979; **12:** 383–85.
1 Rascher W, Dietz R, Schomig A, et al. Modulation of sympathetic vascular tone by prostaglandins in corticosterone-induced hypertension in rats. *Clin Sci* 1979; **57:** 235s–37s.
2. Weeks JR, Sutter DM. An antihypertensive effect of prostacyclin. New York: Raven Press, 1979 253–57.
3 Scoggins BA, Coghlan JP, Denton DA, Mason RT, Whitworth JA. A review of mechanisms involved in the production of steroid induced hypertension with particular reference to ACTH dependent hypertension. In: Mantero F, Biglieri EG, Edwards CRW, eds. Endocrinology of hypertension London: Academic Press, 1982: 41–67.
4. Beilby DS, Coghlan JP, Denton DA, et al. In vivo-modification of angiotensin II pressor responsiveness in sheep by indomethacin. *Clin Exp Pharmacol Physiol* 1981; **8:** 33–37
5. McDougall JG, Barnes AM, Coghlan JP, et al. The effect of corticotrophin (ACTH) administration on the pressor action of angiotensin II, noradrenaline and tyramine in sheep. *Clin Exp Pharmacol Physiol* 1978; **5:** 449–55.
6. Mason RT, Coghlan JP, Denton DA. Do prostaglandins play a role in modulating the haemodynamic effects of ACTH administration? *Proc Endocrinol Soc Aust* 1981; **24:** 7.
7. Coghlan JP, Denton DA, Graham WF, et al. Effect of ACTH administration on the haemodynamic response to arginine-vasopressin in sheep. *Clin Expt Pharmacol Physiol* 1980; **7:** 559–62.

8. Mason RT, Allen KJF, Coghlan JP, Denton, et al. ACTH hypertension modifies the haemodynamic effects of prostacyclin infusions in sheep. *Clin Exp Pharmacol Physiol* 1980; **7:** 469–72.
9. Moncada S, Vane JR. Unstable metabolites of arachidonic acid and their role in hemostasis and thrombosis. *Br Med Bull* 1978; **34:** 129–36.
10. Sinzinger H, Silberbauer K, Winter M. Implanted vascular prostheses generate prostacyclin. *Lancet* 1978; ii: 840–41.
11. Eldor A, Falcone D, Hajjar DP, Minick CR, Weksler BB. Recovery of prostacyclin production by deendothelialized rabbit aorta. *J Clin Invest* 1981; **67:** 735–41.
12. Harker LA, Slichter SJ, Sauvaage LR. Platelet consumption by arterial prostheses: The effect of endothelialization and pharmacological inhibition of platelet function *Ann Surg* 1977; **186:** 594–600.
13. Moncada S, Higgs EA, Vane JR. Human arterial and venous tissue generates prostacyclin (prostaglandin) a potent inhibitor of platelet aggregation. *Lancet* 1977; i: 18–21.
14. Sinzinger H, Schwarz M, Leithner Ch, Hofer R. Labelling of autologous human platelets with indium-111-oxine sulphate for monitoring of human kidney transplants. *Nucl Med Biol (Paris)* 1982; 2752–55.

probable intra-uterine infection; perhaps at the time of birth the duration of the HBV infection in utero had been too short and the babies had not had time to develop anti-HBc.

The active anti-HBs response to the vaccine was excellent, 96–100% of the babies having anti-HBs at the age of one year. Since the geometric mean titre of anti-HBs did not differ significantly between the three treatment groups, it seems that administration of HBIg did not affect anti-HBs response to the vaccine. None of the babies had serious side-effects and our concern about possible induction of immunological tolerance instead of protective immunity was not substantiated. Furthermore, there were no ill-effects in the babies with probable intra-uterine HB virus infections.

Although the heat-inactivated HB vaccine (CLB) may be less pure than other HB vaccines, no serious adverse effects—and notably, no formation of autoimmune antibodies associated with liver disease—have been observed in over 3000 human recipients. Heat inactivation preserves immunogenic potency well, as is indicated by results in patients on chronic haemodialysis.[22] In this trial heat-inactivated HB vaccine (CLB) protected these immunocompromised patients no less well than it did male homosexuals with normal immunoreactivity.[23] Since the processing of this heat-inactivated vaccine is simple[12] and since lower doses may well be equally effective in newborn babies—in adults the CLB vaccine could be diluted 10-fold without losing immunogenic potency[24]—protection of infants against the persistent carrier state should cost much less than it does with other HB vaccines. This is of great importance in the third world countries where hepatitis B has major impact.

We thank the medical and nursing staff of Tsan Yuk Hospital for their cooperation and Mr Kenneth Wong for his technical assistance. We also gratefully acknowledge the help of J. M. Nivard and W. Schaasberg of the Central Laboratory of the Netherlands Red Cross Blood-Transfusion Service in Amsterdam who performed the statistical analysis. This project was supported by the Medical Faculty Research Grant Fund of the University of Hong Kong.

Correspondence should be addressed to V. C. W. W., Department of Obstetrics and Gynaecology, Queen Mary Hospital, Pokfulam road, Hong Kong.

REFERENCES

1. Stevens CE. Viral hepatitis in pregnancy: the obstetrician's role *Clin Obstet Gynaecol* 1982; **25**: 577–84.
2. Wong VCW, Lee AKY, Ip HMH. Transmission of hepatitis B antigens from symptom free carrier mothers to the fetus and the infant. *Br J Obstet Gynaecol* 1980; **87**: 958–65.
3. Prince AM, White T, Pollock N, et al. Epidemiology of hepatitis B infection in Liberian infants. *Infect Immun* 1981; **32**: 675–80.
4. Whittle HC, McLauchlan K, Bradley AK, et al. Hepatitis B virus infection in two Gambian villages. *Lancet* 1983; 1: 1203–06.
5. Beasley RP, Stevens CE. Vertical transmission of HBV and interruption with globulin. In: Vyas GN, Cohen SN, Schmid R, eds. Viral hepatitis. Philadelphia: Franklin Institute Press, 1978; 333–45.
6. Reesink HW, Reerink-Brongers EE, Lafeber-Schut BJT, et al. Prevention of chronic HBsAg carrier state in infants of HBsAg-positive mothers by hepatitis B immunoglobulin. *Lancet* 1979; ii: 436–38.
7. Beasley RP, Hwang LY, Lin CC, et al. Hepatitis B immunoglobulin (HBIg) efficacy in the interruption of perinatal transmission of hepatitis B virus carrier state. *Lancet* 1981; ii: 388–93.
8. Beasley RP, Hwang LY, Stevens CE, et al. Efficacy of hepatitis B immunoglobulin for prevention of perinatal transmission of the hepatitis B virus carrier state: Final report of a randomized double-blind, placebo controlled trial. *Hepatology* 1983; **3**: 135–41.
9. Beasley RP, Hwang LY. Postnatal infectivity of hepatitis B surface antigen-carrier mothers. *J Infect Dis* 1983; **147**: 185–90.
10. Maupas P, Chiron VP, Barin F, et al. Efficacy of hepatitis B vaccine in prevention of early HBsAg carrier state in children. *Lancet* 1981; 1: 289–92.
11. Beasley RP, Hwang LY, Lee GCY, et al. Prevention of perinatally transmitted hepatitis B virus infections with hepatitis B immunoglobulin and hepatitis B vaccine. *Lancet* 1983; ii: 1099–102.
12. Brummelhuis HGJ, Wilson-de Stürler LA, Raap AK. Preparation of hepatitis B vaccine by heat-inactivation. In: Maupas P, Guesry P, eds. Hepatitis B vaccine. Amsterdam: Elsevier/North Holland, 1981: 51–56.

References continued at foot of next column

MATERNAL SERUM ALPHA-FETOPROTEIN MEASUREMENT: A SCREENING TEST FOR DOWN SYNDROME

HOWARD S. CUCKLE   NICHOLAS J. WALD

Department of Environmental and Preventive Medicine, Medical College of St Bartholomew's Hospital, Charterhouse Square, London EC1M 6BQ

RICHARD H. LINDENBAUM

Department of Medical Genetics, Churchill Hospital, Oxford OX3 7LJ

Summary   The median maternal serum alpha-fetoprotein (AFP) level at 14–20 weeks' gestation in 61 pregnancies associated with Down syndrome was 0·72 multiples of the median (MoM) value for a series of 36 652 singleton pregnancies unaffected by Down syndrome or neural-tube defect—a statistically significant reduction. The difference is great enought to form the basis of a screening test. By selecting for amniocentesis women with serum AFP levels ≤0·5 MoM at 14–20 weeks' gestation (excluding any of these that ultrasound cephalometry shows to have been due to the overestimation of gestational age) 21% of pregnancies with Down syndrome would be identified as well as 5% of unaffected pregnancies. If amniocentesis were offered to all women aged 38 years or more and, in addition, to younger women with serum AFP below specified maternal age-dependent cut-off levels (≤1·0 MoM at 37 years, ≤0·9 at 36, ≤0·8 at 35, ≤0·7 at 34, ≤0·6 at 32–33, ≤0·5 at 25–31) 40% of pregnancies with Down syndrome and 6·8% unaffected pregnancies would be selected.

Introduction

IN September, 1983, at the New York State 14th Birth Defects Symposium Merkatz showed that pregnancies with fetal chromosome abnormalities tended to have lower maternal serum alpha-fetoprotein (AFP) levels than unaffected pregnancies.[1] We investigated this further to see whether maternal serum AFP might be a useful screening test

V. C. W. WONG AND OTHERS: REFERENCES—*continued*

13. WHO. Requirements for hepatitis B vaccine. *WHO Tech Rep Ser* no. 658, 1981.
14. Reesink HW, Boer JEG de, Reerink-Brongers EE. Transformation of the Hepanosticon test for the detection of HBsAg into a micro-technique. *Biomedicine* 1976; **25**: 234–36.
15. Hollinger FB, Adam E Heiberg D, et al. Response to hepatitis B vaccine in a young adult population. In: Szmuness W, Alter HJ, Maynard JM, eds. Viral hepatitis Philadelphia: Franklin Institute Press. 1982: 451–66.
16. Mollica R, Musumeci S, Rugolo S, et al. A prospective study of 18 infants of chronic HBsAg mothers. *Arch Dis Childh* 1979; **54**: 750–54.
17. Tada H, Yanagida M, Mishina J, et al. Combined passive and active immunization for preventing perinatal transmission of hepatitis-B virus carrier state. *Pediatrics* 1982; **70**: 613–19.
18. Reesink HW, Duimel WJ, de Boer JEG de, et al. The use of hepatitis B immunoglobulin in the Netherlands. *Devel Biol Standard* 1975; **30**: 310–15.
19. Berkson J, Gage R. Calculation of survival rates for cancer. *Proc Mayo Clin* 1950; **25**: 270.
20. Lee E, Desu M. A computerprogram for comparing K samples with right-censored data. *Comput Programs Biomed* 1972; **2**: 235–321.
21. Low WD Stature and body weight of southern Chinese children. *Z Morph Anthrop* 1971; **63**: 11–45.
22. Desmyter J, Colaeart J, de Groote G, et al. Efficacy of heat-inactivated hepatitis B vaccine in haemodialysis patient and staff. *Lancet* 1983; ii: 1323–27.
23. Coutinho RA, Lelie N, Albrecht-van Lent P, et al. Efficacy of a heat-inactivated hepatitis-B vaccine in male homosexuals: Outcome of a placebo-controlled double blind trial. *Br Med J* 1983; **286**: 1305–08.
24. Lelie PN, Reesink HW, de Jong-van Manen ST, et al. Immunogenicity and safety of plasma-derived heat-inactivated hepatitis-B vaccine (CLB). Studies in volunteers a a low risk of infection with hepatitis-B virus. *Am J Epidem* (in press).

received municipal water, the risk was doubled if the family shared a toilet with at least one other family.

A mass vaccination programme with OPV was undertaken by health authorities. Initially, the programme was directed at children under 5 years of age and, subsequently, at those up to 15 years of age. Following this mass vaccination programme assessments of immunisation levels in the six areas indicated that more than 50% of 12 to 35 month old children had received at least one dose of OPV during the control programme. The mass vaccination programme resulted in an overall coverage of 91 to 99% for two or more doses of OPV. An average of 59% of the children surveyed who had not had poliovaccine previously received at least one dose during the mass campaign.

DISCUSSION

Failure to vaccinate rather than vaccine failure was the most important risk factor for paralytic poliomyelitis. Ensuring that children are vaccinated at the earliest recommended age offers the greatest chance for protection.

The efficacy of OPV has usually been assessed by determining serum antibody response to vaccination, a method that does not give a measure of intestinal immunity. Theoretically, such intestinal immunity may be present even in the absence of systemic antibody response or vice versa. In addition, immune persons may have low levels of systemic antibody that may not be detected by the laboratory method used, and delayed seroconversion may be missed if the serum was collected too early. The best measure of effectiveness of any vaccine is its ability to prevent clinical disease. The clinical efficacy of the vaccine against paralytic disease due to type 1 poliovirus during this outbreak is consistent with levels of seroconversion after vaccination in the United States (92–100 and 97–100% for 2 and 3 doses, respectively) and is considerably higher than serological estimations of efficacy in the developing world.[6] Measurement of clinical efficacy in tropical countries may be a useful adjunct to serological assessment and can be done without sophisticated laboratory support. Clinical efficacy can help in the interpretation of serological findings.

This outbreak shows that major epidemics can occur in places that have been practically free of poliomyelitis for many years and that have high overall community vaccination levels. Overall community vaccination levels can mask the fact that there may be pockets where vaccination levels are considerably lower. The cluster-sampling method may not detect groups of susceptible subjects living within the geographic area being assessed. These groups of unrecognised susceptible subjects may be sufficient to sustain transmission of wild poliovirus in a community. Such susceptible subgroups were responsible for the last two poliomyelitis outbreaks in the United States in 1972 and 1979 and in the Netherlands and Canada in 1978 among religious groups declining vaccination.[7]

The EPI vaccine coverage assessment is a valuable tool for examining immunity levels in a community. When an assessment shows that vaccination levels are low, then additional vaccination efforts are indicated. If, however, the assessment shows that levels are high, it may be appropriate to do additional investigations of subpopulations suspected to be at high risk, especially if the population is heterogeneous.

We thank the following for their help: Dr T. C. Hsu, Dr T. Y. Lee, Mr K. H. Hsu, Dr C. I. Ma, Mr Su Mei Hsu, Mr Shiu Loung Lin, and Miss Fei Fung Lin, Department of Health; Dr T. Y. Kuan, and Dr Y. C. Ko, Taiwan Province Health Department; Dr C. T. Wu, Kao-Hsiung City Health Department; Dr T. H. Wei and Dr C. H. Lee, Taipei City Health Department; Ms L. C. Hsu, National Institute of Preventive Medicine; Prof C. Y. Lee, National Taiwan University College of Medicine; Dr C. L. Chen, Taipei Municipal Women and Children Hospital; Dr H. C. Wang, Veteran General Hospital, Taipei; Dr F. Y. Huang, Mackay Hospital, Taipei; Dr S. L. Chao, Cheng Hsin Rehabilitation Center, Taipei; Rev Georges Massin, St Joseph's Hospital, Lumpei, Yun Lin County; and Dr R. P. Beasley and Dr Lu Yu Huang, University of Washington Medical Research Unit, Taipei. We also thank the many other individuals and institutions in the districts, counties and cities throughout Taiwan who contributed to the collection and analysing of data on clinical cases and vaccine coverage assessments; and Mr J. R. Lilley, Mr S. Brooks, and Ms S. M. Chalmers and their colleagues at the American Institute in Taiwan for their support during our stay in Taiwan; and Ms Connie Keith for preparing the typescript.

Correspondence should be addressed to K. J. B., Surveillance, Investigations and Research Branch, Division of Immunisation, Center for Prevention Services, Centers for Disease Control, Atlanta, Georgia 30333, USA.

REFERENCES

1. Health Statistics I. General Health Statistics 1980. National Health Administration, Taiwan Provincial Health Department, Taipei City Health Department, Kao-Hsiung City Health Department, 1981· 316
2. Chen CL, Chu W, Lee KS. Survey on the incidence of poliomyelitis in Taichung City. Maternal and Child Health in Taiwan, Taiwan Provincial Maternal and Child Health Institute, 1963: 66–73
3. Henderson RH, Sundaresan T. Cluster sampling to assess immunization coverage· a review of experience with a simplified sampling method. Bull WHO 1982, **60:** 253–60.
4. Cox DR. Analysis of binary data. London. Chapman and Hall, 1970 1–142.
5. Bishop Y, Fiemberg S, Holland T Discrete multivariate analysis Cambridge. MIT Press, 1975 401–33
6. Katona P, Jones TS. Operational aspects of the use of oral poliovirus vaccine in developing countries. In: Recent advances in immunization. Pan American Health Organisation, 1983; 18–29.
7. Centers for Disease Control. Poliomyelitis surveillance· Summary 1979 1981; 14–19

Community Health

UNEMPLOYMENT AND MORTALITY IN THE OPCS LONGITUDINAL STUDY

K. A. MOSER   A. J. FOX
D. R. JONES

Social Statistics Research Unit, City University, London EC1V 0HB

Summary   The mortality of men aged 15–64 who were seeking work in the week before the 1971 census was investigated by means of the OPCS Longitudinal Study, which follows up a 1% sample of the population of England and Wales. In contrast to the current position, only 4% of men of working age in 1971 fell into this category. The mortality of these unemployed men in the period 1971–81 was higher (standardised mortality ratio 136) than would be expected from death rates in all men in the Longitudinal Study. The socioeconomic distribution of the unemployed accounts for some of the raised mortality, but, after allowance for this, a 20–30% excess remains; this excess was apparent both in 1971–75 and in 1976–81. The data offer only limited support for the suggestion that some of this excess resulted from men becoming unemployed because of their ill-health; the trend in overall mortality over time and the pattern by cause of death were not those usually associated with ill-health selection. Previous studies have suggested that stress accompanying unemployment could be associated with raised suicide rates, as were again found here. Moreover, the mortality of women whose husbands were unemployed was higher than that of all married women (standardised mortality ratio 120), and this excess also persisted after allowance for their socioeconomic distribution. The results support findings by others that unemployment is associated with adverse effects on health.

THE LANCET, AUGUST 3, 1985

5 days of age. The deficiency may be attributable to an insufficient dietary intake of vitamin K.

Neonatal bleeding can be the result not only of reduced γ-carboxylation due to vitamin K deficiency but also of impaired production of the prothrombin precursor due to immaturity. When the latter is the cause of neonatal bleeding, vitamin K administration will have no effect. Fig 2 shows how improvement in normotest results after vitamin K administration in infants whose vitamin K dependent clotting activity was less than 30%, was significantly related to the pre-treatment level of PIVKA-II. In other words, infants with a prolonged coagulation time but without an increased PIVKA-II level did not have vitamin K deficiency; they had a low coagulation factor level because of impaired protein synthesis. Thus, in terms of assessing vitamin K deficiency, the PIVKA-II level is more useful than the vitamin K dependent coagulation time.

The differences in PIVKA-II levels obtained by various workers might be due to ethnic or socioeconomic differences in the populations studied,[22] or to the sensitivity of the assay method used. The argument against prophylactic administration of vitamin K has been based on the observation that circulating PIVKA-II was not found in the plasma of newborns tested.[8-12] Corrigan suggested that hypoprothrombinaemia in normal term infants was due not to a vitamin K deficiency but rather to immaturity of the system of production of coagulation factor protein.[15] Our sensitive and specific method of detecting vitamin K deficiency clearly shows the high incidence of this deficiency in neonates, which argues for prophylactic administration of vitamin K at birth.

This work was supported by a grant from Eisai Co., Ltd.

Correspondence should be addressed to K. M.

REFERENCES

1 Keenan WJ, Jewett T, Glueck HI. Role of feeding and vitamin K in hypoprothrombinemia of the newborn. *Am J Dis Child* 1971; **121**: 271–77.
2. Sutherland JM, Glueck HI, Gleser G Hemorrhagic disease of the newborn *Am J Dis Child* 1967; **113**: 524–33.
3 Dreyfus M, Lelong-Tissier MC, Lombard C, Tchernia G. Vitamin K deficiency in the newborn *Lancet* 1979; 1: 1351.
4 McNinch AW, Orme RL'E, Tripp JH. Haemorrhagic disease of the newborn returns *Lancet* 1983, 1 1089–90.
5 Glader BE, Buchanan GR. The bleeding neonate *Pediatrics* 1974, **58**: 548–55
6. Editorial. Vitamin K and the newborns. *Lancet* 1978; 11 755–57.
7. Committee on Nutrition of the American Academy of Pediatrics. Vitamin K compounds and the water soluble analogues use in therapy and prophylaxis in pediatrics *Pediatrics* 1961, **28**: 501–07.
8. van Doorm JM, Muller AD, Hemker HC. Heparin-like inhibitor, not vitamin-K deficiency in the newborn. *Lancet* 1977, 1 852–53
9. van Doorm JM, Hemker HC Vitamin-K deficiency in the newborn. *Lancet* 1977; 11: 708–09
10. Malia RG, Preston FE, Mitchell VE Evidence against vitamin K deficiency in normal neonates. *Thromb Haemost* 1980, **44**: 159–60
11. Göbel U, Sonnenschein-Kosenow S, Petrich C, et al Vitamin K deficiency in the newborn. *Lancet* 1977; 11. 187
12. Mori PG, Bisogni C, Odino S, et al Vitamin K deficiency in the newborn. *Lancet* 1977; 11. 188
13. Muntean W, Petek W, Rosanelli K, et al Immunologic studies of prothrombin in newborns *Pediatr Res* 1979; **13**: 1262–65.
14 Corrigan JJ, Kryc JJ Factor II (prothrombin) levels in cord blood. correlation of coagulant activity with immunoreactive protein. *J Pediatr* 1980; **97**: 979–83.
15. Corrigan JJ Vitamin K dependent proteins. *Adv Pediat* 1981, **28**: 57–70.
16. Olson RE The function and metabolism of vitamin K *Ann Rev Nutr* 1984; **4**: 281–37
17. Motohara K, Kuroki Y, Kan H, Endo F, Matsuda I Detection of vitamin K deficiency by use of an enzyme-linked immunosorbent assay for circulating abnormal prothrombin. *Pediatr Res* 1985; **19**: 354–57.
18. Yoshitake S, Imagawa M, Ishikawa E, et al Mild and efficient conjugation of rabbit Fab and horseradish peroxidase using a maleimide compound and its use for enzyme immuno assay *J Biochem* 1982; **92**: 1413–24
19 Oweron PA, Strandi OK. Normotest. *Farmakoteropi* 1969; **25**: 14–26.
20. Shearer MJ, Rahim S, Barkhan P, Stimmler L Plasma vitamin K₁ in mothers and their newborn babies. *Lancet* 1982; 11. 460–63
21. Laurell CB Quantitative estimation of proteins by electro phoresis in agarose gel containing antibodies *Analyt Biochem* 1966; **15**: 45–52
22 Bloch CA, Rothberg AD, Bradlow BA. Mother-infant prothrombin precursor status at birth. *J Pediatr Gastroenterol Nutr* 1984; **3**: 101–03
23 Atkinson PM, Bradlow BA, Moulineaux JD, Walker NP Acarboxy prothrombin in cord plasma from normal neonates *J Pediatr Gastroenterol Nutr* 1984; **3**: 450–53.

Preliminary Communication

CREUTZFELDT-JAKOB DISEASE AFTER ADMINISTRATION OF HUMAN GROWTH HORMONE

JOHN POWELL-JACKSON*   R. O. WELLER†
PHILIP KENNEDY†   M. A. PREECE‡
E. M. WHITCOMBE§   JOHN NEWSOM-DAVIS§

*Royal Hampshire County Hospital, Winchester; †Southampton General Hospital; ‡Institute of Child Health, London WC1; and §National Hospital for Nervous Diseases, London WC1

Summary   A 2-year-old girl had a craniopharyngioma removed in 1964. She received human growth hormone (HGH) twice a week from July, 1972, until July, 1976. In March, 1984, a subacute dementing illness developed with neurological signs that included pronounced cerebellar ataxia. A clinical diagnosis of Creutzfeldt-Jakob disease (CJD) was made. The patient died in February, 1985. Necropsy revealed a spongiform encephalopathy compatible with the transmissible form of CJD. HGH administration may be implicated in the transmission of the disease in this case.

INTRODUCTION

THE transmissible nature of Creutzfeldt-Jakob disease (CJD) was established by Gibbs et al in 1968,[1] placing it in the group of unconventional virus diseases that includes scrapie in sheep and kuru in man. Typical forms of CJD present as subacute dementia evolving over several weeks or months accompanied by pyramidal, extrapyramidal, and cerebellar signs. The mean age at death is 57 years,[2] although cases have been reported in the late teens[3] and early twenties.[4,5] CJD has been transmitted experimentally, not only by intracerebral injection of brain tissue, but also by peripheral routes of inoculation, although the incubation periods are then longer and more variable.[6] Several examples of means of transmission in man have been identified; they include corneal grafting[7] and neurosurgery.[8,9] The natural mode of spread of the CJD agent remains unknown.

The distribution of human growth hormone (HGH) for replacement therapy of growth-hormone-deficient children has recently been halted by the United States Food and Drug Administration and by the United Kingdom Medical Research Council/Department of Health and Social Security joint advisory committee on national pituitary collection, following reports that three patients in the USA died of an illness resembling CJD. The diagnosis was confirmed at necropsy in one case.[10] All patients had received HGH from the late 1960s or early 1970s for a minimum of 5 years.

The withdrawal of HGH has caused concern among physicians treating patients with multiple pituitary hormone deficiencies. Laron and Josefsberg[11] have emphasised the low incidence of complications associated with HGH administration and have called for reports of neurological disease and deaths encountered in subjects so treated. Such a patient is described here; a more detailed account of the pathology will be published elsewhere.

CASE-REPORT

The patient was born in February, 1962. At the age of 2 years she presented with increasing somnolence and was admitted to the Hospital for Sick Children, Great Ormond Street. A craniopharyngioma was removed in September,

The Lancet · Saturday 22 February 1986

EFFECTIVENESS OF INTRAVENOUS THROMBOLYTIC TREATMENT IN ACUTE MYOCARDIAL INFARCTION

GRUPPO ITALIANO PER LO STUDIO DELLA STREPTOCHINASI NELL'INFARTO MIOCARDICO (GISSI)*

Summary   In an unblinded trial of intravenous streptokinase (SK) in early acute myocardial infarction, 11 806 patients in one hundred and seventy-six coronary care units were enrolled over 17 months. Patients admitted within 12 h after the onset of symptoms and with no contraindications to SK were randomised to receive SK in addition to usual treatment and complete data were obtained in 11 712. At 21 days overall hospital mortality was 10·7% in SK recipients versus 13% in controls, an 18% reduction (p=0·0002, relative risk 0·81). The extent of the beneficial effect appears to be a function of time from onset of pain to SK infusion (relative risks 0·74, 0·80, 0·87, and 1·19 for the 0–3, 3–6, 6–9, and 9–12 h subgroups). SK seems to be a safe drug for routine administration in acute myocardial infarction.

Introduction

THE trial of the Italian Group for the Study of Streptokinase in Myocardial Infarction (Gruppo Italiano per lo Studio della Streptochinasi nell'Infarto Miocardico, GISSI) was planned in autumn, 1983. At that time there was a growing consensus on the effectiveness of intracoronary streptokinase (SK) in reopening occluded coronary vessels in around 50–60% of treated patients;[1] and analysis of pooled data suggested that intravenous SK, given in various schedules, could reduce overall mortality in patients treated within 24 h from onset of pain.[2] The clinically relevant challenge was therefore to test in a formal prospective trial whether effective and safe thrombolysis could be achieved with intravenous SK under routine conditions in the majority of patients—in contrast to intracoronary thrombolysis which is practicable only in small numbers of cases.[3]

The participation of the majority of the coronary care units (CCUs) grouped in the National Society of Hospital Cardiologists (Associazione Nazionale Medici Cardiologi Ospedalieri, ANMCO) was sought, to ensure recruitment over an acceptable length of time of the large sample needed to test reliably three key issues: Does intravenous SK infusion produce a clinically relevant benefit in terms of reduction of in-hospital and one-year mortality? Is the effect, if any, dependent on the interval from onset of pain to SK treatment? Are the risks associated with the treatment acceptable?

Steering committee.—F. ROVELLI (chairman), C. DE VITA, G. A. FERUGLIO, A. LOTTO, A. SELVINI, G. TOGNONI.

Coordination and data monitoring.—M. L. FARINA, A. FORESTI, M. G. FRANZOSI, F. MAURI (investigators); S. PAMPALLONA (biostatistician).

Ethics committee.—P. ARMITAGE, A. BERIA DI ARGENTINE, R. BOERI, S. GARATTINI, P. MANTEGAZZA, A. MENOTTI, R. PETO, E. POLLI, M. VERSTRAETE, A. ZANCHETTI.

Scientific advisory board.—Cardiology: C. BELLI, G. BINAGHI, M. BOSSI, F. CAMERINI, E. CRISTALLO, L. DE AMBROGGI, P. F. FAZZINI, F. FURLANELLO, A. L'ABBATE, F. MILAZZOTTO, E. PICCOLO, A. RAVIELE, G. RIGGIO, P. ROSSI, J. A. SALERNO, A. SANTOBONI, P. SOLINAS, C. VECCHIO, P. ZARDINI Haemostasis: M. B. DONATI, P. M. MANNUCCI, G. G. NERI SERNERI.

ECG coding and clinical data reviewing committees.—M. BIRAGHI, E. CHIUINI, M. GASPARINI, A. P. MAGGIONI, M. POGNA. A. VOLPI.

Secretariat.—G. DI BITETTO (secretary); A. COLOMBO, C. MASINI (data input and management).

Regional coordinators.—Piemonte, A. BRUSCA; Lombardia, C. DE VITA; Veneto, E. PICCOLO; Trentino, F. FURLANELLO; Friuli Venezia Giulia, G. A. FERUGLIO; Liguria, E. GATTO; Emilia Romagna, D. BRACCHETTI; Toscana, P. F. FAZZINI; Marche, R. RICCIOTTI; Lazio, F. MILAZZOTTO; Umbria, P. SOLINAS; Abruzzo-Molise, D. DI GREGORIO; Campania, E. CORREALE; Puglia-Basilicata, L. COLONNA; Calabria, F. PLASTINA; Sicilia, A. GALASSI; Sardegna, D. MEREU.

Patients and Methods

The study was planned as a controlled multicentre unblinded trial with central randomisation. Fig 1 summarises the major steps. The only variable distinguishing the treatment group (SK) from the

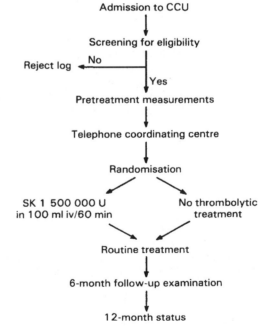

Fig 1—GISSI protocol.

The Lancet · Saturday 24 May 1986

IMPACT OF VITAMIN A SUPPLEMENTATION ON CHILDHOOD MORTALITY
A Randomised Controlled Community Trial

Alfred Sommer   Ignatius Tarwotjo
Edi Djunaedi   Keith P. West, Jr
A. A. Loeden   Robert Tilden
Lisa Mele
AND THE ACEH STUDY GROUP

International Center for Epidemiologic and Preventive Ophthalmology, Dana Center of the Wilmer Institute and School of Public Health, Johns Hopkins University, Baltimore, Maryland; Directorate of Nutrition and National Center for Health Research and Development, Ministry of Health, Government of Indonesia; and Helen Keller International, New York, USA

Summary   450 villages in northern Sumatra were randomly assigned to either participate in a vitamin A supplementation scheme (n=229) or serve for 1 year as a control (n=221). 25 939 preschool children were examined at baseline and again 11 to 13 months later. Capsules containing 200 000 IU vitamin A were distributed to preschool children aged over 1 year by local volunteers 1 to 3 months after baseline enumeration and again 6 months later. Among children aged 12–71 months at baseline, mortality in control villages (75/10 231, 7·3 per 1000) was 49% greater than in those where supplements were given (53/10 919, 4·9 per 1000) (p<0·05). The impact of vitamin A supplementation seemed to be greater in boys than in girls. These results support earlier observations linking mild vitamin A deficiency to increased mortality and suggest that supplements given to vitamin A deficient populations may decrease mortality by as much as 34%.

Introduction

A LONGITUDINAL observational study in rural central Java indicated that children with ocular signs of mild vitamin A deficiency were more likely than neighbourhood controls to die, that mortality was directly related to severity of vitamin A deficiency, and that poor survival was probably attributable, at least partly, to high rates of respiratory disease and diarrhoea.[1-3] We report here the results of a randomised, controlled, community trial of vitamin A prophylaxis in northern Sumatra.

Subjects and Methods

The study was carried out in Aceh Province, which is at the northern tip of Sumatra and where xerophthalmia is prevalent.[4,5] The population is ethnically distinct from that of Java, where the earlier observational study had been conducted.[1-3]

For political and administrative reasons a cluster sampling scheme was employed. The sampling frame consisted of 2048 villages in Aceh Utara and Pidie, two contiguous rural kabupatens (districts) chosen because they had no current or planned development projects or vitamin A supplementation schemes. From a random start, 450 villages were systematically selected for the study; these were then randomised for capsule distribution after the baseline examination (programme villages, n=229) or after the follow-up examination (control villages, n=221). 18 villages from among those still in the sampling frame were substituted for adjacent villages found to have started vitamin A supplementation before the baseline survey.

All members of the two study teams, each consisting of an ophthalmologist (team leader), a nurse, an anthropometrist, a dietary interviewer, five enumerators, and a driver, all fluent in the local dialect received a month's classroom, hospital, and field training. The enumerators, responsible for collecting demographic data, were unaware that mortality was a research question. Standardisation exercises were done before and regularly throughout the study. First, each village was visited to identify households containing children aged 0–5 years and to mark their dwellings. Within 2 days the village was visited by the full team. Enumerators visited every house containing preschool children, collected socioeconomic, demographic, and medical data, and rounded up children at a central point for their clinical examination. Dates of birth were ascertained by reference to local events charted on the Muslim calendar and then translated to their roman equivalent by the use of a specially prepared conversion table. Eyes were examined with a focused light and 2X loupes and diagnoses were made according to standard diagnostic criteria.[5,6] Parents were carefully questioned about the presence of nightblindness.[5,7] They were also asked about a history of diarrhoea (4 or more loose, watery stools per day), of fever or cough lasting at least 24 h in the previous 7 days, and of "ever having" measles.

Recumbent length (if less than 24 months old) or standing height (if 24 months or older) to the nearest 0·1 cm, and weight (using a calibrated Salter scale) to the nearest 0·1 kg, were measured on a 10% subsample of all study children.

All children with active xerophthalmia at baseline examination received at least one large dose of vitamin A and were referred to the local health unit. They were excluded from the analyses of subsequent morbidity and mortality. All children received vitamin A at the follow-up examination 9–13 months later.

Teams first visited villages between September, 1982, and August, 1983, and follow-up visits were made by the same team in the same sequence 9–13 months later. The variation in follow-up time resulted from attempts to minimise the potential confounding influence of the Muslim fasting month and post-fasting holidays.

Standard capsules (supplied by UNICEF) were given to every child aged 1–5 years in programme villages, by a local volunteer trained to do so. The capsule nipple was snipped off and the contents (200 000 IU vitamin A and 40 IU vitamin E) were expressed into the child's mouth. This volunteer kept a list of children treated and issued the household with a distribution card. The first dose was given 1–3 months after the baseline examination and the second 6–8 months later. A distribution monitor visited each village 2–4 weeks after the scheduled distribution and interviewed 10% of eligible households. If coverage was less than 80% the local distributor was encouraged to reach children previously missed.

All data were collected on precoded forms, entered onto diskettes, and shipped to the data management facility at the International Center for Epidemiologic and Preventive Ophthalmology, Johns Hopkins University, where the information was processed with the SIR data management package run on an IBM 4341 computer. Statistical analyses were made with SIR, SAS, and GLIM software. Statistical tests for significance and development of confidence intervals were adjusted for clustering associated with randomisation by village rather than by individual, and for the small number of events expected and observed in any one village by applying poisson regression with extra-poisson variation to account for natural variability in mortality among villages.[8,9] Two-tailed tests were used.

The study was designed to examine overall differences between non-infant preschool-age children in programme versus control villages, on the assumption that mortality would be reduced by at least 20% and allowing for an alpha error of 0·05 and a beta error of

THE LANCET, JANUARY 28, 1989

Occasional Survey

SLEEPING POSITION AND INFANT BEDDING MAY PREDISPOSE TO HYPERTHERMIA AND THE SUDDEN INFANT DEATH SYNDROME

E. A. S. NELSON[1]   B. J. TAYLOR[1]
I. L. WEATHERALL[2]

Department of Paediatrics and Child Health, University of Otago Medical School[1] and Department of Textile Science, University of Otago,[2] Dunedin, New Zealand

Summary   Southern New Zealand has one of the highest postneonatal mortality rates in the developed world (8·1/1000 livebirths) and 77% of these deaths are attributed to the sudden infant death syndrome (SIDS). Both hyperthermia and sleeping position have previously been implicated in SIDS. A theoretical model to estimate the thermal balance of infants used here shows that the head, and particularly the face, becomes the main route for heat loss when thick clothing and bedding are used. This thermoregulatory role could be compromised by the prone sleeping position. It is postulated that particular cultural combinations of infant care practices (sleeping position, clothing, bedding, and room heating) may facilitate hyperthermia and explain widely disparate rates of SIDS in different countries and ethnic groups.

INTRODUCTION

DEATH-SCENE investigations of 26 consecutive sudden infant deaths in New York (1983–85) suggested that in 22, overlying, asphyxia, or hyperthermia was the likely cause of death.[1] It was suggested that old causes of unexpected infant death[2] may have been rediscovered.[3] The widely held belief that a child cannot be suffocated by "ordinary" bedclothes is based on two studies[4,5] that would be considered anecdotal by modern standards.[3,6] The demonstration of microscopic "evidence" of fulminating respiratory infection,[7] combined with these early studies, led to the belief that asphyxia was an unlikely cause of unexpected infant death. This opinion was accepted rapidly and uncritically, perhaps because it had no implications of parental negligence.

INCIDENCE OF SIDS

In New Zealand 67% of postneonatal mortality is attributed to sudden infant death syndrome (SIDS)[8] and the incidence in the south is twice that in the north.[9,10] A detailed review (unpublished) of postmortem data for 1979–84 in southern New Zealand showed that the postneonatal SIDS rate was 6·3/1000 livebirths (77% of all postneonatal deaths—8·1/1000), one of the highest recorded rates in the developed world.[11] Ethnic origin has a strong effect on SIDS incidence in New Zealand (6·5/1000 in Maoris, 3·9/1000 in caucasians, 1·9/1000 in Pacific islanders).[8] However, the percentage Maori population is lower in the south of New Zealand than in the north.[10] In the USA (overall SIDS incidence around 2·0/1000) SIDS incidence is low in Asians (0·5/1000) and high in American Indians (5·9/1000), Alaskan natives (4·5/1000), and poor blacks (5·0/1000).[12] The SIDS incidence in Hong Kong is only 0·3/1000.[13,14]

SLEEPING POSITION AND SIDS

The normal sleeping position for infants in Hong Kong is supine, since the prone position is thought to predispose to suffocation,[13] whereas western mothers do not use the supine position in case their infants vomit and aspirate.[15]

Studies assessing sleeping position in SIDS have shown that the prone position is a risk factor,[16] and adoption of the prone position has coincided with a rise in SIDS rate.[15] Of 42 cases of SIDS in southern New Zealand in 1986–87, 34 (81%) were found prone and 30 (71%) were face-down or with heads covered by bedding (unpublished). In 1983, 46% of New Zealand infants slept prone,[17] and the proportion in southern New Zealand was similar in 1986.[18] However, in other countries where the prone position is advised the SIDS incidence is low (eg, Sweden 0·9/1000[19]), so use of the prone position cannot completely explain New Zealand's high SIDS rate.

HYPERTHERMIA AND SIDS

The infant's thermal environment during health and illness is affected by clothing, bedding, and room heating, which in turn are influenced by weather,[20] socioeconomic status, maternal education,[21] and cultural preferences. Bacon and colleagues[22] suggested that excessive wrapping combined with mild infection could produce heatstroke and sudden unexpected death. Stanton[23] found that 94% of 34 SIDS victims were excessively clothed, in an unusually warm environment, hot and sweaty when found dead, or had an infective illness which would not be expected to cause death. Pre-refrigeration rectal temperatures of over 38°C were noted in 10 of 24 SIDS cases in Sheffield.[24] However, in Hong Kong it is hot and humid in summer, and in the cooler months infants are wrapped warmly if unwell,[14] so hyperthermia cannot be the only factor.

A MODEL OF THERMAL BALANCE

Indoors and under still air conditions, heat loss from the body depends on several interacting variables: body surface area, insulating coverings (including hair), and skin and environmental temperature and vapour pressure. If these variables are known, dry and evaporative heat losses can be estimated[25,26] and calculated separately for each of eleven anterior and eleven posterior body parts.[27] To maintain thermal balance over time, heat loss must match metabolic heat produced.[26] Using this principle, we have developed a theoretical model of thermal balance applicable to infants, dressed and wrapped in blankets, and validated it against published data[28] (see figure). (An appendix detailing the theoretical model is available from the authors.)

Measured and theoretical values for the thermoneutral point (TNP) correlate well (figure). At ambient temperatures below the TNP the measured and theoretical heat loss lines diverge, probably because effects of body posture, vasoconstriction, and falling skin temperature are not considered in the theoretical model. At ambient temperatures above the TNP obligatory heat losses are maintained by raising mean skin temperature above 33°C and by increasing evaporative heat loss with sweating. The model overestimates maximum evaporative losses, which are limited by the infant's ability to sweat.[29] This factor has been allowed for in the figure, in which theoretical evaporative losses are limited to maximum measured values for the first 10 days of life.[29] Respiratory heat loss, which accounts for around 7% of total loss, is not considered in the model.[30]

VOL 335   THE LANCET   241
1989.

MEDICAL SCIENCE

Edinburgh trial of screening for breast cancer: mortality at seven years

M. M. ROBERTS*   F. E. ALEXANDER   T. J. ANDERSON   U. CHETTY
P. T. DONNAN   PATRICK FORREST   W. HEPBURN   A. HUGGINS
A. E. KIRKPATRICK   J. LAMB   B. B. MUIR   R. J. PRESCOTT

Between 1979 and 1981, 45 130 women in Edinburgh aged 45–64 were entered into a randomised trial of breast cancer screening by mammography and clinical examination. The initial attendance rate was 61% but this varied according to age and socioeconomic status and decreased over succeeding years. The cancer detection rate was 6·2 per 1000 women attending at the first visit; the rate fell to around 3 per 1000 in the years when mammography was routinely repeated and to around 1 per 1000 at the intervening visits with clinical examination alone as the screening method. After 7 years of follow-up the mortality reduction achieved was 17% (relative risk = 0·83, 95% CI 0·58–1·18), which was not statistically significant, even when corrected for socioeconomic status. In women aged 50 years and over a mortality reduction of 20% was achieved.

Lancet 1990; **335**: 241–46.

Introduction

Edinburgh was one of the centres in which screening was offered in the UK Trial of the Early Detection of Breast Cancer (TEDBC).[1] In the TEDBC, which was non-randomised, breast cancer mortality in areas in which screening was offered was compared with that in other areas. At the design stage we added a randomised component so that women in Edinburgh aged 45–64 could be allocated to be offered screening or to be controls.[2] Our main objective was to assess the value of screening for breast cancer by mammography and clinical examination in reducing mortality from the disease. We report the 7 year results.

Patients and methods

Recruitment

Detailed methods have been described.[2] The names of all women aged 45–64 in eighty-four general practices in the city were registered. The practices were stratified by number of partners and then randomised, leading to cluster sampling of women in the population. Half the women were invited for screening (study population). The other half formed the control population. Women were entered into the trial between June, 1979, and December, 1981 (survey entry date). All registered women were eligible for study unless they had previously been diagnosed with breast cancer.

Follow-up

For administrative reasons general practices were enrolled in turn. If a practice had control status then the women on its list were allocated survey entry dates. For practices with screening status, however, the date of invitation became the survey entry date. The women who attended underwent mammography (oblique and craniocaudal views) and clinical examination at their initial visit (prevalence screen). Subsequent visits (incidence screens) involved clinical examination alone in years 2, 4, and 6, and clinical examination with mammography (oblique view only) in years 3, 5, and 7. A few women had irregular screening that did not conform to this pattern. The first screen, for instance, therefore occasionally (eg, table IV) refers to a visit several years after the survey entry date.

ADDRESSES: **Edinburgh Breast Screening Centre** (A. Huggins, MB, B B Muir, FRCR), **Medical Statistics Unit** (P T Donnan, MSc, W Hepburn, R. J. Prescott, PhD), **and Pathology Department** (T A Anderson, FRCPath, J Lamb, FRCPath), **University of Edinburgh;** **Leukaemia Research Fund Centre, Pathology Department, University of Leeds** (F E Alexander, PhD); **and University Department of Clinical Surgery** (U Chetty, FRCS, Sir Patrick Forrest, FRCS) **and Department of Radiology** (A. E. Kirkpatrick, FRCPath), **Royal Infirmary of Edinburgh, Edinburgh, UK.** Correspondence to Dr F E Alexander, Leukaemia Research Fund Centre, Department of Pathology, University of Leeds, 17 Springfield Mount, Leeds LS2 9NG, UK

*Dr Roberts, of the Edinburgh Breast Screening Centre, died on June 9, 1989.

THE LANCET

Vol 338   Saturday 30 November 1991   No 8779

ORIGINAL ARTICLES

Swedish Aspirin Low-dose Trial (SALT) of 75 mg aspirin as secondary prophylaxis after cerebrovascular ischaemic events

THE SALT COLLABORATIVE GROUP*

The efficacy of aspirin in daily doses of 300 mg and more as secondary prophylaxis after cerebrovascular events is well established. Since much lower doses of aspirin can inhibit platelet function, and carry a lower risk of adverse effects, the Swedish Aspirin Low-dose Trial (SALT) was set up to study the efficacy of 75 mg aspirin daily in prevention of stroke and death after transient ischaemic attack (TIA) or minor stroke.

1360 patients entered the study 1–4 months after the qualifying event: 676 were randomly assigned to aspirin treatment and 684 to placebo treatment. The median duration of follow-up was 32 months. Compared with the placebo group, the aspirin group showed a reduction of 18% in the risk of primary outcome events (stroke or death; relative risk 0·82, 95% confidence interval 0·67–0·99; log-rank analysis p = 0·02), and reductions of 16–20% in the risks of secondary outcome events (stroke; stroke or two or more TIAs within a week of each other necessitating a change of treatment; or myocardial infarction). Adverse drug effects were reported by 147 aspirin-treated and 123 placebo-treated patients Gastrointestinal side-effects were only slightly more common in the aspirin-treated patients, but that group had a significant excess of bleeding episodes (p = 0·04).

Thus, we have found that a low dose (75 mg/day) of aspirin significantly reduces the risk of stroke or death in patients with cerebrovascular ischaemic events.

Lancet 1991; **338**: 1345–49.

Introduction

Antiplatelet therapy with acetylsalicylic acid (aspirin) is well established as secondary prophylaxis in patients with arterial thrombotic disorders.[1] An overview analysis[2] of patients who have had transient ischaemic attacks (TIAs) or ischaemic strokes showed that a daily dose of 300–1500 mg aspirin reduces the risk of subsequent stroke, myocardial infarction, or vascular death by 22%.

The early trials of antiplatelet therapy used aspirin doses above 900 mg daily, which are needed for the analgesic and anti-inflammatory effects, although it was known even then that a dose equivalent to only 1–2 mg/kg body weight was sufficient to inhibit platelet function in vitro.[3] Subsequent studies have confirmed that platelet cyclooxygenase can be completely inhibited by an aspirin dose as low as 30–75 mg daily.[4 11] A low dose may even be more effective than a high dose, since production of prostacyclin by the vessel wall may be partly preserved.[8] Moreover, both the gastrointestinal side-effects of aspirin and patient compliance with prescription are dose-related.[12,13] The efficacy of aspirin at doses of less than 300 mg as secondary prophylaxis after

*****Coordinating centre:** Division of Clinical Pharmacology, Danderyd Hospital (C-E. Elwin, B. Peterson). **Steering committee:** C. Blomstrand, J-E. Olsson, B. Nilsson, M. von Arbin, M. Britton, C-E. Elwin, C. Helmers, B. Norrving, A. Rosén, K. Samuelsson, K. Strandberg, N. G. Wahlgren. **Adjudication committees:** *Stroke:* K. Samuelsson, C. Blomstrand, A. Gårde, B. Norrving, J-E. Olsson; *Death:* M. Britton; *Myocardial infarction:* M. von Arbin, A. Carlsson, C. Helmers; *Compliance:* C. Blomstrand, C-E. Elwin, A. Rosén, J. Svensson; *Adverse effects:* N. G. Wahlgren. **Safety monitoring committee:** B. Huitfeldt, P. O. Lundberg, L. Wilhelmsen. **Statisticians:** H. Melander, I. Selinus. Correspondence to Dr Bo Norrving, Department of Neurology, University Hospital, S-221 85 Lund, Sweden.

Articles

Concorde: MRC/ANRS randomised double-blind controlled trial of immediate and deferred zidovudine in symptom-free HIV infection

*Concorde Coordinating Committee**

Summary

Concorde is a double-blind randomised comparison of two policies of zidovudine treatment in symptom-free individuals infected with human immunodeficiency virus (HIV): (a) immediate zidovudine from the time of randomisation (Imm); and (b) deferred zidovudine (Def) until the onset of AIDS-related complex (ARC) or AIDS (CDC group IV disease) or the development of persistently low CD4 cell counts if the clinician judged that treatment was indicated.

Between October, 1988, and October, 1991, 1749 HIV-infected individuals from centres in the UK, Ireland, and France were randomly allocated to zidovudine 250 mg four times daily (877 Imm) or matching placebo (872 Def). Follow-up was to death or Dec 31, 1992 (total 5419 person-years; median 3·3 years) and only 7% of the 1749 had not had a full clinical assessment after July 1, 1992. Of those allocated to the Def group, 418 started zidovudine at some time during the trial, 174 (42%) of them at or after they were judged by the clinician to have developed ARC or AIDS (nearly all confirmed subsequently) and most of the remainder on the basis of low CD4 cell counts. Those in the Imm group spent 81% of the time before ARC or AIDS on zidovudine compared with only 16% for those in the Def group.

Despite the large difference in the amount of zidovudine between the two groups and the fact that the number of clinical endpoints (AIDS and death) in Concorde (347) outnumbers the total of those in all other published trials in symptom-free and early symptomatic infection, there was no statistically significant difference in clinical outcome between the two therapeutic policies. The 3-year estimated survival probabilities were 92% (95% CI 90–94%) in Imm and 94% (92–95%) in Def (log-rank p=0·13), with no significant differences overall or in subgroup analyses by CD4 cell count at baseline. Similarly, there was no significant difference in progression of HIV disease: 3-year progression rates to AIDS or

death were 18% in both groups, and to ARC, AIDS, or death were 29% (Imm) and 32% (Def) (p=0·18), although there was an indication of an early but transient clinical benefit in favour of Imm in progression to ARC, AIDS, or death. However, there was a clear difference in changes in CD4 cell count over time in the two groups. Median changes from baseline at 3 months were +20 cells/μL (Imm) and −9 cells/μL (Def), a difference of 29 cells/μL (95% CI 16–42; p<0·0001) which persisted for up to 3 years. Thus such persistent differences in CD4 cell count do not necessarily imply long-term differences in clinical outcome.

6 participants had life-threatening adverse events that were judged to be possibly drug related: 4 occurred on trial capsules before unblinding (3 on zidovudine, 1 on placebo) and 2 occurred on open zidovudine. Despite a daily dose of 1 g of zidovudine, the frequency of severe haematological and other adverse events on trial therapy was low but significantly higher in the Imm group: 16 Imm and 2 Def participants stopped trial drug for haematological events and the estimated proportions with haemoglobin dropping below 10 g/dL were 5% and 1%, respectively, at 1 year and 8% and 2%, respectively, at 3 years. Another 83 (9%) Imm and 36 (4%) Def participants stopped for other adverse events, predominantly gastrointestinal or neurological symptoms (headaches) or malaise.

The results of Concorde do not encourage the early use of zidovudine in symptom-free HIV-infected adults. They also call into question the uncritical use of CD4 cell counts as a surrogate endpoint for assessment of benefit from long-term antiretroviral therapy.

Lancet 1994; **343**: 871–81

See Commentary page 866

*Coordinating Committee: M Seligmann and D A Warrell (joint chairmen), J-P Aboulker, C Carbon, J H Darbyshire, J Dormont, E Eschwege, D J Girling (until 1989), D R James (until 1989), J-P Levy, T E A Peto, D Schwarz, A B Stone, I V D Weller, R Withnall (secretary); K Gelmon (until 1989), E Lafon, A M Swart (trial physicians); the late V R Aber, A G Babiker, S Lhoro, A J Nunn (until 1989), M Vray (statisticians).

Other committees, trials centre staff, and participating centres are listed at the end of the report.

Correspondence to: Dr J H Darbyshire, MRC HIV Clinical Trials Centre, Department of Clinical Epidemiology, National Heart & Lung Institute, Royal Brompton National Heart and Lung Hospital, Sydney Street, London SW3 6NP, UK, and Dr J-P Aboulker, INSERM SC10, 16 Avenue Paul Vaillant Couturier, 94807 Villejuif, France

Introduction

Zidovudine inhibits the human immunodeficiency virus (HIV) reverse transcriptase enzyme and terminates proviral DNA chain synthesis in vitro. In the first placebo-controlled trial of this agent in individuals with advanced AIDS-related complex (ARC) or AIDS, there was a significant reduction in mortality and in the frequency of opportunistic infections over an average follow-up of 4 months.[1] The hope was that use of zidovudine earlier in infection might delay disease progression and therefore further improve survival. In Concorde, a randomised double-blind trial, two policies for use of zidovudine were compared in symptom-free individuals with HIV infection in terms of mortality, progression to ARC or AIDS, and safety and tolerability of the drug. In the immediate group (Imm), zidovudine was given immediately after randomisation; in the deferred group (Def), who received

THE LANCET

in both CJD[4] and Gerstmann-Straussler syndrome,[5] and there is evidence of increased mRNA expression in scrapie.[6] APOE may influence the pathogenesis of prion diseases, perhaps by an interaction with prion protein which affects protein conformation. Whatever the mechanism, the identification of APOE as a determinant of disease phenotype in CJD adds to the evidence for an influence of host genetic factors in human prion diseases. Familial CJD is associated with, and perhaps caused by, mutation of the PRNP gene, and the clinical phenotype in these pedigrees, including age at onset and disease duration, varies with specific PRNP mutations.[7] Homozygosity at codon 129 of the PRNP gene influences susceptibility to both sporadic and iatrogenic CJD,[8,9] and the disease phenotype in association with the codon 178 mutation is determined by the genotype at the 129 locus.[10] Methionine at position 129 produces fatal familial insomnia, while valine at that site results in typical CJD. There is also preliminary evidence of a genetic influence on the neuropathology of CJD, with a relation between a valine at position 129 and prion protein plaques.[11]

Genetic factors, which may now include APOE alleles, influence susceptibility to disease, duration of disease, age at onset of clinical signs, type of clinical presentation, and, perhaps, the distribution and type of lesions in both sporadic and familial CJD. As in scrapie,[12] other areas of the genome may act as determinants of disease susceptibility or expression in human prion diseases, and further definition of susceptibility genes could prove to be important in assessing the risk of exogenous infection (eg, in patients given human pituitary growth hormone). However, clinicopathological variation in CJD may not be determined by genetic factors alone. In scrapie the influence of host genotype on disease is better defined than it is for human disease, and this may allow the selective breeding of low-susceptibility sheep.[13] There are also distinct strains of scrapie agent, with consistent biological characteristics independent of the host genotype, and the existence of similar strains of infectious agent has been suggested in CJD too.

R G Will

National Creutzfeldt-Jakob Disease Surveillance Unit, Western General Hospital, Edinburgh, UK

1   Poirier J, Davignon J, Bouthillier D, Kogan S, Bertrand P, Gauthier S. Apolipoprotein E polymorphism and Alzheimer's disease. *Lancet* 1993; **342:** 697–99.
2   Pickering-Brown SM, Mann DMA, Bourke JP, et al. Apolipoprotein E4 and Alzheimer's disease pathology in Lewy body disease and in other beta-amyloid forming diseases. *Lancet* 1994; **343:** 1155.
3   Hardy J, Crook R, Perry R, Raghavan R, Roberts G. Apo E genotype and Down's syndrome. *Lancet* 1994; **343:** 979–80.
4   Namba Y, Tomonaga M, Kawasaki H, Otomo E, Ikeda K. Apolipoprotein E immunoreactivity in cerebral amyloid deposits and neurofibrillary tangles in Alzheimer's disease and kuru plaque amyloid in Creutzfeldt-Jakob disease. *Brain Res* 1991; **541:** 163–66.
5   Bugiani O, Giaccone G, Frigerio L, Farlow MR, Ghetti B, Tagliavini F. Apolipoprotein E and J immunoreactivity in Gerstmann-Straussler-Scheinker disease. *Neurobiol Aging* 1994; **15** (suppl 1): S156–S157.
6   Diedrich JF, Minnigan H, Carp RI, et al. Neuropathological changes in scrapie and Alzheimer's disease are associated with increased expression of apolipoprotein E and cathepsin D in astrocytes. *J Virol* 1991; **65:** 4759–68.
7   Brown P, Goldfarb L, Gibbs CJ, Gajdusek DC. The phenotypic expression of different mutations in transmissible familial Creutzfeldt-Jakob disease. *Eur J Epidemiol* 1991; **7:** 469–76.
8   Palmer MS, Dryden AJ, Hughes JT, Collinge J. Homozygous prion protein genotype predisposes to sporadic Creutzfeldt-Jakob disease.

Nature 1991; **352:** 340–41.
9   Collinge J, Palmer MS, Dryden AJ. Genetic predisposition to iatrogenic Creutzfeldt-Jakob disease. *Lancet* 1991; **337:** 1441–42.
10 Goldfarb LG, Petersen RB, Tabaton M, Brown P, et al. Fatal familial insomnia and familial CJD: disease phenotype determined by a DNA polymorphism. *Science* 1992; **258:** 806–08.
11 De Silva R, Ironside JW, McCardle L, Esmonde TFG, Bell JE, Will RG. Neuropathological phenotype and "prion protein" genotype correlation in sporadic Creutzfeldt-Jacob disease. *Neurosci Lett* 1994; **179:** 50–52.
12 Carp RI, Callahan SM, Yu Y, Sersen E. Analysis of host genetic control of scrapie-induced obesity. *Arch Virol* 1993; **133:** 1–9.
13 Hunter N, Goldmann W, Benson G, Foster JD, Hope J. Swaledale sheep affected by natural scrapie differ significantly in PrP genotype frequencies from healthy sheep and those selected for reduced incidence of scrapie. *J Gen Virol* 1993; **74:** 1025–31.

Handwashing—the Semmelweis lesson forgotten?

Hospital-acquired infection is still a major cause of morbidity and mortality throughout the world. As hospitals admit more severely ill patients and as use of invasive procedures and devices becomes more frequent, the risk of transmission of pathogens from patient to patient via the hands of health care workers (HCWs) increases. A simple and effective method of preventing this is handwashing. However, studies repeatedly show that doctors, nurses, and others do not always wash their hands before and between all patient contacts. This failure is reminiscent of the situation faced by Ignaz Semmelweis. In 1847 in Vienna, he noted that puerperal fever was more common on a maternity ward where medical students worked than it was on the ward where midwives provided care.[1] He believed that the students were contaminating their hands while dissecting cadavers. He ordered that students wash their hands in chlorinated lime after dissection and before examining patients; the rate of infection fell sharply, as did the mortality rate. When 12 women had puerperal fever on a ward where the students had no contact with cadavers, Semmelweis deduced that infection was also transmitted by living organisms; he then insisted on handwashing with chlorinated lime between all patient examinations. At that time few doctors believed Semmelweis' theory. Unfortunately, he refused to publish his findings. In 1851, and again in 1855, he was appointed to hospitals with high infection and mortality rates—and his hand antisepsis methods resulted in significant decreases in infection and mortality. Only in 1857 did Semmelweis report some of his own findings, but when he died in 1865 his beliefs were still largely ignored by clinicians.

Despite advances in hospital epidemiology and infection control, translating Semmelweis' theory into practice remains a challenge. In the early 1970s hospital infection control programmes were established and they decreased the emphasis on environmental culturing and disinfection and stressed the role of patient-based active surveillance for infection detection and the implementation of prevention measures, notably handwashing. By then we knew the important role that HCWs' hands have in the transmission of nosocomial pathogens,[2–4] and others confirmed the association between handwashing and the reduction in hand microbial flora.[5] These studies showed that handwashing with bland soap at best removes some of the transient microbes mechanically whereas preparations containing

THE LANCET

antiseptic or antibacterial agents not only remove transient microbes mechanically but also chemically killed contaminating and colonising flora and have long-term residual activity.

In the 1980s the US Centers for Disease Control published guidelines that included recommendations on handwashing[6] ("generally considered the most important procedure for preventing nosocomial infections").[6] Despite this recommendation, studies in the USA (the latest evidence comes from an emergency department[7]) found that HCWs, in intensive care units and in outpatient clinics, seldom wash their hands before patient contacts.[7–12] Physicians, it seems, wash their hands no more frequently than nurses do (rates for physicians were 14–59%, while for nurses they were 25–45%, and for other HCWs they were 23–73%). Attempts to improve compliance—eg, by in-service education, distribution of leaflets, lectures, automated dispensers, and feedback on handwashing rates[9–12]—have been associated with at best transient improvement. The most effective measure has been routine observation and feedback,[10,11] but no intervention has had a long-term impact on handwashing practice.

Why do HCWs not comply when handwashing is known to reduce nosocomial infection?[13] Excuses include being too busy, skin irritation, wearing gloves, or not thinking about it.[11] Some HCWs believe that they have washed their hands when necessary even when observations indicate that they have not.[11] Multidrug-resistant pathogens are increasing in frequency and are now a major threat to public health; these pathogens (eg, vancomycin-resistant enterococci) have been recovered from the environment around infected or colonised patients and from the hands of HCWs caring for them. If HCWs cannot be educated to comply perhaps we should tell patients about the importance of handwashing: how many doctors and nurses would ignore a patient's request that they wash their hands first?

William R Jarvis
Hospital Infections Program, National Center for Infectious Diseases, Centers for Disease Control and Prevention, Atlanta, Georgia, USA

1 Semmelweis I. The etiology, the concept, and the prophylaxis of childbed fever. Pest CA: Hartleben's Verlag-Expedition, 1861 (translated by F P Murphy and republished, Classics of Medicine Library, Birmingham, AL, 1981).
2 Salzman TC, Clark JJ, Lkemm L. Hand contamination of personnel as a mechanism of cross-infection in nosocomial infections with antibiotic-resistant *Escherichia coli* and *Klebsiella-Aerobacter. Antimicrob Agents Chemother* 1967; 2: 97–100.
3 Rammelkamp CH Jr, Mortimer EA Jr, Wolinsky E. Transmission of streptococcal and staphylococcal infections. *Ann Intern Med* 1964; 60: 753–58.
4 Casewell M, Phillips I. Hands as a route of transmission of *Klebsiella* species. *BMJ* 1977; ii: 1315–17.
5 Rotter ML. Hygienic hand disinfection. *Infect Control* 1984; 5: 18–22.
6 Garner JS, Simmons BS. Guideline for handwashing and hospital environmental control. *Infect Control* 1986; 7: 231–42.
7 Meengs MR, Giles BK, Chisholm CD, Cordell WH, Nelson DR. Hand washing frequency in an emergency department. *Ann Emerg Med* 1994; 23: 1307–12.
8 Albert RK, Condie F. Hand-washing patterns in medical intensive care units. *N Engl J Med* 1981; 304: 1465–66.
9 Donowitz LG. Handwashing technique in a pediatric intensive care unit. *Am J Dis Child* 1987; 141: 683–85.
10 Graham M. Frequency and duration of handwashing in an intensive care unit. *Am J Infect Control* 1990; 18: 78–81.
11 Dubbert PM, Doice J, Richter W, Miller M, Chapman SW. Increasing ICU staff handwashing: effects of education and group feedback. *Infect

Control Hosp Epidemiol 1990; 11: 191–93.
12 Simmons B, Bryant J, Neiman K, Spencer L, Arheart K. The role of handwashing in prevention of endemic intensive care unit infections. *Infect Control Hosp Epidemiol* 1990; 11: 589–94.
13 Doebbeling BN, Stanley GL, Sheetz CT, et al. Comparative efficacy of alternative handwashing agents in reducing nosocomial infections in intensive care units. *N Engl J Med* 1992; 327: 88–93.

Behavioural science in the AIDS epidemic

Behavioural interventions remain our principal tool for AIDS prevention. This point was driven home once again at the latest International AIDS Conference held in Yokohama in August (*Lancet* 1994; 344: 535). While biological science continues to unravel the secrets of the human immunodeficiency virus (HIV), behavioural science has contributed much to our understanding of its prevalence, incidence, and distribution, the behaviours most implicated in its transmission, possible strategies and options for disease prevention programmes, and the feasibility, cost, and effectiveness of these interventions. In the USA, studies of homosexual men show rapid reductions in high-risk behaviour and falling incidence of infectious diseases, including HIV, as the result of public health interventions.[1–4] Moreover, there is accumulating evidence that public health measures such as outreach programmes for injected-drug users and increased access to supplies of sterile needles have reduced the frequency of behaviours known to transmit bloodborne diseases.[5,6] Other studies have shown a lower incidence of infectious diseases among injected-drug users with ready access to clean syringes. In a Baltimore cohort, diabetic drug users were less likely to seroconvert for HIV than were non-diabetics,[7] and in a Tacoma case-control study, drug users who participated in the syringe exchange scheme were less likely to acquire hepatitis B.[8] A joint National Research Council/Institute of Medicine report on AIDS prevention[9] accords with these findings, and includes a section on mathematical modelling to illustrate reduced HIV incidence through syringe exchange programmes.

Despite such achievements, behavioural science is often viewed with scepticism by practitioners of biomedical science. Studies that rely on "self-reports" of participants and research designs that lack random assignment to isolated conditions are viewed as weaker than true experiments that incorporate biological markers as outcomes.[10] However, traditional experimental methods are often hopelessly inapplicable to studies of risk behaviour as practised and of limited feasibility in the evaluation of fledgling community public health programmes. It is impossible, for example, to draw a truly random sample of injected-drug users owing to the clandestine, illegal, and socially proscribed nature of illicit drug use. The use of biological outcomes (eg, HIV incidence) in prevention research is feasible only in places where there are substantial rates of new infection and large compliant study populations. Behavioural science provides realistic and feasible alternatives to true experimentation with such options as urban ethnography and quasi-experimentation. Moreover, by linking interventions and research, natural experiments can be constructed. When it is done successfully, both prevention and scientific objectives can be simultaneously served.[9,11] Yet the future of intervention research is cloudy. As part of a 1992 reorganisation plan,

Randomised trial of cholesterol lowering in 4444 patients with coronary heart disease: the Scandinavian Simvastatin Survival Study (4S)

Scandinavian Simvastatin Survival Study Group*

Summary

Drug therapy for hypercholesterolaemia has remained controversial mainly because of insufficient clinical trial evidence for improved survival. The present trial was designed to evaluate the effect of cholesterol lowering with simvastatin on mortality and morbidity in patients with coronary heart disease (CHD). 4444 patients with angina pectoris or previous myocardial infarction and serum cholesterol 5·5–8·0 mmol/L on a lipid-lowering diet were randomised to double-blind treatment with simvastatin or placebo.

Over the 5·4 years median follow-up period, simvastatin produced mean changes in total cholesterol, low-density-lipoprotein cholesterol, and high-density-lipoprotein cholesterol of −25%, −35%, and +8%, respectively, with few adverse effects. 256 patients (12%) in the placebo group died, compared with 182 (8%) in the simvastatin group. The relative risk of death in the simvastatin group was 0·70 (95% CI 0·58–0·85, p=0·0003). The 6-year probabilities of survival in the placebo and simvastatin groups were 87·6% and 91·3%, respectively. There were 189 coronary deaths in the placebo group and 111 in the simvastatin group (relative risk 0·58, 95% CI 0·46–0·73), while noncardiovascular causes accounted for 49 and 46 deaths, respectively. 622 patients (28%) in the placebo group and 431 (19%) in the simvastatin group had one or more major coronary events. The relative risk was 0·66 (95% CI 0·59–0·75, p<0·00001), and the respective probabilities of escaping such events were 70·5% and 79·6%. This risk was also significantly reduced in subgroups consisting of women and patients of both sexes aged 60 or more. Other benefits of treatment included a 37% reduction (p<0·00001) in the risk of undergoing myocardial revascularisation procedures.

This study shows that long-term treatment with simvastatin is safe and improves survival in CHD patients.

Lancet 1994; **344**: 1383–89

*Collaborators and participating centres are listed at the end of the report.

Correspondence to: Dr Terje R Pedersen, Cardiology Section, Medical Department, Aker Hospital, N 0514 Oslo, Norway

Introduction

High serum cholesterol is regarded by many as the main cause of coronary atherosclerosis.[1] Several cholesterol-lowering interventions have reduced coronary heart disease (CHD) events in primary and secondary prevention clinical trials.[2-9] Expert panels in Europe and the USA have therefore recommended dietary changes and, if necessary, addition of drugs to reduce high cholesterol concentrations—specifically low-density-lipoprotein (LDL) cholesterol[10-13]—especially in patients with CHD. However, these recommendations have been questioned,[14,15] mainly because no clinical trial has convincingly shown that lowering of cholesterol prolongs life. Furthermore, overviews of these trials have suggested that survival is not improved, particularly in the absence of established CHD, because the observed reduction of CHD deaths is offset by an apparent increase in non-cardiac mortality, including cancer and violent deaths.[14-18]

Simvastatin is an inhibitor of hydroxy-methylglutaryl coenzyme A (HMG-CoA) reductase, which reduces LDL cholesterol[19,20] to a greater extent than that achieved in previous diet and drug intervention trials. The Scandinavian Simvastatin Survival Study (4S) was conceived in April, 1987, to test the hypothesis that lowering of cholesterol with simvastatin would improve survival of patients with CHD. Other objectives were to study the effect of simvastatin on the incidence of coronary and other atherosclerotic events, and its long-term safety.

Patients and methods

Organisation

The study design has been published previously.[21] Patients were recruited at 94 clinical centres in Scandinavia. A steering committee made up of cardiologists, lipidologists, and epidemiologists had scientific responsibility for the study and all reports of the results. One member was the scientific coordinator who worked closely with the study monitors in the Scandinavian subsidiaries of Merck Research Laboratories. Major study events were classified by an independent endpoint classification committee (two experienced cardiologists) without knowledge of treatment allocation. A data and safety monitoring committee performed independent interim analyses of total mortality at prespecified numbers of deaths. The statistician of this committee received information on all deaths directly from the investigators. The study protocol was approved by regional or, if applicable, national ethics committees and by the regulatory agencies in each of the participating Scandinavian countries.

THE LANCET

Donors' attitudes towards body donation for dissection

Ruth Richardson, Brian Hurwitz

Summary

We report a survey in the UK of potential whole-body donors for dissection. 218 people (age range 19–97 years) answered a postal questionnaire, giving information about themselves, their reasons for donation, attitudes towards the dead body, funeral preferences and medical giving and receiving. In addition to altruism, motives included the wish to avoid funeral ceremonies, to avoid waste, and in a few cases, to evade the expense of a funeral. 44% understood that their bodies would be used as teaching material, 42% for experiments. Whilst 69% believed in one or more supernatural phenomena, only 39% said they were religious. 69% requested cremation after dissection; 2% wanted to be buried. The notion of money incentives to promote donation was overwhelmingly rejected.

Lancet 1995; **346:** 277–79

Introduction

Responses of medical students to human dissection have been investigated,[1,2] but how dead bodies arrive in the dissecting-room has received less attention.[3-5] Before the second world war, almost all bodies dissected in UK medical schools were those of the poor, requisitioned from the mortuaries of public institutions such as Poor Law infirmaries and mental hospitals.[4] Nowadays, most bodies dissected in the UK are donated voluntarily.[6]

We report a study to ascertain what sort of people become donors, and their motives for doing so.

Method

The procurement and distribution of bodies for dissection in the medical schools of London is the responsibility of the London Committee of Licensed Teachers of Anatomy. Enquiries are made to a central office, and information packs containing bequest forms are dispatched. There is no central register of future donors. Many information packs are requested for clients by solicitors and other agencies, and are not always used; the enquiry to body-yield ratio is about 5:1.

In 1992, the late John Pegington, Professor of Anatomy at University College, then co-ordinator of distribution of bodies in London, gave permission for a letter explaining our interest in donors' motives to be inserted into information packs. The letter invited recipients to contact us if they were interested in receiving a questionnaire. Anonymity was assured. Between autumn, 1992, and spring, 1993, 800 information packs containing these letters were sent out. Over the next 12 months, 256 requests for questionnaires were received and the same number dispatched. By the summer of 1994, 220 (86%) questionnaires had been returned.

Results

Of the 220 returned questionnaires, 2 were blank: 1 due to the early death of the recipient, the other to family opposition to donation. 218 completed questionnaires were received from 123 women (mean age 66·6 yr), 94 men (mean age 69·8 yr), and one whose sex was unstated. The age range of the whole sample was 19–97 yr.

216 respondents (99%) were UK citizens. Of those who mentioned their social class, 27% described themselves as middle class, and 25% as working class. However, a 2:1 excess of non-manual over manual occupations was evident among those (72%) who told us their occupations (table 1). The sample contained several nurses and other carers, but no doctors.

Eighty per cent of respondents judged their health to be good. Only 10% mentioned a specific medical condition in connection with their wish to donate, usually with the hope that their donation would enable research to protect others from what they themselves had suffered.

Forty five per cent of the sample said they were not religious, 39% that they were, and 11% were unsure. Many with a religious affiliation were lapsed (table 1).

Department of Anatomy, University College, London WC1 6BT, UK
(R Richardson DPhil); **and Department of General Practice,
St Mary's Hospital Medical School, London** (B Hurwitz MD)

Correspondence to: Dr Ruth Richardson

A new variant of Creutzfeldt-Jakob disease in the UK

R G Will, J W Ironside, M Zeidler, S N Cousens, K Estibeiro, A Alperovitch, S Poser, M Pocchiari, A Hofman, P G Smith

Summary

Background Epidemiological surveillance of Creutzfeldt-Jakob disease (CJD) was reinstituted in the UK in 1990 to identify any changes in the occurrence of this disease after the epidemic of bovine spongiform encephalopathy (BSE) in cattle.

Methods Case ascertainment of CJD was mostly by direct referral from neurologists and neuropathologists. Death certificates on which CJD was mentioned were also obtained. Clinical details were obtained for all referred cases, and information on potential risk factors for CJD was obtained by a standard questionnaire administered to patients' relatives. Neuropathological examination was carried out on approximately 70% of suspect cases. Epidemiological studies of CJD using similar methodology to the UK study have been carried out in France, Germany, Italy, and the Netherlands between 1993 and 1995.

Findings Ten cases of CJD have been identified in the UK in recent months with a new neuropathological profile. Other consistent features that are unusual include the young age of the cases, clinical findings, and the absence of the electroencephalogram features typical for CJD. Similar cases have not been identified in other countries in the European surveillance system.

Interpretation These cases appear to represent a new variant of CJD, which may be unique to the UK. This raises the possibility that they are causally linked to BSE. Although this may be the most plausible explanation for this cluster of cases, a link with BSE cannot be confirmed on the basis of this evidence alone. It is essential to obtain further information on the current and past clinical and neuropathological profiles of CJD in the UK and elsewhere.

Lancet 1996; **347:** 921–25

National CJD Surveillance Unit, Western General Hospital, Edinburgh EH4 2XU, UK (R G Will FRCP, J W Ironside MRCPath, M Zeidler MRCP, K Estibeiro BSc); **Department of Epidemiology and Population Science, London School of Hygiene and Tropical Medicine, London, UK** (S N Cousens Dip Math Stat, Prof P G Smith DSc); **INSERM, Hopital de la Salpetriere, Paris, France** (A Alperovitch MD); **Klinik und Poliklinik für Neurologie, Georg-August-Universitat, Gottingen, Germany** (S Poser MD); **Laboratorio di Virologia, Istituto Superiore di Sanità, Rome, Italy** (M Pocchiari MD); **Erasmus University, Rotterdam, The Netherlands** (Prof A Hofman MD)

Correspondence to: Dr R G Will

Introduction

Because of the epidemic of bovine spongiform encephalopathy (BSE) in cattle, surveillance of Creutzfeldt-Jakob disease (CJD) in the UK was reinstituted in May, 1990. The purpose of the surveillance is to identify changes in the pattern of CJD which might indicate an association with BSE. We report ten cases of CJD in the UK with clinical onset of disease in 1994 and 1995. These cases all have neuropathological changes which, to our knowledge, have not been previously reported. They are also unusual in that they occurred in relatively young people, and the clinical course was not typical of cases of sporadic CJD in the UK.

Methods

Since May, 1990, cases of CJD have been identified to the CJD Surveillance Unit, usually by direct referral from professional groups, which include neurologists and neuropathologists. All death certificates in the UK on which CJD is mentioned are obtained and some cases are identified retrospectively in this way; some are identified from other sources. Clinical details are obtained for all cases, and information on potential risk factors for CJD is obtained with a standard questionnaire, usually administered to a close relative of the case. After obtaining informed consent from the relatives or patients, blood is obtained for DNA analysis in most patients. Information on all known cases of CJD in England and Wales since 1970 and in Scotland and Northern Ireland since 1985 is also available from previous surveys of CJD.[1] Parallel studies of CJD have been carried out in France, Italy, Germany, and the Netherlands between 1993 and 1995 with similar methods.[2]

Whenever possible, neuropathological examination is carried out on cases and suspect cases notified to the CJD Surveillance Unit. Such examinations have been done on about 70% of cases notified since May, 1990, either by referral for necropsy in Edinburgh or in cooperation with neuropathologists in other centres who refer cases after diagnosis. Blocks from the frontal, temporal, parietal, and occipital cortex; basal ganglia; thalamus; hypothalamus; cerebellum midbrain; pons; and medulla are fixed in formalin. Blocks are immersed in 96% formic acid for 1 hour before routine processing into paraffin wax. Sections are cut at 5μm and stained by conventional histological techniques and immunocytochemistry for prion protein (PrP). Pretreatments for immunocytochemistry with two monoclonal PrP antibodies (KG9 and 3F4)[3] include incubation in 96% formic acid for 5 min, then 4 mol/L guanidine thiocyanate for 2 hours, and hydrated autoclaving at 121°C for 10 min.

Results

Patients

Of the 207 cases of CJD examined neuropathologically since May, 1990, ten have neuropathological findings that clearly distinguish them from other cases examined by the CJD Surveillance Unit (two have been reported previously[4,5]).

These ten cases (four male) had disease onset from

Articles

Intensive blood-glucose control with sulphonylureas or insulin compared with conventional treatment and risk of complications in patients with type 2 diabetes (UKPDS 33)

UK Prospective Diabetes Study (UKPDS) Group*

Summary

Background Improved blood-glucose control decreases the progression of diabetic microvascular disease, but the effect on macrovascular complications is unknown. There is concern that sulphonylureas may increase cardiovascular mortality in patients with type 2 diabetes and that high insulin concentrations may enhance atheroma formation. We compared the effects of intensive blood-glucose control with either sulphonylurea or insulin and conventional treatment on the risk of microvascular and macrovascular complications in patients with type 2 diabetes in a randomised controlled trial.

Methods 3867 newly diagnosed patients with type 2 diabetes, median age 54 years (IQR 48–60 years), who after 3 months' diet treatment had a mean of two fasting plasma glucose (FPG) concentrations of 6·1–15·0 mmol/L were randomly assigned intensive policy with a sulphonylurea (chlorpropamide, glibenclamide, or glipizide) or with insulin, or conventional policy with diet. The aim in the intensive group was FPG less than 6 mmol/L. In the conventional group, the aim was the best achievable FPG with diet alone; drugs were added only if there were hyperglycaemic symptoms or FPG greater than 15 mmol/L. Three aggregate endpoints were used to assess differences between conventional and intensive treatment: any diabetes-related endpoint (sudden death, death from hyperglycaemia or hypoglycaemia, fatal or non-fatal myocardial infarction, angina, heart failure, stroke, renal failure, amputation [of at least one digit], vitreous haemorrhage, retinopathy requiring photocoagulation, blindness in one eye, or cataract extraction); diabetes-related death (death from myocardial infarction, stroke, peripheral vascular disease, renal disease, hyperglycaemia or hypoglycaemia, and sudden death); all-cause mortality. Single clinical endpoints and surrogate subclinical endpoints were also assessed. All analyses were by intention to treat and frequency of hypoglycaemia was also analysed by actual therapy.

Findings Over 10 years, haemoglobin A_{1c} (HbA_{1c}) was 7·0%

(6·2–8·2) in the intensive group compared with 7·9% (6·9–8·8) in the conventional group—an 11% reduction. There was no difference in HbA_{1c} among agents in the intensive group. Compared with the conventional group, the risk in the intensive group was 12% lower (95% CI 1–21, p=0·029) for any diabetes-related endpoint; 10% lower (−11 to 27, p=0·34) for any diabetes-related death; and 6% lower (−10 to 20, p=0·44) for all-cause mortality. Most of the risk reduction in the any diabetes-related aggregate endpoint was due to a 25% risk reduction (7–40, p=0·0099) in microvascular endpoints, including the need for retinal photocoagulation. There was no difference for any of the three aggregate endpoints between the three intensive agents (chlorpropamide, glibenclamide, or insulin).

Patients in the intensive group had more hypoglycaemic episodes than those in the conventional group on both types of analysis (both p<0·0001). The rates of major hypoglycaemic episodes per year were 0·7% with conventional treatment, 1·0% with chlorpropamide, 1·4% with glibenclamide, and 1·8% with insulin. Weight gain was significantly higher in the intensive group (mean 2·9 kg) than in the conventional group (p<0·001), and patients assigned insulin had a greater gain in weight (4·0 kg) than those assigned chlorpropamide (2·6 kg) or glibenclamide (1·7 kg).

Interpretation Intensive blood-glucose control by either sulphonylureas or insulin substantially decreases the risk of microvascular complications, but not macrovascular disease, in patients with type 2 diabetes. None of the individual drugs had an adverse effect on cardiovascular outcomes. All intensive treatment increased the risk of hypoglycaemia.

Lancet 1998; **352:** 837–53

Introduction

Started in 1977, the UK Prospective Diabetes Study (UKPDS) was designed to establish whether, in patients with type 2 diabetes, intensive blood-glucose control reduced the risk of macrovascular or microvascular complications, and whether any particular therapy was advantageous.

Most intervention studies have assessed microvascular disease: improved glucose control has delayed the development and progression of retinopathy,

*Study organisation given at end of paper

Correspondence to: Prof Robert Turner, UKPDS Group, Diabetes Research Laboratories, Radcliffe Infirmary, Oxford OX2 6HE, UK

COMMENTARY

ELISA) to human putamen, but not to caudate or globus pallidus, were significantly higher among children with Tourette's syndrome than among controls.[13] Western-blot analyses indicated that specific antibodies to the striatum occurred more commonly among patients with Tourette's syndrome than among controls at 83 kDa, 67 kDa, and 60 kDa.[13] Lastly, development of dyskinesias (paw and floor licking, head and paw shaking) and phonic utterances has been reported in rodents after the microinfusion into the striatum of dilute IgG from patients with Tourette's syndrome.[14]

Perlmutter and colleagues have completed a difficult protocol for immunomodulatory therapy. Several key points, some of which they point out, should be emphasised. The inclusion criteria for the study were highly selective, recruitment was nationwide, and initial therapeutic groupings contained only a maximum of ten patients. Hence, it is unclear what proportion of all children with Tourette's syndrome and OCD have an immune-mediated form of the disease and, of these, how many do not improve with standard pharmacotherapy. Immune therapies are not free of medical risks; about two-thirds of individuals receiving active therapy had side-effects. Control populations were limited: there was only an IVIG control group because of the potential risks of sham apheresis. Control comparisons were also limited to the 1-month visit, because children in the sham IVIG group were placed in open trials. Thus the possibility that some neuropsychiatric symptoms, especially the tics, might have spontaneously improved after 1 year cannot be excluded. Overall, the most consistent improvements with active therapies were shown for OCD, anxiety, depression, and global functioning. Although single treatments were reported to produce sustained improvements, psychotropic medications were decreased in dose or discontinued in only about half the patients. Only plasma exchange helped in tic suppression, but the group allocated this form of therapy had the highest baseline severity ratings. In addition, the sham IVIG group that subsequently received open treatment with plasma exchange experienced only a small degree of tic suppression. Finally, explanations are needed for the following: the lack of relation between therapeutic response and the rate of antibody removal; how peripheral changes affect events across the blood-brain barrier; and how the two forms of therapy produce their beneficial response. As Perlmutter and colleagues point out, although potentially promising for the highly selected patient, active immunomodulatory therapy is not ready for routine use. Thus this treatment should be given only as part of controlled double-blind protocols.

Harvey S Singer

Departments of Neurology and Pediatrics, Johns Hopkins University School of Medicine, Baltimore, MD 21287, USA.

1   Selling L. The role of infection in the etiology of tics. *Arch Neurol Psychiatry* 1929; **22:** 1163–71.
2   Matarazzo EB. Tourette's syndrome treated with ACTH and prednisone: report of two cases. *J Child Adolesc Psychopharmacol* 1992; **2:** 215–26.
3   Kiessling LS. Tic disorders associated with evidence of invasive group A beta hemolytic streptococcal disease. *Dev Med Child Neurol* 1989; **31** (suppl 59): 48.
4   Swedo SE, Rapoport JL, Cheslow DL, et al. High prevalence of obsessive-compulsive symptoms in patients with Sydenham's chorea. *Am J Psychiatry* 1989; **146:** 246–49.
5   Cardoso F, Eduardo C, Silva AP, Mota CC. Chorea in fifty consecutive patients with rheumatic fever. *Mov Disord* 1997; **12:** 701–03.
6   Swedo SE, Leonard HL, Garvey M, et al. Pediatric autoimmune neuropsychiatric disorders associated with streptococcal infections (PANDAS): a clinical description of the first fifty cases. *Am J Psychiatry* 1998; **155:** 264–71.
7   Kurlan R. Tourette's syndrome and 'PANDAS': will the relationship bear out? *Neurology* 1998; **50:** 1530–34.
8   Giuliano JD, Zimmerman A, Walkup JT, Singer HS. Prevalence of pediatric autoimmune neuropsychiatric disorders associated with streptococcal infection by history in a consecutive series of community referred children evaluated for tics. *Ann Neurol* 1998; **44:** 556.
9   Husby G, van de Rijn I, Zabriskie JB, et al. Antibodies reacting with cytoplasm of subthalamic and caudate nuclei neurons in chorea and acute rheumatic fever. *J Exp Med* 1976; **144:** 1094–1110.
10 Kiessling LS, Marcotte AC, Culpepper L. Anti-neuronal antibodies in movement disorders. *Pediatrics* 1993; **92:** 39–43.
11 Laurino JP, Hallett J, Kiessling L, Benson M, Pelletier T, Kuhn C. An immunoassay for antineuronal antibodies associated with involuntary repetitive movement disorders. *Ann Clin Lab Sci* 1997; **3:** 230–35.
12 Singer HS, Giuliano JD, Hansen BH, et al. Antibodies against a neuron-like (HTB-10 neuroblastoma) cell in children with Tourette syndrome. *Biol Psychiatry* (in press).
13 Singer HS, Giuliano JD, Hansen BH, et al. Antibodies against human putamen in children with Tourette syndrome. *Neurology* 1998; **50:** 1618–24.
14 Hallett JJ, Harling-Berg CJ, Agrawal JR, et al. Tic-like phonation and dyskinesia in rats after intracaudate microinfusion of sera from children with Tourette syndrome. *FASEB J* 1996; **10:** A1357.

Time to register randomised trials

Every year, national funding agencies, medical research charities, and drug and device manufacturers invest vast sums of money into randomised controlled trials. Although the distribution of this money is not entirely random, the process is certainly chaotic and commonly takes little account of concurrent research. Worse, the piecemeal reporting of these trials is unhelpful for the clinician attempting to obtain an accurate perspective on a particular health intervention. Several case-studies have revealed how the deliberate slicing and subsequent manipulation of trial data can provide a seriously misleading picture of effectiveness.

Two reports have pointed to the harm that can be created when sponsors of trials use data as little more than marketing tools for new drugs.[1,2] In a systematic review of trials of ondansetron for the treatment of postoperative nausea and vomiting, Martin Tramer and colleagues[1] found that "a false impression of ondansetron's efficacy may arise because a quarter of all relevant published reports are duplicates". For the same reason, Patricia Huston and David Moher[2] found it almost impossible to complete a systematic review of risperidone's efficacy in the treatment of schizophrenia. These studies show that those concerned with clinical research have to find better ways of identifying and tracking clinical trials to avoid making erroneous inferences about the effectiveness of new treatments.

The history of this effort shows much good intention but only limited progress. One attempt to link research to practice in the setting of an entire health service began in the UK in 1991 with the launch of the NHS research and development initiative.[3] That programme placed the systematic collection of data from randomised trials at its intellectual centre. The Cochrane Collaboration—an international project to create a database of systematic reviews of the effects of health care across all of medicine—has been its most important and successful partner. The Cochrane Collaboration has focused on published clinical trials. But this approach leaves untackled the large amount of evidence unpublished, mostly because it was regarded as "negative" and, therefore, seemingly unworthy of a drug company's or even an editor's attention.[4] Iain Chalmers has described such under-reporting as scientific misconduct,[5] and publication bias remains a pervasive problem in the medical literature. The medical editors' trials amnesty tried to flush out that evidence, with only partial success.[6]

Rather than treat the problem of hidden research retrospectively, probably a more sensible approach—as suggested by John Simes[7] more than a decade ago—is to prevent the problem in the first place. On the basis of their own investigations of publication bias, Kay Dickersin and Yuan-I Min[8] have argued that one "possibility is to require registration of all clinical trials prior to initiation. While this is widely agreed to be a good approach, widespread registration has not yet been effected . . .Who will take the lead?"

A lead is now being taken in the UK, and a conference to raise greater awareness about this issue and to find ways of fostering trial registration will be held next week in London. The registration of trials is of value not only to those clinicians and investigators wanting to be sure that they have access to all available evidence, but also to patients who may want to know of trials in which they might wish to take part. And research funding agencies need to ensure that their decisions are made in the full knowledge of current work, planned or in progress, to prevent duplication and to promote collaboration.

The conference, organised jointly by the BMJ Publishing Group, Association of the British Pharmaceutical Industry, and *The Lancet*, will bring together patients and people working in research, public health, funding agencies, industry, charities, and publishing. The meeting will review progress being made in trial registration in the USA, Australia, and continental Europe, as well as the UK.

What pointers are there for developing the notion of trial registration into a routine practice? Apart from the NHS national research register and the Cochrane controlled-trials register, the most important recent lead has been taken by the pharmaceutical industry. For example, Schering Health Care and GlaxoWellcome have committed themselves to registering information about randomised phase II, III, and IV (post-licensing) trials. Beginning with the question, "What does it mean to be a modern pharmaceutical company?", Richard Sykes (chairman of GlaxoWellcome) has argued that he and his colleagues understood "the value of information, and we want to create a climate of openness where the evidence for prescribing our products is clear".[9] Not all of those in the pharmaceutical sector agree, and Sykes has been ridiculed by some within the industry who see his step as the creation of a chink in GlaxoWellcome's commercial armour. But how can this be so when all the company is doing is releasing administrative information about current work (objective of the trial, endpoints, numbers, groups, and expected date of closure), not the actual data derived from that work?

Editors also have an important part to play, as Dickersin and Min pointed out. During peer review, editors increasingly find themselves requesting copies of the original trial protocol to check against the final submitted report. That "protocol culture" has led one of us to begin (and the other to start to plan) a protocol registration scheme.[10] Iain Chalmers and Doug Altman have discussed the opportunities that electronic publishing might open up for such protocol registration.[11] Editors are unwilling to fill their journals with promises of what might be. But those same editors can publish these protocols on their websites, perhaps linking them to a central registry.

Publishers could also assist this process by collaborating with one another to construct such a free on-line database. The lead here has been taken by *Current Science*, which launched a meta-register of randomised controlled trials in October, 1998. Trials depend on participation of patients, and many studies are paid for out of taxpayers' money—that is, they are a public good that every member of society already has a stake in. Publishers make a great deal of money out of commercial reprints of clinical trials. To expect publishers to contribute funds to an initiative from which they ultimately benefit is not unreasonable. One might even argue that it is their obligation. A valuable partnership might be with PubMed Central,[12] a project launched by US National Institutes of Health director Harold Varmus to create a free electronic archive of biomedical research.

The pressure to register trials will also rise when research ethics committees, medical research charities, and drug and device manufacturers encourage registration at their respective points of contact with trialists, especially since the decision not to publish results of trials seems to rest more with investigators than with editors.[8] A further challenge is to devise an internationally agreed method for assigning each trial a unique identifier. One such scheme is being piloted in cancer, with the assistance of the Cochrane cancer network.

Taken together, these collective efforts might bring shape to a formless clinical research enterprise. Such a structure should help in the organisation and delivery of high-quality evidence to the clinical setting, with a minimum waste of resources. That target is ambitious, and next week's conference will mark an important step towards its achievement.

A version of this commentary is published in this week's *BMJ* (Oct 2, pp 865–66).

Richard Horton, Richard Smith
The Lancet, London WC1B 3SL, UK; BMJ, London, WC1H 9JR, UK

1   Tramer MR, Moore RA, Reynolds JM, McQuay HJ. A quantitative systematic review of ondansetron in treatment of established postoperative nausea and vomiting. *BMJ* 1997; **314:** 1088–92.

2   Huston P, Moher D. Redundancy, disaggregation, and the integrity of medical research. *Lancet* 1996; **347:** 1024–26.

3   Peckham M. Research and development for the National Health Service. *Lancet* 1991; **338:** 367–71.

4   Easterbrook PJ, Berlin JA, Gopalan R, Matthews DR. Publication bias in clinical research. *Lancet* 1991; **337:** 867–72.

5   Chalmers I. Underreporting research is scientific misconduct. *JAMA* 1990; **263:** 1405–08.

6   Roberts I. An amnesty for unpublished trials. *BMJ* 1998; **317:** 763–64.

7   Simes RJ. Publication bias: the case for an international registry of clinical trials. *J Clin Oncol* 1986; **4:** 1529–41.

8   Dickersin K, Min Y-I. Publication bias: the problem that won't go away. In: Warren KS, Mosteller F, eds. Doing more good than harm: the evaluation of health care interventions. New York: New York Academy of Sciences, 1993.

9   Sykes R. Being a modern pharmaceutical company. *BMJ* 1998; **317:** 1172.

10 McNamee D. Protocol reviews at *The Lancet*. *Lancet* 1997; **350:** 6.

11 Chalmers I, Altman D. How can medical journals help prevent poor medical research? Some opportunities presented by electronic publishing. *Lancet* 1999; **353:** 490–93.

12 Marshall E. NIH's online publishing venture ready for launch. *Science* 1999; **285:** 1466.

Effect of home-based neonatal care and management of sepsis on neonatal mortality: field trial in rural India

Abhay T Bang, Rani A Bang, Sanjay B Baitule, M Hanimi Reddy, Mahesh D Deshmukh

Summary

Background Neonatal care is not available to most neonates in developing countries because hospitals are inaccessible and costly. We developed a package of home-based neonatal care, including management of sepsis (septicaemia, meningitis, pneumonia), and tested it in the field, with the hypothesis that it would reduce the neonatal mortality rate by at least 25% in 3 years.

Methods We chose 39 intervention and 47 control villages in the Gadchiroli district in India, collected baseline data for 2 years (1993–95), and then introduced neonatal care in the intervention villages (1995–98). Village health workers trained in neonatal care made home visits and managed birth asphyxia, premature birth or low birthweight, hypothermia, and breast-feeding problems. They diagnosed and treated neonatal sepsis. Assistance by trained traditional birth attendants, health education, and fortnightly supervisory visits were also provided. Other workers recorded all births and deaths in the intervention and the control area (1993–98) to estimate mortality rates.

Findings Population characteristics in the intervention and control areas, and the baseline mortality rates (1993–95) were similar. Baseline (1993–95) neonatal mortality rate in the intervention and the control areas was 62 and 58 per 1000 live births, respectively. In the third year of intervention 93% of neonates received home-based care. Neonatal, infant, and perinatal mortality rates in the intervention area (net percentage reduction) compared with the control area, were 25·5 (62·2%), 38·8 (45·7%), and 47·8 (71·0%), respectively (p<0·001). Case fatality in neonatal sepsis declined from 16·6% (163 cases) before treatment, to 2·8% (71 cases) after treatment by village health workers (p<0·01). Home-based neonatal care cost US$5.3 per neonate, and in 1997–98 such care averted one death (fetal or neonatal) per 18 neonates cared for.

Interpretation Home-based neonatal care, including management of sepsis, is acceptable, feasible, and reduced neonatal and infant mortality by nearly 50% among our malnourished, illiterate, rural study population. Our approach could reduce neonatal mortality substantially in developing countries.

Lancet 1999; **354:** 1955–61

SEARCH (Society for Education, Action, and Research in Community Health), Gadchiroli, Maharashtra, 442 605, India
(A T Bang MD, R A Bang MD, S B Baitule DHMS, M H Reddy PhD, M D Deshmukh MSc)

Correspondence to: Dr Abhay Bang

Introduction

Nearly 5 millon neonates worldwide die each year, 96% of them in developing countries. Neonatal mortality rate per 1000 live births varies from 5 in developed countries to 53 in the least developed countries.[1,2] Immunisation, oral rehydration, and control of acute respiratory infections have reduced the post-neonatal component of the infant mortality rate. Hence, neonatal mortality now constitutes 61% of infant mortality and nearly half of child mortality in developing countries.[1] For further substantial reduction in infant mortality, neonatal mortality in developing countries must be lowered.

63% of neonates in developing countries, and 83% in rural India, are born at home.[2,3] Standard advice is to admit every ill neonate to hospital,[2,4] but hospitals with facilities for neonatal care are inaccessible for rural populations. Parents may be unwilling to move ill neonates from home because of traditional beliefs and practical difficulties.[5-7] Hence, most neonatal deaths occur at home. Because of serious difficulties in transporting sick neonates to hospitals, those who arrive are generally seriously ill. The estimated cost of hospital-based neonatal care in India is very high.[8,9] Hence, to reduce neonatal mortality, ways to provide neonatal care at home must be developed.

The main causes of neonatal death are prematurity, birth asphyxia or injury, and infections.[2,10,11] Efforts to reduce neonatal mortality by management of birth asphyxia,[12] pre-term births, and low birthweight[13,14] have had varied success, but pneumonia, septicaemia, and meningitis (collectively, sepsis) have not been addressed.

Management of children with pneumonia, diarrhoea, or malaria by health workers is the main strategy of several child-survival programmes and of the Integrated Management of Childhood Illnesses programme.[15] This strategy, however, has not been used for management of sepsis in neonates. Our earlier work in management of pneumonia in neonates with oral co-trimoxazole given by village health workers resulted in 20% reduction in neonatal mortality,[5] and led us to believe that management of neonatal sepsis at home may be possible. We developed a package of home-based neonatal care, including the management of sepsis, and tested it in the field trial, with the hypothesis that the intervention will reduce the neonatal mortality rate by at least 25% in 3 years compared with the control area.

Methods

Study area

Our study was done in the Gadchiroli district of India (Maharashtra state), about 1000 km from the state capital, Mumbai (Bombay, figure 1). This is an extremely underdeveloped district, in which rice cultivation and forestry are the main sources of income. Roads, communications, education, and health services are poor. Government health services in the area comprise a male and a female paramedic worker for every 3000 people, and a primary health centre with

PUBLIC HEALTH

Public health

Insulin for the world's poorest countries

John S Yudkin

In the industrialised world, type 1 diabetes rarely results in death from ketoacidosis. The same is not true in many countries in the developing world where insulin availability is intermittent, and insulin may not even be included on national formularies of essential drugs. The life expectancy for a newly diagnosed patient with type 1 diabetes in some parts of Africa may be as short as 1 year. The World Bank has identified 40 highly indebted poor countries (HIPCs) whose national debt substantially exceeds any possibility of repayment without heavy impact on health and social programmes. Incidence and prognosis of type 1 diabetes in HIPCs are lower than in most industrialised countries, and 0·48% of the world's current use of insulin is estimated to be sufficient to treat all type 1 diabetic patients in these countries. A proposal is made for the major insulin manufacturers to donate insulin, at an estimated cost of US$3–5 million per year, as part of a distribution and education initiative for type 1 diabetic patients in the HIPCs. No type 1 diabetic patient in the world's poorest countries need then die because they, or their government cannot afford insulin.

Three quarters of a century after its discovery, insulin is not routinely available in many parts of the developing world.[1-3] A survey of 25 countries in Africa found that in half insulin was often unavailable in large city hospitals, whereas in only five countries was insulin regularly available in rural areas.[1] In some countries, insulin is not included in the national formulary.[4] In consequence, the life expectancy of a child with newly diagnosed type 1 diabetes in much of sub-Saharan Africa may be as short as 1 year.[5,6]

In the past decade, there has been a substantial decline in health care spending in many parts of the developing world,[7] largely because of heavy demands on government spending for debt repayment. Some countries spend more on interest repayment than on health care and education combined.[8,9] The amount available for health care, and in particular for pharmaceuticals—which have to be purchased with foreign exchange—may be as little as US$2–3 per person per year.[9,10] The World Bank has estimated that the minimum cost of providing basic health care, including essential drugs, for a community is four to five times this amount.[11]

The costs of outpatient health care for type 1 diabetes have been calculated for one African country as around US$229 per person per year, of which some two-thirds (US$156) is for insulin.[12] In a state-funded health care system in developing countries, treating one patient with type 1 diabetes might, in effect, be depriving 75 others of potentially lifesaving chloroquine or antibiotics. The alternative, of patients buying insulin, may cost the equivalent of 6 months salary per year, for continuous treatment.

The World Bank has defined 40 highly indebted poor countries (HIPCs) on the basis that debt repayment greatly exceeds the potential income, and as a consequence, programmes of social investment suffer.[13] The median per capita gross national product for these countries is US$310 per year. Very strict criteria for debt

---

Lancet 2000; **355**: 919–21

Royal Free and University College London School of Medicine, Whittington Hospital, London N19 3UA, UK
(e-mail: j.yudkin@ucl.ac.uk)

rescheduling have been agreed for only seven countries, but Jubilee 2000 is campaigning for cancellation of debt for these 40 countries by the World Bank, the International Monetary Fund, and the bilateral donor countries of the G8.[14] The campaign has gathered wide support in many countries.

My proposal is that the insulin manufacturers guarantee a regular and uninterrupted supply of insulin to the 40 HIPCs, sufficient for treatment of all type 1 diabetic patients. The insulin required is estimated to be less than 0·5% of the world's current use of insulin, and would cost US$3–5 million per year (less than 0·2% of the value of total insulin sales by the three major producers).

Prevalence of type 1 diabetes in highly indebted poor countries

Amos et al[15] reported the prevalence of diabetes in all countries in 1997. Because there are few studies of prevalence in the developing world, and those for all 40 HIPCs are based on but seven studies, these data are subject to substantial guesswork.

African type 1 diabetic patients under 15 years of age can expect to live for just 1 year;[5,6] and this figure has been applied to estimates for all countries where life expectancy for non-diabetics is under 50 years. Proportionately better prognosis has been assumed for people in countries with greater life expectancy in the general population. For type 1 diabetic patients over age 15, even fewer prevalence data are available, and Amos et al[15] assumed an incidence of two-thirds that in children under age 15.

The table shows the estimates[15] of total prevalence of type 1 and type 2 diabetes in 1997 in HIPCs, together with additional estimates for countries for which they did not calculate prevalence because the estimated numbers of type 1 patients was less than 100. Uninterrupted provision of insulin would probably improve greatly the outlook for type 1 diabetic patients, such that life expectancy might be increased about five-fold in those countries whose people have the poorest outlook. Even now, life expectancy for type 1 diabetic patients might be somewhat better than those cited,[16] with a correspondingly higher prevalence of type 1 diabetes (table).

PUBLIC HEALTH

Country	Population (million)*	Type 1 diabetic†	Adjusted type 1 diabetic‡	Type 2 diabetic†	Insulin need (vials)§	Adjusted insulin need (vials)‡§
Angola	30·2	200	1000	30 200	2555	12 775
Benin	5·6	76	380	22 600	971	4854
Bolivia	7·4	800	800	103 000	10 220	10 220
Burkina Fasso	10·2	100	500	43 400	1278	6387
Burundi	6·1	83	415	25 200	1060	5300
Cameroon	13·3	600	3000	42 300	7665	38 325
Central African Rep	3·3	44	220	11 900	562	2811
Chad	6·4	87	435	20 200	1111	5557
Congo Rep	2·3	31	155	8000	396	1980
Congo Dem Repub	43·9	500	2500	135 100	6388	31 938
Côte d'Ivoire	14·8	600	3000	60 200	7665	38 325
Equatorial Guinea	0·4	5	25	1400	64	320
Ethiopia	56·7	700	3500	245 800	8943	44 712
Ghana	17·5	800	800	78 400	10 220	10 220
Guinea	6·7	91	455	30 300	1163	5813
Guinea Bissau	1·1	15	75	5500	192	958
Guyana	0·8	100	100	25 600	1278	1278
Honduras	6·1	900	900	158 100	11 498	11 498
Kenya	31·8	1200	6000	110 500	15 330	76 650
Lao PDR	4·9	66	330	25 400	843	4216
Liberia	2·8	38	190	11 100	485	2427
Madagascar	14·8	200	200	62 800	2556	2556
Mali	8·9	100	500	44 600	1278	6387
Mauritania	2·4	33	155	10 700	422	2108
Mozambique	17·4	200	1000	79 500	2555	12 775
Myanmar	45·1	600	600	287 600	7665	7665
Nicaragua	4·5	700	700	111 700	8943	8943
Niger	9·2	100	500	37 000	1278	6387
Rwanda	8·0	110	550	22 300	1405	7026
Sao Tomé & Principé	0·13	2	2	–	25	25
Senegal	8·6	120	600	35 700	1533	7665
Sierra Leone	4·5	61	305	19 500	779	3896
Somalia	9·1	100	500	40 100	1278	6387
Sudan	26·7	2200	11 000	362 500	28 105	140 525
Tanzania	30·3	400	2000	125 500	5110	25 550
Togo	4·1	100	500	18 100	1278	6387
Uganda	21·3	300	1500	74 700	3833	19 163
Vietnam	73·5	5500	5500	470 900	70 263	70 263
Yemen Republic	15·0	700	700	122 000	8943	8943
Zambia	9·4	200	1000	31 000	2555	12 775
Total	**585·2**	**18 762**	**52 592**	**3 150 400**	**239 691**	**671 995**

*Population in 1995 based on information from Jubilee 2000. †Based on ref 15, estimate for 1997. ‡Assuming life expectancy of 5 years for newly diagnosed type 1 diabetic patient in countries with general population life expectancy below 50 years. §Annual figure, assuming daily insulin dose of 35 U per day for all type 1 diabetic patients.

Estimated prevalence of diabetes in the highly indebted poor countries

The estimates of insulin requirements are based on a daily insulin dose of 35 U per day, and are shown as annual numbers of 10 mL vials of 100U insulin for calculated current prevalence, and for adjusted prevalence consequent upon improved life expectancy. Sufficient insulin to treat all type 1 diabetic patients in the 40 HIPCs would require 671 995 vials per year. This corresponds to only 0·45% of world insulin use, despite the fact HIPCs have 10% of the world population.

Logistics, education, and monitoring

Besides the supply of insulin, secure distribution networks and educational support will also be needed. Nevertheless, the experience of the International Diabetes Federation (IDF) insulin task force suggests that grass-roots health workers in these countries know how to use insulin when it is available. Clearly it would be invidious to prescribe single approaches to insulin delivery and patient education and care in countries with very different health care systems. Attempts to install vertical programmes of health care development in the world's poorest countries, without reference to existing health care systems, have proven costly and ineffective.[17] Firm commitments from ministries of health in the 40 HIPCs as partners to ensure the satisfactory distribution of insulin and education of health workers will be required, and will necessitate coordination between representatives of industry, the IDF, ministries of health, pharmacists, doctors, and others caring for diabetic patients, and the patients and their families.

Several organisations concerned with diabetes, or with pharmaceutical supply, in the developing world already exist. The insulin task force of the IDF consists of volunteers, and does not have the infrastructure to take this on. Other bodies experienced in drug distribution lack the educational and data gathering skills envisaged for the programme, or exist mainly for medical care in emergencies. For this reason, an insulin foundation for developing countries is proposed, to coordinate the programme of supply and education, and to liaise with all partners. The foundation would establish and monitor agreed guidelines for all partners about the supply, distribution, and use of insulin, to obviate possible exploitation of the donations. The foundation would need a small permanent staff with expertise in pharmacy, health care planning, diabetes education, and epidemiology, and a board of trustees, which would include industry representatives. A suggested approach to the programme would be for each manufacturer to donate a proportion (corresponding to estimates of the use of insulin by type 1 diabetic patients) of the average insulin use over the past 5 years. In some countries it might be feasible to establish formulation plants, and to supply insulin in crystalline form.

The introduction of any such programme would need to be accompanied by several measures at country level, both educational and logistic. For an insulin foundation for developing countries to take on such tasks in each of the 40 HIPCs is clearly not feasible, and the role of the foundation would be to provide support, and advice on best practice, to health care planners and practitioners in these countries. The best way for health services to order, store, and distribute insulin, syringes and testing equipment would need to be found. Patients and their families need to understand insulin administration and storage, as well as diabetes self-monitoring. The insulin supplied under the scheme must be used for the purposes intended, rather than for inappropriate treatment of type 2 diabetic patients, or for sale for gain. The guarantee that these measures are instigated and audited should be a condition of the continuation of a country's supply, with breaches being grounds for cancellation.

The local difficulties will differ substantially country by country. Different companies will have particular areas of geographical interest, knowledge, and expertise, as well as clear information about current patterns of insulin use. Support for such a programme from the insulin manufacturers might include some element of redeployment of pharmaceutical company representatives, and producing material for the training of health workers in the management and monitoring of diabetes. The existence of the essential vaccines programme makes the provision of continuously refrigerated supplies possible— even to the most remote health centres and dispensaries in most developing countries.[18] In addition, the programme will encourage collection of reliable data on the prevalence of type 1 diabetes.

Costs of a programme of insulin supply

If manufacturers supply the insulin needs of type 1 diabetic patients in the 40 HIPCs free of charge, would the cost be proportionate to that of requirement—in other words around 0·5% of current world insulin costs? At present, animal insulin is sold at a substantially lower price than human insulin, so that, even at market prices, supplying 0·45% of the world's insulin supply because animal insulin should cost US$3–4 million.[3,19] Costs might be reduced by use of insulin that is being withdrawn from other markets—because of changes in strength, formulation, or species. The costs of drug production are not always tightly related to market price, which includes components for promotion and advertising, and return on investment. Thus the real cost of provision of insulin to type 1 diabetic patients in HIPCs would be only a small proportion of the calculated market cost, besides being offset against the benefits of such a gesture in terms of publicity.

A separate foundation would necessitate additional funding for a central staff and for freight and travel costs. These annual costs, totalling around US$1–2 million per year, could be raised as donations from governmental and charitable organisations in the industrialised countries.

The insulin manufacturers have a long tradition of philanthropy, and indeed Nordisk Insulin Laboratory in Denmark was established as a non-profit company. The insulin manufacturers also continue to support programmes of insulin distribution in the former Soviet Union and elsewhere.[20] The current proposal has parallels in WHO programmes for lymphatic filariasis, supported by SmithKline Beecham,[21] which has led to substantial positive publicity and acclaim for their philanthropy and ethical behaviour.

Acknowledgments
I thank many colleagues for their input and advice, in particular, Ron Raab, Geoff Gill, Jean-Claude Mbanya, and Andrew Swai. Jubilee 2000 can be contacted at P O Box 100, London SE1 7RT, UK, or by telephone ((44)-(0)207-620-4444 ext 2169), fax ((44)-(0)207-620-0719) or e-mail at mail@jubilee2000uk.org.

References

1   McLarty DG, Swai ABM, Alberti KGMM. Insulin availability in Africa: an insoluble problem? *Int Diab Dig* 1994; **5:** 15–17.

2   Savage A. The insulin dilemma: a survey of insulin treatment in the tropics. *Int Diab Dig* 1994; **5:** 19–20.

3   Deeb LC, Tan MH, Alberti KGMM. Insulin availability among International Diabetes Federation member associations. *Diab Care* 1994; **17:** 220–223.

4   Alberti KGMM. Insulin: availability and cost. *World Health Forum* 1994; **15:** 6 (letter).

5   Makame M for the Diabetes Epidemiology Research International Study Group. Childhood diabetes, insulin, and Africa. *Diabet Med* 1992; **9:** 571–73.

6   Castle W, Wicks A. A follow-up of 93 newly diagnosed African diabetics for 6 years. *Diabetologia* 1980; **18:** 121–23.

7   United Nations Development Programme. Human Development Report. New York: UN, 1997.

8   Abbasi K. The World Bank and world health. Under fire. *BMJ* 1999; **318:** 1003–1006.

9   Yudkin JS. Tanzania–still optimistic after all these years? *Lancet* 1999; **353:** 1519–21.

10 Jubilee 2000. The Debt Cutter's Handbook. ISBN 0 9528683 1 8. London, 1996.

11 The World Bank. World Development Report 1993. Investing in Health. Oxford University Press, Oxford, 1993.

12 Chale SS, Swai ABM, Mujinja PGM, McLarty DG. Must diabetes be a fatal disease in Africa? Study of costs of treatment. *BMJ* 1992; **304:** 1215–18.

13 Abbasi K. The World Bank and world health. Changing sides. *BMJ* 1999; **318:** 865–69.

14 Abbasi K. Free the slaves. *Br Med J* 1999; **318:** 1568–69.

15 Amos AF, McCarty DJ, Zimmet P. The rising global burden of diabetes and its complications: estimates and projections to the year 2010. *Diabet Med* 1997; **14** (Suppl 5): S1–S85.

16 Gill GV. Outcome of diabetes in Africa. In Diabetes in Africa. Eds G Gill, J-C Mbanya and G Alberti. FSG Communications Ltd, Cambridge, pp65–71.

17 Decosas J. Developing health in Africa. *Lancet* 1999; **353:** 143–44.

18 Zaffran N. Vaccine transport and storage: environmental challenges. *Dev Biol Stand* 1996; **87:** 9–17.

19 Chantelau E. Diabetes treatment in developing countries. *Lancet* 1993; **342:** 620 (letter).

20 Raab R. The problem of access to insulin, test strips and other diabetes supplies in many countries, and how to improve it. *Practical Diabetes International* 1999; **16:** 58–60.

21 Anonymous. Lymphatic filariasis elimination. WHO, SmithKline Beecham to cooperate on elephantiasis elimination. WHO Division of Control of Tropical Disease. Accessed on: http://158.232.17.12/ctd/html/filariasissb.html, 10 Sept 1999.

RESEARCH LETTERS

Regeneration of cutaneous innervation in a human hand allograft

Jean Kanitakis, Denis Jullien, Bastiaan De Boer, Alain Claudy, Jean Michel Dubernard

On Sept 23, 1998, a human hand allograft was done in our hospital. We followed up the patients for 24 months to assess the skin structure by immunohistology. Most cutaneous structures (including dermal nerves with their Schwann cells and perineurial fibroblasts) were present immediately after surgery and remained detectable throughout the study; from day 464 onwards, axons became detectable within dermal nerves, and their density increased progressively with time. Merkel cells reappeared in the epidermis 12 months after the operation. The regeneration of cutaneous innervation paralleled the recovery of cutaneous sensitivity.

We have previously reported a patient who was given a human hand allograft in our hospital.[1] Sequential histological and immunohistochemical study of skin biopsy samples taken from the allograft at various times in the early period after the operation (up to the third month) enabled us to detect signs of acute graft rejection and to assess the quality of the allografted skin.[2,3]

We report on the regeneration of cutaneous innervation of the allograft that occurred progressively in the mid-term observation period.

To study skin innervation, 4 mm punch biopsy samples were regularly obtained from the skin of the grafted forearm at various days after the operation (day 5–730), fixed in formalin and embedded in paraffin. At day 524 a biopsy sample was taken from the periungual area of the middle finger. The presence and quality of dermal nerves was monitored by routine histology and immunohistochemistry, with a polyclonal antibody to S100 protein that recognises Schwann cells, a monoclonal antibody to the 70, 160, and 210 kDa neurofilaments, and an antibody to epithelial membrane antigen that recognised perineural fibroblasts. Merkel cells were sought with an antibody to keratin 20. Additional antibodies were used to study the presence of cycling cells (MIB1/Ki67), Langerhans cells (Lag), melanocytes (MelanA/MART1), dermal dendrocytes (CD34, factor XIIIa), endothelial cells (CD34, von Willebrand factor), and mast cells (tryptase).

Overall, the structure of the skin remained normal after the initial 3-month period, as reported previously.[3] Several cycling (Ki67+) keratinocytes were found in the basal epidermal layer in all biopsy samples, showing that the epidermis was capable of self-renewal. Epidermal Langerhans cells and melanocytes, dermal dendrocytes, mast cells, eccrine sweat glands, blood

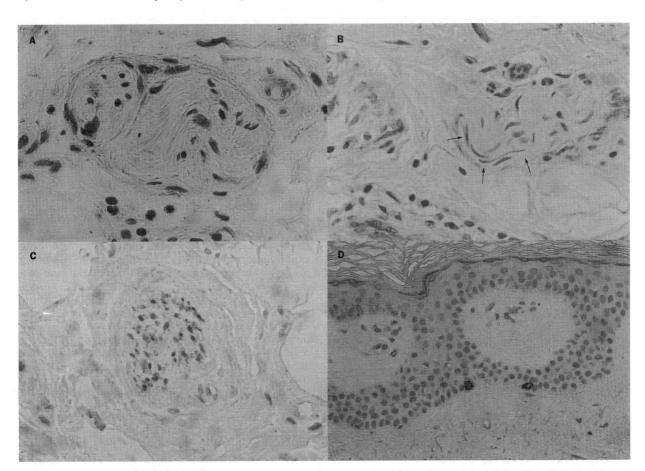

Immunohistochemistry findings at days 85, 465, 566, and 342

A: Day 85, dermal nerves contain perineural fibroblasts and Schwann cells but no axons, as shown by absence of neurofilament immunoreactivity (immunoperoxidase revealed with aminoethylcarbazole 3250). B: Day 464, a slender axon (arrows) is revealed within a dermal nerve (immunoperoxidase shown with aminoethylcarbazole 3400). C: Day 566, several axons are present within a dermal nerve. Note obvious increase of number compared with Panel B (immunoperoxidase revealed with aminoethylcarbazole 3400). D: Day 342, two keratin-20-positive Merkel cells are seen in basal layer of epidermis of allograft (immunoperoxidase revealed with aminoethylcarbazole 3400).

ARTICLES

Parents' accounts of obtaining a diagnosis of childhood cancer

Mary Dixon-Woods, Michelle Findlay, Bridget Young, Helen Cox, David Heney

Summary

Background Quick diagnosis and treatment of cancers is a UK government priority. However, the process of arriving at a diagnosis of childhood cancer has been neglected in comparison with the attention given to cancers in adults. We investigated parents' narratives about the period before their child's diagnosis.

Methods We undertook semistructured interviews with 20 parents whose children (aged 4–18 years) had a confirmed diagnosis of cancer or brain tumour. All interviews were recorded and fully transcribed. Dates of consultations and investigations were noted from children's medical records. Data were analysed by the constant comparison method.

Findings The time before diagnosis is very significant for parents and might affect their adaptation and reaction to their child's diagnosis. Parents were first alerted to their child's illness by a range of signs and symptoms, and by behavioural and affective changes. These early symptoms were often vague, non-specific, and common, and some older children were reluctant to disclose symptoms. Ten families' accounts of this period before diagnosis included a dispute with doctors. Disagreements between parents and doctors about the seriousness of children's symptoms and the need for investigations occurred in both primary and secondary care. Some parents felt that doctors discounted their special knowledge of their child.

Interpretation Parents' accounts offer valuable insights into their experiences of obtaining a diagnosis of childhood cancer and into possible sources of delays in this complex process. If delays are to be avoided or reduced, attention must be given to the different roles of parents, children, general practitioners, hospital specialists, and type of cancer. Our findings have important implications for policy, practice, and research, and for the management of childhood illnesses.

Lancet 2001; **357**: 670–74

Department of Epidemiology and Public Health
(M Dixon-Woods DPhil, B Young PhD) **and Faculty of Medicine and Biological Sciences** (M Findlay BSc), **University of Leicester; and Children's Hospital, Leicester Royal Infirmary, Leicester, UK**
(H Cox MRCP, D Heney MD)

Correspondence to: Dr Mary Dixon-Woods, Department of Epidemiology and Public Health, University of Leicester, Leicester LE1 6TP, UK
(e-mail: md11@le.ac.uk)

Introduction

The UK government has made a commitment to addressing delay in cancer diagnosis and improvement of public awareness and rapid referral of patients with signs and symptoms suggestive of cancer.[1] Children in whom cancer is suspected by their general practitioner (GP) can expect to be seen within 2 weeks by a cancer specialist, but clearly the success of this strategy depends on children presenting with symptoms and on doctors recognising those symptoms as being suggestive of cancer. Much research exists on factors that cause delays in patients' presentation to health services and clinician diagnoses for many cancers in adults.[2,3] Childhood cancers receive less attention than those of adults[4,5] despite recent suggestions that early detection of childhood cancer could reduce mortality.[6] This lack of attention might be partly attributable to the low importance of children's health issues in government policy and research,[7,8] coupled with the rarity of childhood cancer. Nevertheless, when childhood cancer happens, its effects are devastating, and survivors and their families face a lifetime of coping with its aftermath. It is important that parents' experiences of the time before diagnosis are understood.

We examined parents' narratives about the diagnosis of childhood cancer, with the aim of determining how parents felt about the process, how the process affected them, and whether these narratives had implications for early diagnosis and referral of childhood cancers.

Methods

Study design

Over 7 months we undertook semistructured interviews with one or both parents of a child with cancer. This type of interview is an effective method for investigation of parents' experiences of seeking help.[9] We also examined children's medical records to attempt to corroborate parents' accounts and to obtain more precise details of dates, referrals, and investigations. We obtained research ethics committee approval for the project. MF, who did not help to care for any of the children, did the interviews in parents' homes. MF recorded sociodemographic information with a brief questionnaire before interview. Interviews were open-ended, but MF used a prompt guide to ensure that similar topics were discussed every time. We noted the signs and symptoms that parents reported as serious and how they acted on these, their accounts of interactions with health services, and how they perceived the roles of themselves, their children, and health professionals. All interviews were recorded and transcribed verbatim.

Participants

Purposeful sampling is an accepted method in qualitative research and does not aim for statistical representativeness.[10] We included parents of children who had a confirmed diagnosis of leukaemia, malignant solid tumour, or brain tumour. The children were aged between 4 and 18 years and were either receiving treatment or had completed treatment in the previous 4 months at a paediatric oncology unit. To avoid

Articles

Whole genome sequencing of meticillin-resistant *Staphylococcus aureus*

Makoto Kuroda, Toshiko Ohta, Ikuo Uchiyama, Tadashi Baba, Harumi Yuzawa, Ichizo Kobayashi, Longzhu Cui, Akio Oguchi, Ken-ichi Aoki, Yoshimi Nagai, JianQi Lian, Teruyo Ito, Mutsumi Kanamori, Hiroyuki Matsumaru, Atsushi Maruyama, Hiroyuki Murakami, Akira Hosoyama, Yoko Mizutani-Ui, Noriko K Takahashi, Toshihiko Sawano, Ryu-ichi Inoue, Chikara Kaito, Kazuhisa Sekimizu, Hideki Hirakawa, Satoru Kuhara, Susumu Goto, Junko Yabuzaki, Minoru Kanehisa, Atsushi Yamashita, Kenshiro Oshima, Keiko Furuya, Chie Yoshino, Tadayoshi Shiba, Masahira Hattori, Naotake Ogasawara, Hideo Hayashi, Keiichi Hiramatsu

Summary

Background *Staphylococcus aureus* is one of the major causes of community-acquired and hospital-acquired infections. It produces numerous toxins including superantigens that cause unique disease entities such as toxic-shock syndrome and staphylococcal scarlet fever, and has acquired resistance to practically all antibiotics. Whole genome analysis is a necessary step towards future development of countermeasures against this organism.

Methods Whole genome sequences of two related *S aureus* strains (N315 and Mu50) were determined by shot-gun random sequencing. N315 is a meticillin-resistant *S aureus* (MRSA) strain isolated in 1982, and Mu50 is an MRSA strain with vancomycin resistance isolated in 1997. The open reading frames were identified by use of GAMBLER and GLIMMER programs, and annotation of each was done with a BLAST homology search, motif analysis, and protein localisation prediction.

Findings The *Staphylococcus* genome was composed of a complex mixture of genes, many of which seem to have been acquired by lateral gene transfer. Most of the antibiotic resistance genes were carried either by plasmids or by mobile genetic elements including a unique resistance island. Three classes of new pathogenicity islands were identified in the genome: a toxic-shock-syndrome toxin island family, exotoxin islands, and enterotoxin islands. In the latter two pathogenicity islands, clusters of exotoxin and enterotoxin genes were found closely linked with other gene clusters encoding putative pathogenic factors. The analysis also identified 70 candidates for new virulence factors.

Interpretation The remarkable ability of *S aureus* to acquire useful genes from various organisms was revealed through the observation of genome complexity and evidence of lateral gene transfer. Repeated duplication of genes encoding superantigens explains why *S aureus* is capable of infecting humans of diverse genetic backgrounds, eliciting severe immune reactions. Investigation of many newly identified gene products, including the 70 putative virulence factors, will greatly improve our understanding of the biology of staphylococci and the processes of infectious diseases caused by *S aureus*.

Lancet 2001; **357**: 1225–40
See Commentary page 1218

The entire genome sequences of *S aureus* N315 and Mu50 have been deposited in the DDBJ/Genbank/EMBL database under the accession numbers AP003129–AP003138 and AP003358–AP003366, respectively. The plasmid sequences of *S aureus* N315 and Mu50 have been deposited in the DDBJ/Genbank/EMBL database under the accession numbers AP003139 and AP003367, respectively.

Department of Bacteriology, Juntendo University, Tokyo, Japan (M Kuroda PhD, T Baba PhD, H Yuzawa, PhD, L Cui MD, J-Q Lian MD, T Ito PhD, K Hiramatsu MD); **University of Tsukuba, College of Medical Technology and Nursing, Tsukuba** (T Ohta PhD, M Kanamori PhD, H Matsumaru MSc, A Maruyama MSc, H Murakami MSc); **Research Center for Computational Science, Okazaki National Research Institutes, Okazaki** (I Uchiyama MSc); **Division of Basic Medical Sciences, Institute of Medical Science, University of Tokyo, Tokyo** (I Kobayashi PhD, Y Mizutani-Ui MSc, N Kobayashi PhD); **National Institute of Technology and Evaluation** (A Oguchi ASc, K-I Aoki BSc, Y Nagai ASc, A Hosoyama ASc, T Sawano BSc); **Graduate School of Pharmaceutical Sciences, University of Tokyo, Tokyo** (R-I Inoue PhD, C Kaito BSc, K Sekimizu PhD); **Faculty of Agriculture, Kyushu University, Fukuoka** (H Hirakawa PhD, S Kuhara PhD); **Institute for Chemical Research, Kyoto University, Kyoto** (S Goto PhD, J Yabuzaki MSc, M Kanehisa PhD); **School of Science, Kitasato University, Kanagawa** (A Yamashita PhD, K Oshima MSc, K Furuya BSc, C Yoshino BSc, T Shiba PhD, M Hattori PhD); **Human Genome Research Group, RIKEN Genomic Sciences Center, Kanagawa** (M Hattori PhD); **Nara Institute of Science and Technology, Graduate School of Biological Sciences, Nara** (N Ogasawara PhD); **Institute of Basic Medical Sciences, University of Tsukuba, Tsukuba** (H Hayashi MD)

Correspondence to: Dr Keiichi Hiramatsu, Department of Bacteriology, Juntendo University, 2-1-1 Hongo, Bunkyo-ku, Tokyo 113-8421, Japan
(e-mail: hiram@med.juntendo.ac.jp)

Introduction

Staphylococcus aureus is a gram-positive bacterium grouped with *Bacillus* sp on the basis of ribosomal RNA sequences. This immobile coccus grows in aerobic and anaerobic conditions, in which it forms grape-like clusters. Its main habitats are the nasal membranes and skin of warm-blooded animals, in whom it causes a range of infections from mild, such as skin infections and food poisoning, to life-threatening, such as pneumonia, sepsis, osteomyelitis, and infectious endocarditis.[1] The organism produces many toxins and is highly efficient at overcoming antibiotic effectiveness. In 1961 it developed resistance to meticillin, invalidating almost all antibiotics including the most potent β-lactams.[2]

Since the 1970s, meticillin-resistant *S aureus* (MRSA) has become the main cause of nosocomial infection worldwide. Vancomycin was the only antibiotic effective against it, but in 1997, a vancomycin-resistant *S aureus* (VRSA) was also isolated.[3,4] We are now exposed to the threat of MRSA without having developed any antibiotics with greater activity than vancomycin. What is urgently needed is an insight into how the organism generates such

ARTICLES

encoding restriction activity. Some restriction-modification systems essentially stabilise the maintenance of such linked regions, since cells in which the region is deleted are killed as a result of restriction-enzyme activity.[40] A homology search identified an orphan type IC *hsdR* homologue (SA0189) at a location distant from the two islands. This restriction enzyme might therefore be used to form two restriction-modification systems with different target specificities to stabilise maintenance of both islands of the SET-SE family.

Other pathogenic factors
Other pathogenic factors identified in this study are listed in table 4. Among them, a newly identified open reading frame SA0276 encoding a diarrhoeal toxin homologue of *B cereus*[41] is particularly intriguing, because Japanese MRSA strains commonly cause postoperative watery diarrhoea and its cause has not been clearly associated with previously known exotoxins.

Discussion
Acquisition of SCC*mec* has provided *S aureus* with the β-lactam-insensitive cell-wall synthesis enzyme PBP2′, which has made it the most resistant pathogenic organism in hospital-acquired infection. From the genome-research point of view, this acquisition has a major role in the complexity of the *S aureus* genome. For example, we judge that the genome complexity of the first sextant of the *S aureus* genome is at least partly caused by repeated integration and deletion events of SCCs (figure 1). A single integration event of an SCC with a size equivalent to type-II SCC*mec* results in the chimeric structure of the *S aureus* chromosome, in which the first 2% is composed of exogenous DNA. *att*BSCC sequences are reconstituted at the SCC-chromosome junctions every time SCC is integrated,[42] and sequential tandem integration of SCC copies at the reconstituted *att*BSCC site has been shown in vitro (unpublished data).

Besides SCC*mec*, we identified 26 and 28 mobile genetic elements, and three and four pathogenicity or genomic islands in the N315 and Mu50 chromosomes, respectively (table 1). Most of them carry either antibiotic resistance genes or virulence genes that must have been acquired from other bacterial species. In addition, we have found some putative cases of lateral gene transfer from distantly related organisms even among the solitary genes studded within the *S aureus* chromosome. These observations signify not only the extreme complexity of the *S aureus* genome but also its plasticity, the latter of which presumably facilitates the bacterium's ability to adapt to environmental selective pressures such as antibiotics and the human immune system.

Besides vancomycin resistance, Mu50 expresses high-level β-lactam resistance (minimum inhibitory concentration [MIC] of meticillin 512 mg/L). By contrast, N315 is only partly resistant to β-lactam antibiotics (MIC of meticillin 4 mg/L), and is susceptible to vancomycin. However, a two-step selection procedure with β-lactam confers N315 with the high β-lactam resistance expressed by Mu50, and the same procedure with vancomycin makes N315 resistant to vancomycin.[3] The precise genetic events underlying these phenotypic conversions have not been elucidated yet; however, the results of the present study should provide a basis on which to begin these investigations. Aside from the difference in integrated mobile genetic elements, there are fewer than 0·08% overall nucleotide sequence differences between the two strains. Given this close relatedness, detailed sequence comparison and gene expression studies will ultimately identify genes responsible for vancomycin and high β-lactam resistance.

One of the most striking observations in this study is the extreme diversity of superantigens produced by *S aureus*. None of the ten SET homologues had greater than 90% aminoacid identity with the five SET proteins previously found in other strains (figure 4). The presence of three alleles for the *set1* gene has been reported previously,[36] but none of the ten *set* paralogues of N315 or Mu50 belonged to any of the three alleles. This extreme heterogeneity in both gene number and the encoded peptide sequences strongly indicates that the gene cluster is generated by sequential gene duplication in individual strains. Since innumerable *S aureus* strains colonise human beings as natural flora, the diversity of superantigens harboured by *S aureus* is presumably extremely large; perhaps as large as the diversity of human T-cell Vβ and class-II MHC molecules.

Besides the ten SETs, we identified five more new candidates of superantigens (table 4). Including previously identified ones, 25 superantigen homologues were found in the N315 and Mu50 genomes. Production of such an array of superantigens by a single cell reflects the nature of the multiplication strategy of *S aureus* in the human body. Unlike other species of bacteria such as *Neisseria* and *Salmonella*, *S aureus* might not have developed a system of evading the host immune response as the main strategy for survival. On the contrary, *S aureus* seems to challenge host immune response by eliciting regional inflammation and subsequent abscess formation. To be shut in inside the abscess could be advantageous for *S aureus* cells, because the secreted exoenzymes would become concentrated and efficiently destroy white blood cells (with haemolysins and leukocidins) and digest tissues.

Besides toxic-shock syndrome and newly identified inflammatory disease, superantigens are also implicated in the pathogenesis of Kawasaki's disease.[43] An intensive search for the superantigens that cause this disease has been done, but so far none of the previously identified superantigens has been unequivocally correlated with it (T Uchiyama, personal communication). The present study revealed that we are aware of only a fraction of the superantigen diversity that *S aureus* is capable of generating. Searching for new superantigens from clinical *S aureus* strains might shed light on research into Kawasaki's disease and other inflammatory diseases of unknown cause.

Contributors
All investigators contributed to the design of the study and to the writing of the paper. Keiichi Hiramatsu was responsible for experimental design and interpretation of data in both N315 and Mu50 genome projects, and analysed genome complexity. Makoto Kuroda constructed the genomic libraries, and annotated the N315 genome. Toshiko Ohta, Hideo Hayashi, and Naotake Ogasawara designed the experiments on the Mu50 genome project. Ikuo Uchiyama did analyses of codon usage, GC3, and BLAST best hits. Tadashi Baba, Harumi Yuzawa, and Longzhu Cui analysed the genome for pathogenic factors, intermediary metabolism, and repetitive sequences, respectively. Akio Oguchi, Yoshimi Nagai, and Akira Hosoyama did shotgun sequencing of the N315 genome. Ken-ichi Aoki, and Toshihiko Sawano did the BLAST search analysis and illustrations in collaboration with Makoto Kuroda and Keiichi Hiramatsu. Ichizo Kobayashi, Yoko Mizutani-Ui,

Articles

Do women with pre-eclampsia, and their babies, benefit from magnesium sulphate? The Magpie Trial: a randomised placebo-controlled trial

The Magpie Trial Collaborative Group*

Summary

Background Anticonvulsants are used for pre-eclampsia in the belief they prevent eclamptic convulsions, and so improve outcome. Evidence supported magnesium sulphate as the drug to evaluate.

Methods Eligible women (n=10 141) had not given birth or were 24 h or less postpartum; blood pressure of 140/90 mm Hg or more, and proteinuria of 1+ (30 mg/dL) or more; and there was clinical uncertainty about magnesium sulphate. Women were randomised in 33 countries to either magnesium sulphate (n=5071) or placebo (n=5070). Primary outcomes were eclampsia and, for women randomised before delivery, death of the baby. Follow up was until discharge from hospital after delivery. Analyses were by intention to treat.

Findings Follow-up data were available for 10 110 (99·7%) women, 9992 (99%) of whom received the allocated treatment. 1201 of 4999 (24%) women given magnesium sulphate reported side-effects versus 228 of 4993 (5%) given placebo. Women allocated magnesium sulphate had a 58% lower risk of eclampsia (95% CI 40–71) than those allocated placebo (40, 0·8%, vs 96, 1·9%; 11 fewer women with eclampsia per 1000 women). Maternal mortality was also lower among women allocated magnesium sulphate (relative risk 0·55, 0·26–1·14). For women randomised before delivery, there was no clear difference in the risk of the baby dying (576, 12·7%, vs 558, 12·4%; relative risk 1·02, 99% CI 0·92–1·14). The only notable difference in maternal or neonatal morbidity was for placental abruption (relative risk 0·67, 99% CI 0·45–0·89).

Interpretation Magnesium sulphate halves the risk of eclampsia, and probably reduces the risk of maternal death. There do not appear to be substantive harmful effects to mother or baby in the short term.

Lancet 2002; **359**: 1877–90
See Commentary page 1872

*Members listed at end of paper

Correspondence to: Dr Lelia Duley

Resource Centre for Randomised Trials, Institute of Health Sciences, Headington, Oxford OX3 7LF, UK
(e-mail: lelia.duley@ndm.ox.ac.uk)

Introduction

Pre-eclampsia, a multisystem disorder of pregnancy usually associated with raised blood pressure and proteinuria, complicates 2–8% of pregnancies.[1] Although outcome is often good, pre-eclampsia is a major cause of morbidity and mortality for the woman and her child.[2] Eclampsia is defined as the occurrence of one or more convulsions superimposed on pre-eclampsia. In developed countries eclampsia is rare, affecting around one in 2000 deliveries,[3] while in developing countries estimates vary from one in 100 to one in 1700.[4,5] Worldwide an estimated 600 000 women die each year of pregnancy-related causes,[6] with 99% of these deaths occurring in developing countries. Pre-eclampsia and eclampsia probably account for more than 50 000 maternal deaths a year.[7] In places where maternal mortality is high, most of these deaths are associated with eclampsia. Where maternal mortality is lower, a higher proportion will be due to pre-eclampsia. For example, in the UK pre-eclampsia and eclampsia together account for 15% of direct maternal deaths, and two-thirds were related to pre-eclampsia.[2]

For decades anticonvulsant drugs have been given to women with pre-eclampsia, in the belief that they reduce the risk of seizure, and so improve outcome.[8] However, there has been little reliable evidence to support that belief. In 1998, a systematic review[9] of anticonvulsants for women with pre-eclampsia identified four trials (total 1249 women) comparing an anticonvulsant with no anticonvulsant or placebo. This review concluded that magnesium sulphate was the most promising choice for pre-eclampsia, and the priority for further evaluation. Additionally, magnesium sulphate is now the drug of choice for women with eclampsia, with strong evidence that it is better than either diazepam,[10] phenytoin,[11] or lytic cocktail.[12]

The use of magnesium sulphate for pre-eclampsia is increasing,[13] although a range of other anticonvulsant drugs continue to be used, including diazepam and other benzodiazepines, phenytoin, barbiturates, and lytic cocktail. There is also substantial variation in the severity of pre-eclampsia for which a prophylactic anticonvulsant is used. In the USA, for example, magnesium sulphate is given to an estimated 5% of pregnant women before delivery.[14] By contrast, a quarter of UK obstetricians never use any prophylactic anticonvulsants,[13] and those who do often restrict their use to women with severe pre-eclampsia, which is around 1% of deliveries.

The initial question about magnesium sulphate, as a prophylactic anticonvulsant for women with pre-eclampsia, is whether it reduces the risk of eclampsia. Even if it does, reliable information is required before magnesium sulphate can be safely recommended for clinical practice; in particular about the size of any risk reduction, effects on other important outcomes for the woman and child, and disease severity at which benefits outweigh the risks. The Magpie Trial (MAGnesium sulphate for Prevention of Eclampsia) was a large

MRC/BHF Heart Protection Study of antioxidant vitamin supplementation in 20 536 high-risk individuals: a randomised placebo-controlled trial

Heart Protection Study Collaborative Group*

Summary

Background It has been suggested that increased intake of various antioxidant vitamins reduces the incidence rates of vascular disease, cancer, and other adverse outcomes.

Methods 20 536 UK adults (aged 40–80) with coronary disease, other occlusive arterial disease, or diabetes were randomly allocated to receive antioxidant vitamin supplementation (600 mg vitamin E, 250 mg vitamin C, and 20 mg β-carotene daily) or matching placebo. Intention-to-treat comparisons of outcome were conducted between all vitamin-allocated and all placebo-allocated participants. An average of 83% of participants in each treatment group remained compliant during the scheduled 5-year treatment period. Allocation to this vitamin regimen doubled the plasma concentrations of α-tocopherol, increased that of vitamin C by one-third, and quadrupled β-carotene. Primary outcomes were major coronary events (for overall analyses) and fatal or non-fatal vascular events (for subcatergory analyses), with subsidiary assessment of cancer and other major morbidity.

Findings There were no significant differences in all-cause mortality (1446 [14·1%] vitamin-allocated vs 1389 [13·5%] placebo-allocated), or in deaths due to vascular (878 [8·6%] vs 840 [8·2%]) or non-vascular (568 [5·5%] vs 549 [5·3%]) causes. Nor were there any significant differences in the numbers of participants having non-fatal myocardial infarction or coronary death (1063 [10·4%] vs 1047 [10·2%]), non-fatal or fatal stroke (511 [5·0%] vs 518 [5·0%]), or coronary or non-coronary revascularisation (1058 [10·3%] vs 1086 [10·6%]). For the first occurrence of any of these "major vascular events", there were no material differences either overall (2306 [22·5%] vs 2312 [22·5%]; event rate ratio 1·00 [95% CI 0·94–1·06]) or in any of the various subcategories considered. There were no significant effects on cancer incidence or on hospitalisation for any other non-vascular cause.

Interpretation Among the high-risk individuals that were studied, these antioxidant vitamins appeared to be safe. But, although this regimen increased blood vitamin concentrations substantially, it did not produce any significant reductions in the 5-year mortality from, or incidence of, any type of vascular disease, cancer, or other major outcome.

Lancet 2002; **360**: 23–33

*Collaborators and participating hospitals are listed in *Lancet* 2002; 360: xxx–xx.

Correspondence to: Heart Protection Study, Clinical Trial Service Unit and Epidemiological Studies Unit, Radcliffe Infirmary, Oxford OX2 6HE, UK
(e-mail: hps@ctsu.ox.ac.uk)

Introduction

LDL-cholesterol may be rendered more atherogenic by oxidative modification that allows it to accumulate in the artery walls, and antioxidants have been shown to slow the progression of atherosclerosis in animal studies.[1-4] Vitamin E is a major antioxidant in LDL particles, and supplementation with vitamin E substantially prolongs the in-vitro resistance of LDL particles to oxidative damage, and has other potentially protective effects.[3-8] β-carotene, which can also function as a fat-soluble antioxidant in certain physiological circumstances, is carried with vitamin E in the fatty core of LDL particles.[3,4] Vitamin C is a major water-soluble antioxidant in the plasma, and it can help to regenerate oxidised vitamin E.[4,9-11] In several non-randomised observational studies in different populations, dietary intake or plasma concentrations of these antioxidant vitamins were inversely associated with vascular disease incidence and mortality,[12-17] and blood concentrations of autoantibodies to oxidised LDL and the degree of LDL susceptibility to oxidative damage have been associated with atherosclerosis.[18,19] Dietary intake of antioxidant vitamins has also been reported in observational studies to be inversely associated with the incidence of various types of cancer.[16,17,20-23] But, without large-scale randomised evidence, the possibility that these associations merely reflect the effects of other aspects of the diet or lifestyle on disease rates cannot be ruled out.[20,24]

Promising results on the progression of atherosclerosis[25,26] and on the incidence of vascular disease[27,28] have been reported from some small randomised trials of a few years of vitamin E in people with pre-existing vascular disease. But, the available results from much larger randomised trials of several years of vitamin E have been unpromising.[29-34] Similarly, the results thus far available from large long-term randomised trials of β-carotene and of vitamin C have not provided good evidence of benefit.[29,30,34-37] Indeed, the result of some trials have even suggested that these vitamins have adverse effects (in particular on the incidence of haemorrhagic stroke and particular cancers[30,35]), although this observation has not been confirmed by other trials.

The Heart Protection Study provides further evidence about the effects of these three antioxidant vitamins on vascular and non-vascular mortality and major morbidity by a assessing 5 years of their supplementation in large number of high-risk individuals.

Patients and methods

Details of the study objectives, design, and methods are reported elsewhere[38,39] (including the protocol on the study website: www.hpsinfo.org) and are summarised below. As well as comparing antioxidant vitamins versus matching placebo in 20 536 randomised participants (which is the subject of the present report), a "2×2 factorial" design

Articles

⟨ @ Coronavirus as a possible cause of severe acute respiratory syndrome

J S M Peiris, S T Lai, L L M Poon, Y Guan, L Y C Yam, W Lim, J Nicholls, W K S Yee, W W Yan, M T Cheung, V C C Cheng, K H Chan, D N C Tsang, R W H Yung, T K Ng, K Y Yuen, and members of the SARS study group*

Summary

Background An outbreak of severe acute respiratory syndrome (SARS) has been reported in Hong Kong. We investigated the viral cause and clinical presentation among 50 patients.

Methods We analysed case notes and microbiological findings for 50 patients with SARS, representing more than five separate epidemiologically linked transmission clusters. We defined the clinical presentation and risk factors associated with severe disease and investigated the causal agents by chest radiography and laboratory testing of nasopharyngeal aspirates and sera samples. We compared the laboratory findings with those submitted for microbiological investigation of other diseases from patients whose identity was masked.

Findings Patients' age ranged from 23 to 74 years. Fever, chills, myalgia, and cough were the most frequent complaints. When compared with chest radiographic changes, respiratory symptoms and auscultatory findings were disproportionally mild. Patients who were household contacts of other infected people and had older age, lymphopenia, and liver dysfunction were associated with severe disease. A virus belonging to the family *Coronaviridae* was isolated from two patients. By use of serological and reverse-transcriptase PCR specific for this virus, 45 of 50 patients with SARS, but no controls, had evidence of infection with this virus.

Interpretation A coronavirus was isolated from patients with SARS that might be the primary agent associated with this disease. Serological and molecular tests specific for the virus permitted a definitive laboratory diagnosis to be made and allowed further investigation to define whether other cofactors play a part in disease progression.

Lancet 2003; **361:** 1319–25. Published online April 8, 2003
http://image.thelancet.com/extras/03art3477web.pdf
See Commentary pages 1312 and 1313

Introduction

An outbreak of atypical pneumonia in Guangdong Province, People's Republic of China, that has continued since November, 2002, is reported to have affected 792 people and caused 31 deaths.[1] In adjacent Hong Kong, surveillance of severe atypical pneumonia was heightened in the public hospital network under the Hospital Authority of Hong Kong. By the end of February, 2003, clusters of patients with pneumonia were noted in Hong Kong, along with affected close contacts and health-care workers. The disease did not respond to empirical antimicrobial treatment for acute community-acquired typical or atypical pneumonia. Bacteriological and virological pathogens known to cause pneumonia were not identified. Thus, the new disorder was called severe acute respiratory syndrome (SARS). Subsequently, SARS has spread worldwide to involve patients in North America, Europe, and other Asian countries.[1] We investigated patients in Hong Kong to try to identify the causal agent.

Methods

We included in the study 50 patients fitting a modified WHO definition of SARS admitted to three acute regional hospitals in Hong Kong between Feb 26 and March 26, 2003.[2] Briefly, the case definition was fever of 38°C or more, cough or shortness of breath, new pulmonary infiltrates on chest radiography, and a history of exposure to a patient with SARS or absence of response to empirical antimicrobial coverage for typical and atypical pneumonia (β lactams and macrolides, fluoroquinolones, or tetracyclines).

We collected nasopharyngeal aspirates and serum samples from all patients. Paired acute and convalescent sera and faeces were available from some patients. A lung-biopsy tissue sample from one patient was processed for viral culture and reverse-transcriptase PCR (RT-PCR) and for routine histopathological examination and electron microscopy. We used as controls nasopharyngeal aspirates, and faeces and sera submitted for microbiological investigation of other diseases from patients whose identities were masked.

The SARS patients' medical records were reviewed retrospectively by the attending physicians and clinical microbiologists. Routine haematological, biochemical, and microbiological work-up was done, including bacterial culture of blood and sputum, serology, and

*Members listed at the end of paper

Department of Microbiology and Pathology, Queen Mary Hospital, University of Hong Kong, Hong Kong (Prof J S M Peiris DPhil, L L M Poon DPhil, Y Guan PhD, J Nicholls FRCPA, V C C Cheng MRCP, K H Chan PhD, Prof K Y Yuen FRCPath)**; Department of Medicine, Intensive Care and Pathology, Princess Margaret Hospital, Hong Kong** (S T Lai FRCP, W W Yan FRCP, T K Ng FRCPath)**; Government Virus Unit, Department of Health, Hong Kong** (W Lim FRCPath)**; Department of Medicine and Pathology, Pamela Youde Nethersole Eastern Hospital, Hong Kong** (L Y C Yam FRCP, M T Cheung MRCP, R W H Yung FRCPath)**; Department of Medicine, Kwong Wah Hospital, Hong Kong** (W K S Yee MRCP)**; and Department of Pathology, Queen Elizabeth Hospital, Hong Kong Special Administrative Region, China** (D N C Tsang FRCPath)

Correspondence to: Prof J S M Peiris, Department of Microbiology, University of Hong Kong, Queen Mary Hospital, Pokfulam Road, Hong Kong, Special Administrative Region, China
(e-mail: malik@hkucc.hku.hk)

CHILD SURVIVAL I

Child survival I

Where and why are 10 million children dying every year?

Robert E Black, Saul S Morris, Jennifer Bryce

More than 10 million children die each year, most from preventable causes and almost all in poor countries. Six countries account for 50% of worldwide deaths in children younger than 5 years, and 42 countries for 90%. The causes of death differ substantially from one country to another, highlighting the need to expand understanding of child health epidemiology at a country level rather than in geopolitical regions. Other key issues include the importance of undernutrition as an underlying cause of child deaths associated with infectious diseases, the effects of multiple concurrent illnesses, and recognition that pneumonia and diarrhoea remain the diseases that are most often associated with child deaths. A better understanding of child health epidemiology could contribute to more effective approaches to saving children's lives.

Substantial reductions in child mortality occurred in low-income and middle-income countries in the late 20th century, but more than 10 million children younger than 5 years still die every year.[1,2] In this article, the first in a series of five, we consider reasons for these deaths and provide recommendations for how they can be prevented.

Rates of decline in worldwide child mortality peaked in about 1980.[1] In 1990–2001, the number of child deaths fell by 1·1% every year, compared with 2·5% per year during 1960–90.[3] Although this deceleration might be expected in areas that had already achieved low rates of mortality, such slowing has also occurred in high-rate regions. Sub-Saharan Africa had the highest child mortality in 1970–74, but in the years since has had the slowest fall in rate.[1] South Asia also had a high rate of child deaths in the 1970s, and despite a 50% drop in mortality, almost one in ten children in this region still dies before their fifth birthday.[1]

Child mortality varies among world regions, and these differences are large and increasing. In 1990, there were 180 deaths per 1000 livebirths in sub-Saharan Africa and only 9 per 1000 in industrialised countries—a 20-fold difference.[4] In 2000, this gap had increased to 29-fold with mortality rates of 175 and 6 per 1000 children in sub-Saharan Africa and industrialised countries, respectively.[4]

The World Summit for Children in 1990 called for a worldwide reduction in child mortality to below 70 deaths per 1000 livebirths (or a one-third reduction if this yielded a lower mortality rate) by the year 2000.[4] Unfortunately, investments in health systems and interventions necessary to achieve such a reduction in the 1990s were not commensurate with needs. The mortality reduction target was reached for only five of 55 countries with an under-5-year mortality rate of 100 or more in 1990.[4]

In 2002, as part of the millennium development goals for health, nations pledged to ensure a two-thirds reduction in child mortality by 2015, from the base year 1990.[5] In addition to setting such a goal, the global public health community must critically assess how it can be accomplished. A realistic picture of a country's epidemiological profile and the capabilities of its health system is needed before appropriate public health interventions can be developed and implemented.

Development of these interventions also requires an understanding of the determinants of child mortality. These determinants include, at the most distant level, socioeconomic factors, such as income, social status, and education, which work through an intermediate level of environmental and behavioural risk factors.[6] These risk factors, in turn, lead to the proximal causes of death (nearer in time to the terminal event), such as undernutrition, infectious diseases, and injury. In this paper, we will focus on proximal causes of death and on selected environmental and behavioural risk factors. The fourth article in this series will address the socioeconomic determinants of child mortality.

Where do most child deaths occur?

The estimate for global child deaths in 2000 is 10·8 million.[7] In this series, data from 2000 will be used throughout because they are most complete for this period and little has changed in the past 2 years. About 41% of child deaths occur in sub-Saharan Africa and another 34% in south Asia.[7] Because there is substantial variation in death rates within these regions, planning for health interventions should take place at a national level. The incomplete and unreliable nature of these

Lancet 2003; **361:** 2226–34
See Commentary page 2172

Johns Hopkins Bloomberg School of Public Health, Baltimore, MD, USA (Prof R E Black MD); **Department of Epidemiology and Population Health, London School of Hygiene and Tropical Medicine, London, UK** (S S Morris PhD); **and 25 rue du Bugnon, St Genis-Pouilly, 10630 France** (J Bryce EdD)

Correspondence to: Prof Robert E Black, Department of International Health, Johns Hopkins Bloomberg School of Public Health, Baltimore, MD 21205, USA
(e-mail: rblack@jhsph.edu)

Search strategy

The search strategy for the model used to estimate proportionate causes of death has been described.[32] Estimates of the importance of risk factors were taken from published results.[12] For our comorbidity analyses we also contacted researchers and directors of demographic surveillance areas in low-income and middle-income countries.

CHILD SURVIVAL I

Countries ranked by total number of child deaths	Number of child deaths*	Under-5-year mortality-rate rank†	Countries ranked by under-5-year mortality rate	Under-5-year mortality rate (per 1000 births)	Number of child deaths rank
India	2 402 000	54	Sierra Leone	316	36
Nigeria	834 000	17	Niger	270	12
China	784 000	88	Angola	260	11
Pakistan	565 000	43	Afghanistan	257	8
D R Congo	484 000	9	Liberia	235	51
Ethiopia	472 000	21	Mali	233	16
Bangladesh	343 000	57·5	Somalia	225	22
Afghanistan	251 000	4	Guinea-Bissau	215	70
Tanzania	223 000	23	D R Congo	205	5
Indonesia	218 000	76·5	Zambia	202	27
Angola	169 000	3	Chad	200	33
Niger	156 000	2	Mozambique	200	13
Mozambique	155 000	11·5	Burkina Faso	198	20
Uganda	145 000	36	Burundi	190	44
Myanmar	132 000	43	Malawi	188	25
Mali	128 000	6	Rwanda	187	42
Brazil	127 000	92	Nigeria	184	2
Kenya	125 000	39	Mauritania	183	59
Sudan	116 000	45·5	Central African Republic	180	54
Burkina Faso	104 000	13	Guinea	175	41
Iraq	104 000	34	Ethiopia	174	6
Somalia	100 000	7	Côte d'Ivoire	173	24
Yemen	97 000	43	Tanzania	165	9
Côte d'Ivoire	97 000	22	Benin	160	46
Malawi	96 000	15	Equatorial Guinea	156	89
Madagascar	93 000	30·5	Cameroon	154	28
Zambia	88 000	10	Djibouti	146	88
Cameroon	83 000	26	Swaziland	142	85
Philippines	82 000	88	Togo	142	55
South Africa	77 000	66·5	Senegal	139	45
Nepal	76 000	54	Madagascar	139	26
Egypt	76 000	80	Cambodia	135	39
Chad	73 000	11·5	Lesotho	133	73
Iran	71 000	82·5	Iraq	130	21
Mexico	70 000	101·5	Gambia	128	79
Sierra Leone	69 000	1	Uganda	127	14
Turkey	66 000	80	Haiti	125	52
Ghana	65 000	49	East Timor	124	90
Cambodia	63 000	32	Kenya	120	18
Viet Nam	63 000	91	Zimbabwe	117	43
Guinea	62 000	20	Eritrea	114	63
Rwanda	54 000	16	Yemen	110	23

*Number of deaths estimated by multiplying the number of livebirths[8] by the under-5-year mortality rate[7] and by a life-table based adjustment factor that slightly reduces the number of deaths if the yearly number of births has increased over the previous quinquennium and slightly increases it if births have fallen.[9] †Decimal places indicate that two countries were equally ranked.

Table 1: **Countries ranked by total child (under-5-year) deaths or by under-5-year mortality rates in 2000**

data in many countries can make this task difficult, so assessment of the needs and possible interventions for more homogeneous groups of countries is also worthwhile.

A few countries account for a very large proportion of all child deaths. In fact, half of worldwide deaths in children younger than 5 years occur in only six countries, and 90% in 42 countries (table 1).[7–9] However, the order of countries differs when ranked by child mortality rate rather than by number of deaths, in that countries in sub-Saharan Africa with quite small population sizes dominate the highest ranks (table 1); thus, the first 42 countries ranked by mortality rate constitute only 44% of child deaths worldwide.

Figure 1 shows that deaths are concentrated in some regions, in particular south Asia and sub-Saharan Africa. Even within countries, spatial variation in mortality rates can be large. In India, for example, the 1998–99 national family health survey found that mortality rates for children younger than 5 years varied from 18·8 per 1000 births in Kerala to 137·6 per 1000 in Madhya Pradesh.[10]

Although most child deaths in these countries occur in rural areas, urban slum populations can have especially high child mortality rates. For example, children in the slums of Nairobi, Kenya, have mortality rates much higher than rural Kenyan children (150·6 per 1000 livebirths *vs* 113·0, respectively).[11]

Risk factors for child mortality

Unhygienic and unsafe environments place children at risk of death.[2,12] Ingestion of unsafe water, inadequate availability of water for hygiene, and lack of access to sanitation contribute to about 1·5 million child deaths and around 88% of deaths from diarrhoea.[2,12] Other health-related behaviours, such as birth spacing, are also important risk factors for child mortality.[13]

Infants aged 0–5 months who are not breastfed have seven-fold and five-fold increased risks of death from diarrhoea and pneumonia, respectively, compared with infants who are exclusively breastfed.[14] At the same age, non-exclusive rather than exclusive breastfeeding results in more than two-fold increased risks of dying from diarrhoea or pneumonia.[15] 6–11-month-old infants who are not breastfed also have an increased risk of such deaths.[16]

Child deaths are commonly the result of several risk factors. In the future, the joint effects of two or more risk factors on each underlying or associated cause of death should be estimated together.[17] Thus, the total effect of interventions to prevent or mitigate the effects of various sets of risk factors could be established.

Underlying causes of death

WHO's work on the global burden of disease, consistent with the International Classification of Diseases (ICD),

CHILD SURVIVAL I

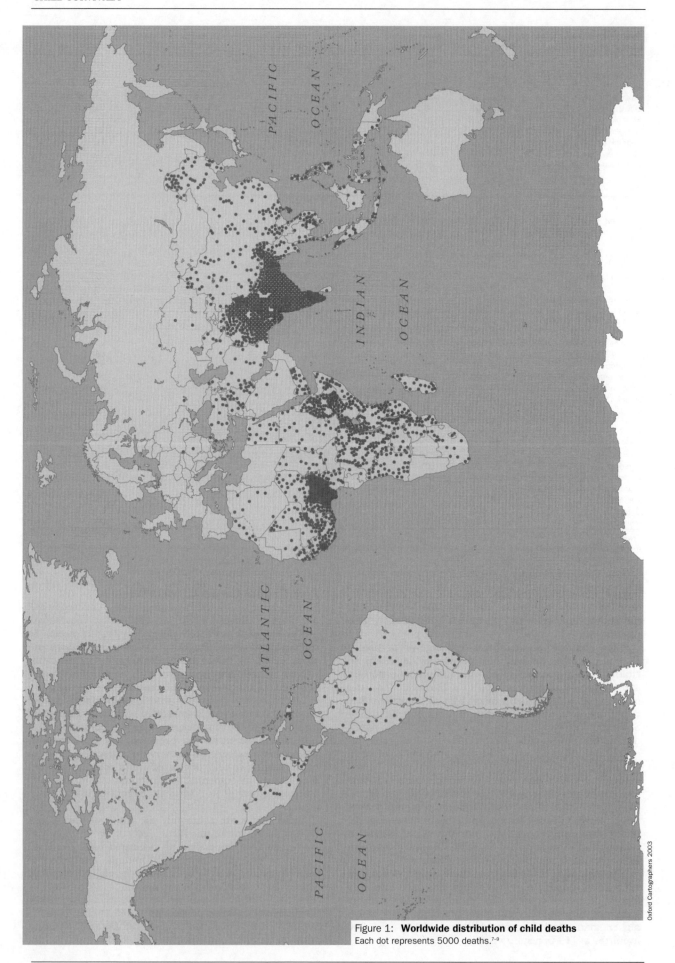

Figure 1: **Worldwide distribution of child deaths**
Each dot represents 5000 deaths.[7-9]

stipulates one cause of death, which is considered to be the "disease or injury which initiated the train of morbid events leading directly to death".[18] This measure ensures that the sum of deaths from all possible causes will not exceed the total number of child deaths. However, such a classification oversimplifies the situation in low-income and middle-income countries where serious illnesses commonly occur sequentially or concurrently before death.

Measles is often complicated by pneumonia or diarrhoea. In studies in Bangladesh, the Philippines, and Uganda it was noted that in children with an illness serious enough to require admission to hospital, 50–79% of measles cases were followed by pneumonia or diarrhoea, which were the reasons for admission.[19–21] Decreases in the immune and non-immune host defences as a consequence of measles lead to a high rate of these subsequent infectious diseases, and also to a higher case fatality rate when they do occur. Likewise, children with AIDS have increased susceptibility to diarrhoea, pneumonia, tuberculosis, and other infections. These diseases also have a higher case fatality rate in people with AIDS compared with those without AIDS. In these examples, measles or AIDS would be judged by ICD rules to be the underlying cause of death and subsequent infections would be associated causes of death.

Underweight status (one SD or more below the weight expected for that age in an international reference population) and micronutrient deficiencies also cause decreases in immune and non-immune host defences, and should be classified as underlying causes of death if followed by infectious diseases that are the terminal associated causes.[22,23] An analysis of ten longitudinal community-based studies of children younger than 5 years showed that being underweight conferred an additional risk of mortality from infectious diseases.[24] The fraction of disease attributable to being underweight was 61% for diarrhoea, 57% for malaria, 53% for pneumonia, 45% for measles, and 53% for other infectious diseases. Fetal malnutrition, manifested in low birthweight, might contribute in a similar way to neonatal mortality.[24] Relative risks for mortality in children younger than 5 years derived from the ten studies assessed have been used to estimate that 53% of all child deaths could be attributed to being underweight (L Caulfield, personal communication). Of these, 35% of all child deaths are due to the effect of underweight status on diarrhoea, pneumonia, measles, and malaria and relative risks of low maternal body-mass index for fetal growth retardation and its risks for selected neonatal causes of deaths.[12,24]

In children with vitamin A deficiency, the risk of dying from diarrhoea, measles, and malaria is increased by 20–24%.[25] Likewise, zinc deficiency increases the risk of mortality from diarrhoea, pneumonia, and malaria by 13–21%.[26] The fraction of these infectious-disease deaths that are attributable to nutritional deficiencies varies with the prevalence of deficiencies; the highest attributable fractions are in sub-Saharan Africa, south Asia, and Andean Latin America.[12] Correct classification of undernutrition and vitamin A and zinc deficiencies as underlying causes of death will permit a true estimate of the importance of these conditions and recognition that interventions can target both the nutritional condition and the resulting terminal infectious diseases.

Clinical causes of death
Classification
All countries need sound epidemiological information to prioritise, plan, and implement public health interventions. Vital event registration that includes cause-of-death data is used to establish the cause structure of mortality in high-income and some middle-income countries, but these are generally not available for the countries where 90% of child deaths take place. Of these countries, only Mexico records more than 95% of causes of death.[27] Where coverage is incomplete, the poorer segments of the population, which have higher mortality and might have different causes of death, are often under-represented.[28] India and China have attempted to establish sample registration systems, but it is not yet clear whether they are truly representative and correctly classify causes of child deaths. Classification of cause of death in vital registration systems is difficult when large proportions of child deaths are not medically attended, and interviews with family members are needed to establish the cause of death.

Alternatives to the reporting of vital events are use of data from nationally-representative surveys and special study populations. With these, ascertainment of death is usually very complete and post-mortem interviews with family members are used to establish causes of death. Although post-mortem interviews have only moderate sensitivity or specificity for some diagnoses, standard methods for data collection and analysis can improve diagnostic accuracy and comparability.[29]

Neonatal disorders
Of the 10·8 million deaths worldwide of children younger than 5 years, 3·9 million occur in the first 28 days of life—ie, the neonatal period. The proportion of deaths that occur in this age interval varies systematically according to the overall rate of mortality. For example, our analysis of results from 44 demographic and health surveys[30] showed that in populations with the highest child mortality rates, just over 20% of all child deaths occurred in the neonatal period, but in countries with mortality rates lower than 35 per 1000 livebirths more than 50% of child deaths were in neonates (figure 2). Regression of the proportion of deaths in the neonatal period on the proportion of child deaths due to AIDS in that country showed a strong association. We used a combination of the natural logarithm of the rate of deaths in children younger than 5 years and the proportion of such deaths attributable to AIDS to predict the proportion of deaths in the neonatal period (r^2=0·76). Predicted deaths were deducted from the neonatal-plus-other category of deaths.

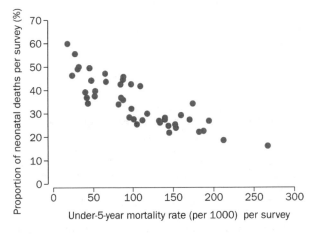

Figure 2: **Relation between under-5-year mortality rate and percentage of these deaths in neonates**
Each dot=one survey.

CHILD SURVIVAL I

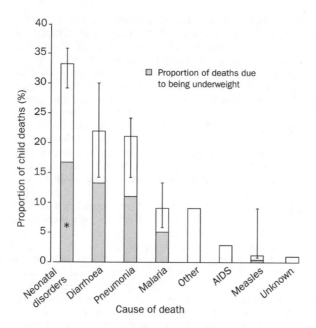

Figure 3: **Distribution of global child deaths by cause**
Bars=uncertainty bounds. *Work in progress to establish the cause-specific contribution of being underweight to neonatal deaths.

There is a paucity of information about the direct causes of neonatal deaths in low-income communities, but it has been estimated that 24% are caused by severe infections, 29% by birth asphyxia, 24% by complications of prematurity, and 7% by tetanus.[31]

Distribution of causes of death globally
We used a prediction model to estimate the distribution of deaths in children younger than 5 years by cause for the 42 countries with 90% of all such deaths in 2000.[32] Estimates and uncertainty bounds were: 22% of deaths attributed to diarrhoea (14–30%), 21% to pneumonia (14–24%), 9% to malaria (6–13%), 1% to measles (1–9%), 3% to AIDS, 33% to neonatal causes (29–36%), 9% to other causes, and fewer than 1% to unknown causes (figure 3). No uncertainty bounds are available for the AIDS estimate because the model did not produce these data (country-level estimates from UNAIDS were used).[33] Figure 3 also shows the fraction of deaths attributed to various causes in which the underlying cause was being underweight.

Comparison with WHO estimates
Estimates of mortality rates in children younger than 5 years in 2000 by cause are published on the WHO website,[34] and are being revised (C Mathers, personal communication). Estimates available at the time of writing attribute 13% of deaths to diarrhoea, 19% to pneumonia, 9% to malaria, 5% to measles, 3% to AIDS, 42% to neonatal causes (birth asphyxia, low birthweight, and disorders arising in the perinatal period), and 9% to miscellaneous other causes, including non-communicable diseases and injury. Uncertainty bounds for the WHO estimates are not available.

Our estimates are not comparable with those of WHO, because WHO's estimates include all WHO member states rather than only 42 countries. Nevertheless, both sets of estimates are generally consistent. WHO and the prediction model identify pneumonia, diarrhoea, and malaria as causing the greatest numbers of deaths in

---

Distribution of causes of death: comparison of WHO mortality database and cause-of-death model

Uniquely, in the 42 countries where 90% of child deaths take place, Mexico has a vital registration system that is considered complete.[27] Therefore, the coverage of the system is 95% or more and implies that there is unlikely to be any substantial selection bias in the proportional distribution of mortality by cause in children younger than 5 years in the vital registration data. We are, therefore, able to validate the predictions of the cause-of-death model using vital registration-based data from Mexico, provided by the Department of Evidence and Information for Policy of WHO (table 2).[34] The following points are of note.

- The model classes all deaths from infectious respiratory illnesses as pneumonia, on the basis that other respiratory illnesses are very rarely fatal, even in young children.
- The model judges undernutrition to be an underlying cause of most infectious illness, and rejects the idea that a few deaths can be singled out as exclusively attributable to nutritional deficiencies. Those deaths ascribed in the WHO mortality database to nutritional deficiencies (3·1%) are therefore reallocated to infectious causes in proportion to their single disease frequencies.
- The model defines neonatal deaths on the basis of a time period (first month of life), which is expected to be roughly equivalent to the sum of deaths from three categories in WHO data—ie, disorders arising during the perinatal period, congenital anomalies, and tetanus. Sepsis deaths in the neonatal period are included in the model but not the WHO estimates, leading to divergence in these values.
- The WHO mortality database does not include a category of deaths due to undetermined causes, because these are reallocated to all causes in proportion to their frequencies. For the model, 0·1% of deaths were in this category.

In the case of Mexico, the WHO mortality database and the cause-of-death prediction model lead to almost identical conclusions about the proportional distribution of deaths by cause in children younger than 5 years. The model results suggest slightly more neonatal deaths (in part because of the difference in definition of this category), and correspondingly fewer deaths from diarrhoea and pneumonia.

---

children younger than 5 years. A comparison of proportional mortality by cause derived from the prediction model with the proportions available for Mexico suggests that our model is predicting reasonably well in this context (panel and table 2).

A careful analysis of the differences between the estimates produced by the two approaches, and the reasons for these, will contribute to an understanding of the relative strengths and weaknesses of different sources of child mortality data and different methodological approaches, for all-cause child mortality and for major causes. Methodological work is underway and is expected to lead to updated estimates and reproducible methods that can be applied regularly as new and better data on the causes of child mortality become available.

	Proportion of deaths	
	WHO	Model
Neonatal	47·9%	52·6%
Diarrhoea	17·5%	14·1%
Respiratory infections	10·4%	8·2%
AIDS	0·1%	0·3%
Other	24·1%	24·7%

Table 2: **Distribution of causes of death in WHO database and cause-of-death model**

CHILD SURVIVAL I

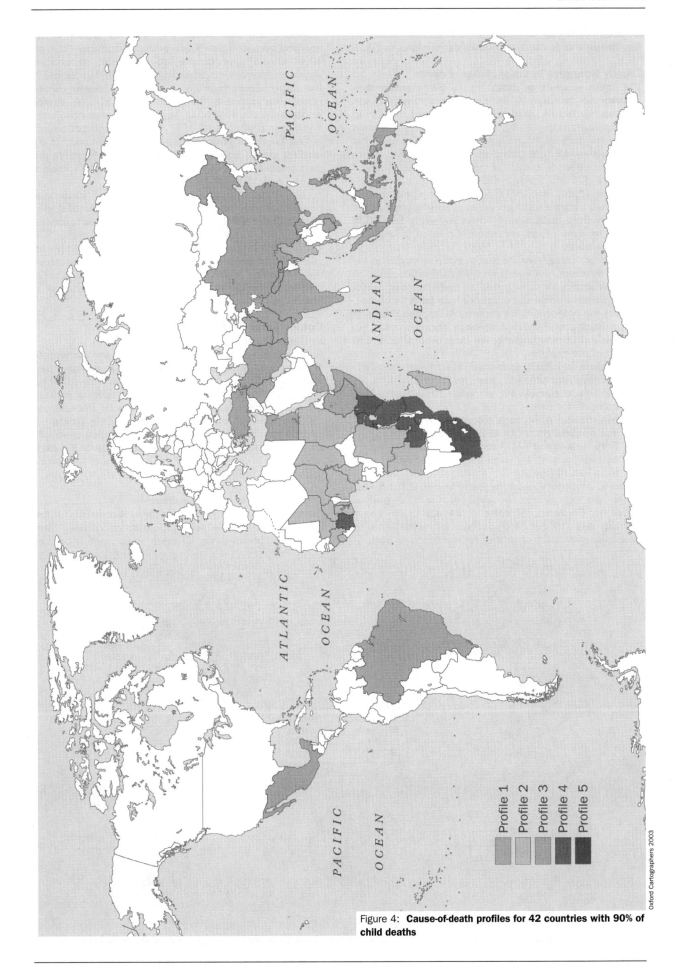

Figure 4: **Cause-of-death profiles for 42 countries with 90% of child deaths**

Profile 1
Profile 2
Profile 3
Profile 4
Profile 5

Oxford Cartographers 2003

CHILD SURVIVAL I

A review of the various models used to estimate under-5-year deaths due to measles is scheduled for later in 2003.

Country typologies by major causes of death

The cause structure of deaths in children younger than 5 years is determined by many environmental and behavioural factors that are often proxied by broad geographical groupings—eg, the countries of sub-Saharan Africa are frequently grouped together. We used the prediction model to estimate that in sub-Saharan Africa the distribution of causes of death would be: neonatal disorders (25%), malaria (22%), pneumonia (21%), diarrhoea (20%), and AIDS (8%). This aggregation is misleading because some countries in sub-Saharan Africa have very little malaria, and others have very few AIDS deaths; whereas others are severely affected by malaria, AIDS, or both.

We propose an alternative way to group countries on the basis of the proportions of death from each major cause. In the 42 countries we considered, the proportions of deaths caused by pneumonia and diarrhoea were fairly consistent, whereas the proportions for malaria, AIDS, and deaths in the neonatal period differed strikingly between countries. The method of grouping is based on causes of death and consists of five profiles.

1. Malaria and AIDS each account for fewer than 10% of deaths and neonatal causes for fewer than 40%.
2. Malaria accounts for at least 10%, but AIDS accounts for fewer than 10%.
3. Malaria and AIDS each account for fewer than 10% and neonatal causes for at least 40%.
4. Both malaria and AIDS account for at least 10%.
5. Malaria accounts for fewer than 10% and AIDS for at least 10% of deaths.

The 42 countries accounting for 90% of all under-5-year deaths are represented in each of the five profiles (figure 4). Countries in profile 1 (average under-5 year mortality rate 109 per 1000) account for most deaths; in these countries, 24% of deaths are attributed to each of diarrhoea and pneumonia and 34% to causes in the neonatal period (figure 5). In profile 2 countries (181 per 1000) 20–26% of deaths are attributed to each of diarrhoea, pneumonia, malaria, and neonatal deaths. In the third largest profile (41 per 1000) diarrhoea and pneumonia account for 23% and 15% of deaths, respectively, but 48% of all deaths are in neonates. Profile 4 (169 per 1000) has 17–19% of deaths attributed to each of diarrhoea and pneumonia and 26% to malaria. In the smallest group, profile 5 (106 per 1000), diarrhoea and pneumonia each account for about 20% of deaths, malaria for 6%, and AIDS for 23%.

Our analysis shows that diarrhoea and pneumonia account for large proportions of deaths in all profiles, even as rates of death fall. Together, they do become somewhat less important at low mortality rates, as in profile 3, in which nearly half of all deaths are in neonates. As mortality rates fall, the proportion of deaths in the neonatal period will increase, which should lead the public health community to increase and improve interventions to prevent deaths in newborns.

Comorbidity in child deaths

Synergy in causes of death

An interaction of two health disorders can have a synergistic effect on mortality—ie, a rate of death that is greater than the sum of the two individual rates of mortality. This has been documented most clearly for the relation between being underweight and infectious diseases.[24,35] For example, children who are mildly underweight ($-2 \leqslant z$ scores<-1) have about a two-fold higher risk of death than those who are better nourished. This risk increases to 5–8 fold in moderately ($-3 \leqslant z$ scores<-2) to severely (<-3 z scores) underweight children.[24]

Co-occurrence of infectious diseases

Another form of comorbidity is the co-occurrence of two infectious diseases, which can occur by chance. More commonly, however, two diseases occur together because

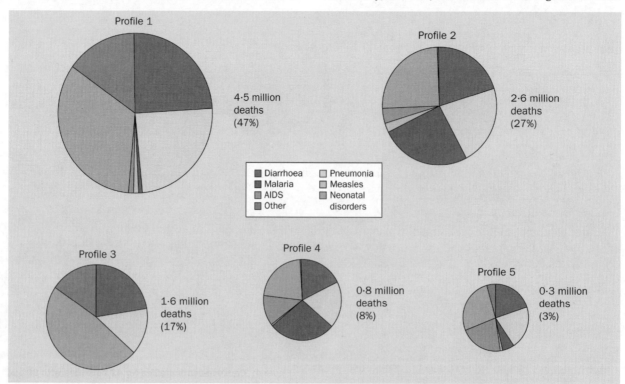

Figure 5: **Distribution of child deaths by cause in five profiles for the 42 countries with 90% of global child deaths in 2000**

they have the same environmental or behavioural risk factors, such as poor sanitation or no breastfeeding in infancy, leading to increased exposure to infections. This comorbidity may also result in synergism, leading to an increased risk of death.

In the past 10 years, it has become more common for studies to include multiple-cause classifications such as diarrhoea plus pneumonia in the causes of death of young children in low-income countries. We did a systematic search for all studies of causes of death of children younger than 5 years in developing countries[32] and identified eight published studies done in Bangladesh, Egypt, the Philippines, and Guinea.[15,36–41] Unpublished studies from Bangladesh and Haiti were also found (H Perry, personal communication). In these studies, reported proportions of deaths attributed to diarrhoea—as a sole cause or in combination with another cause—varied from 15% to 44%. Deaths from pneumonia varied from 20% to 42%, and deaths attributed to two causes in combination varied from 4% to 16%. These proportions can be combined with the overall risk of a child from the same population dying before their fifth birthday to obtain risks of dying from diarrhoea, pneumonia, or both diseases in combination.

To show that comorbidity is an important public health problem, it needs to be established whether deaths from causes in combination are greater than would be expected if each cause acted independently. Multiplication of the risk of death from diarrhoea by the risk from pneumonia allows estimation of the risk of death expected from the random co-occurrence of the two causes, assuming no shared risk factors and no synergy. In the ten studies we assessed, co-occurrence was between 2·7 and 34·2 (median 8·7) times greater than that expected if synergy and risk factors were not present. This finding suggests either that there are shared risk factors for severe diarrhoea and severe pneumonia, or that the two disorders together synergistically provoke death in affected children. Most likely, both mechanisms operate, because even the most powerful shared risk factors, such as not breastfeeding, could not account for such a substantial increase in risk of death with both causes present.

Conclusions

Child health epidemiology is developing and increasingly can provide information useful for public health planning, monitoring, and evaluation. Ideally, information on causes and determinants of death would be available for planning at national or subnational levels. Our epidemiological profiles show the extent of variation between major causes of death even within commonly used regional groupings, which highlights the need for disaggregation at regional and global levels to allow public health intervention efforts to be focused appropriately. The availability of valid epidemiological information at country level will be an important determinant of success in meeting and in measuring progress toward the millennium development goal for child survival.[5] Expanded efforts to build capacity and to improve the completeness and accuracy of available data are needed.

Clearly, pneumonia and diarrhoea will continue to be important causes of child deaths until mortality falls to very low rates. Furthermore, nearly two-thirds of deaths in the 42 countries analysed (and 57% of child deaths worldwide) occur in just 19 countries where the predominant causes are pneumonia, diarrhoea, and neonatal disorders—with very little contribution from malaria and AIDS. On the other hand, malaria plays an important part in child mortality in many countries in sub-Saharan Africa. AIDS accounts for more than 10% of

deaths in just three of the 42 countries; however, in some smaller countries, such as Botswana and Zimbabwe, AIDS causes more than half of child deaths.[33]

Undernutrition is the underlying cause of a substantial proportion of all child deaths, and better information on its determinants is needed. The identification of risk factors, detection of underlying and associated causes of death, and recognition of comorbidity can lead to selection of effective and affordable interventions that are appropriate for national delivery systems.

Contributors
R Black, S Morris, and J Bryce conceived the idea for this article and wrote the paper.

Conflict of interest statement
None declared.

Acknowledgments
Barbara Ewing provided essential help with the preparation of the figures and references. Colin Mathers reviewed earlier drafts of the manuscript and offered useful suggestions on how it could be improved. Members of the Child Health Epidemiology Reference Group (CHERG) who contributed systematic reviews and analyses that have been partly used include Harry Campbell and Igor Rudan (pneumonia); Cynthia Boschi-Pinto, Claudio Lanata, and Walter Mendoza (diarrhoea); Rick Steketee and Alex Rowe (malaria); and Joy Lawn and Zulfiqar Bhutta (neonatal causes). This work was funded by Bill and Melinda Gates Foundation, WHO Department of Child and Adolescent Health and Development, and Johns Hopkins Family Health and Child Survival Cooperative Agreement with the US Agency for International Development. Substantial work was done during a conference supported by the Rockefeller Foundation at the Bellagio Study and Conference Center. The sponsors had no role in these analyses or the preparation of the manuscript. The views represented in this article are those of the individual authors and do not represent the views of their institutions.

References

1 Ahmad OB, Lopez AD, Inoue M. The decline in child mortality: a reappraisal. *Bull World Health Organ* 2000; **78:** 1175–91.
2 WHO. The world health report 2002: reducing risks, promoting healthy life. Geneva: World Health Organization, 2002.
3 UNICEF. State of the world's children 2003. New York: UNICEF, 2002.
4 UNICEF. Progress since the world summit for children: a statistical review. New York: UNICEF, 2001. http://www.unicef.org/pubsgen/wethechildren-stats/sgreport_adapted_stats_eng.pdf (accessed March 24, 2003).
5 UN. General assembly, 56th session. Road map towards the implementation of the United Nations millennium declaration: report of the Secretary-General (UN document no. A/56/326). New York: United Nations, 2001.
6 Mosley WH, Chen LC. An analytical framework for the study of child survival in developing countries. *Popul Develop Rev* 1984; **10** (suppl): 25–45.
7 UNICEF. Child mortality statistics. http://www.childinfo.org/cmr/revis/db2.htm (accessed Feb 20, 2003).
8 United Nations Population Division. World population prospects, the 2000 revision. New York: United Nations Population Division, 2001.
9 Hill K, Pande R, Mahy M, Jones G. Trends in child mortality in the developing world 1960 to 1996. New York: UNICEF, 1998.
10 International Institute for Population Sciences and ORC Macro. 2000 national family health survey (NFHS-2), 1998–99: India, Mumbai. Calverton: ORC Macro, 2000.
11 African Population and Health Research Center. Population and health dynamics in Nairobi's informal settlements. Nairobi, 2002. http://www.aphrc.org/publication/reports4.html (accessed May 21, 2003).
12 Ezzati M, Lopez AD, Rodgers A, Vander Hoorn S, Murray CJL, and the Comparative Risk Assessment Collaborating Group. Selected major risk factors and global and regional burden of disease. *Lancet* 2002; **360:** 1347–60.
13 Setty-Venugopal V, Upadhyay UD. Birth spacing: three to five saves lives. Population Reports, series L, no 13. Baltimore: Johns Hopkins Bloomberg School of Public Health, Population Information Program, 2002.
14 Victora CG, Smith PG, Vaughan JP, et al. Infant feeding and deaths due to diarrhea: a case-control study. *Am J Epidemiol* 1989; **129:** 1032–41.

CHILD SURVIVAL I

15 Arifeen S, Black RE, Antelman G, Baqui A, Caulfield L, Becker S. Exclusive breastfeeding reduces acute respiratory infection and diarrhoea deaths among infants in Dhaka slums. *Pediatrics* 2001; **108:** E 67.

16 WHO Collaborative Study Team on the Role of Breastfeeding on the Prevention of Infant Mortality. Effect of breastfeeding on infant and child mortality due to infectious diseases in less developed countries: a pooled analysis. *Lancet* 2000; **355:** 451–55.

17 Ezzati M, Vander Hoorn V, Rodgers A, Lopez AD, Mathers CD, Murray CJL, and the Comparative Risk Assessment Collaborating Group. Potential health gains from reducing multiple major risk factors: global and regional estimates. *Lancet* (in press).

18 ICD 9 CM. Millennium edition. Vol 1 and 2. Los Angeles: Practice, Management Information Corporation [PMIC], 2000.

19 Kalter HD, Schillinger JA, Hossain M, et al. Identifying sick children requiring referral to hospital in Bangladesh. *Bull World Health Organ* 1997; **75** (suppl 1): 65–75.

20 Kalter HD, Gray RH, Black RE, Gultiano SA. Validation of postmortem interviews to ascertain selected causes of death in children. *Int J Epidemiol* 1990; **19:** 380–86.

21 Kolstad PR, Burnham G, Kalter HD, Kenya-Mugisha N, Black RE. The integrated management of childhood illness in western Uganda. *Bull World Health Organ* 1997; **75** (suppl 1): 77–85.

22 Scrimshaw NS, SanGiovanni JP. Synergism of nutrition, infection, and immunity: an overview. *Am J Clin Nutr* 1997; **66** (suppl): 464–77.

23 Shankar AH, Prasad AS, Zinc and immune function: the biological basis of altered resistance to infection. *Am J Clin Nutr* 1998; **66** (suppl): 447–463.

24 Fishman S, Caulfield LE, de Onis M, et al. Childhood and maternal underweight. In: Ezzati M, Lopez AD, Rodgers A, Murray CJL, eds. Comparative quantification of health risks: global and regional burden of disease attributable to selected major risk factors. Geneva: World Health Organization (in press).

25 Rice AL, West KP, Black RE. Vitamin A deficiency. In: Ezzati M, Lopez AD, Rodgers A, Murray CJL, eds. Comparative quantification of health risks: global and regional burden of disease attributable to selected major risk factors. Geneva: World Health Organization (in press).

26 Caulfield L, Black RE. Zinc deficiency. In: Ezzati M, Lopez AD, Rodgers A, Murray CJL, eds. Comparative quantification of health risks: global and regional burden of disease attributable to selected major risk factors. Geneva: World Health Organization (in press).

27 Lopez AD, Ahmad OB, Guillot M, Inoue M, Ferguson BD, Salomon JA. Life tables for 191 countries for 2000: data, methods, results. GPE discussion paper number 40. Geneva: World Health Organization, 2001.

28 Barreto ICHC, Pontes LK, Corrêa L. Vigilância de óbitos infantis em sistemas locais de saúde: avaliação da autópsia verbal e das informações de agentes de saúde (Portuguese). *Rev Panam Salud Publica* 2000; **7:** 303–12.

29 Anker M, Black RE, Coldham C, et al. A standard verbal autopsy method for investigating cause of death in infants and children. Geneva: World Health Organization, 2001.

30 Demographic and health surveys. STAT compiler. http://www.measuredhs.com (accessed Feb 26, 2003).

31 Save the Children. Report of the state of the world's newborns. http://www.savethechildren.org/mothers/newborns/ (accessed March 31, 2003).

32 Morris SS, Black RE, Tomaskovic L. Predicting the distribution of under-five deaths by cause in countries without vital registration systems. *Int J Epidemiol* (in press).

33 UNAIDS. Global report on HIV/AIDS epidemic. Geneva: UNAIDS, 2002.

34 Mathers CD, Stein C, Fat DM, et al. Global burden of disease 2000: version 2, methods and results. http://www.who.int/evidence (accessed March 14, 2003)

35 Pelletier DL, Frongillo EA, Habicht JP. Epidemiologic evidence for a potentiating effect of malnutrition on child mortality. *Am J Public Health* 1993; **83:** 1130–33.

36 Baqui AH, Black RE, Arifeen S, Hill K, Mitra SN, Sabir AA. Causes of childhood death in Bangladesh: results of a nation-wide verbal autopsy study. *Bull World Health Organ* 1998; **76:** 154–71.

37 Baqui AH, Sabir AA, Begum N, Arifeen SE, Mitra SN, Black RE. Causes of childhood deaths in Bangladesh: an update. *Acta Paediatr* 2001; **90:** 682–90.

38 Becker S, Waheeb Y, El Deeb B, Khallaf N, Black R. Estimating the completeness of under-5 death registration in Egypt. *Demography* 1996; **33:** 329–39.

39 Yassin KM. Incidence and sociodemographic determinants of childhood mortality in rural Upper Egypt. *Soc Sci Med* 2000; **51:** 185–97.

40 Yoon PW, Black RE, Moulton LH, Becker S. The effect of malnutrition on the risk of diarrheal and respiratory mortality in children <2y of age in Cebu, Philippines. *Am J Clin Nutr* 1997; **65:** 1070–77.

41 Scumacher R, Swedberg E, Diallo MO. Mortality study in Guinea: investigating the causes of death for children under 5. Arlington: BASICS II, 2002.

Articles

Breast cancer and hormone-replacement therapy in the Million Women Study

Million Women Study Collaborators

Summary

Background Current use of hormone-replacement therapy (HRT) increases the incidence of breast cancer. The Million Women Study was set up to investigate the effects of specific types of HRT on incident and fatal breast cancer.

Methods 1 084 110 UK women aged 50–64 years were recruited into the Million Women Study between 1996 and 2001, provided information about their use of HRT and other personal details, and were followed up for cancer incidence and death.

Findings Half the women had used HRT; 9364 incident invasive breast cancers and 637 breast cancer deaths were registered after an average of 2·6 and 4·1 years of follow-up, respectively. Current users of HRT at recruitment were more likely than never users to develop breast cancer (adjusted relative risk 1·66 [95% CI 1·58–1·75], p<0·0001) and die from it (1·22 [1·00–1·48], p=0·05). Past users of HRT were, however, not at an increased risk of incident or fatal disease (1·01 [0·94–1·09] and 1·05 [0·82–1·34], respectively). Incidence was significantly increased for current users of preparations containing oestrogen only (1·30 [1·21–1·40], p<0·0001), oestrogen-progestagen (2·00 [1·88–2·12], p<0·0001), and tibolone (1·45 [1·25–1·68], p<0·0001), but the magnitude of the associated risk was substantially greater for oestrogen-progestagen than for other types of HRT (p<0·0001). Results varied little between specific oestrogens and progestagens or their doses; or between continuous and sequential regimens. The relative risks were significantly increased separately for oral, transdermal, and implanted oestrogen-only formulations (1·32 [1·21–1·45]; 1·24 [1·11–1·39]; and 1·65 [1·26–2·16], respectively; all p<0·0001). In current users of each type of HRT the risk of breast cancer increased with increasing total duration of use. 10 years' use of HRT is estimated to result in five (95% CI 3–7) additional breast cancers per 1000 users of oestrogen-only preparations and 19 (15–23) additional cancers per 1000 users of oestrogen-progestagen combinations. Use of HRT by women aged 50–64 years in the UK over the past decade has resulted in an estimated 20 000 extra breast cancers, 15 000 associated with oestrogen-progestagen; the extra deaths cannot yet be reliably estimated.

Interpretation Current use of HRT is associated with an increased risk of incident and fatal breast cancer; the effect is substantially greater for oestrogen-progestagen combinations than for other types of HRT.

Lancet 2003; **362:** 419–27

See Commentary

Correspondence to: Prof Valerie Beral, Cancer Research UK Epidemiology Unit, Gibson Building, Radcliffe Infirmary, Woodstock Road, Oxford OX2 6HE, UK

Introduction

Results from randomised controlled trials and from observational studies show that current and recent use of hormone-replacement therapy (HRT) increases the risk of breast cancer.[1-4] However, the effect of HRT on mortality from breast cancer is unclear[1-5] and use of HRT preparations containing oestrogen-progestagen combinations may be associated with a greater risk of breast cancer than preparations containing oestrogen alone.[6-10] The Million Women Study, a cohort study of a quarter of British women aged 50–64 years, was set up chiefly to investigate the relation between various patterns of use of HRT and breast cancer incidence and mortality.[11]

Methods
Data collection and definitions
The National Health Service Breast Screening Programme (NHSBSP) invites all women in the UK aged 50–64 years for routine screening once every 3 years. From May, 1996, to March, 2001, the NHS breast-screening centres participating in the Million Women Study included the study questionnaire together with their letter of invitation for routine mammography.[11] This letter is generally posted 2–6 weeks before the woman's screening appointment. The questionnaire is returned before women are screened and can be viewed at http://www.millionwomenstudy.org. It contains questions about sociodemographic and other personal factors, including information about use of HRT and menstrual history. The study design, characteristics of the cohort, and patterns of use of HRT have been described elsewhere.[11-13] For a sample of the study population validation studies were done, comparing self-reported data with information in family physicians' records.[14]

Women were classified according to their reported use of HRT, menopausal status, and other relevant factors at recruitment—ie, at baseline. Information collected about use of HRT at baseline included: ever use; current use; age at first and last use; total duration of use; and the name of the proprietary preparation used most recently and duration of its use. The specific constituents and formulations of each proprietary preparation of HRT was obtained from the *British National Formulary*.[15] This information was used to classify the type of preparation used as: oestrogen only; oestrogen-progestagen combination; tibolone, which contains no oestrogen or progestagen; other preparations, including progestagen only, vaginal and other local treatments, and combinations of the above types; or unknown. Users of oestrogen-only preparations were further subdivided according to the specific oestrogen constituent of the HRT (equine oestrogen or oestradiol), its dose, and whether it was administered as an oral, transdermal, or implanted formulation. Users of combined HRT were separated into subgroups by the specific progestagen constituent (medroxyprogesterone acetate, norethis-

Research letters

⊙ Re-emergence of fatal human influenza A subtype H5N1 disease

J S M Peiris, W C Yu, C W Leung, C Y Cheung, W F Ng, J M Nicholls, T K Ng, K H Chan, S T Lai, W L Lim, K Y Yuen, Y Guan

Human disease associated with influenza A subtype H5N1 re-emerged in January, 2003, for the first time since an outbreak in Hong Kong in 1997. Patients with H5N1 disease had unusually high serum concentrations of chemokines (eg, interferon induced protein-10 [IP-10] and monokine induced by interferon γ [MIG]). Taken together with a previous report that H5N1 influenza viruses induce large amounts of proinflammatory cytokines from macrophage cultures in vitro, our findings suggest that cytokine dysfunction contributes to the pathogenesis of H5N1 disease. Development of vaccines against influenza A (H5N1) virus should be made a priority.

Lancet 2004; **363**: 617–19
See Commentary page 582

Highly pathogenic avian influenza (HPAI) virus subtype H5N1 caused disease in 18 patients with six deaths in Hong Kong in 1997. This outbreak was the first documented instance of a purely avian influenza virus causing severe respiratory illness in human beings.[1,2] Here, we report the re-emergence of human H5N1 disease and discuss the possible pathogenesis of the disease.

A family of five from Hong Kong, People's Republic of China, visited Fujian province, mainland China, from Jan 26, to Feb 9, 2003. The 7-year-old daughter developed high fever and respiratory symptoms 2 days after arriving there and died of a pneumonia-like illness 7 days after the onset of symptoms. The exact cause of death could not be ascertained since the girl was buried in mainland China. The family returned to Hong Kong on Feb 9, 2003. The father, a 33-year-old with previous good health, was admitted on Feb 11, 2003, with a 4-day history of fever, malaise, sore throat, cough with blood-stained sputum, and bone pain. He had a lymphocyte count of 0.6×10^9/L (normal range $1.5–4.0 \times 10^9$/L) and radiological evidence of right lower-lobe consolidation. Bacteriological investigations including sputum and blood cultures and acid-fast stain of sputum were unremarkable. Despite treatment with intravenous cefotaxime and oral clarithromycin, clinical and radiological signs showed that the patient was deteriorating. 2 days after admission, oral oseltamivir (75 mg twice daily) was added to his treatment regimen. The patient was electively intubated because of progressive respiratory distress, but his condition worsened and he died 6 days after admission.

Influenza A virus subtype H5N1 was detected by cell-culture methods and by RT-PCR in the nasopharyngeal aspirate collected at day 6 of illness. Serological investigations and cultures to detect other respiratory bacterial and viral pathogens (including RT-PCR for severe acute respiratory syndrome [SARS] coronavirus) were negative.

Autopsy showed features of oedema, haemorrhage, and fibrin exudation in the lung (figure 1). CD68+ macrophages were prominent within alveoli (figure 1) and there were increased numbers of CD3+ T cells in the interstitium. Type-2 pneumocyte hyperplasia was focally present and these pneumocytes showed increased expression of TNF α compared with that in the lung of a patient who died of a non-infective cause (figure 2). We did not detect any viral antigen in cells expressing TNF α. We did note parafollicular reactive histiocytes with haemophagocytosis in the bronchial and hilar lymph nodes. Bone marrow was hypercellular and we identified reactive haemophagocytosis. We did not find evidence of any clinically significant changes in other organs.

With the use of culture and RT-PCR, we detected influenza A in the right and left lung and we noted focal extracellular staining for influenza A antigen (Imagen, DAKO, Cambridge, UK) in cells of the alveolar exudate. Influenza virus was not detectable by RT-PCR or immunofluorescence in other organs.

On Feb 12, 2003, the family's previously healthy 8-year-old son was admitted with a 3-day history of an influenza-like illness. There was radiological evidence of

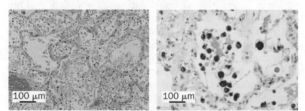

Figure 1: Histological stains of lung tissue from 33-year-old man with H5N1 pneumonia
Left panel: intra-alveolar oedema, haemorrhage, and increased fibrin and alveolar macrophages are evident. Haematoxylin and eosin stain used. Right panel: macrophages were shown by use of immunohistochemical staining with antibody to CD68.

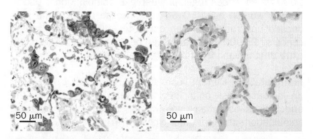

Figure 2: Immunohistochemical staining for TNF α in lung tissue from patient with H5N1 pneumonia and a patient who died from non-infective illness
Stains made with monoclonal antibody SC-7317 (Santa Cruz Biotechnology, Santa Cruz, CA, USA) at a dilution of 1/10 with antigen retrieval. The 33-year-old man with H5N1 pneumonia (left panel) shows greater staining of alveolar epithelial cells than does the control (right panel).

Articles

⊖ Selective serotonin reuptake inhibitors in childhood depression: systematic review of published versus unpublished data

Craig J Whittington, Tim Kendall, Peter Fonagy, David Cottrell, Andrew Cotgrove, Ellen Boddington

Summary

Background Questions concerning the safety of selective serotonin reuptake inhibitors (SSRIs) in the treatment of depression in children led us to compare and contrast published and unpublished data on the risks and benefits of these drugs.

Methods We did a meta-analysis of data from randomised controlled trials that evaluated an SSRI versus placebo in participants aged 5–18 years and that were published in a peer-reviewed journal or were unpublished and included in a review by the Committee on Safety of Medicines. The following outcomes were included: remission, response to treatment, depressive symptom scores, serious adverse events, suicide-related behaviours, and discontinuation of treatment because of adverse events.

Findings Data for two published trials suggest that fluoxetine has a favourable risk-benefit profile, and unpublished data lend support to this finding. Published results from one trial of paroxetine and two trials of sertraline suggest equivocal or weak positive risk-benefit profiles. However, in both cases, addition of unpublished data indicates that risks outweigh benefits. Data from unpublished trials of citalopram and venlafaxine show unfavourable risk-benefit profiles.

Interpretation Published data suggest a favourable risk-benefit profile for some SSRIs; however, addition of unpublished data indicates that risks could outweigh benefits of these drugs (except fluoxetine) to treat depression in children and young people. Clinical guideline development and clinical decisions about treatment are largely dependent on an evidence base published in peer-reviewed journals. Non-publication of trials, for whatever reason, or the omission of important data from published trials, can lead to erroneous recommendations for treatment. Greater openness and transparency with respect to all intervention studies is needed.

Lancet 2004; **363:** 1341–45

Centre for Outcomes Research and Effectiveness, Subdepartment of Clinical Health Psychology, University College London, 1–19 Torrington Place, London WC1E 7HB, UK (C J Whittington PhD, Prof P Fonagy PhD, E Boddington MSc); **Royal College of Psychiatrists' Research Unit, London SW1H 0HW** (T Kendall MRCPsych); **Academic Unit of Child and Adolescent Mental Health, School of Medicine, University of Leeds, Leeds, UK** (Prof D Cottrell FRCPsych); **and Pine Lodge Young People's Centre, Chester, UK** (A Cotgrove MRCPsych)

Correspondence to: Dr Craig Whittington
(e-mail: c.whittington@ucl.ac.uk)

Introduction

Researchers have estimated that 2–6% of children and adolescents in the community suffer from depression,[1,2] and suicide is now the third leading cause of death in 10–19 year olds.[3] There is, therefore, a clear need for safe and effective treatments for this group of people. Although evidence of such treatments for depression in children exists,[4] the lack of efficacy and poor side-effect profile for tricyclic antidepressants[5] leaves selective serotonin reuptake inhibitors (SSRIs) as the only class of antidepressants for pharmacological therapy.

The Expert Working Group of the Committee on Safety of Medicines (CSM) undertook a review of the efficacy and safety of SSRIs in paediatric major depressive disorder. In view of the CSM review, the Medicines and Healthcare products Regulatory Agency (MHRA) released a statement contraindicating the use of all SSRIs other than fluoxetine as new treatment for patients younger than 18 years of age with depressive illness.[6] This advice followed an earlier recommendation by the CSM that both paroxetine and venlafaxine should be contraindicated for use in this context.

The CSM review was initiated because of concerns about the safety of SSRIs; in particular, the possibility that these drugs might be associated with an increased risk of suicidal behaviour and that important withdrawal reactions can happen on stopping treatment.[7] Similar concerns in the USA about the safety of SSRIs prompted reviews by the US Food and Drug Administration[8] and the American College of Neuropsychopharmacology.[9] Although both these organisations raised concerns about the validity of the suicide data and called for further analyses, neither recommended contraindicating SSRIs.

In parallel to the reviews described above, in the UK, the National Collaborating Centre for Mental Health (NCCMH), commissioned by the National Institute for Clinical Excellence (NICE), produced a similar review restricted to published evidence for a national clinical guideline that is being developed for the management of depression in children and young people.

In view of the ongoing debate about publication bias and the serious concerns about withholding unfavourable trial data and under-reporting of adverse events,[10–16] we decided to investigate the risk-benefit profile of individual SSRIs using published data, unpublished data, and the combined dataset.

Methods

The full review protocol is available from the authors and will be published in the full guideline on depression in children (for more information, see http://www.nice.org.uk). Briefly, we searched four electronic bibliographic databases (EMBASE, MEDLINE, PsycINFO, CINAHL) and the Cochrane Library for published trials in which any antidepressant was compared with placebo in participants aged 5–18 years who were diagnosed with depression.

Articles

Association between child and adolescent television viewing and adult health: a longitudinal birth cohort study

Robert J Hancox, Barry J Milne, Richie Poulton

Lancet 2004; 364: 257–62

See Comment page 226

Dunedin Multidisciplinary Health and Development Research Unit, Department of Preventive and Social Medicine, Dunedin School of Medicine, University of Otago, PO Box 913, Dunedin, New Zealand (R J Hancox MD, B J Milne MSc, R Poulton PhD)

Correspondence to:
Dr R J Hancox
bob.hancox@dmhdru.otago.ac.nz

Summary

Background Watching television in childhood and adolescence has been linked to adverse health indicators including obesity, poor fitness, smoking, and raised cholesterol. However, there have been no longitudinal studies of childhood viewing and adult health. We explored these associations in a birth cohort followed up to age 26 years.

Methods We assessed approximately 1000 unselected individuals born in Dunedin, New Zealand, in 1972–73 at regular intervals up to age 26 years. We used regression analysis to investigate the associations between earlier television viewing and body-mass index, cardiorespiratory fitness (maximum aerobic power assessed by a submaximal cycling test), serum cholesterol, smoking status, and blood pressure at age 26 years.

Findings Average weeknight viewing between ages 5 and 15 years was associated with higher body-mass indices (p=0·0013), lower cardiorespiratory fitness (p=0·0003), increased cigarette smoking (p<0·0001), and raised serum cholesterol (p=0·0037). Childhood and adolescent viewing had no significant association with blood pressure. These associations persisted after adjustment for potential confounding factors such as childhood socioeconomic status, body-mass index at age 5 years, parental body-mass index, parental smoking, and physical activity at age 15 years. In 26-year-olds, population-attributable fractions indicate that 17% of overweight, 15% of raised serum cholesterol, 17% of smoking, and 15% of poor fitness can be attributed to watching television for more than 2 h a day during childhood and adolescence.

Interpretation Television viewing in childhood and adolescence is associated with overweight, poor fitness, smoking, and raised cholesterol in adulthood. Excessive viewing might have long-lasting adverse effects on health.

Introduction

Children in developed countries watch a lot of television. Surveys suggest that time spent watching television during childhood and adolescence might even exceed time spent in school.[1] There is increasing concern that the amount of television watched by children could have adverse effects on health. Television viewing might not only displace more energetic activities (contributing to poor fitness and obesity), but also encourage poor dietary habits, violent behaviour, and substance abuse due to the messages conveyed through programme content and advertising.[2]

Studies in children and adolescents have linked television viewing to obesity,[3–6] poor physical fitness,[7,8] lipid abnormalities,[9] and smoking.[10] However, several studies have found the associations to be weak or non-significant,[11–13] and none has addressed the long-term effects of childhood television viewing. In particular, there is no information on whether childhood television viewing affects adult health. To address this issue, we examined the association between child and adolescent television viewing and a range of adult health indicators in a birth cohort of approximately 1000 New Zealanders.

Methods

Participants

Study members were born in Dunedin, Otago province, New Zealand, between April, 1972, and March, 1973.[14] We invited all children who still resided in Otago to participate in the first follow-up assessment at age 3 years. 1037 children (91% of eligible births; 535 [52%] boys, 502 [48%] girls) attended the initial follow-up, constituting the base sample for our study. Further follow-up assessments were undertaken at ages 5 (n=991), 7 (n=954), 9 (n=955), 11 (n=925), 13 (n=850), 15 (n=976), 18 (n=993), 21(n=992), and most recently at age 26 years, when we assessed 980 (96%) of 1019 study members who were still alive. Cohort families represented the full range of socioeconomic status in the South Island, New Zealand, and were mostly of New Zealand European ethnicity. At age 26 years, 73 (7·4%) study members identified themselves as Maori, and 15 (1·5%) as Pacific Islanders. We obtained written informed consent for each assessment. Our study was approved by the Otago Ethics Committee.

Procedures

Information was obtained on television viewing at ages 5, 7, 9, 11, 13, 15, and 21 years. Between ages 5 and 11 years, parents were asked how much time study members spent watching weekday television. At ages 13, 15, and 21 years, study members themselves were asked how long they usually watched television on weekdays and at weekends. Our summary variable was a composite of child and adolescent viewing calculated

Articles

Effect of potentially modifiable risk factors associated with myocardial infarction in 52 countries (the INTERHEART study): case-control study

Salim Yusuf, Steven Hawken, Stephanie Ôunpuu, Tony Dans, Alvaro Avezum, Fernando Lanas, Matthew McQueen, Andrzej Budaj, Prem Pais,
John Varigos, Liu Lisheng, on behalf of the INTERHEART Study Investigators*

Summary

Background Although more than 80% of the global burden of cardiovascular disease occurs in low-income and middle-income countries, knowledge of the importance of risk factors is largely derived from developed countries. Therefore, the effect of such factors on risk of coronary heart disease in most regions of the world is unknown.

Methods We established a standardised case-control study of acute myocardial infarction in 52 countries, representing every inhabited continent. 15152 cases and 14820 controls were enrolled. The relation of smoking, history of hypertension or diabetes, waist/hip ratio, dietary patterns, physical activity, consumption of alcohol, blood apolipoproteins (Apo), and psychosocial factors to myocardial infarction are reported here. Odds ratios and their 99% CIs for the association of risk factors to myocardial infarction and their population attributable risks (PAR) were calculated.

Findings Smoking (odds ratio 2·87 for current vs never, PAR 35·7% for current and former vs never), raised ApoB/ApoA1 ratio (3·25 for top vs lowest quintile, PAR 49·2% for top four quintiles vs lowest quintile), history of hypertension (1·91, PAR 17·9%), diabetes (2·37, PAR 9·9%), abdominal obesity (1·12 for top vs lowest tertile and 1·62 for middle vs lowest tertile, PAR 20·1% for top two tertiles vs lowest tertile), psychosocial factors (2·67, PAR 32·5%), daily consumption of fruits and vegetables (0·70, PAR 13·7% for lack of daily consumption), regular alcohol consumption (0·91, PAR 6·7%), and regular physical activity (0·86, PAR 12·2%), were all significantly related to acute myocardial infarction (p<0·0001 for all risk factors and p=0·03 for alcohol). These associations were noted in men and women, old and young, and in all regions of the world. Collectively, these nine risk factors accounted for 90% of the PAR in men and 94% in women.

Interpretation Abnormal lipids, smoking, hypertension, diabetes, abdominal obesity, psychosocial factors, consumption of fruits, vegetables, and alcohol, and regular physical activity account for most of the risk of myocardial infarction worldwide in both sexes and at all ages in all regions. This finding suggests that approaches to prevention can be based on similar principles worldwide and have the potential to prevent most premature cases of myocardial infarction.

Lancet 2004; **364**: 937–52

Published online
September 3, 2004
http://image.thelancet.com/
extras/04art8001web.pdf

See **Comment** page 912

*Listed at end of report.

Population Health Research
Institute, Hamilton General
Hospital, 237 Barton Street
East, Hamilton, Ontario,
Canada L8L 2X2
(Prof S Yusuf DPhil,
S Ôunpuu PhD, S Hawken MSc,
T Dans MD, A Avezum MD,
F Lanas MD, M McQueen FRCP,
A Budaj MD, P Pais MD,
J Varigos BSc, L Lisheng MD)

Correspondence to:
Prof Salim Yusuf
yusufs@mcmaster.ca

Introduction

Worldwide, cardiovascular disease is estimated to be the leading cause of death and loss of disability-adjusted life years.[1] Although age-adjusted cardiovascular death rates have declined in several developed countries in past decades, rates of cardiovascular disease have risen greatly in low-income and middle-income countries,[1,2] with about 80% of the burden now occurring in these countries. Effective prevention needs a global strategy based on knowledge of the importance of risk factors for cardiovascular disease in different geographic regions and among various ethnic groups.

Current knowledge about prevention of coronary heart disease and cardiovascular disease is mainly derived from studies done in populations of European origin.[2] Researchers are unsure to what extent these findings apply worldwide. Some data suggest that risk factors for coronary heart disease vary between populations—eg, lipids are not associated with this disorder in south Asians,[3] and increases in blood pressure might be more important in Chinese people.[4] Even if the association of a

risk factor with coronary heart disease is similar across populations, prevalence of this factor might vary, resulting in different population attributable risks (PAR)—eg, serum cholesterol might be lower in Chinese populations.[4] On the other hand, these apparent variations between ethnic populations could be attributable to differences between studies in their design and analysis, information obtained, and small sample sizes.

To clarify whether the effects of risk factors vary in different countries or ethnic groups, a large study undertaken in many countries—representing different regions and ethnic groups and using standardised methods—is needed, with the aim to investigate the relation between risk factors and coronary heart disease. Such a study could also estimate the importance of known risk factors on the PAR for acute myocardial infarction. This aim, however, needs either very large cohort trials or case-control studies with many events—eg, several thousands of cases of myocardial infarction in whom all (or most) currently

Articles ▮

Livebirth after orthotopic transplantation of cryopreserved ovarian tissue

J Donnez, M M Dolmans, D Demylle, P Jadoul, C Pirard, J Squifflet, B Martinez-Madrid, A Van Langendonckt

Summary

Background The lifesaving treatment endured by cancer patients leads, in many women, to early menopause and subsequent infertility. In clinical situations for which chemotherapy needs to be started, ovarian tissue cryopreservation looks to be a promising option to restore fertility. In 1997, biopsy samples of ovarian cortex were taken from a woman with stage IV Hodgkin's lymphoma and cryopreserved before chemotherapy was initiated. After her cancer treatment, the patient had premature ovarian failure.

Methods In 2003, after freeze-thawing, orthotopic autotransplantation of ovarian cortical tissue was done by laparoscopy.

Findings 5 months after reimplantation, basal body temperature, menstrual cycles, vaginal ultrasonography, and hormone concentrations indicated recovery of regular ovulatory cycles. Laparoscopy at 5 months confirmed the ultrasonographic data and showed the presence of a follicle at the site of reimplantation, clearly situated outside the ovaries, both of which appeared atrophic. From 5 to 9 months, the patient had menstrual bleeding and development of a follicle or corpus luteum with every cycle. 11 months after reimplantation, human chorionic gonadotrophin concentrations and vaginal echography confirmed a viable intrauterine pregnancy, which has resulted in a livebirth.

Interpretation We have described a livebirth after orthotopic autotransplantation of cryopreserved ovarian tissue. Our findings suggest that cryopreservation of ovarian tissue should be offered to all young women diagnosed with cancer.

Lancet 2004; **364**: 1405–10

Published online
September 24, 2004
http://image.thelancet.com/
extras/04art9230web.pdf

See **Comment** page 1379

Gynaecology Research Unit,
Université Catholique de
Louvain, Brussels, Belgium
(M M Dolmans MD,
D Demylle PhD, C Pirard MD,
B Martinez-Madrid PhD,
A Van Langendonckt PhD); and
Department of Gynaecology,
Cliniques Universitaires St Luc,
Université Catholique de
Louvain, Avenue Hippocrate
10, B-1200 Brussels, Belgium
(Prof J Donnez MD, P Jadoul MD,
J Squifflet MD)

Correspondence to:
Prof Jacques Donnez
donnez@gyne.ucl.ac.be

Introduction

Treatment of childhood malignant disease is becoming increasingly effective. Aggressive chemotherapy and radiotherapy, and bone-marrow transplantation, can cure more than 90% of girls and young women affected by such disorders. However, the ovaries are very sensitive to cytotoxic treatment, especially to alkylating agents and ionising radiation, generally resulting in loss of both endocrine and reproductive function.[1] Moreover, uterine irradiation at a young age reduces adult uterine volume.[2]

By 2010, about one in 250 people in the adult population will be childhood cancer survivors.[3] Several potential options are available to preserve fertility in patients facing premature ovarian failure, including immature and mature oocyte cryopreservation, and embryo cryopreservation.[4,5] For patients who need immediate chemotherapy cryopreservation of ovarian tissue is a possible alternative.[4,6,7] The aim of this strategy is to reimplant ovarian tissue into the pelvic cavity (orthotopic site) or a heterotopic site like the forearm once treatment is completed and the patient is disease-free.[4,8–12]

Oktay and colleagues have reported laparoscopic transplantation of frozen-thawed ovarian tissue to the pelvic side wall,[8] forearm,[9] and beneath the skin of the abdomen. A four-cell embryo was obtained from 20 oocytes retrieved from tissue transplanted to the abdomen, but no pregnancy happened after transfer.[13] Radford and colleagues[12] reported a patient with a history of Hodgkin's disease treated by chemotherapy,

in whom ovarian tissue had been biopsied and cryopreserved 4 years after chemotherapy and later reimplanted. In this case, histological section of ovarian cortical tissue revealed only a few primordial follicles because of the previous chemotherapy. After reimplantation, the patient had only one menstrual period. In 2004, a livebirth after a fresh ovarian tissue transplant in a primate was reported.[14]

In 1995, the Catholic University of Louvain ethics committee approved a protocol to assess the safety and efficacy of cryopreservation of ovarian tissue in women treated with high doses of chemotherapy, which could induce ovarian failure. So far, 146 patients have undergone cryopreservation of ovarian tissue in our department before starting chemotherapy and two patients have undergone reimplantation (one in August, 2004).

Here, we describe the outcome of orthotopic autotransplantation of cryopreserved ovarian tissue in a patient from whom tissue was obtained and frozen before chemotherapy was initiated for Hodgkin's lymphoma.

Methods

Patient

In 1997, a 25-year-old woman presented with clinical stage IV Hodgkin's lymphoma. Ovarian tissue cryopreservation was undertaken before chemotherapy. We obtained written informed consent. By laparoscopy, we took five biopsy samples—about 12–15 mm long and 5 mm wide—from the left ovary. Removal of the whole ovary was not an option because one can never

Articles

Efficacy of the RTS,S/AS02A vaccine against *Plasmodium falciparum* infection and disease in young African children: randomised controlled trial

Pedro L Alonso, Jahit Sacarlal, John J Aponte, Amanda Leach, Eusebio Macete, Jessica Milman, Inacio Mandomando, Bart Spiessens, Caterina Guinovart, Mateu Espasa, Quique Bassat, Pedro Aide, Opokua Ofori-Anyinam, Margarita M Navia, Sabine Corachan, Marc Ceuppens, Marie-Claude Dubois, Marie-Ange Demoitié, Filip Dubovsky, Clara Menéndez, Nadia Tornieporth, W Ripley Ballou, Ricardo Thompson, Joe Cohen

Summary

Background Development of an effective malaria vaccine could greatly contribute to disease control. RTS,S/AS02A is a pre-erythrocytic vaccine candidate based on *Plasmodium falciparum* circumsporozoite surface antigen. We aimed to assess vaccine efficacy, immunogenicity, and safety in young African children.

Methods We did a double-blind, phase IIb, randomised controlled trial in Mozambique in 2022 children aged 1–4 years. The study included two cohorts of children living in two separate areas which underwent different follow-up schemes. Participants were randomly allocated three doses of either RTS,S/AS02A candidate malaria vaccine or control vaccines. The primary endpoint, determined in cohort 1 (n=1605), was time to first clinical episode of *P falciparum* malaria (axillary temperature ⩾37·5°C and *P falciparum* asexual parasitaemia >2500 per μL) over a 6-month surveillance period. Efficacy for prevention of new infections was determined in cohort 2 (n=417). Analysis was per protocol.

Findings 115 children in cohort 1 and 50 in cohort 2 did not receive all three doses and were excluded from the per-protocol analysis. Vaccine efficacy for the first clinical episodes was 29·9% (95% CI 11·0–44·8; p=0·004). At the end of the 6-month observation period, prevalence of *P falciparum* infection was 37% lower in the RTS,S/AS02A group compared with the control group (11·9% vs 18·9%; p=0·0003). Vaccine efficacy for severe malaria was 57·7% (95% CI 16·2–80·6; p=0·019). In cohort 2, vaccine efficacy for extending time to first infection was 45·0% (31·4–55·9; p<0·0001).

Interpretation The RTS,S/AS02A vaccine was safe, well tolerated, and immunogenic. Our results show development of an effective vaccine against malaria is feasible.

Lancet 2004; **364:** 1411–20

See **Comment** page 1380

Centre de Salut Internacional, Hospital Clínic/IDIBAPS, Universitat de Barcelona, Barcelona, Spain
(P L Alonso MD, J J Aponte MD, C Guinovart MD, M Espasa MD, Q Bassat MD, M M Navia PhD, C Menéndez MD); **Centro de Investigação em Saúde de Manhiça, Ministerio de Saúde, CP 1929 Maputo, Mozambique** (P L Alonso, J Sacarlal MD, J J Aponte, E Macete MD, I Mandomando VetMed, C Guinovart, M Espasa, Q Bassat, P Aide MD, M M Navia, C Menéndez, R Thompson PhD); **Faculdade de Medicina, Universidade Eduardo Mondlane, Maputo, Mozambique** (J Sacarlal); **Instituto Nacional de Saúde and Direcção Nacional de Saúde, Ministerio de Saúde, Maputo, Mozambique** (E Macete, I Mandomando, P Aide, R Thompson); **GlaxoSmithKline Biologicals, Rixensart, Belgium** (A Leach MRCPCH, B Spiessens PhD, O Ofori-Anyinam PhD, S Corachan BSc, M Ceuppens MD, M-C Dubois MSc, M-A Demoitié MSc, N Tornieporth MD, W R Ballou MD, J Cohen PhD); **and Malaria Vaccine Initiative, PATH, Rockville, MD, USA** (J Milman MPH, F Dubovsky MD)

Correspondence to:
Dr Pedro L Alonso,
Centre de Salut Internacional, Hospital Clínic, Villarroel 170, 08036 Barcelona, Spain
palonso@clinic.ub.es

Introduction

During the 20th century, economic and social development and antimalarial campaigns have resulted in eradication of malaria from large swathes of the planet, reducing the world's malarious surface from 50% to 27%. Nonetheless, in view of expected population growth, by 2010, half the world's population—nearly 3·5 billion people—will be living in areas where malaria is transmitted.[1] Current estimates suggest that more than 1 million deaths are attributable to malaria every year, and the economic costs for Africa alone are equivalent to US$12 billion annually.[2] These figures highlight the desperate global malaria crisis and the profound challenges to the international health community and countries of sub-Saharan Africa. The reasons for this crisis are many and include emergence of widespread resistance to available, affordable, and previously highly effective drugs, breakdown and inadequacy of health systems, and lack of resources. Unless we find ways to control this disease, global efforts to improve health and child survival, reduce poverty, increase security, and strengthen the most vulnerable societies will fail.

At the beginning of the 21st century, emerging scientific knowledge and new impetus for malaria research

provide opportunities to develop an effective malaria vaccine that could greatly contribute to control of this devastating disease.[3] RTS,S/AS02A is one of the most advanced malaria vaccine candidates in development.[4] This vaccine specifically targets the pre-erythrocytic stage of *Plasmodium falciparum* and confers protection against infection by *P falciparum* sporozoites delivered via laboratory-reared infected mosquitoes in malaria-naive adult volunteers and against natural exposure in semi-immune adults.[5–7]

In 2000, GlaxoSmithKline (GSK) and the Malaria Vaccine Initiative (MVI) Programme for Appropriate Technology in Health (PATH) entered into a partnership to develop RTS,S/AS02A as a vaccine to prevent severe malaria disease in infants immunised in the context of the Expanded Programme on Immunisation (EPI). Consecutive phase I studies undertaken in The Gambia of children aged 6–11 years and 1–5 years showed that the vaccine was safe, well tolerated, and immunogenic (Bojang KA, unpublished data). Subsequently, a paediatric vaccine dose was selected and studied in a phase I trial of Mozambican children aged 1–4 years, in which it was found to be safe, well tolerated, and immunogenic (Macete E, unpublished data).

Series

Neonatal Survival 1

4 million neonatal deaths: When? Where? Why?

Joy E Lawn, Simon Cousens, Jelka Zupan, for the Lancet Neonatal Survival Steering Team*

The proportion of child deaths that occurs in the neonatal period (38% in 2000) is increasing, and the Millennium Development Goal for child survival cannot be met without substantial reductions in neonatal mortality. Every year an estimated 4 million babies die in the first 4 weeks of life (the neonatal period). A similar number are stillborn, and 0·5 million mothers die from pregnancy-related causes. Three-quarters of neonatal deaths happen in the first week—the highest risk of death is on the first day of life. Almost all (99%) neonatal deaths arise in low-income and middle-income countries, yet most epidemiological and other research focuses on the 1% of deaths in rich countries. The highest numbers of neonatal deaths are in south-central Asian countries and the highest rates are generally in sub-Saharan Africa. The countries in these regions (with some exceptions) have made little progress in reducing such deaths in the past 10–15 years. Globally, the main direct causes of neonatal death are estimated to be preterm birth (28%), severe infections (26%), and asphyxia (23%). Neonatal tetanus accounts for a smaller proportion of deaths (7%), but is easily preventable. Low birthweight is an important indirect cause of death. Maternal complications in labour carry a high risk of neonatal death, and poverty is strongly associated with an increased risk. Preventing deaths in newborn babies has not been a focus of child survival or safe motherhood programmes. While we neglect these challenges, 450 newborn children die every hour, mainly from preventable causes, which is unconscionable in the 21st century.

Lancet 2005; 365: 891–900

See **Comment** pages 821, 822, 825, and 827

Published online March 3, 2005 http://image.thelancet.com/ extras/05art1073web.pdf

*Lancet Neonatal Survival Steering Team listed at end of article

Saving Newborn Lives/Save the Children-USA, and International Perinatal Care Unit, Institute of Child Health, London, Cape Town, South Africa (J E Lawn MRCP); London School of Hygiene and Tropical Medicine, London, UK (Prof S Cousens DipMathStat); and Department of Reproductive Health and Research, WHO, Geneva, Switzerland (J Zupan MD)

Correspondence to: Dr Joy E Lawn, Saving Newborn Lives/Save the Children-USA, and International Perinatal Care Unit, 11 South Way, Pinelands, Cape Town 7405, South Africa joylawn@yahoo.co.uk

Of the 130 million babies born every year, about 4 million die in the first 4 weeks of life—the neonatal period.[1] A similar number of babies are stillborn—dying in utero during the last 3 months of pregnancy. Most neonatal deaths (99%) arise in low-income and middle-income countries, and about half occur at home. In poor communities, many babies who die are unnamed and unrecorded, indicating the perceived inevitability of their deaths. By contrast, the 1% of neonatal deaths that arise in rich countries are the subject of confidential inquiries and public outcry if services are judged substandard. Most trials of neonatal interventions focus on these few deaths in rich countries. The inverse care law, first described in the UK in the 1960s, remains valid: "The availability of good medical care tends to vary inversely with the need for it in the population served."[2] For newborn babies, this law could appropriately be renamed the inverse information and care law: the communities with the most neonatal deaths have the least information on these deaths and the least access to cost-effective interventions to prevent them.

In this report, the first in a series of four on neonatal survival, we present epidemiological data to help guide efforts to reduce deaths of newborn children in countries where most of these deaths take place. This series follows the Bellagio child survival series,[3] which emphasised the need for further work into neonatal deaths. It will also focus on strengthening of health systems (including community level) to provide care for newborn children in the highest mortality settings, and the costs of doing so. Our emphasis on neonatal survival is deliberate.[4] We believe stillbirths, maternal morbidity and mortality, and neonatal morbidity are of great public-health importance. However, doing justice to all of these topics is not possible

in one series. We believe that increased attention to improving health systems around the time of childbirth will also reduce maternal deaths and stillbirths.

MDGs and newborn babies

The Millennium Development Goals (MDGs) represent the widest commitment in history to addressing global poverty and ill health.[5] The fourth goal (MDG-4) commits the international community to reducing mortality in children aged younger than 5 years by two-thirds between 1990 and 2015. Between 1960 and 1990, the risk of dying in the first 5 years of life was halved—a major achievement in child health.[6] However, achieving MDG-4 will depend on mortality reductions even greater in percentage terms than those achieved in the past (figure 1). A decade before the target date of 2015, many are already predicting the goal will not be met.[7] Challenges include AIDS[5] and increasing poverty, particularly in Africa, as well as a lack of global investment in child survival,[8] despite 10·6 million deaths every year.[9]

Another challenge, less frequently identified in policy analysis, is the slow progress in reducing global neonatal mortality (figure 1). Child survival programmes in the developing world have tended to focus on pneumonia, diarrhoea, malaria, and vaccine-preventable conditions, which are important causes of death after the first month of life. Between 1980 and 2000, child mortality after the first month of life—ie, from month 2 to age 5 years—fell by a third, whereas the neonatal mortality rate (NMR) was reduced by only about a quarter. Hence, an increasing proportion of child deaths is now in the neonatal period; estimates for 2000[1] show that 38% of all deaths in children younger than age 5 years happen in the first month of life. Deaths in the first week of life have shown the least

INDEX

Notes

Dates in brackets refer to publication year.

Page numbers in brackets indicate a reference not immediately obvious in the text.

Page numbers suffixed by E indicate a *Lancet* editorial.

Double surnames appear under the last name unless hyphenated.

A

abdominal masses, ultrasound detection, 229, 332–333
abdominal resection, rectal cancer, 273
Abercrombie, G F (1953), 228, 321–322
abortion, early foetal death, 233, 384–385
    see also pregnancy
Abrahams, A (1919), 111–112
Abrams, L D (1958), 229, 334
abscess, liver, 32
accidents
    railway, 102
    road, 227, 305–307
    secondary effects, 102
    see also artificial respiration, emergency, injury
accoucheurs, face-masks for, 239
acetonuria, 200
Achong (1964), 341, 363
acidosis, 200
acid reflux, *H. pylori* and, 345, (409–411)
acrylic intra-ocular lenses, 228, 316–319
ACTH-dependent hypertension, vasodilator prostaglandins, 411
actinomycete infections, Farmer's lung, 341, 362
acute hæmorrhagic fever, new virus in Zaire, 393–395
acute respiratory insufficiency, treatment, 320
acyclovir, herpes virus infection trial, 344, 404
Addenbrooke, Bertram (1906), 173
Addison's disease, 238
adenomatous polyps, epidemiology, 377
adolescents, television viewing and adult health effects, 348, 452
adrenalin, as vaso-motor/cardiac stimulant, 116, 172–173
adrenergic beta-receptor antagonist, first, 341, 364–365
adrenocorticotrophic hormone-dependent hypertension, vasodilator prostaglandins, 411
adulteration of foods *see* food
aetiology of disease, (1888), 136
agglutination tests (blood-group antigens), 228, 328
    foetal, 228, 329
agnosia, finger, 287
ague, treatment, 166
Aide, Pedro (2004), 455
AIDS *see* HIV infection/AIDS
Airey, Richard (1866), 109
air pollution, 228, 322–323
air-raids
    civilian psychiatric casualties, 226, 281
    emotivity measurement, 118, 215
Albert, Prince Consort, illness and death of, 20, 98, 114
albinism of hair, 83
Alexander, F E (1990), 418
Alexander, Frederick W (1910), 117, 186
alimentary system, force feeding effects, 192
alkalis, acidosis treatment, 230
alkaptonuria, 116
Allard, Dr (1885), 135
allergic contact dermatitis, 234
allografts, cutaneous nerve regeneration, 433
Alonso, Pedro L (2004), 349, 455
Alperovich, A (1996), 425

alpha-fetoprotein (AFP) measurement
    anencephaly diagnosis, 343, 388–389
    Down syndrome diagnosis, 345, 412
alum, adulteration in bread, 86, 102–103
Alwall, Nils (1948), 227, 297–299
amaurosis, 33–34
p-aminobenzene-sulphonamide, puerperal infection treatment, 254
p-aminosalicylic acid, tuberculosis treatment, 226–227, 289–290, 304
amnesia, shell-shock, 197
amniocentesis, 342–343, 367
amniotic-fluid cells, chromosome analysis, 342, 367
amputation, 4, 113, 120–122
    phantom limbs, 226, 287
    post-surgical treatment, 125
Amussat, M (1834), (54)
anaemia
    aplastic, 242
    operative shock, 195
    in pregnancy, 260
anaesthesia, 19
    brain cell exhaustion, 195
    chloroform, 19–20, 81–82, 87E
    closed method, 250
    ether (sulphuric), 19, 75–78
    eucaine, 156
    local, 156
    neuromuscular blockade, 224, (244–246)
    operative shock, 194–195
    pre-medication, 117, (194–196)
    shock prevention, 194–195
    spinal, caesarian section, 237
analytical chemistry
    aspirin, 115, 161
    bread, adulteration, 21, 86, 102–103
    cognac, 161
    iron water, 161
    poisoned confectionery, 18, 45–47
    potash water, 161
    prussic acid analysis, 42–44
    vasogens, 161
    whisky, 161
Analytical Records (*Lancet* section), (1899), 161
Anand, J K (1961), 360
anastomoses, 194
anatomical supplies
    body-snatching/murder, 17, 35–38E
    donation, 346, 424
anatomy demonstrations, public, 17, 31–32
Garrett Anderson, Louisa (1916), 118, 200–201
Anderson, T J (1990), 418
Andover workhouse scandal, 6
Andrews, James (1969), 378
anencephaly diagnosis, AFP measurement, 343, 388–389
aneurysm, treatment of, 144
angina pectoris
    amyl nitrite, 113
    balloon angioplasty, 344, 396